MW01641074

Shackelford's

Surgery of the ALIMENTARY TRACT

CoEditors

MARK B. ORRINGER
and
RICHARD HEITMILLER

Volume I

Esophagus

DANIEL T. DEMPSEY

Volume II

Stomach and Duodenum
Incisions

JEREMIAH G. TURCOTTE

Volume III

Pancreas
Biliary Tract
Liver and Portal Hypertension
Spleen

JOHN H. PEMBERTON

Volume IV

Colon
Rectum and Anus

KEITH D. LILLEMOE

Volume V

Mesenteric Circulation
Hernia
Small Intestine

Fifth Edition

Shackelford's

Surgery of the ALIMENTARY TRACT

GEORGE D. ZUIDEMA, M.D.
Professor of Surgery and Vice Provost for Medical Affairs, Emeritus
The University of Michigan
Ann Arbor, Michigan

CHARLES J. YEO, M.D.
Professor of Surgery and Oncology
The Johns Hopkins University School of Medicine
Baltimore, Maryland

W.B. SAUNDERS COMPANY
A Harcourt Health Sciences Company
Philadelphia London New York St. Louis Sydney Toronto

W.B. SAUNDERS COMPANY
A Harcourt Health Sciences Company

The Curtis Center
Independence Square West
Philadelphia, Pennsylvania 19106

Library of Congress Cataloging-in-Publication Data

Shackelford's surgery of the alimentary tract / [edited by] George D. Zuidema, Charles J. Yeo.—5th ed.

p. ;cm.

Rev. ed. of: Shackelford's surgery of the alimentary tract / [edited by] George D. Zuidema. 4th ed. c1996.

Includes bibliographical references and indexes.

ISBN 0–7216–8203–0 (5 vol. set)

1. Alimentary canal—Surgery. I. Zuidema, George D. II. Yeo, Charles J. III. Shackelford's surgery of the alimentary tract. [DNLM: 1. Digestive System Surgical Procedures—methods. 2. Digestive System Diseases—surgery. WI 900 S9617 2001]

RD540.S476 2001 617.4′3—dc21

DNLM/DLC 00-030058

Acquisitions Editor: Lisette Bralow
Developmental Editor: Hazel Hacker
Illustration Specialist: Walter Verbitski
Book Designer: Karen O'Keefe Owens

ISBN Volume I 0-7216-8204-9
Volume II 0-7216-8205-7
Volume III 0-7216-8206-5
Volume IV 0-7216-8207-3
Volume V 0-7216-8208-1
SHACKELFORD'S SURGERY OF THE ALIMENTARY TRACT—5th ed. Five-volume set 0-7216-8203-0

Printed in the United States of America.

Last digit is the print number: 9 8 7 6 5 4 3 2 1

To our wives, Joan and Theresa, to our mentors in the science of surgery, and to our many colleagues whose work has made this fifth edition possible.

George D. Zuidema
Charles J. Yeo

To my wife, Susan, for her years of support and personal self-sacrifice for my career and to my colleagues on the faculty of the University of Michigan Section of Thoracic Surgery and our Thoracic Surgery Residents, who have contributed so greatly to the care of our patients.

Mark B. Orringer

Contributors

HENRY D. APPELMAN, M.D.
Professor of Pathology, University of Michigan, Medical School, Ann Arbor, Michigan
Barrett's Esophagus: Morphologic Considerations

RALPH W. AYE, M.D.
Clinical Assistant Professor of Surgery, University of Washington; Head, Thoracic Oncology Group, Swedish Medical Center, Seattle, Washington
The Hill Repair

RONALD BELSEY, M.D.
Former Professor Emeritus, Department of Surgery, The University of Chicago Pritzker School of Medicine, Chicago, Illinois
The Belsey Mark IV Antireflux Procedure

ARNOLD G. CORAN, M.D.
Professor of Surgery and Head of the Section of Pediatric Surgery, University of Michigan Medical School; Surgeon-In-Chief, C. S. Mott Children's Hospital, Ann Arbor, Michigan
Congenital Abnormalities of the Esophagus

ABE DEANDA, JR., M.D.
Assistant Professor, Division of Cardiothoracic Surgery, Medical College of Virginia, Richmond, Virginia
Miscellaneous Conditions of the Esophagus

TOM R. DEMEESTER, M.D.
Professor and Chairman, Department of Surgery, University of Southern California School of Medicine, Los Angeles, California
Physiologic Diagnostic Studies

CLAUDE DESCHAMPS, M.D.
Associate Professor of Surgery and Consultant, General Thoracic Surgery, Mayo Clinic and Foundation, Rochester, Minnesota
Surgical Management of Esophageal Diverticula

ANDRÉ DURANCEAU, M.D.
Professor of Surgery, Department of Surgery, Université de Montreal Faculty of Medicine, Chair, Division of Thoracic Surgery, Université de Montreal Academic Centre, Montreal, Quebec, Canada
Anatomy and Embryology; Physiology of the Esophagus

FREDERIC E. ECKHAUSER, M.D.
Professor of Surgery, University of Michigan Medical Center, Ann Arbor, Michigan
Esophageal Varices

THOMAS R. EUBANKS, D.O.
Assistant Professor, University of Washington; Attending Surgeon, University of Washington Medical Center, Seattle, Washington
Laparoscopic Esophageal Surgery

MARK K. FERGUSON, M.D.
Professor of Surgery, Department of Surgery, The University of Chicago Pritzker School of Medicine, Chicago, Illinois
Endoscopic Evaluation of the Esophagus; Carcinoma of the Esophagus and Cardia

ELLIOT K. FISHMAN, M.D.
Professor of Radiology and Oncology, The Russell H. Morgan Department of Radiology and Radiological Science, The Johns Hopkins University School of Medicine, Baltimore, Maryland
Radiologic Evaluation of the Esophagus

ARLENE A. FORASTIERE, M.D.
Professor, Department of Oncology, The Johns Hopkins University School of Medicine, Baltimore, Maryland
Multimodality Therapy for Esophageal Carcinoma

CARROLL M. HARMON, M.D., Ph.D.
Assistant Professor of Surgery, University of Michigan Medical School; Attending Surgeon, C. S. Mott Children's Hospital, Ann Arbor, Michigan
Congenital Abnormalities of the Esophagus

RICHARD F. HEITMILLER, M.D.
Associate Professor of Surgery and Oncology and Chief, Division of General Thoracic Surgery, The Johns Hopkins Medical Institutions, Baltimore, Maryland
Benign Tumors and Cysts of the Esophagus

CLEMENT A. HIEBERT, M.D.
Chairman Emeritus, Department of Surgery, Maine Medical Center, Portland, Maine; Clinical Assistant in Surgery, Harvard Medical School, Boston, Massachusetts; Clinical Professor of Surgery, University of Vermont College of Medicine, Burlington, Vermont
Overview: Hiatal Hernia, Gastroesophageal Reflux, and Their Complications

LUCIUS D. HILL, M.D.†
Clinical Professor of Surgery, University of Washington; Chairman, Gastrointestinal Center, Swedish Hospital, Seattle, Washington
The Hill Repair

KAREN M. HORTON, M.D.
Assistant Professor of Radiology, The Russell H. Morgan Department of Radiology and Radiological Science, The Johns Hopkins Medical Institutions, Baltimore, Maryland
Radiologic Evaluation of the Esophagus

MARK D. IANNETTONI, M.D.
Associate Professor of Surgery, Section of General Thoracic Surgery, University of Michigan Medical School, Ann Arbor, Michigan
Esophageal Trauma

†Deceased

BRONWYN JONES, M.B.B.S., F.R.C.R., F.R.A.C.P.
Professor of Radiology, The Russell H. Morgan Department of Radiology, and Radiological Science, The Johns Hopkins University School of Medicine, Baltimore, Maryland
Radiologic Evaluation of the Esophagus

LAWRENCE R. KLEINBERG, M.D.
Assistant Professor, Radiation Oncology, The Johns Hopkins University School of Medicine, Baltimore, Maryland
Radiation Therapy in Curative and Palliative Therapy of Esophageal Cancer

JAMES A. KNOL, M.D.
Associate Professor of Surgery, University of Michigan Medical School, Ann Arbor, Michigan
Esophageal Varices

STEFAN J. M. KRAEMER, M.D.
Surgeon, Ryan Hill Research Foundation, Seattle, Washington
The Hill Repair

DOROTHEA LIEBERMANN-MEFFERT, M.D., PH.D.
Professor, Department of Surgery, Chirurgische Klinik and Poliklinik, Klinikum Rechts der Isar, Technical University of Munich, Munich, Germany; Professor, Department of Surgery, Kantonsspital University Hospital, Basel, Switzerland
Anatomy and Embryology; Physiology of the Esophagus

ALEX G. LITTLE, M.D.
Professor and Chairman, Department of Surgery, University of Nevada School of Medicine; Chief of Surgery, University Medical Center, Las Vegas, Nevada
Functional Disorders of the Esophagus

RODNEY J. MASON, M.D., PH.D.
Assistant Professor of Surgery, University of Southern California; Attending Surgeon, University of Southern California University Hospital, Los Angeles, California
Physiologic Diagnostic Studies

DOUGLAS J. MATHISEN, M.D.
Professor of Surgery, Harvard Medical School; Chief of Thoracic Surgery, Massachusetts General Hospital, Boston, Massachusetts
Techniques of Esophageal Reconstruction

BARBARA J. MCKENNA, M.D.
Associate Professor of Pathology, Albany Medical Center, Albany, New York
Barrett's Esophagus: Morphologic Considerations

TIMOTHY T. NOSTRANT, M.D.
Professor of Medicine, University of Michigan Medical School; University of Michigan Hospitals, Ann Arbor, Michigan
Esophageal Dilatation

MARK B. ORRINGER, M.D.
John Alexander Distinguished Professor and Head, Section of Thoracic Surgery, University of Michigan Medical Center, Ann Arbor, Michigan
Reflux Stricture and Short Esophagus; Transhiatal Esophagectomy Without Thoracotomy; Complications of Esophageal Surgery; Esophageal Trauma; Miscellaneous Conditions of the Esophagus

HIRAM C. POLK, JR., M.D.
Ben A. Reid, Sr. Professor and Chairman, Department of Surgery, University of Louisville School of Medicine, Louisville, Kentucky
The Nissen Fundoplication: Operative Technique and Clinical Experience

PETER C. PAIROLERO, M.D.
Professor of Surgery and Chair, Department of Surgery, Consultant, Division of General Thoracic Surgery, Mayo Clinic and Foundation, Rochester, Minnesota
Surgical Management of Esophageal Diverticula

CARLOS A. PELLEGRINI, M.D.
Professor and Chairman, Department of Surgery, University of Washington; Attending Surgeon, University of Washington Medical Center, Seattle, Washington
Laparoscopic Esophageal Surgery

JOHN C. RABINE, M.D.
Fellow, Division of Gastroenterology, University of Michigan Hospital, Ann Arbor, Michigan
Esophageal Dilatation

CAROLYN E. REED, M.D.
Professor of Surgery, Medical University of South Carolina; Director, Hollings Cancer Center, Charleston, South Carolina
Esophageal Carcinoma: Palliation with Intubation and Laser

THOMAS W. RICE, M.D.
Head, Section of General Thoracic Surgery, Department of Thoracic and Cardiovascular Surgery, Cleveland Clinic Foundation, Cleveland, Ohio
Endoscopic Esophageal Ultrasonography

GEORGE A. SAROSI, M.D.
Assistant Professor of Surgery, University of Texas, Southwestern Medical School; Staff Physician, Veterans Affairs Medical Center, Dallas, Texas
Esophageal Varices

HUBERT J. STEIN, M.D.
Private Docent, Department of Surgery, Technische University of Munich; Chief, General and Thoracic Surgery, Klinikum Rechts der Isar, Munich, Germany
Anatomy and Embryology

VICTOR F. TRASTEK, M.D.
Professor of Surgery and Chair, Department of Surgery, Consultant, Division of General Thoracic Surgery, Mayo Clinic-Scottsdale, Scottsdale, Arizona
Barrett's Esophagus: Surgical Implications; Surgical Management of Esophageal Diverticula

RICHARD I. WHYTE, M.D.
Associate Professor and Head, Division of Thoracic Surgery, Stanford University School of Medicine, Stanford, California
Miscellaneous Conditions of the Esophagus

EARLE W. WILKINS, JR., M.D.
Clinical Professor of Surgery Emeritus, Harvard Medical School; Senior Surgeon, Massachusetts General Hospital, Boston, Massachusetts
Techniques of Esophageal Reconstruction

MARK A. WILSON, M.D., PH.D.
Associate Professor of Surgery, University of Louisville; Director, Price Institute of Surgical Research, University of Louisville, Louisville, Kentucky
The Nissen Fundoplication: Operative Technique and Clinical Experience

GREGORY ZUCCARO, JR., M.D.
Head, Section of Gastrointestinal Endoscopy, Cleveland Clinic Foundation, Cleveland, Ohio
Endoscopic Esophageal Ultrasonography

Preface

We are pleased to present the fifth edition of *Shackelford's Surgery of the Alimentary Tract,* an encyclopedic five-volume set that has served as an invaluable source of information on alimentary tract surgery for thousands of practicing general surgeons and residents over the past decades. The first edition of *Surgery for the Alimentary Tract* was edited by Dr. Richard T. Shackelford and published in 1955. Following the success of the first edition, the W.B. Saunders Company urged Dr. Shackelford to produce a second edition. Between 1978 and 1986, this was accomplished as a five-volume set, expanded substantially from the first edition, with Dr. George D. Zuidema joining Dr. Shackelford as a coeditor, and with the help of many faculty members at The Johns Hopkins University School of Medicine.

The third edition, edited by Dr. Zuidema, appeared in 1991 and proved to be an important step forward, as the field of alimentary tract surgery had advanced as a result of many surgical research findings and emerging technologies. It was in the third edition that Dr. Zuidema enlisted the help of a guest editor for each of the five volumes of the series.

The fourth edition was published in 1996, and it instantly became a classic reference text, well known to surgeons worldwide specializing in the field of alimentary tract surgery. The edition also found a place in many libraries and has served as a reference source for internists, gastroenterologists, and others.

This fifth edition has been accomplished with the help of colleagues who have served as guest editors for each of the five volumes. The publication of this edition is particularly timely, for numerous dramatic changes in surgical practice, operative approaches, molecular biology, and noninvasive therapies have occurred in the past few years. Each volume retains extensive sections on anatomy and physiology, then directs attention to the appropriate surgical issues. The fifth edition presents an enormous amount of new knowledge and many innovations, and it includes the contributions of many new authors and several new volume editors.

Volume I (Esophagus) is edited by Dr. Mark B. Orringer, aided by Dr. Richard F. Heitmiller. The volume covers esophageal anatomy, physiology, and surgery in depth, adding a new chapter entitled "Laparoscopic Esophageal Surgery." New fundamentals of antireflux surgery, oncologic esophageal surgery, and multimodality therapy for esophageal carcinoma are also discussed in depth.

Dr. Daniel T. Dempsey assumes volume editor duties for Volume II (Stomach and Duodenum, Incisions). Dr. Dempsey has created an almost entirely new volume, with numerous new contributors. New chapters cover "Mechanical and Motility Disorders of the Stomach and Duodenum" and "Laparoscopic Surgery of the Stomach and Duodenum." Further, the section on "Incisions" provides one of the most comprehensive descriptions of alimentary tract incisions, wound drainage, wound closure, and gastrointestinal suturing.

For Volume III (Pancreas, Biliary Tract, Liver and Portal Hypertension, Spleen), Dr. Jeremiah G. Turcotte continues as the volume editor. All chapters are updated, many by new contributors, and many new concepts and techniques are illustrated. In addition, a chapter on "Laparoscopic Splenectomy" is now included.

Dr. John H. Pemberton is the new editor of Volume IV (Colon, Rectum and Anus). The vast majority of chapters in this volume are newly written, with first-time contributors bringing fresh concepts to the field. Chapters new to this volume include "Laparoscopic Colon and Rectal Surgery," "Operations for Colorectal Cancer: Coloanal Anastomosis," "Recurrent and Metastatic Colorectal Cancer," "Resection and Ablation of Metastatic Colorectal Cancer of the Liver," "Evaluation and Management of Constipation and Pelvic Floor Disorders," "Rectovaginal Fistula," "Surgery in the Immunocompromised Patient," and "Reoperative Pelvic Surgery."

The new editor for Volume V is Dr. Keith D. Lillemoe. Updated chapters are included in the sections on Mesenteric Circulation and Hernia, with many new authors in the section on Small Intestine. For example, Crohn's disease is now covered in two chapters, the first dealing with "General Considerations" and the second dealing with "Surgical Management."

This edition would have been impossible without the hard work of each of the volume editors. They have each been helped immensely by their colleagues, staff, and chapter contributors. We would like to thank each of the volume editors for their help with this important project. It has been a pleasure to work with each of them.

We would like to express our appreciation to the many individuals who have contributed chapters to these five volumes. We understand how much work is involved in producing superb chapters, and we wish to recognize these individuals and thank them for their dedication and commitment. The many contributors to this fifth edition are clearly leaders in their fields, and we are deeply indebted to them all for sharing their knowledge and enthusiasm, culminating in an outstanding work.

The vast majority of the correspondence, mailings, and editorial oversight originated in the Department of Surgery at The Johns Hopkins University School of Medicine. Donna Adelsberg has provided tremendous support and assistance and deserves much praise.

We would also like to thank Lisette Bralow, Hazel Hacker, and Betty Taylor of the W.B. Saunders Company for their efforts in bringing this project to its fruition. They have been tremendous to work with, and have served as an inspiration during all phases of preparation of this edition.

CHARLES J. YEO
GEORGE D. ZUIDEMA

Acknowledgment

I would be remiss in not acknowledging the tremendous source of knowledge, inspiration, and direction that Drs. George D. Zuidema and John L. Cameron have provided to me during my career in surgery. Commencing as a medical student at Johns Hopkins (when Dr. Zuidema was the Chief of Surgery), carrying through to my years on the house staff at Johns Hopkins (under first Dr. Zuidema and then Dr. Cameron) and now as a faculty member (under Dr. Cameron), I have been privileged to work with these two special surgical educators. I am indebted to Dr. Zuidema for the opportunity to become involved with this book, and to work with true professionals every step along the way.

CHARLES J. YEO

Contents

VOLUME IV

COLON

VOLUME V

MESENTERIC CIRCULATION

VOLUME

I

Anatomy, Embryology, Physiology, and Congenital Abnormalities of the Esophagus

CHAPTER

1 Anatomy and Embryology

DOROTHEA LIEBERMANN-MEFFERT • ANDRÉ DURANCEAU
HUBERT J. STEIN

ANATOMY OF THE ESOPHAGUS

MACROSCOPIC FEATURES

Configuration

The esophagus is the narrowest tube of the intestinal tract. It ends by widening into its most voluminous part, the stomach. At rest, the esophagus is collapsed; it forms a soft muscular tube that is flat in its upper and middle parts, with a presenting diameter of 2.5 × 1.6 cm. The lower esophagus is rounded, and its diameter is 2.5 × 2.4 cm.[51]

Compression or constriction by adjacent organs, vessels, or muscles causes narrowing, which can be visualized by means of fluoroscopy and endoscopy.[51,55] The aortic compression, which is left-sided and anterolateral, is caused by the crossing of the aortic arch, the left atrium, and the left principal bronchus at a location 22 cm from the incisors. Occasionally, a mechanical imprint of the diaphragm exists, but more apparent are two functional muscular constrictions: the upper and the lower esophageal sphincters. They can be defined manometrically, respectively, at the esophageal opening, between 14 and 16 cm from the incisors, and at the entrance into the stomach, between 40 and 45 cm from the incisors (Fig. 1-1).

Length

The length of the esophagus is defined anatomically as the distance between the cricoid cartilage and the gastric orifice. In the adult, it ranges from 22 to 28 cm (24 ± 5 standard deviations), 3 to 6 cm of which are located in

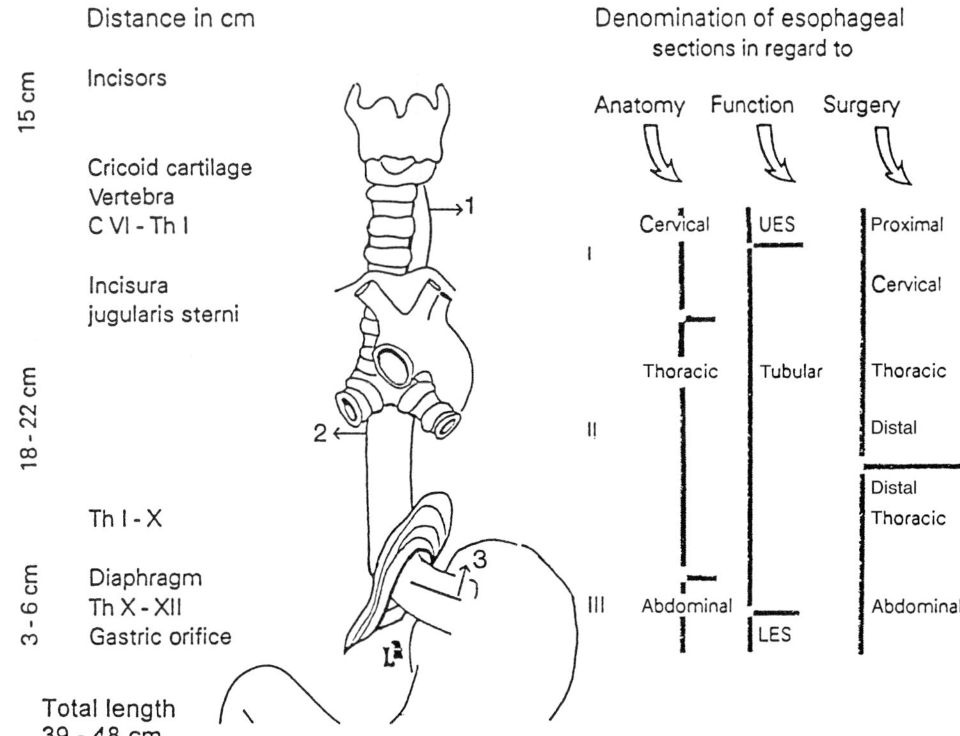

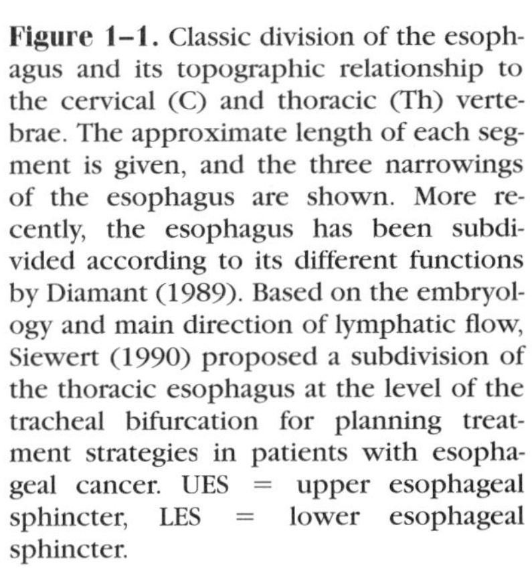
Figure 1–1. Classic division of the esophagus and its topographic relationship to the cervical (C) and thoracic (Th) vertebrae. The approximate length of each segment is given, and the three narrowings of the esophagus are shown. More recently, the esophagus has been subdivided according to its different functions by Diamant (1989). Based on the embryology and main direction of lymphatic flow, Siewert (1990) proposed a subdivision of the thoracic esophagus at the level of the tracheal bifurcation for planning treatment strategies in patients with esophageal cancer. UES = upper esophageal sphincter, LES = lower esophageal sphincter.

the abdomen.[17,32,67] In contrast to Lerche,[32] Liebermann-Meffert et al.[35] found the length of the esophagus to be related to the subject's height rather than sex.

The identification and marking of the cricoid cartilage is rather difficult. For practical reasons, clinicians measure the distance between both ends of the esophagus by including the oropharynx and the pharynx and use the incisors as a direct macroscopic landmark during endoscopic procedures.[12,51,55] These distances are shown in Figure 1-1.

Orthotopic and Non-anatomic Bypass

On measuring the differences in length required for esophageal replacement, the shortest distance between the cricoid cartilage and the celiac axis was found to be the orthotopic route in the posterior mediastinum (30 cm). The retrosternal location (32 cm) and the subcutaneous route (34 cm) proved to be longer.[47] There were no differences between men and women.

Periesophageal Tissue Compartments

Unlike the general structure of the digestive tract, the esophagus has neither mesentery nor serosal coating. Its position within the mediastinum and a complete envelope of loose connective tissue allows the esophagus extensive transverse and longitudinal mobility. Respiration may induce craniocaudal movement over a few millimeters, and swallows may result in excursion over as much as the height of one vertebral body.[12] There are surgical implications to this observation. It is because the esophagus is surrounded by loose areolar connective tissue (Fig. 1-2) that it may be subjected to a blunt stripping from the mediastinum when there are no periesophageal contraindications to the use of this technique, such as fixation or invasion by malignant tumor.[2,21,35,48]

Another anatomic peculiarity is of clinical interest: The esophagus is enclosed between well-defined fascial planes. Connective tissues in which the esophagus and the trachea are embedded are bounded by the pretracheal

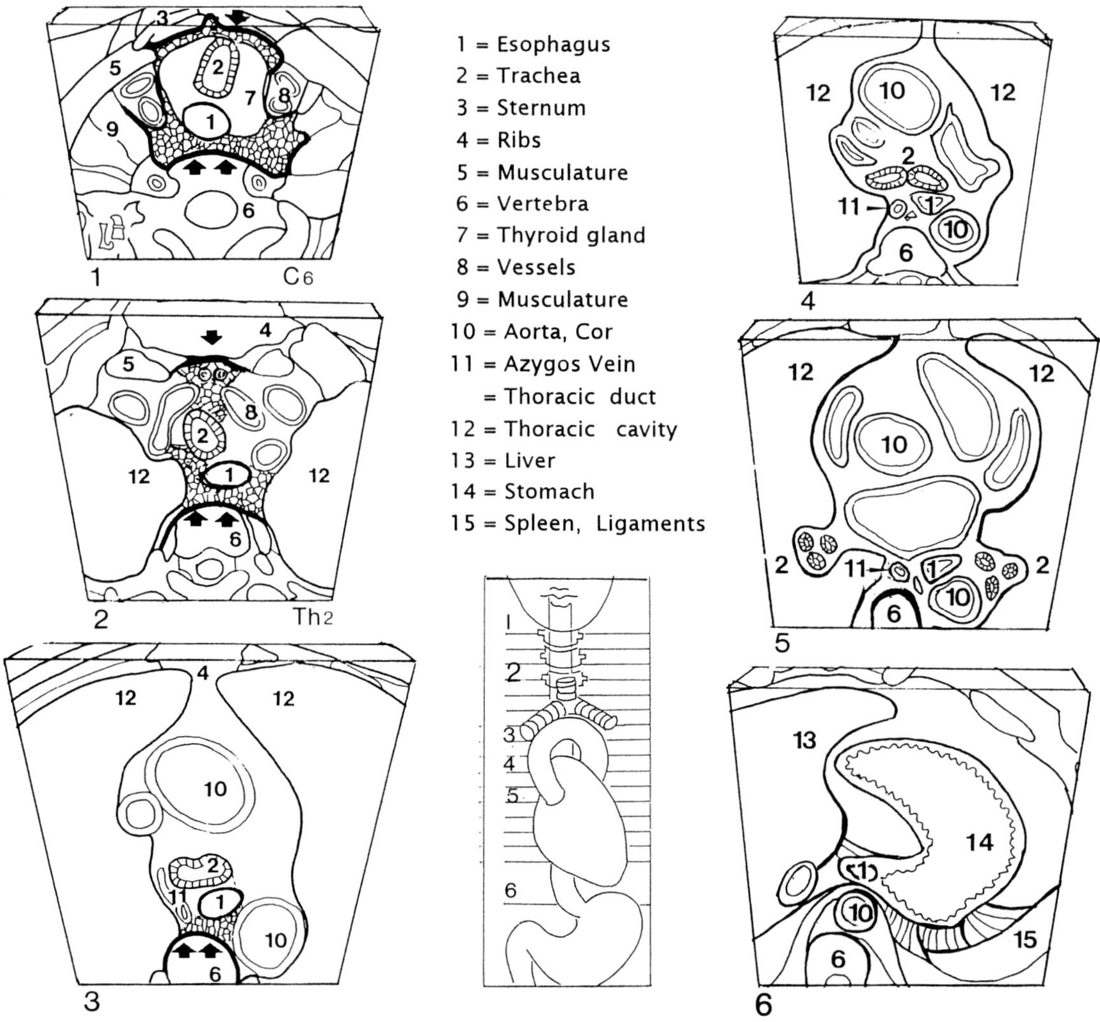

Figure 1-2. Topographic anatomy of the esophagus shown from the cervical level (1) to the esophagogastric junction (6). Transverse section through the mediastinum shows the esophagus and its surrounding structures in the CT aspect. The close positional relationship among the esophagus, trachea, and vertebrae and the fascial planes is displayed. The thick dark lines are the prevertebral and previsceral fascia *(arrows)*; the net-like pattern represents the respective areolar connective tissue. (Modified after Wegener, O.H.: Neuromuscular organization of esophageal and pharyngeal motility. Arch. Intern. Med., *136*:524, 1976, with permission.)

fascia anteriorly and the prevertebral fascia posteriorly. In the upper chest, both fascias unite to form the carotid sheath. Thus, the anterior and posterior spaces between these fascias form a communicating compartment between the neck and the chest, and this provides a plane for the rapid spread of infection through the mediastinum (see Fig. 1-2).

The previsceral or pretracheal space surrounds the vascular structures of the mediastinum and is limited distally by the fibrous tissue of the pericardium. Infections spreading from anterior lesions of the esophagus may follow this route. The retrovisceral or prevertebral space extends commonly from the base of the skull to the diaphragm. This space is formed by the buccopharyngeal fascia spreading downward by a sheath that separates the esophagus from the prevertebral fascia. Below the level of the tracheal bifurcation, this space may be obliterated. The retrovisceral space is clinically more important than is the previsceral space, because most instrument perforations of the upper digestive tract with subsequent outflow of esophageal content occur above the narrowing of the cricopharyngeal sphincter in the posterior hypopharynx.[55] At this level, as in the chest, there is no barrier to the spread of infection into the mediastinum. Rupture of the esophagus or leakage of an esophageal anastomosis also may result in descending mediastinitis along these planes. Prompt diagnosis is vital for the patient, because the prognosis for esophageal perforation depends on the rapidity with which treatment is initiated.

Supporting and Anchoring Structures

The esophagus, both proximally and distally, is stabilized by bony, cartilaginous, or membranous structures (Fig. 1-3). At the cranial end, the exterior esophageal musculature is firmly inserted on the posterior plane (i.e., on the ridge of the cricoid cartilage), with the help of the cricoesophageal tendon (Fig. 1-4).

The claim that broad fibrous tissue or muscle strings connect trachea, esophagus, and pleura as pictured by Laimer[28] and adopted in Netter's atlas[46] could not be substantiated by the authors' studies.[40,41] Instead, the authors found that between the neck and the tracheal bifurcation are numerous delicate, slightly undulated membranes; these are 170 μm thick and approximately 3 to 5 mm long, extend up to 1.5 cm in a craniocaudal direction, and anchor the esophageal wall to the trachea, pleura, prevertebral fascia, and surrounding tissue of the posterior mediastinum (Figs. 1-3, 1-5*A*, and 1-5*B*). The membranes consist of collagen and elastic fiber elements (see Fig. 1-5*A*) and occasional interpositioned sparse muscle fibers, are stretchable to some extent, and accumulate around the tracheal bifurcation.[41] Although most membranes can be torn easily, pull-through dissection of the esophagus may eventually cause tears to the connected structures, because some individuals possess membranes of up to 700 μm thickness together with firm intramural insertions (see Fig. 1-5*A*). Because the possibility for tearing is unpredictable, mediastinoscopic dissection of the membranes close to the wall of the upper half of the esophagus—instead of blunt transhiatal

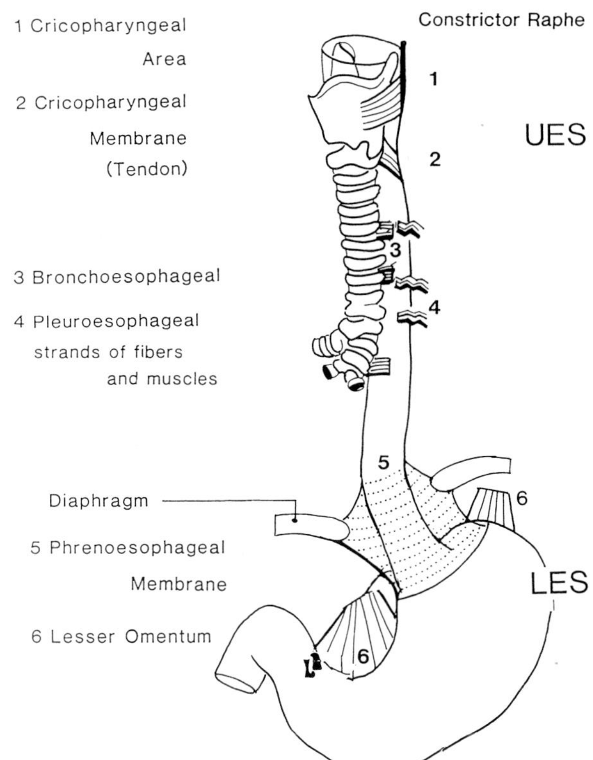

Figure 1-3. Attachments of the esophagus. The upper end of the esophagus obtains a firm anchorage by the insertion of its longitudinal muscle into the cartilaginous structures of the hypopharynx (1) via the cricoesophageal tendon (2). The circular muscle is stabilized by its continuity with the inferior laryngeal constrictor muscles (1), which insert via the raphe to the sphenoid bone. Tiny membranes connect the esophagus with the trachea, bronchi, pleura, and prevertebral fascia (3 and 4). The attachment at the lower end by the phrenoesophageal membrane (5) is rather mobile, whereas the posterior gastric ligaments, such as the gastrosplenic, phrenicolienal, and phrenicogastric ligaments (6) and the lesser omentum (6), yield a tight adherence. UES = upper esophageal sphincter, LES = lower esophageal sphincter.

pull-through esophagectomy—appears to be advisable to reduce the risk of tracheopleural tears and chylothorax.[6,40,41]

The distal esophagus traverses the diaphragm through the esophageal hiatus, which is bounded by the two diaphragmatic crura. The configuration of these structures has been extensively reviewed by Postlethwait[51] and in *Gray's Anatomy*.[66] Their insertion on the anterolateral surfaces of the first three or four lumbar vertebrae and the organization of their fibers may give a varying shape to the hiatus. This shape is influenced by respiration, swallowing, and altered thoracoabdominal pressure.

The diaphragm is inserted on the lumbar vertebrae, the ribs, and the sternum and has a large membranous central portion. This central tendon consists of decussating strands of fibrous tissue. The membranous portion is frequently larger than that described in the literature, and the left crus of the diaphragm may consist of membranous tissue rather than a significant muscular mass (Fig. 1-6).[41,66] The subdiaphragmatic and the endothoracic aponeuroses blend at the central margin of the diaphragm to constitute the phrenoesophageal membrane, also known as Laimer's ligament or Allison's membrane (Fig.

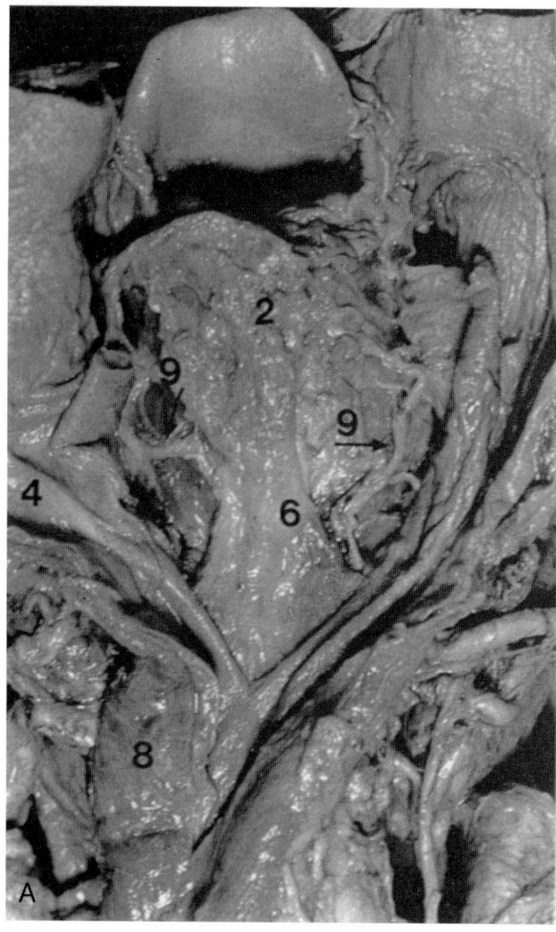

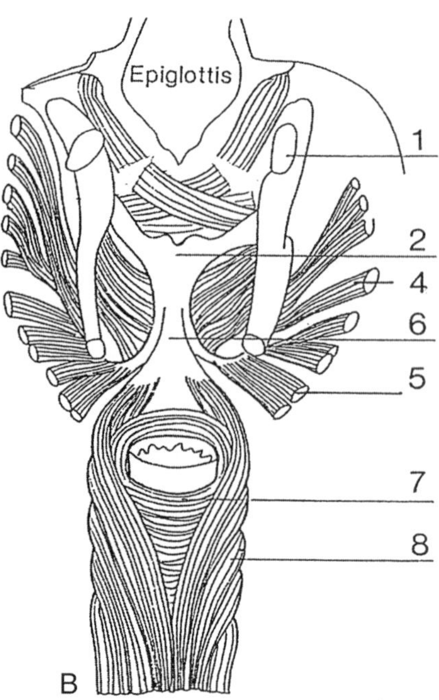

Figure 1–4. The posterior walls of the pharynx (4) and the esophagus (7 and 8) have been cut open in the midline. This is shown in a specimen *(A)* and half-schematically *(B)*. The structures of the hypopharynx are exposed by retracting the overlying incised tissue and removing the mucosa. In the center lies the cricoesophageal tendon (6), which attaches at the longitudinal muscle layer of the esophagus (8) to the cricoid cartilage (2). The terminal branches of the left laryngeal recurrent nerve (9) are dissected and are seen lateral to the cricoesophageal tendon. Thyroid cartilage (1). (Specimen and photo courtesy of Liebermann-Meffert, Munich.)

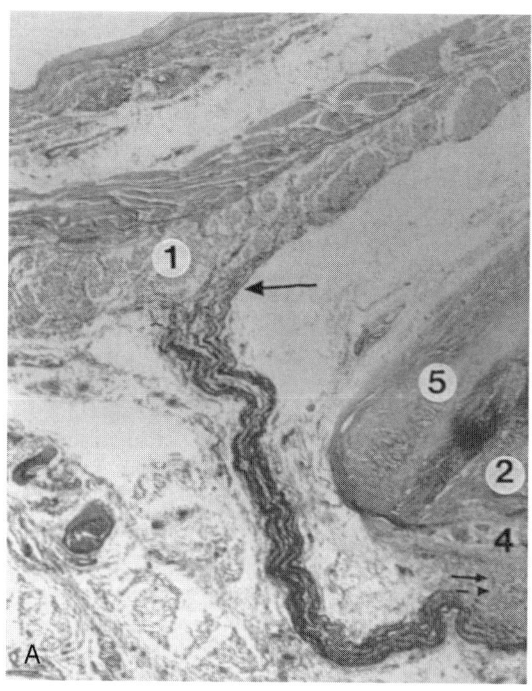

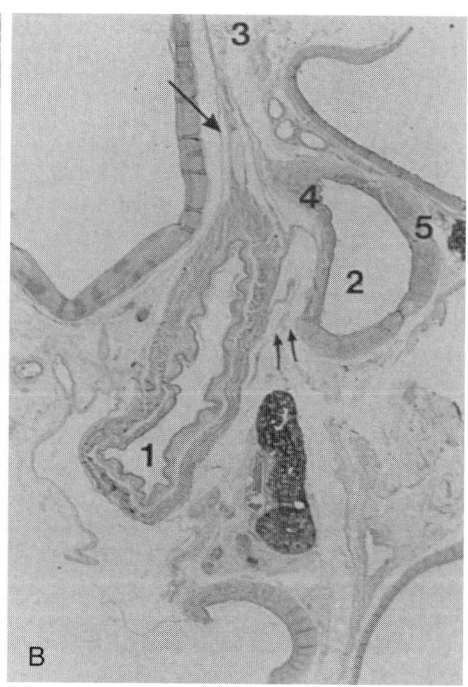

Figure 1–5. *A* and *B*, Example of the tiny fiber membranes that connect esophagus (1), trachea (2), pleura (3), tracheal membrane (4), and cartilaginous structures (5). At their insertions, the fiber elements fan out to deep finger-shaped extensions between the muscular bundles of the esophagus *(arrow)* and into the membranous part of the trachea *(double arrows)*. This texture, in conjunction with the elasticity of the membranes, certainly provides adequate adjustment during the movements of the esophagus. In case of rapid pull, the fibers eventually tear off the tissues in which they are anchored. (Human esophagus, transverse section, hematoxylin and eosin.) (Courtesy of Huber, Haeberle, and Liebermann-Meffert, Munich.)

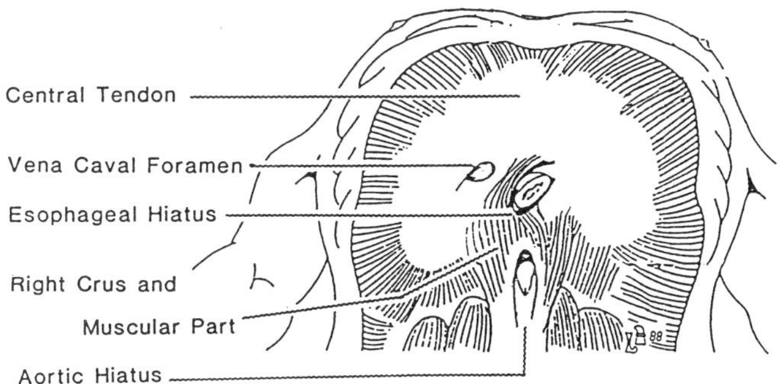

Figure 1–6. Diaphragm and esophageal hiatus viewed from the abdominal aspect.

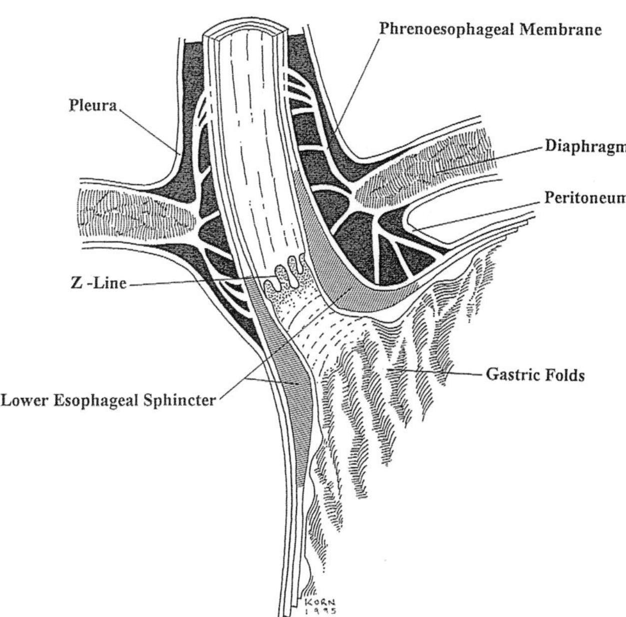

Figure 1–8. Diagram of the tissue organization and the supporting structures at the esophagogastric junction. The esophagus is opened alongside the greater and lesser curvatures. The luminal aspect is displayed from the left side. The fiber elements that attach the phrenoesophageal membrane to the muscle wall of the terminal esophagus are shown. The fibers are similar to those shown in Figure 1–5. (Courtesy of Dr. Owen Korn, Munich and Santiago di Chile.)

1–7). Macroscopically, the phrenoesophageal membrane can be recognized by its well-defined lower edge and its slightly yellow color, even in the presence of severe periesophagitis. The membrane is composed of, in equal proportions, elastic and collagenous fiber elements, which guarantee sufficient pliability. Owing to its origin from fascia, the phrenoesophageal membrane in general is relatively strong. It splits into two sheets (Fig. 1–8). One sheet extends upward 2 to 4 cm through the hiatus, where its elastic and collagenous fibers traverse the esophageal musculature to insert on the submucosa.[15] The other sheet passes down across the cardia to the level of the gastric fundus to blend into the gastric serosa, the gastrohepatic ligament, and the dorsal gastric mesentery (see Figs. 1–2, 1–3, and 1–7). Although there are some attachments by loose connective tissue, the phrenoesophageal membrane is clearly separated from the esophageal musculature of the gastroesophageal junction, which is wrapped by the membrane as by a wide collar (see Fig. 1–7). This structural arrangement allows the terminal esophagus and the junction to move in relation with the diaphragm and to "slip through the hiatus like in a tendon sheath."[23] With advancing age, the elastic fibers are replaced by inelastic collagenous tissue, and the adhesion of the phrenoesophageal membrane to the lower esophagus becomes looser.[15] This leads to a loss of pliability. Disruption of the anchoring structures of the cardia and proximal stomach in conjunction with a wide hiatus may result in protrusion of the gastroesophageal junction and the cardia, or even parts of the stomach, into the mediastinum. Abnormal anchoring of the phrenoesophageal membrane in youth and pathologic accumulation of adipose tissue in the separating connective tissue space between the phrenoesophageal membrane and the cardia musculature are considered to contribute to the development of a hiatal hernia.[15]

REGIONAL ANATOMY

General Aspects

The esophagus is a midline structure lying on the anterior surface of the spine. It descends through three compartments: the neck, the chest, and the abdomen. This pro-

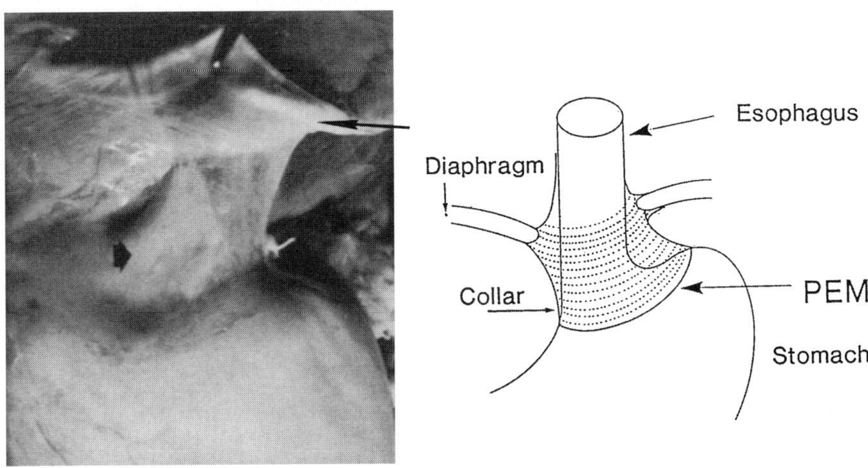

Figure 1–7. The phrenoesophageal membrane (PEM). The lower component of the membrane inserts on the gastric fundus. On the left, the diaphragm is held with a forceps. Diaphragmatic decussating fibers *(long arrow)* and a submembranous inlay of adipose tissue *(short arrow)* are seen. The PEM wraps the esophagogastric junction with a wide membranous collar. (Specimen and photo: Liebermann-Meffert, Munich.)

gression has led to its classic division into cervical, thoracic, and abdominal segments (see Fig. 1-1). Two more useful subdivisions have been proposed (see Fig. 1-1). The one by Diamant[10] refers to functional aspects and makes the distinction between the esophageal body and the upper and lower sphincters. The other, by Siewert et al.,[59] refers to oncosurgical concepts and distinguishes between the proximal and distal esophagus, using the tracheal bifurcation as a partition. This concept integrates the features of embryologic development, in particular the differently oriented pathways of lymphatic drainage (see the section "Lymphatic Drainage" later in this chapter).

The topographic relationships of the esophagus have been studied extensively using different technical approaches[32,50,65,66] (see also Fig. 1-2). The conclusions are as follows.

As the next structure after the pharynx (see Fig. 1-4), the esophagus begins at the cricoid cartilage opposite the sixth cervical vertebra. It passes into the chest at the level of the sternal notch and travels within the chest cavity on the anterior limit of the posterior mediastinum. Between the thoracic inlet and the diaphragm, it remains in close relationship with the spine. It ends at the esophagogastric junction, opposite the twelfth thoracic vertebra. Three minor deviations are present along its trajectory. The first one is toward the left at the base of the neck (Figs. 1-2 and 1-9). This makes the surgical approach to the esophagus easier from the left than from the right in performing intestinal-cervical esophageal anastomoses after esophagectomy. The second deviation is observed at the level of the seventh thoracic vertebra, where the esophagus turns slightly to the right of the spine. On radiologic evaluation, however, the esophageal axis is virtually straight. Unaffected by scoliotic curves of the vertebral column the esophagus preserves the normal straight course; this differs from the behavior of the large vascular structures, which follow the abnormality of the spine.[45] Vascular anomalies or mediastinal masses, however, may displace, bow, or indent the esophagus, but any distortion of its axis strongly suggests mediastinal invasion and retraction, usually by a malignancy.[2]

Owing to the third deviation of the terminal portion of the esophagus, the esophagogastric junction or cardia is positioned slightly lateral to the xiphoid process of the sternum and is found to the left of the spine. At this point, the fundus and the proximal stomach extend anterolateral to the body of the vertebra; therewith the greater curvature faces the posterior subdiaphragmatic space and the anterior gastric wall faces lateral. This topographic dimension is not well displayed in standard anatomy textbooks but is excellently obtained from computed tomographic studies.[65] A better understanding of the events leading to herniation of the cardia and the interpretation of pressure measurement data of the lower esophageal sphincter (LES) will result.

Topographic Relations

Ventral to and in direct local contact with the cervical esophagus lies the flat fibrous membrane of the trachea (see Fig. 1-9). This feature deserves special attention

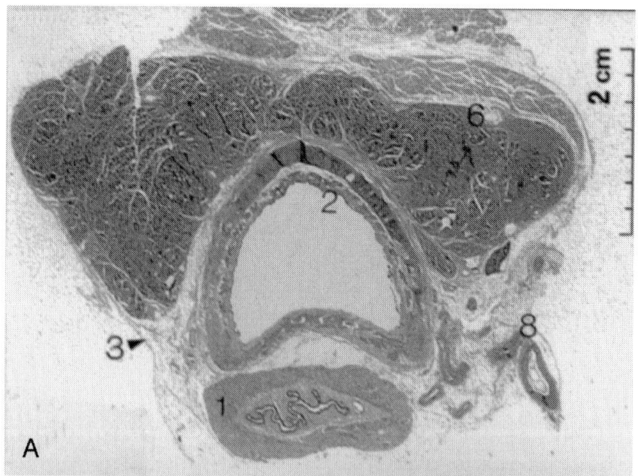

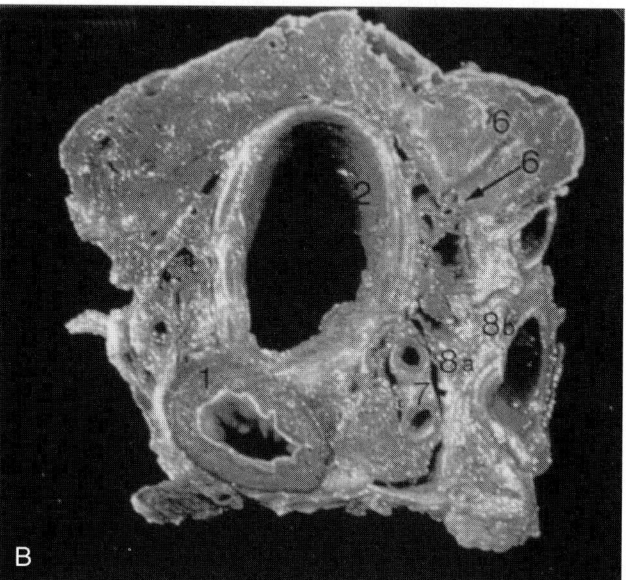

Figure 1-9. Transverse section through the neck and upper chest of a human autopsy specimen viewed from a cranial aspect. 1 = esophagus, 2 = trachea, 3 = pleura, 6 = thyroid gland and vessels *(arrow)*, and 8 = vessels. The histologic section shows the esophagus still in midline posterior position *(A)*, whereas in the more distal level of the macroscopic cut surface *(B)*, the esophagus has shifted toward the left. Note the intimate local relationship between the esophagus and the trachea. (From Liebermann-Meffert, D: *In* Fuchs, K.H., Stein, H.J., Thiede, A. [eds.]: Gastrointestinale Funktionsstörungen. Berlin, Springer, 1997, with permission.)

because, as far as the tracheal bifurcation, only a thin layer of loose connective tissue separates the two structures (see Fig. 1-9). Any malignant tumor may easily spread from one to the other. The development of a tracheoesophageal fistula following either esophagectomy or irradiation in this inherently weak area is a catastrophic problem for both patient and physician.[3,18] The posteromedial aspects of both thyroid lobes cover the cranial 2 to 3 cm of the esophagus on both sides. The vascular structures and the innervation are discussed later in this chapter.

Between the thoracic inlet and the tracheal bifurcation, at the level of the fifth thoracic vertebra, the esophagus retains its intimate relationship to the trachea ventrally and to the prevertebral fascia posteriorly (see Fig.

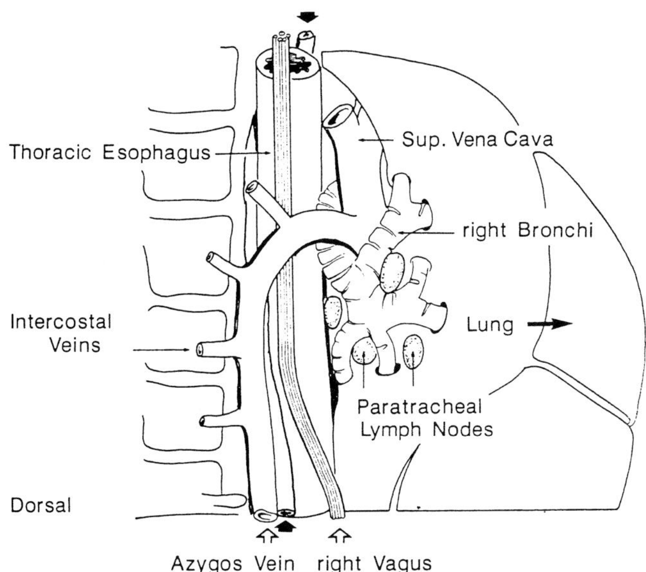

Figure 1–10. The position and relationships of the azygos vein, the thoracic duct, and the vagus nerve are shown from a right lateral aspect.

1-2). Lateral on both sides are the mediastinal pleura and the lungs and their hilus. On the right lies the subclavian artery and the azygos vein, which arches over the right principal bronchus to end in the superior vena cava (Fig. 1-10). In performing transthoracic esophagectomy, surgical access for safe removal of the esophagus is preferably through the right chest,[59] where the azygos vein must usually be divided before the esophagus can be dissected free. The primarily right-side-positioned thoracic duct crosses behind the esophagus just above the arch of the azygos vein at the level of T4 to T5. Structures on the left of the esophagus are the aortic arch and the aorta, which subsequently turns to the midline toward posterior behind the esophagus. In front of the esophagus are the lung hilum and the heart. The vessels and nerves that supply the esophagus and the adjacent organs are discussed later in this chapter. The pleura on the left side of the mediastinum occasionally may extend behind the esophagus. Both vagi accompany the esophagus while it passes through the hiatus at the level of the tenth thoracic vertebra.

In the abdomen, part of the left lobe of the liver lies ventral to the esophagus. Both diaphragmatic crura are lateral and posterior. The inferior vena cava is lateral to the right crus, whereas the aorta is found posterior to the left crus. The cranial pole of the spleen is in close relationship to the terminal esophagus (see Fig. 1-2).

Tissue Organization of the Esophagus

The overall tissue structure of the esophagus parallels the basic tissue organization of the digestive tract (Fig. 1-11). It comprises an external fibrous layer (tunica adventitia), a muscular layer (tunica muscularis), a submucous layer (tela submucosa), and an internal mucous layer (tunica mucosa).

Tunica Adventitia

The tunica adventitia is a thin layer composed of loose connective tissue. It envelops the esophagus, connects it with adjacent structures, and contains small vessels, lymphatic channels, and nerve fibers.

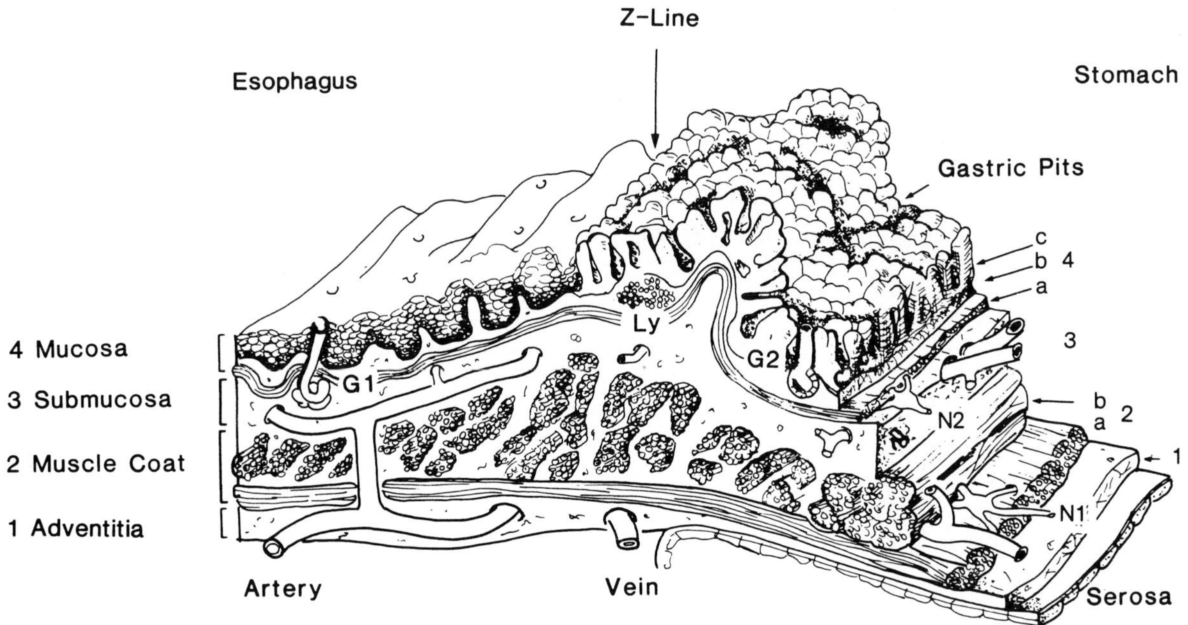

Figure 1–11. Wall structure at the esophagogastric junction. The tunica muscularis is composed of both a longitudinal and a circular layer. (a = muscularis mucosae, b = lamina propria, c = epithelium, G1 = esophageal glands, G2 = gastric glands, Ly = lymph vessels, N1 = myenteric plexus, N2 = submucous nerve plexus.)

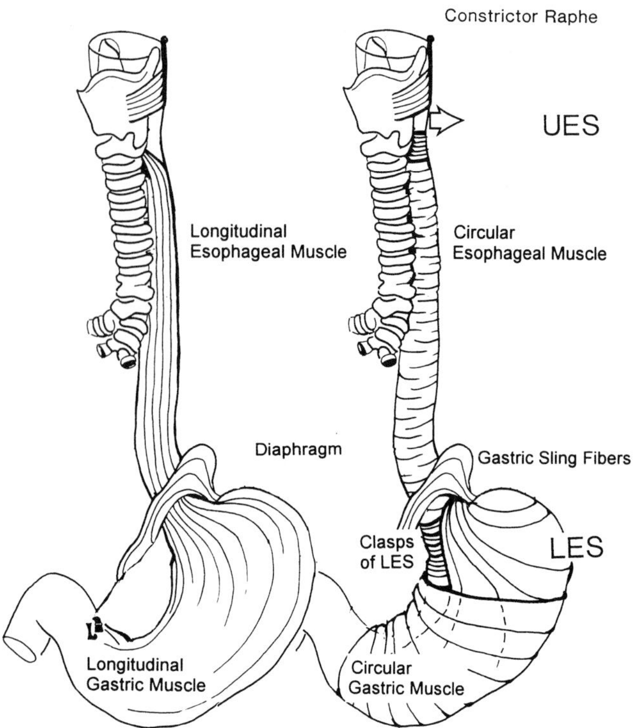

Figure 1-12. Architecture of the longitudinal and circular muscle layers across the esophagus, the stomach, and the respective junctions. (UES = upper esophageal sphincter, LES = lower esophageal sphincter.)

Tunica Muscularis

This layer consists of two complete muscle coats, each with a different orientation of muscle fibers (Fig. 1-12). The outer muscle layer parallels the longitudinal axis of the esophagus, whereas the muscle fibers of the inner layer are superimposed on a horizontal axis. For this reason, these muscle layers are classically called *longitudinal* and *circular*, respectively.

Esophageal Body

The longitudinal layer originates from the small tendon at the dorsal plane of the cricoid cartilage as shown in Figure 1-4. After leaving the larynx, the muscular bundles fan out posteriorly, leaving vacant an area of exterior muscle (Laimer's triangle) before they wrap the esophagus entirely (Figs. 1-13 and 1-14). As long bundles, they course straight down the esophagus to cross the gastric inlet, where the majority of the fibers change their arrangement,[33] as shown in Figures 1-12 and 1-15.

The circular layer continues the cricopharyngeus muscle and begins at the level of the cricoid cartilage, possibly as an independent sheet (see Fig. 1-13).[32,33,39] In their descent, the fibers of the inner muscular layer form imperfect circles with overlapping ends. Approximately 3 cm above the junction with the stomach, the muscle fibers increase in number, causing a stepwise thickening of the inner musculature.[33,40] This is consistent with the rearrangement of the muscle fibers of the inner layer (see Figs. 1-12 and 1-15). As shown in Figure 1-12, the bundles on the side of lesser curvature retain their orientation and form short muscle clasps, whereas those on the greater curvature change to become the oblique gastric sling fibers. It has been suggested that the myotomy for achalasia preferably should be performed between the muscle clasps and sling fibers to preserve sphincter competence.[4]

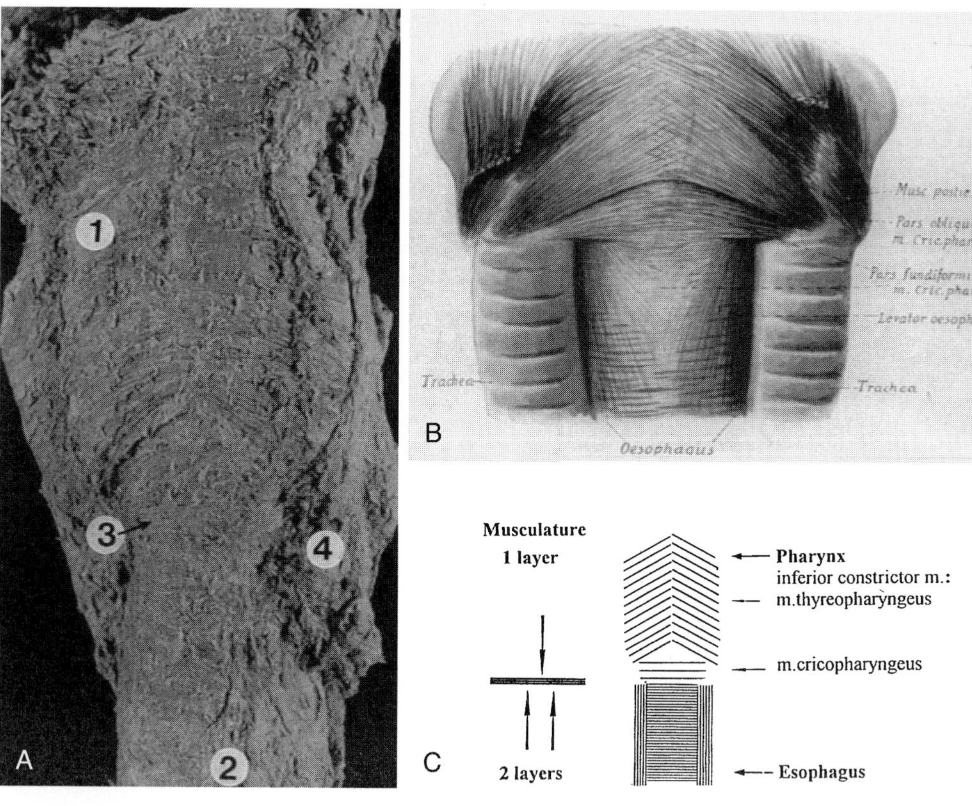

Figure 1-13. Structures at the pharyngoesophageal junction viewed from a posterior aspect. These are shown *(A)* in a human dried-fiber specimen (by Liebermann-Meffert), *(B)* in a schematic drawing of an anteriorly opened and unfolded specimen (by Killian), and *(C)* in a simplified diagram of the muscle organization. The muscular arrangement of the inferior constrictor of the pharynx (1) confirms Killian's observation of the tile-shaped arrangement of the bundles of the inferior constrictor muscle (Killian, G.: Z. Ohrenheilk, *55*:1, 1908.). With respect to the junction, two features should be emphasized: the change of one muscle layer at the pharynx (1) into two at the esophagus (2) just below the cricopharyngeal muscle (3) (UES), the cricopharyngeal muscle being part of the pharynx by position and anatomic characteristics. Residual tissue from the removed thyroid gland (4). (From Liebermann-Meffert, D: *In* Fuchs, K.-H., Stein, H.J., Thiede, A. [eds.]: Gastrointestinale Funktionsstörungen, Berlin, Springer, 1997, with permission.)

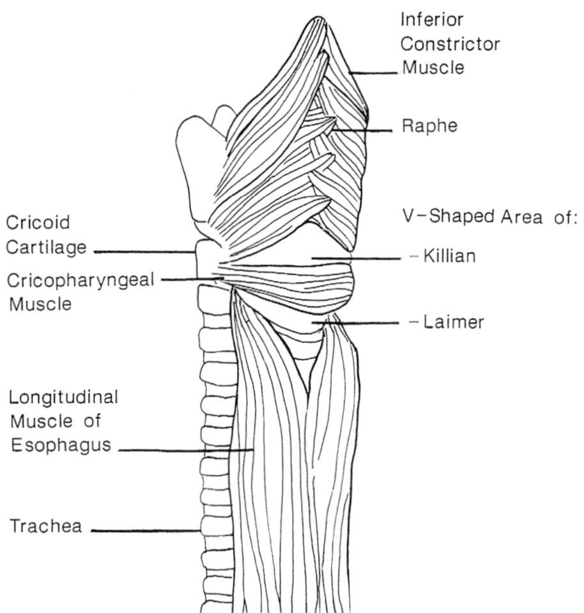

Figure 1–14. Schematic drawing of the structures at the pharyngoesophageal junction seen from the posterior aspect. The location of Killian's and Laimer's triangles is indicated; Zenker's diverticula develop cranial to the cricopharyngeal muscle, the upper esophageal sphincter is located at the V-shaped area of Killian.

A question has been raised about the exact distribution of the striated and smooth muscle in the esophagus.[36] Looking at serial sections through 15 human esophagi, Liebermann-Meffert and Geissdörfer noted that in the most proximal portion of the esophagus almost all the muscle fibers of both layers are striated.[36] In the following 6 to 8 cm, the tunica muscularis contains in both the external and the internal layers progressively more and more fascicles of smooth muscle (Fig. 1–16). The transition between both types is neither abrupt nor confined to individual muscle bundles and lacks any distinct anatomic separation.[36,40,41] Below the tracheal bifurcation, the striated muscle is completely replaced by smooth muscle.[36,44] The muscularis mucosa, however, is composed uniquely of smooth muscle fibers throughout the entire esophagus.

Upper Esophageal Sphincter

This sphincter lies at the end of the pharynx. It is manometrically a zone of elevated pressure, 2 to 4 cm in length,[69] and marks the entrance into the esophagus. The high pressure may result mainly from the effect of the cricopharyngeus muscle, which loops around the hypopharynx (see Figs. 1–13 and 1–14) and inserts on both cricoid processes. Although it is not a true sphincter in the anatomic sense, the cricopharyngeus muscle behaves like one.[14] During its sling-like contraction, the muscle closes the esophageal opening by exerting its effects ventrally against the "bony" plane of the cricoid cartilage. This accounts for the asymmetric pressure profile in manometric measurements.[69]

Lower Esophageal Sphincter

Whether or not the structure at the gastroesophageal junction is a true anatomic sphincter has long been de-

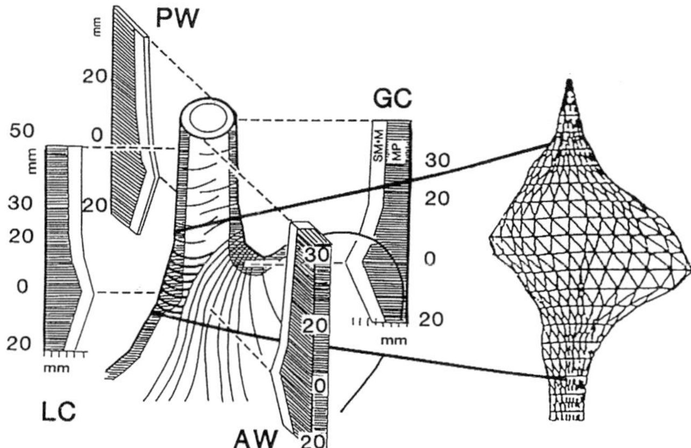

Figure 1–15. Schematic drawing showing the correlation between radial muscle thickness *(left)* and three-dimensional manometric pressure image *(right)* at the gastroesophageal junction. Muscle thickness across the gastroesophageal junction at the posterior gastric wall (PW), greater curvature (GC), anterior gastric wall (AW), and lesser curvature (LC) is shown in mm. Radial pressures at the gastroesophageal junction (in mmHg) are plotted around an axis representing atmospheric pressure. Note the marked radial and axial asymmetry of both the muscular thickness and the manometric pressure profile.

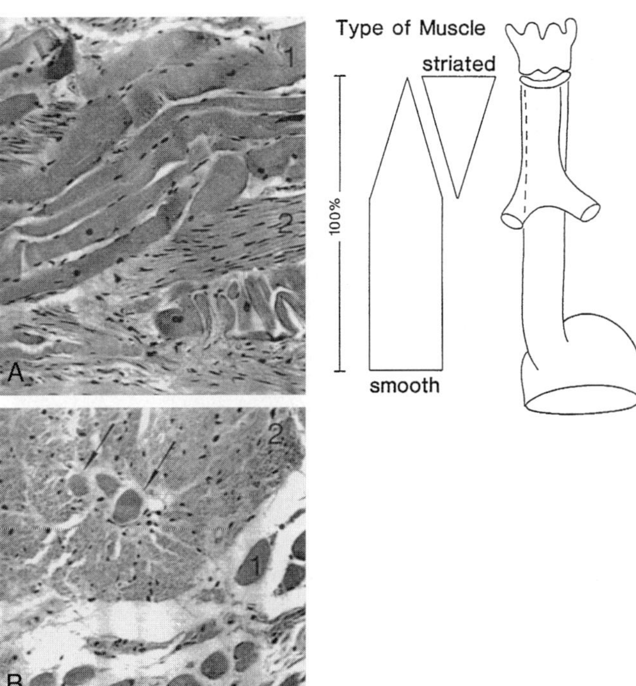

Figure 1–16. Histologic specimens of the human esophagus taken in the transverse *(A)* and the longitudinal *(B)* sections 4 cm above the tracheal bifurcation at the transition between striated (1) and smooth muscle (2). Individual striated muscle fibers are interspersed among smooth muscle strands *(arrows)*. The diagram shows the distribution of striated and smooth muscle in adult esophagus as evaluated from consecutive serial histologic sections of 13 esophagi. (Specimen and photo courtesy of Liebermann-Meffert, Geissdörfer, and Winter, Munich.)

bated.[11,19,31] Manometrically, there is a zone of elevated pressure, 3 to 5 cm in length, immediately above the junction of the esophagus with the stomach, the muscle of which behaves differently from the muscle above and below it.[52,58] With the use of small markers in a simultaneous radiomorphologic study, it has been shown that this high-pressure zone correlates with the thickened musculature at this site.[33,34] The specific arrangement of the musculature, as shown in Figures 1-12 and 1-15, also accounts for sphincter asymmetry.[27,33,34] Asymmetry of the high-pressure zone at this position also has been proven manometrically.[68] The manometric pressure image of the lower esophageal high-pressure zone, obtained by the recently developed technique of the three-dimensional computerized vector diagram, matches the muscular asymmetry at the human cardia (see Fig. 1-15).[60-62] Surgical removal of these structures by partial or total myectomy was shown to reduce significantly the specific sphincter pressure values of this muscle arrangement as recorded on manometry.[4,54,58,63] Dissection of the diaphragm or of the phrenoesophageal membrane produced no effect on the pressure values of the sphincter.[34]

Tela Submucosa

The tela submucosa connects the muscular coat and the mucosa. It contains elastic and collagenous fibers, a meshwork of blood vessels (see Fig. 1-11), abundant lymph vessels, nerves, and mucous glands. The deep esophageal glands are small branching glands of a mixed type, and their ducts pierce the muscularis mucosae.

Tunica Mucosa

This inner layer is made up of the muscularis mucosae, the tunica propria, and a stratified squamous epithelium without keratinization (see Fig. 1-11). The muscularis mucosae, when contracted, creates the folds of the mucosa. These long folds run in the longitudinal axis of the esophagus and also show small transverse rippled folds at the end of the esophagus.[13,33] All these folds disappear on distention of the esophageal lumen. The fibrous tunica propria projects into the epithelium, thus forming the papillae. It contains lymph channels in the lowermost level of the mucosa, occasional mononuclear cells, clusters of inflammatory cells, lymphocytes, and, in the distal esophagus, focal superficial (mucous) glands that resemble cardiac glands.

Clinically, the surface of the esophageal mucosa is reddish in its cranial portion and becomes paler toward the lower third of the esophagus. The smooth esophageal mucosa can be distinguished easily from the dark mamillated gastric mucosa. The mucosal transition at the squamocolumnar junction is an objectively recognizable reference point for the endoscopist.[55] On fresh anatomic specimens, it is characterized by an abrupt demarcation line, called the Z-line. This serrated line is located at or immediately above the gastric orifice. Any proximal extension of a gastric- or intestinal-type columnar epithelium is pathologic and is attributable to long-standing gastroesophageal reflux that causes chronic, severe esophageal mucosal and submucosal damage.[25,55]

STRUCTURES SUPPLYING THE ESOPHAGUS

Arterial Supply

A few investigators have discussed the macroscopic aspects of human esophageal vascularization.[37,56] Yet some details remain unclear and debatable. Angiograms do not outline the arterial pattern well because of the overlying arteries associated with other structures. Large en bloc

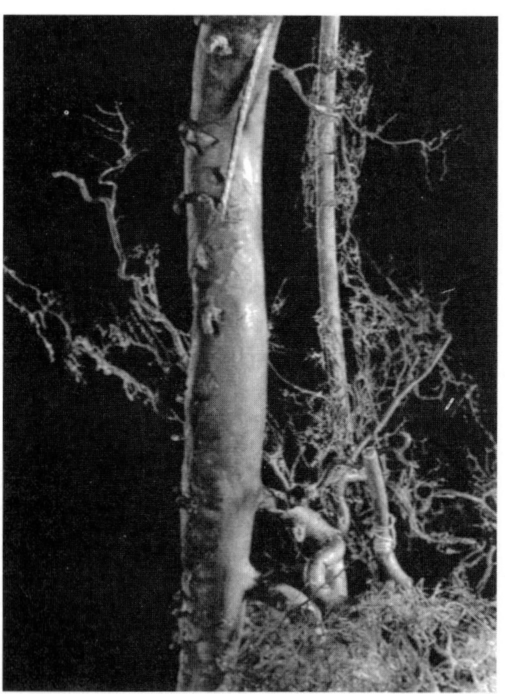

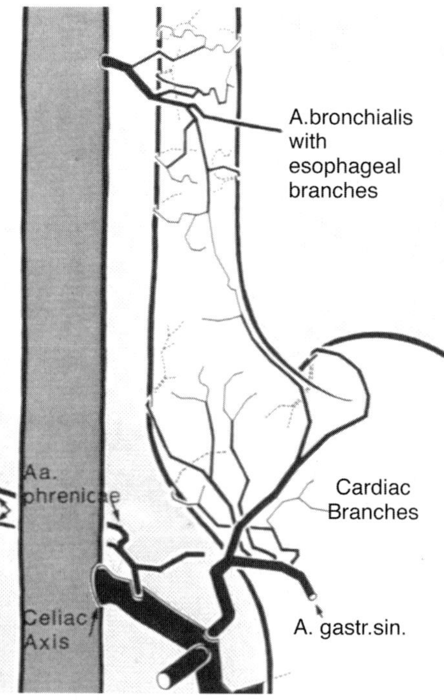

Figure 1-17. Arterial cast showing the vascular supply to the middle and lower esophagus. Note that the esophageal branch derives from the bronchial artery. In esophageal resections, it should be ligated close to the esophageal wall so as not to jeopardize the blood supply of the left main bronchus. In this context, it should be mentioned that the esophagus shares its blood supply with other organs: the thyroid gland, the trachea, the stomach, and the spleen.

corrosion casts, however, produce realistic three-dimensional replicas of the vascular system and display clearly both the large extraparietal arterial sources (Fig. 1-17) and the details of their microvascular connections (Fig. 1-18). There are three principal arterial sources for the esophagus (Fig. 1-19). In the neck, the upper superior and inferior thyroid arteries send small descending arteries to the cervical esophagus. At the level of the aortic arch, a group of three to five tracheobronchial arteries arise from the concavity of the arch and give rise to several esophageal tributaries. Occasionally, one or two eosophageal arteries proper arise from the anterior wall of the thoracic aorta. At the esophagogastric junction, the left gastric artery gives off up to 11 larger ascending branches that supply mostly the anterior and the right aspects of the lower esophagus[35,37] (see Fig. 1-17). Vessels from the splenic artery supply the posterior esophageal wall and parts of the greater curvature. Some larger branches run upward through the diaphragmatic hiatus before they enter the esophageal wall (see Figs. 1-17 and 1-19). Because the branches of the principal vessels anastomose, it is difficult to distinguish the proportion and percentage of blood distributed from each individual artery.

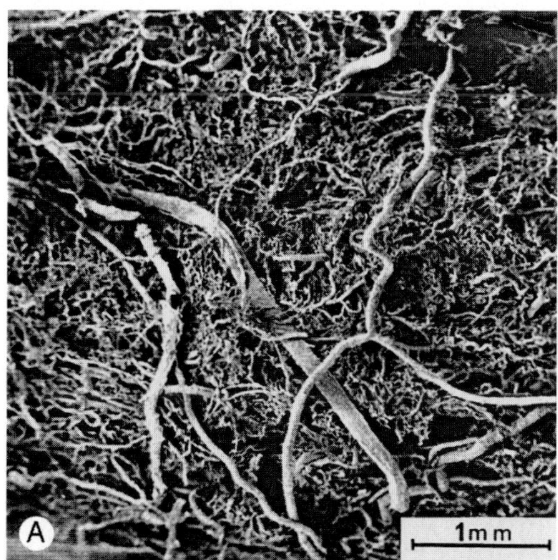

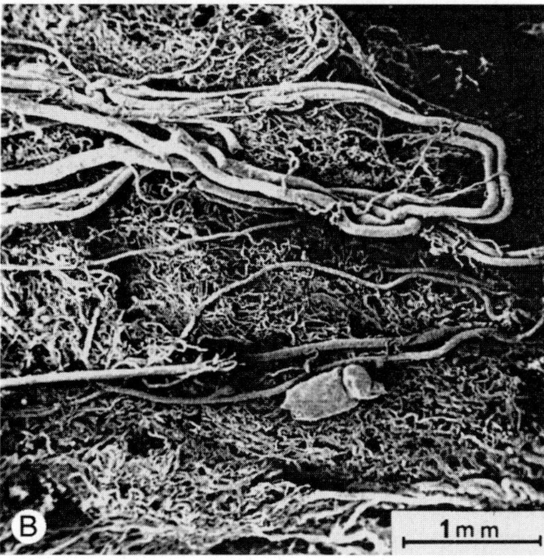

Figure 1-18. Scanning electron micrographs (SEMs) of complete vascular casts using a specially created resin without particles. The microvascular supply in the esophageal submucosa in the mid-esophagus *(A)* and in the cardia *(B)* is displayed. The vessels form a polygonal meshwork overlying the mucosa. (SEMs by Dr. Duggelin, Basel.)

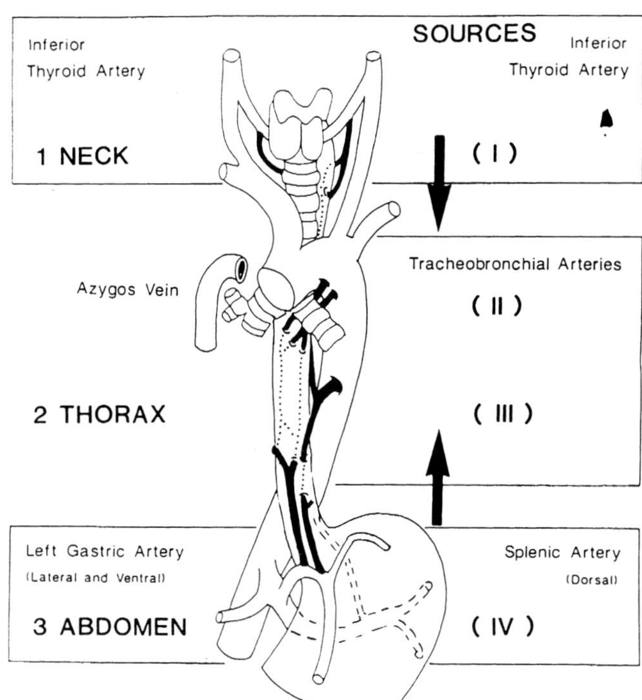

Figure 1-19. Extravisceral sources of arterial blood supply to the esophagus, intramural anastomoses *(dotted line)*, and topographic relationship of the azygos vein to the esophagus and tracheal bifurcation. The arrows indicate the direction of flow.

Two facts became obvious through Liebermann-Meffert's studies[35] that had not been appreciated before: All major arterial vessels divide into minute branches at some distance from the esophageal wall. It appears that such small esophageal tributaries, when torn, have the benefit of contractile hemostasis. Previous claims that essential nutritional vessels arise from the intercostal or phrenic arteries or directly from the aorta could not be confirmed.[35]

Further points of surgical importance need to be emphasized. The extraesophageal branches enter the esophageal wall, pass through the tunica muscularis, and give off a small number of branches to the muscle before they form a wide vascular plexus within the submucosa and mucosa (see Fig. 1-18). The evident continuity of the vessels and the rich anastomosing intramural vascularity[1,33,38] explain why, on the one hand, the mobilized esophagus retains an excellent blood supply over a long distance[67] and why, on the other hand, ligation of the left gastric artery in creation of a gastric substitute after esophagectomy most of the time does not compromise the surgical anastomosis.[38] The extremely small caliber of the nutritional vessels may also explain the failure of esophagointestinal anastomosis after any mechanical damage to the microvascular circulation.

The blunt pull-through esophagectomy without thoracotomy for esophageal cancer proposed in 1913 by Denk[9] and in 1935 by Grey Turner[21] has found an increasing number of advocates.[2,29,33,48,59] It is described as a relatively safe procedure[35,48] that involves relatively low blood loss, provided that the dissection is undertaken close to the esophagus. When hemorrhage occurred after stripping of the esophagus, it was most often from the site of malignant tumor fixation and, in particular, from injury to the azygos vein.

Venous Drainage

The most comprehensive macroscopic description of esophageal venous drainage presumably was presented by Butler[7] in 1951. He classified the esophageal veins as *intrinsic* or *extrinsic* veins, referring to intraesophageal and extraesophageal wall veins. The intraesophageal veins include a subepithelial plexus in the lamina propria mucosa close to the epithelium. This plexus receives its blood from the adjacent capillaries. It drains into the submucous plexus, which comprises vessels that unite to form small communicating veins; these are arranged mainly in the longitudinal axis.[64] Aharinejad et al.[1] studied the human microvasculature of the esophagus in detail. They described two small veins that usually accompany the circumferential arteries in the lamina submucosa as perforating veins that originate from the small communicating veins of the submucous plexus and pierce the muscular wall of the esophagus together with the perforating arteries. They receive tributaries from the muscle coats and then form the extramural, extrinsic veins at the surface of the esophagus.[1,7,64] No valves were found within the esophageal venous circulatory system.[1,7,64] The extrinsic veins drain into the locally corresponding large vessels; these are the inferior and superior thyroid veins, which empty into the brachiocephalic and jugular veins, the azygos and hemiazygos veins, and the gastric and splenic veins.

As was well shown in 1918 by Elze and Beck[16] there are two clearly delineated venous plexuses within the extremely thin submucosa beneath the mucosa of the hypopharynx (Fig. 1–20). This is exactly at the level of the pharyngoesophageal junction. One plexus lies on the dorsal aspect of the inferior constrictor muscle, and the other is in the midline posterior to the cricoid cartilage (see Fig. 1–20). In the ten specimens studied by Liebermann-Meffert,[39,43] both plexuses were of similar size, approximately 2 to 3 cm broad and 4 cm long, and consisted of several veins up to 4 mm thick and of mostly longitudinal orientation, which were joined by several transverse anastomoses. These veins receive the blood from the mucosa of the hypopharynx, larynx, and esophagus and drain into the thyroid and jugular veins.[16] The venous plexuses may account for a postcricoid impression on the esophagus[16] and may be involved in the "globus sensation" in case of venous stasis and tissue swelling.[16,26] The plexuses may contribute to some extent to the competence and action of the upper esophageal sphincter.

It may be of clinical interest that a specialized venous arrangement, clearly documented by Vianna et al.,[64] is present at the terminal esophagus (Fig. 1–21). It has been suggested that these venous anastomoses possibly constitute a communication between the azygos and the portal systems. The intermediate "palisade zone" (see Fig. 1–21) may act as a high-resistance watershed between both systems, providing bidirectional flow.[64] Moreover, anastomoses between the systemic and the portal systems are found in the submucosa and lamina propria of

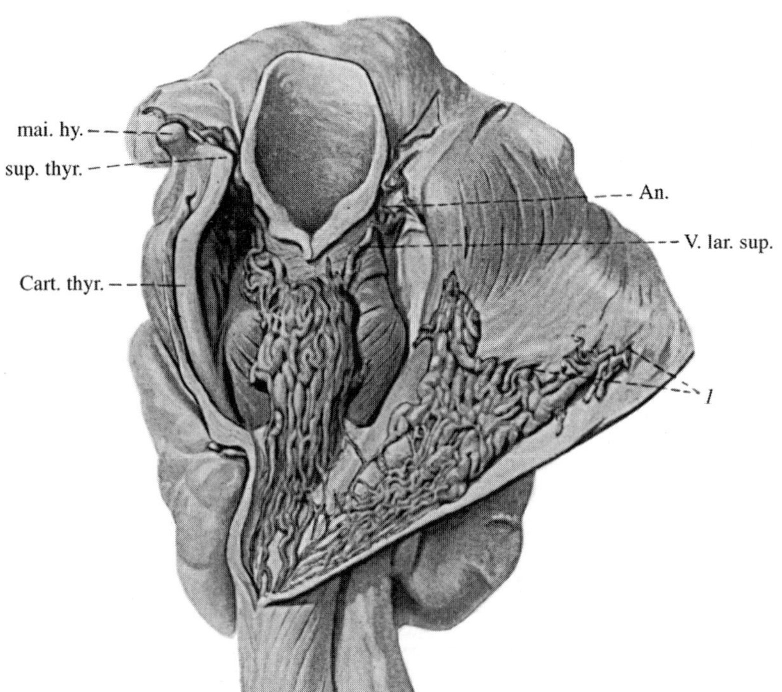

Figure 1–20. The hypopharygeal-esophageal venous plexuses, which are located just underneath the mucosa. Original drawing. (From Elze, C., and Beck, K., Die venösen Wundernetze des Hypopharynx. Z. Ohrenheilk., 77:185, 1918.)

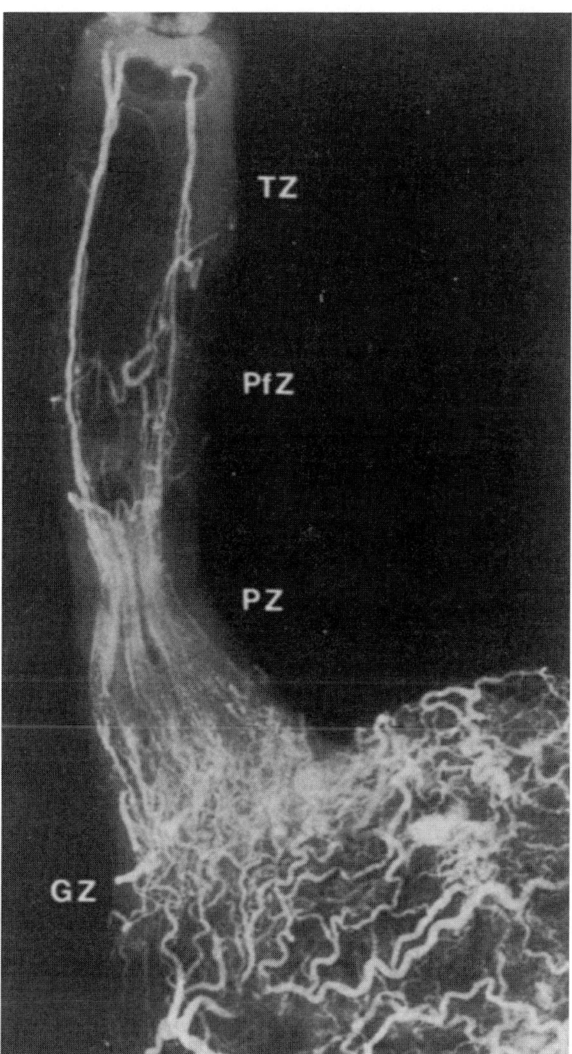

Figure 1–21. Radiograph of the venous circulation at the esophagogastric junction and the esophagus after injection with barium gelatin. This example shows the various zones of different venous architecture, such as the gastric zone (GZ), the palisade zone (PZ), the perforating zone (PfZ), and the truncal zone (TZ), as well as the irregular polygonal network of the proper gastric veins. (From Vianna, A., Hayes, P.C., Moscoso, G., et al.: Normal venous circulation of the gastroesophageal junction: A route of understanding varices. Gastroenterology, *93*:876, 1987, with permission.)

the lower end of the esophagus. The thin-walled superficial veins may enlarge in portal venous obstruction to form varices.[7,64]

A few more points are of surgical interest. Because of its proximity to the hilus of the lung and its lymph nodes, the azygos vein is one of the initial structures to become involved during the extramural spread of tumors of the midesophagus (see Fig. 1–10). In this situation, the azygos vein may be injured easily during esophageal resection. In particular during blunt pull-through dissection, this vein represents a high-risk factor in causing fatal hemorrhage. Collateral circulation between the azygos vein and the hemiazygos vein is well known.[46,66] However, the hemiazygos, the accessory hemiazygos, and the superior intercostal trunks may also form a vessel that does not connect with the azygos vein.[46] The hemiazygos vein, if not dissected out, can be a source of severe bleeding when the esophagus is resected through a right thoracotomy.

Lymphatic Drainage

Presumably due to the considerable technical difficulty in identifying the minute channels both in vivo and post mortem, the anatomic knowledge of the lymphatic system of the esophagus is extremely poor, and previous accounts so far have not been substantiated.[40,41] Nevertheless, one may accept that the lymphatic system of the esophagus comprises the lymph ducts and lymph nodes, as has been described for other parts of the gut.[30,49,50,53]

Lymph capillaries may commence in the tissue spaces as a network of endothelial channels or as blind endothelial sacculations (Fig. 1–22) similar to those found in mesenteric tissues.[30] The submucosa of the human stomach contains a network of numerous lymph vessels in parallel orientation with the longitudinal organ axis (Fig. 1–23). The plexuses give off occasional branches to the collecting subadventitial and surface trunks.[30,53] Different from the esophageal veins, all these channels possess valves (see Fig. 1–23).

Our own studies of autopsy specimens examined with electron-microscopic techniques imply that a similar pattern is present in the esophagus. Initial lymphatics appear to originate exclusively in the region between the mucosa and the submucosa to form longitudinally arranged collecting channels in the submucosa.

Lymphatic Ducts and Lymph Nodes

The lymphatic ducts at the surface of the esophagus may empty into the regional lymph nodes. As has been postulated,[46,50,57,66] the esophagus drains into the paratracheal, tracheobronchial, carinal, juxtaesophageal, and intra-aorticoesophageal lymph nodes, and the abdominal esophagus empties into the superior gastric, pericardiac, and inferior diaphragmatic lymph nodes (Fig. 1–24). However, the classic chain of lymph nodes surrounding the esophagus as it is described in textbooks and illustrated by Netter[46] could not be substantiated by the authors' examinations under normal conditions. In 17 noncancerous autopsy specimens, the authors found only a few small periesophageal lymph nodes. This observation coincides with the report of Wirth and Frommhold,[70] who found mediastinal lymph nodes in only 5% of 500 normal lymphograms.

Although tiny lymph nodes with a diameter less than 1 mm are not visible macroscopically, many small nodes can be detected microscopically, for example, in the tracheoesophageal groove. It is conceivable that such small lymph nodes increase in size, thus augmenting the number of visible nodes. Also regional differences potentially prevail. Lymph nodes, which are occasionally large and numerous, may be concentrated around the tracheal bifurcation (i.e., the carina of the trachea).[43] Most of them studied by the authors contained black coal particles; however, the authors could not determine by the available techniques whether these nodes drain the esophagus

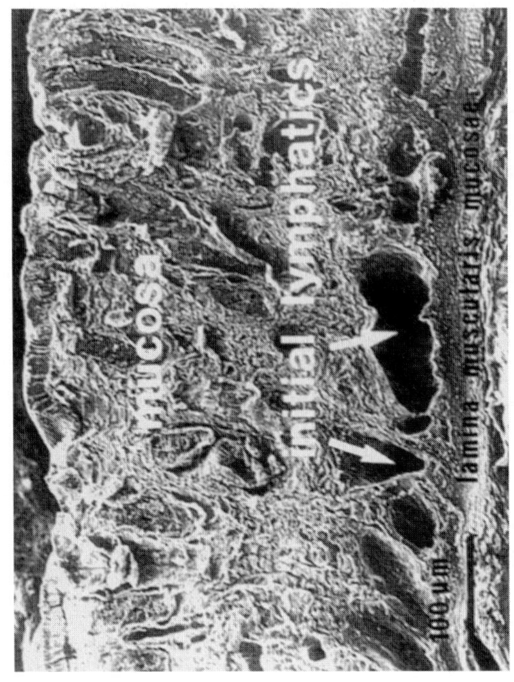

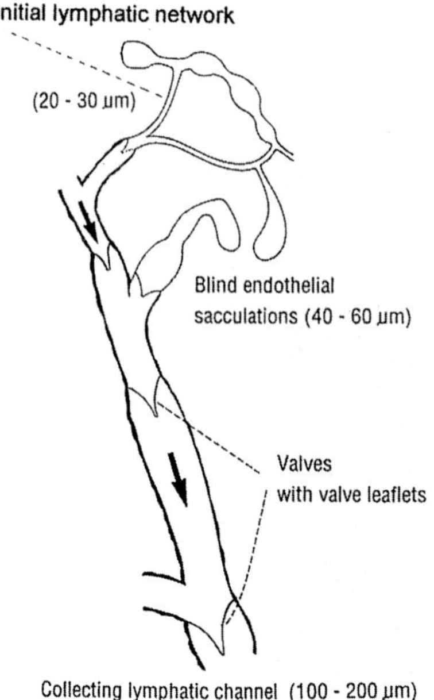

Figure 1–22. Initial lymphatics *(arrows)* between the lower border of the tunica mucosa and the tela submucosa seen on a histologic photomicrograph *(A)* and in a schematic drawing *(B)*. This view is taken from the gastric wall, but also seems to be of relevance for the esophagus. (From Lehnert et al.: Lymph and blood capillaries of the human gastric mucosa. Gastroenterology, *89*:939, 1985.)

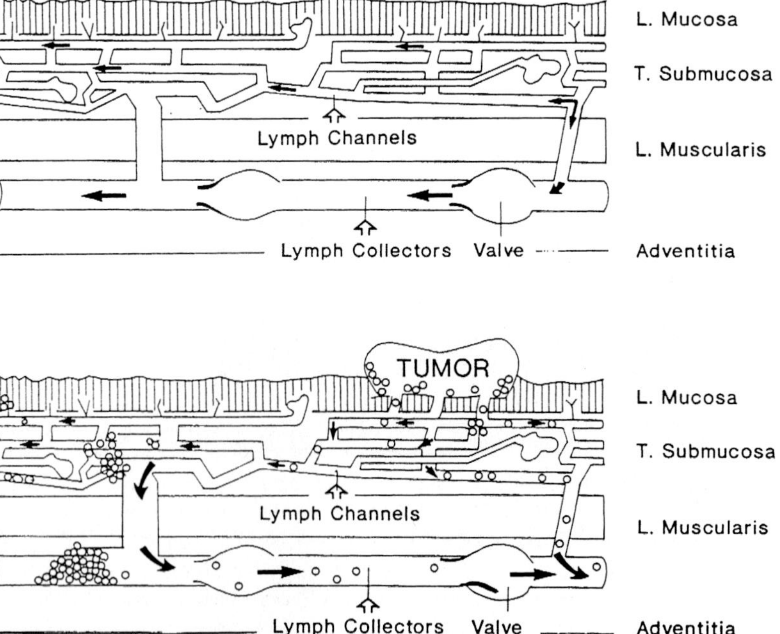

Figure 1–23. Lymphatic pathways in the esophageal wall. The suggested pattern of lymph flow is shown to explain the possible local and distal spread of tumor cells, including block of distal lymphatics. The embryologic development and the presence and alignment of valves suggest this pattern of lymph flow, although it has never been substantiated experimentally up to now.

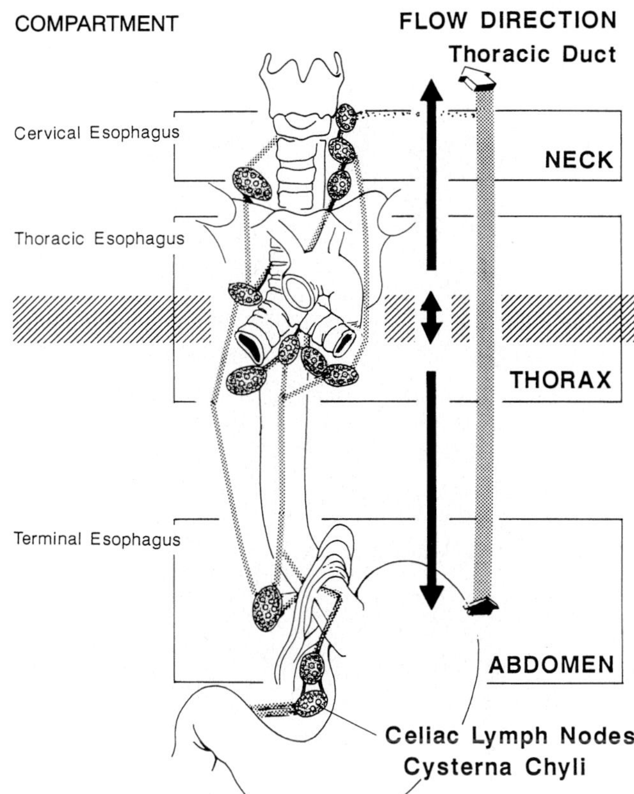

Figure 1–24. A knowledge of the direction of lymph flow and the position of major lymph nodes is essential in understanding the potential spread of an esophageal malignancy. Lymph from areas above the tracheal bifurcation drains mostly toward the neck, and that below the tracheal bifurcation flows preferentially toward the celiac axis. Lymph flow at the bifurcation appears to be bidirectional. The dimensions of the lymph nodes are out of scale. In the normal, nonmalignant condition, esophageal and mediastinal lymph nodes are difficult to discern because of their small diameter of only 3 to 7 mm. Lymph nodes that drain the lung are usually bigger and can be easily visualized by their carbon particle content.

or the lungs, or both, or whether they transport proximally or distally.[43]

Lymph nodes in the lateral and ventral mediastinum are mostly located in the upper third of the thorax, whereas the nodes in the dorsal mediastinum are mostly found in the lower third of the thorax. This parallels to some extent the findings of Lam and associates,[29] who found in a large series of patients that most metastases of esophageal tumors were located at the cardia and in the neck.

The concept that lymph flows in the submucosal channels more readily longitudinally than through the few transverse connections in the muscle (see Fig. 1–23) and that only finally does lymph flow through the subadventitial lymphatics and small ducts into the mediastinal lymph nodes is supported by the clinical observation that initial tumor spread follows the longitudinal axis of the esophagus within the submucosa, rather than extending in a circular manner. A paucity of lymphatics within the lamina mucosa and the abundance of submucosal lymphatic channels[30,40,41,43] may explain why intramural cancer spreads predominantly within this layer. Unappreciated malignant mucosal lesions may be accompanied by extensive tumor spread underneath an intact mucosa, and tumor cells may follow the lymphatic channels for a considerable distance before they pass the muscular coat to empty into the lymph nodes. Tumor-free margin at the resection line, as confirmed by the anatomic point of view, does not guarantee radical tumor removal. This feature may be consistent with the relatively high postoperative recurrence rate at the resection line, including satellite tumors and metastases in the submucosa far distant from the primary tumor,[2,59] even if the margins at the resection line were previously tumor free.

From clinical observations in cancer patients,[2,22,29,40,59] one may deduct (see Fig. 1–24) that lymph from above the carina flows toward cranial into the thoracic duct or subclavian lymph trunks, whereas lymph from below the carina flows mainly toward the cysterna chyli via the lower mediastinal, left gastric, and celiac lymph nodes. Flow may, however, change under pathologic conditions.[30,43] When lymph vessels become blocked and dilated owing to tumor invasion, the valves become incompetent and the flow reverses[71] (see Fig. 1–23). This explains the retrograde, unexpected spread of some malignant tumors but limits the value of establishing pathways of normal flow.

Thoracic Duct

The thoracic duct begins at the proximal end of the cysterna chyli, at the level of the twelfth thoracic vertebra, and passes up through the diaphragm via the aortic foramen. It then ascends through the posterior mediastinum, between the aorta on its left and the azygos vein on its right aspect, and continues left dorsal to the esophagus (Figs. 1–10 and 1–25). At the level of the fifth thoracic vertebra and just above the arch of the azygos vein, the thoracic duct inclines to the left to become left-side-positioned with regard to the esophagus and spine.[50,57,70,71] Then it ascends lateroposterior parallel to the trachea and esophagus to convey the lymph into the bloodstream, terminating at the confluence between the left subclavian and jugular veins. There are, however, a

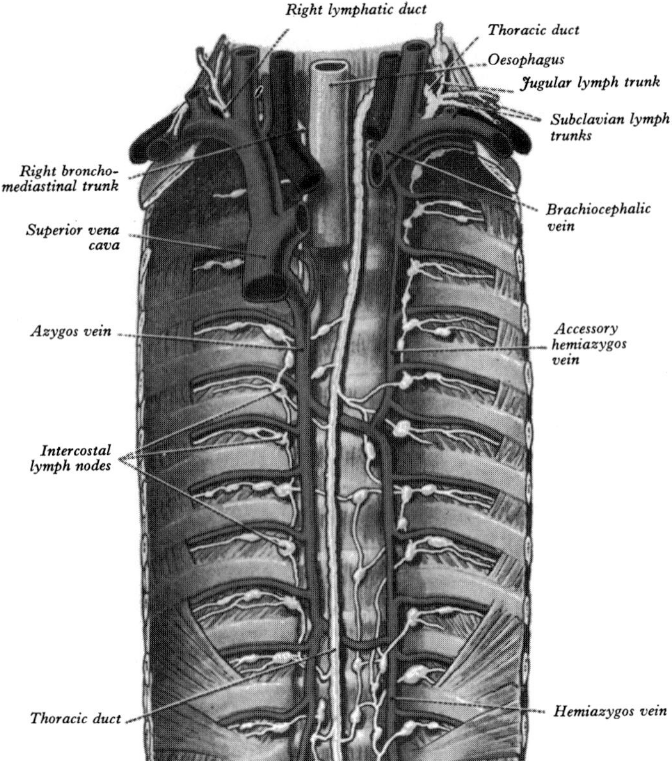

Figure 1–25. The upper thoracic and right lymphatic ducts. (From Warwick R., and Williams RL [eds.]: Gray's Anatomy, 35th ed. Edinburgh, Longman, 1973, p. 727.)

great number of anatomic variations.[5,24,46,50,57,66,70,71] The close local relationship of the delicate thoracic duct to the esophagus and trachea accounts for the occasional injury during esophagectomy and cervical anastomosis, causing chylothorax.[48]

Innervation

The innervation of the esophagus is through the visceral (splanchnic) component of the autonomic nervous system. It consists of two parts, the sympathetic and the parasympathetic systems, that exert antagonistic influences on the viscera. The various pathways have been described in detail.[8,20,66] The nerve trunks and the principal branches are composed of parallel nerve bundles that contain efferent or afferent axons. The epineurium, a dense connective tissue sheath, surrounds the nerve trunk.

Extramural Innervation

According to the classic description, the sympathetic nerve supply is through the cervical and thoracic sympathetic chain, which runs downward lateral to the spine (Fig. 1–26). The other sources of sympathetic supply to the middle and lower esophagus are the cardiobronchial and the periesophageal splanchnic nerves, deriving from the celiac plexus.[46] Interconnecting with fibers of the parasympathetic cervical and thoracic plexus, the sympathetic nervous system also uses the vagus nerve as a carrier for some of its fibers.[20,46,66]

The vagus nerve is the tenth cranial nerve, deriving from the dorsal vagal nucleus. The fibers that supply the striated musculature in the pharynx and esophagus, however, arise in the nucleus ambiguus. The vagus is a mixed nerve and also carries sensory fibers from the superior ganglion and the inferior ganglion (nodose ganglion). As thick trunks, the right and left vagus nerves descend bilaterally (see Fig. 1–26); they reduce their diameters by giving off fibers to the superior laryngeal nerve (SLN), which innervates the pharynx and larynx. The right inferior (recurrent) laryngeal nerve (RLN) leaves the vagus to turn dorsally around the subclavian artery (see Fig. 1–26). The left RLN leaves the vagus and circles around the aortic arch. On both sides, the RLNs ascend as slack cords that sinuously pass upward toward the neck[42] (Figs. 1–27 and 1–28). They course in intimate local relationship within the lateral peritracheal or periesophageal tissue or, less frequently, in the tracheoesophageal groove[42] (see Fig. 1–27). The left RLN lies closer to the wall of the esophagus than does the right one. Both RLNs are 2 to 3 mm thick and give off in equal distribution 8 to 14 branches to the esophagus and trachea.[42] Beneath the thyroid glands, the thyroid vessels, in an unpredictable manner, encircle the RLNs, which are still more than 1 mm thick when they enter the hypopharynx laterocaudal to the cricopharyngeal muscle (Figs. 1–28 and 1–29; see also Fig. 1–4*A*). On both sides, the RLNs continue in the groove lateral to the posterior arytenoid muscle (see Fig. 1–4*A*). Except for the cricothyroids, they innervate all the muscles of the larynx via small branches.[42]

The vagal trunks, at the level of the tracheal bifurcation and posterior to the lung hilus, give off numerous branches to form pulmonary plexuses. More distally, the vagal trunks separate into the coarse network of the anterior and posterior esophageal plexuses (see Fig. 1–26). Before they cross the diaphragm through the esophageal hiatus, these plexuses join again to form the anterior and posterior vagus nerves. The anterior branch shows a number of anatomic variants and is usually found on the anterior esophageal wall, where it is visible below the phrenoesophageal membrane. The posterior vagus nerve is usually at some distance from the esophagus and to its right.

Intramural Innervation

The fine structure of the esophageal innervation is composed of a dense network of nerve fibers containing numerous groups of ganglia. The ganglia are located either between the longitudinal and the circular muscle layers (Auerbach's plexus) or in the submucosa (Meissner's plexus). The ganglia of Auerbach's plexus are scattered, with a variable number of cells, within the entire esophagus. However, the concentration of the ganglion cells is greatest in the terminal esophagus and at the gastroesophageal junction.[13,46,66]

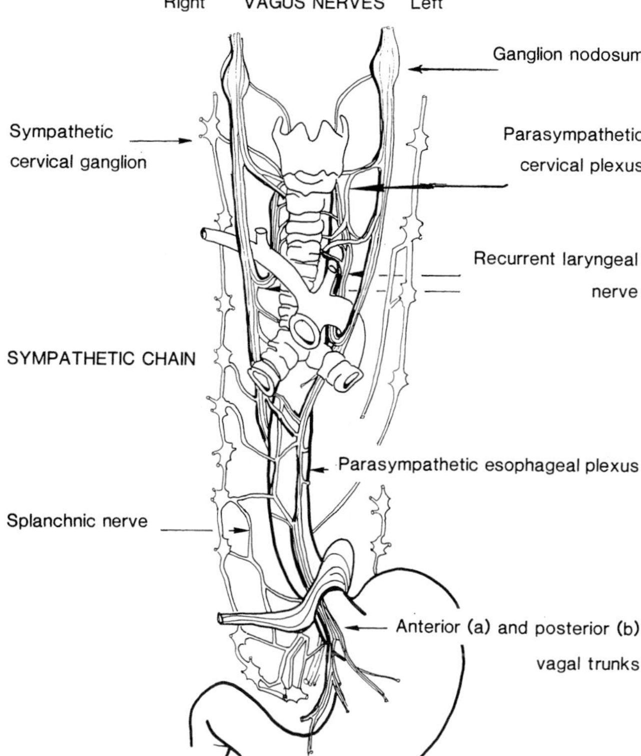

Figure 1–26. Sympathetic and parasympathetic nerve systems. The sympathetic system forms a chain of ganglia from the base of the skull to the coccyx. In the neck, the sympathetic chain is posterior to the carotid sheath. In the chest, it is found anterolateral to the bodies of the vertebrae. Both vagus nerves carry the parasympathetic innervation and travel along the esophagus. The locations of the right and left superior and inferior recurrent laryngeal nerves are shown.

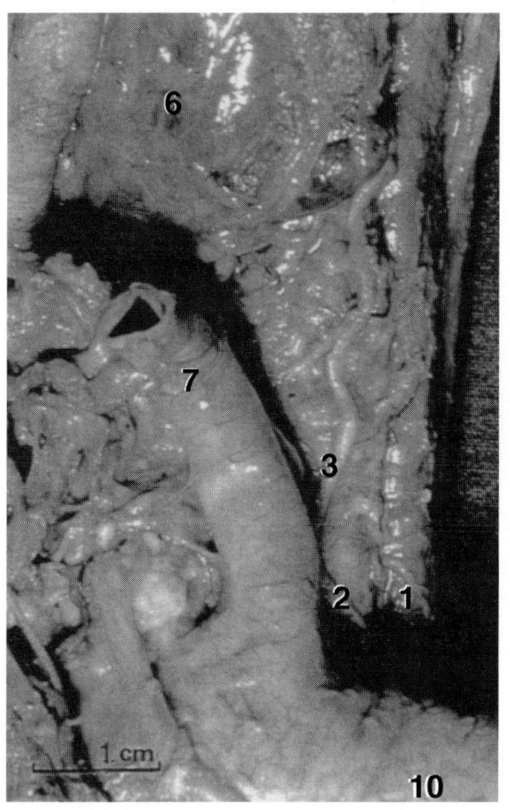

Figure 1–27. Meandering course of the left recurrent laryngeal nerve (3) shown before its dissection from the underlying peritracheal tissues (2). The thyroid gland (6) is still in place. Esophagus (1), aorta (10), left common carotid artery (7).

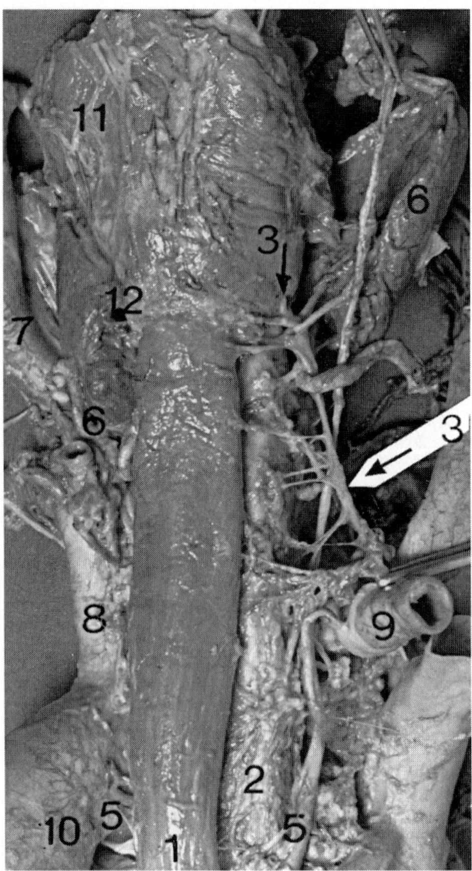

Figure 1–28. Posterior aspect of the muscular wall of the esophagus (1) and pharynx (11). The right recurrent laryngeal nerve (3) largely removed from its peritracheal tissue bed is pulled down toward lateral behind its turning point (forceps) around the subclavian artery (9). The rami of the recurrent laryngeal nerve enter the lateral wall of the esophagus (1) and trachea (2). The left thyroid gland (6) is in its natural position, the right is displaced toward posterior. Underneath the lower lobe the thyroid artery and its branches encircle the recurrent laryngeal nerves. The turning point of the left recurrent laryngeal nerve is seen under the aortic arch (10). Esophagus (1), common carotid artery (7), brachiocephalic trunk (8). Note the venous network on top of the pharyngeal muscle (11), the upper esophageal sphincter (12), and the phrenic nerve (13).

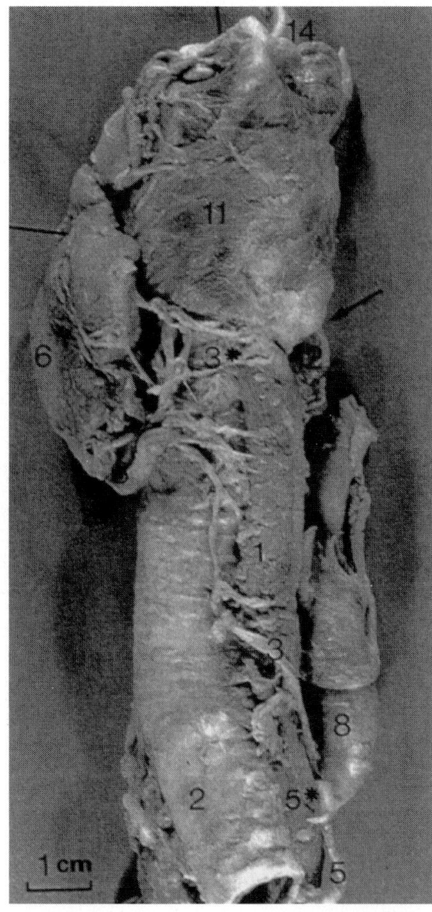

Figure 1–29. The course of the left recurrent laryngeal nerve (3) between the turning point from the vagus nerve (5) and its entry into the larynx is photographed from the lateral aspect after removal from the peritracheal tissues. The attachments of the thyroid gland (6) are removed, and the gland is shifted posteriorly to display the recurrent laryngeal nerve (3) and the vascular arrangement underneath. Esophagus (1), trachea (2), inferior constrictor muscle of the pharynx wall (11)—that is, the upper esophageal sphincter (12). Note the Zenker's diverticulum on the right *(arrow)*.

References

1. Aharinejad, S., Böck, P., and Lametschwandtner, A.: Scanning electron microscopy of esophageal microvasculature in human infants and rabbits. Anat. Embryol., *186:*33, 1992.
2. Akiyama, H.: Surgery for carcinoma of the esophagus. Curr. Probl. Surg., *17:*53, 1980.
3. Bartels, H., Stein, H. J., and Siewert, J. R.: Tracheobronchial lesions following oesophagectomy: Predisposing factors, respiratory management and outcome. Br. J. Surg., *85:*403, 1998.
4. Bombeck, C. T., Nyhus, L. M., and Donahue, Ph. E.: How far should the myotomy extend on the stomach? *In* Giuli, R., McCallum, R. W., and Skinner, D. B. (eds.): Primary Motility Disorders of the Esophagus. Paris, Libbey Eurotext, 1991, p. 455.
5. Bruna, J.: Types of collateral lymphatic circulation. Lymphology, *7:*61, 1974.
6. Bumm, R., Hölscher, A. H., Feussner, H., et al.: Endodissection of the thoracic esophagus. Ann. Surg., *218:*97, 1993.
7. Butler, H.: The veins of the esophagus. Thorax, *6:*276, 1951.
8. Cunningham, E. T., and Sawchenko, P. E.: Central neural control of esophageal motility: A review. Dysphagia, *5:*35, 1990.
9. Denk, W.: Zur Radikaloperation des Oesophaguskarzinoms. Z. Chir., *40:*1065, 1913.
10. Diamant, N. E.: Physiology of esophageal motor function. Gastroenterol. Clin. North Am., *18:*179, 1989.
11. Didio, L. J. A., and Anderson, M. C.: The Sphincters of the Digestive System: Anatomical, Functional and Surgical Considerations. Baltimore, Williams & Wilkins, 1968.
12. Dodds, W. J., Stewart, E. T., Hodges, D., et al.: Movement of the feline esophagus associated with respiration and peristalsis. J. Clin. Invest., *52:*1, 1983.
13. Eckardt, V. F., and LeCompte, P. M.: Esophageal ganglia and smooth muscle in the elderly. Dig. Dis. Sci., *23:*443, 1978.
14. Ekberg, O., and Lindström, C.: The upper esophageal sphincter area. Acta Radiol., *28:*173, 1987.
15. Eliska, O.: Phreno-oesophageal membrane and its role in the development of hiatal hernia. Acta Anat. (Basel), *86:*137, 1973.
16. Elze, C., and Beck, K.: Die venösen Wundernetze des Hypopharynx. Z. Ohrenheilk., *77:*185, 1918.
17. Enterline, H., and Thompson, J. J.: Pathology of the Esophagus. New York, Springer, 1984.
18. Ferguson, M. K., and Altorki, N. K.: Malignant esophagorespiratory fistula. Postgr. Gen. Surg., *5:*107, 1993.
19. Friedland, G. W.: Historical review of the changing concepts of lower esophageal anatomy, 430 B.C.–1977. Am. J. Roentgenol., *131:*373, 1978.
20. Goyal, R. K., and Cobb, B. W.: Motility of the pharynx, esophagus and esophageal sphincters. *In* Johnson, L. R. (ed.): Physiology of the Gastrointestinal Tract. New York, Raven Press, 1981.
21. Grey Turner, G.: Carcinoma of the esophagus: The question of its treatment by surgery. Lancet, *18:*130, 1936.
22. Haagensen, C. D., Feind, C. R., and Herter, F. P.: The Lymphatics in Cancer. Philadelphia, W.B. Saunders, 1972.
23. Hayek, H. V.: Die Kardia und der Hiatus Oesophagus des Zwerchfells. Z. Anat. Entwickl. Gesch., *100:*218, 1933.
24. Idanov, D. A.: Anatomie du canal thoracic et des principaux collecteurs lymphatiques du tronc chez l'homme. Acta Anat., *37:*20, 1959.
25. Ismail-Beigi, F., Horton, P. F., and Pope, C. E.: Histological consequences of gastroesophageal reflux in man. Gastroenterology, *58:*163, 1970.
26. Killian, G.: Über den Mund der Speiseröhre. Z. Ohrenheilk. *55:*1, 1908.
27. Korn, O., Stein, H. J., Richter, T. H., et al.: Gastroesophageal sphincter: A model. Dis. Esophagus, *10:*105, 1997.
28. Laimer, E.: Beitrag zur Anatomie des Oesophagus. Med. Jb. (Wien), 333, 1883.
29. Lam, K. H., Cheung, H. C., Wong, J., et al.: The present state of surgical treatment of carcinoma of the esophagus. J. R. Coll. Surg. Edinb., *27:*315, 1982.
30. Lehnert, T. H., Erlandson, A., and Decosse, J. J.: Lymph and blood capillaries of the human gastric mucosa: A morphologic basis for metastasis in early gastric carcinoma. Gastroenterology, *89:*939, 1985.
31. Lendrum, F. C.: Anatomic features of the cardiac orifice of the stomach. Arch. Intern. Med., *59:*474, 1937.
32. Lerche, W.: The Esophagus and Pharynx in Action: A Study of Structure in Relation to Function. Springfield, IL, Charles C Thomas, 1950.
33. Liebermann-Meffert, D., Allgöwer, M., Schmid, P., et al.: Muscular equivalent of the lower esophageal sphincter. Gastroenterology, *76:*31, 1979.
34. Liebermann-Meffert, D., Heberer, M., and Allgöwer, M.: The muscular counterpart of the lower esophageal sphincter. *In* DeMeester, T. R., and Skinner, D. B. (eds.): Esophageal Disorders: Pathology and Therapy. New York, Raven Press, 1985.
35. Liebermann-Meffert, D., Lüscher, U., Neff, U., et al.: Esophagectomy without thoracotomy: Is there a risk of intramediastinal bleeding? A study on blood supply of the esophagus. Ann. Surg., *206:*184, 1987.
36. Liebermann-Meffert, D., and Geissdörfer, K.: Is the transition of striated into smooth muscle precisely known? *In* Giuli, R., McCallum, R. W., and Skinner, D. B. (eds.): Primary Motility Disorders of the Esophagus: 450 Questions—450 Answers. Paris, Libbey Eurotext, 1991.
37. Liebermann-Meffert, D., and Siewert, J. R.: Arterial anatomy of the esophagus: A review of literature with brief comments on clinical aspects. Gullet, *2:*3, 1992.
38. Liebermann-Meffert, D., Meier, R., and Siewert, J. R.: Vascular anatomy of the gastric tube used for esophageal reconstruction. Ann. Thorac. Surg., *54:*1110, 1992.
39. Liebermann-Meffert, D.: The pharyngoesophageal segment: Anatomy and innervation. Dis. Esophagus, *8:*242, 1995.
40. Liebermann-Meffert, D., and Duranceau, A.: Anatomy and embryology. *In* Orringer, M. B., and Zuidema, G. D. (eds.): Shackelford's Surgery of the Alimentary Tract: The Esophagus, Vol. I, 4th edition. Philadelphia, W.B. Saunders, 1996.
41. Liebermann-Meffert, D.: Funktionsstörungen des pharyngo-ösophagealen Übergangs: a) Funktionelle und chirurgisch orientierte Anatomie, b) Mobilitätsstörungen des tubulären Ösophagus. *In* Fuchs, K. H., Stein, H. J., and Thiede, A. (eds.): Gastrointestinale Funktionsstörungen, Diagnose, Operationsindikation, Therapie. Berlin, Springer, 1997.
42. Liebermann-Meffert, D., Walbrun, B., Hiebert, C. A., et al.: Recurrent and superior laryngeal nerves—a new look with implications for the esophageal surgeon. Ann. Thorac. Surg., *67:*212, 1999.
43. Liebermann-Meffert, D.: Anatomy, embryology, and histology. *In* Pearson, F. G., Cooper, J. D., Delauriers, J., et al. (eds.): Esophageal Surgery, 2nd ed, Philadelphia, W.B. Saunders, 2000.
44. Meyer, G. W., Austin, R. M., Brady, C. E., et al.: Muscle anatomy of the human esophagus. J. Clin. Gastroenterol., *8:*131, 1986.
45. Nathan, H.: Relations of the soft structures of the posterior mediastinum in the scoliotic spine. Acta Anat. (Basel), *133:*260, 1988.
46. Netter, F. H.: The Ciba Collection of Medical Illustrations, Vol. 3: Digestive System. Part 1: Upper Digestive Tract. New York, Ciba Pharmaceutical Embassy, 1971.
47. Ngan, S. Y. F., and Wong, J.: Lengths of different routes for esophageal replacement. J. Thorac. Cardiovasc. Surg., *91:*790, 1986.
48. Orringer, M. B., and Orringer, J. S.: Esophagectomy without thoracotomy: A dangerous operation? J. Thorac. Cardiovasc. Surg., *85:*72, 1983.
49. Partsch, H. (ed.): Progress in Lymphology. Vol. XI. Amsterdam, Exerpta Medica, 1988.
50. Pernkopf, E.: Topographische Anatomie des Menschen. Lehrbuch und Atlas der regionär-stratigraphischen Präparation. 1. Band: Allgemeines, Brust und Brustgliedmaβe. Berlin, Urban und Schwarzenberg, 1937.
51. Postlethwait, R. W.: Surgery of the Esophagus, Norwalk, CT, Appleton-Century-Crofts, 1987.
52. Preiksaitis, H. G., Tremblay, L., and Diamant, N. E.: Regional differences in the in vitro behaviour of muscle fibers from the human lower esophageal sphincter. J. Gastrointest. Motility, *3:*195, 1991.
53. Sakata, K.: Ueber die Lymphgefäβe des Oesophagus und über seine regionalen Lymphdrüsen mit Berücksichtigung der Verbreitung des Carzinoms. Mitt. Grenzgebiete Med. Chir., *11:*634, 1903.

54. Samuelson, S. L., Bombeck, C. T., and Nyhus, L. M.: Lower esophageal sphincter competence: Anatomic-physiologic correlation. *In* DeMeester, T. R., and Skinner, D. B. (eds.): Esophageal Disorders: Pathophysiology and Therapy. New York, Raven Press, 1985.
55. Savary, M., and Miller, G.: The Esophagus: Handbook and Atlas of Endoscopy. Switzerland, Gassmann, 1978.
56. Shapiro, A. L., and Robillard, G. L.: The esophageal arteries: Their configurational anatomy and variations in relation to surgery. Ann. Surg., *131*:171, 1950.
57. Shdanow, D. A.: Die Kollaterallymphwege der Brusthöhle des Menschen. Anat. Anz., *82*:417, 1936.
58. Siewert, J. R., Jennewein, H. M., and Waldeck, F.: Experimentelle Un-tersuchungen zur Funktion des unteren Oesophagussphinkters nach Intrathorakalverlagerung, Myotomie und zirkulärer Myektomie. Bruns Beitr. Klin. Chir., *22*:818, 1973.
59. Siewert, J. R., Liebermann-Meffert, D., Fekete, F., et al.: Oesophaguscarcinom. *In* Siewert, J. R., Harder, F., Allgöwer, M., et al. (eds.): Chirurgische Gastroenterologie, Band 2, 2. Auflage. Berlin, Springer, 1990.
60. Stein, H. J., DeMeester, T. R., Naspetti, R., et al.: Three-dimensional imaging of the lower esophageal sphincter in gastroesophageal reflux disease. Ann. Surg., *214*:374, 1991.
61. Stein, H. J., Liebermann-Meffert, D., DeMeester, T. R., et al.: Three-dimensional pressure image and muscular structure of the human lower esophageal sphincter. Surgery, *117*:692, 1995.
62. Stein, H. J., Korn, O., and Liebermann-Meffert, D.: Manometric vector volume analysis to assess the lower esophageal sphincter function. Ann. Chir. Gynaecol., *84*:151, 1995.
63. Vandertoll, D. J., Ellis, F. H., Schlegel, J. F., et al.: An experimental study of the role of gastric and esophageal muscle in gastroesophageal competence. Surg. Gynecol. Obstet., *122*:579, 1966.
64. Vianna, A., Hayes, P. C., Moscoso, G., et al.: Normal venous circulation of the gastroesophageal junction: A route of understanding varices. Gastroenterology, *93*:876, 1987.
65. Wegener, O. H.: Whole Body Computerized Tomography. Basel, Karger, 1983.
66. Williams, P. L., and Warwick, R.: Gray's Anatomy. Edinburgh, Churchill Livingstone, 1980.
67. Williams, D. B., and Payne, W. S.: Observations on esophageal blood supply. Mayo Clin. Proc., *57*:448, 1982.
68. Winans, C. S.: Manometric asymmetry of the lower esophageal high pressure zone. Gastroenterology, *62*:830, 1972.
69. Winans, C. S.: The pharyngoesophageal closure mechanism: A manometric study. Gastroenterology, *63*:768, 1972.
70. Wirth, W., and Frommhold, H.: Der Ductus thoracicus und seine Variationen. Lymphographische Studie. Fortschr. Roentgenstr., *112*:450, 1970.
71. Zschiesche, W.: Kompensationsmechanismen des menschlichen Ductus thoracicus bei Lymphabflußstörungen. Fortschr. Med., *81*:869, 1963.

ORGANOGENESIS OF THE ESOPHAGUS

The first stages of life constitute the embryonic period, which extends from fertilization to the fetal period. The fetal period starts at the ninth week of gestation and ends at birth. The age of the embryo is estimated by the number of somites present during the early stages and by the crown-rump (CR) length when this measure becomes adequate at the end of the fifth week.[11] The planes of section used in this chapter to describe the development of the embryo are illustrated in Figure 1-30. The progression of events that take place during the various stages of esophageal development is shown in Table 1-1. The information presented in the following pages is based on the teaching of established textbooks of embryology[4,5,9,10,13,32,38,41,42] as well as on Liebermann-Meffert's personal studies.[28-30]

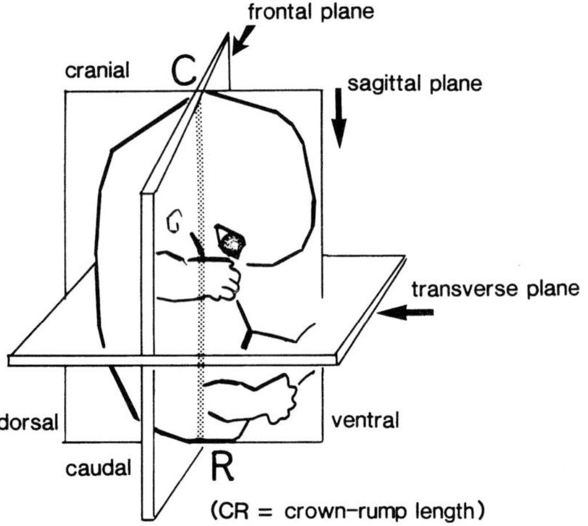

Figure 1-30. Planes of section used to study embryos and fetuses. The sagittal and transverse planes are shown; they refer to the longitudinal and horizontal descriptions frequently used in the literature.

FORMATION OF THE PRIMITIVE DIGESTIVE SYSTEM

The digestive tube derives from two germ layers, the endoderm and the mesoderm. The endoderm is recognizable by the eighth day of the embryonic period, when it rapidly forms the lining of the yolk sac (Fig. 1-31*A*). Until the fourteenth or fifteenth day, the embryo displays a bilaminar disk of ectoderm and endoderm. The third embryonic layer, which appears on the fifteenth day to develop between the two initial layers, is the mesoderm. It provides the material necessary for the connective tissues, the muscle coats of the gut, and the serous coverings. By the twenty-first day, the mesoderm has thickened to form longitudinal masses, the paraxial mesoderm, which segments progressively in a cranial to caudal direction into cubes of tissue, which are the somites (Fig. 1-32). This process ends with the formation of 33 to 35 somites by the thirty-first embryonic day. The separation of the endoderm and the ectoderm by the mesoderm allows the endoderm to undergo the extensive changes needed for the establishment of the primitive gut, which forms during the fourth week.[10] Head, tail, and lateral folds compress the dorsal part of the yolk sac, which becomes incorporated as a rim (see Fig. 1-31*A* and *B*). Successive compression with formation of a "body cylinder" at about the twenty-eighth day divides the yolk sac into an extraembryonic part (which regresses and disappears at about the twelfth week) and an intraembryonic part, which represents the origin of the digestive tract and its accessory glands (Fig. 1-31*C* and Fig. 1-33). Initially, a buccopharyngeal membrane separates the upper endodermal tube from the stomodeal cavity (see Figs.

Table 1–1. Progression of Various Stages of Esophageal Development

STAGES	
SHAPE OF EMBRYO	Elongated ➡ Flexion ➡ C-Shape ➡ Deflexion ➡ Elongation
GENERAL EVENTS	Nidation; Gastrulation; Branchial Arches; Somite Segmentation
CROWN-RUMP LENGTH (mm)	1,5 ⇨ 2,5 ⇨ 4 ⇨ 7 ⇨ 11 ⇨ 13 ⇨ 15 ⇨ 21 ⇨ 24
AGE (weeks)	1, 2, 3, 4, 5, 6, 7, 8
AGE (days)	10, 20, 30, 40, 50, 60
APPEARANCE OF TISSUES, ORGANS AND STEPS IN FORMATION OF FOREGUT	Endoderm; Mesoderm; Folding of Gut from Yolk Sac; Mucosa (Columnar Cells); Primitive Gut, Intraembryonic Coelom; Tracheal Groove, Gastric Dilation; Aortic Arch Arteries, Vagal Innervation; Buccopharyngeal Membr. degenerates; Trachea, Primary Bronchi; Lung Buds, Sympathetic Innervation; Celiac axis; Circular Muscle; Neuroblasts form Periesophageal Net; Esophagus + Sept. transv. innervated; Esophageal Elongation; Veins, Lymphatics, Diaphragm completed; Mucosal (Vacuolization begins); Topographical Relationships completed; Longitudinal Muscle

1-31*B* and *C*, 1-32*B*, and 1-33). The early digestive system at this point is divided into the foregut, the midgut, and the hindgut (Fig. 1-34).

DEVELOPMENT OF THE FOREGUT AND ITS DERIVATIVES

The primitive foregut is initially uniform in shape (see Fig. 1-33*A*). It then gives rise to sacculations by which develop the pharynx and its derivatives, the esophagus, the trachea and lungs, the stomach and duodenum, the choledochal duct, the liver, the biliary system, and the pancreas (see Fig. 1-34).

Both the larynx and the trachea originate from the cranial part of the foregut, from the endodermal lining of the laryngotracheal sacculation, and from the surrounding mesenchyme, which derives from the fourth and sixth pairs of bronchial arches. Therewith, connective tissue, cartilage, muscle, and blood and lymphatic vessels originate from the splanchnic mesoderm on the ventral surface of the foregut into which the lower respiratory system subsequently extends.

The primordium of the laryngeal aditus is bounded by the hypobranchial eminence. At a later stage, this becomes the epiglottis. Caudal to the primitive aditus, arytenoid swellings develop in a T-shaped pattern from the anterior pharyngeal wall to constrict the lumen. The swellings fuse with the lateral margins of the epiglottis, forming the aryepiglottic folds. Cranial to the tracheal sacculation, the laryngeal cartilages develop in the branchial mesoderm during the seventh week. The early development of the lower respiratory system is marked by the sacculation of a median ventral diverticulum of the foregut (Fig. 1-35), called the tracheal bud, which also shapes the tracheoesophageal groove.[10,23,33] This protrusion of the anterior endodermal wall is the primordium of the trachea and the lungs and appears at the 25-somite stage on the twenty-first day[39] (Fig. 1-36). It rapidly elongates downward and bifurcates into two lateral protrusions, the lung buds (see Fig. 1-36). The elongating tracheal tube immediately approaches the esophagus, but never fuses with it.[44] By the end of the seventh week, distinct rings of cartilage are seen along the trachea (Fig. 1-37*A* and *B*).

The differentiation process of the ventral trachea and of the dorsal esophagus has been detailed in two anatomic and scanning electron microscope (SEM) studies (see Fig. 1-35) of this area that were performed in the chick embryo.[23,24] The work of these investigators elegantly contradicts the classical concept initiated in 1887

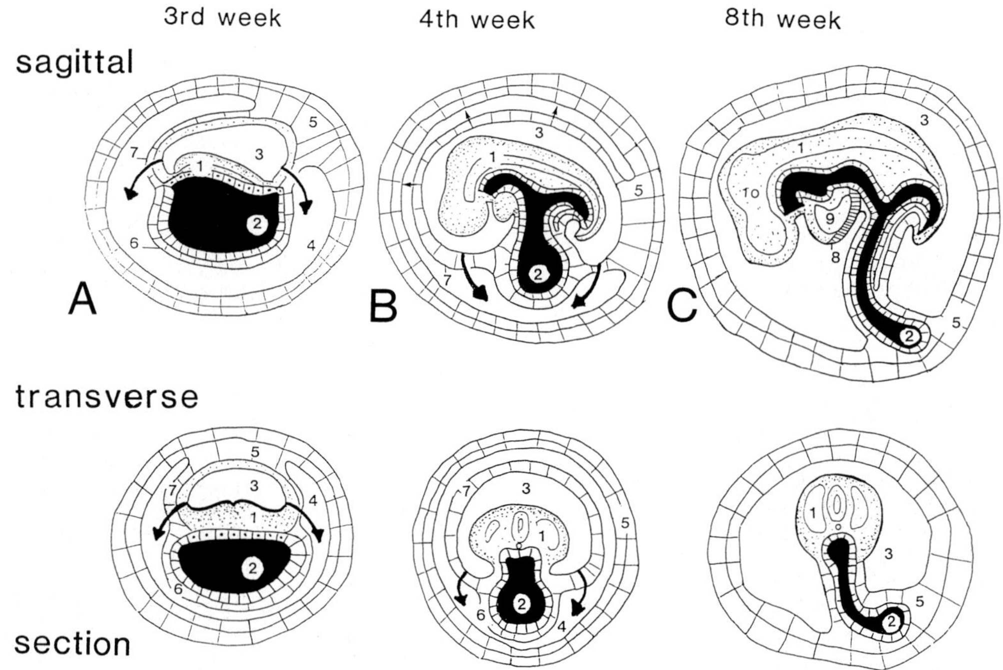

Figure 1–31. The primitive intestinal tube is shown at three stages of its development *(A–C)* during the third, fourth, and eighth weeks of gestation. Before the formation of the head fold, during the third week the yolk sac is an ovoid cavity. Its roof is the endoderm, which is the underlayer of the embryonic disk. With the formation of the head fold during the fourth week, a portion of the yolk sac becomes included within the embryo. This results in an endodermal tube dorsal to the pericardial cavity and the septum transversum; it adopts a medial position. The tissues of the cranial foregut form the buccopharyngeal membrane, which separates the future digestive tube from the primitive mouth, the stomodeum. Laterally, the foregut is bounded by the bronchial mesoderm. Rapid growth of the brain with transverse and sagittal folding during the fifth week results in the apparent flexion of the embryo. Simultaneous constriction at the junction between the embryo and the yolk sac separates the primitive midgut from the yolk sac remnant. The amniotic cavity expands and obliterates the extraembryonic coelom. (1 = embryo, 2 = yolk sac cavity, 3 = amniotic cavity, 4 = extraembryonic coelom, 5 = cytotrophoblast and extraembryonic mesenchyme, 6 = somatopleure, 7 = splanchnopleure, 8 = septum transversum, 9 = cardiac tube.)

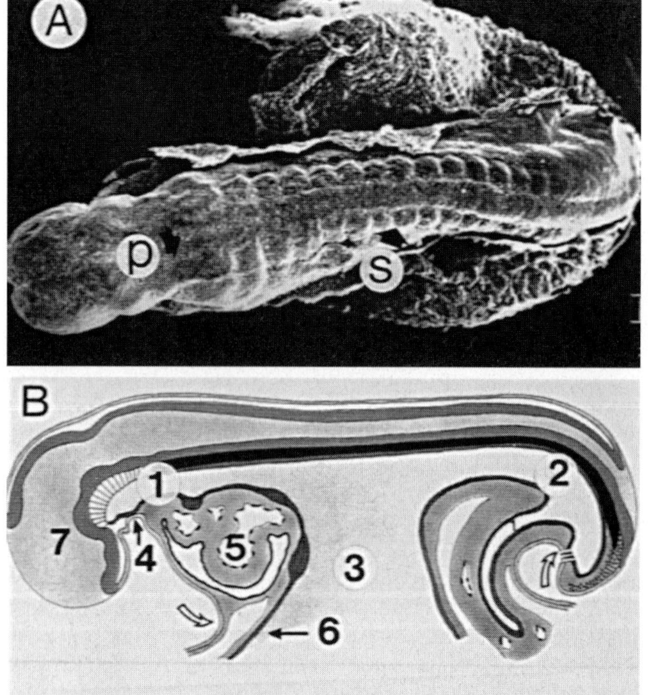

Figure 1–32. Formation of the gut in the human embryo, 3-mm CR length, at the end of the first month of gestation. *A,* Scanning electron micrograph showing an embryo with paired somites (s), which develop from the mesenchymal plate (p). *B,* Schematic counterpart in the sagittal plane, which shows the developing structures: 1 = foregut, 2 = hindgut, 3 = yolk sac cavity, 4 = stomodeum and buccopharyngeal membrane, 5 = developing heart, 6 = septum transversum, and 7 = brain. (Part *A* from Jirásek, J.E.: Atlas of Human Prenatal Morphogenesis. Boston, Nijhoff, 1983, with permission. Part *B* from Hinrichsen, K.V.: Human Embryologie. Heidelberg, Springer-Verlag, 1990, with permission. Modified from Liebermann-Meffert, D.: Anatomy, embryology, and histology. *In* Pearson, F.G., Delauriers, J., Ginsberg, R.J., et al. [eds.]: Esophageal Surgery. New York, Churchill Livingstone, 1995, with permission.)

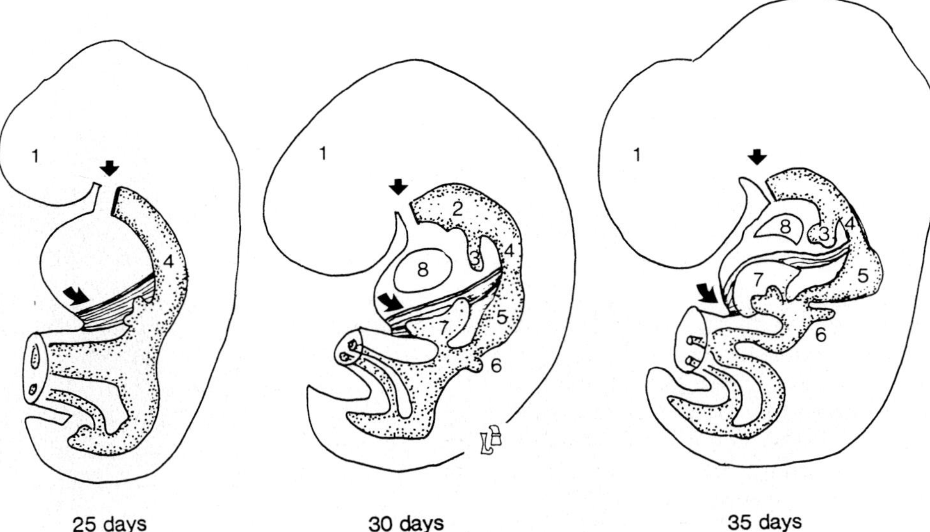

Figure 1–33. Sagittal section diagram through human embryos of different stages. The digestive tract and its accessory glands undergo rapid development between the twenty-fifth and the thirty-fifth days. (1 = head, 2 = pharynx, 3 = tracheal bud, 4 = esophagus, 5 = stomach, 6 = pancreas, 7 = liver, 8 = heart, a = foregut, b = midgut, c = hindgut.) The septum transversum and the buccopharyngeal membrane are indicated by short and curved arrows, respectively.

DERIVATIVES OF

Head and Neck Material

Pharyngeal Pouches (a)
Branchial Arches (b)
Upper Foregut (c)

Body Material

Paraxial Mesoderm
Trunk Somites (g)
including Mesenchyme
Axial and visceral Muscle
Lower Foregut (d)
Midgut (e)
Hindgut (f)

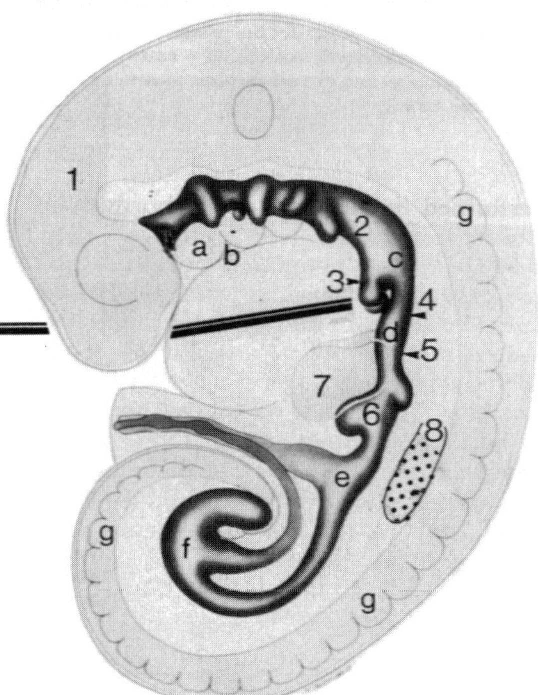

PRIMORDIUM OF

1 Head
2 Pharynx / Larynx
3 Trachea
4 Esophagus
5 Stomach
6 Pancreas
7 Liver
8 Upper Limb

Figure 1–34. Schematic drawing of a sagittal section through the body of a 28-day-old human embryo. Foregut, midgut, and hindgut are differentiated. The stomach, however, still presents as an asymmetric tubal segment. The initially elongated body bends, owing to the increasing number of somites and to the prominence of the head. This gives the embryo a C shape. The horizontal line at the left indicates the limits between the branchial derivatives and those of the somites. The dotted area in the gut marks the caudal border of the foregut, which is disproportionately large when compared with the midgut and hindgut. (After Hinrichsen, K.V.: a. Intestinaltrakt, b. peripheres Nervensystem, c. Venen. *In* Hinrichsen K.V. [ed.]: Human Embryologie: Lehrbuch und Atlas der vorgeburtlichen Entwicklung des Menschen. Berlin, Springer-Verlag, 1990, pp. 105, 449, 516, with permission.)

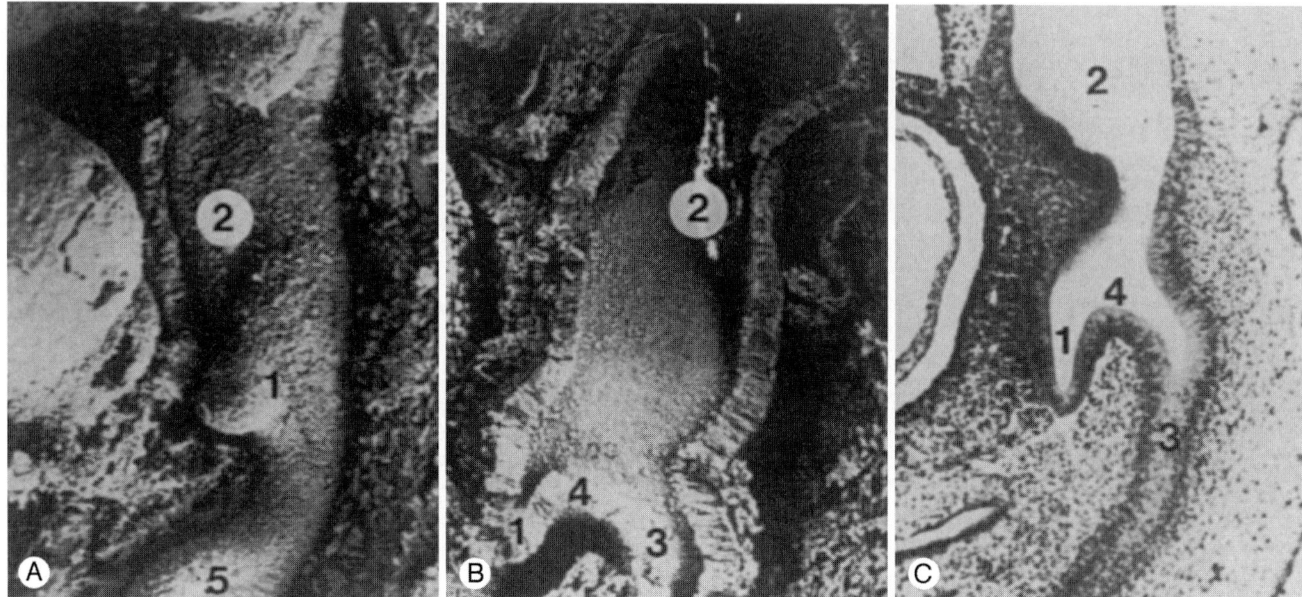

Figure 1–35. Sprouting of the tracheal bud (1) from the foregut. The primitive pharynx (2), esophagus (3), tracheoesophageal fold (4), and stomach (5) are shown. Although this photograph is of a chick embryo, it strongly resembles the wax plate reconstructions of 3- to 5-mm CR human embryos studied by Zwa-Tun,[44] who used the material of the Carnegie collection. Sagittal sections. SEM from the external *(A)* and internal *(B)* aspects and histologic section *(C)*. (Courtesy of D. Kluth, M.D., Hamburg.)

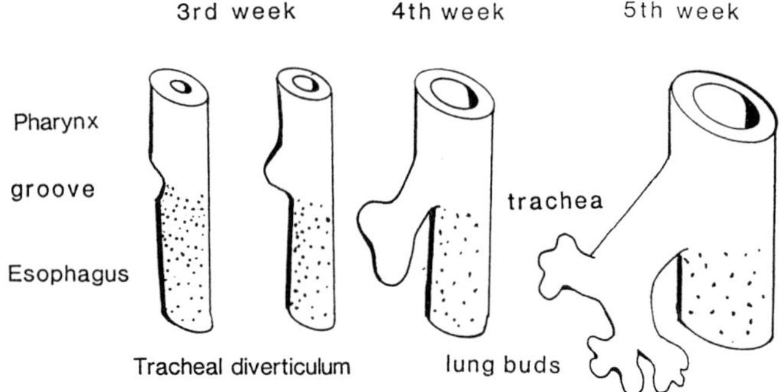

Figure 1–36. Diagram showing the event of separation of the trachea from the foregut. Following the formation of the primitive foregut, the appearance and downward elongation of the tracheal and lung bud make the trachea and esophagus two different entities. Both structures become intimately positioned but do not fuse. Sagittal sections. The tracheal groove will become the tracheal diverticulum, trachea, and lungs.

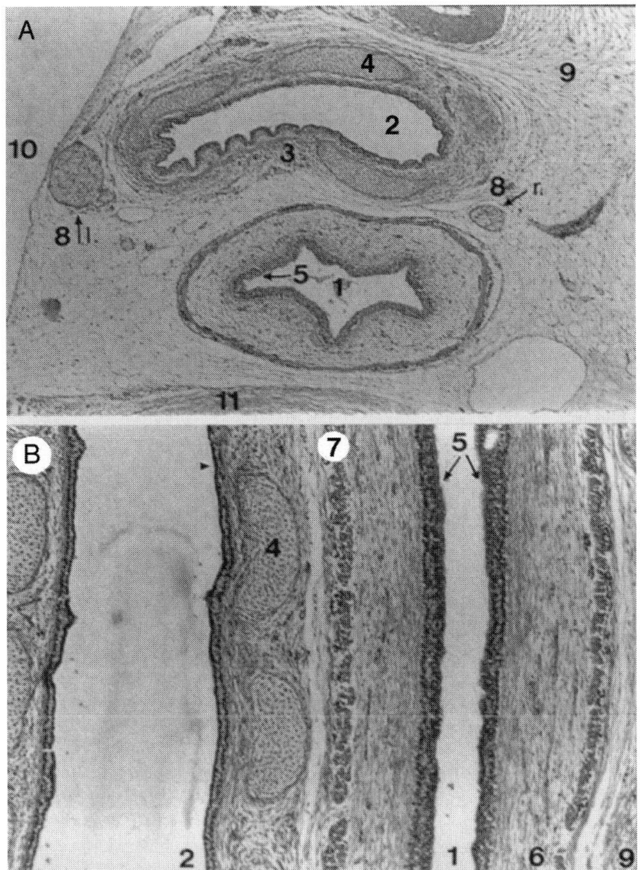

Figure 1–37. Histologic sections, hematoxylin and eosin preparation, 5 μm, through two human embryos of similar age, 44-mm *(A)* and 46-mm *(B)* crown-rump length, and similar level, which is at the entry into the chest. *A* is in the transverse plane, viewed from caudal, and *B* is in the sagittal plane viewed from the left. The esophagus is in the posterior position. Both slices show primitive, developing tissues but definite adult organ relationships, such as the intimate location of the esophagus (1) relative to the trachea (2). 3 = tracheal membrane, 4 = tracheal cartilages, 5 = developing mucosa (note the difference of the cell layers between 1 and 2), 6 = esophageal submucosa (note the dimension of the tissue portion when compared with 7), 7 = muscle coat with large circular and small longitudinal layer, 8 = future inferior laryngeal (recurrent) nerves (r = right, l = left), 9 = primitive mediastinum with undifferentiated tissue of the previsceral and retrovisceral spaces, 10 = pleural cavities (coelom), 11 = primitive vertebral fascia. (From the collection of Liebermann-Meffert.)

by His,[14] who taught that the trachea became separated from the esophagus by the formation of a septum caused by lateral folding that "pinched off" the primitive foregut.[9,20,22,35] This teaching was accepted for years. Smith[39] in 1956 was presumably the first to deny this interpretation, and as already mentioned, in 1987 Kluth developed the concept of an independent formation of the trachea from a protrusion of the primitive hypopharynx.

The esophagus is initially very short. It extends from the tracheal groove to the dilatation of the foregut, which is to become the stomach (Figs. 1-38 and 1-39). Shortly after the formation of the tracheal bud, the primitive esophagus extends rapidly. This lengthening is caused by two factors: the extensive growth of the embryonic "cranium" and the unbending of the body away from the pericardium.[33,34] The movement of the head and body away from the heart at this stage is responsible for the classic misinterpretation that organs migrate upward or downward. In reality, elongation of the distal esophagus becomes more pronounced than that of the proximal and middle parts, and through additional rapid growth of its wall, the esophagus reaches the definite topographic relationships with its surrounding structures by the end of the seventh week (18- to 22-mm CR length).

At the time when the tracheal bud extends, a fusiform dilatation of the foregut, the primitive stomach, appears dorsal and caudal to the septum transversum (see Figs. 1-33 and 1-38). The locations of the later cardia and of the pylorus are definitely determined by the celiac and pancreatic vessel stalks (see Figs. 1-38 and 1-39). The asymmetric growth of the gastric wall[3,28] would suggest positional changes of the stomach,[28,29] but, in fact, there is no evidence of any esophageal[19] or gastric mechanical rotation.[11,29] As the embryo grows, the left side of the primitive stomach enlarges progressively and forms the shape of the greater curvature.[3,29] Compared with the right side, which is to become the lesser curvature, this enlargement is found to coincide with increased local mitotic activity in the wall of the greater curvature, in particular in the area of the future gastric fundus.[3] The growth processes of the fundus delineate the initially ill-defined gastroesophageal junction (Fig. 1-38*A* through *D*).[27,29,33,34] Individual variations in the height of the fundus and the acuteness of the angle of His (cardiac angle) persist during the subsequent fetal period.

FORMATION AND DIVISION OF THE INTRAEMBRYONIC BODY CAVITY

From the intraembryonic portion of the coelom (see Fig. 1-31) arise the principal cavities of the trunk. They appear in the lateral and cardiogenic mesoderm in the 21-day-old embryo. Partial degeneration of the ventral mesenchyme results in fusion of the paired cavities. The coelom enlarges to extend from the thorax to the pelvis. The common body cavity can be subdivided into three parts: the pericardial cavity; the channel-like pericardioperitoneal cavities, which will give rise to the pleural cavity; and the peritoneal cavity. The mesothelium derived from the somatic mesoderm lines the parietal wall, and the mesothelium from the splanchnic mesoderm lines the visceral wall.

ANCHORING STRUCTURES OF THE ESOPHAGUS AND DIAPHRAGM

The caudal part of the foregut, the midgut, and the hindgut are suspended in the peritoneal cavity by the dorsal mesentery, which develops from the dorsal body mesenchyme. The cranial part of the foregut, however, lies in the broad mesenchymal mass of embryonic connective tissue that extends from the sternum to the spine. This forms the primitive ventral and dorsal mediastinum. Caudally, the ventral part is bound by a transverse mesen-

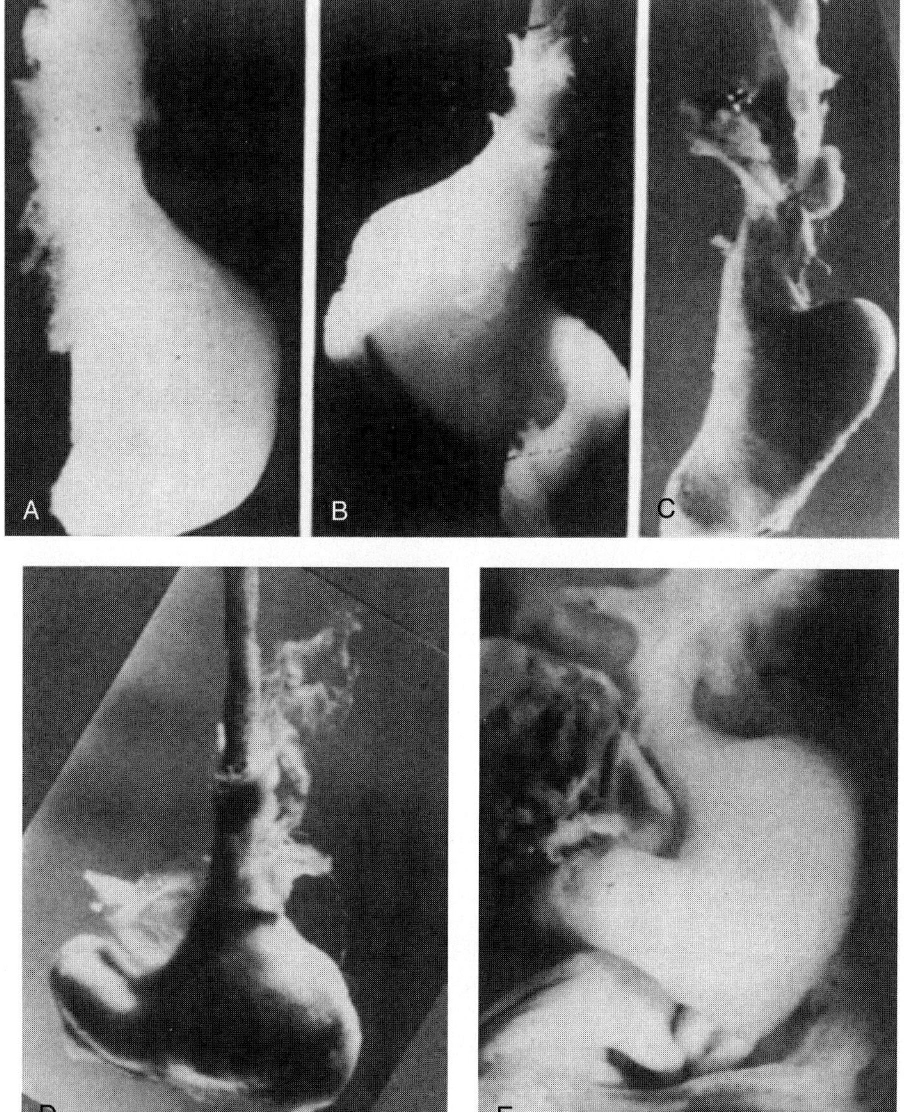

Figure 1–38. *A-E*, Macroscopic view of human stomachs of embryos between 8- and 22-mm CR lengths. Owing to localized cell proliferation, the greater curvature undergoes extensive growth during the 5- through 25-mm stages, which will also form the gastric fundus, the cardiac angulation, and the esophagogastric junction. Both cardia and pylorus are connected by the stalk of the celiac and superior mesenteric vessels. Therewith, growth processes will occur mainly at the free margin of the stomach, at the greater curvature. The lesser curvature does not join this excessive growth stimulation, which, finally, causes the gastric asymmetry. This event is illustrated by the series of human embryos of different CR length (A = 8 mm, B = 14 mm [posterior view], C = 18 mm, D = 19 mm, E = 22 mm).

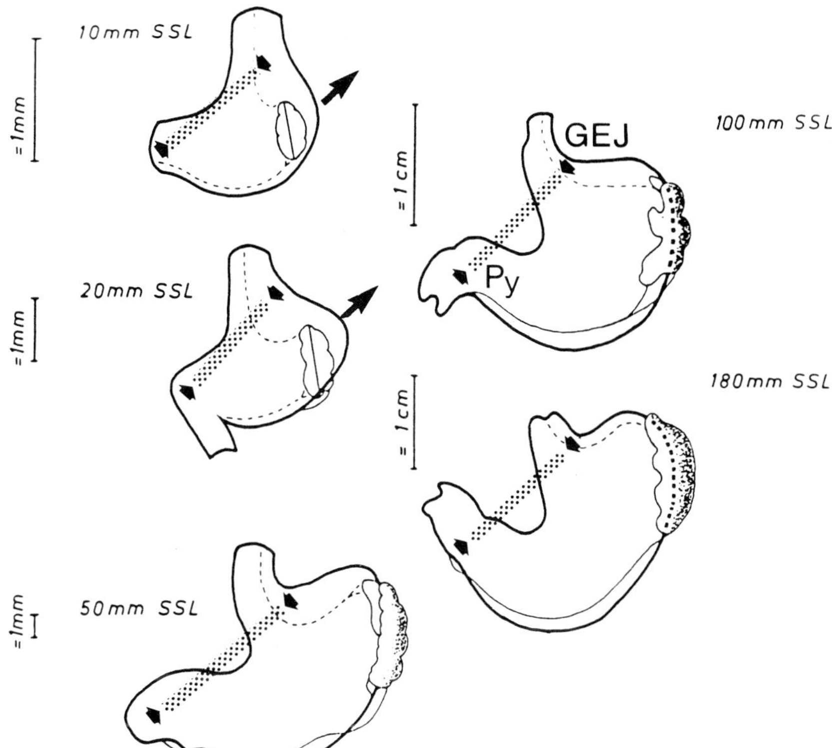

Figure 1–39. The changes in gastric shape are due to an asymmetric growth process involving mostly the greater curvature by great mitotic activity within the wall.[3,29] The cardia and the pylorus remain in place anterior to the spine, where they are held because of their firm dorsal attachment (GEJ and Py) and their relationship to the vessel stalks. SSL = Crown-rump length of the embryo, i.e., fetus. GEJ = gastroesophageal junction.

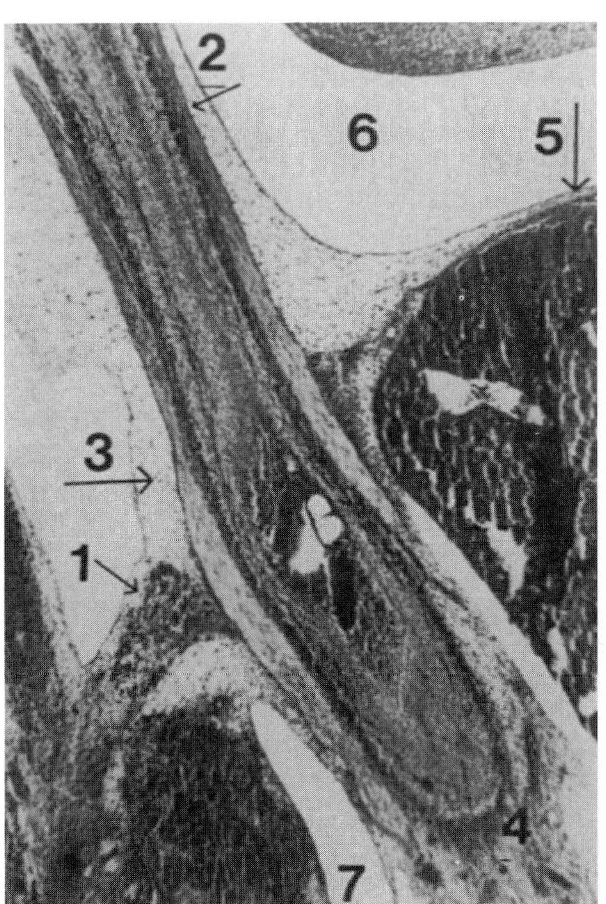

Figure 1–40. Anchoring structures above the esophagogastric junction (sagittal section through a 15-mm CR human embryo). The section parallels but does not cut the esophageal and gastric lumen. (1 = diaphragm, 2 = esophagus, 3 = phrenoesophageal membrane, 4 = stomach, 5 = liver, 6 = pleural cavity, 7 = abdominal cavity, 8 = vacuoles in the mucosa.) The small arrows show the differentiating muscular wall. (Courtesy of Fernandez de Santos, M.D., Madrid.)

chymal plate separating the primordium of the heart from the liver. This is the septum transversum (see Figs. 1-31 and 1-34). In the umbilical cord and near the septum transversum lie the omphaloenteric and umbilical veins.

The lung buds grow into the mesenchyme surrounding the pericardioperitoneal spaces. These small channels expand, splitting the tissues of the lateral body wall into mesenchymal bulges.[39] During the sixth week, these bulges extend from a dorsolateral position toward a ventral and medial orientation. They develop mesentery-type folds that later become membranes. By the end of the sixth week, the free ends of these membranes fuse with the mesoderm ventral and dorsal to the esophagus and with the septum transversum (see Fig. 1-33). Supported by the rapid growth of the liver, the partitions that will become the diaphragm isolate the caudal part of the pericardioperitoneal channel, thus separating the pleural and peritoneal cavities (Fig. 1-40).

Occasionally, and mainly on the left, the pleuroperitoneal cavity remains open, creating the congenital foramen of Bochdalek, which allows a free communication between the chest and the abdomen. The abdominal contents may then herniate into the thorax and cause neonatal problems. The rare persistence of the foramen of Morgagni is the result of a persisting gap from the costosternal origin of the diaphragm: It permits herniation into the anterior mediastinum. Incomplete development of the musculature deriving from the lateral body wall may lead to congenital eventration of the diaphragm.

The diaphragm develops from four sources[20,43] (Fig. 1-41). The largest portion derives from the septum transversum, which has already fused with the ventral mesenchyme of the esophagus. It eventually forms the central tendon of the diaphragm. The median portion derives from the dorsal mesenchyme of the esophagus and gives rise to the crura of the diaphragm. The crura are formed at a point where the septum transversum and the pleuroperitoneal membrane fuse. The peripheral muscular diaphragm originates from the dorsolateral portion of the body wall tissue. Enlargement of the pleural cavity results in a splitting of this tissue with subsequent membrane formation. What is initially the largest portion of the primitive diaphragm eventually forms the small intermediate muscular portion of the diaphragm. This is derived from the pleuroperitoneal membranes at the point where they have fused with the dorsal mesenchyme of the esophagus and the septum transversum. Rapid growth of the dorsal body of the embryo, as opposed to the slower growth of the pericardium, causes an apparent descent of the diaphragm.[43] By the end of the sixth week, the diaphragm is complete and is located at the level of the thoracic somites. By the end of the seventh week, it reaches its final position at the level of the first lumbar vertebra. The diaphragm can be easily identified by its distinctive musculature at the 15-mm CR stage (see Fig. 1-40). It is assumed that the musculature of the diaphragm originates from the cervical myotomes. The larger part, however, is more likely derived from thoracic myotomes when the lateral body wall enlarges owing to expansion of the pleural cavities. The phrenoesophageal membrane, which holds the esophagus in place within its diaphragmatic hiatus (see Fig. 1-40), differentiates after esophageal muscle specialization.

By the end of the embryonic period, in the early ninth week, the definite shapes of all the main organ systems have been established. The external appearance of the organs is now less affected by further development. During the fetal period, beginning with the ninth week, maturation and growth of the various tissues and organs take place.

TISSUE ORGANIZATION OF THE FOREGUT

Musculature

The esophageal musculature develops from myoblasts in the mesoderm that surrounds the primitive gut. These cells derive from the mesenchymal cells. Two types of muscle tissue appear in specific locations in the foregut. These are skeletal striated muscle in the pharynx, larynx, and upper esophagus and visceral smooth muscle in the mid- and lower esophagus and the gut. The striated mus-

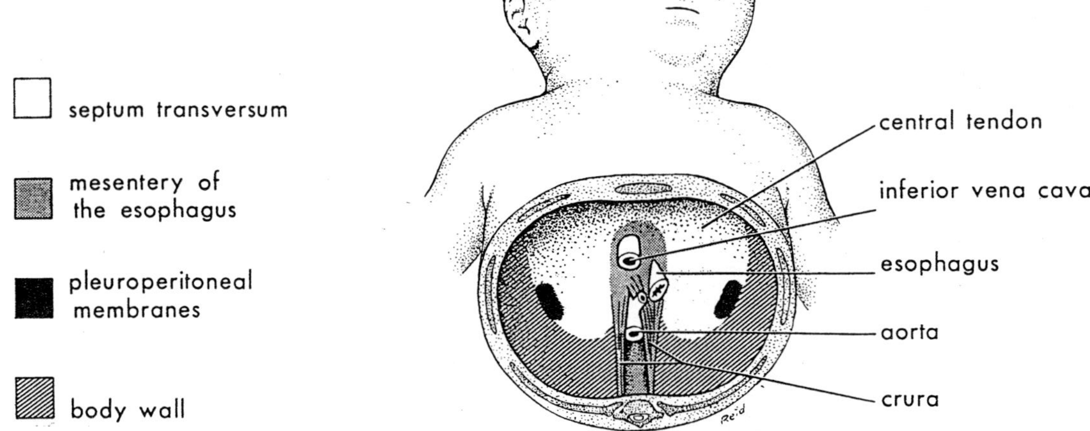

Figure 1-41. Tissue origin of the diaphragm and its four sources. (From Moore, K.L.: The Developing Human, Philadelphia. W.B. Saunders, 1988, with permission.)

cle is derived from the caudal branchial arches and is innervated by the branchiomotor branches of the vagus nerves. The smooth foregut muscle is derived from the visceral splanchnopleuric mesoderm and is innervated by the sympathetic nervous system. The mesenchymal cells that give rise to the musculature are all morphologically similar before the myoblasts differentiate into striated and smooth muscle cells. Both muscle types appear simultaneously on the outer aspect of the esophageal tube as a ring-shaped condensation of elongated nuclei in the 8- to 10-mm CR embryo (Figs. 1–42*A* and 1–43). These cells constitute the circular muscle layer of the lamina muscu-

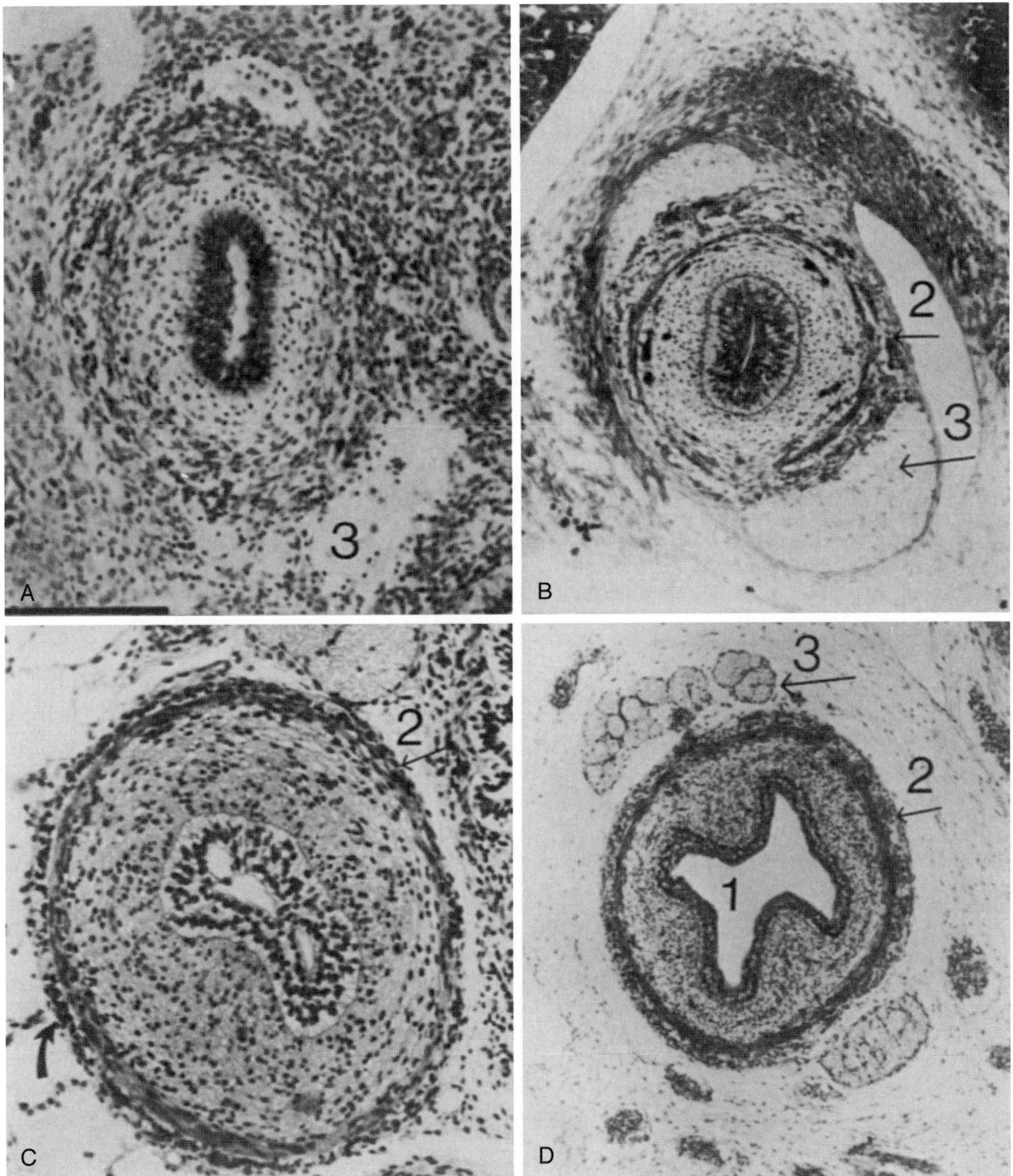

Figure 1–42. Transverse section through the esophagus in embryos of 8.5-mm *(A)*, 12.5-mm *(B)*, 20-mm *(C)*, and 40-mm *(D)* CR length. The mucosal epithelium lining the lumen (1) is stratified columnar in the 8.5-mm CR embryo and will become vacuolized between 12.5 and 20 mm CR and multilayered columnar in the 40-mm CR stage. The tissue that surrounds the mucosal epithelium consists mainly of undifferentiated mesenchyme in the 8.5-mm CR embryo. Differentiation of the inner muscle coat is identified by the cell condensation around the mucosal ring seen in *A* (2). Pale areas of neural cells as precursors to the recurrent laryngeal nerves are seen exterior to the foregut tube (3). In the 12-mm and 20-mm CR stages, the inner muscular layer is further advanced. The outer longitudinal muscle layer and the muscularis mucosae, however, can be identified only at the 40-mm CR length. During this development, the extrinsic innervation, and in particular the recurrent laryngeal nerve, has become of conspicuous size (3). The developmental changes in luminal diameter and shape of the esophagus are seen. (*A*, *B*, and *D* from the collection of Liebermann-Meffert; *C* from Enterline, H., and Thompson, J.: Pathology of the Esophagus. Heidelberg, Springer, 1984, with permission.)

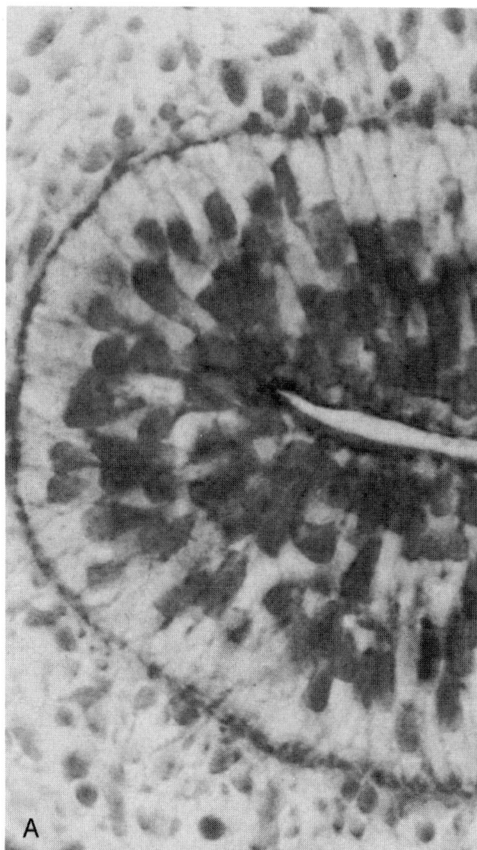

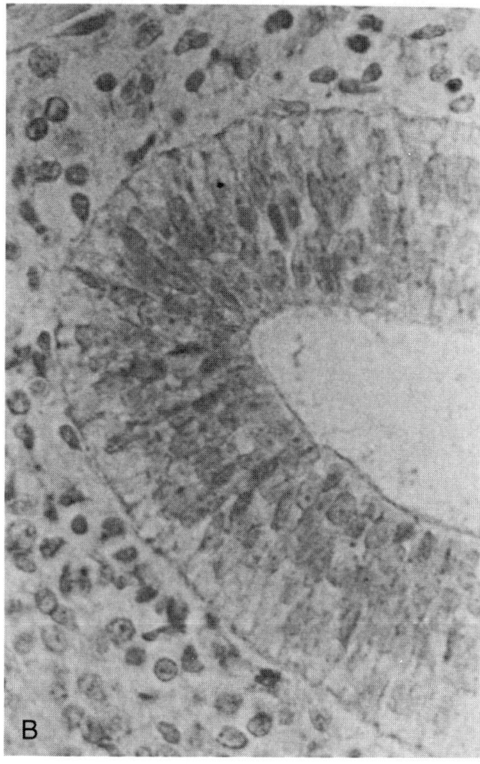

Figure 1–43. Comparison of transverse sections through the esophagus *(A)* and stomach *(B)* in the 8.5-mm CR embryo. Consisting of three layers, the esophageal epithelium is stratified and columnar; it shows a basal layer of cells with large oval nuclei. The basement membrane seen here may not yet be distinct in all embryos at this stage of development. The stomach shows an epithelium that has fewer layers and a distinct basement membrane. (From the collection of Liebermann-Meffert.)

laris. No such arrangement exists in the gastric wall at this stage. The longitudinal muscle layer is ill-defined but is differentiated in the 15-mm CR embryo. Both the circular and the longitudinal layers are developed and form a complete sheet around the esophagus at the 20-mm CR stage (see Fig. 1–42*B*). However, at this stage the musculature forms a very thin sheet of tissue compared to the thickness of the submucosa and mucosa. By the 24-mm CR stage, the muscularis mucosae becomes apparent, and it is well defined in the 65-mm CR stage (see Fig. 1–42*C* and *D*).

The muscle bundles of the esophagus can be distinguished macroscopically in the 76- to 90-mm fetus.[34] The fiber arrangement of the muscle layers in the esophagus and at the esophagogastric junction is comparable at that point with the arrangement seen in the adult.[28,29]

Lamina Mucosa and Esophageal Lumen

Discussion about the developmental changes of the mucosa of the esophagus dates back to the turn of the twentieth century.[1,17,25,27,35,37] The description in this chapter is based on the early studies and more recent investigations.[6,16,36,39] They also include the studies of Liebermann-Meffert (Table 1–2).

The differentiation of the mucosa from the endoderm has been identified in the 2.5-mm CR embryo at about the third week of gestation (see Table 1–1). The foregut is lined with two or three layers of pseudostratified columnar epithelium, which is uniformly thick along the entire esophagus and is surrounded by undifferentiated mesenchymal cells (Figs. 1–42, 1–43, and 1–44). This pseudostratified aspect of the mucosa lasts until the 12- to 13-mm CR stage.[16,33] At that time, the mucosa becomes multilayered and thicker owing to cell proliferation (see Fig. 1–42 and Table 1–2). When the embryo is 12 mm CR long, tiny, thin-walled hollow spaces start to appear in the basal level of the epithelium (Figs. 1–44 and 1–45*A* and Table 1–2). Subsequently, when the embryo is about 25 mm CR long, it is seen that the thin spaces represent vacuoles. These increase in number and may become much larger than the esophageal lumen itself (see Fig. 1–45) and are most conspicuous in the 25- to 29-mm CR stage. The vacuoles are located between the columnar cells or close to the luminal surface (see Figs. 1–42 and 1–45). Condensation and size vary individually, but the vacuoles are largest and most numerous at levels close to the tracheal bifurcation. Most of the larger vacuoles contain a somewhat fibrous material (see Fig. 1–45*A* and *B*). With the disappearance of the vacuoles, which is complete in the 75-mm CR fetus, the esophageal lumen, which was narrow until this period and closely resembled a vacuole (see Fig. 1–45), starts to widen (see Fig. 1–42 and Table 1–2). It has been suggested that rupture of the vacuoles would increase the width of the esophageal lumen.[1,21] However, the events during vacuolization and the reasons for the appearance and rupturing of the vacuoles have never been explained satisfactorily,[32] and the significance of vacuolization remains unclear.

Large, dark cells appear in the basal epithelial cell layer of the 30- to 40-mm CR embryo. The stratified columnar

Table 1–2. Prenatal Development of the Mucosa in the Human Esophagus

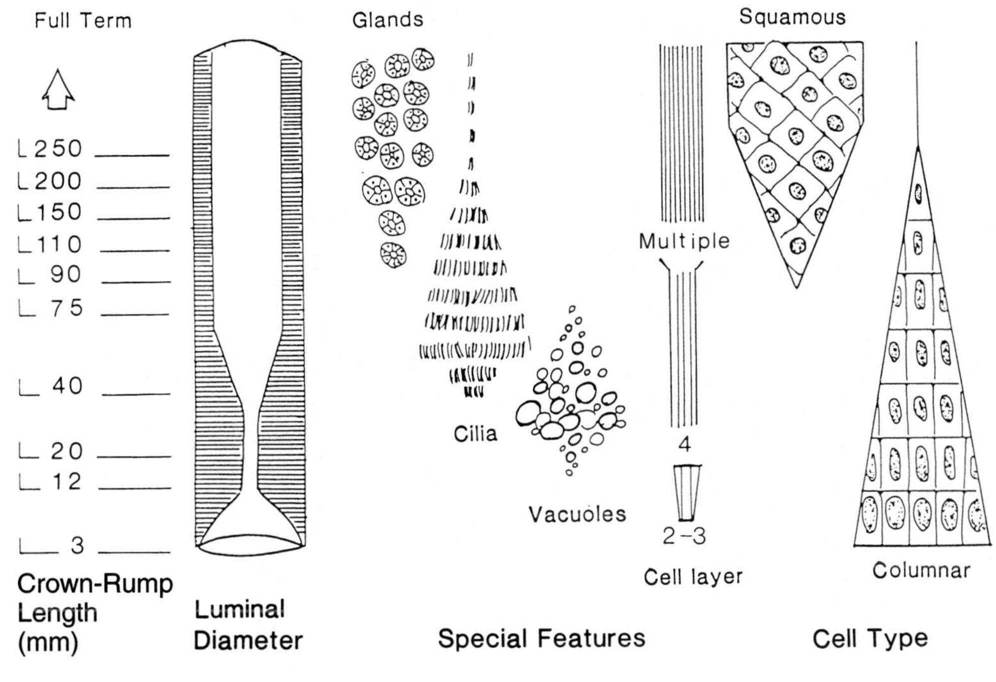

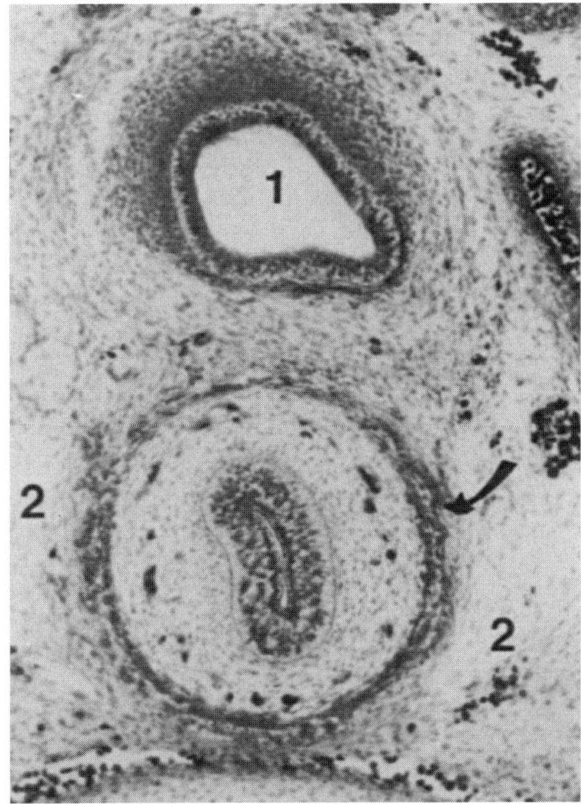

Figure 1–44. Transverse section through the upper esophagus of a 12.5-mm CR embryo above the level of the developing tracheal bifurcation with narrowing of the lumen owing to cell proliferation. The arrow shows the differentiating circular muscle layer of the esophagus (1 = primordium of the trachea, 2 = recurrent laryngeal nerve). (From the collection of Liebermann-Meffert.)

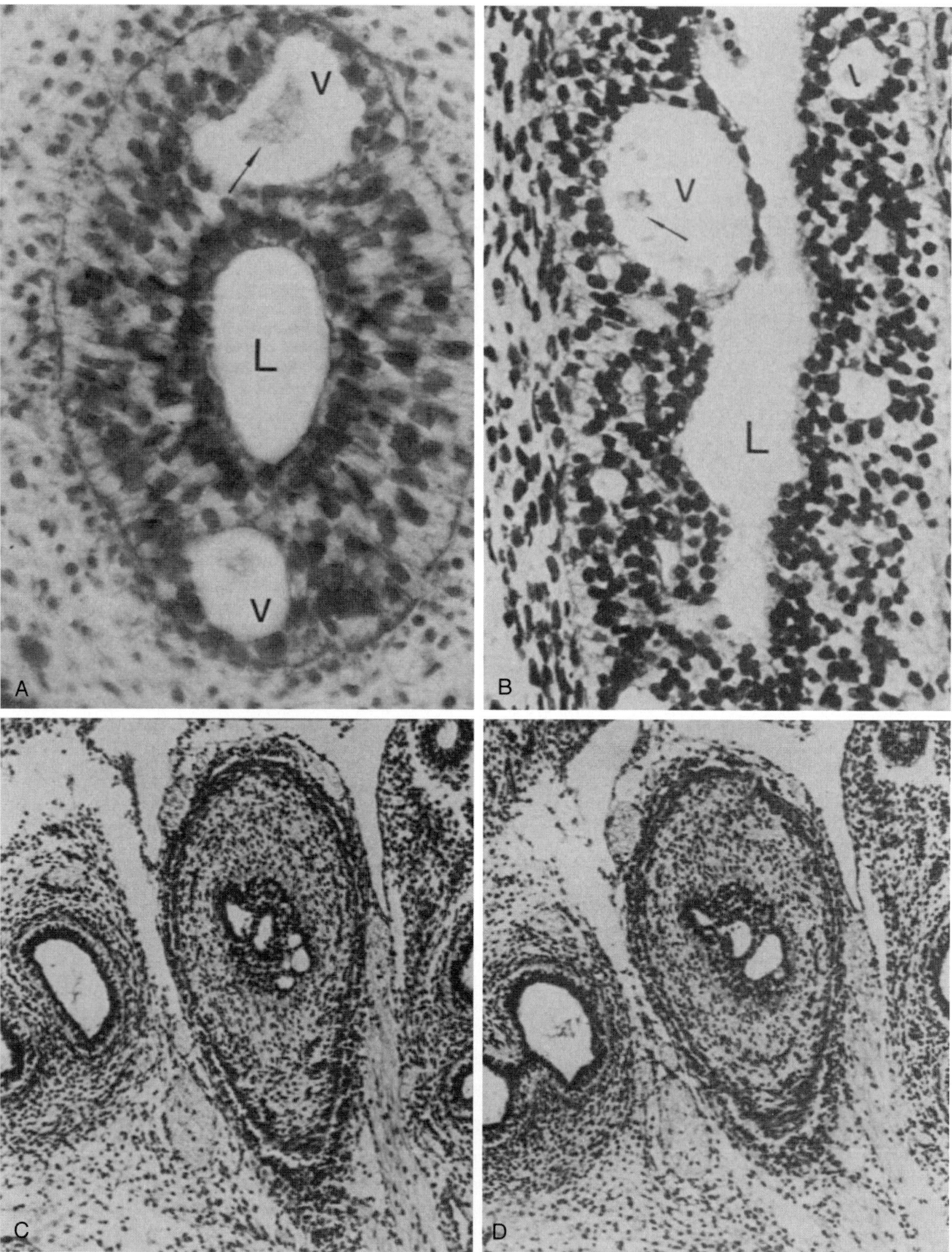

Figure 1–45. Transverse section of the middle esophagus at the vacuolated stages of the mucosa in 12.5-mm CR *(A),* 20-mm CR *(B),* and 40-mm CR (*C* and *D*) embryos. The vacuoles are located between the epithelial cells. Some are large with a diameter occasionally greater than that of the esophageal lumen. Serial sections suggest that some of the vacuoles may even be multichambered (*C* and *D*). Small stretched epithelial cells form partitions that separate from the esophageal lumen *(C).* Some of the vacuoles contain aggregated fiber material (*arrows* in *A* and *B*). (L = esophageal lumen, V = vacuole). (*A* from the collection of Liebermann-Meffert; *B* from Enterline, H., and Thompson, J.: Diseases of the Esophagus. Heidelberg, Springer-Verlag, 1984, with permission; *C* and *D* courtesy of Fernandez de Santos, M.D., and Tello Lopez, M.D., Madrid.)

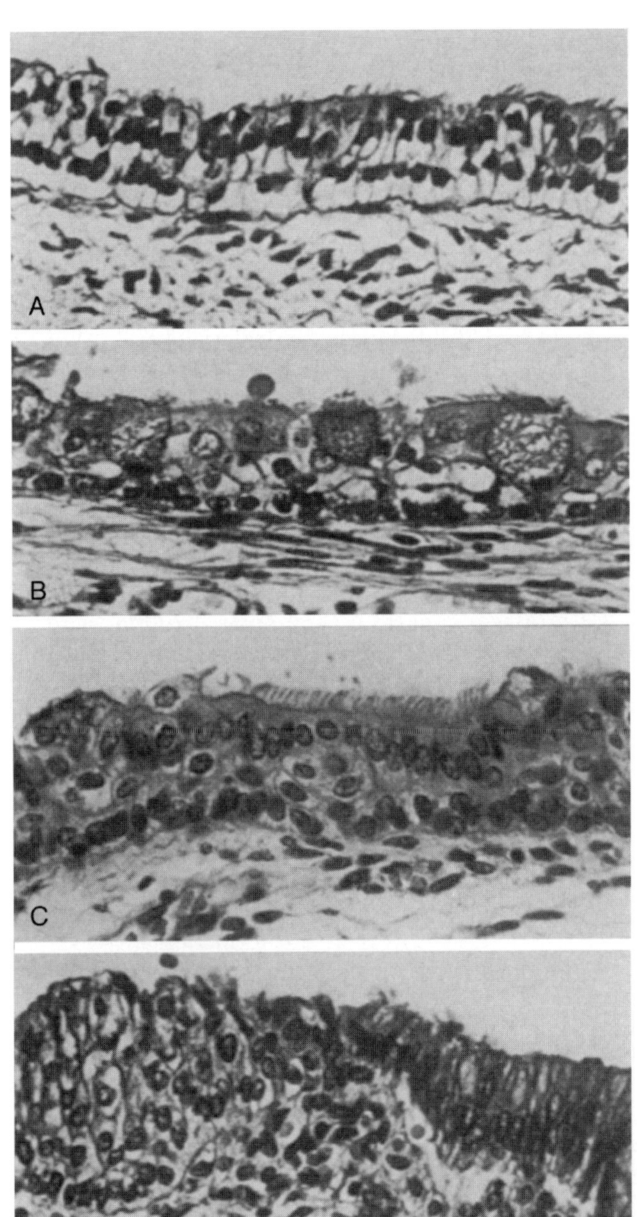

Figure 1–46. Transverse sections through the esophagus at different stages of mucosal development. *A,* Ciliated pseudostratified columnar epithelium at the 28-mm CR stage. *B,* Ciliated columnar cells. Goblet cells are present on top of several layers of polygonal cells that represent early squamous replacement found in the 190- to 230-mm CR fetus. *C,* A later stage in the process of squamous replacement in which patchy remnants of ciliated epithelium may remain until birth. *D,* A residual island of mucin-secreting cells in the esophagus of a newborn. (From Enterline, H., and Thompson, J.: Diseases of the Esophagus. Heidelberg, Springer-Verlag, 1984, with permission.)

epithelium is generally four cells deep (see Fig. 1–45*A*). The basal epithelial cells project toward the lumen to become ciliated columnar cells (Fig. 1–46*A* and Table 1–2). These cells progress from the middle third of the esophagus in a cranial and caudal direction. Ciliated cells line the entire mucosa of the esophagus of the 60-mm CR embryo, except for the upper and lower ends. Here, the epithelium consists of a single layer of large columnar cells[17,34,35] containing mucin-bearing cells (goblet cells). In the approximately 200-mm CR fetus, the area of these cells, which are in continuity with the gastric mucosa, is reduced (see Fig. 1–46*B* and *C*) and is lost at about the 240-mm CR stage.

An interesting aspect of the mechanisms of the developing esophageal mucosa was studied by Menard and Arsenault.[31] These investigators were able to study explants of the esophagus from early-stage human fetuses maintained in organ culture. Using this fresh material, they followed the ultrastructural changes that occurred in esophageal epithelialization during maturation of the tissue. They observed that during the replacement of the epithelium, islets of ciliated cells actually developed epithelium.

The stratified squamous epithelium appears in the 90- to 130-mm CR fetus (see Fig. 1–46*C*). Again, this epithelium migrates from the middle third of the esophagus, spreading cranially and caudally until squamous epithelium has progressively and almost completely replaced the ciliated columnar epithelium in the 250-mm CR fetus. Some patches of ciliated columnar cells, however, occasionally remain until birth and are usually found in the proximal esophagus.

The first superficial glands have been observed during the 160-mm CR stage (see Table 1–2). They contain acini. These glands are numerous in the esophagus of 210-mm CR fetuses and are located mostly at the level of the cricoid cartilage and at the lower end of the esophagus.[16,34] During the last 3 months of gestation, the downgrowth of the surface epithelium begins to generate submucosal glands (Fig. 1–47).

The formation of the esophageal lumen is greatly influenced by the development of the mucosa. Owing to cell proliferation and to the appearance of the vacuoles between the 10- and 21-mm CR stages, the initially slitlike (see Figs. 1–42 and 1–44) or elliptic lumen becomes narrow and asymmetric and then assumes a bizarre configuration (see Fig. 1–42*A* to *C*). This phenomenon is more pronounced at levels between the esophageal opening and the tracheal bifurcation and is caused by cell proliferation (see Fig. 1–44). As the process of vacuoliza-

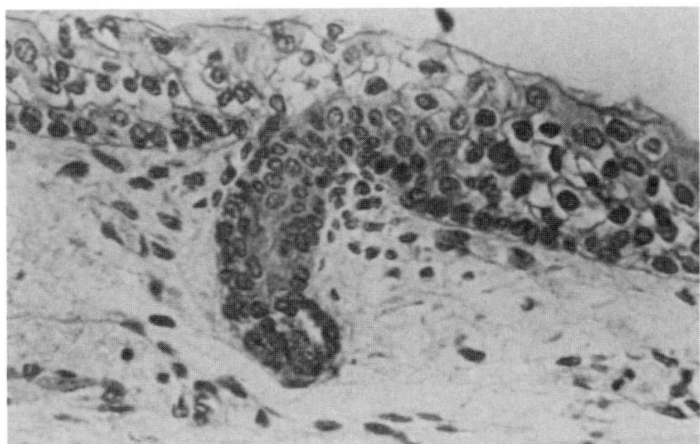

Figure 1–47. During the last trimester of fetal development, downgrowth of the surface epithelium begins to generate future submucosal glands. A few ciliated cells are present on the surface above the squamous epithelium. (From Enterline, H., and Thompson, J.: Diseases of the Esophagus. Heidelberg, Springer-Verlag, 1984, with permission.)

tion continues and larger vacuoles appear, the narrowing of the entire esophageal lumen becomes apparent. During this period of vacuolization, when slices of the esophageal wall are taken in the thickest part of the wall, an image of solid lumen occlusion may result (Figs. 1-44 and 1-48). This picture is probably what led Kreuter[25] in 1905 to suggest, erroneously, that a physiologic solid occlusion of the esophageal lumen takes place during this stage of development. He concluded that esophageal atresia could result if recanalization of the lumen did not occur by vacuolization. Although no subsequent investigator reconfirmed Kreuter's ideas, his opinion still appears in a number of current surgery and anatomic textbooks. Vacuolization of the esophageal mucosa occurs during a period in which the trachea and lungs are already fully developed. From this observation, it was suggested that atresia of the esophagus is mostly due to a growth defect of the esophagus and trachea, combined with an overgrowth of the epithelium, which bulges into the foregut.[7,25]

With the disappearance of the vacuoles, the esophageal lumen enlarges. Owing to the growth processes in the submucosa, four to five large folds have developed (see Fig. 1-42*D*). These folds parallel the longitudinal axis of the esophagus and constitute the definite configuration of the esophageal lumen.

VASCULARIZATION OF THE FOREGUT

The vessels are formed in the early somite stage in the somatopleural mesenchyme of the body wall. Two major arterial sources supply the foregut. One is located in the mesenchyme of the fourth to the sixth pharyngeal arches and represents the arterial system of the aortic arches that partly encircle the pharynx (Fig. 1-49). These vessels also supply the upper and middle foregut. At the end of the somite period (5-mm CR length), a pair of pharyngeal arch arteries develops in the mesenchyme of the sixth branchial arch, giving rise to vascular branches that descend to supply the region of the trachea and the lung buds. The third major source develops in the mesenchyme around the primitive midgut, where the initially paired dorsal aortas fuse caudally to form a single midline vessel. The visceral vessels of the infradiaphragmatic aorta fuse to form the celiac axis, which gives off tributaries to the lower portion of the foregut and to the superior and inferior mesenteric arteries (see Fig. 1-49).

Thus, a number of changes alter the primitive vascular pattern and result in establishment of the final arterial pattern. However, vessels deriving from the branchial region, even after deflexion of the embryo and elongation of the esophagus, have a distal flow direction, whereas the vessels deriving from the celiac axis contribute the vascular supply to the esophagus in a cranial flow direction (see Fig. 1-49). The feature that deserves special attention is that venous drainage and lymphatic drainage follow the same bidirectional pattern of flow but with a reverse orientation (Fig. 1-50). This orientation never changes from the fetal throughout adult life.

One must keep in mind that the esophagus originates from two different tissue sources: the head and neck material and the body mesenchyme (see Figs. 1-31 and 1-34). This origin results in the formation of two areas that develop simultaneously while maintaining a common

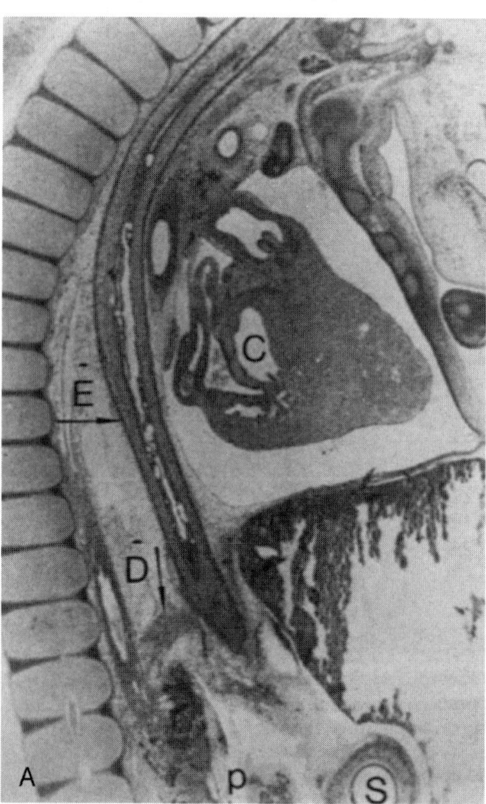

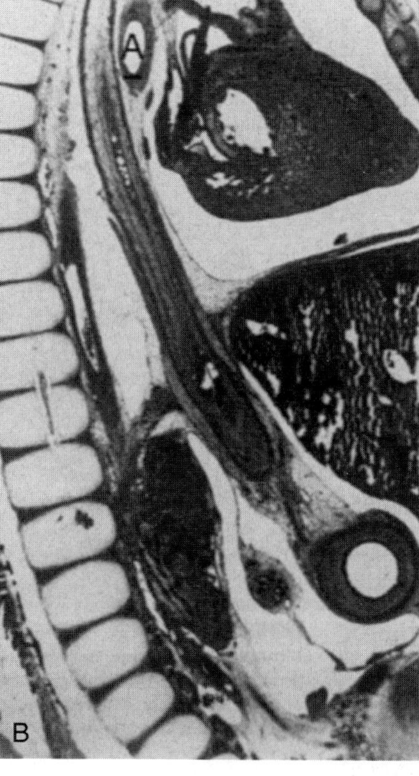

Figure 1-48. Sagittal sections through the esophagus of a 15-mm CR embryo at two consecutive levels. *A,* The esophageal musculature is cut at its peripheral limits. The lumen appears to be obliterated by musculature mimicking a solid structure. *B,* A deeper slice through the esophageal wall displays the vacuolated but patent esophageal lumen. (A = aorta, E = esophagus, D = diaphragm, p = pancreas, S = stomach.) (Courtesy of Fernandez de Santos, M.D., and Tello Lopez, M.D., Madrid.)

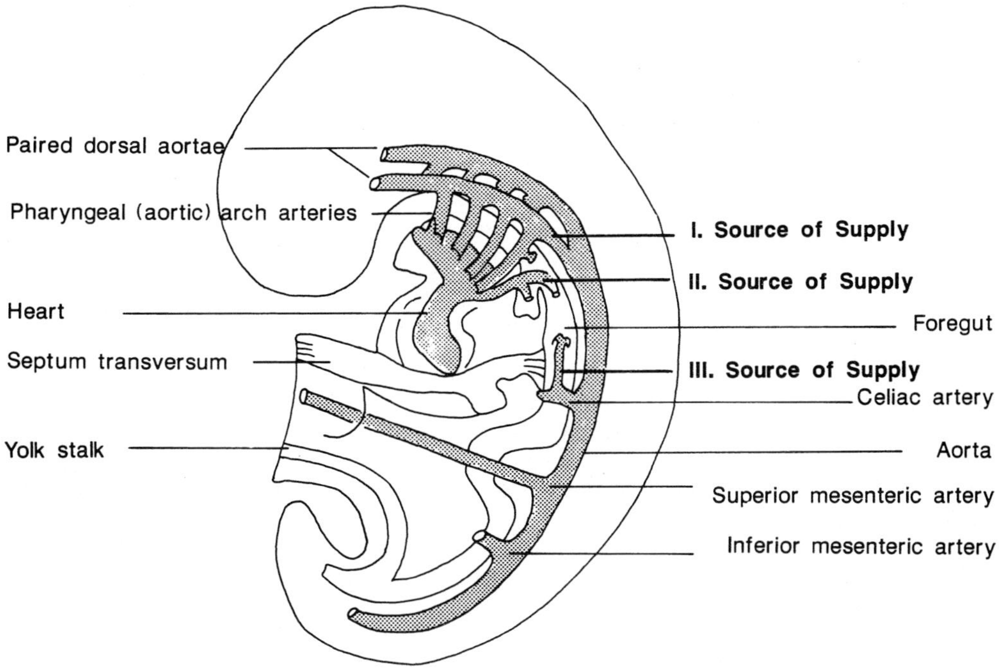

Figure 1–49. Schematic drawing of a sagittal section through the foregut. As shown, two of the three main sources of the adult blood supply are derived from branchial arch arteries. These are the esophageal branches from I, the later thyroid arteries, and from II, the tracheobronchial arteries. The third source (III) derives from the gastric and splenic branches of the celiac artery. (Modified from Moore, K.L.: The Developing Human, Philadelphia, W.B. Saunders, 1988, with permission.)

delimitation at the level of the tracheal bifurcation (see Fig. 1-50). This fact has some significance for the direction of lymphatic flow and, in particular, for esophageal malignancies.

The lymphatic system itself appears concurrently with the venous system 2 weeks after the cardiovascular system. Lymph sacculations develop in the jugular region (Fig. 1-51), and definitive lymph vessels are identified in the 11-mm CR embryo during the sixth week, supplying the foregut and the trachea.[8,32]

INNERVATION OF THE FOREGUT

The vagus nerve is formed by the early fusion of nerves from the last three branchial arches (Fig. 1-52). Large efferent and afferent general components are distributed to the whole foregut.[2,9,13,15] The efferent fibers arise from the specialized dorsal motor nucleus, whereas the afferent fibers derive from neuroblasts of the neural crest. Removal of the neural crest at an early stage of development results in an absence of ganglia in the esophagus.[13,18]

The phrenic nerve, which is responsible for the innervation of the developing diaphragmatic muscle, is formed from the anterior primary rami of the third to the fifth cervical nerves.[39]

The cells of the sympathetic nervous system migrate along the rami of the thoracic spinal nerves in the late somite stage.[26] The nerve fibers then leave their medial position to pass behind the corresponding aorta, where

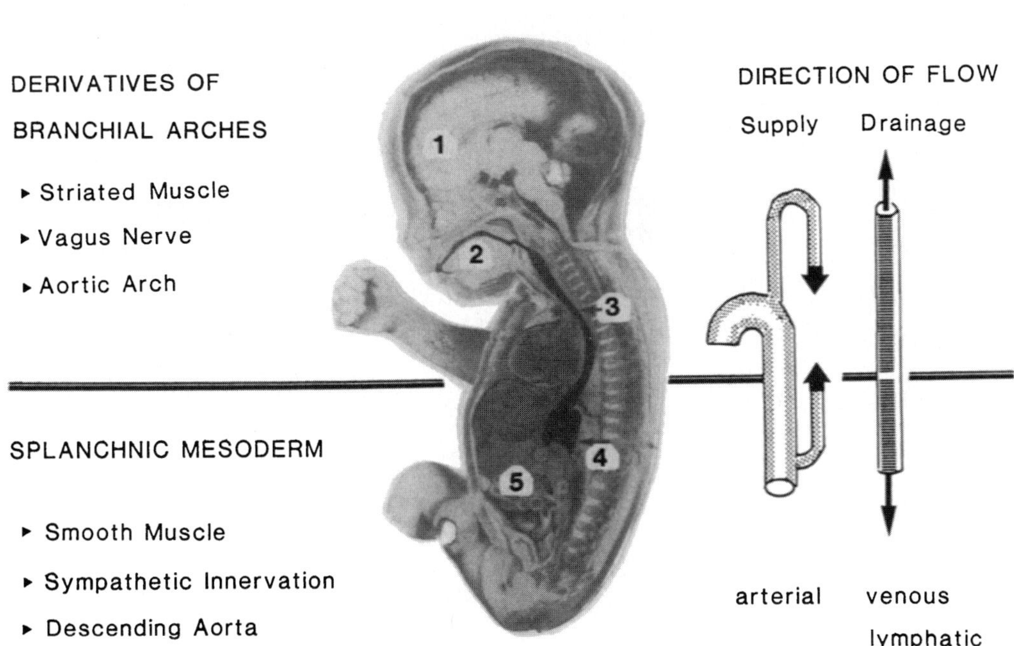

Figure 1–50. The esophagus in the fetus and its topographic development. Structures above the line of the tracheal bifurcation (vessels, nerves, and lymphatics) originate from the tissue of the branchial arches and pharyngeal pouches. Below this line, the structures derive from the lateral plate of the body mesenchyme. This border, located at the level of the tracheal bifurcation, permanently defines the direction of vascular flow. (1 = head, 2 = oral cavity and pharynx, 3 = esophagus, 4 = stomach, 5 = bowel.)

they form the primordium of the sympathetic nervous system. The precise origin of these cells is not yet clarified. Smith and Taylor[40] reviewed the subject of vagal system development, emphasizing the diverse opinions that exist on the matter. Liebermann-Meffert identifies the two vagal trunks in the 8.5-mm CR embryo.[29] The same is true for the inferior laryngeal (recurrent) nerves (see Fig. 1–42*A*). They are already large at the 12- to 20-mm CR stage (see Figs. 1–42 and 1–44). Both vagal nerves (see Fig. 1–52) and the recurrent laryngeal nerves adopt their definite position alongside the esophagus at the early stage of development when the embryonal body straightens.[18,41]

Campenhout[2] observed that neuroblasts from the periesophageal plexus enter the esophageal wall very early in development; that is, before the embryo has reached 10-mm CR length. The neuroblasts form a complete periesophageal network at the outer limits of the circular muscle layer of the esophagus before the longitudinal muscle is differentiated. In the 40-mm CR embryo, 8 to 12 nerve bundles cover the esophagus. By the time the embryo reaches 65 mm CR, the periesophageal plexus consists of large, interlacing vagal bundles that contain ganglia. The myenteric plexus is identifiable in the 10-week-old fetus.[12,13,40] At this stage, ganglion cells are not positively identifiable but are represented by numerous pale areas in the myenteric plexus. The number of cells, the cell size, and the nerve density peak at the sixteenth to twentieth weeks of gestation.[15] Sparse submucosal nerve fibers can be discerned in the 35-mm CR embryo. These fibers become the submucosal plexus. According to Hewer,[12] this plexus is not well developed until the 67-mm CR stage, but it is complete in the 80-mm CR fetus.[40] In the 90-mm CR fetus, the submucosal plexus is extensive and consists of fine nerve fibers and ganglia. The innervation of the muscularis mucosae is particularly rich in the fetus at the 140-mm CR stage.

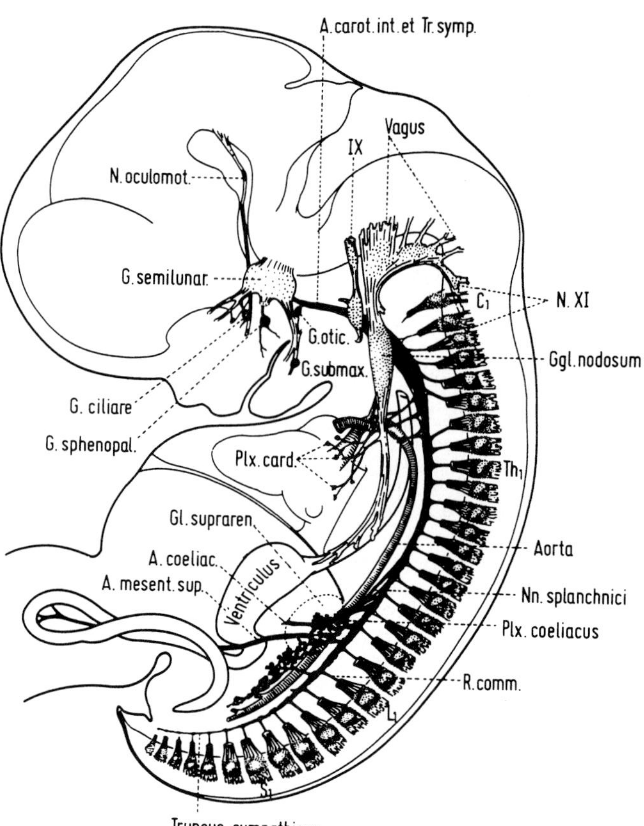

Figure 1–52. The parasympathetic and sympathetic nervous systems in relation to the foregut in a human embryo of 18 mm CR. (From Hinrichsen, K.V.: a. Intestinaltrakt, b. peripheres Nervensystem, c. Venen. *In* Hinrichsen, K.V. [ed.]: Human Embryologie: Lehrbuch und Atlas der vorgeburtlichen Entwicklung des Menschen. Berlin, Springer-Verlag, 1990, pp. 305, 449, 516, with permission.)

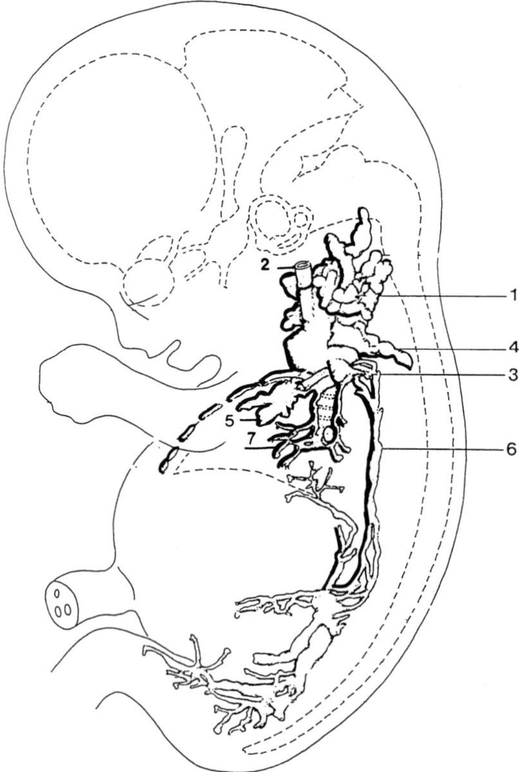

Figure 1–51. Schematic illustration of the saccular lymphatic system at the 30-mm CR stage, eighth week of gestation. The branchiogenic part into which the upper foregut drains is far more voluminous than that of the lower foregut, midgut, and hindgut. The saccus jugularis (1); the jugular vein (2); the suprascapular (3); supraclavicular (4); and axillar lymphatic protrusions (5); the thoracic duct (6); and the bronchoesophagomediastinal lymphatics (7) are seen. (After Gaudecker, B. von: Lymphatische Organe. *In* Hinrichsen, K.V. [ed.]: Human Embryologie: Lehrbuch und Atlas der vorgeburtlichen Entwicklung des Menschen. Berlin, Springer-Verlag, 1990, p. 340, with permission.)

References

1. Boerner-Patzelt, D.: Die Entwicklung der Magenschleimhautinseln im oberen Anteil des Oesophagus von ihrem ersten Auftreten bis zur Geburt. Anat. Anz., *55:*162, 1922.
2. Campenhout, E. van: Le développement du système nerveux sympathique chez le poulet. Arch Biol. (Paris), *42:*479, 1931.
3. Dankmeijer, J., and Miete, M.: Sur le développement de l'estomac. Acta Anat., *47:*384, 1961.
4. David, G., and Haegel, P.: Embryologie: Traveaux Practiques et Enseignement Dirigé. Paris, Masson, 1968.
5. England, M. A.: Farbatlas der Embryologie. Deutsche Ausgabe, Lütjen-Drecoll, E. (ed.). Stuttgart, Schattauer, 1985.

6. Enterline, H., and Thompson, J.: Pathology of the Esophagus. New York, Springer, 1984.
7. Forssner, H.: Die angeborene Darm- und Oesophagusatresie. Arb. Anat. Inst. Wiesbaden, *34:*1, 1907.
8. Gaudecker, B. von: Lymphatische Organe. *In* Hinrichsen, K. V. (ed.): Human Embryologie. Lehrbuch und Atlas der vorgeburtlichen Entwicklung des Menschen. Berlin, Springer, 1990, p. 340.
9. Gray, S. W., and Skandalakis, J. E.: Embryology for Surgeons. The Embryological Basis for the Treatment of Congenital Defects. Philadelphia, W.B. Saunders, 1972, p. 63.
10. Hamilton, W. J., and Mossman, H. W.: Hamilton, Boyd and Mossman's Human Embryology. Prenatal Development of Form and Function, 4th ed. London, Macmillan, 1978.
11. Heuser, C. H., and Corner, G. W.: Developmental horizons in human embryos—age groups xi to xxiii. Collected papers from the Contributions to Embryology. Washington, Carnegie Institution of Washington, 1951.
12. Hewer, E.: Development of nerve endings in the foetus. J. Anat. (Lond.), *69:*369, 1934.
13. Hinrichsen, K. V.: a) Intestinaltrakt, b) peripheres Nervensystem, c) Venen. *In* Hinrichsen, K. V. (ed.): Human Embryologie. Lehrbuch und Atlas der vorgeburtlichen Entwicklung des Menschen. Berlin, Springer, 1990, pp. 516, 449, 305.
14. His, W.: Zur Bildungsgeschichte der Lungen beim menschlichen Embryo. Arch. Anat. Entwickl. Gesch., *17:*89, 1887.
15. Hitchcock, R. J. I., Pemble, M. J., Bishop, A. E., et al.: Quantitative study of the development and maturation of human oesophageal innervation. J. Anat., *180:*175, 1992.
16. Johns, B. A. E.: Developmental changes in the esophageal epithelium in man. J. Anat. (Lond.), *86:*431, 1952.
17. Johnson, F. D.: The development of the mucous membrane of the esophagus, stomach and small intestine in the human embryo. Am. J. Anat., *10:*521, 1910.
18. Jones, D. S.: Origin of the vagi and the parasympathetic ganglion cells of the viscera of the chick. Anat. Rec., *82:*185, 1942.
19. Kanagasuntheram, R.: Development of the human lesser sac. J. Anat. (Lond.), *91:*188, 1957.
20. Keith, A.: The nature of the mammalian diaphragm and pleural cavities. J. Anat. (Lond.), *39:*243, 1905.
21. Keith, A.: Human Embryology and Morphology, 5th ed. London, Arnold, 1933, p. 303.
22. Keith, A., and Spicer, J. E.: Three cases of malformation of the tracheo-oesophageal septum. J. Anat. Physiol., *41:*52, 1906.
23. Kluth, D., and Habenicht, R.: The embryology of usual and unusual types of esophageal atresia. Pediatr. Surg. Int., *2:*223, 1987.
24. Kluth, D., Steding, G., and Seidl, W.: The embryology of foregut malformations. J. Pediatr. Surg., *22:*389, 1987.
25. Kreuter, E.: Die angeborenen Verschliessungen und Verengerungen des Darmkanals im Lichte der Entwicklungsgeschichte. Dtsch. Z. Chir., *79:*1, 1905.
26. Kuntz, A.: The role of the vagi in development of the sympathetic nervous system. Anat. Anz., *35:*381, 1909.
27. Lewis, E. T.: The form of the stomach in human embryos with notes upon the nomenclature of the stomach. Am. J. Anat., *13:*477, 1912.
28. Liebermann-Meffert, D.: Die Muskelarchitektur der Magenwand des menschlichen Föten im Vergleich zum Aufbau der Magenwand des Erwachsenen. Morphol. Jb., *108:*391, 1966.
29. Liebermann-Meffert, D.: Form und Lageentwicklung des menschlichen Magens und seiner Mesenterien. Acta Anat., *72:*376, 1969.
30. Liebermann-Meffert, D.: Die Frühentwicklung der Milz menschlicher Feten mit Befunden zur Problematik der Erythropoese. Embryonic development of the human spleen and erythropoiesis. *In* Lennert, K., and Harms, D. (eds.): Die Milz/The Spleen. Berlin, Springer, 1970, pp. 222–236.
31. Menard, D., and Arsenault, P.: Maturation of human fetal esophagus maintained in organ culture. Anat. Rec., *217:*348, 1987.
32. Moore, K. L.: The Developing Human: Clinically Oriented Embryology, 4th ed. Philadelphia, W.B. Saunders, 1988.
33. Mueller-Botha, G. S.: Organogenesis and growth of the gastroesophageal region in man. Anat. Rec. *133:*219, 1959.
34. Neumann, J.: Die Metaplasie des foetalen Oesophagusepithels. Fortschr. Med., *15:*366, 1897.
35. Rosenthal, A. H.: Congenital atresia of the esophagus with tracheo-esophageal fistula: Report of eight cases. Arch. Pathol., *12:*756, 1931.
36. Sakai, N., Suenaga, T., and Tanaka, K.: Electron microscopic study on the esophageal mucosa in human fetuses. Auris Nasus Larynx (Tokyo), *16:*177, 1989.
37. Schridde, H.: Ueber die Epithelproliferationen in der embryonalen menschlichen Speiseröhre. Virchows Arch. Pathol. Anat., *191:*178, 1908.
38. Skandalakis, J. E., and Gray, S. W. (eds.): Embryology for Surgeons: The Embryological Basis for the Treatment of Congenital Anomalies, 2nd ed. Baltimore, Williams & Wilkins, 1994.
39. Smith, E. I.: The early development of the trachea and esophagus in relation to atresia of the esophagus and tracheoesophageal fistula. Contrib. Embryol. Carnegie Inst., *36:*43, 1956.
40. Smith, R. B., and Taylor, J. M.: Observations on the intrinsic innervation of the human fetal esophagus between the 10-mm and 140-mm crown-rump length stages. Acta Anat., *81:*127, 1972.
41. Stephens, T. D.: Atlas of Human Embryology. New York, Macmillan, 1980.
42. Tuchmann-Duplessis, H., and Haegel, P.: Illustrated Human Embryology, Vol. II: Organogenesis. New York, Springer, 1972.
43. Wells, L. J.: Development of the human diaphragm and pleural sacs. Contrib. Embryol. Carnegie Inst., *24:*93, 1954.
44. Zwa-Tun, H. A.: The tracheo-esophageal septum—fact or fantasy? Acta Anat. (Basel), *114:*1, 1982.

CHAPTER

2 Physiology of the Esophagus

ANDRÉ DURANCEAU • DOROTHEA LIEBERMANN-MEFFERT

PHARYNX

When a swallow is initiated, an organized sequence of events occurs involving a sweeping action of the tongue, closing of the nasopharynx by the velopharyngeal muscles, and subsequent sequential contractions of the superior, medial, and inferior constrictor muscles. This sequence is difficult to evaluate because of the rapidity and variety of the events that take place.[18]

Neurogenic Events and Control

Tactile receptors in the pharynx elicit a series of reflex muscle activities that pull the pharynx up, elevate the hyoid bone, and bring the pharynx forward and upward. Respiration ceases, and the larynx is closed by the false and true vocal cords while the epiglottis hides the laryngeal additus. At the same time, the muscles of the upper middle and lower constrictors, which form a continuous sheet of muscle, are activated sequentially as the inferior constrictor remains inhibited during most pharyngeal muscle activity (Fig. 2–1).

Pharyngeal Swallowing

Pharyngeal swallowing is divided into six phases:

1. When the bolus is in the oral cavity, the soft palate is opposed to the posterior portion of the tongue, closing the oropharynx.
2. Elevation of the soft palate and of the hyoid bone occurs while the whole pharynx is raised in a piston-like motion.
3. Active compression of the tongue on the bolus pushes it against and along the hard palate toward the entrance of the oropharynx. The soft palate elevates posteriorly and opposes the constrictor wall, closing the nasopharynx. When the bolus passes the limits of the oropharynx, involuntary deglutition occurs, and the descending wave of peristalsis begins.
4. The hyoid bone reaches maximal elevation, and the larynx elevates to approach the hyoid. At this point, the laryngeal vestibule closes, and the epiglottis tilts downward while pharyngeal peristalsis descends toward the hypopharynx.
5. With pharyngeal contraction, approximation of the pharyngeal wall, soft palate, and posterior tongue creates a closed chamber where the bolus is squeezed into the hypopharynx and through the open cricopharyngeal sphincter.
6. The pharyngeal airway reopens, and the soft palate, tongue, larynx, and hyoid bone return to their resting positions. The epiglottis springs back to a vertical position, and the laryngeal airway reopens when the pharyngoesophageal junction closes and resumes its elevated resting pressure.[16]

Sokol and associates studied simultaneous cineradiographic and manometric activity of the pharynx and hypopharynx in asymptomatic subjects using continuous perfusion techniques.[44] At rest, the resting pressures in the pharyngeal cavity are equal to atmospheric pressure.

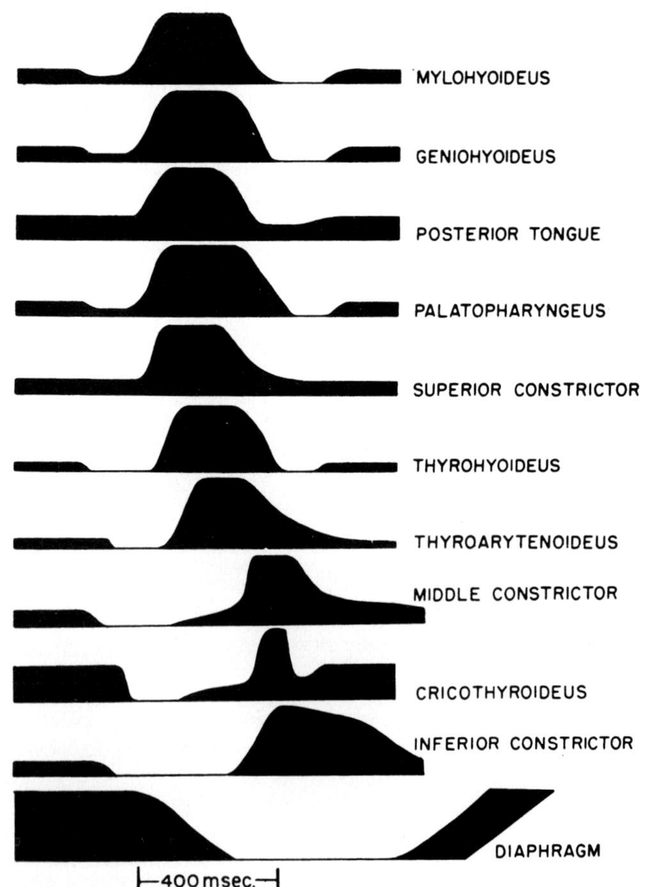

Figure 2–1. Segmental activation of the muscles forming the upper, middle, and lower pharyngeal constrictors. (From Doty, R.W., and Bosma, J.F.: Electromyographic activity of pharyngeal muscles during swallowing. J. Neurophysiol., *19*:44, 1956, with permission.)

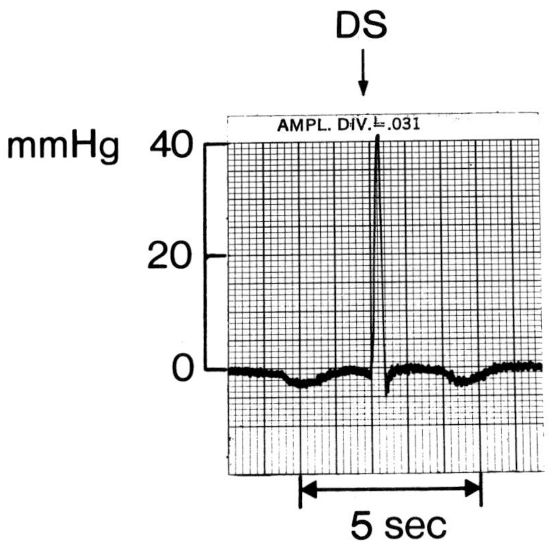

Figure 2–2. Pharyngeal contraction. A powerful single-peak contraction is produced with a duration of 0.4 second. This wave progresses at a speed of 9 to 25 cm/sec. (DS, dry swallow.)

In the hypopharynx, when the pharyngeal wall is collapsed and no air column exists, resting pressures increase progressively to a maximal pressure at the level of the cricopharyngeal muscle. On swallowing, pressure recordings show an initial double pressure peak corresponding to the elevation of the laryngopharynx and the simultaneous thrust of the tongue (E waves and I waves). Peak pharyngeal contraction follows these two initial waves; it is a peristaltic sequence starting radiologically as a stripping wave with closure of the velopharyngeal muscles, and it empties the pharyngeal content toward the hypopharynx. In the hypopharynx, the same small double peak is identified on swallowing and is attributed to the upward laryngeal movement, the tongue thrust, and the progression of trapped air or the advancing bolus.

Accurate recording of pharyngeal motor events is not possible using a water-filled or a water-perfused system. For these reasons, Dodds and associates studied human pharyngeal motor function in 12 recordings using an intraluminal strain gauge system.[14] They observed that the pressure was highest in the hypopharynx with pressure amplitudes on contraction averaging 200 mmHg. Peak contractions reached 600 mmHg in one subject. Contraction pressures averaged 100 mmHg in the oropharynx and 150 mmHg in the nasopharynx. The wave duration decreased progressively from nasopharynx to hypopharynx from 1.0 to 0.3 second, and the peristaltic wave speed ranged between 9 and 25 cm/sec (Fig. 2–2). Observations by Kahrilas and associates[30,31] and Castell and colleagues[5] confirm the difficulties in obtaining precise information on pharyngeal function.

Upper Esophageal Sphincter

Sokol and co-workers reported that between the end of the air column of the pharynx and the negative intrathoracic pressure there is a high-pressure zone 2.5 to 4.5 cm in length.[44] Within this zone is a shorter high-pressure zone 1 cm long of maximally elevated pressure that corresponds to the location of the cricopharyngeus muscle (Fig. 2–3). The cricopharyngeus is a muscle sling attached posteriorly to both laminae of the cricoid cartilage. It exerts its maximal pressure in an anteroposterior direction, closing the pharyngoesophageal junction and form-

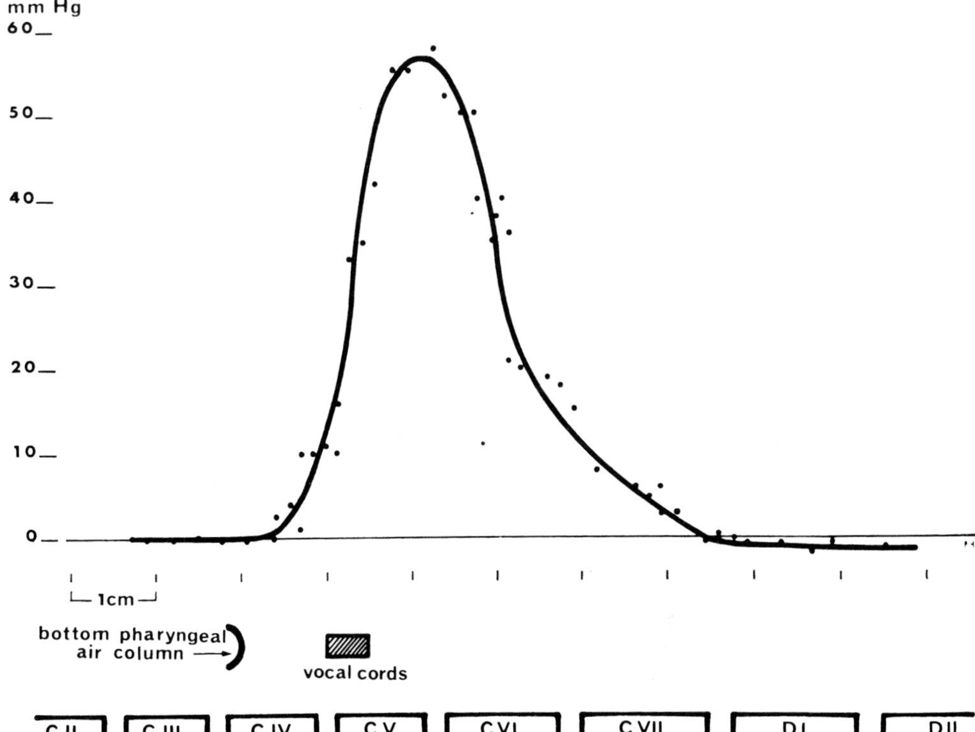

Figure 2–3. Relationship of the pharyngoesophageal high-pressure zone to the spine. (From Sokol, E.M., Hellmann, P., Wolf, B.S., et al.: Simultaneous cineradiographic and manometric study of the pharynx, hypopharynx and cervical esophagus. Gastroenterology, *51*:960, 1966, with permission.)

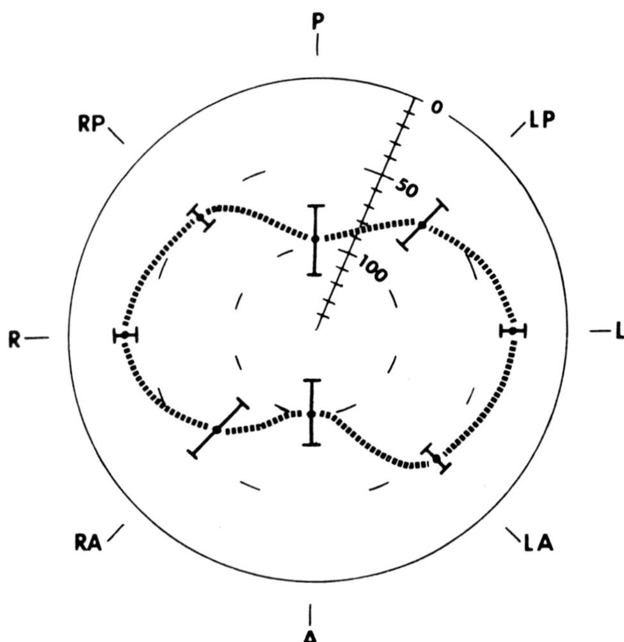

Figure 2–4. Asymmetry of the upper esophageal sphincter. (A, anterior; L, left; LA, left anterior; LP, left posterior; P, posterior; R, right; RA, right anterior; RP, right posterior.) (From Winans, C.S.: The pharyngoesophageal closure mechanism: A manometric study. Gastroenterology, *63*:768, 1972, with permission.)

ing a crescentic slit seen at rigid esophagoscopy as the upper limit of the esophagus.

Winans studied the pharyngoesophageal high-pressure zone of 18 human subjects.[48] He used a special eight-lumen recording catheter with recording orifices spaced around the circumference of the catheter. He observed significant pressure differences related to the position of the recording port, and this led to the concept of sphincter asymmetry. In the upper esophageal sphincter, the greatest pressures (averaging 100 mmHg) were recorded from the anterior and posterior orifices. Asoh and Goyal showed that the upper esophageal sphincter is a high-pressure zone created mainly by the cricopharyngeus and the inferior pharyngeal constrictor.[2] They observed that its asymmetry is not only radial but also axial (Fig. 2–4).

Control Mechanisms

The high-pressure zone of the upper esophageal sphincter is attributable to continuous active muscle contraction and to the elasticity of the surrounding structures. At rest, the cricopharyngeus is a striated muscle that receives its motor nerves from the vagal nuclei through the vagi and without synaptic interruption. The nerve endings come into direct contact with the motor end plates, and a continuous vagal discharge maintains the tonus of the sphincter at rest.[2,8]

On swallowing, a sequence of relaxations involving pharyngoesophageal muscle groups is caused by disappearance of the action potentials in the muscle fibers. The forward and upward displacement of the larynx is also involved in the opening mechanism of the sphincter. Although there is general agreement that the cricopharyngeus is the major component of the upper esophageal sphincter (UES), its wider pressure zone as observed by Sokol,[44] Winans,[48] and Welch[47] must be explained by other factors: the passive elastic forces may maintain a closed UES. If the nervous supply to the sphincter is removed, residual closing pressures remain.[2] The circular muscle of the pharyngoesophageal junction may also play a role.[51]

Pressure Profile

On swallowing, the UES high-pressure zone falls to resting atmospheric pressure and remains open to accommodate bolus transport through the sphincter area. This relaxation is brought about by cessation of vagal nerve stimulation and by a vertical upward displacement of the larynx, which pulls the upper sphincter for about 2 cm. Full sphincter relaxation is observed for 0.5 to 1.2 seconds, and with passage of the hypopharyngeal contraction, the sphincter closes with a contraction that creates a pressure that is often twice as high as the resting pressure in the sphincter (Figs. 2–5 and 2–6).

Recording problems exist with UES evaluation. A single side-hole catheter recording must take into account the sphincter asymmetry. The eight-lumen circumferential recording catheter does not follow the upward movement of the sphincter on swallowing. Rapid pull-through techniques record a higher anteroposterior basal tone.[20,47] A manometric recording device[15] was proposed by Dent[11] and adapted to the upper sphincter by Kahrilas[28]; it is a sleeve concept that is thought to record UES pressure behavior despite its movement during deglutition. However, evaluation of relaxation and coordination with pharyngeal contraction remain difficult. Castell and co-workers proposed positioning the recording sensor above the high-pressure zone of the sphincter for that purpose, allowing the opened sphincter, in its upward excursion, to be studied.[5,6]

Kahrilas and colleagues used this sleeve sensor to mon-

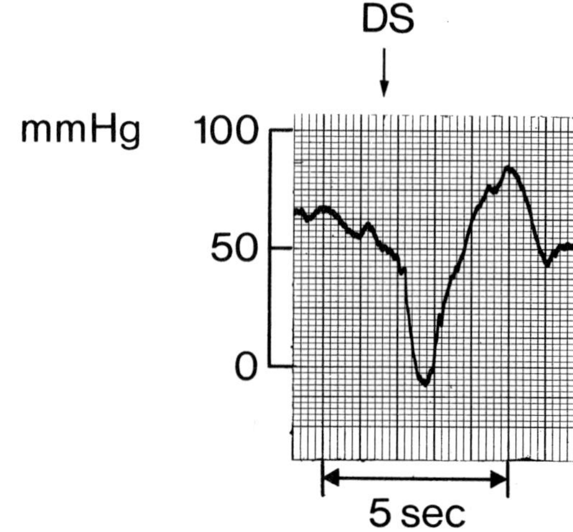

Figure 2–5. The high-pressure zone of the upper esophageal sphincter is caused by continuous active contraction of the cricopharyngeus muscle. (DS, dry swallow.)

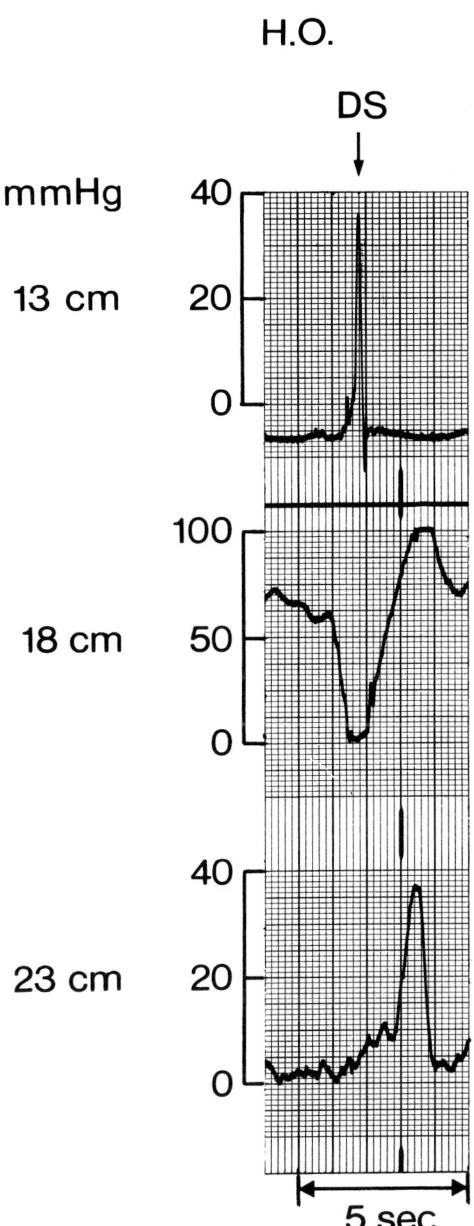

Figure 2–6. Pharynx, upper esophageal sphincter, and cervical esophagus in action. During the rapid single contraction of the pharynx (13 cm), the high-pressure zone of the upper esophageal sphincter (18 cm) falls to ambient pressure. Passage of the contraction in the hypopharynx closes the sphincter, and the wave continues into the cervical esophagus (23 cm). (DS, dry swallow.)

itor anterior and posterior pressures in the UES for prolonged periods of time.[29] Compared with conventional manometric recordings, the sleeve method showed lower UES pressures and less variability between subjects, thus suggesting that the sleeve method for recording creates less stimulation to the sphincter during recording. The sleeve recording of UES function also showed less susceptibility to axial movement. During these long-term recordings, the basal resting pressures of the UES showed a range of from 16 to 118 mmHg, with an overall mean of 42 mmHg. Pressures before a meal (45 mmHg) did not vary from pressures after a meal (43 mmHg). From these values, resting UES pressures fell to 20 mmHg during stage I sleep and decreased further to 8 mmHg during deep sleep. Arousal is associated with an abrupt increase in UES resting pressure. Similarly, sleep decreases the swallowing rate from a mean of 1.6/min during wakefulness to 0.24/min during stage I sleep and to 0.06/min during deep sleep. The use of a circumferential pressure-sensing transducer permits recording in a sitting position. It provides direct measure of the circumferential squeeze by the sphincter.[5]

Kahrilas and associates, when studying the belching mechanism, documented that the UES responded to esophageal body distention in two distinct ways: abrupt relaxation occurred when the esophagus was distended with air boluses, and a pressure increase was seen when fluid boluses were used to distend the esophagus.[27]

Gerhardt and co-workers showed that the UES responds to the stimulus of intraesophageal volume.[20] They also showed that it responds to an intraluminal acid stimulus to a degree greater than can be explained by its volume effect alone. UES pressure is not altered by changes in osmolality of the infused fluids during short-term infusion. UES pressure response to intraesophageal acid infusion is dose dependent: acid delivered at increasing rates into the esophagus evoked incremental increases in the UES resting pressure.

ESOPHAGEAL BODY

Innervation and Control Mechanisms

Function of the esophageal body is dependent on activity of the longitudinal and circular layers of muscle. These two muscle layers show a striated arrangement in the proximal esophagus and a smooth muscle organization in the distal two thirds of the organ. The striated part of the esophagus receives direct innervation from vagal nuclei nerves, which end in striated muscle cell motor units. The smooth muscle of the esophageal body is innervated by sympathetic and parasympathetic nerves that ramify in intramural plexuses, both myenteric and submucosal. Motor nerves for the smooth muscle portion are different from those for striated muscle, but coordination of the movements of the entire esophagus is centrally controlled.[8] Activation of the striated part of the muscle is by excitatory cholinergic nerves, which are central in origin. This activation is prevented by curare and succinylcholine.[9] The smooth muscle esophagus shows contractions that will act as homogeneous entities with its striated portion. Excitatory cholinergic nerves acting through muscarinic receptors are the only kind of motor nerves in the longitudinal muscle layer. In the circular layer, a single nerve excitation exists, but there is a different response of the muscle to stimuli: a brief contraction of the muscle follows the end of the period of nerve stimulation. The response of the circular muscle is thus organized so that direct stimulation of the muscle by dilatation is followed, above the point of distention, by an "on" response, a burst of action potentials in the muscle cells. Immediately after cessation of this stimula-

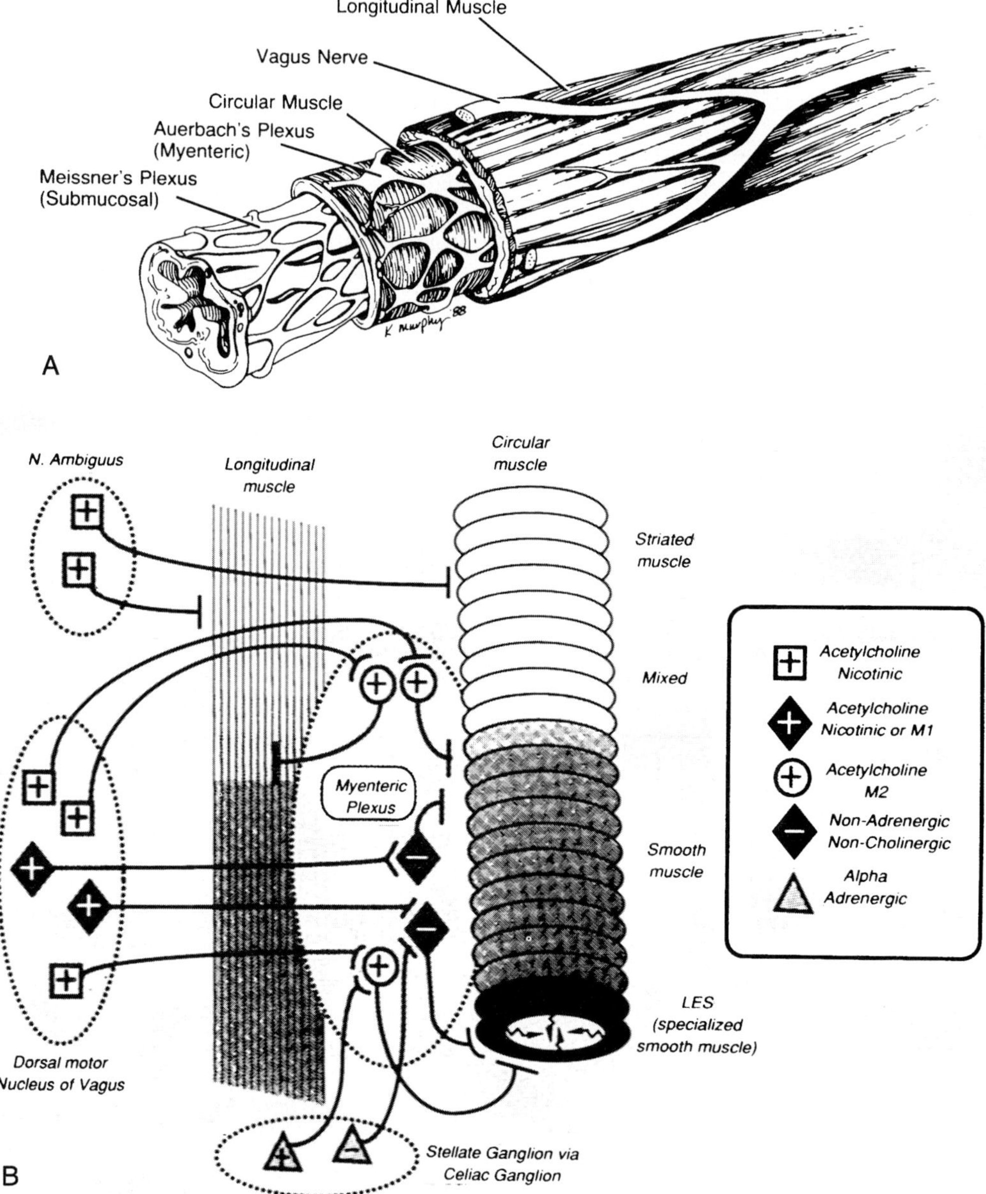

Figure 2–7. Control mechanisms of the esophageal body and lower esophageal sphincter. *A*, Intrinsic nervous plexuses of the esophagus. *B*, Intrinsic and extrinsic innervation of the esophagus. (LES, lower esophageal sphincter.) (From Castell, D.O.: The Esophagus. Boston, Little, Brown, 1992, with permission.)

tion, an "off" response appears, which is a burst of action potentials in the muscle cells below the point of stimulation and occurring over a long segment of esophagus with caudad propagation.[7] The "on" response is probably a direct response of the muscle to stretch, whereas the "off" response is a noncholinergic neural excitation. Sugarbaker and associates showed that on swallowing and on vagal stimulation, the longitudinal muscle contracts initially and for a longer duration, whereas the circular muscle is inhibited, showing hyperpolarization before its own contraction.[45] The integrating mechanisms for both layers that are the basis for normal esophageal contractions have not been clarified (Fig. 2–7).

Pressure Responses

Three types of pressure waves are seen in the esophageal body. Primary peristalsis is a well-organized propulsive wave triggered by voluntary deglutition. Secondary peristalsis refers to peristaltic waves that are not controlled by swallowing: they usually appear after esophageal dilatation either from a retained bolus or from active distention of the esophagus. Tertiary contractions are nonpropulsive and are observed after voluntary swallows or spontaneously between swallows (Fig. 2–8).

Primary peristalsis is triggered by swallowing and thereafter is not under voluntary control. A different response is observed when the swallow is dry than when a liquid bolus is given (wet swallow). Complete contraction responses are seen in only about two thirds of "dry" voluntary swallows.[13] Water boluses of 2 to 10 ml should produce complete peristaltic sequences in more than 96% of all swallows.[17]

With closure of the proximal esophageal sphincter, the esophageal contraction travels down the esophageal body at a speed of 2 to 5 cm/sec.[17,26,35,40] This velocity is slower in the proximal half and accelerates significantly in the distal half before slowing as it approaches the area immediately above the lower esophageal sphincter (LES). It contracts for a duration of 2 to 6 seconds and traverses the whole esophagus in 8 to 10 seconds (Fig. 2–9).

Pressure values obtained in the esophageal body after swallowing may be influenced by the recording method, the rate of swallowing, and the site of contraction in the esophageal body (Table 2–1).[24,37,43] In the proximal esophagus, immediately under the proximal sphincter, the pressure amplitude reaches a mean value of 53 mmHg. Peak contraction pressures are maximal in the lower third of the esophagus, with pressures reaching 69 mmHg[26] (Fig. 2–10). These authors also confirmed the presence of a pressure trough at the junction of the proximal and middle thirds, between 15 and 20 cm from the LES. The amplitude of the contractions at that level was significantly lower than that seen in the rest of the esophagus (see Fig. 2–2). This pressure trough is best explained by the variation in muscle response at the transition zone from striated muscle to smooth muscle. Hollis and Castell observed that in individuals older than 80 years, a marked decline in the amplitude of esophageal contractions occurred without an increase in abnormal spontaneous motility.[25] This decline is probably due to a weakening of the esophageal smooth muscle without an alteration in innervation. In a large population of healthy volunteers, longer double-peaked contractions are considered to be a variant of normal and are confined to the smooth muscle segment of the distal esophagus. Triple-peaked waves are not seen in healthy subjects.[39]

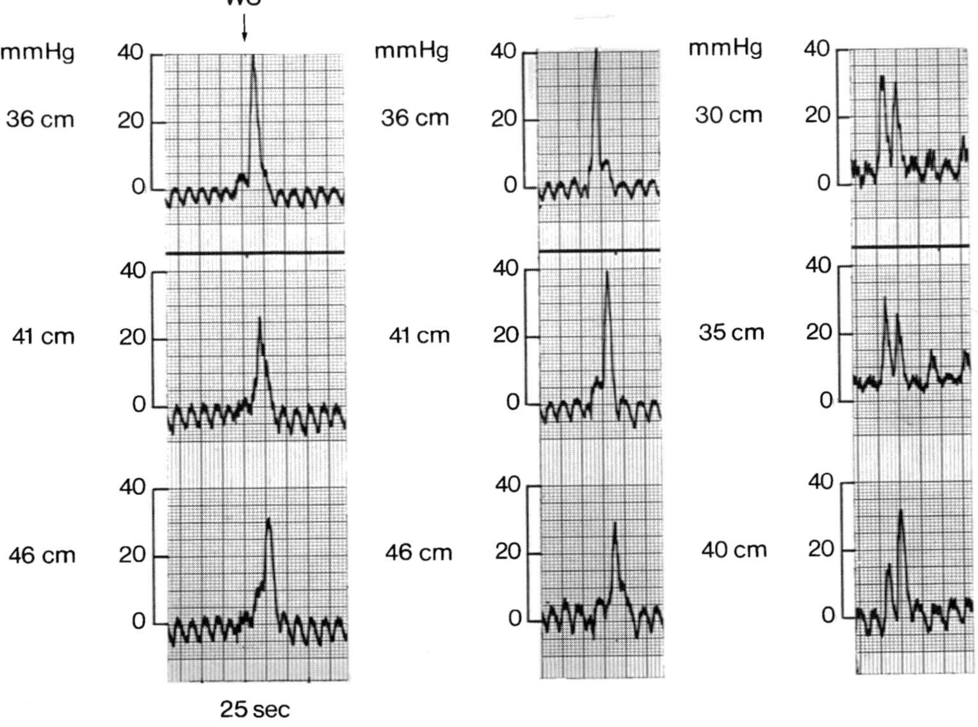

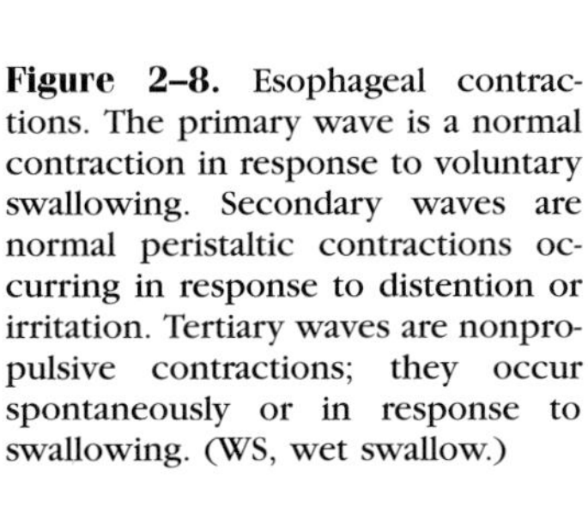
Figure 2–8. Esophageal contractions. The primary wave is a normal contraction in response to voluntary swallowing. Secondary waves are normal peristaltic contractions occurring in response to distention or irritation. Tertiary waves are nonpropulsive contractions; they occur spontaneously or in response to swallowing. (WS, wet swallow.)

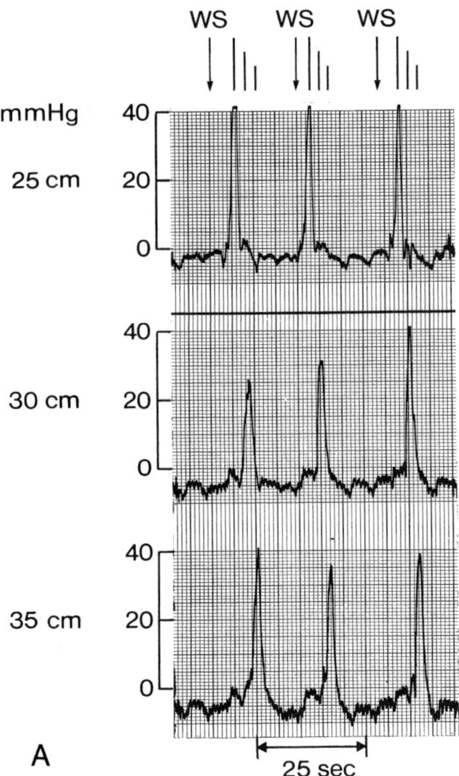

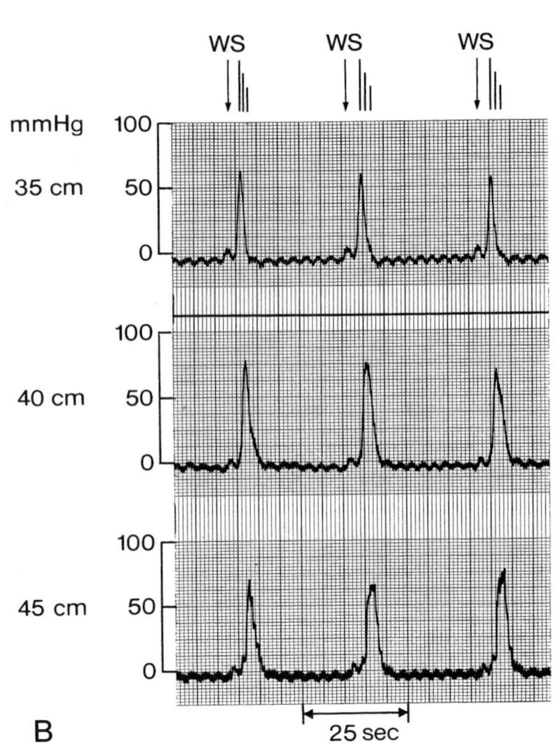

Figure 2–9. *A*, Normal peristalsis in response to swallowing in the proximal 10 cm of the esophagus. (WS, wet swallow.) *B*, The same primary wave in the distal 10 cm of the esophageal body shows a stronger and slightly longer contraction.

Secondary peristalsis refers to propulsive waves sweeping the esophagus in response to distention or irritation. No swallowing is recorded before these contractions. When an acid bolus is injected into the esophagus, a transient pressure rise of 20 to 60 mmHg is generally followed within 5 to 15 seconds by a secondary peristaltic sequence, which reduces the intraesophageal acid volume to a minimum[23] (Fig. 2–11). When acid is reduced to a small residual amount, neutralization occurs by active swallowing with saliva, restoring intraesophageal pH to normal. Secondary peristalsis is modulated by a peripheral and local neuromuscular mechanism. Rapid distention of the esophagus also evokes secondary peristalsis with a contraction starting above the area of distention and progressing with identical force and velocity as for primary contractions.

Tertiary contractions occur after voluntary deglutition or spontaneously between swallows (Figs. 2–12 and 2–13). Three to 4% of all swallows are followed by nonpropulsive contractions. Spontaneous tertiary activity on a motility tracing occurs with a frequency of 40 to 50 total contractions per hour (0.84/min). The peak pressure generated by these spontaneous contractions is 10 to 13 mmHg, and there seems to be a strong psychological influence on this type of activity.[17] Robin also suggested a relationship between abnormal contractions and the emotional state of the patient during recording.

LOWER ESOPHAGEAL SPHINCTER

It has been known since the beginning of the century that the esophagogastric junction is normally closed at

Table 2–1. Esophageal Pressures Generated With Swallowing

Investigators	Recording Method	Pressures in Esophageal Body (mmHg) Proximal	Middle	Distal
Nagler-Spiro (1961)	Water-filled, unperfused	—	20–90	—
Vantrappen-Hellemans (1967)	Water-filled, unperfused	28	35	37
Pope (1970)	Water-perfused	20–50	30–90	35–100
Duranceau (1983)	Water-perfused	48–59	—	55–74
Siet et al. (1974)	Microtransducers	51	—	74
Hollis-Castel (1972)	Microtransducers	—	—	58–219
Humphries-Castell (1977)	Microtransducers	35	53	69

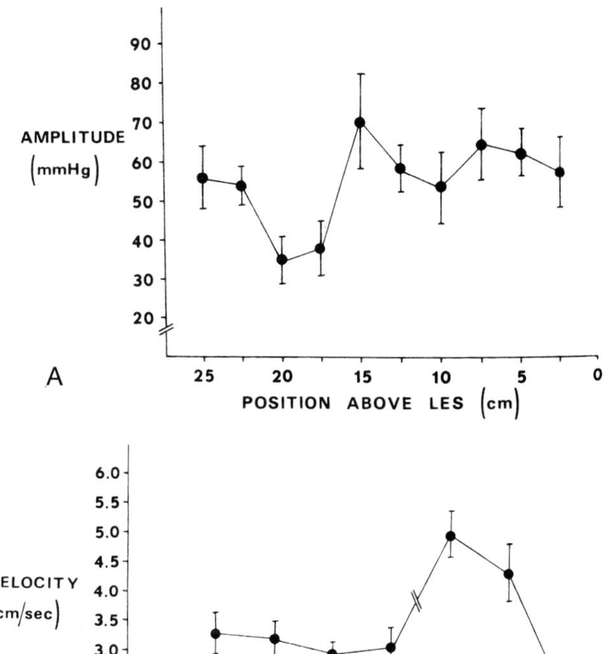

Figure 2–10. *A*, Pressure profile of esophageal peristalsis along the esophagus of normal humans as measured by direct intraesophageal transducers. (LES, lower esophageal sphincter.) *B*, Esophageal wave velocity in the human esophageal body. (From Humphries, T.J., and Castell, D.O.: Pressure profile of esophageal peristalsis in normal humans as measured by direct intraesophageal transducers. Digest. Dis., *22*:641, 1977, with permission.)

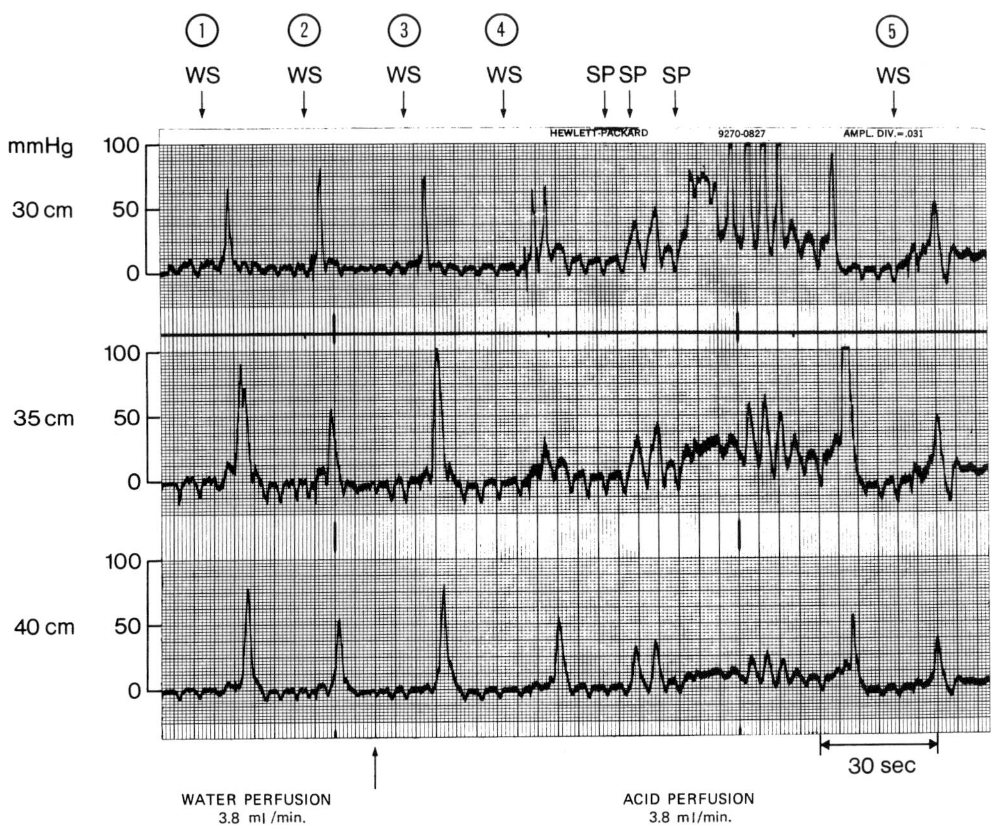

Figure 2–11. Primary peristalsis appears after voluntary deglutitions (wet swallow [WS] 1-3). When the esophagus is perfused with acid, spontaneous tertiary activity (SP) appears with a longer repetitive contraction that ends by a secondary contraction. A voluntary swallow under acid perfusion is followed by a tertiary wave response (WS 5).

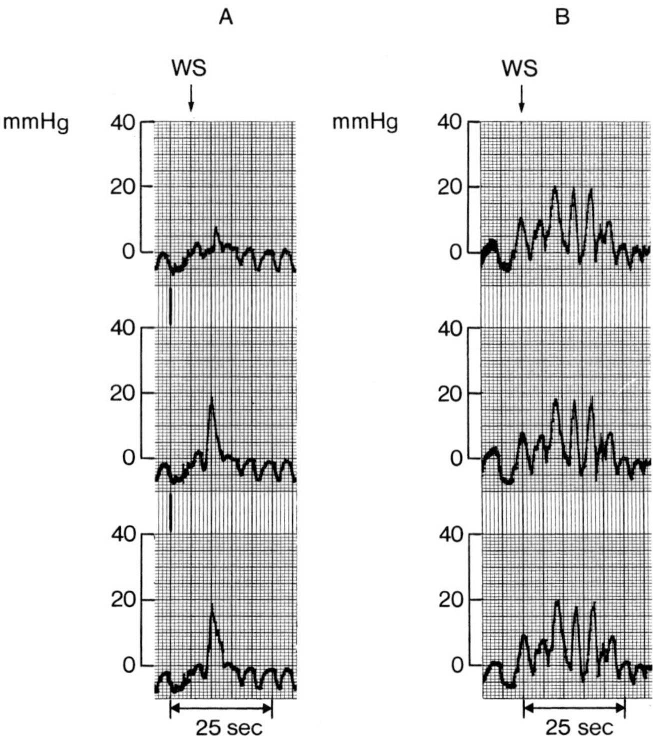

Figure 2–12. *A* and *B*, Tertiary contractions appear in response to deglutition. These contractions are abnormal. (WS, wet swallow.)

rest and relaxes with swallowing, belching, and vomiting. A physiologic sphincter that maintains a basal tone above that of the intragastric pressure, relaxes with swallowing, and contracts when the peristaltic wave passes through was clearly identified in the 1950s.[4,19,42] Improvement in manometric recording of esophageal pressures led to greater accuracy and comprehension of LES behavior.[36,50] The use of a sleeve catheter allows long-term recording of pressure events in the LES region.[11]

Control Mechanisms

The control mechanisms used for maintaining a basal sphincter tone are still unclear. Tonic contraction of the LES is demonstrated in small strips of muscle cut from the region of the sphincter, whereas similar strips cut a short distance above and below this region do not demonstrate this tonus.[9] This tonic contraction arises from the circular muscle layer at this level, possibly from special intrinsic properties of the muscle itself with associated neurohormonal control. Muscle of the junction contracts with excitation of cholinergic receptors but is inhibited by beta-adrenergic receptors. Relaxation of the sphincter muscle is also confined to this specialized area when it is stimulated deliberately. The same stimulation in adjacent regions causes contraction. It is possible that relaxation is activated by the swallowing center in the vagal nuclei with local mechanoreceptors acting to modulate it.

Pressure Profile

The pressure profile of the LES shows considerable radial asymmetry. The highest pressures are recorded in a left posterior orientation[49] (Fig. 2–14*B*). On swallowing, the sphincter relaxes to allow passage of luminal contents being propelled toward the stomach by peristaltic activity (Fig. 2–14*A*). This relaxation is seen in more than 98% of all swallows, and the LES remains open for 6 to 9 seconds.[17] LES relaxation is also present when esophageal body distention is produced or when gastric fundus distention occurs. Transient LES relaxation lasting for 5 to 30 seconds was observed by Dent.[11,12] This relaxation may be an important factor in permitting both physiologic and pathologic reflux.[15] Gastric distention leading to nonadrenergic, noncholinergic inhibition of LES tone is a possible mechanism that explains these transient relaxations.

The level of basal tone recorded in the LES is variable and is influenced by catheter orientation within the sphincter, esophageal movement with respiration and swallowing, the method of recording, the time elapsed since the last meal, and the recording equipment being used.[34] The LES is also affected by a large number of neurohumoral and pharmacologic agents (Table 2–2). The normal resting pressure of the LES varies from 13 to 26 mmHg.[22] Richter reported mean LES pressures of 29 mmHg when a rapid pull-through method was used.[38] In the same group of normal volunteers, the LES showed a mean resting pressure of 24 mmHg when studied by a standard pull-through technique. The pressure gradient between the negative intrathoracic pressure and the posi-

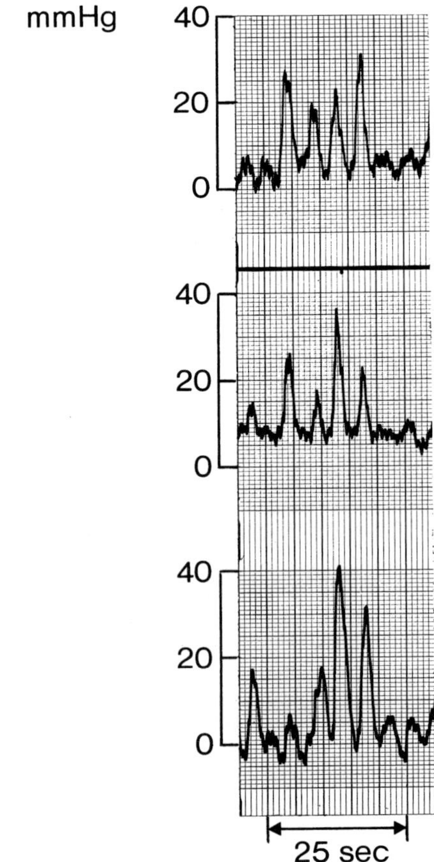

Figure 2–13. Spontaneous tertiary activity. These contractions may represent abnormal activity. They also may be strongly influenced by psychological factors.

tive intragastric pressure represents the pressure values that oppose the reflux of gastric contents toward the esophagus. This pressure barrier provided by the sphincter is seen as correlating linearly with the propensity toward reflux.[1] Haddad also observed a significant correlation of LES pressure with reflux.[21] Other reports do not agree with such a correlation.[3,33] Moreover, a protective reflex against reflux has been proposed after observing that an increase in intra-abdominal pressure led to an increase in LES pressure regardless of the position of the sphincter.[10,32]

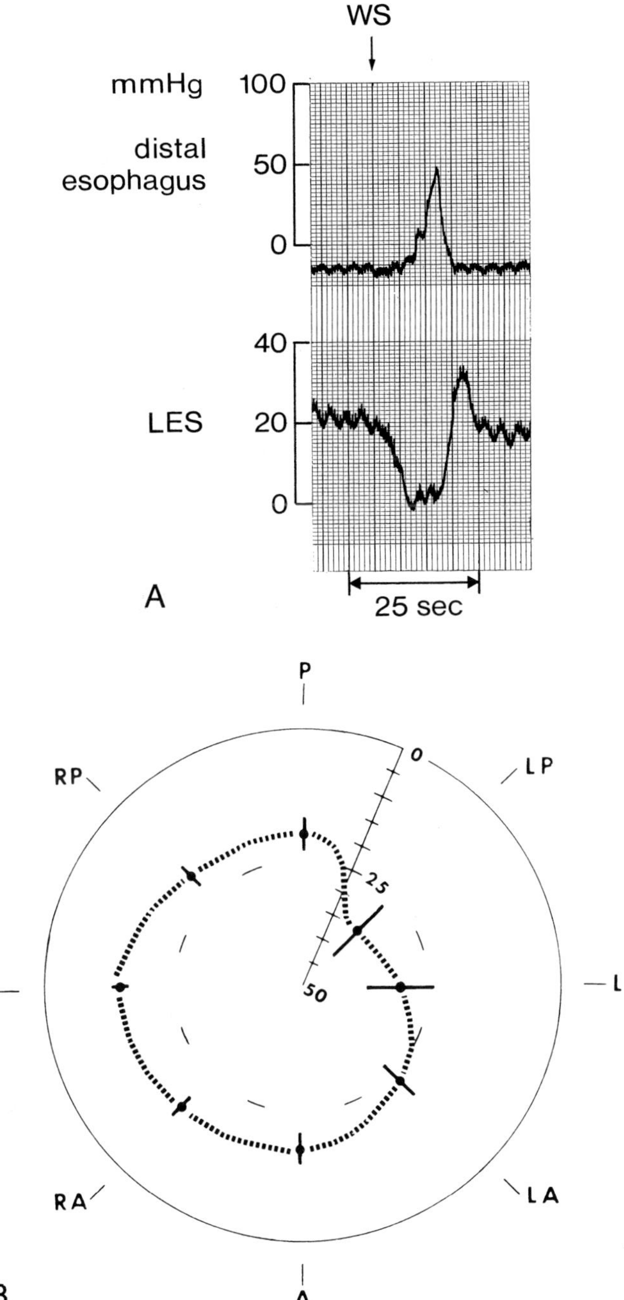

Figure 2–14. *A*, Normal lower esophageal sphincter (LES) upon swallowing. (WS, wet swallow.) The resting pressure falls to the level of intragastric pressure. The relaxation period is coordinated with the contraction in the distal esophagus. The passage of the peristaltic wave through the sphincter area closes the esophagogastric junction after the bolus is in the stomach. The sphincter then returns to its normal resting pressure. *B*, Radial configuration of the lower esophageal sphincter. (A, anterior; L, left; LA, left anterior; LP, left posterior; P, posterior; R, right; RA, right anterior; RP, right posterior.) (From Winans, C.S.: Manometric asymmetry of the lower esophageal high pressure zone. Digest Dis., *22*:348, 1977, with permission.)

Table 2–2. Influences on Lower Esophageal Sphincter Pressure

Factors Decreasing LES Pressure	Factors Increasing LES Pressure
Ingestants	
Alcohol	Antacids
Fatty foods	Protein meal
Chocolate	
Peppermint	
Coffee, tea	
Drugs	
Anticholinergic agents	Cholinergic agents (e.g., bethanechol)
Diazepam	Domperidone
Morphine	Guaiacol
Adrenergic blockers	
Calcium-blocking agents	
Hormones	
Progesterone	Gastrin
Secretin	
Cholecystokinin (CCK)	
Glucagon	
Miscellaneous	
Increased H^+	Increased intragastric pressure
Fundic gas distention	
Smoking	

After relaxation, the lower sphincter contracts with the passage of peristalsis. This contraction is long lasting and of low amplitude when it occurs above the pressure inversion point. Below this point, relaxation is simply followed by restoration of the resting tone.

References

1. Ahtaridis, G., Snape, W.J., and Cohen, S.: Lower esophageal sphincter pressure as an index of gastroesophageal acid reflux. Dig. Dis. Sci., *26*:993, 1981.
2. Asoh, R., and Goyal, R.K.: Manometry and electromyography of the upper esophageal sphincter in the uposum. Gastroenterology, *74*:514, 1978.
3. Bennett, J.R., and Stancin, C.: Correlation between a physiological test of gastroesophageal reflux and sphincter squeeze. Rendicond. Gastroenterol., *5*:132, 1973.
4. Botin, J.W., Olsen, A.M., Muersch, H.J., et al.: A study of esophageal pressure in normal persons and patients with cardiospasm. Gastroenterology, *23*:278, 1953.
5. Castell, J.A., Dalton, C.B., and Castell, D.O.: Pharyngeal and upper esophageal sphincter manometry in humans. Am. J. Physiol., *21*:G173, 1990.
6. Castell, J.A., and Dalton, C.B.: Esophageal manometry. *In* Castell, D.O. (ed.): The Esophagus. Boston, Little, Brown, 1992, p. 143.
7. Christensen, J.: Patterns and origin of some esophageal responses to stretch and electrical stimulation. Gastroenterology, *59*:909, 1970.
8. Christensen, J.: The controls of oesophageal movement. Clin. Gastroenterol., *5*:15, 1976.

9. Christensen, J.: The innervation and motility of the oesophagus. Front. Gastrointest. Res., *3:*18, 1978.
10. Cohen, S., and Harris, L.D.: Lower esophageal pressure as an index of lower esophageal sphincter strength. Gastroenterology, *58:*157, 1970.
11. Dent, J.A.: A new technique for continuous sphincter pressure measurement. Gastroenterology, *71:*2637, 1976.
12. Dent, J., Dodds, W.J., Friedman, R., et al.: Mechanisms of gastroesophageal reflux in recumbent asymptomatic human subjects. J. Clin. Invest., *65:*256, 1980.
13. Dodds, W.J., Hogan, W.E.J., Reid, D.P., et al.: A comparison between primary esophageal peristalsis following wet swallows. J. Appl. Physiol., *35:*851, 1973.
14. Dodds, W.J., Hogan, W.J., Lyndon, S.B., et al.: Quantification of pharyngeal motor function in normal human subjects. J. Appl. Physiol., *39:*692, 1975.
15. Dodds, W.J., Dent, J., Hogan, W.J., et al.: Mechanism of gastroesophageal reflux in patients with reflux esophagitis. N. Engl. J. Med., *307:*154, 1982.
16. Donner, M.W., Bosma, J.F., and Robertson, D.L.: Anatomy and physiology of the pharynx. Gastrointest. Radiol., *10:*196, 1985.
17. Duranceau, A.C., Devroede, G., Lafontaine, E., et al.: Esophageal motility in asymptomatic volunteers. Surg. Clin. North Am., *63:*777, 1983.
18. Ergun, G.A., Kahrilas, P.J., and Logemann, J.A.: Interpretation of pharyngeal manometric recordings: Limitations and variability. Dis. Esophagus, *6:*11, 1993.
19. Fyke, F.E., Code, C.F., and Schlegel, F.J.: The gastroesophageal sphincter in healthy human beings. Gastroenterologia, *86:*135, 1956.
20. Gerhardt, D.C.: Human upper esophageal sphincter: Response to volume, usmotic and acid stimuli. Gastroenterology, *75:*268, 1978.
21. Haddad, J.R.: Relaxation in gastroesophageal reflux to yield sphincter pressures. Gastroenterology, *58:*175, 1970.
22. Hellemans, J., and Vantrappen, G.: Manometric measurements of the resting pressure in the lower esophageal sphincter. *In* Hellemans, J., and Vantrappen, G. (eds.): Diseases of the Esophagus. New York, Springer-Verlag, 1974, p. 48.
23. Helm, F.H., Dodds, W.J., Pelc, L.R., et al.: Effect of esophageal emptying and saliva on clearance of acid from the esophagus. N. Engl. J. Med., *310:*284, 1984.
24. Hollis, J.B., and Castell, D.O.: Amplitude of esophageal peristalsis as determined by rapid infusion. Gastroenterology, *63:*417, 1972.
25. Hollis, J.B., and Castell, D.O.: Esophageal function in elderly men: A new look at "presbyesophagus." Ann. Intern. Med., *80:*371, 1974.
26. Humphries, I.J., and Castell, D.O.: Pressure profile of esophageal peristalsis in normal humans as measured by direct intraoesophageal transducers. Dig. Dis., *22:*641, 1977.
27. Kahrilas, P.J., Dodds, W.J., Dent, J., et al.: Upper esophageal sphincter function during belching. Gastroenterology, *91:*133, 1986.
28. Kahrilas, P.J., Dent, J., Dodds, W.J., et al.: A method for continuous monitoring of upper esophageal sphincter pressure. Dig. Dis. Sci., *32:*121, 1987.
29. Kahrilas, P.J., Dodds, W.J., Dent, J., et al.: Effect of sleep, spontaneous gastroesophageal reflux, and a meal on upper esophageal sphincter pressure in normal human volunteers. Gastroenterology, *92:*466, 1987.
30. Kahrilas, P.J., Dodds, W.J., and Dent, J., et al.: Upper esophageal sphincter function during deglutition. Gastroenterology, *95:*52, 1988.
31. Kahrilas, P.J., Logemann, J.A., Lin, S., and Ergun, G.A.: Pharyngeal clearance swallow: A combined manometric and video fluoroscopic study. Gastroenterology, *103:*128, 1992.
32. Lind, J.F., Warrian, W.G., and Wankling, W.J.: Responses of the gastroesophageal junctional zone to increases in abdominal pressure. Can. J. Surg., *9:*32, 1966.
33. MacLaurin, C.: The intrinsic sphincter in the prevention of gastroesophageal reflux. Lancet, *2:*801, 1963.
34. Meyer, G.W., and Castell, D.O.: In support of the clinical usefulness of lower esophageal sphincter pressure determination. Dig. Dis. Sci., *26:*1028, 1981.
35. Nagler, R., and Spiro, H.M.: Serial esophageal motility studies in asymptomatic young subjects. Gastroenterology, *41:*371, 1961.
36. Pope, C.E.: A dynamic test of sphincter strength: Its application to the lower esophageal sphincter. Gastroenterology, *52:*779, 1967.
37. Pope, C.E.: Effect of infusion on force of closure measurements in the human esophagus. Gastroenterology, *58:*616, 1970.
38. Richter, J.E.: Normal values for esophageal manometry. Chap. 6. *In* Castell, D.U., Richter, J.E., and Bohg Dalton, U. (eds.): Esophageal Motility Testing. New York, Elsevier Science Publishing, 1987, pp. 79–90.
39. Richter, J.E., Chi-Li Wu, W., and Castell, D.O.: Double-peaked contraction waves in a variant of normal. Gastroenterology, *89:*479, 1985.
40. Richter, J.E.. Chi-Li Wu, W., Johns, D.N., et al.: Esophageal manometry in 95 healthy adult volunteers. Dig. Dis. Sci., *32:*583, 1987.
41. Robin, J., Nagler, R., Spiro, H., et al.: Measuring the effect of emotions on esophageal motility. Psychosom. Med., *24:*170, 1962.
42. Sanchez, G.C., Draer, P., and Ingelfinger, P.J.: Motor mechanisms of the esophagus, particularly of its distal portion. Gastroenterology, *25:*321, 1953.
43. Siet, J.J., Dodds, W.J., Hogan, W.J., et al.: Intraluminal esophageal manometry: An analysis of variables affecting recording fidelity of peristaltic pressure. Gastroenterology, *67:*221, 1974.
44. Sokol, E.M., Hellmann, P., Wolf, B.S., et al.: Simultaneous cineradiographic and manometric study of the pharynx, hypopharynx and cervical esophagus. Gastroenterology, *51:*960, 1966.
45. Sugarbaker, D.J., Ratian, S., and Goyal, R.K.: Mechanical and electrical activity of esophageal smooth muscle during peristalsis. Am. J. Physiol., *246:*G145, 1984.
46. Vantrappen, G., and Hellemans, J.: Studies on the normal deglutition complex. Am. J. Dig. Dis., *12:*255, 1967.
47. Welch, R.W., Lockmann, K., Ricks, P.M., et al.: Manometry of the normal upper esophageal sphincter and its alterations in laryngectomy. J. Clin. Invest., *63:*1036, 1979.
48. Winans, C.S.: The pharyngoesophageal closure mechanism: A manometric study. Gastroenterology, *63:*768, 1972.
49. Winans, C.S.: Manometric asymmetry of the lower esophageal high pressure zone. Am. J. Dig. Dis., *22:*348, 1977.
50. Winans, C.S., and Harris, L.D.: Quantification of lower esophageal sphincter competence. Gastroenterology, *52:*773, 1967.
51. Zaino, C., Jacobson, H.G., Lepow, H., et al.: The Pharyngo-Esophageal Sphincter. Springfield, IL, Charles C Thomas, 1970.

CHAPTER

3 Congenital Abnormalities of the Esophagus

CARROLL M. HARMON • ARNOLD G. CORAN

The major congenital anomalies of the esophagus are esophageal atresia (EA) and tracheoesophageal fistula (TEF). This chapter focuses mainly on these two anomalies and includes a brief description of the other congenital anomalies occasionally encountered: laryngotracheoesophageal cleft (LTEC), congenital stenosis of the esophagus (CES), esophageal duplication, and congenital vascular obstruction of the esophagus. A short description of esophageal replacement in children is also given.

ESOPHAGEAL ATRESIA AND TRACHEOESOPHAGEAL FISTULA

History

The common form of EA, EA with distal TEF, was first described in 1697 by Thomas Gibson.[1] William Durston had previously reported in 1670 the first description of congenital EA.[2] Management by nonsurgical means resulted in 100% mortality rates during the next 250 years.

A surgical approach to this entity awaited the development of thoracic surgery as a specific discipline in the 1920s. In 1929, Vogt[3] described the various types of esophageal malformations, which provided a basis for the subsequent clinical classifications of the anomaly. In 1936, Lanman[4] first attempted a primary repair of EA-TEF, and in 1940 he reported the Boston Children's Hospital experience with 30 infants who were treated surgically, of whom all died. The first survivors with the anomalies were patients who were admitted on successive days in late 1939, reported independently by William Ladd[5] of Boston and Logan Leven[6] of Minneapolis. Both patients were managed using a staged approach with initial gastrostomy, secondary fistula ligation or division with cervical esophagostomy, and the creation of an antethoracic skin tube conduit from the esophagostomy to the gastrostomy.

The first reported patient with EA at the University of Michigan was seen in 1935 and was managed unsuccessfully with gastrostomy alone. In 1939, Cameron Haight first attempted a primary repair.[7] After four failed attempts to achieve survival with primary repair, there was little enthusiasm when the next patient with this disorder was transferred to the University of Michigan Hospital in early 1941. The infant was an "unusually robust" 12-day-old child weighing 8 lb 4 oz on admission. The first successful primary repair of EA with TEF was accomplished in this patient using a left extrapleural approach and a single-layer anastomosis. Postoperatively, the patient developed an anastomotic leak, which was managed nonoperatively. She later developed a stricture at the anastomosis, which responded to a single dilatation.

In 1943, Haight revised his procedure to a right extrapleural approach because he thought that better exposure of the distal segment was obtained from this side. Between 1939 and 1969, Haight cared for more than 280 infants with EA and reported a 52% survival rate.[8] Many of Haight's initial teachings continue to guide the current management of the infant with congenital atresia of the esophagus.

Embryology

The pathogenesis of EA and associated TEFs is uncertain, in large part because the details of normal esophageal and tracheal embryology are still undetermined. Wilhelm His, Sr., the founder of the study of human embryology, was the first to describe the development of the respiratory system.[9] He believed that the division of the foregut was the result of the fusion of invaginating lateral longitudinal ridges, which would create a septum that divides the foregut into a dorsal digestive tract and a ventral respiratory system. Most modern theories of the division of the foregut, as well as the theories of pathogenesis of the anomalies of the esophagus, have been based on this description.[10-14] However, more recent reports suggest that the ingrowth of lateral foregut wall ridges does not occur in the human embryo; therefore, different theories have been put forth to describe the pathogenesis of esophagotracheal anomalies.

In scanning electron microscopy studies of chick embryo morphology, Kluth et al.[15] found that the esophagus and trachea normally develop and separate as a result of cranial, ventral, and dorsal folds that arise in the foregut. The descending paired cranial folds represent the primitive larynx. The caudal ascending ventral fold, which appeared to correspond to the tracheoesophageal septum in earlier reports, separates the trachea from the esophagus. The dorsal pharyngoesophageal fold demarcates the primitive pharynx from the esophagus. EA with distal fistula is proposed to result from excessive ventral invagination of the pharyngoesophageal fold, creating an upper esophageal pouch and preventing the cranial folds from descending to meet the ventral fold, thus maintaining a connection between esophagus and trachea. Kluth et al. proposed that isolated atresia may be explained by developmental disorders of the esophageal circulation as seen with intestinal atresia.

O'Rahilly and Muller[16] proposed an alternate hypothesis for the normal and abnormal development of the respiratory and esophageal tracts based on the examination of more than 100 human embryos in the Carnegie Collection. The yolk sac, from which most of the digestive tract develops, is noted between 9 and 13 postovulatory days, and by day 20, most embryos possess a foregut.[16] By day 22, a longitudinal median pharyngeal groove develops in the ventral aspect of the foregut, and by day 26, the lung bud forms from this sulcus. On day 28, the lung bud is clearly separated from the digestive tract, quickly becomes paired, and descends caudally into the mesenchyme ventral to the foregut. The part of this mesenchyme that comes to lie between the respiratory and digestive tubes constitutes the tracheoesophageal septum, which is believed to be necessary for the normal separation of the two tubes.[16] According to O'Rahilly and Muller, there is no cephalad extension of this separation point as postulated by many authors, but instead the most cranial limit of this septum remains fixed as the trachea and its bifurcation descend in a caudal and dorsal direction. Because the tracheoesophageal separation point is rostral at approximately the C2 level and because most TEFs occur at or near the tracheal bifurcation, this theory argues against the notion that a failure of the division of a common channel into respiratory and digestive tubes is the origin of TEF. Rather, it should be considered that a fistula is created by an abnormal epithelium-lined connection that develops between the two originally separate tubes. The most probable timing of this event would be at approximately 33 days, when the region of the tracheal bifurcation achieves its closest relationship to the esophagus. These observations might account for isolated TEF without EA but do not account for EA, either alone or in combination with TEF. O'Rahilly and Muller support the theory of Politzer,[17] which suggests that isolated EA occurs because the considerable growth of the esophageal mesenchymal coat outpaces the cellular division in its epithelial lining, resulting in the epithelium becoming stretched and then interrupted.

Recently, Diez-Pardo et al.[18] reported on a potentially important animal model for EA-TEF and VACTERL (***V***ertebral, ***A***norectal, ***C***ardiac, ***T***racheoesophageal, ***R***enal, and radial ***L***imb anomalies) association that involves the use of the glycosidic anthracyclin antibiotic Adriamycin (doxorubicin) as a teratogen in 8- to 9-day-old rat fetuses. Many investigators have subsequently used this model to study the pathogenesis of EA and TEF. Using embryonic microdissection techniques, Crisera et al.[19] suggested that in this animal model, the TEF is formed as a middle branch of a tracheal trifurcation with distal fistulization into the stomach, suggesting that the primary defect lies at the level of the respiratory tract and not the gastrointestinal tract.

Candidate genes responsible for EA may belong to the HOX D group, which is involved in pattern formation of the limbs and foregut and may be linked to the VACTERL association.[20] Insight into the cellular, biochemical, and genetic signals responsible for normal cell–cell and cell-matrix interactions, migration, and subsequent organogenesis is required to more clearly understand the pathogenesis of esophagotracheal and associated anomalies.

Epidemiology

The reported incidence of EA varies widely from 1:2,440 in Finland[21] to 1:4,500 in the United States[22] and Australia.[23] Harris et al.[24] summarized data from three large congenital malformation databases, described the epidemiology of intestinal atresia, and reported a significantly lower rate of EA among nonwhite populations (0.55 per 10,000 births) compared with the white population (1.0 per 10,000 births) in California. Overall, the average rate of EA is 2.4 per 10,000 births.

Population studies have reported a slight, but statistically significant, increased preponderance for EA in males, in nonwhites, and in firstborn infants and an association with increasing maternal age.[24] The rate of twinning among infants with EA is high and occurs in approximately 6% of cases compared with 1% in the general population.[24] Chromosomal anomalies are also relatively frequent, occurring in 6.6% of infants with EA, and include trisomy 13 and 18 in addition to the well-described VACTERL association.[24]

Environmental teratogens have been implicated in the pathogenesis EA as well, with EA noted in infants born to mothers with prolonged exposure to contraceptive pills,[25] thalidomide,[26] and methimazole.[27]

EA is most commonly a sporadic occurrence and appears to be heterogeneous with respect to cause. It is occasionally present in individuals with the DiGeorge sequence, polysplenia sequence, Holt-Oram syndrome, and the Pierre-Robin sequence.[28] There are a number of studies that have described transverse and vertical familial cases of all varieties of EA.[28-34] For the counseling of families, based on the literature to date there is a 0.5 to 2% empiric risk of recurrence for parents of a single affected child, rising to 20% if more than one sibling is affected.[28] The empiric risk of an affected child born to an affected parent is 3 to 4%.[28] The evidence to date suggests both nongenetic maldevelopment and genetic causes.

Associated Anomalies

Other congenital anomalies are often (50 to 70%) associated with EA, and it is often that the associated anomaly significantly alters treatment and affects survival (Table 3-1).[35] The anomalies are most common in cases of EA without TEF and least common in cases of H-type fistula.[36] Cardiovascular anomalies occur most frequently (11 to 49%), followed by genitourinary (20 to 25%),[37,38] gastrointestinal (10 to 24%),[38,39] and skeletal (13 to 55%) anomalies.[40,41] Associated neurologic anomalies include neural tube defects (2.3%), hydrocephalus (5.2%), holoprosencephaly (2.3%), and anophthalmia or microphthalmia (3.7%).[24] Other anomalies include choanal atresia (5.2%), facial cleft (7.2%), abdominal wall defects (4.3%), and diaphragmatic hernia (2.9%).[24]

Table 3–1. Incidence of Associated Anomalies

Anomaly	Incidence (%)
Cardiovascular	35
Genitourinary	20
Gastrointestinal	24
Neurologic	10
Skeletal	13
VACTERL association	25
Overall	50 to 70

Table 3–2. Incidence of Anomalies

Type	Incidence (%)	Gross Type
1. Esophageal atresia with distal tracheoesophageal fistula	85.8	C
2. Esophageal atresia without tracheoesophageal fistula	7.8	A
3. Tracheoesophageal fistula without esophageal atresia	4.2	E
4. Esophageal atresia with fistula to both pouches	1.4	D
5. Esophageal atresia with proximal tracheoesophageal fistula	0.8	B

Significant gastrointestinal anomalies include anorectal atresia (9%), duodenal atresia (5%), ileal atresia, malrotation (4%), and annular pancreas and pyloric stenosis.[42] Genitourinary defects are varied and include hypospadias, undescended testes, renal agenesis or hypoplasia, cystic renal disease, hydronephrosis, vesicoureteral reflux, uterine duplication, pelviureteral and vesicoureteral obstruction, urachal anomalies, ambiguous genitalia, and cloacal or bladder extrophy.[24,37,43]

Most of the deaths associated with EA are related to complex cardiac anomalies. The risk of death for an infant with an EA associated with a major cardiac anomaly is reported to be 30%.[44] The most common single anomaly is a ventricular septal defect, which has a 16% associated mortality rate. Other common cardiac anomalies include tetralogy of Fallot, patent ductus arteriosus, and atrial septal defects. Coarctation of the aorta is found in 1 to 5% of infants with EA, TEF or both.[45]

In 1973, a broad spectrum of associated malformations were described that appear together and are associated with EA.[46] The association was referred to by the acronym VATER (***V***ertebral defects, ***A***nal atresia, ***T***racheoesophageal fistula, ***E***sophageal atresia, and ***R***enal defects). As the phenotype expanded, the acronym was changed to **VACTERL** association.[47] The high incidence of urinary tract anomalies that should be considered in the renal category includes megalourethra, urethral duplication, urethra valves, stricture, and hypospadias. Infants who have EA with the VACTERL association have a high mortality rate (25%), with cardiovascular anomalies being the principal cause of death.[48]

EA is also found in conjunction with the **CHARGE** association (***C***oloboma, ***H***eart defects, ***A***tresia choanae, developmental ***R***etardation, ***G***enital hypoplasia, and ***E***ar deformities [deafness]).[49] Although infrequent, EA has also been reported in the **Schisis** association (omphalocele, neural tube defects, cleft lip and palate, and genitalia hypoplasia),[50] trisomy 18, cerebral hypoplasia, and Potter's syndrome (bilateral renal agenesis).[51,52]

In addition to a TEF, there are other pulmonary and tracheobronchial anomalies associated with EA, including pulmonary agenesis, ectopic or absent right upper lobe bronchus, congenital bronchial stenosis, and a decreased ratio of circumferential cartilaginous trachea to membranous trachea.[53] Other syndromes that have been reported in association with EA are Down's syndrome, Fanconi constitutional anemia, Townes-Brock syndrome, Bartsocas-Papas syndrome, and McKusick-Kaufman syndrome.[28,54–58]

Classification

On the basis of a summary of more than 2,200 cases of various esophageal anomalies from six large series, the incidence of the various types of anomalies is given in Table 3–2.[52,59–63]

Numerous classification schemes have been proposed and used in describing EA; however, the most useful and practical classification may be simple anatomic descriptions as listed earlier. A large number of institutions still use the Gross classification (Fig. 3–1).

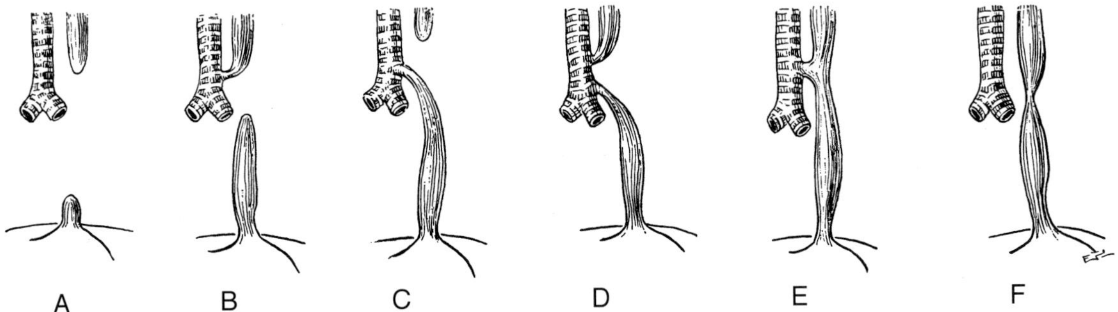

Figure 3–1. Gross classification. Anatomic patterns of esophageal atresia. *A*, Esophageal atresia without tracheoesophageal fistula. This malformation is almost invariably associated with a "long gap." *B*, Atresia with proximal tracheoesophageal fistula. It is an uncommon anomaly: the abdomen is airless, and the diagnosis may be missed unless contrast studies are used. *C*, Esophageal atresia with distal tracheoesophageal fistula; this is the most frequently encountered form of esophageal anomaly. *D*, Atresia with double (proximal and distal) fistula. Although rare, this form is found more often than originally thought. *E*, Tracheoesophageal fistula without atresia (H-type fistula). This anomaly may be missed in the newborn period because swallowing is possible. It is associated with recurrent cough, pneumonia, and abdominal distention. *F*, Esophageal stenosis. (From Gross, R.E.: The Surgery of Infancy and Childhood. Philadelphia, WB Saunders, 1953, p. 76.)

In addition to the previously given descriptive classification, infants with EA have been stratified according to survival. Waterston's 1962 classification, which is based on risk factors, placed infants with EA and TEF into groups based on birth weight, pneumonia, and associated congenital anomalies. Infants in the "good-risk" category (A) were typically managed with immediate surgical repair, "moderate-risk" infants (B) were managed with delayed repair, and "high-risk" infants (C) were managed with staged repair. Although the Waterston classification continues to be used to compare results between centers, many investigators have questioned its validity regarding care for these infants.[35,44,51,64] With modern neonatal critical care, more low-birth-weight infants are surviving, and more treatment options are available for the infant with multiple congenital anomalies. As a result, a search for modern criteria for prognosis and survival has produced several new classification schemes ranging from broad overall physiologic status of the infant[64] to the measured length of the esophageal gap.[65] Other prognostic classifications have been proposed. Poenaru et al.[51] put forward the Montreal classification, in which only severe pulmonary dysfunction with preoperative mechanical ventilation requirement and severe associated anomalies are independent predictors of survival. In a review of 357 patients with EA who were cared for at the Hospital for Sick Children in London between 1980 and 1992, Spitz et al.[52] identified birth weight and major cardiac disease as important predictors of survival (Table 3-3). The Montreal and Spitz classifications are most commonly used.

Diagnostic and Clinical Findings

Prenatal sonography has a positive predictive value of 56% in the detection of EA.[66,67] The sonographic finding of an anechoic area observed in the middle of the fetal neck in association with polyhydramnios and a small stomach size may increase the accuracy of prenatal diagnosis of EA.[68]

Most infants with EA are symptomatic in the first few hours of life, with early clinical signs being excessive salivation as secretions pool in the posterior pharynx and regurgitation of the first feeding, often associated with choking and coughing. Other features are cyanosis with or without feeding, respiratory distress, inability to swallow, and inability to pass a tube through the mouth or nose into the stomach. If a distal fistula is present, the abdomen distends as inspired air passes through the fistula into the stomach. Pulmonary compromise can be significant as gastric fluid passes upward through the TEF and spills into the trachea and lungs, leading to chemical pneumonitis. As the abdomen distends with air, the diaphragm elevates and the pulmonary status worsens. Aspiration of saliva from the upper pouch into the trachea further exacerbates the pulmonary compromise. The larger the distal TEF, the greater are the intestinal distention and subsequent respiratory compromise. In addition, if an associated distal congenital obstruction of the intestine is present, such as duodenal atresia or imperforate anus, then the proximal intestinal distention is even greater and the respiratory compromise is worse.

The diagnosis of EA can be confirmed by passing a firm catheter through the mouth into the esophagus to the point where resistance is met. A few milliliters of air can be injected through the tube and used as a contrast agent to distend the upper esophageal pouch as a frontal and lateral film is obtained. If necessary, 0.5 to 1.0 ml of diluted barium can be used as a contrast agent and injected into the upper pouch to confirm the diagnosis. Under carefully controlled fluorography, barium may also be used to detect a proximal TEF; however, under the usual circumstance of a portable film performed in the neonatal unit, barium identified in the tracheobronchial tree more likely represents contrast material aspirated through the larynx rather than through a proximal TEF. Nevertheless, a very small upper blind pouch suggests the presence of a proximal TEF. Air in the stomach and bowel confirms the presence of a distal TEF. The absence of air in the abdomen typically represents isolated EA without TEF (Fig. 3-2). The diagnosis of TEF without EA is more difficult and requires a high index of suspicion based on clinical symptoms. The diagnosis can be made with barium esophagography with the patient in the prone position; however, bronchoscopy and esophagoscopy are often required to confirm the diagnosis.

Because the incidence of other congenital defects associated with EA is between 50 and 70%, clinical evidence of these other anomalies should be considered in the diagnostic evaluation for EA. In addition to a physical examination focused to evaluate for known associated defects, such as those of the VACTERL and CHARGE association, additional testing usually includes echocardiography, renal sonography, and chromosomal analysis. In fact, it is not unusual for the finding of an anorectal malformation, for instance, to proceed the clinical signs and symptoms of EA.

Table 3-3. Predictors of Survival in Cases of Esophageal Anomalies

Group	Total No. of Patients	No. of Patients Who Died	Survival Rate (%)
I Birthweight >1500 g without major congenital heart disease	293	10	97
II Birthweight <1500 g or major congenital heart disease	70	29	59
III Birthweight <1500 g and major congenital heart disease	9	7	22

Preoperative Treatment

Pneumonitis is the most critical problem that requires attention in the immediate preoperative period, and it results from aspiration of the pharyngeal contents and from reflux of the gastric juice through the TEF into the tracheobronchial tree. Preoperative treatment involves both the prevention of further aspiration and reflux and

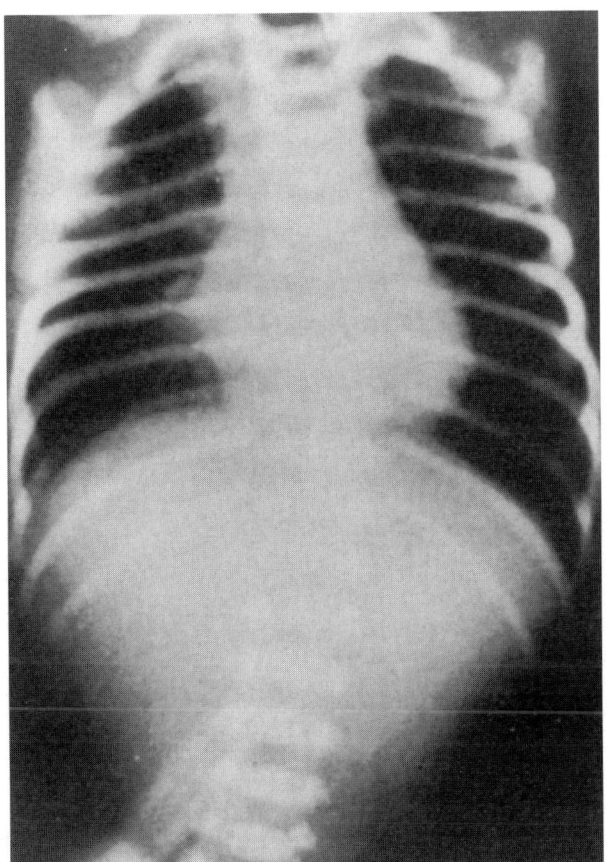

Figure 3–2. Gasless abdomen confirms the diagnosis of isolated esophageal atresia.

the treatment of any pneumonitis that may be present. A double-lumen, sump catheter should be positioned into the upper esophageal pouch to continuously aspirate saliva under low-pressure suction (Fig. 3–3). The "Replogle type" of catheter is best for this purpose, because the perforations along the side of the catheter are located only near the tip of the catheter, minimizing the possibility of suctioning oxygenated air away from the larynx.

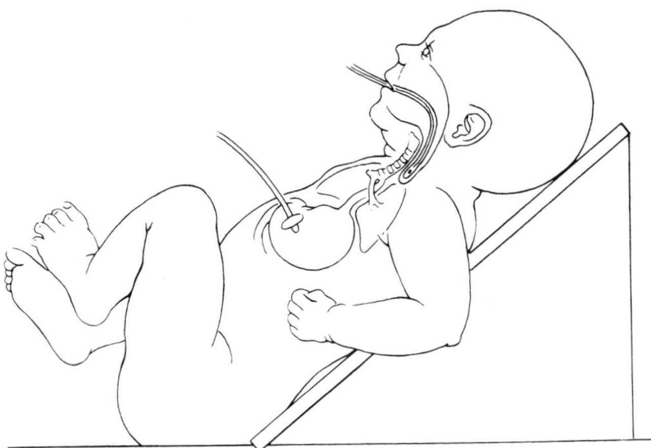

Figure 3–3. The infant is kept in the upright position until definitive surgery is carried out. A gastrostomy tube is not routinely placed preoperatively.

The infant should be positioned to minimize reflux of gastric fluid up through the TEF. Traditionally, an upright sitting position has been advocated; however, there are those who argue that the head-up, prone position is most effective at minimizing reflux. Broad-spectrum antibiotic coverage and pulmonary physiotherapy are also initiated. Intravenous fluid therapy should be started with 10% dextrose and hypotonic saline to maintain fluid, electrolyte, and glucose balance. Vitamin K analog should also be administered before surgery. Routine endotracheal intubation should be avoided because of the risk of gastric perforation and worsening respiratory distress as the abdomen becomes distended from ventilation through the TEF.

Surgical Treatment

The operative approach to the infant with EA depends greatly on the specific type of anomaly present and the occurrence of associated anomalies.

Esophageal Atresia With Distal Tracheoesophageal Fistula

Immediate surgery for EA with distal TEF is seldom necessary, and a period of 24 to 48 hours between diagnosis and surgery allows for a full assessment of the infant and treatment of pulmonary insufficiency, including atelectasis and pneumonitis. In an otherwise healthy baby without major associated anomalies or significant prematurity, division of the fistula and primary anastomosis of the esophagus is possible and is the operative procedure of choice.

The infant is typically positioned for a standard right posterolateral thoracotomy with the right arm extended above the head and the head slightly flexed (Fig. 3–4). If a right-sided aortic arch is identified on a preoperative echocardiogram, then a left-sided thoracotomy is typically preferred. A curved skin incision is made around the lower border of the scapula extending from the anterior axillary line posteriorly to the paravertebral region. The thorax is entered through the fourth intercostal space by dividing the intercostal muscles, with care taken to avoid incision of the pleura. Most pediatric surgeons continue to advocate the extrapleural approach for EA/TEF repair because a significant anastomotic leak does not result in an empyema but merely causes an esophagocutaneous fistula, which typically closes over 1 to 2 weeks. With

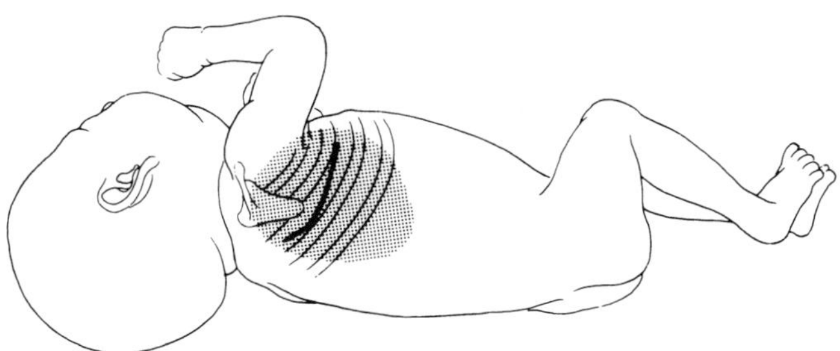

Figure 3–4. A right posterolateral thoracotomy is used.

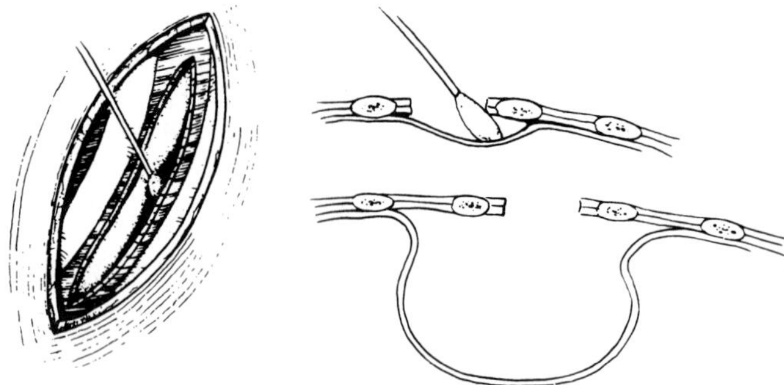

Figure 3–5. Wet cotton-tipped applicators aid in the extrapleural dissection.

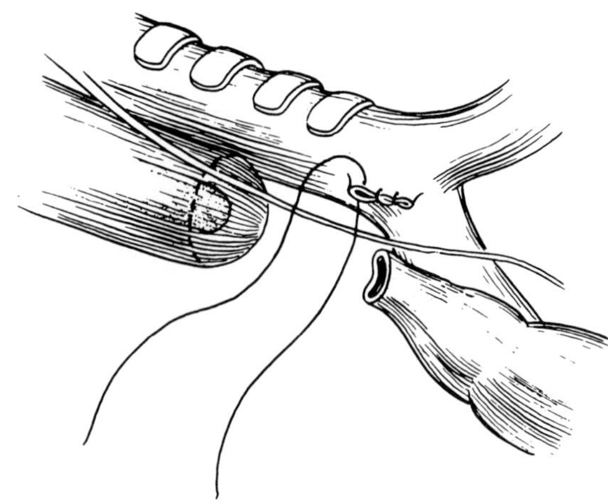

Figure 3–7. The tracheal end of the fistula is closed with interrupted 5-0 or 6-0 silk or Prolene.

the extrapleural approach, the pleura is gently pushed away from the chest wall, allowing the insertion of a rib-spreading retractor (Fig. 3–5). Moist pledgets, tissue applicators, or gauze can be used to dissect the pleura anteromedially as the rib spreader is sequentially opened and the azygos vein is exposed and divided. When the posterior mediastinum is exposed, the upper pouch, distal TEF, trachea, and vagus nerve are identified (Fig. 3–6). The lower esophagus is dissected circumferentially at the level of the fistula, and every effort is made to preserve vagal fibers that supply the distal esophagus. Traction on a heavy silk, tape, or vesiloop passed around the distal esophagus controls gas flow and affords exposure for fistula closure typically using 5-0 or 6-0 silk, or polypropylene, suture in interrupted fashion (Fig. 3–7).

The extent of distal mobilization should be minimized to avoid damage to vagal branches as well as the segmental blood supply. However, if distal mobilization is necessary to ensure a primary anastomosis, it should be carried out. Next, the upper esophageal pouch is identified by having the anesthesiologist push down on the sump tube. A traction suture can be placed through the tip of the pouch to assist in proximal dissection and to avoid the trauma of repeated forceps application to the proximal pouch (Fig. 3–8). Mobilization of the upper pouch should be sufficient to bring the upper pouch down to the distal esophageal segment. This usually means dissection all the way to the thoracic inlet. Extensive circumferential dissection of the proximal pouch also allows the identification of an undiagnosed proximal TEF. Great care must be taken during the dissection between the esophagus and the membranous trachea to avoid inadvertently opening the trachea.

The tip of the upper pouch is excised at its lowest point to a diameter corresponding to the distal esophageal lumen. An end-to-end anastomosis is begun by placing interrupted 5-0 or 6-0 sutures in the back wall with the knots tied on the inside of the lumen (Fig. 3–9). Great care is taken to include full-thickness esophageal wall that includes mucosa and muscularis. Unless the two ends of the esophagus are very close, it is best to place the entire back row of sutures before tying them. A small feeding tube can then be passed and advanced across the anastomosis into the stomach to ensure distal esophageal patency and for early postoperative enteral feeding if desired.[69–71] The anterior layer of the anastomosis is then completed over the tube with the knots tied on the outside. Typically, a chest tube or closed suction drain is placed in the retropleural space and secured with a loose absorbable suture to the lateral chest wall somewhat away from the anastomosis.

Particular attention must be given to infants with EA and a large distal TEF with severe respiratory distress syndrome. Under these circumstances, preoperative endotracheal intubation is often necessary; however, high-

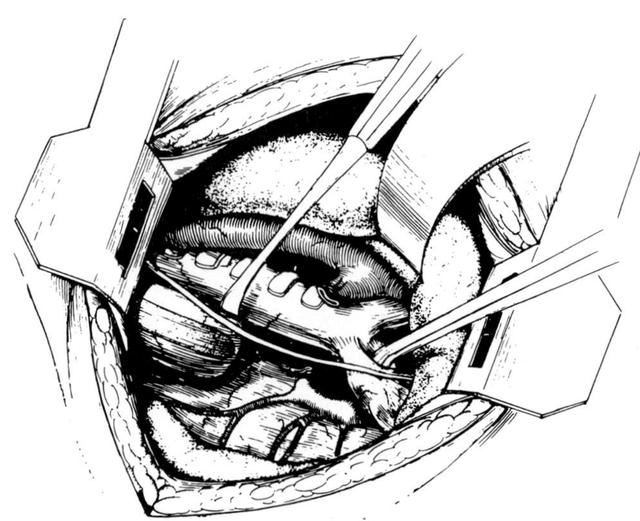

Figure 3–6. The divided azygos vein with the tracheoesophageal fistula under it is seen in this diagram.

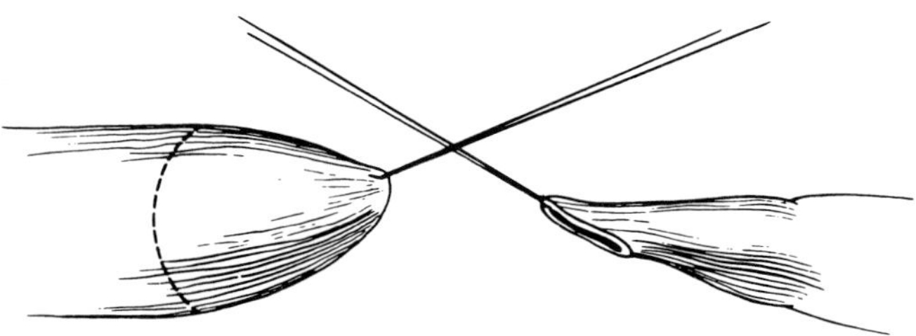

Figure 3–8. The feasibility of the primary anastomosis between the two esophageal segments is assessed.

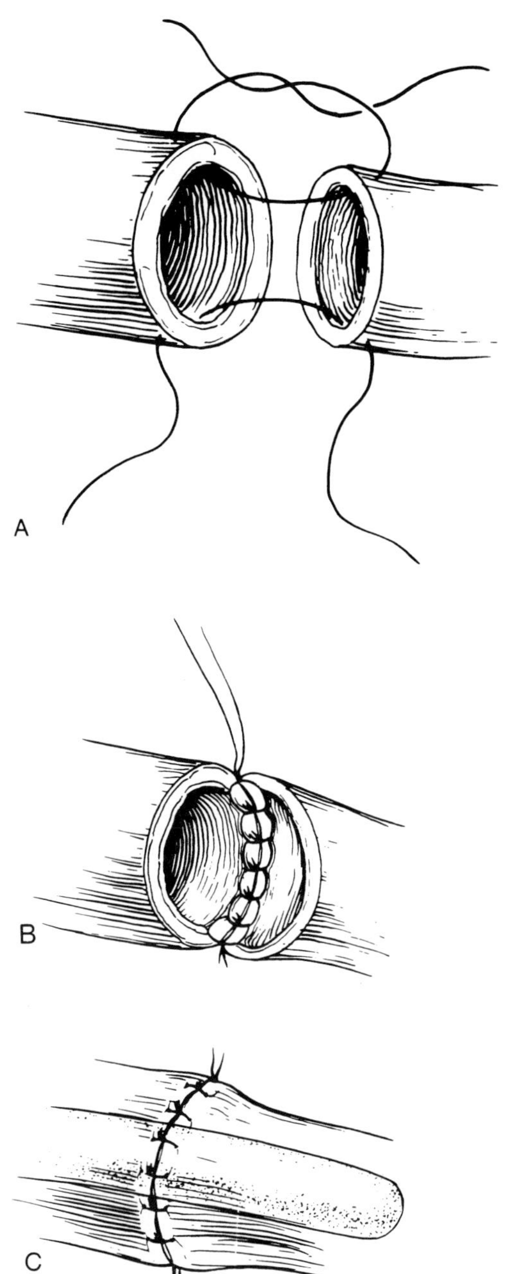

Figure 3–9. The anastomosis is performed as a single layer with the knots on the inside posteriorly *(A)* and on the outside anteriorly *(B)*. The anterior row is performed over a tube *(C)*.

pressure ventilation may worsen lung ventilation and abdominal distention as inspired air is diverted through the TEF into the stomach, thus exacerbating respiratory compromise. In this circumstance, the infant may require emergent surgical intervention to stabilize the pulmonary status and to avoid gastric perforation, which is often fatal under these circumstances. Several preoperative maneuvers have been described to palliate this situation, including positioning of the tip of the endotracheal tube below the fistulous orifice[72] and bronchoscopic placement of a balloon-tip catheter through the fistula to ablate the flow of ventilated air through the fistula.[73] Several emergency transabdominal operative approaches have been described to deal with this problem, including gastric division,[74] banding of the gastroesophageal junction,[75] and emergency gastrostomy to decompress the air-filled stomach and small bowel. The latter approach, although relatively rapid, places the infant at risk of pulmonary collapse as each ventilator breath volume bypasses the lung by preferentially passing through the TEF and escaping via the low-resistance gastrostomy tube. Placing the gastrostomy tube on underwater seal may increase air resistance and lessen runoff through the fistula. We, as well as Templeton et al.[76] and Spitz,[20] recommend early thoracotomy and fistula division in the infant with severe respiratory distress syndrome requiring high-pressure ventilation as the most expeditious and effective approach to improving pulmonary failure. In many circumstances, the infant improves remarkably after emergency fistula ligation, allowing primary repair of the esophagus and thus eliminating the need for a second operation.

Long-Gap Esophageal Atresia

Occasionally in infants with EA/TEF and typically in infants with isolated EA, the upper pouch is high and the distance between upper and lower esophageal segments limits the ability to complete a tension free, end-to-end esophagoesophagostomy with relative ease. Although much has been said and written about the subject, there is no precise definition of *long-gap esophageal atresia*. The measurement of gap length can be biased by the method used to measure the distance between the proximal and distal ends of the esophagus. Some use preoperative measurement of the gap by placing a radiopaque tube or bougie in the upper pouch and contrast or a flexible endoscope into the distal pouch through a previously placed gastrostomy tube.[77] Other definitions of gap length are based on intraoperative measurements either before or after mobilization of the proximal pouch and, on occasion, the proximal and distal pouches.

In the case of isolated EA, in which a "long gap" is expected, most pediatric surgeons would proceed with the operative placement of a gastrostomy tube, a period of observation, and an attempted delayed primary repair. It is well documented that during the first several months of life, the gap between the two ends of the esophagus tends to lessen because of spontaneous growth, making a primary repair more feasible.[78,79] In addition, many preoperative, mechanical techniques have been described to facilitate narrowing of the esophageal gap. The most commonly used method is that of upper pouch bougienage. A weighted bougie is passed per os into the upper pouch with forward pressure applied on a daily or twice-daily basis for 6 to 12 weeks before a delayed primary repair is attempted.[80,81] The use of preoperative upper and lower pouch (via the gastrostomy tube site) bougienage to lessen the gap length has also been described.[20]

A variety of innovative preoperative and operative methods to deal with long-gap EA have been advocated. In addition to preoperative attempts to elongate the esophagus, a variety of intraoperative techniques have been used to establish a primary esophageal anastomosis, either at an initial operation in the newborn period or at the time of a delayed operation after use of the elongation

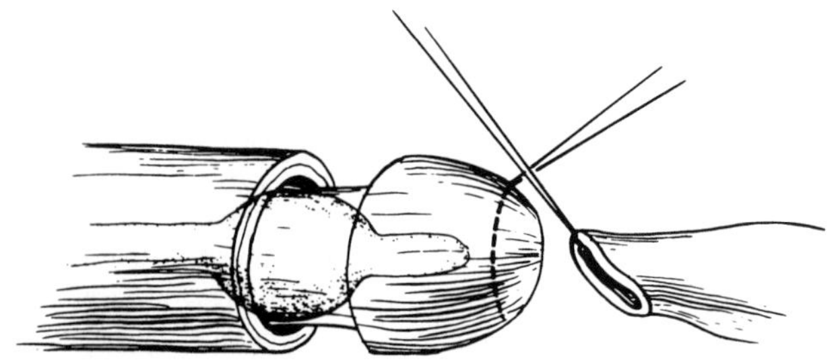

Figure 3–10. This diagram shows the use of a proximal esophagomyotomy to gain additional length.

methods described earlier. One of the most commonly used techniques to lessen the gap between the upper and lower pouch and to decrease anastomotic tension is the upper pouch circular myotomy as described by Livaditis and co-workers[82–84] and others.[85–92] A balloon catheter can be inflated in the upper esophageal pouch to assist in mobilization and the myotomy (Fig. 3–10).[85,93–95]

A number of technical modifications of the single circumferential myotomy have been described to gain additional esophageal length. Several upper pouch myotomies can be performed, even with the addition of a right cervical incision to mobilize the upper esophageal pouch up and out of the neck and to perform a more proximal second or third circular myotomy.[96] In addition to proximal esophageal pouch myotomy, Lai et al.[97] reported experience with five infants who underwent distal circular esophageal myotomy in addition to proximal myotomy. The use of a spiral upper pouch myotomy with oblique suture closure of the muscular layer has also been advocated to minimize the risk of postoperative complications as well as to theoretically improve motility.[98,99] Another modification of the esophageal myotomy that has been described is the use of circumferential incisions of the upper pouch muscle layer with short horizontal myotomies in rows so that when pulled distally, the upper pouch lengthens and narrows, allowing a better fit for the smaller distal esophageal segment.[100] Another method to elongate the upper pouch involves the creation of a full-thickness anterior flap of the upper pouch wall, which when folded distally can be rolled into a tube and attached to the lower esophageal segment.[101–104] Another method described to facilitate esophageal lengthening is a multistaged, extrathoracic elongation technique in which the upper esophagus is mobilized and brought out initially as an end-cervical esophagostomy. Every 2 to 3 weeks, the esophagus and its cutaneous stoma are operatively mobilized and translocated down the anterior chest wall until a sufficient length is achieved to perform an end-to-end esophageal anastomosis.[105]

Complications that relate to the commonly used circular myotomy have been described; they include full-thickness esophagotomy with esophageal leak, long-term food particle impaction,[87] and ballooning at the myotomy site, resulting in an esophageal pseudodiverticulum formation. The latter has been reported to be a potential serious complication in a few patients, resulting in tracheal compression and respiratory distress; however, this serious problem typically occurs in the setting of a distal anastomotic stricture.[85,87,106] In addition to pseudodiverticulum formation, it has been suggested that circular myotomy results in esophageal dysmotility.[87,107] A number of studies have suggested that esophageal motility is abnormal in children who have undergone myotomy and primary repair of EA.[108–111] However, EA results in abnormal motility, and Sumitomo et al.[112] reported no difference in a number of motility parameters in a comparison of patients with or without a myotomy.

There are occasions when at the time of attempted initial or delayed primary repair, the esophageal segments do not reach together even though one or more of the methods described earlier have been tried. Several additional techniques have been described to facilitate an esophageal anastomosis. Despite the long-held opinion that the blood supply to the distal esophagus is tenuous and may be compromised by mobilization, many surgeons have found that the distal esophagus can be, and often is, mobilized to facilitate a primary anastomosis. We have had success in achieving primary end-to-end esophageal anastomosis by completely mobilizing the distal esophagus down to, and even through, the esophageal hiatus of the diaphragm. By this approach, a portion of the fundus of the stomach can be brought up into the chest to facilitate anastomosis[96] (Fig. 3–11). Taking this concept further, Schärli[113] described a combined abdominal and thoracic procedure in which distal esophageal elongation was achieved through ligation and division of the left gastric artery, transverse or diagonal division of the lesser curvature of the stomach, and mobilization of the gastric cardia and upper fundus into the chest to achieve primary esophageal anastomosis. A partial fundoplication is recommended to treat the anticipated gastroesophageal reflux (GER). With a similar approach, a Collis gastroplasty has also been described as a means of lengthening the distal esophagus to avoid esophageal replacement.[114]

In addition to the surgical techniques discussed here to facilitate saving and using the native esophagus as the conduit of choice for the repair of long-gap EA, the use of postoperative head flexion, paralysis, and mechanical ventilatory support have been strongly advocated by some to minimize the risk of anastomotic disruption in cases where the esophageal anastomosis is under significant tension.[20,39,115] The rationale for this approach is the prevention of disruptive forces at the anastomosis through flexion of the neck and paralysis of the striated muscles in the proximal esophagus.[20]

Esophageal Atresia Without Tracheoesophageal Fistula

Infants born with isolated EA have almost no esophagus in the thorax. It is important to be aware of this fact to institute an appropriate treatment plan and to avoid fruitless exploratory thoracotomy. The preoperative and operative treatment of this lesion was discussed extensively in the preceding section on long-gap esophageal atresia. Associated congenital anomalies are more frequent in EA without TEF as noted in a review of 69 infants with isolated EA treated during a 50-year period of time. Ein and Shandling[116] reported a 52% incidence of prematurity,

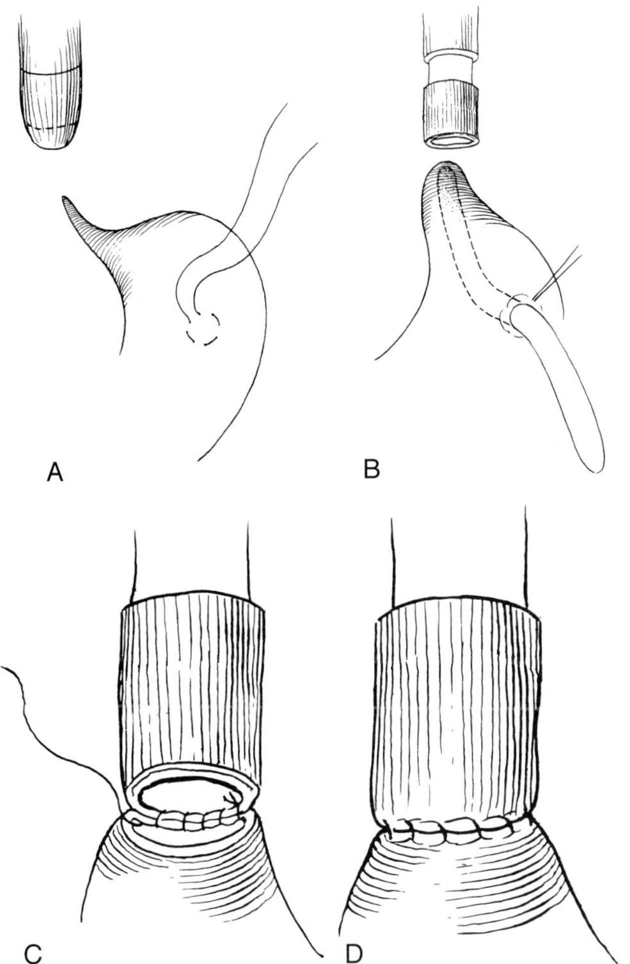

Figure 3–11. The stomach is mobilized into the chest *(A)*, a proximal esophagomyotomy is performed *(B)*, and the anastomosis (*C* and *D*) is performed as described in Figure 3–14 *A* and *B*.

a 10 to 20% incidence of Down's syndrome, and a 10% incidence of duodenal atresia. The clinical presentation of an infant with isolated EA is similar to that of EA with TEF in terms of inability to swallow; however, the abdomen is typically scaphoid, and there is no air in the gastrointestinal tract on plain films of the abdomen. An upper pouch sump tube is placed immediately, and a gastrostomy tube should be placed within the first 24 hours of life, and an attempt to achieve a delayed primary repair should be undertaken using the various methods previously discussed. The gastrostomy tube placement allows the early institution of enteral feedings, which leads to subsequent enlargement of the diminutive stomach. This allows the stomach to be used as an esophageal substitute if necessary. At the time of placement, a contrast imaging study can be obtained to evaluate the unusual possibility of a coexisting duodenal atresia, as well as an occluded, but present, distal esophageal fistula to the trachea, which might suggest the potential for early esophageal repair. A period of observation and enteral nutritional support is instituted with or without daily upper pouch bougienage. When no further elongation progress is evident beyond 10 to 12 weeks or when the two ends of the esophagus can be brought to close proximity, surgery is undertaken. Occasionally, an infant can be cared for at home; however, it is not unusual to have occasional respiratory symptoms when the upper pouch sump tube becomes obstructed, resulting in oropharyngeal aspiration.

Thoracotomy with retropleural dissection and mobilization of the proximal and distal esophageal segments is undertaken in an attempt at primary anastomosis, with circular myotomy and opening of the esophageal hiatus for more distal mobilization, if necessary. If these efforts do not allow a primary anastomosis, proximal pouch flap esophagoplasty or the addition of an abdominal approach to mobilize a portion of or the entire stomach to pull up into the chest (or neck) can be undertaken. Under circumstances where the two ends of the esophagus are clearly too distant for a primary esophageal anastomosis, despite preoperative attempts at elongation, then we have proceeded with a primary gastric transposition to the cervical esophagus without a thoracotomy. Under these latter circumstances, some surgeons, especially in the past but even today, will proceed to a cervical esophagostomy, preferably on the left side, with plans for a future esophageal replacement procedure. When the patient is 6 months to 1 year old, a gastric transposition, coloesophagoplasty, or gastric tube interposition is usually performed.

Postoperative complications after the repair of isolated EA are similar to those in infants with repaired EA with TEF and principally include anastomotic leak and stricture, dysphagia, and GER. Perhaps surprisingly, infants with EA without TEF have been reported to have significant tracheomalacia (TM), which is consistent with the reports that tracheobronchial anomalies occur in association with EA.[116,117]

Isolated (H-Type) Tracheoesophageal Fistula

Congenital TEF without EA, or "H" (perhaps more anatomically accurate as "N") type of TEF occurs with approximately 4% of esophageal anomalies reported. This anomaly usually presents in the first few days of life when the neonate chokes on attempts to feed or has unexplained cyanotic spells. Older infants and children are more likely to present with recurrent bouts of pneumonia, typically involving the right upper lobe. Because these are nonspecific symptoms, a high index of suspicion is necessary to consider isolated TEF as a diagnosis.

The diagnosis of isolated TEF can be suspected on the basis of plain chest radiographs that show evidence of aspiration pneumonitis with gastric distention. A reliable method of establishing the diagnosis is with a prone tube videoesophagogram that involves the use of a small nasogastric tube passed into the distal esophagus, with contrast medium gradually injected as the tube is slowly withdrawn. It is crucial that the radiologist who performs the study is familiar with this diagnostic approach, because more than 50% of H-type fistulas may be missed on routine esophageal contrast swallows. Bronchoscopy with esophagoscopy can confirm the diagnosis and, if performed immediately before the operation to divide the fistula, allows for the passage of a fine catheter

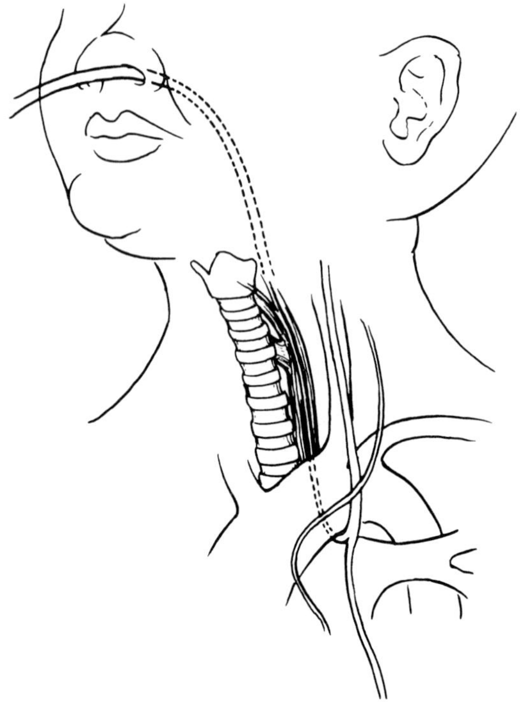

Figure 3–12. A cervical approach is used for an isolated tracheoesophageal fistula. This shows a left cervical approach, which can be used, although I prefer a right cervical incision.

through the fistula to aid in subsequent identification at surgical exploration.

The majority of isolated TEFs can be successfully divided through a right-sided cervical approach (Fig. 3–12). The sternocleidomastoid muscle is retracted posteriorly, dividing the sternal head if necessary, and dissection proceeds medially to the carotid sheath. The identification of the trachea and esophagus is facilitated by palpation of the endotracheal and nasogastric tubes. The recurrent laryngeal nerve must be identified and preserved. Identification of the fistula is facilitated by encircling the esophagus with slings; however, it is important to be aware that the contralateral recurrent laryngeal nerve can be damaged during this maneuver. Once the fistula is identified, often higher-than-expected traction stitches should be placed close to the esophagus through the superior and inferior extent of the fistula to avoid posterior rotation of the esophagus after division of the fistula. On the tracheal side, 5-0 polypropylene or silk sutures are placed at the superior and inferior limits of the fistula. The fistula is now divided close to the esophagus, and interrupted 5-0 polypropylene or silk sutures are placed on the tracheal side to close the fistula (Fig. 3–13). The esophageal end of the fistula is closed with interrupted fine silk or absorbable polyglycolic acid sutures. Some surgeons advocate the interposition of muscle tissue between the two opposing suture lines to reduce the likelihood of recurrence of the fistula. A right thoracotomy is best used on the rare occasion when the fistula is identified to be well down within the thorax or when a recurrent fistula from a previous EA repair is being approached.

Postoperative complications include respiratory distress secondary to edema of the trachea or injury to the recurrent laryngeal nerves. The degree of preexisting lung disease and concerns about tracheal edema may warrant leaving the endotracheal tube in place postoperatively for several days. Esophageal leak and recurrence of isolated TEF are rare.

Esophageal Atresia With Upper Pouch Fistula

The incidence of a fistula between the upper esophageal pouch and the trachea is variably reported.[52,59–61,63,118–120] The exact incidence of this type of fistula has probably been underestimated in that some initially unrecognized proximal pouch fistulas have been reported as recurrent TEFs after the repair of EA with distal TEF.[120] There are two versions of this anomaly: (1) proximal pouch fistula in association with distal TEF (double fistula) with an incidence of 1.4% and (2) proximal pouch fistula without distal TEF with an incidence of 0.8% (averaged from several large reports). Even though the occurrence of this type of fistula is rare, it is important to identify and treat it early to avoid ongoing pulmonary aspiration with recurrent pneumonia. The diagnosis should be made by a preoperative proximal pouch contrast study, preferably performed by a skilled pediatric radiologist, under optimum conditions in the radiology suite with fluoroscopy and videotape recording. This study will usually show a small upper pouch in addition to identification of the fistula. A frequent point of confusion during and in the interpretation of this study is the occurrence of the spillover of contrast material from the pouch up into the larynx and down into the trachea. Because of the potential for inaccurate interpretation, many surgeons rely on preoperative bronchoscopy with esophagoscopy to make or confirm the diagnosis of proximal pouch fistula. Unfortunately, a small proximal fistula can be missed with

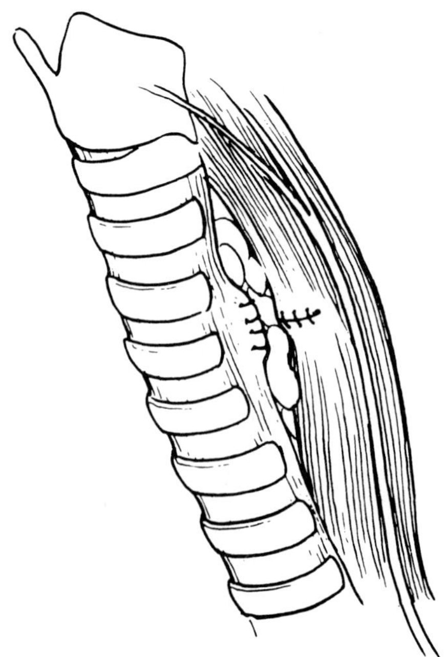

Figure 3–13. The fistula is divided and both sides are closed with interrupted sutures of 5-0 or 6-0 silk.

endoscopy as well. Another common approach to the diagnosis of this anomaly is to completely mobilize the upper pouch during the repair of the EA to localize and repair an unsuspected upper pouch fistula. As with the other diagnostic modalities mentioned, proximal pouch fistulas have gone unrecognized during surgical exploration as well, in part because of the extreme proximal nature of some of these fistulas. A proximal pouch fistula should be suspected and sought if the upper pouch is unusually narrow or short at the time of exploration, suggesting decompression through a fistula.

Once identified, a proximal fistula should be surgically ligated and divided as with a distal TEF. If an upper pouch fistula is diagnosed after the initial repair of EA with or without distal TEF, then often a cervical approach can be used as previously described for an H-type TEF.

Postoperative Treatment

The postoperative care of an infant after the repair of EA with or without a TEF is often modified by the complexity of the surgical procedure. Many infants with EA/TEF without associated anomalies are placed in an erect infant seat after surgery, and a premeasured nasogastric tube is taped to the child's incubator so that if suctioning is needed, the tube will be passed no further than a point proximal to the esophageal anastomosis. The tube is measured at the time of the surgery. Antibiotics are continued until the chest tube is removed, and intravenous fluids are maintained until gastrostomy feedings are begun. Peripheral intravenous nutrition is started on the first postoperative day. If the child is stable and there is no evidence of saliva leaking through the chest tube, gastrostomy feedings are sometimes begun on the fourth postoperative day. On the 5th to 10th postoperative day, an Hypaque swallow is performed; if no leak is seen, this is followed by a barium swallow to visualize the anastomosis completely. Formula feedings are begun immediately after radiographs show no evidence of a leak, and the chest tube is removed.

Results

Survival rates for infants with EA with or without TEF have improved dramatically since the 1950s, with reviews that report 85 to 95% overall survival rates compared with less than 40% in the pre-1950 era.[20,59,60,62,63,121] However, there remain subsets of infants with EA who have a poorer prognosis. Waterston's risk classification scheme historically helped to identify infants with EA at particular risk for poor outcome and as such helped direct treatment options.[122] Newer risk classification schemes have been proposed. It appears that infants with EA at high risk include those with (1) birth weight of less than 1,500 g, (2) major congenital heart disease, (3) severe associated anomalies and ventilator dependency, and possibly (4) a long gap length between the two ends of esophagus.[20,51,65]

Early Complications

Anastomotic Leak

Anastomotic leak at the esophagoesophagostomy occurs in approximately 14 to 16% of patients. The vast majority are clinically insignificant and can be managed with adequate drainage and nutritional support. When a retropleural approach is undertaken and a mediastinal drain is in place and patent, up to 95% of anastomotic leaks will close spontaneously.[60,63] Even when transthoracic repair is followed by disruption and the pleural space is contaminated, adequate drainage can usually be achieved, which allows for spontaneous closure of the leak. Breakdown of the anastomosis is frequently followed by the formation of a stricture at the site of the leak and on occasion is associated with a recurrent TEF. Major disruptions of the esophageal anastomosis account for only 3 to 5% of postoperative leaks and are typically recognized early (24 to 48 hours) after the initial repair, as the infant frequently deteriorates from tension pneumothorax or mediastinitis uncontrolled by drainage and antibiotics. Factors that contribute to anastomotic leak include poor surgical technique, ischemia of the esophageal ends, and excessive tension at the anastomotic site. In this setting, reoperation for the control of sepsis with adequate drainage and attempted repair of the anastomotic leak are warranted. Pleural or pericardial patch, with or without intercostal muscle flap buttress, may be helpful to secure anastomotic closure.[123,124] If the esophageal anastomosis is not repairable, cervical esophagostomy and delayed esophageal replacement may be required.

Esophageal Stricture

Esophageal stricture is a common complication after anastomosis of the esophagus in EA; however, the reported incidence varies widely depending on the criteria used to define a stricture. In large series, the rate of stricture that requires dilation is reported to be as high as 40%.[39,63] Spitz and Hitchcock[125] proposed that the definition of stricture be that the patient experiences symptoms (dysphagia, recurrent respiratory problems from aspiration or foreign body obstruction) *and* a narrowing noted at endoscopy or on contrast esophagography. The factors that have been implicated in the pathogenesis of esophageal stricture include poor anastomotic technique (excessive tension, two-layered anastomosis, silk suture material), ischemia at the ends of the esophagus, GER, and anastomotic leak. The treatment of a clinically significant narrowing at the site of the esophageal anastomosis is dilation, with antegrade or retrograde bougienage. The use of Savary-type dilators that are passed prograde over a guide wire has demonstrated advantages in our experience, because this method allows fluoroscopic assessment during sequential dilations and the ability to use contrast injection during the dilation session and typically eliminates the need for rigid esophagoscopy. The use of Grunzig-type balloon catheters to dilate esophageal strictures, including after EA repair, has been reported and has the theoretical advantage of producing a uniform and radial force at the site of the stricture, rather than the shearing axial force applied using traditional bougienage.[126,127] Many strictures respond to one to three dilations (53%) in the first months after esophageal repair. However, occasionally a recalcitrant stricture is resistant to repeated dilations and requires resection and reanastomosis or even esophageal replacement. It is crucial to determine whether esophageal stricture is associated with GER through investigation with contrast esophagography, pH monitoring, or both. Many strictures will not be responsive to dilation attempts if severe GER persists in bathing the stricture with acid. Often, the stricture resolves after antireflux surgery.

Recurrent Tracheoesophageal Fistula

Recurrent TEF occurs in 3 to 14% of patients after initial operative division or ligation.[39,59,60,63,128,129] Recurrent TEF has been attributed to anastomotic leak with local inflammation and erosion through the previous site of TEF repair. Techniques that have been described to minimize the likelihood of recurrent TEF include the use of a pleural flap,[63] vascularized pericardial flap,[123,130,131] and azygos vein flap[132] interposed between the esophageal and tracheal suture lines. Although a recurrent TEF typically occurs in the early postoperative period, it may not be recognized for months to years. Symptoms can be typical of those of a congenital H-type TEF, including coughing and choking or cyanosis with feedings; however, less obvious symptoms, such as recurrent pulmonary infections, are more common. The diagnosis may be suggested by an air-filled esophagus on plain radiographs of the chest. Routine contrast swallows will miss as many as 50% of recurrent fistulas. As with a congenital H-type fistula, esophagography performed in the prone position under videofluoroscopy is a reliable method of establishing the diagnosis. Bronchoscopy with cannulation of the fistula with a No. 2 to 3 French catheter is also a reliable diagnostic approach and is invaluable in locating the fistula during the operative procedure. A recurrent TEF rarely closes spontaneously and typically requires operative repair. Thoracotomy with fistula ligation and division is the operation of choice. To minimize the chance of recurrent fistulization, which has been reported in 10 to 20% of patients with a first-time TEF recurrence, pleura, intercostal muscle or pericardium should be interposed between the esophagus and trachea.[133] Endoscopic eradication of TEF using various chemicals or diathermy has been reported,[134-136] and fibrin glue was used for this purpose with success in one case report.[137]

Late Complications

Gastroesophageal Reflux

GER in infants with repaired EA is common, and the incidence appears to be increasing in reports as suspicion and diagnostic investigation have been more common. The magnitude of the problem is reflected in the findings that GER occurs in 40 to 70% of patients after the repair of EA.[60,63,138,139] The cause of GER in this group of infants probably relates to the shortening of the intra-abdominal esophagus due to anastomotic tension or esophageal motor dysfunction, either acquired secondary to operative manipulation or intrinsic to the congenital anomaly itself.[139-141] The diagnosis of pathological GER is suspected with symptoms of vomiting, dysphagia, and recurrent anastomotic stenosis, which is occasionally associated with the impaction of a foreign body or food bolus. In addition, respiratory symptoms such as stridor, cyanotic spells, recurrent pneumonia, and reactive airway disease may indicate GER as opposed to other conditions such as TM. Esophagitis is frequently observed in these patients, and Barrett's esophagus was identified in older children and adolescents on long-term follow-up of patients with EA.[139,142-145] There has been one case of esophageal adenocarcinoma reported in a 20-year-old patient who had undergone repair of a TEF as an infant.[146]

The diagnosis of pathologic GER in infants and children after repair of EA is suggested on an upper gastrointestinal contrast study. The 24-hour pH probe data, although not as standardized for children as it is for adults, typically documents pathologic reflux.[139] Extensive esophageal manometric studies have consistently documented abnormal esophageal peristalsis and decreased lower esophageal sphincter pressures after EA repair; as a result, this test is probably not helpful in the diagnosis of GER.

In infants and children with pathologic GER, aggressive medical management is typically undertaken with thickening of feeds, positioning of the infant in the prone or upright posture, and the use of acid-reduction agents such as H_2-blockers such as cimetidine or ranitidine and prokinetic agents such as cisapride or metaclopromide. However, 45 to 75% of these infants ultimately undergo antireflux operations because of failed medical management, refractory anastomotic stricture, or development of a distal esophageal stricture.[60,63,138] The choice of antireflux operation is controversial. The Nissen fundoplication has typically been considered to be the best option[140,147,148]; however, complications and debilitating dysphagia have been a common problem after the 360-degree wrap.[60,138,149,150] The proposed reason for the comparative poorer results of Nissen fundoplication in infants and children with EA is that the dyskinetic esophagus does not generate sufficient coordinated propulsive force to overcome the increased lower esophageal resistance resulting from the circumferential wrap. In our experience with 21 patients who underwent Nissen fundoplication after EA repair, only 8 had an uncomplicated course with elimination of GER and no dysphagia.[138] Prolonged dysphagia was common, and wrap disruption and recurrent GER occurred in 33% compared with 10% of infants and children with GER without EA. Due to the general poor results with Nissen fundoplication in this setting, we have been using the anterior, Thal fundoplication, in these patients or a modification of the Nissen fundoplication with an ultrashort, very floppy wrap (1.0 to 5 cm over a large dilator).

Tracheomalacia

Significant respiratory symptoms that occur after the repair of EA with TEF can be due to TM. TM affects approximately 10 to 20% of infants after repair of EA with TEF, of whom approximately half require surgical correction.[151] It is often difficult to clinically distinguish these symptoms from those of recurrent TEF, anastomotic leak, or GER.[152] TM is defined as generalized or localized weakness of the trachea that allows the anterior and posterior tracheal walls to come together during expiration or coughing. In infants with associated TEF, structural anomalies of the trachea were identified in 75% of 40 infants at autopsy, suggesting that embryologic events leading to TEF perhaps contribute to the development of TM.[153] The cartilage was shown to be shorter than normal, thereby failing to provide the support necessary to maintain a patent airway.[153] In addition, the trachea may be easily compressed between the aorta anteriorly and the often-dilated upper esophagus posteriorly in infants after the repair of EA with TEF, and this has been considered a significant cause of TM. Support for the notion that the primary etiology of TM is related to intrinsic esophageal weakness is found in the report of Kimura et al.,[154] who studied TM by using cine computed tomography. It is interesting that in one series, there was no evidence of TM in infants with EA alone, suggesting that EA and TM have a separate pathogenesis.[155] The level of collapse is usually in the region of or just above the original site of the TEF in the distal third of the trachea.

The clinical presentation of TM is broad, ranging from a "brassy" or "barking" cough in mild cases to recurrent pneumonia or acute life-threatening apneic spells. Often, infants with TM have a reluctance to feed because of difficulty in breathing during feeding or cyanotic attacks. These symptoms usually appear when the infant is a few months old.[156] Life-threatening apneic spells were noted in 27 of 32 children with TM reported by Filler et al. in 1992.[157] Typically, these spells occur during or within 5 to 10 minutes of a meal and are characterized by cyanosis progressing to apnea, bradycardia, and, ultimately, cardiorespiratory arrest if not interrupted. The diagnosis is established with bronchoscopy, which reveals a slit-like lumen of the trachea at the involved area.

The treatment of TM remains controversial. Most infants with mild to moderate symptoms of TM do not require operative intervention, because symptoms tend to improve with time. In infants with severe symptoms, including acute life-threatening events, the operative treatment of choice is an aortopexy.[158,159] This operation is typically performed through a lateral thoracotomy; the ascending aorta and arch are sutured up to the posterior surface of the sternum. Lifting the aorta up in this manner lifts the anterior wall of the trachea up as well and opens the tracheal lumen.[156,160,161] A modification of this operation has been proposed that uses a flap of pericardium based at the root of the aorta to be sutured to the sternum in cases in which the aortic arch would not reach the posterior sternum without undue tension.[162] The role of various stents in the treatment of TM after the repair of EA, although successful in case reports, has yet to be validated as a standard treatment method.[163-165] Filler et al.[157] recommends consideration of an airway stent for children in whom aortopexy does not relieve tracheal collapse. Tracheostomy is a final treatment option.

Disordered Peristalsis

As previously discussed, the esophagus of an infant with EA has abnormal peristaltic activity that is secondary to the congenital defect itself as well as perhaps the operative repair of the lesion. This disorder is clinically very significant in that it is responsible for many long-term symptoms after EA repair, including dysphagia and recurrent respiratory problems. Although these symptoms may improve with time, early problems with feeding intolerance and food bolus obstruction can lead to failure to thrive.

LARYNGOTRACHEOESOPHAGEAL CLEFT

LTEC is a rare congenital anomaly consisting of a midline communication between the larynx, trachea, and esophagus. The malformation was possibly first described in 1792 by Richter in his doctoral thesis in which he described an infant who choked and vomited upon feeding. No autopsy was performed, however, leaving the diagnosis unconfirmed.[166] The next description of an infant with LTEC is in 1949 by Finlay.[167] In 1955, the first successful correction of a laryngotracheoesophageal cleft was performed by Pettersson.[168]

As with EA and TEF, the embryogenesis of LTEC is not completely understood. The long-held theory is that there is an arrest of the cranial extension of the tracheoesophageal septum, allowing for the persistence of an esophagotrachea.[9,11,169] Studies suggests that as with TEF, there is initial normal development followed by a far-reaching fusion of the trachea and esophagus.[16] Although there is no consistent pattern of inheritance, sporadic familial associations have been described,[170] and LTEC is reported with the "G" and Pallister-Hall syndromes.[171] The sex incidence of LTEC favors males with a ratio of 5:3.[172]

A variety of associated congenital anomalies occur in the setting of LTEC, including gastrointestinal, genitourinary, and cardiac malformations.[172] EA with TEF occurs in 20 to 37% of patients with LTEC.[172-174] Other associated gastrointestinal malformations include anal defects (21%), malrotation or defects of intestinal fixation (13%), and meconium ileus (8%).[172,175] Genitourinary anomalies occur with an incidence of 14 to 44% and include hypospadias, inguinal hernias, undescended testes, and renal agenesis.[172,175] Cardiovascular anomalies have been identified in 16 to 33% of patients and include ventricular septal defects, coarctation of the aorta, and transposition of the great vessels.[172]

To more adequately delineate therapy, several classification schemes have been described. In reporting the first surgical repair in 1955, Pettersson[168] described three types of clefts: type I, limited to the larynx and involving part, or all, of the cricoid plate; type II, extending beyond the cricoid lamina to the cervical trachea; and type III, involving the entire trachea down to the carina. A type IV was suggested by Ryan et al.[176] in 1991 in which the cleft extends beyond the carina to involve one or both main stem bronchi.

Symptoms of LTEC vary depending on the extent of the cleft; however, most patients present immediately after birth with respiratory distress aggravated by feeding. Additional symptoms can include a characteristic toneless or hoarse cry, cyanosis, choking, increased secretions, and recurrent aspiration pneumonia. It is not unusual for the severity of associated anomalies to obscure the presence of LTEC, especially if it is a minimal type I or II lesion. We treated an infant with imperforate anus who was noted to have a type II LTEC after repeat bouts of respiratory distress. Based on the common symptoms of LTEC, the diagnostic evaluation typically proceeds along the lines of the more commonly suspected diagnosis of EA/TEF or TM. Contrast esophagography demonstrates rapid confluence of contrast material in the upper esophagus and trachea; however, it is often difficult to know whether this is secondary to spillover at the level of the larynx or passage of contrast through a cleft. Endoscopy is the definitive method for diagnosis of LTEC; but it can still be difficult to identify a cleft unless the index of suspicion is high and the frequent mucosal infolding at the level of the subglottic region is pushed open to reveal the cleft.

The management of infants with LTEC begins by maneuvers to minimize aspiration and to stabilize the airway. Donahoe and Hendren[174] recommended avoiding endotracheal intubation if possible in the preoperative period; however, it is often necessary to intubate the trachea and to perform tube gastrostomy before undertaking definitive surgical repair. Operative procedures for the repair of LTEC vary depending on the severity of the cleft. Asymptomatic type I clefts may require no operative intervention, and those that are symptomatic have been successfully repaired endoscopically.[172] Type II LTEC can be approached via a lateral pharyngotomy, posterior pharyngotomy, or anterior laryngofissure. The lateral exposure has been most often reported; it permits easy access to the cleft and allows for asymmetric incisions in the mucosa, thereby avoiding contiguous suture lines. The major disadvantage to this approach is risk to the recurrent laryngeal nerves. The anterior laryngeal approach provides exposure of the larynx and upper trachea and has no risk of recurrent laryngeal nerve injury. Concerns regarding postoperative laryngeal stability have been raised, and some surgeons recommend the use of stents during the healing process.[172,177]

Operative management for type III and IV LTEC requires a combined cervical and thoracic approach. Donohoe and Hendren[174] described the use of a specifically designed bifurcated endotracheal tube with flanged ends that can be positioned during bronchoscopy and suspension anteriorly of the trachea with a ureteral catheter sling (Fig. 3-14). This endotracheal tube allows for confident airway control during the multiple position changes frequently required during the operation. A right thoracotomy is performed and the tracheoesophageal cleft is exposed retropleurally. The tracheoesophageal groove is incised on the right and opened from the carina to the thoracic inlet. Separation of the two tubes is completed by incising along the left side of the esophagotracheal common wall, leaving an approximately 1-cm flap of esophagus running the length of the trachea to assist in creation of the neomembranous portion of the trachea. It is important to size the esophageal flap correctly to avoid stenosis or a floppy posterior wall, which can result in TM. As the dissection proceeds, it is also important to push away and thus protect the left vagus and recurrent laryngeal nerves. The closure of the trachea and the esophagus is begun in a caudal-to-cranial fashion, with running polypropylene for the esophagus and interrupted polypropylene for the trachea. A right cervical incision now exposes the upper portion of the esophagus and trachea, pharynx, and larynx, and the repair is continued, including a three-layer repair of the larynx and placement of a tracheostomy tube, which can be custom designed to avoid undue pressure against the posterior tracheal repair. Some surgeons prefer an anterior approach that divides the larynx and trachea in the midline, as described for type II defects.

Postoperative survival continues to be rather poor, averaging about 75%, depending on the severity of the malformation. Anastomotic leaks are reported to occur in approximately 50% of repairs and typically require reoperation via a different approach.[172] In addition, inability to wean from the ventilator, pharyngoesophageal dysfunction, and GER are common postoperative complications. Reduction in morbidity and mortality rates depends in part on earlier recognition to prevent secondary complications.

CONGENITAL STENOSIS OF THE ESOPHAGUS

True CES is a rare condition and historically has been confused with esophageal strictures secondary to inflammation and GER in particular. CES has been reported to occur once in every 25,000 to 50,000 births,[178,179] and as of 1995 only 500 cases have been described in the world literature.[180] For unknown reasons, the incidence of CES appears to be higher in Japan than other parts of the world.[181] The incidence of other anomalies in association with CES is reported to be 17 to 33% and includes EA with or without TEF; H-type TEF; cardiac anomalies; intestinal atresia; midgut malrotation; anorectal malformations; hypospadias; malformations of the head, face, and limbs; and chromosomal anomalies.[179]

Classification schemes for CES have been numerous and confusing, in part because of the difficulty in differentiating congenital from acquired lesions. The definition and classification proposed by Nihoul-Fekete et al.[179] are perhaps the most clear. CES is defined as an intrinsic stenosis of the esophagus that is present at birth and is caused by congenital malformation of esophageal wall architecture.[179] Three forms of CES are described: (1) a membranous web or diaphragm, (2) fibromuscular thickening, and (3) that secondary to tracheobronchial remnants in the wall of the esophagus.

Congenital membranous web or *diaphragm* is reported as the rarest of the three forms of CES.[180] It has been considered to represent a missed form of EA[182] and may be analogous to membranes in other parts of the gastrointestinal tract. It usually is a partially obstructing lesion that is typically located in the mid or lower portion of the esophagus. The membrane is covered on both

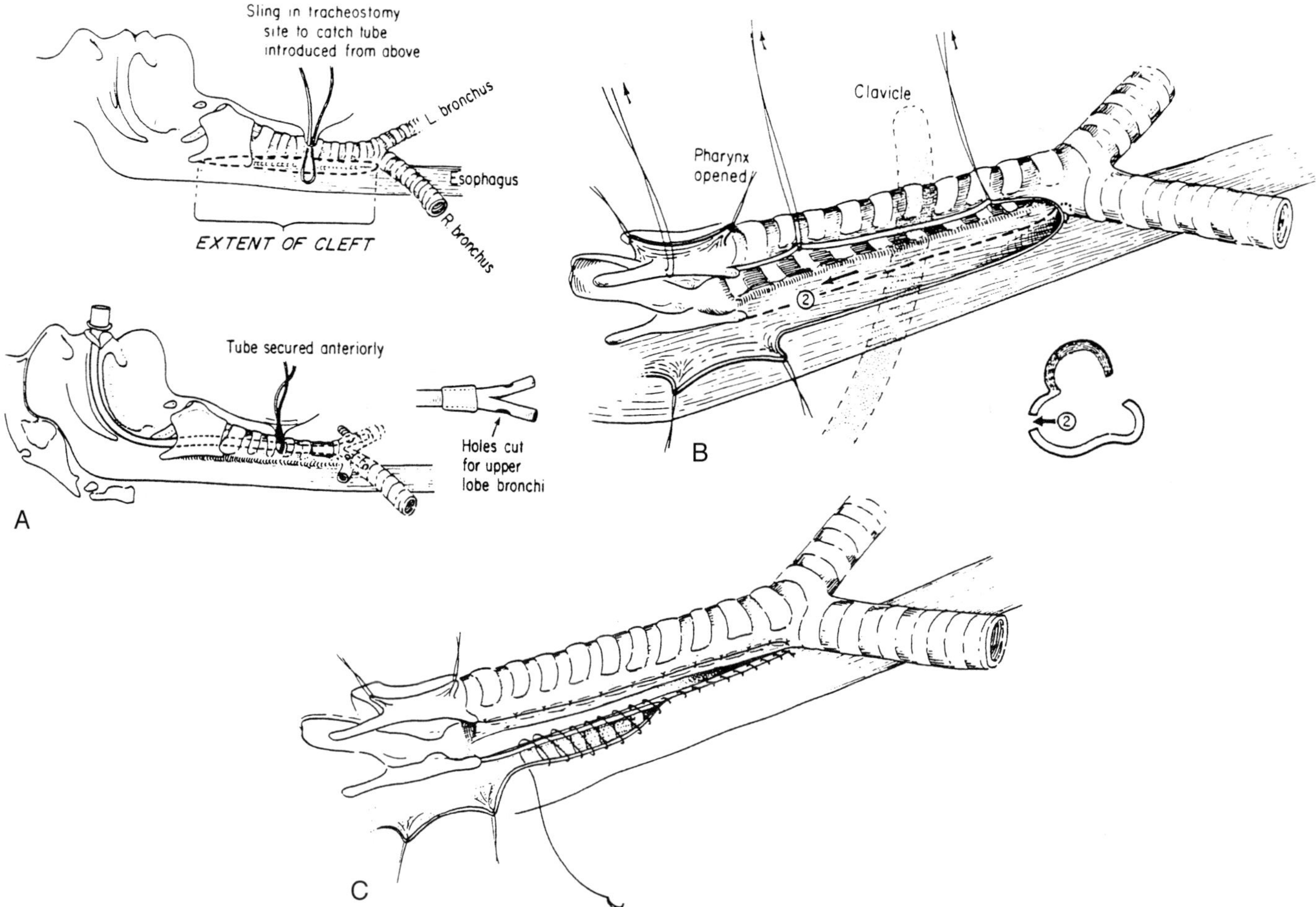

Figure 3–14. Repair of a type III LTEC. *A*, Stabilization of a bifurcated endotracheal tube is performed at bronchoscopy using a loop passed through a tracheotomy, which draws the endotracheal tube forward. *B*, A cervical and thoracic approach allows retropleural exposure of the cleft. A longitudinal incision is made in the right tracheoesophageal groove below the tracheal rings. The incision is extended inferiorly and across the esophagus and up the left side, leaving approximately 1 cm of esophageal wall attached to the trachea to allow adequate tissue to close the trachea. *C*, The trachea has been closed with interrupted sutures, and the esophagus is closed in a running fashion up to the thoracic inlet. Closure of the laryngeal portion of the cleft and the lateral pharyngeal wall is not yet accomplished. (From Donahoe PK, and Gee PE: Complete laryngotracheal cleft: management and repair. J Pediatr Surg *19:*143, 1984. Used with permission.)

sides with squamous epithelium and typically has an eccentric opening. Symptoms usually occur at several months of age as the infant begins taking solid food.

The second type of CES has been termed *idiopathic muscular hypertrophy* or *fibromuscular stenosis*, and it is the most common form of CES in some reports.[179] Histologically, these lesions appear to show submucosal proliferation of smooth muscle fibers and fibrous connective tissue with normal overlying squamous epithelium.[179] A resemblance to hypertrophic pyloric stenosis has been suggested[179,183]; however, there is no clear embryologic or pathogenic explanation for these lesions.

CES due to tracheobronchial remnants is described as the most common type of CES in some reports, and certainly it is the most described and understood of the three types of CES. It is believed that CES due to tracheobronchial remnants occurs as part of a spectrum of anomalies, including EA/TEF, related to the separation of the foregut from the respiratory tract around the 25th embryonic day.[184] Tracheobronchial tissue is believed to become sequestered in the wall of the esophagus, residing in the typical distal location because of the higher growth rate of the esophagus compared with the tracheobronchial tree.

CES due to tracheobronchial remnants was first reported in 1936 by Frey and Duschel[185] in a 19-year-old girl who died with the diagnosis of achalasia. In 1964, Holder et al.[36] noted three cases of distal esophageal stenosis in their review of 1,058 infants with EA, TEF, or both. After several additional reports,[186,187] Spitz[188] first demonstrated in 1973 a clear congenital basis for this disorder. Up to 1991, fewer than 50 cases of CES secondary to tracheobronchial remnants had been reported in the English- and German-language literature.[184] In addition, 71 cases had been reported in the Japanese literature as of 1981,[181] and of a total of 76 cases of CES in 1987, 6 were from the Chinese-language literature.[189]

Diagnosis

Symptoms of CES usually begin in infancy with progressive dysphagia and vomiting, typically after the introduction of semisolid or solid foods around the age of 6 months. There are, however, case reports of severe symptoms of regurgitation and respiratory distress in the newborn.[179] In some patients, a foreign body in the esophagus may be the first symptom noted.[190] It is frequently difficult to establish the correct diagnosis. Contrast esophagography typically reveals an abrupt distal esophageal narrowing, most often interpreted as a stricture related to GER. Stenosis secondary to fibromuscular hypertrophy can demonstrate a more tapered narrowing (see Fig. 3-16). CES caused by webs or fibromuscular hypertrophy can on occasion present as mid or even upper esophageal stenosis.[191] Over time, the esophagus proximal to the stenosis can dilate, and contrast study results can be interpreted as achalasia.[192] Additional studies that are helpful in the differentiation of CES from achalasia and strictures due to GER include esophageal manometry and pH monitoring. Esophagoscopy typically will demonstrate esophageal narrowing with normal-appearing mucosa at the level of the stenosis in cases of CES.

Treatment

The treatment of CES should allow for relief of the symptoms of stenosis and maintenance of antireflux mechanism of the gastroesophageal junction. Bougienage has been typically successful in the treatment of CES secondary to fibromuscular hypertrophy. Antegrade and retrograde tapered dilators have been the traditional form of bougienage, but hydrostatic balloon dilation has been successful.[179,192] A series of dilatations may be required for resolution of the stenosis. Membranous webs have on occasion been adequately treated with dilations, and there is one report of the successful endoscopic excision of a congenital web.[193]

Most membranous webs and CES secondary to tracheobronchial remnants must be treated through surgical excision, either as the primary approach or after unsuccessful attempts at dilation. It is important to clearly identify the location of the stenosis preoperatively with contrast esophagography to plan the operative approach. A right thoracotomy is typically used for stenosis in the midesophagus, and a left thoracotomy is used for stenosis in the lower esophagus. An abdominal approach should be used for CES in the abdominal portion of the esophagus. At exploration, the exact extent of the stenosis can be difficult to determine, and the use of a balloon catheter passed beyond the stenosis, inflated, and pulled back against the stenosis has been suggested as a helpful technique.[194] In most cases, the stenosis is less than 3 cm, and segmental resection and end-to-end esophageal anastomosis can be accomplished, with care taken to preserve the phrenic and vagal nerves. In cases of long fibromuscular hypertrophy with failed dilation attempts, resection and esophageal replacement with colon, stomach, or jejunum might be necessary. If the stenosis is near the gastroesophageal junction, most surgeons advocate segmental resection with esophageal anastomosis and an antireflux procedure to prevent postoperative reflux. Modified Hill gastropexy and Nissen fundoplication, with or without pyloroplasty, have been most commonly used[179,194]; however, a Collis gastroplasty in combination with a Nissen fundoplication has been reported to be effective in dealing with esophageal shortening and postoperative GER.[195]

Results

Good long-term results have been reported for dilation and operative resection.[179] Patients who have undergone distal esophageal CES resection without an antireflux procedure have developed significant GER that requires a subsequent antireflux operation. Reported complications from treatment by dilation include esophageal leakage and failure of therapy. Complications after resection and anastomosis include esophageal leak with mediastinitis, which can typically be successfully treated with mediastinal drainage.

ESOPHAGEAL DUPLICATIONS

A variety of epithelium-lined cysts appear in the mediastinum. Enterogenous cysts or esophageal duplications account for one fourth of these mediastinal cysts. These cysts are found in the posterior mediastinum and are covered by an intestinal muscular wall. They are lined by intestinal epithelium, most commonly gastric epithelium. Occasionally, these cysts may be lined by ciliated respiratory epithelium.[196] Associated cervical and upper thoracic vertebral anomalies, such as hemivertebra, are very common.[197-201] Not infrequently, abdominal intestinal duplications are also present in the same patient. In fact, some of the esophageal duplications pass through the diaphragm and connect with duplications in the jejunum or with the jejunum itself.[202-204] Occasionally, the cysts may be attached to or communicate with the spinal canal; in this situation, they are termed *neurenteric cysts*.[200,201]

In general, these cysts are closely connected to the esophagus, but they may be readily dissected away during removal. They usually have no communication with the lumen of the esophagus and are generally filled with mucoid material. The high incidence of gastric-lined epithelium can lead to peptic ulceration of these cysts with resultant substernal pain, erosion into the bronchus or esophagus, and pulmonary hemorrhage.[196]

These cysts cause symptoms due to their size and location and to peptic ulceration. In general, they should be completely excised, keeping in mind the possible extension of the enteric cyst through the diaphragm into the abdomen.

VASCULAR RINGS

Vascular rings are a relatively rare cause of esophageal obstruction that result from faulty embryologic development of the aortic arch. These rings are either complete or incomplete and result in obstruction of the trachea, the esophagus, or both.[205-208]

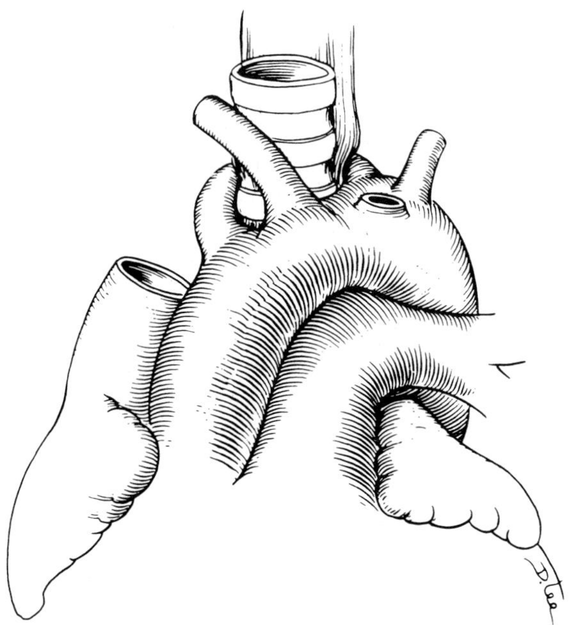

Figure 3–15. Typical anatomy in double aortic arch. Here, the anterior arch is larger, but in some instances the posterior arch is more important.

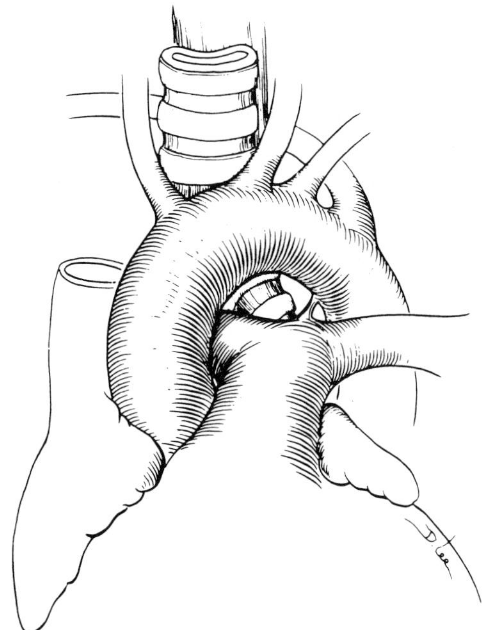

Figure 3–16. Typical anatomy in aberrant right subclavian artery.

Complete Rings

The double aortic arch represents the most common type of complete vascular ring (Fig. 3–15). It results from persistence of both the right and left embryologic aortic arches. The double aortic arch arises from the ascending aorta and then bifurcates, with one branch going to the right and behind the trachea and esophagus and the other branch passing to the left and in front of the trachea. These two branches join again to form the descending aorta. Each arch gives rise to a common carotid and subclavian artery; the innominate artery is usually absent. The ductus arteriosus may be on the left, on the right, or bilateral. The size of the arch varies, but the anterior, left arch is usually smaller.

The other complete ring is a right aortic arch with a left ligamentum arteriosum or ductus arteriosus. A complete ring is formed by the ascending aorta and pulmonary artery anteriorly, the aortic arch on the right, and either the ductus arteriosus or the ligamentum arteriosum and left subclavian artery on the left.

Incomplete Rings

An aberrant right subclavian artery is the most common vascular anomaly of the aorta, and it occurs in about 0.5% of the population. The aberrant artery arises as the last branch of the aortic arch and passes behind the esophagus to reach the right arm (Fig. 3–16). This anomaly is rarely symptomatic but may cause dysphagia (dysphagia lusoria) (Fig. 3–17).

A pulmonary artery sling, which results from an aberrant left pulmonary artery arising from the right pulmonary artery posteriorly and passing over the right main stem bronchus, causing compression of the right main stem bronchus and the distal trachea, is a rare anomaly that does not cause esophageal compression. Likewise, an anomalous innominate artery, which arises more distally than normal from the aorta, causes only tracheal compression.[209]

Clinical Picture

The symptoms caused by vascular rings result from compression of the trachea, the esophagus, or both. The

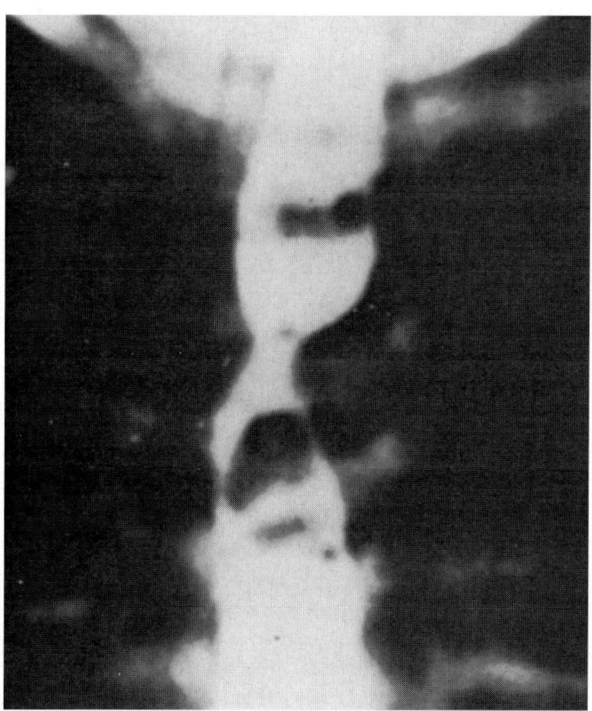

Figure 3–17. Barium esophagogram reveals typical lateral indentations.

child with a double aortic arch in general has the most symptoms early in infancy. The typical clinical picture is one of inspiratory wheezing, coughing, noisy breathing, shortness of breath, stridor, and frequent bouts of pneumonia. Feeding problems become apparent when solid foods are started. The diagnosis can be made with a barium swallow; however, the definitive diagnostic test is a computed tomography scan with intravenous contrast. Angiography and endoscopy are not usually needed to make a definitive diagnosis.

Treatment

Any patient who has symptoms that result from a vascular ring should be treated surgically.[210,211] Most vascular rings can be approached through a left anterolateral thoracotomy in the third or fourth interspace. In the case of a double aortic arch, the ductus arteriosus or ligamentum arteriosum is divided, and the smaller arch is then divided either distal to the origin of the left subclavian artery when the anterior (left) arch is hypoplastic or near its junction with the descending aorta when the posterior (right) arch is hypoplastic. If the arches are equal in size, the right or posterior arch is divided preferentially. After division of the arch, the fibrous tissue around the esophagus and trachea must be divided completely to free up these two structures. A right aortic arch with a left ligamentum arteriosum is managed by dividing the ligament and performing appropriate lysis of the fibrous tissue around the esophagus and trachea. A symptomatic aberrant right subclavian artery should be divided at its takeoff from the aorta through a left posterolateral thoracotomy. An anomalous innominate artery is managed by an aortopexy, in which the aortic arch is sutured to the undersurface of the sternum to open up the tracheal lumen.

ESOPHAGEAL REPLACEMENT IN CHILDREN

A brief discussion of esophageal replacement in children is warranted. This subject is covered much more extensively in Chapters 24 and 25. In the past, esophageal replacement in children was required for wide-gap EA with or without TEF, severe caustic injury to the esophagus, esophageal varices, peptic strictures due to GER, and esophageal destruction secondary to candidiasis in the immunologically suppressed patient. However, the frequency with which these indications occur is markedly diminished. Most surgeons make a vigorous attempt to stretch the upper blind esophageal pouch[212] and create upper pouch myotomies[83,213] to perform a primary anastomosis in a patient with a long-gap EA. This method of treatment has resulted in a marked decrease in the need for esophageal replacement in patients with this anomaly. Likewise, the need for esophageal replacement for severe caustic injuries has significantly decreased due to the success of vigorous initial management of this injury and the decreased incidence of this type of accident. The introduction of endosclerosis[214] and the high success rate of portosystemic shunts in children have eliminated the use of esophageal replacement for the management of esophageal varices in children.[215,216] Although esophageal replacement is occasionally required for a severe distal esophageal stricture secondary to peptic esophagitis resulting from GER, the prompt recognition of this abnormality in children has resulted in the occurrence of fewer of these types of strictures.[217]

Various tissues have been used for esophageal substitution, starting with antethoracic skin tubes (which were used for the first survivors of EA by Ladd,[5] Lanman,[4] and Gross[218]) and including jejunal segments, various parts of the colon,[219-222] gastric tubes, gastric pull-ups, and free jejunal grafts. The most commonly used esophageal substitutes are (1) the right or transverse colon,[223-232] (2) gastric tubes,[233-237] and (3) the gastric pull-up.[238,239] In each case, the substitute acts as a pure conduit, and there is no evidence of peristaltic activity. In most cases, gastric reflux into the conduit is minimal; if it does occur, the conduit is usually resistant to the effects of the acid. In a patient with EA who has been treated with a cervical esophagostomy and gastrostomy in the newborn period, the ideal age for esophageal replacement is about 1 year, when the child weighs about 20 lb.

Right colon substitution is performed through a laparotomy and cervical incision, in which the right colic and ileocolic arteries are divided and the blood supply of the right colon conduit is based on the middle colic artery.[240] The right colon is placed retrosternally in an isoperistaltic manner with the cecum anastomosed to the cervical esophagostomy in the neck. The lower end of the colon is anastomosed to the stomach.

A more popular colon substitute is the transverse colon based on the left colic artery,[223,226,227] as originally described by Waterston.[222] The operation is performed through a left thoracoabdominal incision through the seventh intercostal space, with circumferential division of the diaphragm to expose the intra-abdominal contents. The vascular supply of the transverse colon conduit is based on the left colic artery, and the middle colic artery is divided for mobilization. The conduit is brought up behind the pancreas and stomach to lie in the chest posterior to the hilus of the left lung. The proximal part of the conduit is placed posterior to the subclavian vessels and lateral to the carotid sheath, where it is anastomosed to the cervical esophagostomy. The distal end of the conduit is connected to the distal esophageal remnant or stomach in patients with EA and the stomach in patients with caustic injuries.

The results of colon interposition are in general very good. Death almost never occurs, and the complications are reasonable. The most common complication is an anastomotic leak in the neck, which usually closes spontaneously. This leak may result in a stricture at the cervical anastomosis, which is easily dilated. Occasionally, total ischemia of the conduit occurs because of inadequate arterial blood supply or venous obstruction. The inadequate arterial blood supply may also be secondary to undue tension. This is not very common but does require immediate removal of the conduit. The long-term follow-up of these children indicates that most grow and develop normally with good nutrition.

The gastric tube is an excellent alternative to colon interposition in patients with anomalies of the colon such as a high imperforate anus or failure of a previous colon interposition. After the introduction of the gastric tube by Gavriliu and Heimlich for esophageal substitution in adults, the procedure became popularized in children by Burrington and Stephens.[234] In 1973, Anderson and Randolph[233] reported their experience with 23 children with excellent results. The approach is made through an abdominal and cervical incision. The gastrocolic omentum is divided a safe distance from the gastroepiploic vessels. The right gastroepiploic artery is divided at the point of origin of the gastric tube, a site that is carefully selected to avoid narrowing of the pyloric outlet. This is usually 2 cm proximal to the pylorus. The GIA stapler (United States Surgical Corporation) is placed 2 cm from the greater curvature encompassing both anterior and posterior gastric walls, using a No. 18 to 24 French chest tube in the stomach along the greater curvature as a guide for the stapler and to ensure an appropriately sized gastric tube. The spleen is preserved after division of the short gastric vessels. The staple lines are reinforced with nonabsorbable sutures. The gastric tube can be brought to the neck either through a substernal tunnel or behind the hilus of the left lung through a small thoracotomy. The distal end of the gastric tube is anastomosed to the cervical esophagostomy. The mortality rate for this operation is similar to that with colon interposition. The complication rates are also about the same. The most common complication is a leak at the cervical anastomosis, which usually closes spontaneously. The other complications include ischemic stricture of the conduit itself, pyloric outlet obstruction that requires pyloroplasty, and early leak into the chest from the gastric tube suture line. Although follow-up with this operation is not as long as that with the colon interposition, most series report excellent growth and development in children who have undergone this operation in infancy and early childhood.

The latest operation for esophageal replacement in children is the gastric pull-up.[238,239] Although there is extensive experience with this operation in adults with carcinoma of the esophagus, there has been great concern about the physiologic effect of this procedure on young children. The two concerns are the effect on nutrition of a stomach placed in the thoracic cavity and the potential compression of the lung by the intrathoracic stomach. In fact, neither of these has been a problem in the children who have been treated with this procedure to date. The operation can be done either through a cervical and abdominal approach or by using a left thoracoabdominal exposure along with a cervical incision. The Hospital for Sick Children at Great Ormond Street in London has had significant experience with this operation (>100 cases), with excellent results.[239] In fact, their results with this operation appear to be better than their extensive experience with the Waterston coloesophagoplasty, which was developed at that institution.

References

1. Gibson, T.: The Anatomy of Humane Bodies Epitomized, 5th ed. London, Awnsham and Churchill, 1697.
2. Durston, W.: Philosophical Transaction of the Royal Society. 1670.
3. Vogt, E.C.: Congenital atresia of the esophagus. Am. J. Roentgenol., *22:*463, 1929.
4. Lanman, T.H.: Congenital atresia of the esophagus: A study of thirty-two cases. Arch. Surg., *41:*1060, 1940.
5. Ladd, W.E.: The surgical treatment of esophageal atresia and tracheoesophageal fistulas. N. Engl. J. Med., *230:*625, 1944.
6. Leven, N.L.: Congenital atresia of the esophagus with tracheoesophageal fistula. J. Thorac. Surg., *648*, 1940.
7. Haight, C., and Towsley, H.: Congenital atresia of the esophagus with tracheoesophageal fistula: Extrapleural ligation of fistula and end-to-end anastomosis of esophageal segments. Surg. Gynecol. Obstet., *76:*672, 1943.
8. Haight, C.: Congenital esophageal atresia and trachesophageal fistula. *In* Mustard, W.T., et al. (eds.): Pediatric Surgery. Chicago, Year-Book Medical Publishers, 1969, p. 357.
9. His, W.: Zur Bildungsgeschischte der Lungen beim menschlischen Embryo. Arch. Anat., *89*, 1887.
10. Grosser, O., Lewis, F.T., and McMurrich, J.P.: The development of the intestinal tract and respiratory organs. *In* Keibel, F., and Mall, F.P. (eds.): Manual of Human Embryology. Philadelphia, J.B. Lippincott, 1912, p. 291.
11. Smith, E.I.: The early development of the trachea and esophagus in relation to atresia of the esophagus and tracheoesophageal fistula. Embryol. Carnegie Inst., *36:*41, 1957.
12. Rosenthal, A.H.: Congenital atresia of the esophagus with tracheoesophageal fistula: Report of eight cases. Arch. Pathol., *12:*756, 1931.
13. Streeter, G.L.: Development horizons in human embryos: Description of age groups XV, XVI, XVII, XVIII. Contr. Embryol. Carnegie Inst., *32:*133, 1945.
14. Skandalakis, J.E., and Gray, S.W.: Embryology for Surgeons. Philadelphia, W.B. Saunders, 1994, p. 65.
15. Kluth, D., Steding, G., and Seidl, W.: The embryology of foregut malformations. J. Pediatr. Surg., *22:*389, 1987.
16. O'Rahilly, R., and Muller, F.: Chevalier Jackson lecture. Respiratory and alimentary relations in staged human embryos: New embryological data and congenital anomalies. Ann. Otol. Rhinol. Laryngol., *93:*421, 1984.
17. Politzer, G.: Die formale Benese der kongenitalen atresia des darmes beim Menschen. Roux'Arch Entwicklungsmechanik, *147:*119, 1954.
18. Diez-Pardo, J.A., et al.: A new rodent experimental model of esophageal atresia and tracheoesophageal fistula: Preliminary report. J. Pediatr. Surg., *31:*498, 1996.
19. Crisera, C., et al.: TTF-1 and HNF-3b in the developing tracheoesophageal fistula: Further evidence for the respiratory origin of the 'distal esophagus.' J. Pediatr. Surg., *34:*1322, 1999.
20. Spitz, L.: Esophageal atresia: Past, present, and future. J. Pediatr. Surg., *31:*19, 1996.
21. Kyyronen, P., and Hemminki, K.: Gastro-intestinal atresias in Finland in 1970–79, indicating time-place clustering. J. Epidemiol. Commun. Health, *42:*257, 1988.
22. Haight, C.: Some observations on esophageal atresias and tracheoesophageal fistulas of congenital origin. J. Thorac. Surg., *34:*141, 1957.
23. Myers, N.A.: Oesophageal atresia: The epitome of modern surgery. Ann. R. Coll. Surg. Engl., *54:*277, 1974.
24. Harris, J., Kallen, B., and Robert, E.: Descriptive epidemiology of alimentary tract atresia. Teratology, *52:*15, 1995.
25. Szendrey, T., Danyi, G., and Czeizel, A.: Etiological study on isolated esophageal atresia. Hum. Genet., *70:*51, 1985.
26. Chen, H., Goei, G.S., and Hertzler, J.H.: Family studies in congenital esophageal atresia with or without tracheoesophageal fistula. In Epstein, C.J., et al. (eds.): Risk, Communication, and Decision Making in Genetic Counseling, Vol. BD:OAS XV(5C). New York, Alan R. Liss for the National Foundation March-of-Dimes, 1979, p. 27.
27. Johnsson, E., Larsson, G., and Ljunggren, M.: Severe malformations in infant born to hyperthyroid woman on methimazole. Lancet, *350:*1520, 1997.
28. Pletcher, B.A., et al.: Familial occurrence of esophageal atresia with and without tracheoesophageal fistula: report of two unusual kindreds. Am. J. Med. Genet., *39:*380, 1991.
29. Grieve, J.G., and McDermott, J.G.: Congenital atresia of the oesophagus in two brothers. Can. Med. Assoc. J., *41:*185, 1939.

30. Engel, P.M., et al.: Esophageal atresia with tracheoesophageal fistula in mother and child. J. Pediatr. Surg., *5*:564, 1970.
31. Forrester, R.M., and Cohen, S.J.: Esophageal atresia associated with an anorectal anomaly and probably laryngeal fissure in three siblings. J. Pediatr. Surg., *5*:674, 1970.
32. Warren, J., Evans, K., and Carter, C.O.: Offspring of patients with tracheo-oesophageal fistula. J. Med. Genet., *16*:338, 1979.
33. Van-Staey, M., et al.: Familial congenital esophageal atresia: Personal case report and review of the literature. Hum. Genet., *66*:260, 1984.
34. Lipson, A.H., and Berry, A.B.: Oesophageal atresia in father and daughter. Aust. Paediatr. J., *20*:329, 1984.
35. Dunn, J.C., Fonkalsrud, E.W., and Atkinson, J.B.: Simplifying the Waterston's stratification of infants with tracheoesophageal fistula. Am. Surg., *65*:908, 1999.
36. Holder, T.M., et al.: Esophageal atresia and tracheoesophageal fistula: A survey of its members by the surgical section of the American Academy of Pediatrics. Pediatrics, *34*:542, 1964.
37. Beasley, S.W., et al.: Urinary tract abnormalities in association with oesophageal atresia frequency, significance, and influence on management. Pediatr. Surg. Int., *7*:94, 1992.
38. Rejjal, A.: Congenital anomalies associated with esophageal atresia: Saudi experience. Am. J. Perinatol., *16*:239, 1999.
39. Spitz, L., et al.: Management of esophageal atresia. World J. Surg., *17*:296, 1993.
40. German, J.C., Mahour, G.H., and Woolley, M.M.: Esophageal atresia and associated anomalies. J. Pediatr. Surg., *11*:299, 1976.
41. Xia, H., et al.: Skeletal malformations associated with esophageal atresia: Clinical and experimental studies. J. Pediatr. Surg., *34*:1385, 1999.
42. Cieri, M.V., Arnold, G.L., and Torfs, C.P.: Malrotation in conjunction with esophageal atresia/tracheo-esophageal fistula. Teratology, *60*:114, 1999.
43. Cord-Udy, C.L., Wright, V.M., and Drake, D.P.: Association of ambiguous genitalia with VATER anomalies and its significance in management. Pediatr. Surg. Int., *11*:50, 1996.
44. Spitz, L.: Esophageal atresia and tracheoesophageal fistula in children. Curr. Opin. Pediatr., *5*:347, 1993.
45. Tsang, T.M., Tam, P.K.H., and Westaby, S.: Management of coexisting coarctation of the aorta and oesophageal atresia. Pediatr. Surg. Int., *11*:107, 1996.
46. Quan, L., and Smith, D.W.: The VATER association: Vertebral defects, anal atresia, T-E fistula with esophageal atresia, radial and renal dysplasia: A spectrum of associated defects. J. Pediatr., *82*:104, 1973.
47. Baumann, W., et al.: VATER oder ACTERL syndrom. Klin. Pediatr., *188*:328, 1976.
48. Iuchtman, M., et al.: Morbidity and mortality in 46 patients with the VACTERL association. Isr. J. Med. Sci., *28*:281, 1992.
49. Kutiyanawala, M., et al.: CHARGE and esophageal atresia. J. Pediatr. Surg., *27*:558, 1992.
50. Chittmittrapap, S., et al.: Oesophageal atresia and associated anomalies. Arch. Dis. Child., *64*:364, 1989.
51. Poenaru, D., et al.: A new prognostic classification for esophageal atresia. Surgery, *113*:426, 1993.
52. Spitz, L., et al.: Esophageal atresia: At-risk groups for the 1990s. J. Pediatr. Surg., *29*:723, 1994.
53. Steadland, K.M., et al.: Unilateral pulmonary agenesis, esophageal atresia, and distal tracheoesophageal fistula. Ann. Thorac. Surg., *59*:511, 1995.
54. Perel, Y., et al.: Oesophageal atresia, VACTERL association: Fanconi's anaemia related spectrum of anomalies. Arch. Dis. Child., *78*:375, 1998.
55. Ein, S.H., et al.: Esophageal atresia with distal tracheoesophageal fistula: Associated anomalies and prognosis in the 1980s. J. Pediatr. Surg., *24*:1055, 1989.
56. Parent, P., et al.: Clinical heterogeneity of Townes-Brocks syndrome. Arch. Pediatr., *2*:551, 1995.
57. Hennekam, R.C., Huber, J., and Variend, D.: Bartsocas-Papas syndrome with internal anomalies: Evidence for a more generalized epithelial defect or new syndrome? Am. J. Med. Genet., *53*:102, 1994.
58. Pul, N., Pul, M., and Gedik, Y.: McKusick-Kaufman syndrome associated with esophageal atresia and distal tracheoesophageal fistula: A case report and review of the literature. Am. J. Med. Genet., *49*:341, 1994.
59. Louhimo, I., and Lindahl, H.: Esophageal atresia: Primary results of 500 consecutively treated patients. J. Pediatr. Surg., *18*:217; discussion 225, 1983.
60. Manning, P.B., et al.: Fifty years' experience with esophageal atresia and tracheoesophageal fistula: Beginning with Cameron Haight's first operation in 1935. Ann. Surg., *204*:446, 1986.
61. Randolph, J.G.: Esophageal atresia and congenital stenosis—Esophageal atresia and associated malformations, including laryngotracheoesophageal cleft. *In* Welch, M.D., et al. (eds.): Pediatric Surgery. Chicago/London, Year-Book Medical Publishers, Inc., 1986, p. 682.
62. Beasley, S.W., et al.: Developments in the management of oesophageal atresia and tracheo-oesophageal fistulas. Med. J. Aust., *150*:501, 1989.
63. Engum, S.A., et al.: Analysis of morbidity and mortality in 227 cases of esophageal atresia and/or tracheoesophageal fistula over two decades. Arch. Surg., *130*:502; discussion 508, 1995.
64. Randolph, J.G., Newman, K.D., and Anderson, K.D.: Current results in repair of esophageal atresia with tracheoesophageal fistula using physiologic status as a guide to therapy. Ann. Surg., *209*:526; discussion 530, 1989.
65. Brown, A.K., and Tam, P.K.: Measurement of gap length in esophageal atresia: A simple predictor of outcome. J. Am. Coll. Surg., *182*:41, 1996.
66. Stringer, M.D., et al.: Prenatal diagnosis of esophageal atresia. J. Pediatr. Surg., *30*:1258, 1995.
67. Farrant, P.: The antenatal diagnosis of oesophageal atresia by ultrasound. Br. J. Radiol., *53*:1202, 1980.
68. Satoh, S., et al.: Antenatal sonographic detection of the proximal esophageal segment: Specific evidence for congenital esophageal atresia. J. Clin. Ultrasound, *23*:419, 1995.
69. Sweed, Y., Bar-Maor, J.A., and Shoshany, G.: Insertion of a soft Silastic nasogastric tube at operation for esophageal atresia: A new technical method. J. Pediatr. Surg., *27*:650, 1992.
70. Shandling, B.: The insertion of a soft Silastic nasogastric tube at an operation for an esophageal atresia. J. Pediatr. Surg., *28*:280, 1993.
71. Moriarty, K.P., et al.: Transanastomotic feeding tubes in repair of esophageal atresia. J. Pediatr. Surg., *31*:53, 1996.
72. Salem, M.R., et al.: Prevention of gastric distention during anesthesia for newborns with tracheoesophageal fistulas. Anesthesiology, *38*:82, 1973.
73. Filston, H.C., et al.: The Fogarty balloon catheter as an aid to management of the infant with esophageal atresia and tracheoesophageal fistula complicated by severe RDS or pneumonia. J. Pediatr. Surg., *17*:149, 1982.
74. Randolph, J.G., Tunell, W.P., and Lilly, J.R.: Gastric division in the critically ill infant with esophageal atresia and tracheoesophageal fistula. Surgery, *63*:496, 1968.
75. Leininger, B.J.: Silastic banding of esophagus with subsequent repair of esophageal atresia and tracheosesophageal fistula. J. Pediatr. Surg., *7*:404, 1972.
76. Templeton, J., Jr., et al.: Management of esophageal atresia and tracheoesophageal fistula in the neonate with severe respiratory distress syndrome. J. Pediatr. Surg., *20*:394, 1985.
77. Chan, K.L., and Saing, H.: Combined flexible endoscopy and fluoroscopy in the assessment of the gap between the two esophageal pouches in esophageal atresia without fistula. J. Pediatr. Surg., *30*:668, 1995.
78. Puri, P., et al.: Delayed primary anastomosis for esophageal atresia: 18 months' to 11 years' follow-up. J. Pediatr. Surg., *27*:1127, 1992.
79. Ein, S.H., Shandling, B., and Heiss, K.: Pure esophageal atresia: Outlook in the 1990s. J. Pediatr. Surg., *28*:1147, 1993.
80. Howard, R., and Myers, N.A.: Esophageal atresia: A technique for elongating the upper pouch. Surgery, *58*:725, 1965.
81. Mahour, G.H., Woolley, M.M., and Gwinn, J.L.: Elongation of the upper pouch and delayed anatomic reconstruction in esophageal atresia. J. Pediatr. Surg., *9*:373, 1974.
82. Livaditis, A.: End-to-end anastomosis in esophageal atresia: A clinical and experimental study. Scand. J. Thorac. Cardiovasc. Surg., *2*:Suppl 2:7, 1969.
83. Livaditis, A., Radberg, L., and Odensjo, G.: Esophageal end-to-end anastomosis. Reduction of anastomotic tension by circular myotomy. Scand. J. Thorac. Cardiovasc. Surg., *6*:206; discussion 209, 1972.
84. Livaditis, A.: Esophageal atresia: A method of over-bridging long segmental gaps. Z. Kinderchir., *13*:298, 1973.

85. Eraklis, A.J., Rossello, P.J., and Ballintine, T.V.N.: Circular esophagomyotomy of the upper pouch in primary repair of long segment esophageal atresia. J. Pediatr. Surg., *11*:709, 1976.
86. Kontor, E.J.: Esophageal atresia with wide gap: Primary anastomosis following Livaditis procedure. J. Pediatr. Surg., *11*:583, 1976.
87. Slim, M.S.: Circular myotomy of the esophagus: Clinical application in esophageal atresia. Ann. Thorac. Surg., *23*:62, 1977.
88. Vizas, D., Ein, S.H., and Simpson, J.S.: The valve of circular myotomy for esophageal atresia. J. Pediatr. Surg., *13*:357, 1978.
89. de Lorimer, A.A., and Harrison, M.R.: Long gap esophageal atresia. J. Thorac. Coardiovasc. Surg., *79*:138, 1980.
90. Janik, J.S., et al.: Long-term follow-up of circular myotomy for esophageal atresia. J. Pediatr. Surg., *15*:835; discussion 840, 1980.
91. Hoffman, D.G., and Moazam, F.: Transcervical myotomy for wide-gap esophageal atresia. J. Pediatr. Surg., *19*:680, 1984.
92. Lindahl, H., and Louhimo, I.: Livaditis myotomy in long-gap esophageal atresia. J. Pediatr. Surg., *22*:109, 1987.
93. Schwartz, M.Z.: An improved technique for circular myotomy in long-gap esophageal atresia. J. Pediatr. Surg., *18*:833, 1983.
94. Lindahl, H.: Esophageal atresia: A simple technical detail aiding the mobilization and circular myotomy of the proximal segment. J. Pediatr. Surg., *22*:113, 1987.
95. De Carvalho, J.L., Maynard, J., and Hadley, G.P.: An improved technique for in situ esophageal myotomy and proximal pouch mobilization in patients with esophageal atresia. J. Pediatr. Surg., *24*:872, 1989.
96. Coran, A.G.: Ultra-long-gap esophageal atresia: How long is long? Ann. Thorac. Surg., *57*:528, 1994.
97. Lai, J.Y., et al.: Experience with distal circular myotomy for long-gap esophageal atresia. J. Pediatr. Surg., *31*:1503, 1996.
98. Kimura, K., et al.: A new approach for the salvage of unsuccessful esophageal atresia repair: A spiral myotomy and delayed definitive operation. J. Pediatr. Surg., *22*:981, 1987.
99. Rossello, P.J., Lebron, H., and Franco, A.A.: The technique of myotomy in esophageal reconstruction: An experimental study. J. Pediatr. Surg., *15*:430, 1980.
100. Lindell-Iwan, L.: Modification of Livaditis' myotomy for long gap oesophageal atresia. Ann. Chir. Gynaecol., *79*:101, 1990.
101. Gough, M.: Esophageal atresia—Use of an anterior flap in the difficult anastomosis. J. Pediatr. Surg., *15*:310, 1980.
102. Ten Kate, J.: A method of suturing in operations for congenital oesophageal atresia. J. Arch. Chir. Neder., *4*:43, 1952.
103. Bar-Maor, J.A., Shoshany, G., and Sweed, Y.: Wide gap esophageal atresia: A new method to elongate the upper pouch. J. Pediatr. Surg., *24*:882, 1989.
104. Davenport, M., and Bianchi, A.: Early experience with oesophageal flap oesophagoplasty for repair of oesophageal atresia. Pediatr. Surg. Int., *5*:332, 1990.
105. Kimura, K., and Soper, R.T.: Multistaged extrathoracic esophageal elongation for long gap esophageal atresia. J. Pediatr. Surg., *29*:566, 1994.
106. Otte, J.B., et al.: Diverticulum formation after circular myotomy for esophageal atresia. J. Pediatr. Surg., *19*:68, 1984.
107. Siegel, M.J., et al.: Circular esophageal myotomy simulating a pulmonary or mediastinal pseudocyst. Pediatr. Radiol., *136*:365, 1980.
108. Shepard, R., Fenn, S., and Sieber, W.K.: Evaluation of esophageal function in postoperative esophageal atresia and tracheoesophageal fistula. Surgery, *59*:608, 1966.
109. Duranceau, A., et al.: Motor function of the esophagus after repair of esophageal atresia and tracheoesophageal fistula. Surgery, *82*:116, 1977.
110. Orringer, M.B., Kirsh, M.M., and Sloan, H.: Long-term esophageal function following repair of esophageal atresia. Ann. Surg., *186*:436, 1977.
111. Wearlin, S.L., et al.: Esophageal function in esophageal atresia. Dig. Dis. Sci., *26*:796, 1981.
112. Sumitomo, K., Ikeda, K., and Nagasaki, A.: Esophageal manometrical assessment after esophageal circular myotomy for wide-gap esophageal atresia. Jpn. J. Surg., *18*:218, 1988.
113. Schärli, A.F.: Esophageal reconstruction in very long atresias by elongation of the lesser curvature. Pediatr. Surg. Int., *7*:101, 1992.
114. Evans, M.: Application of Collis gastroplasty to the management of esophageal atresia. J. Pediatr. Surg., *30*:1232, 1995.
115. MacKinlay, G.A., and Burtles, R.: Oesophageal atresia: Paralysis and ventilation in management of the wide gap. Pediatr. Surg. Int., *2*:10, 1987.
116. Ein, S.H., and Shandling, B.: Pure esophageal atresia: A 50-year review. J. Pediatr. Surg., *29*:1208, 1994.
117. Usui, N., et al.: Anomalies of the tracheobronchial tree in patients with esophageal atresia. J. Pediatr. Surg., *31*:258, 1996.
118. Beasley, S.W., Auldist, A.W., and Myers, N.A.: Current surgical management of oesophageal atresia and/or tracheo-oesophageal fistula. Aust. A.Z. J. Surg., *59*:707, 1989.
119. Dudgeon, D.L., Morrison, C.W., and Woolley, M.M.: Congenital proximal tracheoesophageal fistula. J. Pediatr. Surg., *7*:614, 1972.
120. Johnson, A.M., et al.: Esophageal atresia with double fistula: The missed anomaly. Ann. Thorac. Surg., *38*:195, 1984.
121. O'Neill, J., Jr., G. Holcomb, Jr., and Neblett, W.D.: Recent experience with esophageal atresia. Ann. Surg., *195*:739, 1982.
122. Waterston, D.J., Bonham-Carter, R.E., and Aberdeen, E.: Esophageal atresia: tracheo-oesophageal fistula: A study of survival in 218 infants. Lancet, *819*, 1962:
123. Wheatley, M.J., and Coran, A.G.: Pericardial flap interposition for the definitive management of recurrent tracheoesophageal fistula. J. Pediatr. Surg., *27*:1122, 1992.
124. Chavin, K., et al.: Save the child's esophagus: Management of major disruption after repair of esophageal atresia. J. Pediatr. Surg., *31*:48, 1996.
125. Spitz, L., and Hitchcock, R.: Oesophageal atresia and tracheo-oesophageal fistula. *In* Freeman, N.V., et al. (eds.): Surgery of the Newborn. New York, Churchill Livingstone, 1994, p. 22.
126. Tam, P.K., et al.: Endoscopy-guided balloon dilatation of esophageal strictures and anastomotic strictures after esophageal replacement in children. J. Pediatr. Surg., *26*:1101, 1991.
127. Allmendinger, N., et al.: Balloon dilation of esophageal strictures in children. J. Pediatr. Surg., *31*:334, 1996.
128. Ein, S.H., et al.: Recurrent tracheoesophageal fistulas: Seventeen-year review. J. Pediatr. Surg., *18*:436, 1983.
129. McKinnon, L.J., and Kosloske, A.M.: Prediction and prevention of anastomotic complications of esophageal atresia and tracheo-esophageal fistula. J. Pediatr. Surg., *25*:778, 1990.
130. Coran, A.G.: Pericardioesophageoplasty: A new operation for partial esophageal replacement. Am. J. Surg., *125*:294, 1973.
131. Botham, M.J., and Coran, A.G.: The use of pericardium for the management of recurrent tracheoesophageal fistula. J. Pediatr. Surg., *21*:164, 1986.
132. Kosloske, A.M.: Azygous flap technique for reinforcement of esophageal closure. J. Pediatr. Surg., *25*:793, 1990.
133. Spitz, L.: Recurrent tracheoesophageal fistula. *In* Pediatric Surgery, 5th ed. Spitz, L., and Coran, A.G. (eds.): London, Chapman & Hall Medical, 1995, p. 4.
134. Gdanietz, K., and Krause, I.: Plastic adhesives for closing esophago-tracheal fistulae in children. Z. Kinderchir., *17*:137, 1975.
135. Pompino, H.J.: Endoscopic closure of tracheo-esophageal fistulae. Z. Kinderchir., *27*:90, 1979.
136. Rangecroft, L., et al.: Endoscopic diathermy obliteration of recurrent tracheoesophageal fistulae. J. Pediatr. Surg., *19*:41, 1984.
137. Gutierrez, C., et al.: Recurrent tracheoesophageal fistula treated with fibrin glue. J. Pediatr. Surg., *29*:1567, 1994.
138. Wheatley, M.J., Coran, A.G., and Wesley, J.R.: Efficacy of the Nissen fundoplication in the management of gastroesophageal reflux following esophageal atresia repair. J. Pediatr. Surg., *28*:53, 1993.
139. Tovar, J.A., et al.: Ambulatory 24-hour manometric and pH metric evidence of permanent impairment of clearance capacity in patients with esophageal atresia. J. Pediatr. Surg., *30*:1224, 1995.
140. Jolley, S.G., et al.: Patterns of gastroesophageal reflux in children following repair of esophageal atresia and distal tracheoesophageal fistula. J. Pediatr. Surg., *15*:857, 1980.
141. Ashcraft, K.W., et al.: Early recognition and aggressive treatment of gastroesophageal reflux following repair of esophageal atresia. J. Pediatr. Surg., *12*:317, 1977.
142. Tibboel, D., et al.: Prospective evaluation of postoperative morbidity in patients with esophageal atresia. Pediatr. Surg. Int., *4*:252, 1988.
143. Parker, A.F., Christie, D.L., and Cahill, J.L.: Incidence and significance of gastroesophageal reflux following repair of esophageal atresia and tracheoesophageal fistula and the need for anti-reflux procedures. J. Pediatr. Surg., *14*:5, 1979.
144. Tovar, J.A., et al.: Barrett's oesophagus in children and adolescents. Pediatr. Surg. Int., *8*:389, 1993.
145. Cooper, J.E., Spitz, L., and Wilkins, B.M.: Barrett's esophagus in

children: A histologic and histochemical study of 11 cases. J. Pediatr. Surg., *22:*191, 1987.
146. Adzick, N.S., et al.: Esophageal adenocarcinoma 20 years after esophageal atresia repair. J. Pediatr. Surg., *24:*741, 1989.
147. Fonkalsrud, E.W.: Gastroesophageal fundoplication for reflux following repair of esophageal atresia: Experience with nine patients. Arch. Surg., *114:*48, 1979.
148. Spitz, L., Kiely, E., and Brereton, R.J.: Esophageal atresia: Five year experience with 148 cases. J. Pediatr. Surg., *22:*103, 1987.
149. Lindahl, H., Rintala, R., and Louhimo, I.: Failure of the Nissen fundoplication to control gastroesophageal reflux in esophageal atresia patients. J. Pediatr. Surg., *24:*985, 1989.
150. Corbally, M.T., Muftah, M., and Guiney, E.J.: Nissen fundoplication for gastro-esophageal reflux in repaired tracheo-esophageal fistula. Eur. J. Pediatr. Surg., *2:*332, 1992.
151. Filler, R.M., Rossello, P.J., and Lebowitz, R.L.: Life-threatening anoxic spells caused by tracheal compression after repair of esophageal atresia: correction by surgery. J. Pediatr. Surg., *11:*739, 1976.
152. Delius, R.E., Wheatley, M.J., and Coran, A.G.: Etiology and management of respiratory complications after repair of esophageal atresia with tracheoesophageal fistula. Surgery, *112:*527, 1992.
153. Wailoo, M.P., and Emery, J.L.: The trachea in children with tracheo-oesophageal fistula. Histopathology, *3:*329, 1979.
154. Kimura, K., et al.: Aortosternopexy for tracheomalacia following repair of esophageal atresia: Evaluation by cine-CT and technical refinement. J. Pediatr. Surg., *25:*769, 1990.
155. Rideout, D.T., et al.: The absence of clinically significant tracheomalacia in patients having esophageal atresia without tracheoesophageal fistula. J. Pediatr. Surg., *26:*1303, 1991.
156. Kiely, E.M., Spitz, L., and Brereton, R.: Management of tracheomalacia by aortopexy. Peidatr. Surg. Int., *2:*13, 1987.
157. Filler, R.M., Messineo, A., and Vinograd, I.: Severe tracheomalacia associated with esophageal atresia: Results of surgical treatment. J. Pediatr. Surg., *27:*1136; discussion 1140, 1992.
158. Gross, R.E., and Neuhauser, E.B.D.: Compression of the trachea by an anomalous innominate artery. Am. J. Dis. Child., *75:*570, 1945.
159. Schwartz, M.Z., and Filler, R.M.: Tracheal compression as a cause of apnea following repair of tracheoesophageal fistula: Treatment by aortopexy. J. Pediatr. Surg., *15:*842, 1980.
160. Benjamin, B., Cohen, D., and Glasson, M.: Tracheomalacia in association with congenital tracheoesophageal fistula. Surgery, *79:*504, 1976.
161. Cohen, D.: Tracheopexy—Aorto-tracheal suspension for severe tracheomalacia. Aust. Paediatr. J., *17:*117, 1981.
162. Applebaum, H., and Woolley, M.M.: Pericardial flap aortopexy for tracheomalacia. J. Pediatr. Surg., *25:*30, 1990.
163. Vinograd, I., Filler, R.M., and Bahoric, A.: Long-term functional results of prosthetic airway splinting in tracheomalacia and bronchomalacia. J. Pediatr. Surg., *22:*38, 1987.
164. Johnston, M.R., et al.: External stent for repair of secondary tracheomalacia. Ann. Thorac. Surg., *30:*291, 1980.
165. Bousamra, M., et al.: Wire stent for tracheomalacia in a five-year-old girl. Ann. Thorac. Surg., *61:*1239, 1996.
166. Richter, C.F.: Dissertatio Medica de Infanticido in Artis Obstetricae. Leipzig, 1792.
167. Finlay, H.V.L.: Familial congenital stridor. Arch. Dis. Child., *24:*219, 1949.
168. Pettersson, G.: Inhibited separation of the larynx and the upper part of the trachea from the esophagus in a newborn: Report of a case successfully operated upon. Acta Chir. Scand., *10:*250, 1955.
169. Blumberg, J.B., et al.: Laryngotracheo-esophageal cleft, the embryologic implications: Review of the literature. Surgery, *57:*559, 1965.
170. Phelan, P.D., et al.: Familial occurrence of congenital laryngeal clefts. Arch Dis. Child., *48:*275, 1973.
171. Greenberg, C.R., and Schraufnagel, D.: The G syndrome: A case report. Am. J. Med. Genet., *3:*59, 1979.
172. DuBois, J.J., et al.: Current management of laryngeal and laryngotracheoesophageal clefts. J. Pediatr. Surg., *25:*855, 1990.
173. Welch, R.G., and Husain, O.A.N.: Atresia of the oesophagus with common tracheo-oesophageal tube. Arch. Dis. Child., *367*, 1958.
174. Donahoe, P.K., and Hendren, W.H.: The surgical management of laryngotracheoesophageal cleft with tracheoesophageal fistula and esophageal atresia. Surgery, *71:*363, 1972.
175. Tyler, D.C.: Laryngeal cleft: Report of eight patients and review of the literature. Am. J. Genet., *21:*61, 1990.
176. Ryan, D.P., et al.: Laryngotracheoesophageal cleft (type IV): Management and repair of lesions beyond the carina. J. Pediatr. Surg., *26:*962; discussion 969, 1991.
177. Bell, D.W., et al.: Laryngotracheoesophageal cleft: The anterior approach. Ann. Otol. Rhinol. Laryngol., *86:*616, 1977.
178. Valerio, D., Jones, P.F., and Stewart, A.M.: Congenital oesophageal stenosis. Arch. Dis. Child., *52:*414, 1977.
179. Nihoul-Fekete, C., et al.: Congenital esophageal stenosis: A review of 20 cases. Pediatr. Surg. Int., *2:*86, 1987.
180. Murphy, S.G., Yazbeck, S., and Russo, P.: Isolated congenital esophageal stenosis. J. Pediatr. Surg., *30:*1238–1241, 1995.
181. Nishina, T., Tsuchida, Y., and Saito, S.: Congenital esophageal stenosis due to tracheobronchial remnants and its associated anomalies. J. Pediatr. Surg., *16:*190, 1981.
182. Kluth, D.: Atlas of esophageal atresia. J. Pediatr. Surg., *11:*901, 1976.
183. Todani, T., et al.: Congenital oesophageal stenosis due to fibromuscular thickening. Z. Kinderchir., *39:*11, 1984.
184. Yeung, C.K., et al.: Congenital esophageal stenosis due to tracheobronchial remnants: A rare but important association with esophageal atresia. J. Pediatr. Surg., *27:*852, 1992.
185. Frey, E.K., and Duschel, L.: The cardiospasms. Ergeb. Chirur. Orthop., *29:*637, 1936.
186. Tuqan, N.A.: Annular stricture of the esophagus distal to the congenital tracheoesophageal fistula. Surgery, *52:*394, 1962.
187. Mahour, G.H., et al.: Congenital esophageal stenosis distal to esophageal atresia. Surgery, *69:*936, 1971.
188. Spitz, L.: Congenital esophageal stenosis distal to associated esophageal atresia. J. Pediatr. Surg., *8:*973, 1973.
189. Liu, Y.X., and Xue, F.: Congenital esophageal stenosis due to tracheobronchial cartilage. Int. J. Pediatr. Otorhinolaryngol., *14:*95, 1987.
190. Bluestone, C.D., Kerry, R., and Sieber, W.K.: Congenital esophageal stenosis. Laryngoscope, *79:*1095, 1969.
191. Grabowski, S.T., and Andrews, D.A.: Upper esophageal stenosis: Two case reports. J. Pediatr. Surg., *31:*1438, 1996.
192. Neilson, I.R., et al.: Distal congenital esophageal stenosis associated with esophageal atresia. J. Pediatr. Surg., *26:*478; discussion 481, 1991.
193. Sharma, A.K., et al.: Congenital esophageal obstruction by intraluminal mucosal diaphragm. J. Pediatr. Surg., *26:*213, 1991.
194. Ohi, R., and Tseng, S.W.: Congenital oesophageal stenosis. *In* Puri, P. (ed.): Newborn Surgery. London, Butterworth-Heinemann, 1996.
195. Chahine, A.A., Campbell, A.B., and Hoffman, M.A.: Management of congenital distal esophageal stenosis with combined Collis gastroplasty-Nissen fundoplication. Pediatr. Surg. Int., *10:*23, 1995.
196. Macpherson, R.I., Reed, M.H., and Ferguson, C.C.: Intrathoracic gastrogenic cysts: A cause of lethal pulmnary hemorrhage in infants. J. Can. Assoc. Radiol., *24:*362, 1973.
197. Bentley, J.F.R., and Smith, J.R.: Developmental posterior enteric remnants and spinal malformations: The split notochord syndrome. Arch. Dis. Child, *35:*76, 1960.
198. Elwood, J.S.: Mediastinal duplication of the gut. Arch. Dis. Child., *35:*474, 1959.
199. Fallon, M., Gordon, A.R.G., and Lendrum, A.C.: Mediastinal cysts of foregut origin associated with vertebral abnormalities. Br. J. Surg., *41:*520, 1954.
200. Holmes, G.L., Trader, S., and Ignatiadis, P.: Intraspinal enterogenous cysts. Am. J. Child., *132:*906, 1978.
201. Mann, K.S., et al.: Spinal neurenteric cyst: Association with vertebral anomalies, diastematomyelia, dorsal fistula. Surg. Neurol., *32:*358, 1984.
202. Leider, H.J., Snodgrass, J.J., and Mishridk, A.S.: Intrathoracic alimentary duplications communicating with small intestine. Arch. Surg., *71:*203, 1955.
203. Pokorny, W.J., and Goldstein, I.R.: Enteric thoracoabdominal duplication in children. J. Thorac. Cardiovasc. Surg., *87:*821, 1984.
204. Shepherd, M.P.: Thoracic, thoraco-abdominal and abdominal duplication. Thorax, *20:*82, 1965.
205. Arciniegas, E., et al.: Surgical management of congenital vascular ring. J. Thorac. Cardiovasc. Surg., *77:*721, 1979.
206. Binet, J.P., and Langlois, J.: Aortic arch anomalies in children and infants. J. Thorac. Cardiovasc. Surg., *73:*248, 1977.
207. Edwards, J.E.: Anomalies of the derivatives of aortic arch system. Med. Clin. North Am., *32:*925, 1948.

208. Park, C.D., et al.: Tracheal compression by the great arteries in the mediastinum. Arch. Surg., *103:*626, 1971.
209. Gross, R.E., and Neuhauser, E.B.D.: Compression of the trachea by an anomalous innominate artery: An operation for its relief. Am. J. Dis. Child., *75:*570, 1948.
210. Richardson, J.V., et al.: Surgical management of vascular ring. Ann. Surg., *31:*426, 1981.
211. Roesler, M., et al.: Surgical management of vascular ring. Ann. Surg., *197:*139, 1983.
212. Woolley, M.M.: Esophageal atresia and tracheoesophageal fistula: 1939 to 1979. Am. J. Surg., *139:*771, 1980.
213. Ricketts, R.R., Luck, S.R., and Raffensperger, J.G.: Circular esophagomyotomy for primary repair of long-gap esophageal atresia. J. Pediatr. Surg., *16:*365, 1981.
214. Lilly, J.R., VanStiegmann, A., and Stellin, A.: Esophageal endosclerosis in children with portal vein thrombosis. J. Pediatr. Surg., *17:*571, 1982.
215. Altman, R.P.: Portal decompression by interposition mesocaval shunt in patients with biliary atresia. J. Pediatr. Surg., *11:*809, 1976.
216. Clatworthy, H.W., Jr., and Boles, E.J.: Extrahepatic portal bed block in children: Pathogenesis and treatments. Ann. Surg., *150:*371, 1959.
217. Skinner, D.B., and DeMeester, T.R.: Gastroesophageal reflux. Curr. Probl. Surg., ***131,*** 1976.
218. Gross, R.E.: The Surgery of Infancy and Childhood. Philadelphia, W.B. Saunders, 1955.
219. Othersen, H.B., and Clatworthy, H.W.: Functional evaluation of esophageal replacement in children. J. Thorac. Cardiovasc. Surg., *53:*53, 1967.
220. Schiller, M., Frey, T.R., and Boles, E.T.: Evaluation of colonic replacement of the esophagus in children. J. Pediatr. Surg., *6:*753, 1971.
221. Singh, A., and Rickham, P.P.: Subtotal colonic replacement of the esophagus in infancy. Br. J. Surg., *58:*377, 1977.
222. Waterston, D.: Colonic replacement of esophagus (intrathoracic). Surg. Clin. North Am., *44:*1441, 1964.
223. Azar, H., Crispin, A.R., and Waterston, D.J.: Esophageal replacement with transverse colon in infants and children. J. Pediatr. Surg., *6:*3, 1971.
224. Blanchard, H., et al.: Retrosternal esophageal replacement in children. Can. J. Surg., *15:*137, 1972.
225. Campbell, J.R., et al.: Esophageal replacement in infants and children by colon interposition. Am. J. Surg., *144:*29, 1982.
226. Freeman, N.V., and Cass, D.T.: Colon interposition: A modification of the Waterston technique using the normal esophageal route. J. Pediatr. Surg., *17:*17, 1982.
227. German, J.C., and Waterston, D.J.: Colon interposition for the replacement of the esophagus in children. J. Pediatr. Surg., *11:*227, 1976.
228. Gross, R.E., and Firestone, F.N.: Colonic reconstruction of the esophagus in infants and children. Surgery, *61:*955, 1967.
229. Kelly, J.P., Shackelford, G.D., and Rober, C.L.: Esophageal replacement with colon in children: Functional results and long-term growth. Ann. Thorac. Surg., *36:*634, 1983.
230. Longino, L.A., Woolley, M.M., and Gross, R.E.: Esophageal replacement in infants and children with use of a segment of colon. J.A.M.A., *171:*1187, 1959.
231. Neville, W.E., and Closes, G.H.A., Jr.: Colon replacement of the esophagus in children for congenital and acquired disease. J. Thorac. Cardiovasc. Surg., *40:*507, 1960.
232. Neville, W.E., and Najem, A.Z.: Colon replacement of the esophagus for congenital and benign disease. Ann. Thorac. Surg., *36:*626, 1983.
233. Anderson, K.D., and Randolph, J.G.: The gastric tube for esophageal replacement in infants and children. J. Thorac. Cardiovasc. Surg., *66:*33, 1973.
234. Burrington, J.D., and Stephens, C.A.: Esophageal replacement with a gastric tube in infants and children. J. Pediatr. Surg., *3:*246, 1968.
235. Cohen, D.H., Middleton, A.W., and Fletcher, J.: Gastric tube esophagoplasty. J. Pediatr. Surg., *9:*451, 1974.
236. Ein, S.H.H., et al.: A further look at the gastric tube as an esophageal replacement in infants and children. J. Pediatr. Surg., *8:*859, 1973.
237. Lindahl, H., Louhimo, I., and Virkola, K.: Colon interposition or gastric tube? Follow-up study of colon-esophagus and gastric tube esophagus patients. J. Pediatr. Surg., *18:*58, 1983.
238. Coran, A.G.: Gastric pull-up for esophageal replacement in infants and children. Movie presented at annual meeting of American College of Surgeons, October 1986.
239. Spitz, L., Kiely, E., and Sparnon, T.: Gastric transposition for esophageal replacement in children. Ann. Surg., *206:*69, 1987.
240. Mahoney, E.B., and Sherman, C.D.: Total esophagoplasty using intrathoracic right colon. Surgery, *35:*936, 1954.

VOLUME

I

Radiologic and Endoscopic Evaluation, Physiologic Studies, and Ultrasonography

CHAPTER

4 Radiologic Evaluation of the Esophagus

KAREN M. HORTON • BRONWYN JONES • ELLIOT K. FISHMAN

Endoscopic studies are often considered the diagnostic modality of choice for the evaluation of esophageal pathology. However, radiologic studies continue to play a vital role in the diagnosis of many benign and malignant diseases of the esophagus. Although upper endoscopy can be used to evaluate the esophageal lumen and mucosa, it cannot be used to detect extrinsic disease and provides limited functional information. Contrast esophagography allows real-time visualization of esophageal peristalsis, thereby providing both functional and anatomic information. Nuclear scintigraphy allows evaluation and quantification of esophageal peristalsis and gastroesophageal reflux. Computed tomography (CT) is used to image the esophageal lumen and adjacent structures.

This chapter reviews a variety of radiologic imaging studies commonly performed for the evaluation of esophageal pathology. Techniques, protocols, and radiographic findings are discussed and illustrated.

CONTRAST STUDIES

With the increasing availability and popularity of upper endoscopy, the number of upper gastrointestinal contrast studies that are performed annually continues to decline. However, contrast studies play a vital role in the diagnosis of many esophageal diseases and in the follow-up after surgery or other interventions. The contrast esophagogram is the main contrast study performed for imaging of the esophagus.

TECHNIQUE

Contrast esophagography can be performed with a variety of contrast agents and techniques, depending on the clinical indication.

The most sensitive method for examination of the esophageal mucosa is the *double-contrast esophagogram*. The technique allows visualization of processes that affect the esophageal mucosa, such as esophageal ulcers, early carcinomas, Barrett's esophagus, esophagitis, and others. During this examination, the patient is standing and at a slightly oblique angle. He or she swallows 4 to 6 g of effervescent granules with 10 ml of water and then immediately gulps approximately 50 to 75 ml of high-density (thick) barium (250% wt/vol). The effervescent granules will release carbon dioxide in the esophagus and stomach; the esophagus will therefore be distended and coated with the thick barium (Fig. 4-1). The distention is only transient, so the radiologist must quickly obtain the necessary spot films of the esophagus while it is maximally distended.

In patients who are unable to stand or who are unable to tolerate the effervescent granules, a *single-contrast* examination of the esophagus can be performed with a dilute (thin) barium suspension. To obtain single-contrast views of the esophagus, the patient is typically in the prone, right oblique position and drinks contrast medium

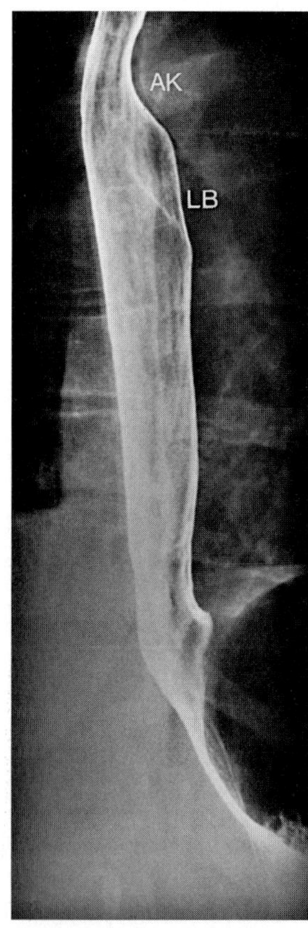

Figure 4-1. Normal double-contrast esophagogram demonstrates good esophageal distention and coating. The extrinsic impressions from the aortic knob (AK) and left main stem bronchus (LB) are normal.

quickly through a straw. If the patient is unable to lie prone, he or she can lie in the supine oblique position. With the single-contrast technique, the esophageal lumen is filled with the contrast material and appears as a continuous column (Fig. 4–2). Single-contrast examinations with thin barium are preferred in patients with suspected stricture, rings, or obstruction and are most sensitive for demonstrating hiatal hernias. Esophageal peristalsis is also best assessed in the prone, right anterior oblique position with a thin barium suspension. However, subtle mucosal abnormalities, such as shallow ulcers, superficial carcinomas, and mild esophagitis, are not reliably detected with the single-contrast technique. For complete evaluation of the esophagus, both double-contrast and single-contrast examinations are performed.

If esophageal perforation is suspected, a single-contrast esophagogram should be performed with a water-soluble contrast agent. These agents include Gastrografin or Omnipaque and are readily absorbed from the mediastinum, pleural spaces, and peritoneal cavity. However, these agents do not coat the esophagus well, and subtle mucosal abnormalities will not be appreciated. Also, certain water-soluble agents, such as Gastrografin, should not be used in patients with suspected aspiration. This agent is hyperosmolar to serum and other body fluids, and if aspirated, even in small amounts, it can induce laryngospasm, pulmonary edema, and death.[15,90]

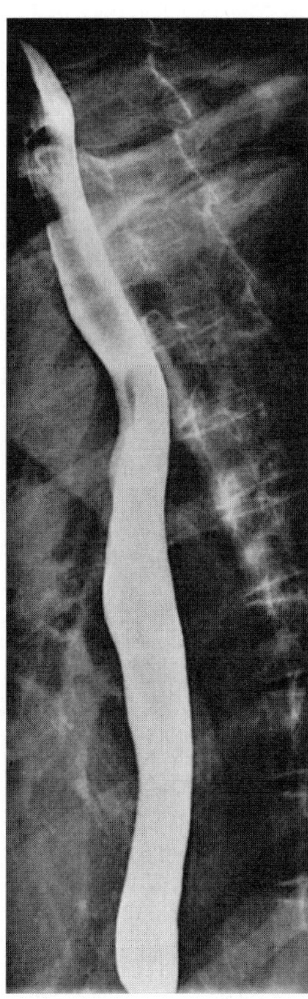

Figure 4–2. Normal single-contrast esophagogram. The esophagus appears as a continuous column filled with thin barium.

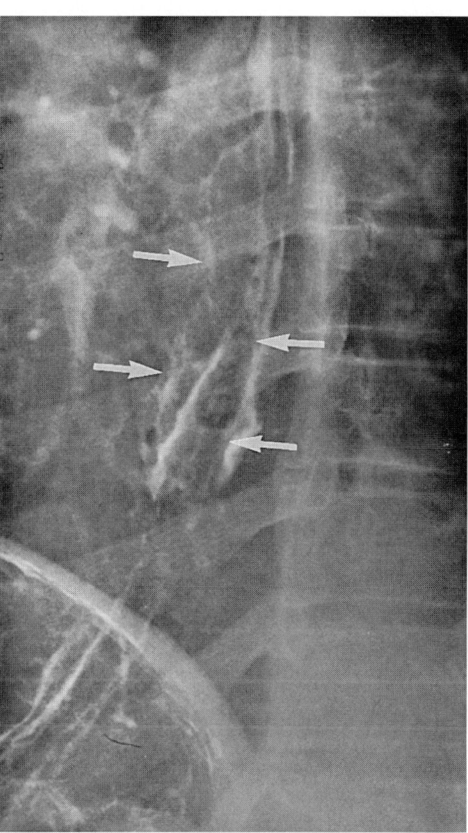

Figure 4–3. Esophagogram with barium paste according to the mucosal relief technique demonstrates multiple serpiginous filling defects *(arrows)* in the mid and distal esophagus, compatible with esophageal varices. With this technique, the esophagus is collapsed and coated with barium paste.

Supplemental Techniques

The mucosal relief technique allows visualization of the coated mucosal folds in a relaxed, collapsed esophagus and is especially effective at demonstrating esophageal varices.[18] It is achieved when the patient swallows barium paste in several small swallows, to result in good coating, and then stops swallowing for several minutes, to suspend peristalsis. The patient should be provided a basin in which to expectorate during this time. Spot films are then obtained of the relaxed, coated esophagus. This technique can demonstrate even small varices (Fig. 4–3), but it is not commonly used because varices are well demonstrated by CT and endoscopy.

In patients with dysphagia, various solid or semisolid materials can be administered; these include barium paste, barium mixed with applesauce, barium graham cracker, barium marshmallow, or barium pills.

In certain patients, abnormal esophageal motility may be provoked by specific types of food. For instance, some patients develop spasm only with solid foods and have normal motility with liquids. In special clinical situations, acid may be added to barium in an attempt to recreate the patient's reported symptoms and to aid in the diagnosis of esophagitis.[27] In addition, the barium solution may be chilled. Because cold liquids decrease esophageal peristalsis, this may help improve distention of the lower esophagus.[84]

NORMAL RADIOLOGIC ANATOMY OF THE ESOPHAGUS

The esophagus begins at the C5-6 vertebral body level, just inferior to the cricopharyngeus muscle. The esophagus continues inferiorly into the thorax, posterior to the trachea, to reach the gastroesophageal junction. Some normal structures cause extrinsic impressions on the esophagus, such as the aortic arch on the left side of the thoracic esophagus, the left main stem bronchus that is lower, and the left atrium on the distal esophagus (see Fig. 4-1). There also usually is a narrowing of the distal esophagus as it passes through the diaphragmatic hiatus, usually around the T10 vertebral body level. A small segment of the distal thoracic esophagus (the vestibule) may be slightly wider than the remainder of the esophagus and should not be mistaken for a hiatal hernia. There is a portion of the esophagus that is infradiaphragmatic: the submerged segment.

On contrast esophagography, the normal esophageal mucosa appears featureless. Normal esophageal folds should not measure more than 1 to 2 mm in diameter and should be smooth in contour.

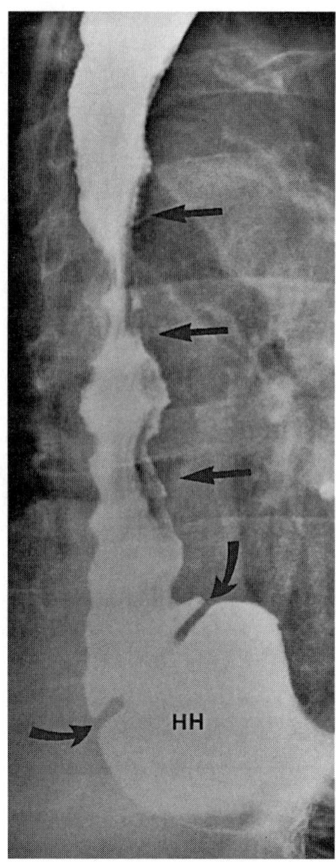

Figure 4–4. Single-contrast esophagogram demonstrates a hiatal hernia (HH). A nonstenotic Schatzki ring *(curved arrows)* with a diameter of 2.5 cm is also present. The patient was asymptomatic. There is a moderate hiatal hernia. Spasm is present in the lower esophagus *(straight arrows)*.

HIATAL HERNIA AND GASTROESOPHAGEAL REFLUX

Contrast esophagography is sensitive for the evaluation of hiatal hernia. The most sensitive technique involves a single-contrast upper gastrointestinal series with the patient in the prone, right oblique position with a bolster (Fig. 4-4). The bolster increases intra-abdominal pressure and maximizes distention of the hernia. The relationship of hiatal hernia to gastroesophageal reflux remains controversial. In a series of 13 patients with hiatal hernia, Ott et al.[84] correlated the presence of a hiatal hernia with the results of pH monitoring during a 24-hour period. Abnormal results of pH monitoring were found in 31% of patients with a hiatal hernia compared with 18% of patients without a hiatal hernia.[84] Therefore, the presence or absence of hiatal hernia does not correlate well with the results of pH monitoring. However, patients with larger hiatal hernias were more likely to have abnormal findings on pH monitoring.

Although esophageal pH monitoring is the most sensitive test for the diagnosis of gastroesophageal reflux, this is expensive and not always readily available. There is continued controversy over the role of barium studies in the detection of reflux. During the standard double- and single-contrast upper gastrointestinal series, the fluoroscopist observes the gastroesophageal junction while the patient changes position. This may demonstrate spontaneous reflux. Additional maneuvers can be performed to increase the sensitivity for the detection of reflux, including straight leg raise or coughing to increase intra-abdominal pressure. Also, the water siphon test can be performed. In this study, the patient is positioned in the right oblique supine position, so the fundus and cardia are filled with contrast medium. Then the patient takes a few swallows of water through a straw. The fluoroscopist observes the gastroesophageal junction. When the water crosses through the gastroesophageal junction, this creates a siphon effect and reflux may be detected. In a series of 117 subjects reported by Thompson et al.,[107] the findings of a pH probe were correlated with barium examination. The barium examination included change in position, coughing, and the water siphon test. In this series, the standard barium study showed unprovoked reflux in only 26% of the subjects proved to have reflux by the pH study. However, when the water siphon test was used, the sensitivity of the barium examination increased to 70%. Overall, in this series, the water siphon test was shown to have a specificity of 74% and a positive predictive value of 80%.[107]

BARRETT'S ESOPHAGUS

Because patients with Barrett's esophagus are predisposed to the development of esophageal carcinoma, early

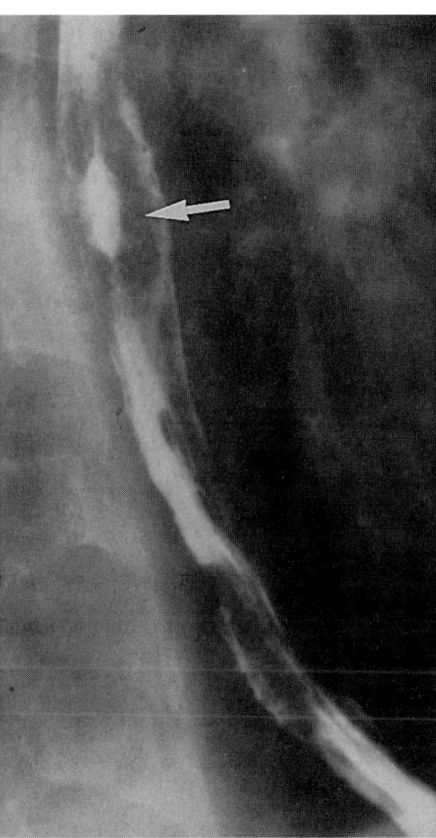

Figure 4–5. Double-contrast esophagogram demonstrates a large ulcer *(arrow)* in a patient with Barrett's esophagus. (From Wall, S.D., and Jones, B.: Gastrointestinal tract in the immunocompromised host: Opportunistic infections and other complications. Radiology, *185*:327, 1992.)

identification of these patients is important so routine surveillance can be performed. The double-contrast barium esophagogram is the most sensitive radiographic study for the detection of Barrett's esophagus. However, the radiographic findings can often be subtle and can be difficult to detect unless the technique is optimal. Contour defects, subtle alterations in esophageal mucosal patterns, or ulcerations are typical[14,36,37] (Fig. 4–5). In addition, the presence of a stricture in the mid esophagus in association with a mucosal reticular pattern or deep ulceration may suggest the diagnosis. Other findings, such as hiatal hernia, thickened mucosal folds, and gastroesophageal reflux, are also frequent findings but are not specific. In a series of 29 cases of Barrett's esophagus confirmed with endoscopy, barium studies revealed thickened and irregular mucosal folds in 28 of 29 patients, hiatal hernia in 26 of 29 patients, esophageal stricture in 25 of 29 patients, ulceration in 20 of 29 patients, and granular mucosal pattern in 16 of 24 patients.[14] However, there is no specific sign of Barrett's esophagus on contrast studies, and therefore endoscopy is necessary for definitive diagnosis.

ESOPHAGITIS

Esophagitis is the most common disorder encountered during radiologic examination of the esophagus.[60] The radiologist's objective is to detect esophagitis at its early stages and to attempt to distinguish among the various causes. This requires careful attention to technique.

The double-contrast esophagogram is the most sensitive technique for the detection of subtle abnormalities that occur early in esophagitis. This is usually combined with single-contrast views of the esophagus in the prone oblique position during continuous drinking. The patient turns to the supine position, and the gastroesophageal junction is monitored for reflux of the contrast medium back into the esophagus.

Radiologic features of esophagitis on contrast esophagography include erosions, ulcers, plaques, spasm, and fold thickening or transverse ridging.[60] Careful analysis of these findings, along with the clinical history, may help suggest the specific cause of the esophagitis.

Infectious Esophagitis

Infectious esophagitis is not uncommon and may be caused by a variety of agents. Certain infections may produce characteristic findings on the contrast esophagogram that allows the radiologist to suggest the etiologic agent.

For instance, candidal (monilial) esophagitis typically demonstrates discrete longitudinally oriented plaque-like lesions in the esophagus, which correspond to the white plaques seen during endoscopy[65] (Fig. 4–6). The interven-

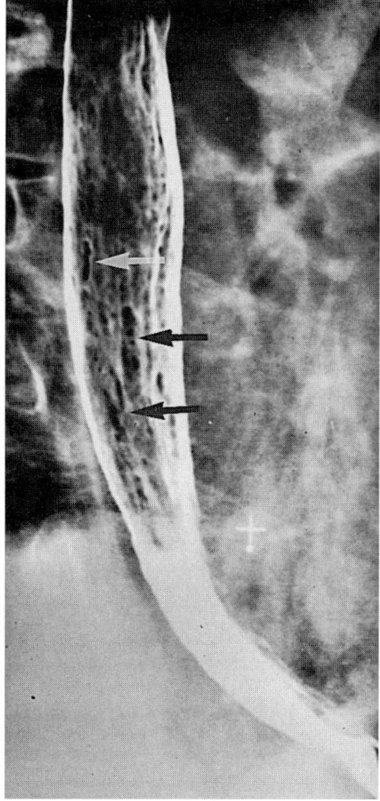

Figure 4–6. Double-contrast esophagogram demonstrates multiple oval and linear filling defects *(arrows)*, compatible with plaques due to *Candida* esophagitis. (From Jones, B., and Braver, J.M. (eds.): Essentials of Gastrointestinal Radiology. Philadelphia, W.B. Saunders, 1982.)

ing mucosa usually appears normal. Ulcerations can occur, usually in association with the plaques. In severe cases of candidal esophagitis, the esophagus has a "shaggy" contour, resulting from barium trapped between coalescent mucosal plaques[60] (Fig. 4-7). This radiographic appearance is very suggestive of *Candida*. The sensitivity of double-contrast esophagography in the diagnosis of candidal esophagitis is approximately 90%.[65]

In contrast to *Candida*, herpes esophagitis typically demonstrates discrete superficial ulcers in the mid esophagus on a background of normal mucosa. These ulcers can be detected in more than 50% of patients with endoscopically proved disease.[64] Although herpes esophagitis classically occurs in immunocompromised patients, it has been reported in a group of young healthy men.[103]

Cytomegalovirus (CMV) may demonstrate an identical pattern of superficial ulceration on normal mucosa.[2] However, in other patients with CMV esophagitis, there may be one or more large (>1 to 2 cm), relatively flat ulcers (Fig. 4-8). This is very suggestive of CMV, because herpetic ulcers are rarely this large.

In addition to CMV and herpes simplex, HIV infection of the esophagus has been reported to cause esophagitis and a giant esophageal ulcer. In a series of four patients described by Levine et al.,[63] all four patients had a large esophageal ulcer. Endoscopy was performed, and the patients were negative for CMV or herpes simplex. In a series of 21 HIV-positive patients studied by Sor et al.,[104] 16 of the patients had ulcers caused by HIV, 3 had ulcers caused by CMV, and 2 had ulcers caused by both CMV and HIV. It was not possible to differentiate the HIV from the CMV ulcers on the basis of clinical or radiographic criteria. Endoscopy is necessary for definitive diagnosis. In cases of a single large esophageal ulcer, HIV should be considered as possible cause when biopsies reveal the absence of CMV or herpes simplex.

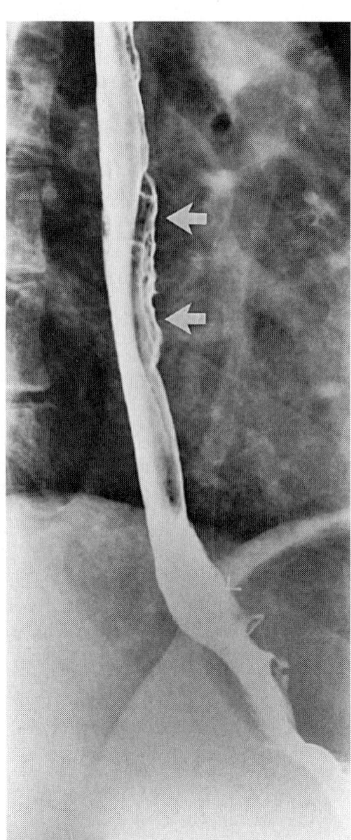

Figure 4–8. Contrast esophagogram demonstrates a large ulcer *(arrows)* compatible with a CMV ulcer. An HIV ulcer could have an identical appearance. Endoscopy is necessary with biopsy to differentiate. (From Jones, B., and Braver, J.M. (eds.): Essentials of Gastrointestinal Radiology. Philadelphia, W.B. Saunders, 1982.)

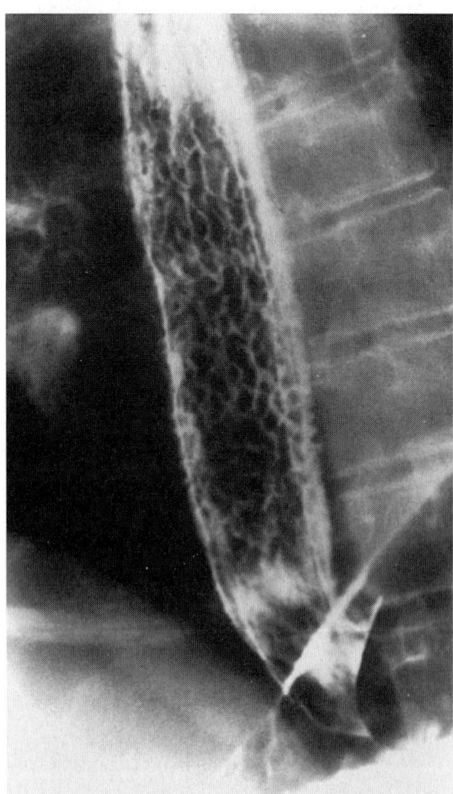

Figure 4–7. Double-contrast esophagogram demonstrates multiple intersecting linear and horizontal ulcers with intervening areas of edema, resulting in a shaggy, cobblestone appearance. This is severe candidal esophagitis. (From von Heuck, F.: Klinische Radiologie Diagnotik mit bildgebenden Verfahren. *In* von Fuchs, H.-F., and Donner, M.W. [eds.]: Gastrointestinaltrakt. Berlin, Springer-Verlag, 1990.)

Reflux Esophagitis

The radiographic appearance of esophagitis caused by gastroesophageal reflux varies. In patients with mild reflux esophagitis, subtle mucosal granularity or nodularity may be present as a result of mucosal inflammation[60] (Fig. 4-9). Reflux esophagitis is the most common cause of ulceration in the esophagus. One or more ulcerations or erosion is characteristically present in the distal esophagus or at the gastroesophageal junction and occurs on a background of mucosal disease and esophageal fold thickening.[60] Hiatal hernia or reflux of contrast may also be demonstrated during the radiologic examination. Transverse ridging was first reported in the pediatric population but is also seen as a sign of esophagitis in the adult.

Chronic long-term reflux can result in scarring or strictures, usually beginning at the gastroesophageal junction

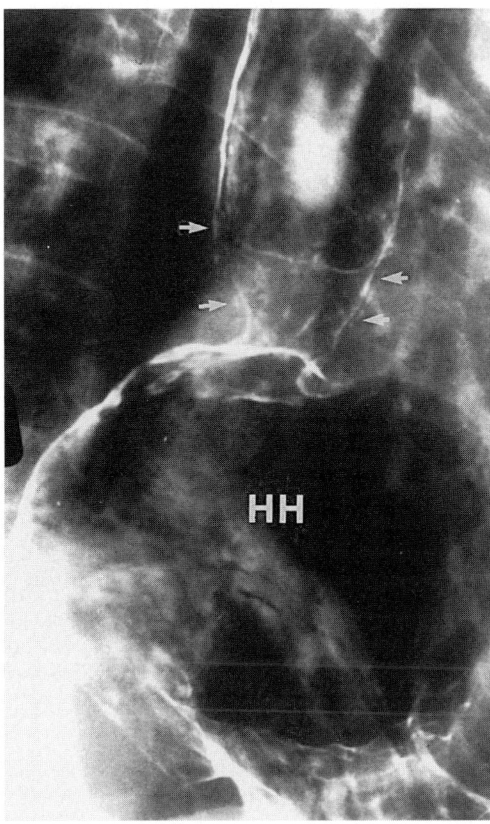

Figure 4–9. Double-contrast upper GI series demonstrates a large hiatal hernia (HH) with minimal narrowing at the gastroesophageal junction. In the distal esophagus, there are many small collections of barium due to ulceration *(arrows)*. This is an example of esophagitis. (From von Heuck, F.: Klinische Radiologie Diagnotik mit bildgebenden Verfahren. *In* von Fuchs, H.-F., and Donner, M.W. [eds.]: Gastrointestinaltrakt. Berlin, Springer-Verlag, 1990.)

and extending superiorly (Fig. 4–10). Chronic reflux may also occur in the setting of prolonged nasogastric intubation, and alternative methods of feeding, such as gastrostomy or jejunostomy, should be considered.

Other Causes of Esophagitis

Drugs such as tetracycline, doxycycline, potassium chloride, quinidine, and aspirin can result in esophagitis, especially if taken without water or immediately before going to bed[51] (Figs. 4–11 and 4–12). Prolonged contact to the esophageal mucosa can produce a focal esophagitis, typically in the mid esophagus at the level of the aortic arch or left main stem bronchus.[51] Radiation, caustic ingestion, and Crohn's disease can also result in an acute esophagitis. In these instances, there usually is a supporting clinical history.

INTRAMURAL PSEUDODIVERTICULOSIS

Intramural pseudodiverticulosis represents dilated submucosal glands in the esophagus. On esophagograms, these appear as tiny (1 to 3 mm) flask-like outpouchings from the esophagus (Fig. 4–13). These may be diffuse or segmental and should not be mistaken for ulcers. Unlike ulcers, when viewed in profile, the pseudodiverticula do not appear to communicate with the esophageal lumen.[13] More than 90% of patients with intramural pseudodiverticulosis have an associated stricture, most frequently in the upper third of the esophagus.[11,17] The condition is thought to represent a sequela of long-term gastroesophageal reflux.[66] There also is some evidence of an association between intramural pseudodiverticulosis and candidal infection.[11,17] In addition, in a study by Plavsic et al.,[87] there was a significantly increased prevalence of intramural pseudodiverticulosis in patients with esophageal carcinoma. Therefore, regular screening contrast esophagography or endoscopy in patients with intramural diverticulosis should be considered.

ESOPHAGEAL VARICES

Although esophageal varices can be detected on contrast esophagography, this is not a sensitive technique. The detection of esophageal varices on contrast studies requires careful attention to technique.[10] If the esophagus is distended, varices are easily obscured and flattened by contrast medium within the lumen. In addition, varices can collapse if the esophagus is well distended. Although

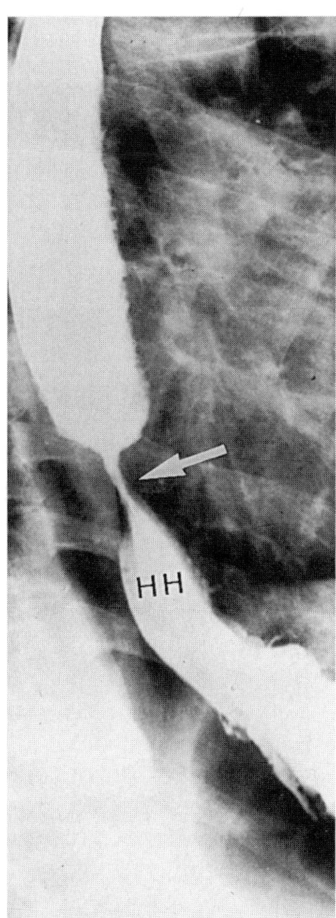

Figure 4–10. Single-contrast esophagogram demonstrates a distal esophageal stricture *(arrow)* due to gastroesophageal reflux. There is also a small hiatal hernia (HH). (From Jones, B., Ravich, W.J., and Donner, M.V.: Dysphagia in systemic disease. Curr. Imaging, *3*:158, 199.)

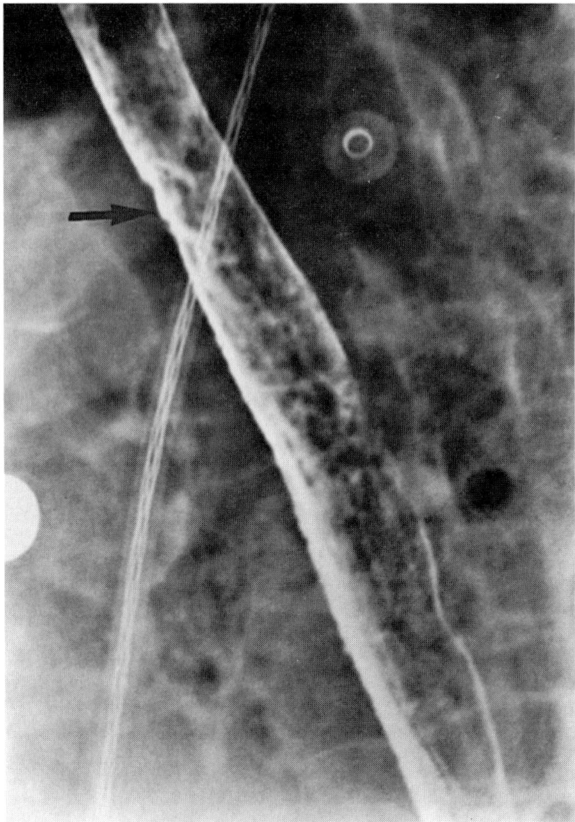

Figure 4–11. Double-contrast esophagogram demonstrates an acute esophagitis with a 1 cm ulcer *(arrow)*. This was due to quinidine.

the mucosal relief views are helpful in demonstrating the presence of esophageal varices, varices can also be missed with this technique if esophageal peristalsis is not suspended.[61] Therefore, if an esophagogram is performed to evaluate for possible esophageal varices, the study should be single contrast in addition to the mucosal relief view. Also, the administration of anticholinergic agents (e.g., propantheline bromide or hyoscine *N*-butylbromide) can be helpful by decreasing esophageal peristalsis.[23]

Esophageal varices due to liver disease and portal hypertension are most prominent in the distal third or lower half of the esophagus and appear as serpiginous filling defects or nodular scalloped longitudinal filling defects within the esophagus (see Fig. 4–3). Because varices may distend and/or collapse during peristalsis and with varying degrees of esophageal distention, the changing appearance of the varices at fluoroscopy helps to differentiate this from other inflammatory or neoplastic conditions that could have a similar nodular appearance.

When esophageal varices are detected in the upper esophagus, this is typically a result of superior vena caval obstruction. These varices in the proximal thoracic esophagus are usually termed *downhill varices*, because the venous blood is flowing down from the head and upper extremity via collateral vessels to return to the heart. Varices in the distal esophagus are commonly referred to as *uphill varices*, because the collateral vessels are flowing up from the abdomen to join the azygos vein to return to the heart.

BENIGN STRICTURES

An esophageal stricture is a focal or diffuse region of luminal narrowing due to scarring. This is best evaluated with single-contrast esophagograms. Measurements of stricture length and diameter are usually made with spot films. However, these measurements will be affected by magnification, which can be up to 30%. More accurate measurement of the lumen of the strictured segment can be made using a solid bolus of a known diameter, such as a barium pill or marshmallow.[28]

The appearance, length, and location of the stricture may be helpful in suggesting the cause. For instance, peptic strictures typically occur in the distal esophagus and are associated with hiatal hernia and gastroesophageal reflux[72] (see Fig. 4–10). Strictures that occur secondary to long-term nasogastric intubation usually appear as long, smooth areas of narrowing that involve the lower and mid esophagus[4,115] (Fig. 4–14). In contrast, strictures associated with Barrett's esophagus usually appear tapered or ring-like and occur in the mid esophagus, usually at the squamocolumnar junction and sometimes associated with adjacent mucosal abnormalities.[57] Similarly, radiation strictures or strictures due to oral medications such as potassium chloride tend to occur in the mid esophagus at areas of anatomic hold-up such as at the aortic arch or at the level of the left main stem bronchus.[58] Other causes, including dermatologic conditions

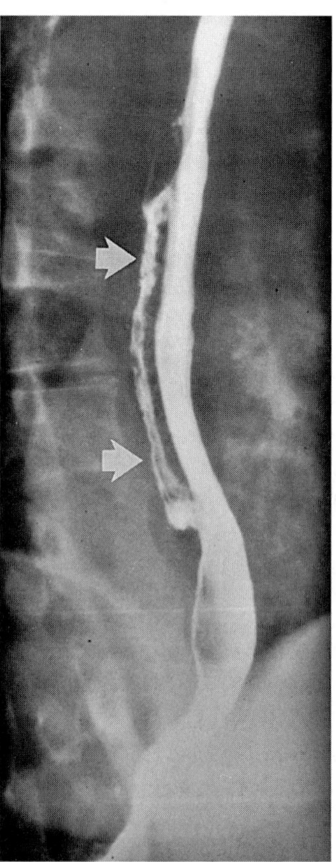

Figure 4–12. Single-contrast esophagogram in a patient taking ferrous sulfate demonstrates narrowing of the esophageal lumen and intramural extention of contrast *(arrows)*.

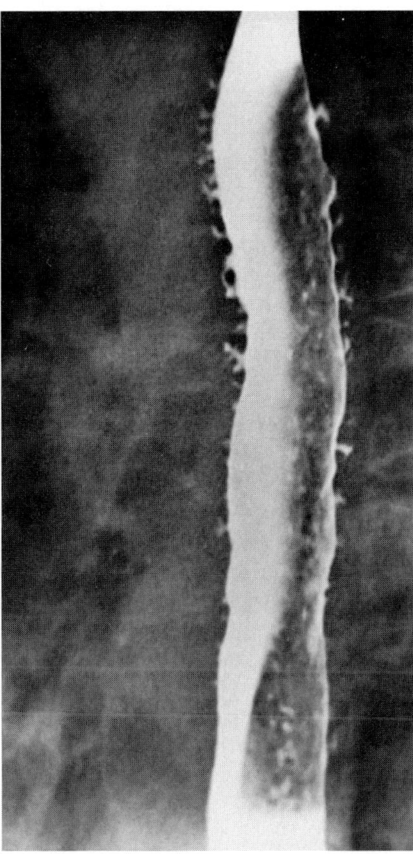

Figure 4–13. Double-contrast esophagogram demonstrates multiple flask-like outpouchings of the esophagus. This is actually filling of the submucosal glands. This is an example of intramural pseudodiverticulosis. (From von Heuck, F.: Klinische Radiologie Diagnotik mit bildgebenden Verfahren. *In* von Fuchs, H.-F., and Donner, M.W. [eds.]: Gastrointestinaltrakt. Berlin, Springer-Verlag, 1990.)

such as epidermolysis bullosa or benign mucous membrane pemphigoid and lichen planus, may also result in benign esophageal strictures or webs.[76,81] In these cases, there is usually a clinical history that can help in determination of the cause.

Crohn's disease also is a potential cause of esophageal disease, including ulcers and strictures.[35] However, there usually is a history of advanced Crohn's disease that involves the small bowel or colon at the time the esophageal disease presents.

CAUSTIC INJURY

The ingestion of common household chemicals can cause severe injury to the esophagus. Although more common in children due to accidental ingestion, caustic ingestion by adults may occur during attempted suicide. The most severe injuries are caused by the ingestion of household cleaners that contain caustic soda lye. This produces severe esophageal injury and necrosis.[39] The ingestion of acids may also cause necrosis, but this tends to be more superficial.[78]

The radiographic findings on esophagogram after caustic ingestion vary depending on the chemical and the severity and acuteness of the injury. In the acute stages, there may be abnormal esophageal motility such as spasm or loss of peristalsis, and the esophageal contour is irregular and shaggy due to mucosal ulceration and sloughing of the mucosa.[33] Extravasation into intramural tracts or even fistulas may be found. In the subacute and chronic stages, a long esophageal stricture is the most common finding. This often appears to very irregular and may cause significant narrowing of the esophageal lumen.[61] In severe cases, the entire esophagus may have a thin, thread-like appearance (Fig. 4–15). This is very suggestive of a stricture caused by caustic ingestion, in that other causes of esophageal stricture rarely result in such significant diffuse esophageal narrowing. When the esophagus is examined after caustic ingestion, the stomach should also be carefully evaluated, because approximately 20% of patients with esophageal injury after alkaline ingestion have gastric involvement. This is often manifested by narrowing, fold thickening, or ulceration that involves the gastric antrum.[79]

WEBS AND RINGS

A *web* is a thin mucosal fold that is most frequently located along the anterior aspect of the upper esophagus, usually at the junction of the hypopharynx and cervical esophagus.[29,109] However, webs may also occur in the

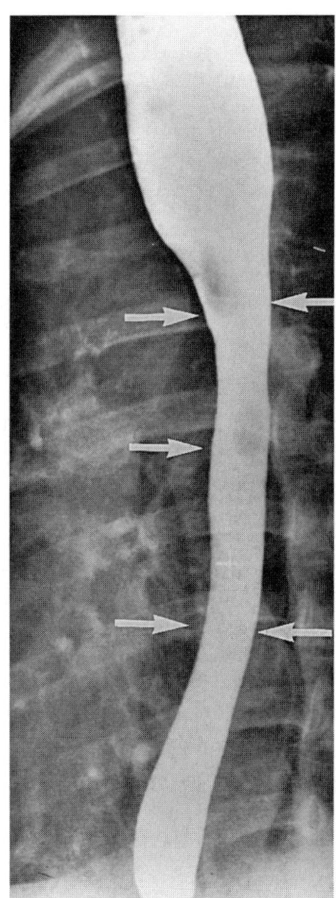

Figure 4–14. Single-contrast esophagogram demonstrates a long smooth stricture involving the mid and distal esophagus with minimal dilatation of the upper esophagus. This is a result of long-term nasogastric tube intubation.

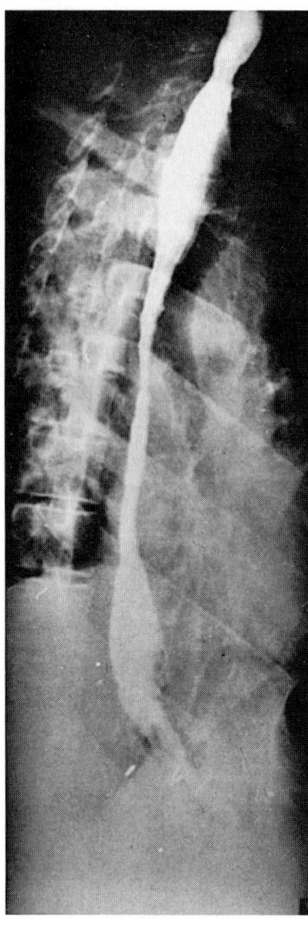

Figure 4–15. Single-contrast esophagogram demonstrates a long, smooth stricture of the lower esophagus with tapered margins. This is an example of a lye stricture. (From Jones, B., and Braver, J.M. (eds.): Essentials of Gastrointestinal Radiology. Philadelphia, W.B. Saunders, 1982.)

distal esophagus. On contrast esophagogram, a web appears as a discrete shelf-like defect, typically measuring between 1 and 2 mm in thickness (Fig. 4–16). In the cervical esophagus, the web is most commonly found only along the anterior aspect of the esophagus. However, a web may be circumferential and therefore can cause luminal narrowing and dysphagia. If the web results in significant luminal narrowing, a jet effect can be produced. This is a *flow phenomenon*, which occurs as the contrast medium flows rapidly through the narrowed segment. Radiographic detection of webs is related to the bolus size and may be evident only on maximal distention. Therefore, a web may be demonstrated only when a solid bolus is administered.

There is a relationship between cervical webs and iron deficiency anemia. This was first reported in 1921 by Vinson,[114] and the association has subsequently become known as the *Plummer-Vinson syndrome*. In Europe, the association is known as the *Paterson-Kelly syndrome*. There is some indication that patients with Plummer-Vinson syndrome are at an increased risk for developing carcinoma of the pharynx or esophagus.[61]

Webs that occur in the lower esophagus can be caused by scarring from gastroesophageal reflux.[74] These webs occur above the level of the gastroesophageal junction, allowing differentiation of these webs from a Schatzki ring.[116]

Webs usually have smooth contours and appear unchanged on repeated swallows. Often, these webs are difficult to detect under real-time fluoroscopy. The use of cine or video recording may be helpful for detection. Also, in the postcricoid region, there may be redundant mucosa, which can give the radiographic appearance of a web. However, this finding is thought to be a normal variant and is usually transient, rather than reproducible.

Schatzki's ring is a well-defined annular indentation of the distal esophagus first described by Templeton in 1944[106] and subsequently reported by Schatzki in 1953[99] in combination with dysphagia. This ring is a mucosal ring located at the junction of the esophagus and stomach (see Fig. 4–4). The major symptoms related to the ring are dysphagia or food impaction. Lower esophageal rings can be present in up to 18% of patients undergoing routine upper gastrointestinal series.[49] Typically, symptoms do not occur unless the ring is narrowed. In Schatzki's original report, patients were typically symptomatic when the luminal diameter measured less than 14 mm, and patients may or may not have been symptomatic with lumens of 14 to 18 mm. Other authors have reported symptoms with a diameter of 11 mm or less, especially if inflamed.[74] To best demonstrate the presence of a lower esophageal ring, the patient should be in the prone oblique position over a bolster or during Valsalva.[96]

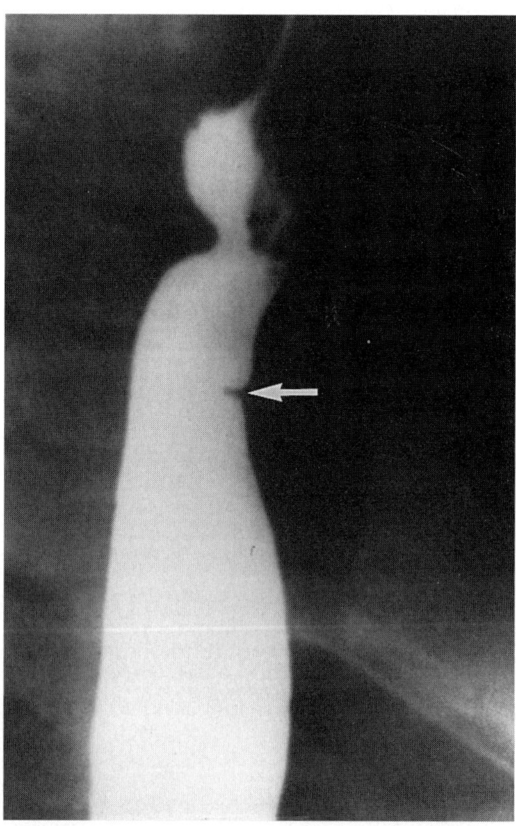

Figure 4–16. Single-contrast oblique view of the pharynx and upper esophagus demonstrating a thin horizontal linear filling defect on the anterior wall, compatible with a web. (From Taveras, J.M., and Ferrucci, J.T. [eds.]: Radiology Diagnosis: Imaging and Intervention. Volume 4. Philadelphia, J.B. Lippincott, 1992, p. 12.)

Single-contrast examination is preferred to complete filling of the lumen of the esophagus and stomach to better demonstrate the presence of hiatal hernia and/or Schatzki's ring. A solid bolus such as a barium marshmallow or pill can be administered for accurate measurements of the diameter of the ring, if necessary.

DIVERTICULA

Diverticula form at three distinct levels in the esophagus: at the pharyngoesophageal segment, in the middle third of the esophagus, and in the distal esophagus, just proximal to the esophageal hiatus. Contrast esophagography plays a role in the detection of these diverticula as well as postoperative follow-up.

Zenker's Diverticulum

A Zenker's diverticulum develops in an anatomically weak area on the posterior wall of the pharynx between the horizontal and oblique fibers of the cricopharyngeus muscle.[61] This region is known as *Killian's triangle* or *dehiscence*. On contrast pharyngoesophagography, a Zenker's diverticulum appears as an extraluminal contrast collection at the C5-6 level, above the level of the cricopharyngeus (Fig. 4-17). It is found along the posterior wall of the pharynx and typically flops to the left. There may be preferential filling of the diverticulum and retention of contrast medium in the diverticulum between swallows. Video examination may demonstrate reflux of contrast from the diverticulum back into the pharynx. This can predispose to aspiration. Enlargement of the cricopharyngeus muscle is often an associated finding, and both manometric and contrast studies have demonstrated premature closure of the cricopharyngeus in these patients.[53,118] Most patients with Zenker's diverticulum have other associated radiographic findings such as gastroesophageal reflux, hiatal hernia, or Schatzki's ring.[61] Contrast studies can be performed after surgical or endoscopic resection of Zenker's diverticulum to evaluate for complications such as extravasation or recurrence of the diverticulum.

Midesophageal Diverticulum

Diverticula can also form in the midesophagus. Traditionally, these were considered traction diverticula, usually resulting from scarring or inflammation in the mediastinum in conditions such as tuberculosis.[109] These traction diverticula often are triangular due to scarring and extrinsic pulling from mediastinal fibrosis. More recently, midesophageal pulsion-type diverticula were described in association with esophageal motor disorders[100] (Fig. 4-18).

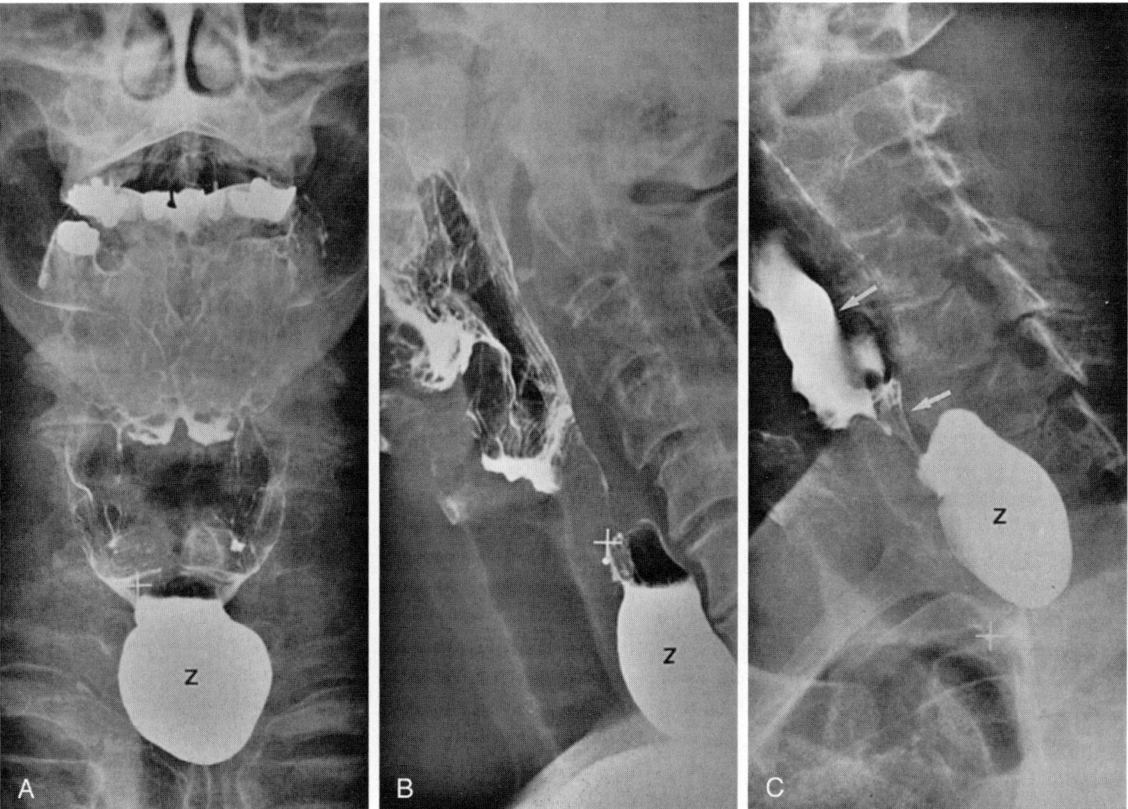

Figure 4-17. Spot films from videopharyngogram in the *(A)* frontal, *(B)* lateral, and *(C)* oblique projections demonstrate a 4.5 × 3 × 4.5 cm Zenker's diverticulum (Z). This fills with contrast and is seen above the level of the cricopharyngeus. Contrast within the diverticulum refluxes back into the pharynx *(arrows)*.

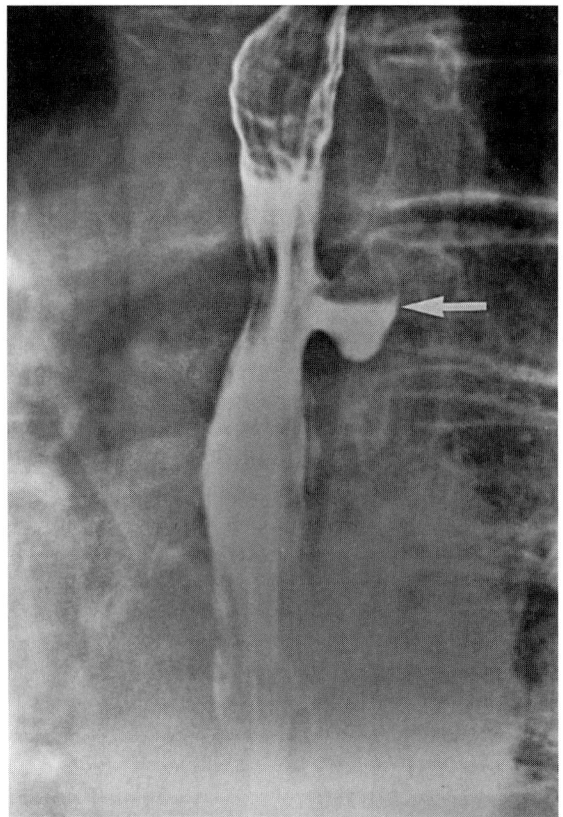

Figure 4–18. Double-contrast esophagogram demonstrates a 2 cm diverticulum *(arrow)* in the midesophagus with a small air fluid level.

Epiphrenic Diverticulum

An epiphrenic diverticulum forms in the distal esophagus, usually superior to the esophageal hiatus (Fig. 4–19). These usually extend to the left of midline and can vary in size. They usually measure between 1 and 10 cm. Epiphrenic diverticula are considered pulsion diverticula and most likely occur secondary to motor disorders of the lower esophageal sphincter.[31] Therefore, epiphrenic diverticulum can been seen in conditions such as achalasia.

FOOD IMPACTION

In patients with acute esophageal obstruction due to food impaction, the contrast esophagogram can be therapeutic as well as diagnostic. Usually, a single-contrast study is performed with barium or water-soluble contrast medium. The esophagogram typically demonstrates a mobile intraluminal mass of food. This may be causing a partial or even complete obstruction of the esophageal lumen (Fig. 4–20). In these cases, the radiologist may attempt to relieve the obstruction by using intravenous glucagon, effervescent granules, water, or sometimes high-density barium. In a series of 43 patients described by Robbins and Shortsleeve,[94] the use of intravenous glucagon, effervescent granules, and water relieved the obstruction in 69% of patients, thereby avoiding endoscopy.[94] Because there is a theoretical risk of esophageal perforation by abrupt distention of the esophagus with effervescent agents, they should not be administered if the obstruction has been present for more than 24 hours.[61] Also, it is important to restudy these patients with an esophagogram after the obstruction has been relieved. This may identify an underlying cause for the impaction, such as a ring or stricture. The practice of administering proteolytic digestive agents such as meat tenderizer in patients with obstructing food is no longer advised due to reported complications such as perforation, mediastinitis, and death.[1,46]

ESOPHAGEAL PERFORATION

Perforation of the esophagus is a potentially life-threatening event. The diagnosis can be suggested on chest radiography by the presence of mediastinal or subcutaneous air. For confirmation, a contrast esophagogram is typically performed and usually shows extravasated contrast (Fig. 4–21) or, in cases of contained tear, intramural extension of the contrast (see Fig. 4–12). Water-soluble contrast medium is the medium of choice for demonstrating esophageal perforation, because unlike barium, it is readily absorbed from the mediastinum. However, false-negative results in as many as 25% have been reported

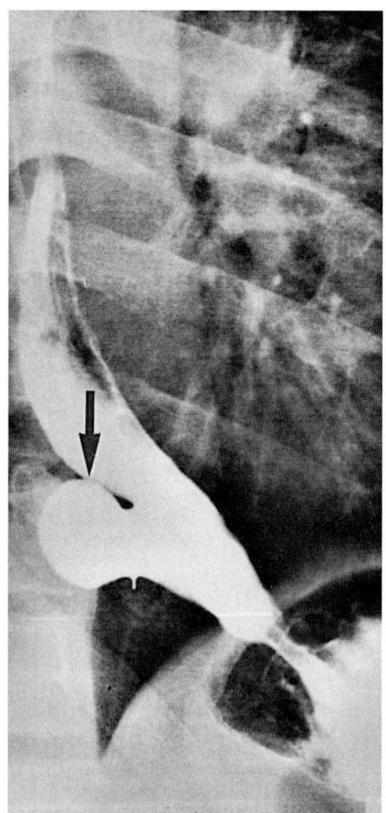

Figure 4–19. Single-contrast esophagogram demonstrates an epiphrenic diverticulum in the distal esophagus *(arrow)*. (From von Heuck, F.: Klinische Radiologie Diagnotik mit bildgebenden Verfahren. *In* von Fuchs, H.-F., and Donner, M.W. [eds.]: Gastrointestinaltrakt. Berlin, Springer-Verlag, 1990.)

with contrast examinations.[117] When a gastrointestinal perforation is suspected, if no leak is seen with water-soluble contrast medium, then barium should be administered. This leads to greater accuracy, because the barium is more radiopaque. In a series of patients reported on by Foley et al.,[32] six mucosal tears or perforations of the esophagus were diagnosed with the use of barium after negative studies were obtained with water-soluble contrast medium. In a larger study of 67 patients by Buecker et al.,[12] in 4 of 18 patients without evidence of extravasation with the use of water-soluble contrast medium, perforation was subsequently detected with barium. In a study by Brick and Palmer,[10] follow-up studies performed with barium in 26 patients did not yield additional important information. In general, when there is a high suspicion of esophageal perforation, water-soluble contrast medium should be used. If this does not reveal a leak, barium should be administered for greater sensitivity. Although theoretically, there is a risk of barium mediastinitis, this is very slight. In a study by Gollub and Bains,[41] of 29 esophageal perforations diagnosed in 12 patients using barium, no cases of mediastinitis were reported.[41]

Boerhaave's syndrome is a spontaneous esophageal perforation that is life threatening and requires early diagnosis as well as aggressive treatment to prevent fulminant mediastinitis, sepsis, and death. Approximately 40% of patients with spontaneous esophageal rupture present with a history of alcoholism or heavy alcohol use.[8] Spontaneous perforations of the esophagus typically appear just above the gastroesophageal junction. Chest radiographs may demonstrate a left pleural effusion or pneumomediastinum. On contrast esophagography, these perforations tend to be present on the left side of the distal esophagus, where there may be an intrinsic weakness.[70] The perforations are typically 1 to 4 cm in length and vertically oriented. Pneumomediastinum or pneumopericardium may also be present.[95] Small perforations are recognized by localized collections of extravasated contrast medium. Larger perforations may appear as free extravasation of contrast medium into the mediastinum. Video recordings may also be helpful to better recognize subtle perforations.

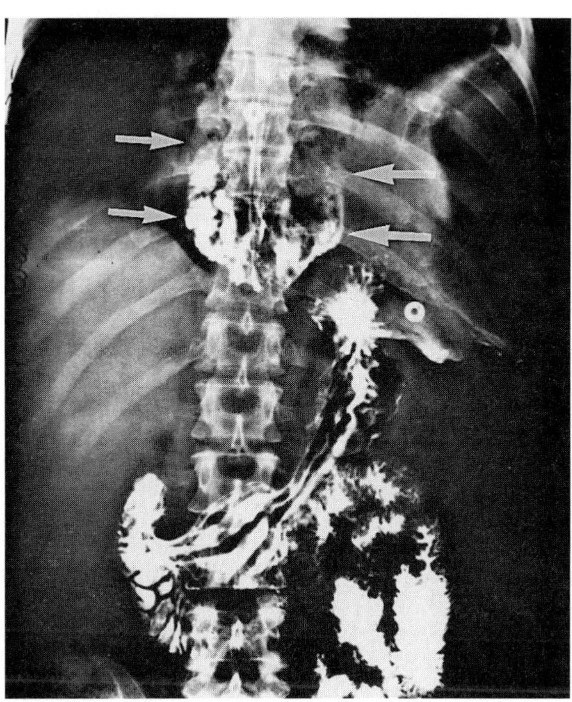

Figure 4–21. Contrast upper GI series in a patient with Boerhaave's syndrome demonstrates free extravasated contrast into the mediastinum adjacent to the esophagus. (From Jones, B., and Braver, J.M. (eds.): Essentials of Gastrointestinal Radiology. Philadelphia, W.B. Saunders, 1982.)

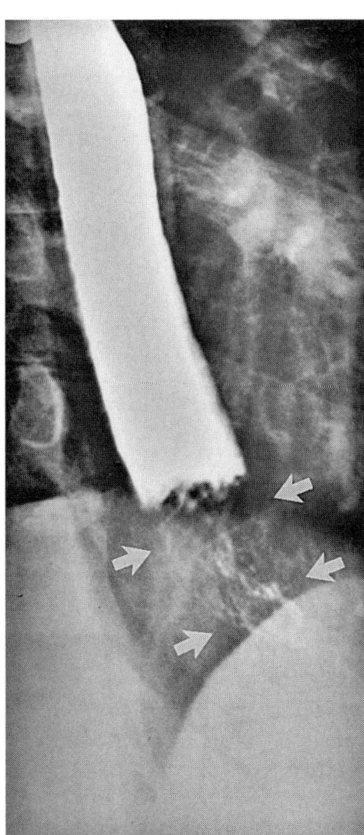

Figure 4–20. Single-contrast esophagogram in a 12-year-old boy complaining of dysphagia after a large meal. There is minimal dilatation of the upper and midesophagus with an abrupt change in caliber in the distal esophagus *(arrows)*, compatible with food impaction. Only minimal contrast trickles through the obstruction into the stomach. Endoscopy was necessary for removal of the impacted meat. An infiltrating esophageal carcinoma could have a similar appearance.

Mallory-Weiss tears represent a mucosal tear only, presenting classically with hematemesis after a vomiting episode. The contrast esophagogram is typically negative, and the diagnosis is made at endoscopy. Intramural rupture of the esophagus will demonstrate intramural dissection of contrast medium with or without a mucosal flap.

ESOPHAGEAL MOTILITY DISORDERS

Contrast studies of the esophagus can provide functional as well as anatomic information. Usually, a combination of spot films and videofluorography is optimum to evaluate esophageal peristalsis. With the patient in a prone oblique position, one swallow of contrast can be followed through the esophagus. Normal peristalsis is visualized as a progressive peristaltic wave that clears all contrast medium from the esophagus. The lower esophageal sphincter is closed between swallows and opens to allow the bolus to pass.

Esophageal Spasm

During the contrast esophagogram, nonpropulsive simultaneous contractions (spasm) can be visualized. Spasm is a nonperistaltic contraction that may occur spontaneously or in response to swallowing (see Fig. 4-4). This can be subtle or severe, obliterating the esophageal lumen. Esophageal spasm may be transient or persistent, causing a hold-up of contrast medium in the esophagus or even retrograde movement of contrast. Spasm may occur in a variety of conditions, including reflux and esophagitis. Some patients develop spasm only with a solid bolus, the "solid-induced spasm."

Diffuse esophageal spasm is a condition characterized by chest pain and dysphagia. Usually, spasm is detected on at least 10% of swallows.[93] The radiographic diagnosis of diffuse esophageal spasm requires the demonstration of normal peristalsis at some time during the examination (Fig. 4-22). This helps distinguish esophageal spasm from other conditions, such as vigorous achalasia. In some patients, the symptoms of chest pain are provoked when cold liquids are swallowed, and in those patients, the barium can be chilled before the examination. Some researchers believe that diffuse esophageal spasm may be within the same spectrum as achalasia.[69,101]

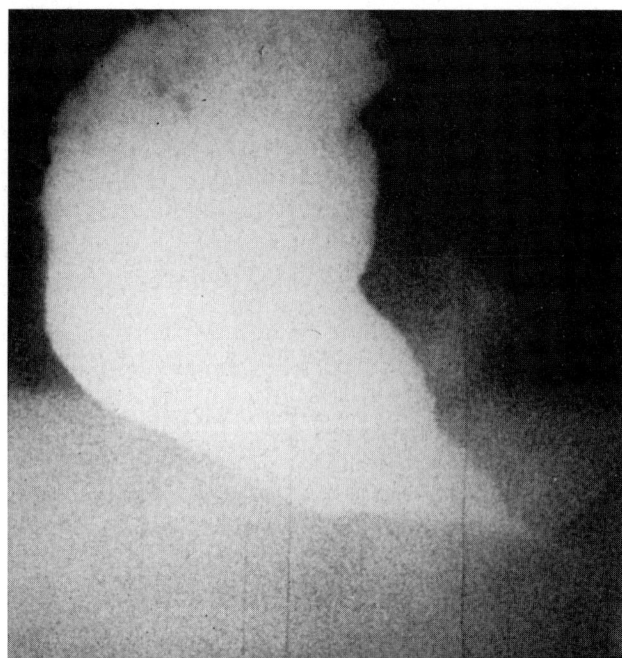

Figure 4-23. Single-contrast esophagogram in a patient with achalasia demonstrates the characteristic tapering of the distal esophagus. This is referred to as a "bird's beak."

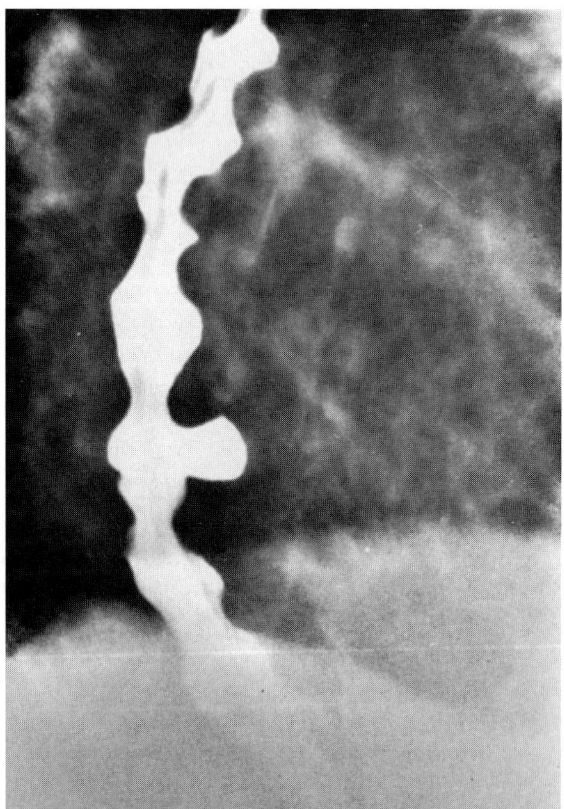

Figure 4-22. Single-contrast esophagogram demonstrates diffuse esophageal spasm. Spasm can result in partial or complete obliteration of the esophageal lumen. This can result in pseudodiverticula between adjacent areas of spasm. (From von Heuck, F.: Klinische Radiologie Diagnotik mit bildgebenden Verfahren. *In* von Fuchs, H.-F., and Donner, M.W. [eds.]: Gastrointestinaltrakt. Berlin, Springer-Verlag, 1990.)

The "nutcracker esophagus" is a controversial condition in which the peristaltic waves have increased duration and amplitude and are associated with chest pain.[111] The contrast esophagogram is usually normal in the nutcracker esophagus. The relationship between nutcracker esophagus and diffuse esophageal spasm is not well understood. It is possible that this condition is a precursor of diffuse esophageal spasm.[19,80]

Achalasia

The radiologic diagnosis of achalasia is usually characteristic in advanced cases. The esophagogram typically demonstrates dilatation of the esophagus with retained fluid and food. The distal esophagus typically appears smooth and tapered, producing a beak-like configuration (Fig. 4-23). This deformity occurs in the region of the lower esophageal sphincter. Under fluoroscopic observation, this relaxes intermittently, allowing small quantities of contrast medium to squirt through the sphincter into the stomach. This is best demonstrated when the patient is in an upright oblique position. In patients with early achalasia, the radiographic diagnosis can be difficult, because there may be only minimal dilatation of the esophagus and minimal narrowing at the gastroesophageal junction. The key to diagnosis is observation of intermittent opening of the lower esophageal sphincter and absence of normal peristalsis. Vigorous achalasia is typically diagnosed when there also is severe spasm.[7] However, the distinction between classic and vigorous achalasia as separate entities has been questioned.[38,110]

Esophageal emptying can be evaluated in patients with achalasia using a timed barium swallow. This technique was described by de Oliveira et al.[24] Patients were given 100 to 200 ml of barium, and spot films were obtained at 1, 2, and 5 minutes after ingestion. This examination served as a baseline study and was repeated and compared with examination after the injection of botulinum toxin. This is an example of how the contrast study can provide quantitative information in addition to anatomic detail.

Scleroderma

Esophageal involvement in patients with scleroderma is common.[34] The earliest finding on contrast esophagography is a decrease in or absence of normal esophageal motility.[61] This is typically apparent in the lower and distal esophagus, because only smooth muscle is affected. Also, in patients with scleroderma, the esophagus is usually dilated and the lower esophageal sphincter is incompetent. This leads to significant gastroesophageal reflux and may eventually lead to severe esophagitis and stricture formation.[34] Esophageal involvement by scleroderma may also lead to the development of Barrett's esophagus and adenocarcinoma.[89]

BENIGN MASSES

Benign esophageal tumors can be detected on routine contrast esophagograms. The most common benign tumor of the esophagus is a leiomyoma.[40] These are typically detected in the mid and distal esophagus and vary in size (Fig. 4–24). Because leiomyomas are located within the wall of the esophagus, they appear on contrast studies as round smooth masses covered by smooth intact mucosa, or there may be central ulceration.[61] When large, leiomyomas may be difficult to distinguish from extrinsic masses. Other benign intramural tumors, such as lipoma, hamartoma, or neuromas, can have a similar smooth appearance. However, these are less common. Congenital esophageal cysts can have an identical appearance on contrast studies. In these cases, a CT scan can be helpful in demonstrating the water attenuation of a congenital cyst versus the smooth muscle attenuation of a leiomyoma. Similarly, a lipoma can be diagnosed definitively with CT by demonstrating the fat attenuation.

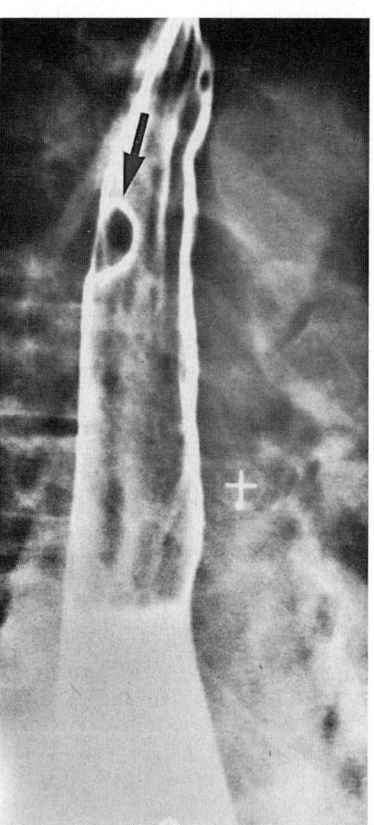

Figure 4–24. Double-contrast esophagogram demonstrates a 1.5 cm smooth intramural (submucosal) mass *(arrow)* in the upper esophagus, compatible with a leiomyoma. (From von Heuck, F.: Klinische Radiologie Diagnotik mit bildgebenden Verfahren. *In* von Fuchs, H.-F., and Donner, M.W. [eds.]: Gastrointestinaltrakt. Berlin, Springer-Verlag, 1990.)

ESOPHAGEAL CANCER

Double-contrast esophagography is the most sensitive radiologic technique for the diagnosis of esophageal cancer. The radiologic appearance of esophageal cancer depends on location and stage. Early esophageal cancer can result in subtle changes on the double-contrast esophagogram (Fig. 4–25). It may appear as small polypoid lesions or flat plaque-like lesions.[54,62] In addition, there may be focal deformity, ulceration, or nodularity of the mucosa.[62] Early lesions may produce subtle changes on double-contrast esophagograms that would be invisible if single-contrast technique were performed. Although most early esophageal cancers appear as focal lesions, superficial spreading carcinoma of the esophagus may involve a large area. More advanced esophageal cancers typically result in luminal narrowing with raised margins and ulcerated mucosa (Fig. 4–26). There often is an abrupt transition between the normal esophagus and the carcinoma. Esophageal cancers, which are infiltrating, can have tapered borders that may mimic the appearance of benign strictures. Complications of advanced esophageal carcinoma can also be detected on contrast studies; these include perforation, esophageal obstruction, and tracheoesophageal fistula.

When esophageal carcinoma is detected in the distal esophagus, a careful examination of the gastric cardia and fundus is necessary to detect tumor infiltration through the lower esophageal sphincter. Gastric adenocarcinomas arising in the gastric fundus can extend superiorly to involve the lower esophagus, thereby mimicking primary esophageal carcinoma. Usually, endoscopy and biopsy are necessary to distinguish the two.

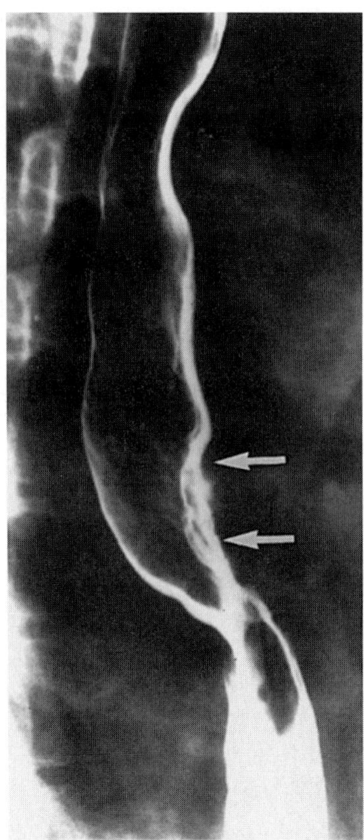

Figure 4–25. Double-contrast esophagogram demonstrates a 5-cm infiltrating lesion involving the left lateral wall of the esophagus *(arrows)*. This was biopsy-proven squamous cell carcinoma. (From von Heuck, F.: Klinische Radiologie Diagnotik mit bildgebenden Verfahren. *In* von Fuchs, H.-F., and Donner, M.W. [eds.]: Gastrointestinaltrakt. Berlin, Springer-Verlag, 1990.)

COMPLICATIONS AFTER TRANSHIATAL ESOPHAGECTOMY

Transhiatal esophagectomy is routinely performed for the treatment of benign and malignant esophageal disease. The procedure involves creating a new conduit using the stomach (preferably) or colon. A wide spectrum of complications can occur after these procedures, many of which can be detected with contrast studies of the pharynx and esophagus.

Leak at the surgical anastomosis of the remaining esophagus to the pull-up occurs in up to 15% of patients and can be detected on fluoroscopic studies with water-soluble contrast.[50] A leak appears as extraluminal collections of contrast medium that typically occurs near the esophagogastric anastomosis (Fig. 4–27). This use of videotaping, which allows review in slow motion, will increase the detection of subtle leaks.

Aspiration pneumonia after esophagectomy is a major source of complications and death, regardless of the surgical approach. It occurs in up to 15% of patients. The routine use of videofluorography in patients after esophagectomy is a sensitive and accurate technique for evaluating oral and pharyngeal function and thereby identifying patients with or at risk for aspiration (Fig. 4–28). Factors that may contribute to aspiration include pharyngeal or vocal cord paralysis, reflux through the gastric pull-up, and colonic interposition and cricopharyngeal obstruction. If aspiration is detected on videofluorography, the necessary dietary modifications and swallowing rehabilitation can be instituted. One series found that transient laryngeal penetration or aspiration occurred in 47% of patients after transhiatal esophagectomy.[45] The majority had improved or resolved by 1 month.

Tracheoesophageal fistula is an uncommon complication of esophagectomy.[75] During esophagectomy, injury to the trachea can occur, usually resulting from blunt dissection of a large tumor with tracheal adherence or as a result of hyperinflation of the endotracheal tube. Damage to the trachea along with other factors, such as radiation therapy or anastomotic leak, may result in the formation of a fistula between the trachea and esophagus, usually at the esophagogastric anastomosis. On contrast studies, this appears as a linear contrast tract that extends from the anastomosis to the airway. If a tracheoesophageal fistula is suspected clinically, Omnipaque or thin barium should be administered. Hypertonic solutions such as Gastrografin should not be administered due to the risk of pulmonary edema.

The development of a benign stricture at the esophagogastric anastomosis is a significant cause of complications and death in patients after esophagectomy and gastric pull-up (Fig. 4–29). The reported frequency of the complication averages 15%.[47] Stricture appears as a smooth narrowing of the anastomotic lumen.

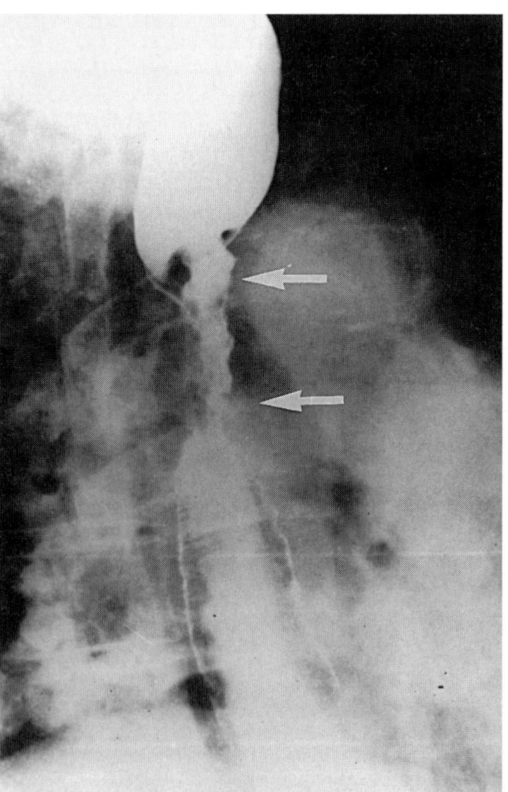

Figure 4–26. Single-contrast esophagogram demonstrates moderate luminal narrowing of the esophagus with overhanging edges *(arrows)*. This was biopsy-proven adenocarcinoma.

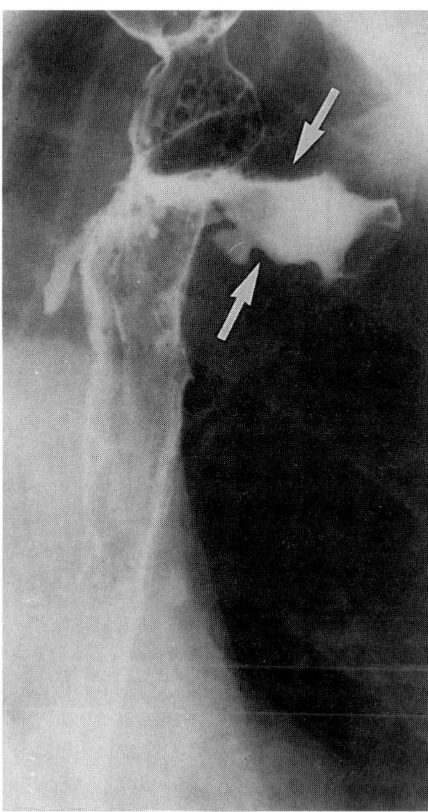

Figure 4–27. Contrast esophagogram in a patient after esophagectomy and gastric pull-up demonstrates extravasation of contrast *(arrows)* at the anastomotic site.

GASTROESOPHAGEAL SCINTIGRAPHY

Gastroesophageal scintigraphy is an alternative screening test for the presence of gastroesophageal reflux. The procedure is noninvasive and well tolerated. The patient drinks technetium sulfur colloid water. A gamma camera is used to detect and quantify the reflux of gastric contents back into the esophagus. The patient is typically supine and is monitored for 20 to 30 minutes. Compared with esophageal pH monitoring, gastroesophageal scintigraphy has a sensitivity ranging between 75 and 90% and a specificity ranging between 90 and 95%.[6,71,98] Scintigraphy is more sensitive than pH monitoring in the detection of buffered gastric contents.[102]

Esophageal transit scintigraphy can also be performed using technetium sulfur colloid water and is especially helpful when esophageal manometry is unavailable or equivocal.[52] This test permits the measurement and quantification of the movement of liquids through the esophagus. The patient is imaged immediately after ingestion of the radiotracer. Images are obtained every second for 20 to 30 seconds. The transit of radiotracer can be visually evaluated and can be quantified with computer software. This technique can be valuable when evaluating the response to treatment in patients with achalasia.[67] The examination can also be performed with a solid bolus, consisting of technetium sulfur colloid–labeled egg sandwich.

An exciting application of nuclear medicine studies in patients with esophageal cancer is the use whole body positron emission tomography (PET). In a case report by Yasuda et al.,[120] (^{18}F)-2-fluoro-2-D-deoxyglucose was administered to a patient, and scans were obtained 1 hour later. The whole body PET images detected not only the primary esophageal cancer but also multiple areas of nodal metastasis in the mediastinum and abdomen, which were subsequently confirmed with CT scanning. This is an exciting potential application of PET imaging and may come to play a useful role in the detection and staging of esophageal cancer.

COMPUTED TOMOGRAPHY

Overview

Although the contrast esophagogram is often considered to be the best radiologic modality for esophageal imaging, it visualizes only the esophageal mucosa and, to a lesser extent, intramural pathology. Contrast esophagography provides limited information regarding the extraluminal spread of esophageal disease. However, CT can be used to image the esophageal lumen, the wall, and adjacent structures and to assess for the presence of lymphadenopathy as well as to simultaneously detect distant metastases. Therefore, CT has come to play an important role in the evaluation of a variety of esophageal conditions.

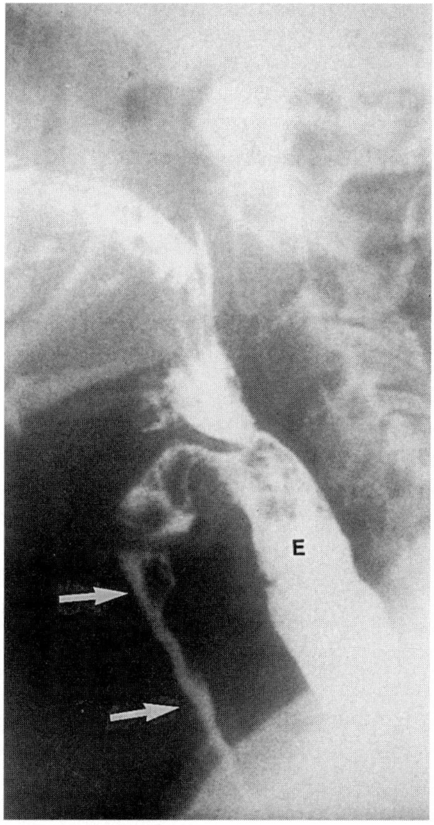

Figure 4–28. Lateral spot film of pharynx obtained during videopharyngogram in a patient after esophagectomy and gastric pull-up demonstrates moderate aspiration *(arrows)*. E, Esophagus.

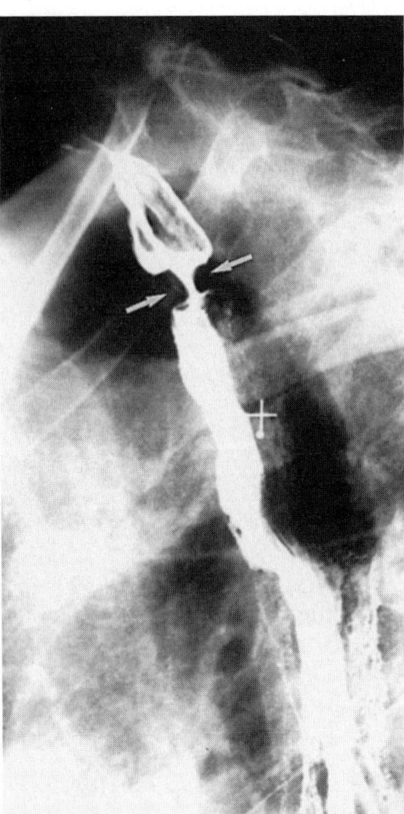

Figure 4–29. Spot film taken during videopharyngoesophagogram in a patient after esophagectomy and gastric pull-up demonstrates a severe anastomotic stricture *(arrows)*.

Spiral CT offers distinct advantages over conventional CT for imaging esophageal pathology. Spiral CT combines subsecond scanning, rapid intravenous contrast administration, narrow collimation, and close interscan spacing. In addition, three-dimensional data manipulation and display capabilities are now widely available, making spiral CT an important adjunct to barium studies and endoscopy for the evaluation of both benign and malignant disease of the esophagus.

Examination Technique

Accurate imaging of the esophagus requires careful attention to technique. For optimal imaging of the esophagus, the administration of both oral and intravenous contrast medium is necessary.

When esophageal disease is suspected, we routinely administer 750 ml of a 3% oral Hypaque (Hypaque; Nycomed, Princeton, NJ) solution approximately 30 to 60 minutes before the scan to fully opacify the stomach and proximal small bowel. An additional 250 ml of oral contrast agent is administered immediately before scanning to ensure maximal gastric distention. A special barium paste (Esoph-o-CAT; E-Z-M Co., Westbury, NY) is administered immediately before the start of the scan, after the patient is positioned on the CT table. This results in good opacification of the esophagus without creating streak artifacts through the mediastinum.[20] If additional esophageal distention is desired, effervescent Citrocarbonate granules (4 to 6 g) can be given with 30 ml of water, immediately before the start of scanning. This will distend the esophagus with air.

The administration of intravenous contrast medium is essential for the complete evaluation of esophageal disease, especially in patients with known or suspected esophageal cancer. We routinely administer 110 to 120 ml of Omnipaque 350 (Omnipaque; Nycomed, Princeton, NJ) intravenously, at a rate of 2 to 3 ml/sec with the use of a mechanical injector. Scanning should be performed during the portal venous phase, approximately 45 seconds after the start of the injection, to maximize the detection of liver metastases in patients with esophageal cancer. Images should be obtained from above the thoracic inlet through the liver, to ensure complete imaging of the esophagus as well as potential metastasis in the chest, liver, or adenopathy near the celiac axis. We routinely perform 5-mm collimation with a table speed of 8 mm/sec and a reconstruction interval of 5 mm. In select cases, narrower collimation (i.e., 3 mm) may be useful to evaluate suspected local tumor extension. In addition, imaging at deep inspiration with a single breath hold is optimum, because this results in better distention of the posterior wall of the trachea, which is useful when assessing possible tracheal invasion by an adjacent esophageal tumor.[119]

Advances in computer technology allow the interactive three-dimensional display of CT data sets. The three-dimensional data can be manipulated using different orientations and cut planes and by adjusting window level, center, brightness, and opacity to best demonstrate esophageal pathology. The data are especially helpful when assessing possible local extension of esophageal cancer or for evaluation of tracheoesophageal fistula.

Normal Esophagus

On CT scanning, the esophagus is easily identified due to the surrounding natural contrast provided by the lung and mediastinal fat (Fig. 4–30). In normal patients, the esophagus is usually collapsed, although a small amount of intraluminal air is considered normal, especially in anxious patients.[26] However, air-fluid levels or a fluid-filled esophagus is abnormal. A luminal diameter of more than 10 mm is usually abnormal and may indicate a distal obstruction or esophageal dysmotility. The normal esophageal wall is very thin, usually less than 3 mm, when the lumen is well distended.[92] The wall may appear thicker (up to 5 mm) when the esophagus is collapsed or at the level of the lower esophageal sphincter.[26] This should not be confused with pathologic thickening.[73] If necessary, effervescent granules can be administered and the scan repeated to better distend collapsed segments.

Esophageal Cancer

Although the initial diagnosis of esophageal cancer is typically made with endoscopy or contrast esophagography, CT plays a valuable role in surgical and treatment

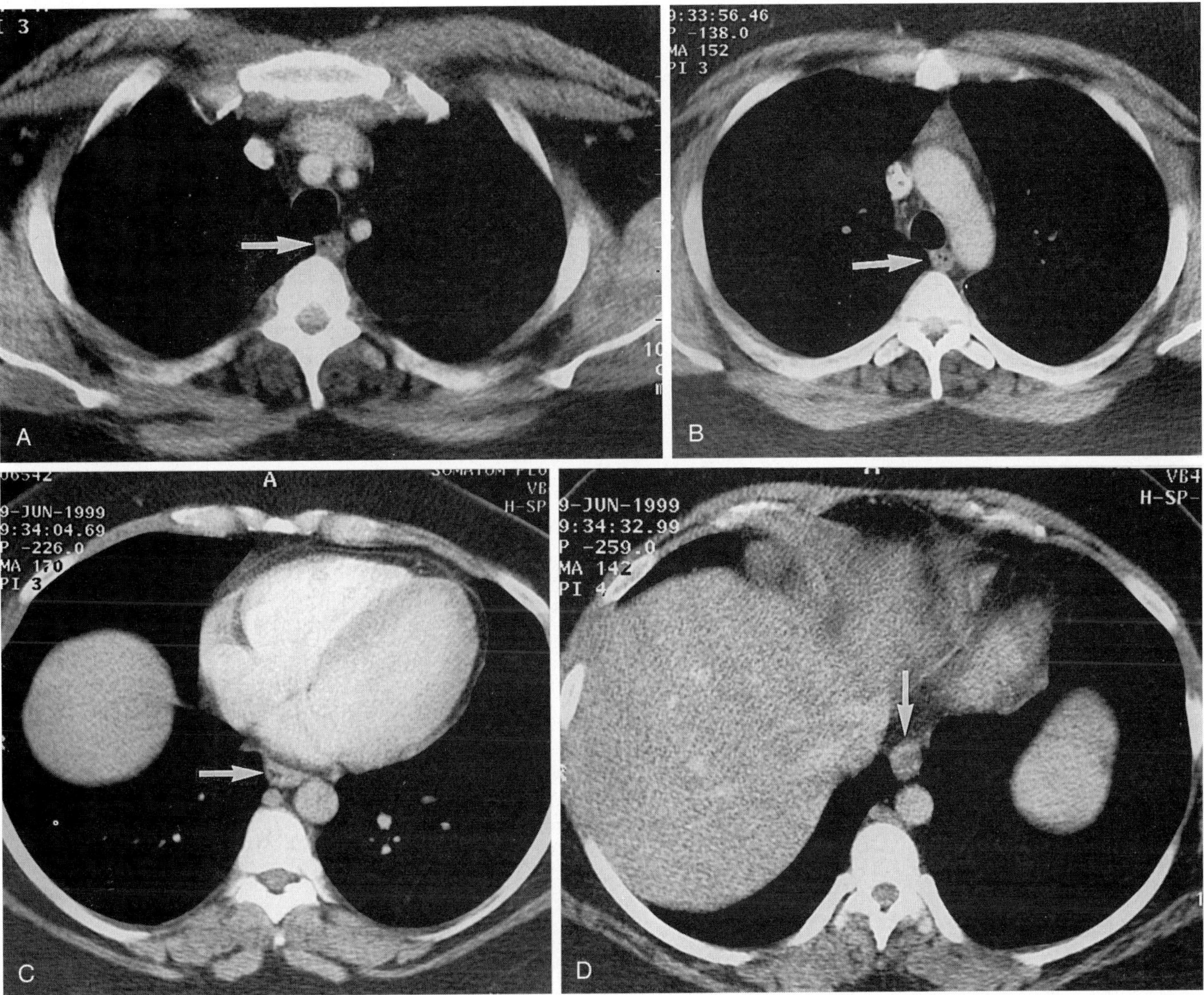

Figure 4–30. Normal esophagus *(arrow)* on CT at the level of *(A)* the great vessels, *(B)* the aortic arch, *(C)* the heart, *(D)* the diaphragm. The normal esophagus is collapsed and surrounded by periesophageal fat planes.

planning as well as a limited role in staging. Preoperative CT can demonstrate tumor size, local extension, invasion of adjacent organs, and the presence of distant metastases.

Primary Tumor

Because most malignant esophageal tumors are at an advanced stage at the time of diagnosis (TMN stage III), the primary tumor is typically visible on CT scanning in untreated patients. Very little has been reported about CT evaluation of early-stage esophageal tumors.[30,42] A limitation of CT staging of esophageal tumors is its inability to determine the exact depth of tumor infiltration of the esophageal wall, which is important for staging early carcinoma. Endoscopic ultrasound offers a distinct advantage over CT in patients with tumor confined to the esophageal wall, restaging of tumor depth after chemoradiation therapy and in detection of anastomotic recurrence.[68]

The CT appearance of primary esophageal carcinoma can include (1) discrete intraluminal mass, (2) focal or segmental eccentric wall thickening, or (3) focal or segmental circumferential wall thickening (Figs. 4–31 through 4–33). CT is accurate in the evaluation of tumor width, which is important, because there is a correlation between a lesion of more than 3.0 cm wide on CT and the presence of periesophageal spread.[59,85] However, CT evaluation of tumor length may not be as accurate, especially in patients after chemoradiation therapy and in tumors of the distal esophagus, where spread into the stomach may be difficult to accurately define with axial CT.[59] The use of multiplanar reconstruction or three-dimensional imaging may improve evaluation of tumor length and extension into the gastric cardia (Fig. 4–34).

The CT appearance of esophageal cancer can overlap with inflammatory conditions of the esophagus such as esophagitis. Therefore, when unsuspected esophageal pathology is detected on CT, endoscopy is recommended for further evaluation and biopsy if necessary.

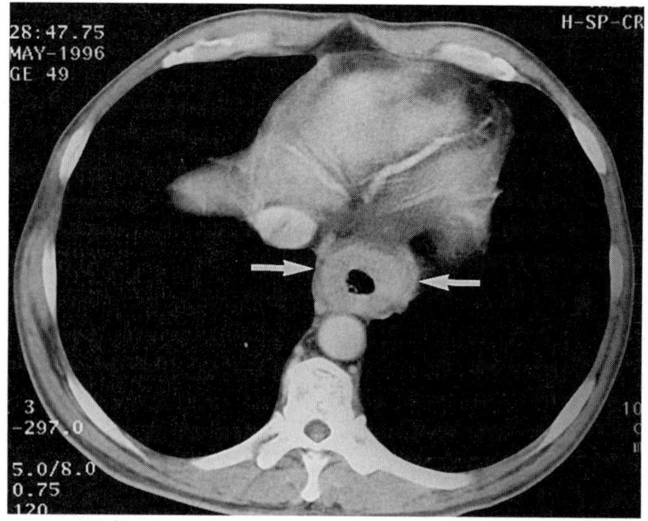

Figure 4–31. Contrast-enhanced spiral CT of the chest in a 53-year-old man with chest pain demonstrates marked circumferential thickening of the distal esophagus *(arrows)* measuring 1.5 cm in thickness. Esophageal cancer was confirmed at endoscopy.

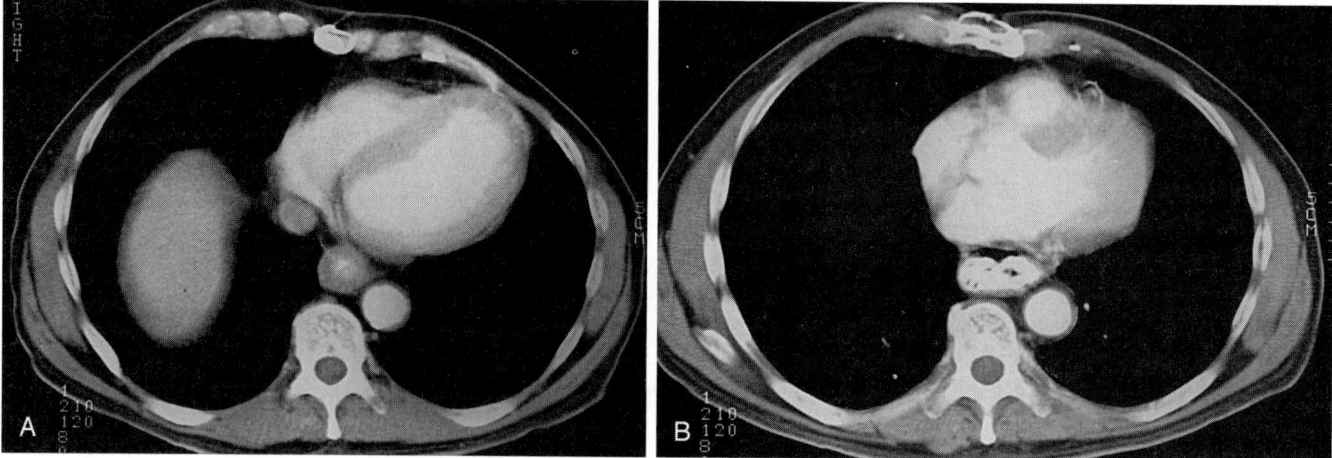

Figure 4–32. *A,* Spiral CT with intravenous and oral contrast in a 63-year-old man with newly diagnosed esophageal cancer reveals an area of circumferential thickening in the distal esophagus, at the gastroesophageal junction. *B,* A scan of the upper chest demonstrates dilatation of the proximal esophagus, which is filled with oral contrast *(arrow)*. This is compatible with partial obstruction by the tumor.

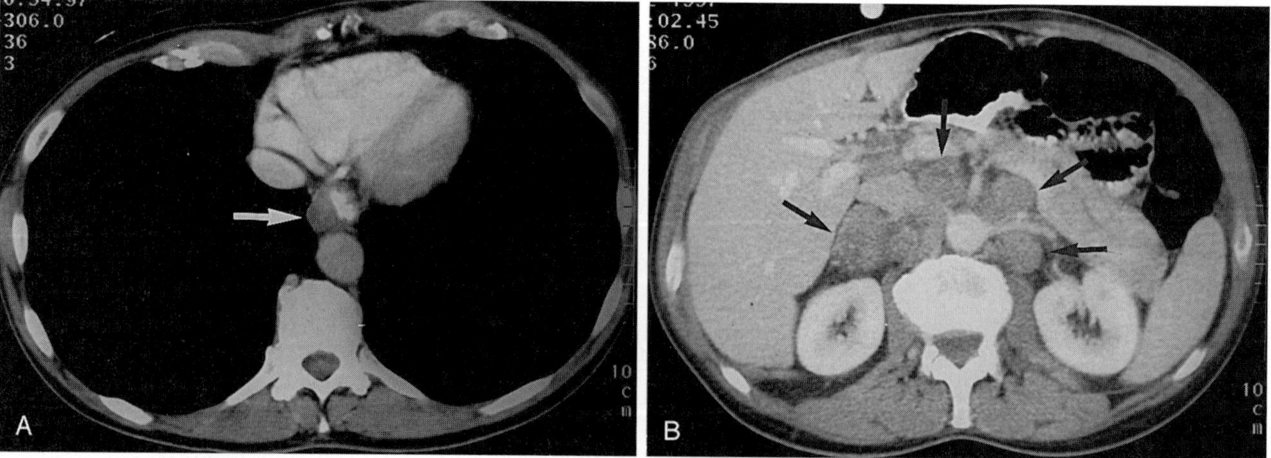

Figure 4–33. Contrast-enhanced spiral CT of the chest in a 67-year-old man with esophageal cancer demonstrates *(A)* a 1.5 cm mass along the right wall of the distal esophagus *(arrow)*. *B,* A scan of the upper abdomen in the same patient reveals adenopathy around the celiac axis and in the periportal region *(arrows)*.

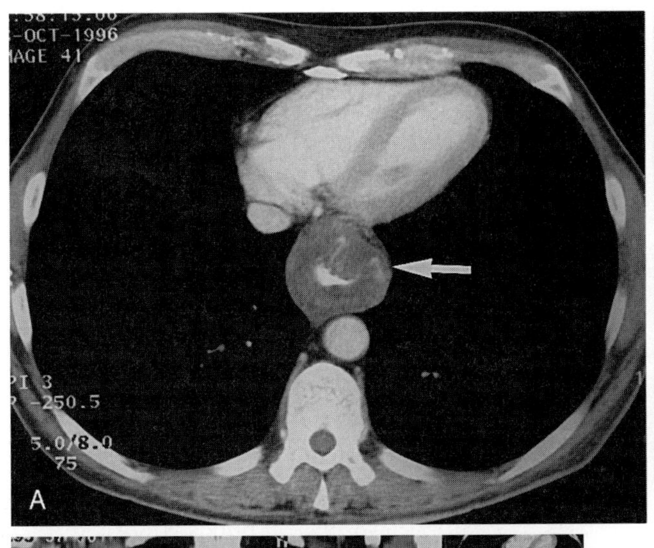

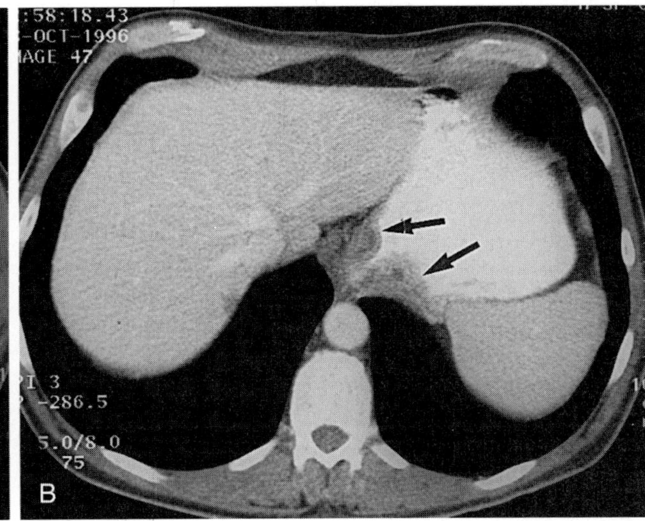

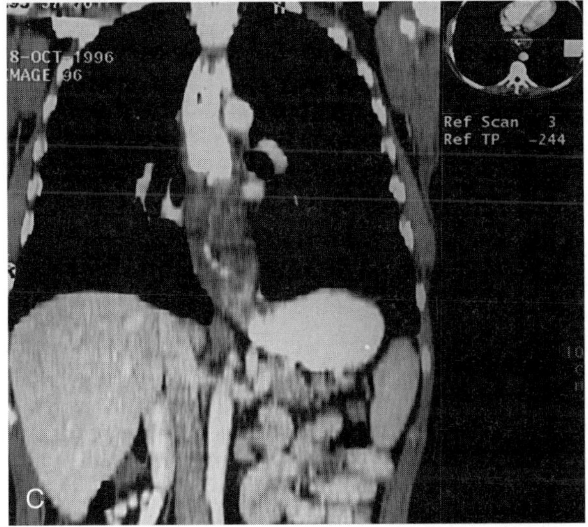

Figure 4–34. *A,* Contrast-enhanced spiral CT of the chest reveals marked circumferential thickening of the esophagus compatible with esophageal cancer *(arrow). B,* There is also thickening at the level of the gastroesophageal junction, indicating extension into the gastric cardia *(arrows). C,* A coronal reconstruction nicely demonstrates the extent of tumor involvement.

Local Extension

Advanced tumors are characterized by mediastinal extension of tumor with or without local adenopathy. Mediastinal invasion can involve the periesophageal fat, aorta, tracheobronchial tree, pericardium, or diaphragm.

Although CT cannot determine the intramural tumor depth, CT can often detect transmural spread of tumor into the periesophageal fat. The periesophageal fat normally demonstrates low (fat) attenuation on CT. In patients with esophageal cancer, early periesophageal invasion may appear as increased attenuation of the fat surrounding the esophagus.[21] This appearance is not specific for tumor invasion and can occur in patients with esophagitis or in patients with esophageal cancer after chemoradiation.

There normally is a distinct fat plane between the esophagus and other mediastinal organs. In patients with esophageal cancer, the loss of this fat plane between the aorta and esophagus, especially if 90 degrees or more of contact is allowed, is highly suggestive of tumor invasion of the aorta[85] (Fig. 4–35). Similarly, the loss of a discrete fat plane between the esophagus and pericardium suggests tumor invasion. CT does not accurately detect diaphragmatic invasion,[112] although this typically does not preclude attempt at surgical resection. Although the loss of specific mediastinal fat planes is an important CT feature for the detection of local invasion, the absence of all fat planes throughout the mediastinum can occur as a normal variant in cachectic patients or in patients who have received radiation therapy or surgery.[82,108]

Tracheobronchial tree involvement is suspected when the posterior wall of the trachea or main stem bronchus is displaced, compressed, or directly invaded by the adjacent tumor mass[85,108] (Figs. 4–36 and 4–37). Malignant tracheoesophageal fistulas can be detected with CT. When tracheoesophageal fistula is suspected, thin (2-mm) collimation should be performed. Three-dimensional imaging is especially helpful for visualization of the fistula and for surgical planning[55] (Fig. 4–37).

Overall, the reported sensitivity of CT for the detection of mediastinal invasion in patients with esophageal carcinoma ranges from 88 to 100% with a specificity ranging between 85 and 100%.[21,22,44,85,108] In a study by Takashima et al.[105] of 35 patients with esophageal cancer, MRI and CT demonstrated similar accuracy in predicting resectability, demonstrating an accuracy of 87% and 84%, respectively.

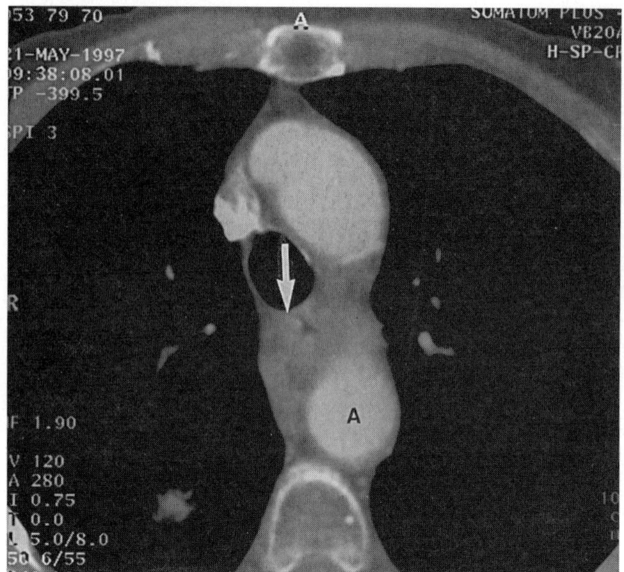

Figure 4–35. Contrast-enhanced spiral CT of the chest for staging in a 63-year-old man with esophageal carcinoma reveals circumferential thickening of the esophagus *(arrow)*. The periesophageal fat is hazy with increased attenuation and there is loss of the normal fat plane between the esophagus and the descending aorta (A). This is compatible with local tumor extension.

Adenopathy

In patients with esophageal cancer, the presence of nodal metastases is a strong prognostic indicator and significantly decreases the 5-year survival rate.[113] The sensitivity of CT for the detection of mediastinal lymphadenopathy is approximately 85%, because metastatic involvement of periesophageal nodes may not result in significant nodal enlargement.[112] In a study by Picus et al.,[85] almost all of the periesophageal nodes that contained tumor measured less than 7 mm and were indistinguishable on CT from uninvolved nodes. Inflammatory nodes in the mediastinum commonly measure up to 1 cm in short axis.

The accuracy of CT for the prediction of abdominal lymph node involvement ranges between 83 and 87%.[119] CT is especially accurate in the detection of metastatic nodes in the celiac and gastrohepatic ligament, a common site of nodal disease (Fig. 4-38; see Fig. 4-33). Celiac axis nodes that measure more than 5 to 6 mm in short axis are suggestive of tumor involvement.

The primary limitation of CT is its inability to distinguish benign from metastatic nodes, based only on size criteria. Change in the CT attenuation of involved nodes, such as central low density of necrosis, is a helpful CT sign of metastatic involvement but is present in only a minority of cases.

Although patients with localized nodal spread may experience a decreased postoperative survival rate, metastases to small periesophageal nodes is not always considered a contraindication to surgical resection.[43,97]

Distant Metastases

The liver is a common site for metastases from esophageal cancer, and thus accurate liver imaging is crucial for accurate staging. The demonstration of liver metastases can avoid needless surgery and can guide treatment to palliation instead of cure. Contrast-enhanced spiral CT is considered the preferred technique for liver imaging and is more sensitive than conventional scanning for the detection of metastatic disease. A study of the detection of hepatic masses by Kuszyk et al.[56] using spiral CT demonstrated a greater than 90% sensitivity for detecting liver lesions of more than 1 cm and a 56% sensitivity for detecting lesions less than 1 cm. This represents an improvement compared with traditional non-spiral CT scanning.

The accuracy of dynamic enhanced CT and unenhanced MRI in the detection of metastatic liver disease

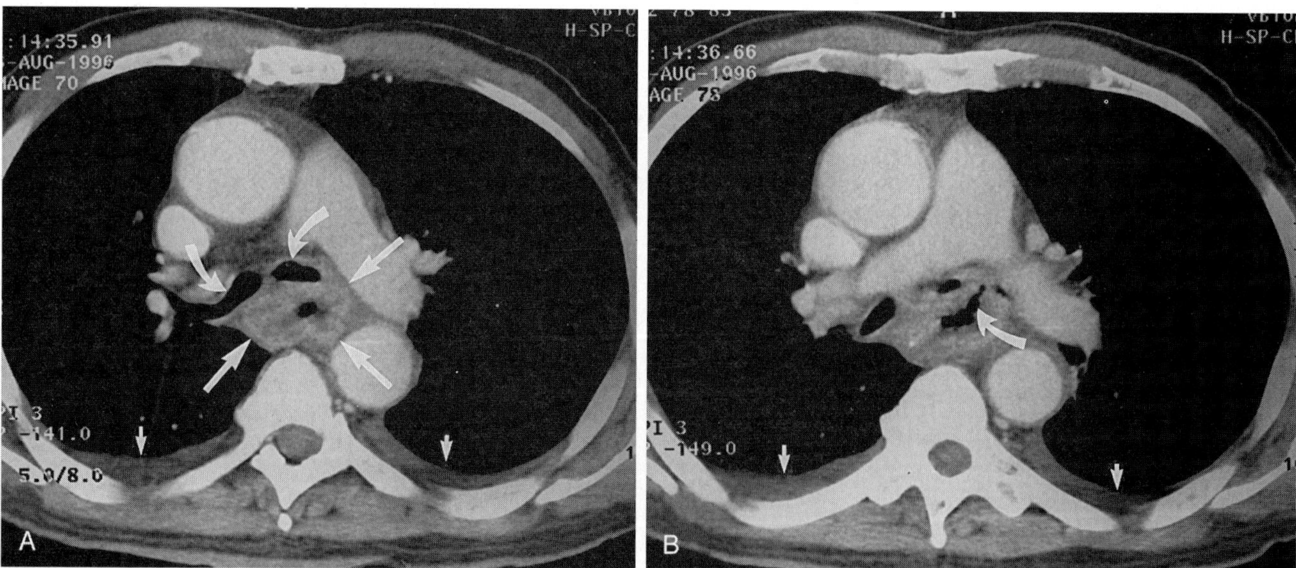

Figure 4–36. Contrast-enhanced spiral CT in an 83-year-old man with esophageal cancer demonstrates *(A)* moderate circumferential esophageal thickening *(straight arrows)* at the level of the main stem bronchi *(curved arrows)*. *B,* A tracheoesophageal fistula *(curved)* is identified extending from the tumor to the left mainstem bronchus.

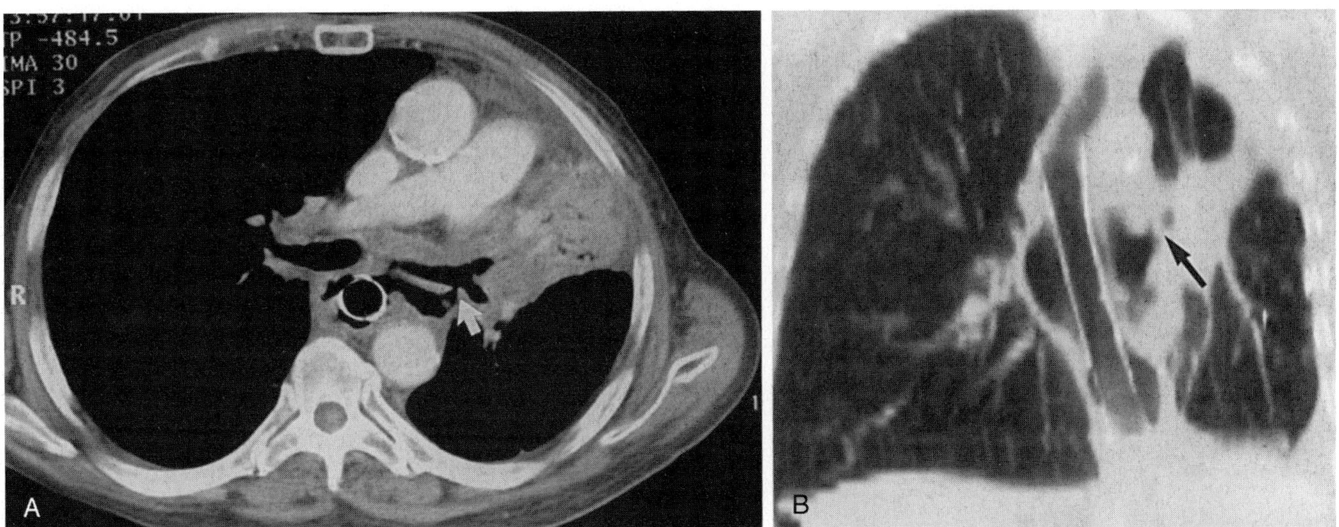

Figure 4–37. *A,* Contrast-enhanced spiral CT in a patient with unresectable esophageal cancer, following esophageal stent placement. There is marked circumferential thickening of the esophagus with increased density of the adjacent mediastinal fat, compatible with local invasion. A fistula is present between the esophageal mass and the left main stem bronchus *(arrow)*. This results in atelectasis and infiltrate in the left lung. *B,* 3D image in the coronal projection nicely demonstrates the esophageal stent and the communication between the esophagus and airway/lung *(arrow)*.

appears to be equal at 85%.[121] In a series of 478 patients with colorectal cancer, the specificity for both CT (97%) and MRI (94%) for the detection of liver metastases was similar to that of most published series.[121] The sensitivity of the two techniques in this study was 62% and 70%, respectively. Although MRI can detect smaller lesions than CT, these tiny lesions cannot be definitively characterized as benign or malignant and usually require continued follow-up to assess for growth in size or number.

On CT, liver metastases usually appear as hypodense lesions (Fig. 4–39). Most metastases are best visualized during the portal venous phase of liver enhancement, and therefore, careful coordination of contrast injection and the timing of data acquisition is crucial for maximum sensitivity. Metastases are usually multiple and vary in size. If only one lesion is detected, CT or ultrasound-guided biopsy can be performed to obtain pathologic confirmation.

Benign Esophageal Tumors

Benign esophageal tumors such as leiomyoma, lipoma, fibroma, neurofibroma, hamartoma, and hemangioma may be incidental findings on CT. These tumors are typically intramural and smooth in contour (Figs. 4–40 and 4–41). Only large tumors (>1 to 2 cm) will be detected on CT. In some cases, CT may allow definite diagnosis or be used as a problem-solving tool. For instance, the diagnosis of lipoma can be confidently made with CT, which

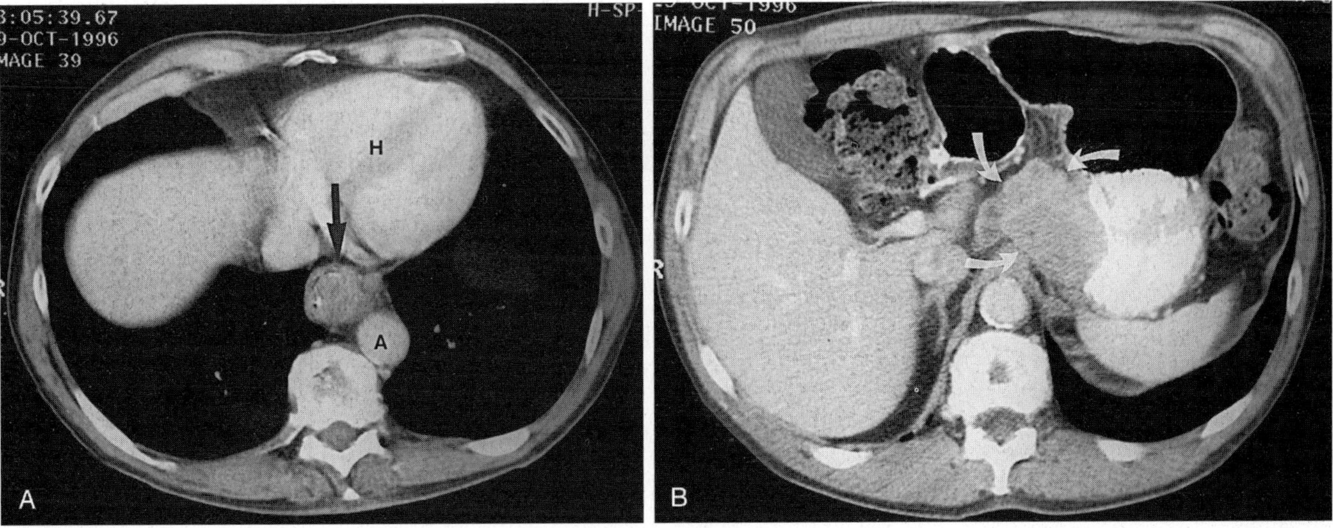

Figure 4–38. *A,* Contrast-enhanced spiral CT in a 60-year-old man with dysphagia reveals a 3-cm mass in the distal esophagus *(arrow)*. There is a good fat plane demonstrated between the esophageal mass and the aorta (A) and heart (H). *B,* CT scan of the upper abdomen in the same patient demonstrates a 4 × 6 cm nodal mass *(curved arrows)* in the gastrohepatic ligament. Squamous cell carcinoma of the esophagus was diagnosed at endoscopy.

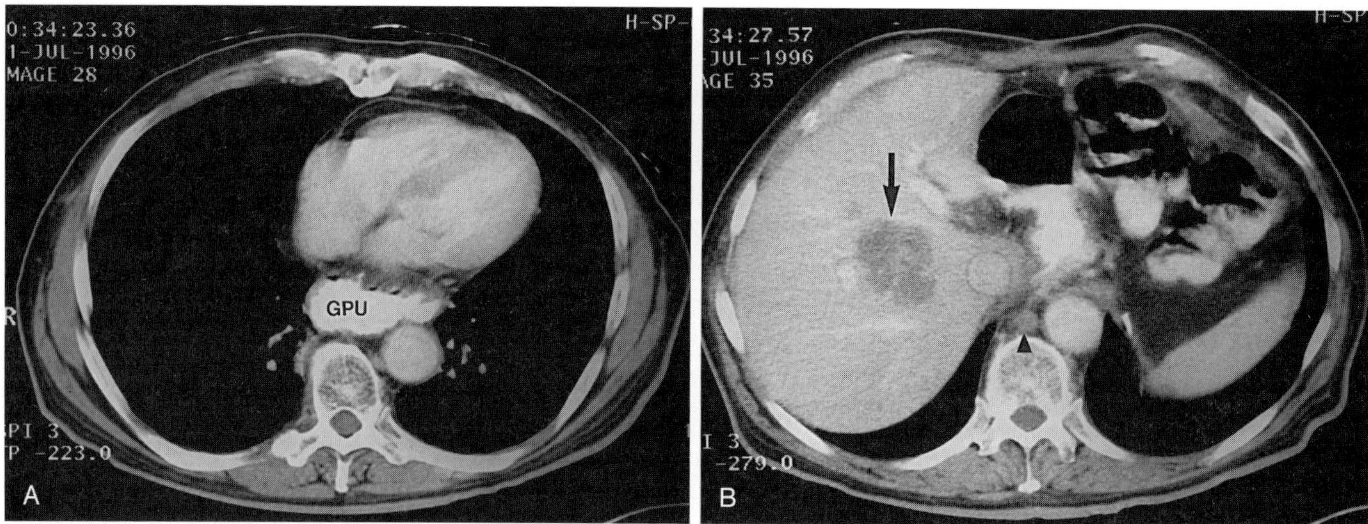

Figure 4–39. Contrast-enhanced spiral CT in a patient with esophageal carcinoma after esophagectomy and gastric pull-up. *A,* The CT demonstrates a contrast filled intrathoracic stomach, compatible with gastric pull-up (GPU). *B,* There is a 4 cm low attenuation mass within the liver *(arrow)* compatible with metastasis.

will demonstrate characteristic fat attenuation. Similarly, esophageal cysts, such as congenital duplication cysts or acquired retention cysts, may demonstrate water attenuation on CT, depending on the contents of the cyst.

Postoperative Esophagus

CT plays an important role in patients after transhiatal esophagectomy. This surgical procedure is complex and can result in a number of postsurgical complications. CT has an especially valuable role in the assessment of postoperative complications such as perforation, mediastinal abscess, chylothorax, or lymphocele.[91]

Mediastinal abscess is an important potential complication of esophagectomy that usually results from an anastomotic leak. It can be suspected by the development of fever, leukocytosis, and chest pain. On CT, a mediastinal abscess appears as a loculated fluid collection in the mediastinum and typically demonstrates an enhancing wall and may contain gas or an air-fluid level (Fig. 4–42).

Chylothorax also is a well-recognized complication of transhiatal esophagectomy, occurring in between 0.8 and 3% of patients. Chylothorax results from injury to the thoracic duct.[83,91] During esophagectomy, the thoracic duct may be injured, usually between the diaphragmatic hiatus and the carina, where the duct is a prevertebral structure that courses behind the esophagus before crossing to the left of the spine at the T4–5 level. On CT, a persistent or increasing pleural effusion is demonstrated. CT can sometimes distinguish a chylous from nonchylous effusion by noting a fat-fluid level in the chylous effusion. However, in most cases, correlation with thoracentesis and laboratory analysis is necessary for specific diagnosis.

A lymphocele is another complication that results from injury to the thoracic duct during surgery. It represents a more localized fluid collection on CT (Fig. 4–43) compared with a layering and free flowing chylothorax. After

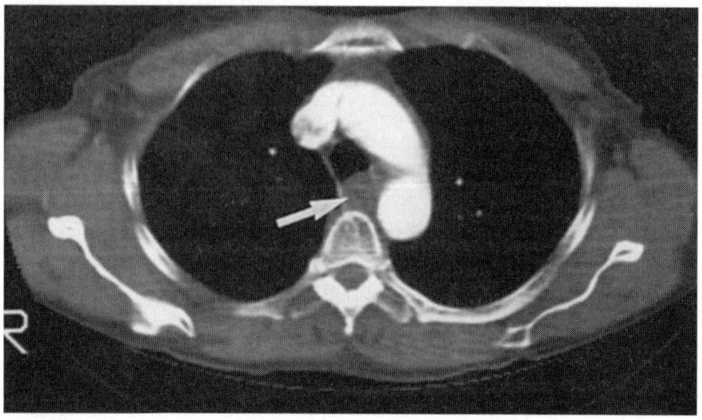

Figure 4–40. Contrast-enhanced spiral CT in a 51-year-old woman with a submucosal lesion noted on barium esophagogram demonstrates a low density mass in the esophagus *(arrow)*. This is a biopsy-proven leiomyoma.

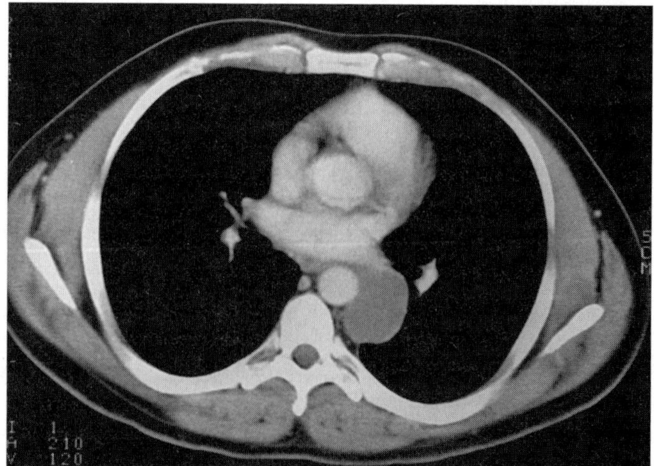

Figure 4–41. Contrast-enhanced spiral CT in a 33-year-old man with incidental mass noted on chest x-ray demonstrates a low attenuation cystic mass which is intimately related to the esophagus, compatible with a duplication cyst.

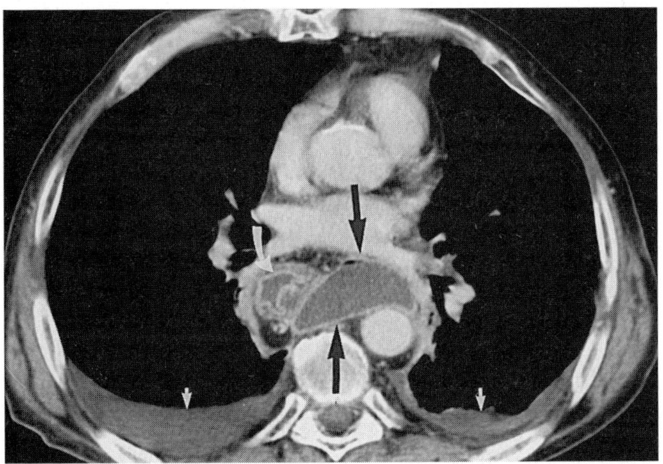

Figure 4–42. Contrast-enhanced spiral CT in 64-year-old male after esophagectomy and gastric pull-up for esophageal cancer demonstrates 6 × 4 cm fluid collection in the mediastinum *(arrow)* adjacent to the gastric pull-up *(curved arrow)*. There is a small amount of air within the collection. This CT appearance is compatible with abscess. There are also small bilateral pleural effusions *(small arrows)*.

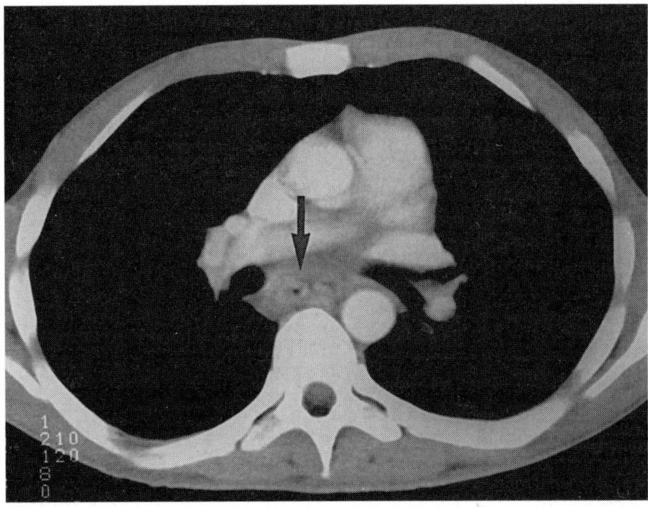

Figure 4–44. Contrast-enhanced spiral CT in a 33-year-old HIV-positive man with chest pain demonstrates moderate circumferential thickening of the esophagus *(arrow)* which is low in density, compatible with edema. There is also increased density within the adjacent mediastinal fat compatible with inflammation. These findings are most compatible with esophagitis in this clinical setting. This was confirmed at endoscopy. Locally invasive esophageal cancer could have a similar CT appearance.

esophagectomy, a lymphocele may occur in the thorax or upper abdomen.[91]

Benign Esophageal Pathology

Esophagitis

Although CT is not typically performed for the diagnosis or evaluation of esophagitis, it may be detected in patients undergoing CT for the evaluation of chest pain or vague gastrointestinal complaints.

Esophagitis appears as circumferential esophageal wall thickening on CT. In severe cases, the esophageal wall may demonstrate low density due to significant edema and inflammation.[82] In addition to esophageal wall thickening, esophageal ulceration, intramural dissection, or fistula can occasionally be present, especially in patients with unusual infections, such as tuberculosis.[25] In patients with severe esophagitis and inflammatory stranding in the mediastinal fat, the CT findings may mimic invasive esophageal carcinoma (Fig. 4–44). In these cases, endoscopy is recommended, because the CT appearance of esophageal cancer and esophagitis can overlap.

Overall, the CT findings in patients with esophagitis are nonspecific. CT can suggest the diagnosis, but in most cases, the CT findings do not indicate the specific cause of the esophagitis. CT is useful to evaluate compli-

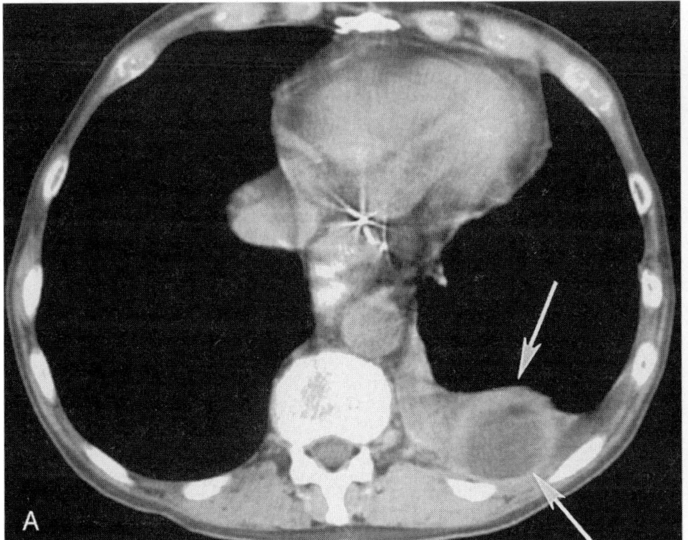

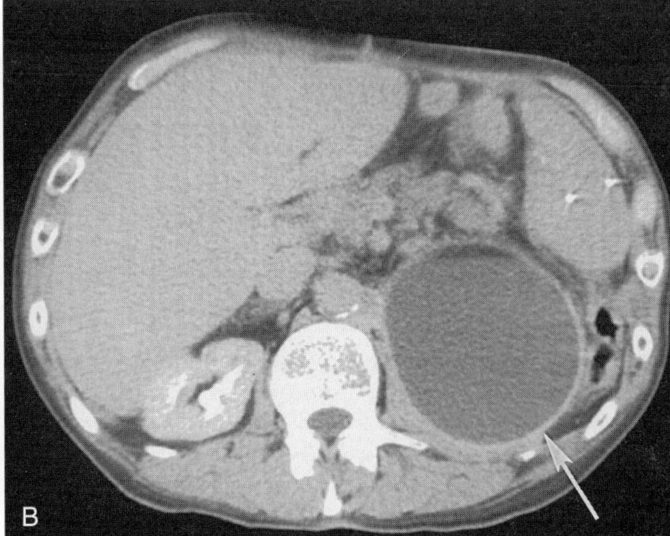

Figure 4–43. Contrast-enhanced CT in a patient after esophagectomy with gastric pull-up demonstrates a 12 × 10 × 20 cm lymphocele *(arrows)*, which extends from the posterior left chest *(A)* into the retroperitoneum *(B)*.

cations of severe esophagitis, such as esophageal perforation.

Barrett's Esophagus

The role of CT in patients with Barrett's esophagus is not well known. Although the diagnosis of Barrett's esophagus requires either barium esophagography or endoscopy, CT may play a role in the surveillance of patients with known Barrett's esophagus and high-grade dysphasia. In a study of 15 patients by Pietras et al.,[86] CT scans were reviewed and compared with pathologic specimens after esophagectomy for Barrett's esophagus with high-grade dysplasia. In this series, CT was used to correctly predict the presence or absence of esophageal cancer in 10 of the 15 patients. A correct prediction was made in 5 of 7 patients with cancer and 5 of 8 patients without cancer.[86] CT criteria for esophageal cancer included wall thickening, mass, celiac adenopathy, or liver metastasis. Therefore, in patients with Barrett's esophagus and high-grade dysplasia, surveillance endoscopy and biopsies are typically performed. However, because the diagnosis of carcinoma is difficult to determine on biopsy specimens in these patients, CT may also play a role in surveillance as well.

Foreign Bodies

Swallowed foreign bodies such as chicken or fish bones are often well demonstrated on plain films or contrast studies of the pharynx or esophagus. However, CT can be performed if these other modalities are equivocal or when the foreign body is small and only faintly radiopaque. CT can easily demonstrate the present of foreign bodies due to its excellent contrast and spatial resolution and can simultaneously assess for associated wall perforation.[9]

Gastroesophageal Varices

The CT appearance of esophageal varices depends on the size and extent of involvement. Usually, on unenhanced scans, small esophageal varices appear as thickening of the distal esophageal wall or gastric cardia.[16] Large varices can simulate adenopathy in the posterior mediastinum on noncontrast scans, which is a potential pitfall. Therefore, when gastroesophageal varices are suspected, intravenous contrast medium is essential. With intravenous contrast agents, esophageal varices will appear as enhancing vessels at the gastroesophageal junction[3] (Fig. 4–45).

Three-dimensional CT angiography can also be used to better evaluate portosystemic collateral vessels and to clearly demonstrate esophageal venous collateral vessels and their relationship to the portal and systemic venous systems (Fig. 4–46). Despite rapid contrast injection and fast scanning, at this time, spiral CT cannot be used to routinely detect active variceal bleeding.

Achalasia

Although the diagnosis of achalasia is usually made with barium studies and endoscopy with manometry, CT may be the first imaging modality performed in patients with nonspecific complaints or in patients in whom a mediastinal mass has been detected on a chest radiograph. In patients with achalasia, CT demonstrates moderate to marked dilatation of the esophagus, which will often contain a moderate amount of retained food and mucus, which mix with the oral contrast agent (Fig. 4–47). The mean esophageal diameter in patients with achalasia undergoing CT is 4.5 cm at the level of the carina, with an abrupt transition at the level of the lower esophageal sphincter.[88] The esophageal wall will typically be of normal thickness. CT can be performed in patients after pneumostatic dilatation if a complication such as perforation is suspected.

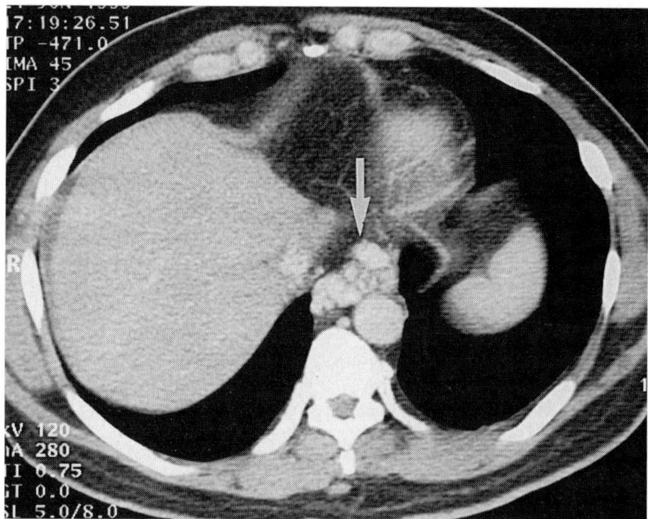

Figure 4–45. Contrast-enhanced spiral CT in a patient with cirrhosis and portal hypertension demonstrates enhancing esophageal varices.

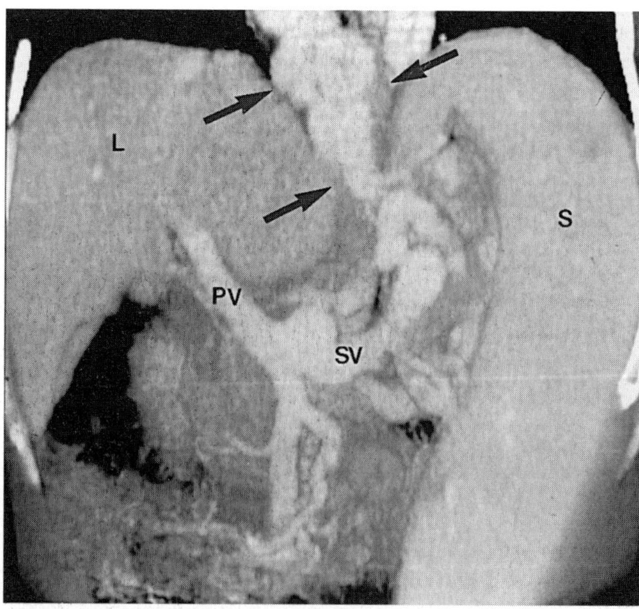

Figure 4–46. Coronal 3D image from contrast-enhanced spiral CT in a patient with cirrhosis and portal hypertension demonstrates large gastroesophageal varices *(arrows)*. There is moderate splenomegaly. L, liver; S, spleen; PV, portal vein; SV, splenic vein.

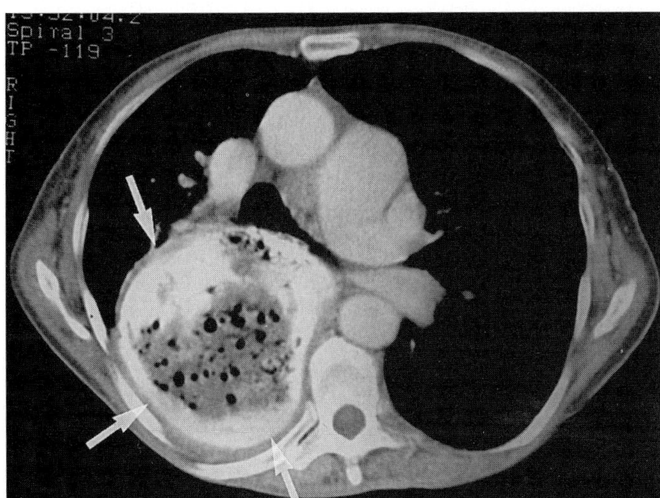

Figure 4–47. Spiral CT of the chest with oral and intravenous contrast in a patient with a large right lung mass identified on chest radiograph demonstrates marked dilatation of the esophagus with retained food mixed with oral contrast. This degree of dilatation is compatible with achalasia.

Esophageal Perforation

Perforation of the esophagus may occur spontaneously or as a result of chest trauma, foreign body aspiration, esophageal neoplasms, or endoscopic procedures. The condition can be life threatening and must be recognized early. Although contrast radiography is considered to be the radiographic standard for the evaluation of patients with suspected esophageal perforation, up to 10% of patients with esophageal perforation may have false-negative findings on contrast esophagography.[5] In addition, if the clinical symptoms are atypical, CT may be performed early in the clinical course and may be the first to suggest the diagnosis.[117] Therefore, recognition of the CT findings in esophageal perforation is important. Also, CT can detect extraluminal complications of perforation such as pneumomediastinum, mediastinal abscess, and empyema.

CT is useful on the diagnosis of esophageal perforation and may help direct surgical management. Extraluminal air is the most useful CT finding, occurring in more than 90% of cases[117] (Fig. 4–48). Although mediastinal air is a sensitive indicator of esophageal perforation, it is not specific. Patients with pneumothorax or pneumoperitoneum may have extension of air into the mediastinum, without esophageal injury. Other CT findings include the presence of mediastinal fluid, pleural fluid, or esophageal wall thickening. Extravasated oral contrast may be demonstrated, when the perforation is transmural. In cases of contained intramural perforation, CT will demonstrate intramural air and/or contrast.

In patients with esophageal carcinoma as the cause of the perforation, CT can evaluate the location of the mass and assess for local extension and distant metastases. In patients with suspected esophageal injury and/or perforation after ingestion of a caustic substance, CT can be performed, because there is a risk of perforation of the acutely inflamed esophagus during endoscopy.

Anomalous Vessels

Anomalies of the thoracic aorta and great vessels are not uncommon and can result in esophageal compression and dysphagia. Enhanced spiral CT with three-dimensional reconstruction is an excellent modality to identify these complex anomalies and to demonstrate their effect on adjacent mediastinal structures. MRI with its multiplanar capability and lack of ionizing radiation is also able to demonstrate these vascular anomalies.

The most common congenital anomaly of the aorta is an isolated aberrant right subclavian artery. On CT, the aberrant vessel can be identified arising distal to the left subclavian artery and crossing the mediastinum behind the esophagus.[77] Mass effect on the esophagus can cause dysphagia (Fig. 4–49). A right aortic arch with an aberrant left subclavian artery is less common but may also result in esophageal compression.[48] A pulmonary sling occurs when an aberrant left pulmonary artery arises from the right pulmonary artery and passes between the trachea and the esophagus. Compression of both the trachea and esophagus can occur. This anomaly can also be reliably detected with contrast-enhanced CT.[77]

CONCLUSION

Since the 1980s, radiologic studies have come to play a critical role in imaging of the gastrointestinal tract. Contrast studies continue to provide important information about both anatomy and function of the esophagus and often serve as a valuable adjunct to endoscopy. With its ability to visualize the esophageal lumen, wall, and adjacent mediastinal organs, CT is useful in the evaluation of both benign and malignant diseases of the esophagus. With continued advances in CT technology, contrast

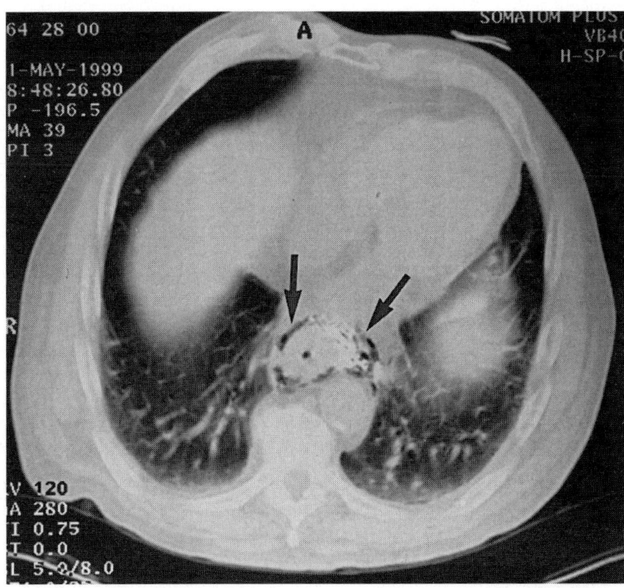

Figure 4–48. Spiral CT of the chest in a patient with esophageal cancer complaining of chest pain after esophageal stent placement. The CT demonstrates extraluminal air and contrast in the mediastinum *(arrows)* compatible with perforation.

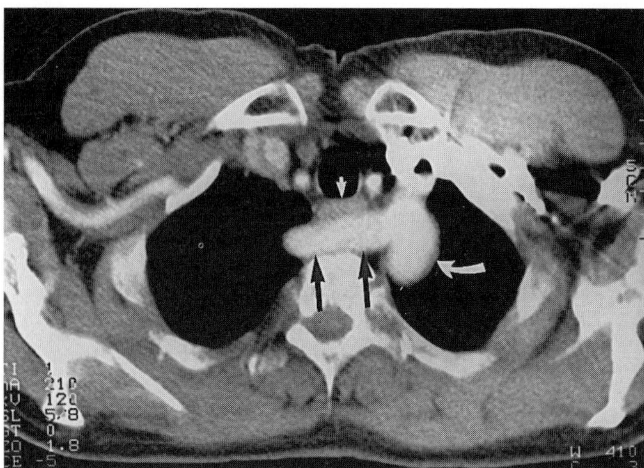

Figure 4–49. Contrast-enhanced spiral CT in a 64-year-old man with dysphagia demonstrates a large aberrant right subclavian artery *(straight arrows)* arising from a left aortic arch *(curved arrow)*. The aberrant vessel crosses behind the esophagus *(small arrow)* causing extrinsic compression. This is an example of dysphagia lusoria.

agents, and computer applications, the role of CT in esophageal imaging will likely increase.

References

1. Andersen, H.A., Bernatz, P.E., and Grindlay, J.H.: Perforation of the esophagus after use of a digestive agent: Report of a case and experimental study. Ann. Otol. Rhinol. Laryngol., *68:*890, 1959.
2. Balthazar, E.J., Megibow, A.J., Hulnick, D., et al.: Cytomegalovirus esophagitis in AIDS: Radiographic features in 16 patients. Am. J. Radiol., *149:*919, 1987.
3. Balthazar, E.J., Naidich, D.P., Megibow, A.J., and Lefleur, R.S.: CT evaluation of esophageal varices. Am. J. Radiol., *148:*131, 1987.
4. Banfield, W.J., and Hurwitz, A.L.: Esophageal stricture associated with nasogastric intubation. Arch. Intern. Med., *134:*1083, 1974.
5. Bladergroen, M.R., Lowe, J.E., and Postlethwait, R.W.: Diagnosis and recommended management of esophageal perforation and rupture. Ann. Thorac. Surg., *42:*235, 1986.
6. Blumhagen, J.D., Rudd, T.G., and Christie, D.L.: Gastroesophageal reflux in children: Radionuclide gastroesophagography. Radiology, *135:*1001, 1980.
7. Bondi, J.L. Godwin, D.H., and Garrett, J.M.: "Vigorous achalasia": Its clinical interpretation and significance. Am. J. Gastroenterol., *58:*145, 1972.
8. Brauer, R.B., Liebermann-Meffert, D., Stein, H.J., et al.: Boerhaave's syndrome: Analysis of the literature and report of 18 new cases. Dis. Esophagus, *10:*64, 1997.
9. Braverman, I., Gomori, J.M., Polv, O., and Saah, D.: The role of CT imaging in the evaluation of cervical esophageal foreign bodies. J. Otolaryngol., *22:*311, 1993.
10. Brick, I.B., and Palmer, E.D.: Comparison of esophagoscopic and roentgenologic diagnosis of esophageal varices in cirrhosis of the liver. Am. J. Radiol., *73:*387, 1955.
11. Bruhlmann, W.F., Zollikofer, C.L., Maranta, E., et al.: Intramural pseudodiverticulosis of the esophagus: Report of seven cases and literature review. Gastrointest. Radiol., *6:*199, 1981.
12. Buecker, A., Wein, B.B., Neuerburg, J.M., and Guenther, R.W.: Esophageal perforation: Comparison of use of aqueous and barium-containing contrast media. Radiology, *202:*683, 1997.
13. Castillo, S., Aburashed, A., Kimmelman, J., and Alexander, L.C.: Diffuse intramural esophageal pseudodiverticulosis: New cases and review. Gastroenterology, *72:*541, 1977.
14. Chen, Y.M., Gelfand, D.W., Ott, D.J., and Wu, W.C.: Barrett esophagus as an extension of severe esophagitis: Analysis of radiologic signs in 29 cases. Am. J. Radiol., *145:*275, 1985.
15. Chiu, C.L., and Gambach, R.R.: Hypaque pulmonary edema: A case report. Radiology, *111:*91, 1974.
16. Cho, K.C., Patel, Y.D, Wachsberg, R.H., and Seeff, J.: Varices in portal hypertension: Evaluation with CT. Radiographics, *15:*609, 1995.
17. Cho S.R., Sanders M.M., Turner M.A., et al.: Esophageal intramural pseudodiverticulosis. Gastrointest. Radiol., *6:*9, 1981.
18. Cockrill, E.M., Miller, R.E., Chernish, S.M., et al.: Optimal visualization of esophageal varices. Am. J. Radiol., *126:*512, 1976.
19. Cole, M.J., Paterson, W.G., Beck, I.T., and DaCosta, L.R.: The effect of acid and bethanechol stimulation in patients with symptomatic hypertensive peristaltic (nutcracker) esophagus: Evidence that this disorder may be a precursor to diffuse esophageal spasm. J. Clin. Gastroenterol., *8:*223, 1986.
20. Conces, D.J., Jr., Tarver, R.D., and Lappas, J.C.: The value of opacification of the esophagus by low denisty barium paste in computed tomography of the thorax. J. Comput. Assist. Tomogr., *12:*202, 1988.
21. Coulomb, M., Lebas, J.F., Sarrazin, R., and Geindre, M.: Oesophageal cancer extension: Diagnostic contribution and effects of therapy of computed tomography (French). J. Radiol., *62:*475, 1981.
22. Daffner, R.H., Halber, M.D., Postlethwait, R.W., et al.: CT of the esophagus. II. Carcinoma. Am. J. Radiol., *133:*1051, 1979.
23. Dalinka, M.K., Smith, E.H., Wolfe, R.D., et al.: Pharmacologically enhanced visualization of esophageal varices by Pro-Banthine. Radiology, *102:*281, 1972.
24. de Oliveira, J.M., Birgisson, S., Doinoff, C., et al.: Timed barium swallow: A simple technique for evaluating esophageal emptying in patients with achalasia. Am. J. Radiol., *169:*473, 1997.
25. de Silva, R., Stoopack, P.M., and Raufman, J.P.: Esophageal fistulas associated with mycobacterial infection in patients at risk for AIDS. Radiology, *175:*449, 1990.
26. Desai, R.K., Tagliabue, J.R., Wegryn, S.A., and Einstein, D.M.: CT evaluation of wall thickening in the alimentary tract. Radiographics, *11:*771, 1991.
27. Donner, M.W., Silbiger, M.L., Hookman, B., and Hendrix, T.R.: Acid-barium swallows in the radiographic evaluation of clinical esophagitis. Radiology, *87:*220, 1966.
28. Dyet, J.F., Bennett, J.R., Buckton, G., and Ashworth, D.: The radiological measurement of oesophageal stricture diameter. Clin. Radiol., *34:*647, 1983.
29. Ekberg, O., and Nylander, G.: Webs and web-like formations in the pharynx and cervical esophagus. Diagn. Imaging, *52:*10, 1983.
30. Endo M., Takemoto, T., and Shirakabe, H.: Minute lesions of esophageal cancer. Semin. Surg. Oncol., *2:*177, 1986.
31. Ferraro P., and Durnanceau, A.: Esophageal diverticula. Chest Surg. Clin. North Am., *4:*741, 1994.
32. Foley, M.J., Ghahremani, G.G., and Rogers, L.F.: Re-appraisal of contrast media used to detect upper gastrointestinal perforations: Comparison of ionic water soluble media with barium sulfate. Radiology, *144:*231, 1982.
33. Franken E.A., Jr.: Caustic damage of the gastrointestinal tract: Roentgen features. Am. J. Radiol., *118:*77, 1973.
34. Fulp, S.R., and Castell, D.O.: Scleroderma esophagus. Dysphagia, *5:*204, 1990.
35. Gheorghe, C., Aposteanu, G., Popescu, C., et al.: Long esophageal stricture in Crohn's disease: A case report. Hepatogastroenterology, *45:*738, 1998.
36. Glick, S.N.: Barium studies in patients with Barrett's esophagus: Importance of focal areas of esophageal deformity. Am. J. Radiol., *163:*65, 1994.
37. Glick, S.N., Teplick, S.K., and Amenta, P.S.: The radiologic diagnosis of Barrett esophagus: Importance of mucosal surface abnormalities on air-contrast barium studies. Am. J. Radiol., *157:*951, 1991.
38. Goldenberg, S.P., Burrell, M., Fette, C.G., et al.: Classic and vigorous achalasia: A comparison of manometric, radiographic, and clinical findings. Gastroenterology, *101:*743, 1991.
39. Goldman, L.P., and Weigert, J.M.: Corrosive substance ingestion: A review. Am. J. Gastroenterol., *79:*85, 1984.
40. Goldstein, H.M., Zornoza, J., and Hopens, T.: Intrinsic disease of the adult esophagus: Benign and malignant tumors. Semin. Roentgenol., *3:*183, 1981.
41. Gollub, M.J., and Bains, M.S.: Barium sulfate: A new (old) contrast agent for diagnosis of postoperative esophageal leaks. Radiology, *202:*360, 1997.

42. Guanrei, Y., Songliang, Q., He, H., and Guizen, F.: Natural history of early esophageal squamous carcinoma and early adenocarcinoma of the gastric cardia in the People's Republic of China. Endoscopy, *20:*95, 1988.
43. Gunnlaugsson, G.H., Wychulis, A.R., Roland, C., and Ellis, F.H., Jr.: Analysis of records of 1,657 patients with carcinoma of the esophagus and cardia of the stomach. Surg. Gynecol. Obstet., *130:*997, 1970.
44. Halvorsen, R.A., Jr., and Thompson, W.M.: Computed tomographic staging of gastrointestinal malignancies. Part I. Esophagus and stomach. Invest. Radiol., *22:*2, 1987.
45. Heitmiller, R.F., and Jones, B.: Transient diminished airway protection after transhiatal esophagectomy. Am. J. Surg., *162:*442, 1991.
46. Holsinger, L.W., Jr., Fuson, R.L., and Sealy, W.C.: Esophageal perforation following meat impaction and papain ingestion. J.A.M.A., *203:*734, 1968.
47. Honkoop, P., Siersema, P.D., Tilanus, H.W., et al.: Benign anastomotic strictures after transhiatal esophagectomy and cervical esophagogastrostomy: Risk factors and management. J. Thorac. Cardiovasc. Surg., *111:*1141, 1996.
48. Jaffe, R.B.: Radiographic manifestations of congenital anomalies of the aortic arch. Radiol. Clin. North Am., *29:*319, 1991.
49. Johnson, A.C., Lester, P.D., Johnson, S., et al.: Esophagogastric ring: Why and when we see it and what it implies: A radiologic-pathologic correlation. South Med. J., *85:*946, 1992.
50. Katariya, K., Harvey, J.C., Pina, E., and Beattie, E.J.: Complications of transhiatal esophagectomy. J. Surg. Oncol., *57:*157, 1994.
51. Kikendall, J.W., Friedman, A.C., Oyewole, M.A., et al.: Pill-induced esophageal injury: Case reports and review of the medical literature. Dig. Dis. Sci., *28:*174, 1983.
52. Klein, H.A.: Esophageal transit scintigraphy. Semin. Nucl. Med., *25:*306, 1995.
53. Knuff, T.E., Benjamin, S.B., and Castell, D.O.: Pharyngoesophageal (Zenker's) diverticulum: A reappraisal. Gastroenterology, *82:*734, 1982.
54. Koehler, R.E., Moss, A.A., and Margulis, A.R.: Early radiographic manifestations of carcinoma of the esophagus. Radiology, *119:*1, 1976.
55. Kozuka, T., Minaguchi, K., Yamaguchi, R., et al.: Three dimensional imaging of the tracheobronchial system using spiral CT. Comput. Methods Prog. Biomed., *57:*133, 1998.
56. Kuszyk, B.S., Bluemke, D.A., Urban, B.A., et al.: Portal-phase contrast enhanced helical CT for the detection of malignant hepatic tumors: Sensitivity based on comparison with intraoperative and pathologic findings. Am. J. Radiol., *166:*91, 1996.
57. Lackey, C., Rankin, R.A., and Welsh, J.D.: Stricture location in Barrett's esophagus. Gastrointest. Endosc., *30:*331, 1984.
58. Lambert, J.R., and Newman, A.: Ulceration and stricture of the esophagus due to oral potassium chloride (slow release tablet) therapy. Am. J. Gastroenterol., *73:*508, 1980.
59. Lefor, A.T., Merino, M.M., Steinberg, S.M., et al.: Computerized tomographic prediction of extraluminal spread and prognostic implications of lesion width in esophageal cancer. Cancer, *62:*1287, 1988.
60. Levine, M.S.: Radiology of esophagitis: A pattern approach. Radiology, *179:*1, 1991.
61. Levine, M.S.: Radiology of the Esophagus. Philadelphia, W.B. Saunders, 1988.
62. Levine, M.S., Dillon, E.C., Saul, S.H., and Laufer, I.: Early esophageal cancer. Am. J. Radiol., *146:*507, 1986.
63. Levine, M.S., Loercher, G., Katzka, D.A., et al.: Giant, human immunodeficiency virus-related ulcers in the esophagus. Radiology, *180:*323, 1991.
64. Levine, M.S., Loevner, L.A., Saul, S.H., et al.: Herpes esophagitis: Sensitivity of double-contrast esophagography. Am. J. Radiol., *151:*57, 1988.
65. Levine, M.S., Macones, A.J., Jr., and Laufer, I.: *Candida* esophagitis: Accuracy of radiographic diagnosis. Radiology, *154:*581, 1985.
66. Levine, M.S., Moolten, D.N., Herlinger, H., and Laufer, I.: Esophageal intramural pseudodiverticulosis: A reevaluation. Am. J. Radiol., *147:*1165, 1986.
67. Lichtenstein, G.R.: Esophageal scintigraphy in achalasia and achalasia-like disorders. J. Nucl. Med., *33:*590, 1992.
68. Lightdale, C.J., and Botet, J.F.: Esophageal carcinoma: Pre-operative staging and evaluation of anastomotic recurrence. Gastrointest. Endosc., *36:*11, 1990.
69. Longstreth, G.F., and Foroozan, P.: Evolution of symptomatic diffuse esophageal spasm to achalasia. South Med. J., *75:*217, 1982.
70. Love, L., and Berkow, A.E.: Trauma to the esophagus. Gastrointest. Radiol., *2:*305, 1978.
71. Malmud, L.S., and Fisher, R.S.: Gastroesophageal scintigraphy. Gastrointest. Radiol., *5:*195, 1980.
72. Marks, R.D., and Richter, J.E.: Peptic strictures of the esophagus. Am. J. Gastroenterol., *88:*1160, 1993.
73. Marks, W.M., Callen, P.W., and Moss, A.A.: Gastroesophageal region: Source of confusion on CT. Am. J. Radiol., *136:*359, 1981.
74. Marshall, J.B., Kretschmar, J.M., and Diaz-Arias, A.A.: Gastroesophageal reflux as a pathogenic factor in the development of symptomatic lower esophageal rings. Arch. Intern. Med., *150:*1669, 1990.
75. Marty-Ane, C.H., Prudhome, M., Fabre, J.M., et al.: Tracheoesophagogastric anastomosis fistula: A rare complication of esophagectomy. Ann. Thorac. Surg., *60:*690, 1995.
76. Mauro, M.A., Parker, L.A., Hartley, W.S., et al.: Epidermolysis bullosa: Radiographic findings in 16 cases. Am. J. Radiol., *149:*925, 1987.
77. McLoughlin, M.J., Weisbrod, G., Wise, D.J., and Yeung, H.P.: Computed tomography in congenital anomalies of the aortic arch and great vessels. Radiology, *138:*399, 1981.
78. Muhletaler, C.A., Gerlock, A.J., Jr., de Soto, L., and Halter, S.A.: Acid corrosive esophagitis: Radiographic findings. Am. J. Radiol., *134:*1137, 1980.
79. Muhletaler, C.A., Gerlock, A.J., Jr., de Soto, L., and Halter, S.A.: Gastroduodenal lesions of ingested acids: Radiographic findings. Am. J. Radiol., *135:*1247, 1980.
80. Narducci, F., Bassotti, G., Gaburri, M., and Morelli, A.: Transition from nutcracker esophagus to diffuse esophageal spasm. Am. J. Gastroenterol., *80:*242, 1985.
81. Naylor, M.F., MacCarty, R.L., and Rogers, R.S., 3rd: Barium studies in esophageal cicatricial pemphigoid. Abdom. Imaging, *20:*97, 1995.
82. Noh, H.M., Fishman, E.K., Forastiere, A.A., et al.: CT of the esophagus: Spectrum of disease with emphasis on esophageal carcinoma. Radiographics, *15:*1113, 1995.
83. Orringer, M.B., Bluett, M., and Deeb, G.M.: Aggressive treatment of chylothorax complicating transhiatal esophagectomy without thoracotomy. Surgery, *104:*720, 1988.
84. Ott, D.J., Gelfand, D.W., Munitz, H.A., and Chen, Y.M.: Cold barium suspensions in the clinical evaluation of the esophagus. Gastrointest. Radiol., *9:*193, 1984.
85. Picus, D., Balfe, D.M., Koehler, R.E., et al.: Computed tomography in the staging of esophageal carcinoma. Radiology, *146:*433, 1983.
86. Pietras, E.S., Fishman, E.K., Jones, B., and Heitmiller, R.F.: Carcinoma of the esophagus arising in Barrett esophagus: Value of CT. Appl. Radiol., *25:*26, 1996.
87. Plavsic, B.M., Chen, M.Y., Gelfand, D.W., et al.: Intramural pseudodiverticulosis of the esophagus detected on barium esophagograms: Increased prevalence in patients with esophageal carcinoma. Am. J. Radiol., *165:*1381, 1995.
88. Rabushka, L.S., Fishman, E.K., and Kuhlman, J.E.: CT evaluation of achalasia. J. Comput. Assist. Tomogr., *15:*434, 1991.
89. Recht, M.P., Levine, M.S., Katzka, D.A., et al.: Barrett's esophagus in scleroderma: Increased prevalence and radiographic findings. Gastrointest. Radiol., *13:*1, 1988.
90. Reich, S.B.: Production of pulmonary edema by aspiration of water-soluble nonabsorbable contrast media. Radiology, *92:*367, 1969.
91. Reichle, R.L., Fishman, E.K., Nixon, M.S., et al.: Evaluation of the postsurgical esophagus after partial esophagogastrectomy for esophageal cancer: Normal postoperative appearance and complications. Invest. Radiol., *28:*247, 1993.
92. Reinig, J.W., Stanley, J.H., and Schabel, S.I.: CT evaluation of thickened esophageal walls. Am. J. Radiol., *140:*931, 1983.
93. Richter, J.E., and Castell, D.O.: Diffuse esophageal spasm: A reappraisal. Ann. Intern. Med., *100:*242, 1984.
94. Robbins, M.I., and Shortsleeve, M.J.: Treatment of acute esophageal food impaction with glucagon, an effervescent agent, and water. Am. J. Radiol., *162:*325, 1994.
95. Rogers, L.F., Puig, W., Dooley, B.N., and Cuello, L.: Diagnostic considerations in mediastinal emphysema: A pathophysiologic-roentgenologic approach to Boerhaave's syndrome and spontaneous pneumomediastinum. Am. J. Radiol., *115:*495, 1972.

96. Rohrmann, C.A., Jr.: When is a Schatzki ring clinically significant and what is the best maneuver to demonstrate it on barium swallow? Does the abnormality progress if it is not treated? Am. J. Radiol., *163:*215. 1994.
97. Rosenberg, J.C., and Franklin, R.Z.S.: Squamous cell carcinoma of the thoracic esophagus: An interdisciplinary approach. Curr. Probl. Cancer, *5:*1, 1981.
98. Rudd, T.G., and Christie, D.L.: Demonstration of gastroesophageal reflux in children by radionuclide gastroesophagography. Radiology, *131:*483, 1979.
99. Schatzki, R.G.J.: Dysphagia due to diaphragm-like localized narrowing in the lower esophagus (lower esophageal ring). Am. J. Radiol., *70:*911, 1953.
100. Schima, W., Schober, E., Stacher, G., et al.: Association of mid esophageal diverticula with oesophageal motor disorders: Videofluoroscopy and manometry. Acta Radiol., *38:*108, 1997.
101. Shah, S.W., Khan, A.A., Alam, A., et al.: Diffuse esophageal spasm: Transformimg into achalasia. J. Pakistan Med. Assoc., *48:*58, 1998.
102. Shay, S.S., Abreu, S.H., and Tsuchida, A.: Scintigraphy in gastroesophageal reflux disease: A comparison to endoscopy, LESp and 24-h pH score, as well as to simultaneous pH monitoring. Am. J. Gastroenterol., *87:*1094, 1992.
103. Shortsleeve, M.J., and Levine, M.S.: Herpes esophagitis in otherwise healthy patients: Clinical and radiological findings. Radiology, *182:*859, 1992.
104. Sor, S., Levine, M.S., Kowalski, T.E., et al.: Giant ulcers of the esophagus in patients with human immunodeficiency virus: Clinical, radiographic, and pathologic findings. Radiology, *194:*447, 1995.
105. Takashima, S., Takeuchi, N., Shiozaki, H., et al.: Carcinoma of the esophagus: CT vs MR imaging in determining resectability. Am. J. Radiol., *156:*297, 1991.
106. Templeton, F.E.: X-Ray Examination of the Stomach: A Description of the Roentgenologic Anatomy, Physiology and Pathology of the Esophagus, Stomach and Duodenum. Chicago, University of Chicago Press, 1944.
107. Thompson, J.K., Koehler, R.E., and Richter, J.E.: Detection of gastroesophageal reflux: Value of barium studies compared with 24-hr pH monitoring. Am. J. Radiol., *162:*621, 1994.
108. Thompson, W.M., Halvorsen, R.A., Foster, W.L., Jr., et al.: Computed tomography for staging esophageal and gastroesophageal cancer: reevaluation. Am. J. Radiol., *141:*951, 1983.
109. Tobin, R.W.: Esophageal rings, webs, and diverticula. J. Clin. Gastroenterol., *27:*285, 1998.
110. Todorczuk, J.R., Aliperti, G., Staiano, A., and Clouse, R.E.: Reevaluation of manometric criteria for vigorous achalasia? Is this a distinct clinical disorder? Dig. Dis. Sci., *36:*274, 1991.
111. Traube, M., Albibi, R., and McCallum, R.W.: High-amplitude peristaltic esophageal contractions associated with chest pain. J.A.M.A., *250:*2655, 1983.
112. van Overhagen, H., Lameris, J.S., Berger, M.Y., et al.: CT assessment of resectability prior to transhiatal esophagectomy for esophageal/gastroesophageal junction carcinoma. J. Comput. Assist. Tomogr., *17:*367, 1993.
113. van Overhagen, H., Lameris, J.S., Berger, M.Y., et al.: Supraclavicular lymph node metastases in carcinoma of the esophagus and gastroesophageal junction: Assessment with CT, US, and US-guided fine-needle aspiration biopsy. Radiology, *179:*155, 1991.
114. Vinson, P.O.: Hysterical dysphagia. Minn. Med., *5:*107, 1921.
115. Waldman, I., and Berlin, L.: Stricture of the esophagus due to nasogastric intubation. Am. J. Radiol., *94:*321, 1965.
116. Weaver, J.W., Kaude, J.V., and Kamlin, D.J.: Webs of the lower esophagus: A complication of gastroesophageal reflux. Am. J. Radiol., *142:*289, 1984.
117. White, C.S., Templeton, P.A., and Attar, S.: Esophageal perforation: CT findings. Am. J. Radiol., *160:*767, 1993.
118. Winans, C.S.: The pharyngoesophageal closure mechanism: A manometric study. Gastroenterology, *63:*768, 1972.
119. Wolfman, N.T., Scharling, E.S., and Chen, M.Y.: Esophageal squamous carcinoma. Radiol. Clin. North Am., *32:*1183, 1994.
120. Yasuda, S., Raja, S., and Hubner, K.F.: Application of whole-body positron emission tomography in the imaging of esophageal cancer: Report of a case. Surg. Today, *25:*261, 1995.
121. Zerhouni, E.A., Rutter, C., Hamilton, S.R., et al.: CT and MR imaging in the staging of colorectal carcinoma: Report of Radiology Diagnostic Oncology Group II. Radiology, *200:*443, 1996.

CHAPTER

5 Endoscopic Evaluation of the Esophagus

MARK K. FERGUSON

ENDOSCOPIC ANATOMY OF THE ESOPHAGUS

The length of the esophagus is related directly to the height of the individual and averages 25 cm in the adult. The cricopharyngeus lies 15 to 18 cm from the incisors, whereas the lower esophageal sphincter is found about 40 cm from the incisors. The internal diameter of the esophagus is 1.5 to 2.5 cm and is maximal in the distal portion. Compression of the lumen on the left lateral portion by the aortic arch is found approximately 25 cm from the incisors, and compression from the left main stem bronchus is often evident just distal to this. Anterior impressions resulting from cardiac structures, particularly the left atrium, are often found more distally. The lower esophageal sphincter is typically less distensible than the remainder of the esophagus and measures 2 to 2.5 cm in length. The diaphragm is usually located 2 cm proximal to the esophagogastric junction. The true end of the esophagus can be identified endoscopically by the location of the lower esophageal sphincter or by visualizing the termination of the tubular peristaltic wave.

The mucosal surface is arranged in longitudinal columns 2 to 4 mm wide except under conditions of maximum distention. These run distally to converge in the "cardiac rosette" at the level of the diaphragm. The esophageal squamous mucosa is typically a translucent pink and has an easily identified submucosal vascular network that runs longitudinally. At the level of the gastroesophageal junction, the squamous esophageal mucosa changes abruptly to columnar mucosa, which is an orange-red color. The mucosal junction may have a serrated edge, frequently referred to as the Z-line, and may lie up to 2 cm proximal to the lower esophageal sphincter.

INDICATIONS FOR ESOPHAGOSCOPY

Diagnostic esophagoscopy is performed to make a thorough visual examination of the entire esophagus and relevant portions of the stomach and duodenum, to discover all significant abnormalities, and to take samples of lesions for biopsy when appropriate. It is generally indicated when the endoscopic findings influence patient management or when an empiric trial of therapy for an esophageal disease is unsuccessful (Table 5-1).[4]

Esophagoscopy should be performed when upper abdominal discomfort is associated with signs of organic disease, including anorexia or weight loss, or when it persists despite a trial of appropriate therapy. Dysphagia or odynophagia should always be evaluated endoscopically. Symptoms of gastroesophageal reflux disease that persist or progress in spite of proper therapy warrant endoscopic evaluation. Esophagoscopy is also indicated to confirm radiographic findings suggesting a neoplastic lesion, a gastric or esophageal ulcer, or an obstructing stricture or mass in the esophagus. Periodic esophagoscopy should be performed in all patients with Barrett's esophagus for surveillance for malignant degeneration and for follow-up of large ulcers on Barrett's esophagus to demonstrate healing. Esophagoscopy is used as the initial method of evaluation in most cases of acute gastrointestinal bleeding as an alternative to x-ray studies. Esophagoscopy is also indicated when surgical treatment of such bleeding is under consideration or for evaluation of iron deficiency anemia that is presumed to be caused by chronic blood loss. The initial evaluation of the extent of acute injury following caustic ingestion is also performed endoscopically.

FLEXIBLE ESOPHAGOGASTRODUODENOSCOPY

Equipment

Flexible esophagogastroduodenoscopy (EGD) is the technique most commonly used for endoscopic examination of the esophagus and related organs. The endoscopes range in size from 6 to 13.2 mm in outer diameter (Table 5-2). They typically have an 8-cm distal section that bends upward 210 degrees, downward 90 degrees, right 100 degrees, and left 100 degrees. Scope tip bending is controlled manually by means of two control wheels mounted near the head of the scope. The usual working length of such a scope is about 103 cm, with an overall length of 135 cm. Standard optical systems provide a 0-degree direction of view (forward viewing) with a field of view of 100 to 120 degrees and a depth of field of 3 to 100 mm. Instrumentation channels range in diameter from 2 to 3.7 mm, allowing use of a wide range of biopsy forceps (Fig. 5-1), cytology brushes, and irrigation catheters.

Table 5–1. Indications for Endoscopic Examination of the Esophagus*

1. Upper gastrointestinal distress associated with symptoms suggesting serious organic disease (e.g., anorexia and weight loss)
2. Dysphagia or odynophagia
3. Esophageal reflux symptoms that are persistent or recurrent despite appropriate therapy
4. For confirmation and histologic diagnosis of radiographically demonstrated esophageal mass, stricture, or ulcer
5. Gastrointestinal bleeding
6. Periodic surveillance of Barrett's esophagus
7. Cirrhotic patients in whom prophylactic sclerotherapy is considered
8. Assessment of acute injury after caustic ingestion

*From the American Society for Gastrointestinal Endoscopy: Appropriate Use of Gastrointestinal Endoscopy. Manchester, MA, American Society for Gastrointestinal Endoscopy, 1992, p. 5, with permission.

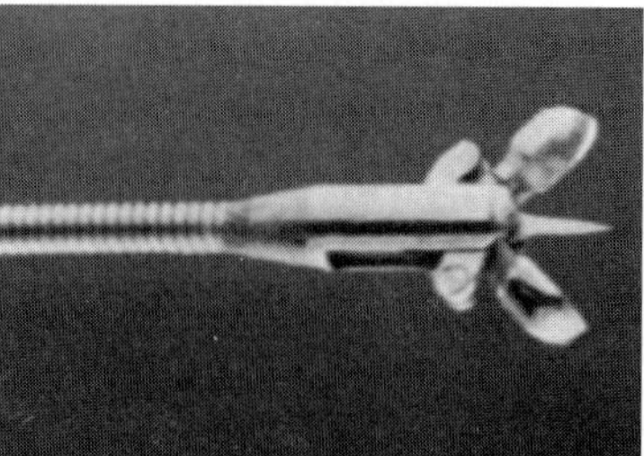
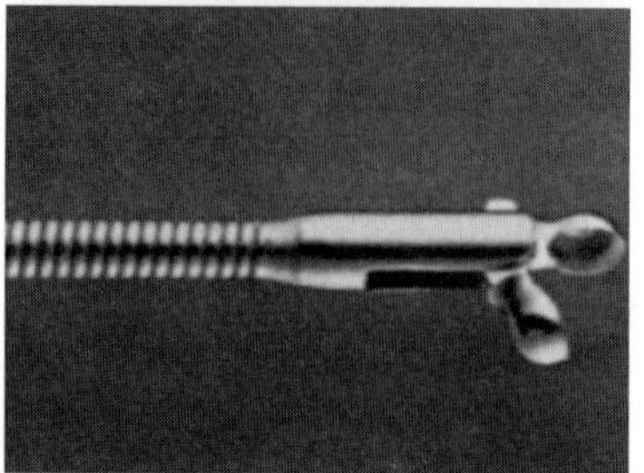
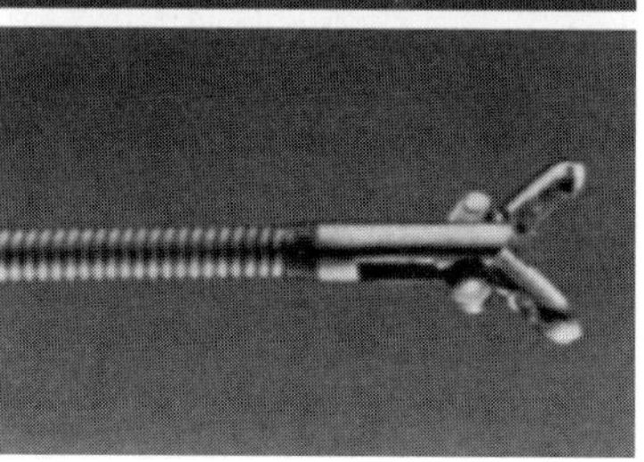

Figure 5–1. Biopsy forceps for flexible endoscopes come in many varieties, including the cup biopsy forceps with needle *(top),* the right-angled cup biopsy forceps *(middle),* and the ellipsoid biopsy forceps *(bottom).*

Technique

Preparation of the Patient

As with all procedures performed on patients, the indications for the procedure, the conduct of the procedure, and its possible complications are explained to maximize the patient's understanding and cooperation and to minimize as much as possible the patient's fear and anxiety. The patient is instructed to ingest nothing by mouth (including medications) for a minimum of 6 hours before the examination. A formal informed consent form is presented to the patient and a signature is obtained. Initial vital signs, including blood pressure and pulse rate, are recorded. The electrocardiogram is monitored and oxygen saturation is continuously determined using a pulse oximeter.

Bacteremia is a common occurrence following upper gastrointestinal endoscopy. For most procedures the incidence ranges from 0 to 10%, but esophageal dilation and endoscopic sclerotherapy may have rates as high as 50%.[9,51] Prophylactic antibiotics should be administered to those patients who have a prosthetic heart valve, a surgically constructed systemic pulmonary shunt, or a history of endocarditis. The use of prophylactic antibiotics is controversial for patients with valvular heart disease accompanied by a murmur. The standard regimen recommended by the American Heart Association includes ampicillin and gentamicin parenterally 30 to 60 minutes prior to the procedure. In patients who are allergic to penicillin, vancomycin is substituted.[5,16]

A topical anesthetic is applied to the posterior oropharynx. Some endoscopists also apply simethicone in an effort to reduce foaming of fluids in the endoscopic field. Most endoscopists administer an intravenous sedative to increase the patient's comfort, most commonly diazepam or midazolam in a dose sufficient to produce mild lethargy. Additional premedication with meperidine given intramuscularly before the procedure or intravenously accompanying the sedative is also sometimes used. The benefit of this additional medication is unproven.[19] Some endoscopists also administer atropine in an effort

Table 5–2. Dimensions of Flexible Esophagoscopes*

Instrument	External Diameter (mm)	Instrument Channel Diameter (mm)	Bending Range (°)		
			Up	*Down*	*Right, Left*
GIF N230	6	2	180	180	160
GIF XP240	7.7	2.2	210	90	100
GIF P140	8.7	2.2	210	90	100
GIF XQ140	9.4	2.8	210	90	100
GIF Q140	10.5	2.8	210	90	100
GIF LT100	13.2	2.8, 3.7	210	90	100

*Olympus brand.

to decrease oral secretions and gastric motility, although there is likewise no proven benefit with this drug.

Instrumentation

The choice of flexible endoscopes for use in examining the esophagus, stomach, and duodenum is based on a number of factors. Scopes with the largest diameter (11 to 13 mm) are generally used for therapeutic endoscopy; they provide one or sometimes two instrumentation channels of large caliber. Most diagnostic EGDs can be performed with an intermediate-caliber (9 to 11 mm) endoscope, which has a single instrumentation channel that is 2.8 mm in diameter. This scope accommodates all but the largest forceps, all cytology brush catheters, and most irrigation tubing. In elderly patients, in patients with a deformity of the upper gastrointestinal tract, and in pediatric patients, scopes with the smallest diameter (6 to 9 mm) should be employed to minimize discomfort and maximize the likelihood of a complete examination.

Examination

The patient is placed in the left lateral position with the torso elevated and the knees flexed for comfort. During intubation of the hypopharynx, the neck is flexed so that the chin approaches the chest wall, maximizing the space between the cricoid cartilage and the posterior wall of the hypopharynx. A bite block is placed in the patient's mouth to avoid damage to the scope from the patient's teeth. The tip of the scope is inserted through the bite block and is deflected along the base of the tongue under direct vision. Blind intubation is used by some endoscopists, but this procedure risks intubation of the glottis or injury to the glottis, hypopharynx, or esophagus, particularly in patients with a cervical diverticulum. Moreover, narrow-diameter instruments often do not possess sufficient rigidity to pass through the cricopharyngeus during blind intubation, thereby increasing the risk of tracheal intubation.

The endoscopist follows the base of the tongue to the epiglottis and posterior to this point visualizes the glottic structures and the posterior hypopharynx. The cricoid cartilage is found toward the 6-o'clock position and normally impinges on the posterior wall of the hypopharynx. In elderly patients, cervical spine disease may further compromise the lumen of the posterior hypopharynx. In these and most other patients, it is most convenient to deflect the scope into the left or right piriform sinus and then return it to the midline as it passes into the cricopharyngeus.

The cricopharyngeus is found in the midline or just to the left of center, 15 to 18 cm from the incisors; it is recognized as a confluence of several folds. Asking the patient to swallow while visualizing this structure often allows easy intubation of the esophagus under direct vision. However, it is often difficult to examine this region carefully during insertion of the endoscope because displacement of hypopharyngeal structures during swallowing results in loss of the view of the cricopharyngeus. In such situations, gentle pressure is exerted on the scope when the cricopharyngeus is in view, and the pressure is gently increased as the patient swallows. Using this technique, the esophagus is almost always entered without trauma or discomfort to the patient.

After passing through the cricopharyngeus, the scope is slowly advanced through the esophagus. Gentle insufflation of air maintains luminal patency. Primary peristaltic waves can be seen following a swallow, and secondary peristaltic waves frequently are visible following air insufflation. Between 23 and 25 cm from the incisors, an indentation in the left anterolateral surface of the esophagus marks the point of contact of the esophagus with the aortic arch. Excessive compression or mucosal irregularities in this region may signal the presence of an aortic aneurysm, aortic dissection, or aortoesophageal fistula. Just below this point, a diagonal impression is seen on the esophagus extending from its superomedial aspect to its inferolateral aspect anteriorly; this impression is caused by the left main stem bronchus. Distal to this point, double pulsations are seen on the anteromedial esophageal wall that are due to contractions of the left atrium.

Special attention is paid to the most distal 5 to 10 cm of the esophagus and the gastroesophageal junction. Mucosal abnormalities, including columnar lining of the esophagus (Barrett's esophagus) and esophagitis, are most likely to be found in this region. The distances of both the squamocolumnar junction and the gastroesophageal junction from the incisors are measured. It is also useful to note the level of the diaphragmatic hiatus, which is distinctly visualized by asking the patient to inhale sharply through the nose, a maneuver commonly called the "sniff test." During sharp inhalation, the crura indent the esophagus sharply on its medial and lateral sides.

Unless the stomach and duodenum have been recently examined during a previous endoscopic procedure, it is recommended that these organs be routinely examined during any EGD procedure because there is a high incidence of unsuspected abnormal findings in this region. Once the endoscope has entered the stomach, the control head and scope are rotated clockwise 60 to 90 degrees to align the scope with the longitudinal axis of the stomach. The scope is gently advanced as air is insufflated to expand the stomach.

The gastric angle (angulus) is a mucosal crescent found between the 3- and 9-o'clock positions that marks the junction between the stomach body and the antrum. After passing the angulus, the pyloric channel and pylorus can be visualized and intubated. Occasionally, a high-lying pylorus requires upward deflection of the scope for visualization.

Once the pyloric channel is entered, the duodenal bulb is examined beginning with insufflation of air to inflate the bulb. The descending duodenum can be intubated by direct entry or by torquing the shaft an additional 90 degrees and aligning the tip with the medial wall of the duodenum. In this situation, advancement of the scope allows indirect intubation of the descending portion of the duodenum to its junction with the third portion.

Inspection of the duodenal lumen reveals concentric mucosal rings, or Kerckring folds, as well as the duodenal

(Wirsung's) papilla on the medial wall and the accessory (Santorini's) papilla 2 cm proximal to it. Gradual withdrawal of the scope is accompanied by a thorough visualization of all mucosal surfaces. A second close inspection of the duodenal bulb is performed to eliminate the possibility of an overlooked ulcer or growth. The pyloric channel is carefully examined during gradual withdrawal. After re-entry of the tip of the scope into the stomach, a systematic examination of all gastric mucosal surfaces is undertaken. The antrum is examined carefully, using arc-like swings of the scope tip during its gradual withdrawal.

The fundus and the gastric side of the cardia can be adequately visualized and examined only by means of retroflexion maneuvers. A J-type retroflexion maneuver may be performed by deflecting the tip maximally in the up position along the lesser curvature, producing a 180-degree retroflexion. The scope can be withdrawn gradually until the cardia and fundus are viewed, occasionally rotating the instrument counterclockwise to move the tip along the greater curve. Better visualization of these structures may be obtained by performing a U-type retroflexion. The scope is aligned along the esophageal axis rather than the gastric axis by rotating it 60 to 90 degrees in a counterclockwise direction when the tip is at the junction of the body and the fundus. The tip is deflected upward and the scope is blindly advanced, the retroflexion being aided by impaction of the scope along the greater curvature of the stomach. The instrument is gradually withdrawn in the retroflexed position, occasionally using deflection to the right of the tip to obtain an adequate view of the fundus and cardia.

The endoscope is straightened, and as much insufflated air is evacuated from the stomach as possible to maximize the patient's comfort. Re-examination of the diaphragmatic hiatus, the gastroesophageal junction, the squamocolumnar junction, and the distal esophagus is performed. The scope is again gradually withdrawn to the region just below the cricopharyngeus. A careful examination of this area is undertaken during slow withdrawal to ensure that no pathologic lesion was missed during intubation. The scope is removed, and the patient is observed until he or she adequately recovers from the intravenous sedation.

Proper techniques of endoscopic biopsy and brushing and specimen processing are critical to a successful diagnostic EGD. In general, the largest biopsy forceps that fits through the instrumentation channel should be used. Large biopsy forceps (No. 8 French) with a central bayonet can be used with biopsy channels larger than 2.6 mm in diameter. Jumbo forceps (3.6-mm diameter) require a biopsy channel of 3.7 mm. Careful identification of the level of the biopsy (distance from the incisors) and its orientation circumferentially within the esophagus or by region within the stomach or duodenum is important. Unless an immediate diagnosis is desired by means of a frozen section, the tissue should be gently teased from the forceps cup with a needle and placed in a fixative.

Needle aspiration cytology can be performed in pathologic sites by passing a retractable needle into the lesion and aspirating it manually with a syringe. A more common cytologic technique is targeted brushing, which is performed by passing a sheathed brush through the instrumentation channel of the endoscope into the area in question, extending the brush, and vigorously passing it against the mucosal surface before resheathing and removing it. Brushing should be the final examination performed to eliminate possible histologic abnormalities found in subsequent biopsy specimens taken from the same site and to eliminate bleeding as a source of error in directed biopsies. The typical cytology specimen should be placed on a glass slide and immersed immediately in a fixative to prevent drying. It is then examined by the cytologist following staining by the usual Papanicolaou technique.

RIGID ESOPHAGOSCOPY

Until the 1970s, rigid esophagoscopy was the most common technique used in endoscopic evaluation of the esophagus. Its role was limited by the frequent need for general anesthesia, insufficient lighting, a narrow angle of vision at the end of the long hollow tube, and, in some cases, by cervical spine disease. The development of a rod-lens system in the 1960s and the application of this technology to telescopes for the rigid endoscopes greatly improved the viewing angle and the image quality. At the same time, fiberoptic light sources enhanced image brightness. Although flexible EGD is currently the technique of choice for most endoscopic examinations of the esophagus, the rigid scope systems continue to find application today. Specific indications for rigid esophagoscopy include removal of foreign bodies, dilation of strictures under certain circumstances, a need for larger or deeper biopsies than those obtainable through a flexible endoscope, and evacuation of rapid bleeding with large suction devices.

Equipment

Esophagoscope tubes for adult use are approximately 50 cm long with a maximum outer diameter of 10 or 12 mm for round tubes or 16 mm for oval tubes (Table 5-3). The tips are typically rounded and beveled to minimize trauma and maximize viewing of the mucosal surface. Pediatric scopes range from 20 to 45 cm in length and from 3.5 to 10 mm in diameter. The proximal portion of the beveled tip may be slotted for variceal sclerotherapy. Illumination of the tube is accomplished through a proximal prismatic light deflector or through a rigid fiberoptic light carrier inserted through the scope. An external magnifying lens can be adapted to the esophagoscope tube to improve image size. The rigid tubes typically have an adaptor for air insufflation, usually accomplished with a bulb. Optical telescopes are available for most rigid tubes, with forward-viewing (0 degrees), angled-viewing (30 degrees), and side-viewing (90 degrees) distal lenses. These telescopes can be incorporated into optical biopsy forceps or grasping forceps.

Technique

Patient Preparation

As with flexible esophagoscopy, the patient should be given a detailed explanation of the indications for and

Table 5–3. Dimensions of Rigid Esophagoscopes

Manufacturer	Style	Diameter (mm)	Length (cm)
Pediatric			
Pilling	Holinger	3.5	25, 30
		4	30
		6	30, 45
		7	30, 45
		8	45, 53
		9	30, 45, 53
		10	53
Storz		4.8	20
		5.6	20
		6.7	30
		7.7	30
		8.2	30
	Benjamin	7 × 8	22
		9 × 10	22
		10 × 12	27
Wolf		4	17
		5	22
		5.5	27
		6.5	32
Adult			
Pilling	Jackson	7 × 10	25
		8 × 12	50
		9 × 13	25
		10 × 14	30, 40, 50
		12 × 16	50
		12 × 18	35
Storz	Optical	12	51
		13	51
	Roberts-Jesberg	7 × 10	30
		8 × 12	30, 50
		10 × 14	30, 50
		12 × 16	30, 50
	Benjamin	12 × 14	37
		16 × 18	37
		18 × 20	47
Wolf		6 × 8	25, 35
		8 × 12	25, 45
		10 × 14	30, 40, 50

possible complications of the planned procedure to minimize anxiety and achieve maximum cooperation. The patient should have nothing to eat for at least 6 to 8 hours before the procedure. An electrocardiogram, chemistry profile, and coagulation profile are sometimes obtained preoperatively. The recommendations regarding antibiotic prophylaxis for endocarditis outlined earlier are also applicable for patients undergoing rigid endoscopy.

Examination

Rigid esophagoscopy is performed with the patient under general anesthesia in most circumstances. Modern anesthetic techniques have eliminated many of the risks of general anesthesia and provide greater patient comfort than when the procedure is attempted using topical anesthesia with sedation. The major drawback of a general anesthetic with a muscle relaxant is loss of muscle tone with collapse of the hypopharyngeal structures posteriorly, causing occasional difficulty in cricopharyngeal identification and intubation. It is sometimes best if the patient is able to maintain spontaneous ventilation during the procedure.

The patient is placed in supine position with the head and shoulders on a movable headrest, which allows flexion and extension of the patient's neck when desired by the endoscopist. After a general anesthetic has been administered and endotracheal intubation achieved, the patient's esophagus is intubated. The fingers of the endoscopist's guiding hand (usually the nondominant hand) are used to prevent injury to the patient's teeth or alveolar ridge, while the thumb and forefinger of the guiding hand support the scope. The scope is advanced through the right side of the mouth and used to elevate the tongue and epiglottis. After identifying the right arytenoid cartilage, the tip of the scope is passed posteriorly into the right piriform sinus. Using the guiding hand, the tip of the scope is gently advanced and elevated until the cricopharyngeus is visualized. It is critical that the axis of the scope be aligned with the esophageal axis at this point.

Because of the relationship of the cricopharyngeus with the posterior portion of the cricoid cartilage and the cervical spine, the highest risk of perforation of the esophagus occurs during intubation of the cricopharyngeus. Gentle pressure is used to insinuate the scope through the cricopharyngeus.

With the scope in the esophagus, the neck is extended and maintained in this position as the instrument is advanced into the distal esophagus. The scope is never advanced unless the lumen of the esophagus is clearly visible. Air insufflation aids in opening the lumen and provides a better view of the esophageal mucosa. The scope is advanced mainly with the operating hand, while the guiding hand is always in place to protect the teeth or alveolar ridge.

As the cardia is reached, the neck is extended further, and the head is turned rightward to orient the esophagoscope diagonally from right to left in a cephalocaudal direction to allow passage through the cardia and diaphragmatic hiatus into the stomach. A small amount of proximal stomach can be examined in a relatively cursory fashion.

COMPLICATIONS OF ESOPHAGOSCOPY

Although mortality and morbidity related to endoscopy are low, the actual number of complications associated with it is not negligible because of the great number of procedures performed. The major complications include perforation, bleeding, cardiopulmonary problems, reactions to medications, and infections (Table 5–4).[6,33,36,41,47,50,53] The incidence and severity of these vary according to whether diagnostic or therapeutic endoscopy is performed and whether flexible or rigid scope systems are used. The overall incidence of morbidity ranges from 0.1 to 1.5%, and mortality ranges from 0.01 to 0.5%.[33,50]

Perforation

Perforation of the esophagus during esophagoscopy occurs in 0.05 to 2.5% of patients.[36,42,47] Although rare, this

Table 5–4. Complications of Esophagoscopy*

	Incidence (per 1,000 cases)	
Complication	***Flexible Endoscopy***	***Rigid Endoscopy***
Perforation	0.1	2.5
Bleeding	0.07	0.04
Aspiration	0.5	0.7
Arrhythmia	1.2	1.4
Death	0.3	0.4

From references 6, 33, 36, 41, 47, 50:

Ancona E, and Gayet B: Esophageal perforations. I: Etiology, diagnosis, localization and symptoms. *In* Siewert, J.R., and Holscher, A.H. (eds.): Diseases of the Esophagus. Berlin, Springer-Verlag, 1988, p. 1327.

Maroy, B., and Moullot, P.: Safety of upper gastrointestinal endoscopy with intravenous sedation by the endoscopist at office: 17,963 examinations performed in a community center by two endoscopists over 17 years. J. Clin. Gastroenterol., *27*:368, 1998.

Nashef, S.A.M., and Pagliero, K.M.: Instrumental perforation of the esophagus in benign disease. Ann. Thorac. Surg., *44*:360, 1987.

Quine, M.A., Bell, G.D., McCloy, R.F., et al: Prospective audit of upper gastrointestinal endoscopy in two regions of England: Safety, staffing, and sedation methods. Gut, *36*:462, 1995.

Sarr, M.G., Pemberton, J.H., and Payne, W.S.: Management of instrumental perforations of the esophagus. J. Thorac. Cardiovasc. Surg., *84*:211, 1982.

Shamir, M., and Schuman, B.M.: Complications of fiberoptic endoscopy. Gastrointest. Endosc., *26*:86, 1980.

can be a devastating complication because disruption of the intrathoracic esophageal wall bathes the mediastinal tissues with highly contaminated oral secretions and, frequently, gastric contents. Thus, both a chemical mediastinitis and a superimposed infection owing to anaerobic and aerobic organisms are rapidly established. Although cervical perforation often results in a more limited leak and can sometimes be controlled by conservative measures, an unrecognized perforation in this area can also have fatal consequences. The site of perforation is the cervical esophagus in 40% of patients, the midesophagus in 25%, and the distal esophagus in 35%.[47] Females appear to be more likely to have cervical perforations, whereas male patients more commonly develop perforations in the thoracic esophagus. Rigid esophagoscopes account for relatively more perforations than do flexible scopes (80% of the total in one series), although the actual distribution varies according to the frequency with which each technique is used. Cervical spine disease is a risk factor for perforation, particularly in patients undergoing rigid esophagoscopy, as are inflammation and stricture.

Bleeding

Significant bleeding following flexible or rigid esophagoscopy is uncommon, occurring in 0.01 to 0.1% of cases. It arises more commonly in the stomach than in the esophagus and is usually secondary to an aggressive biopsy, injury to pre-existing varices, or, in some cases, a Mallory-Weiss tear during or shortly after esophagoscopy.

Cardiopulmonary Complications

Cardiopulmonary complications arising from endoscopy include aspiration pneumonia, cardiac arrhythmias, hypoxemia, respiratory arrest, and cardiac arrest. The latter three complications may also be ascribed to errors in administration of sedation. Stimulation of the glottis may lead to a vagally induced bradycardia. Other arrhythmias encountered include sinus tachycardia, ventricular and atrial premature beats, and, occasionally, ischemic changes. Some arrhythmias are due to sympathetic discharge during the procedure, and others may be related to hypoxia, which can develop in the presence of a partially obstructed airway.[20] Routine monitoring of oxygen saturation, easily accomplished with a pulse oximeter, is recommended.[17]

SPECIFIC ABNORMALITIES

Peptic Esophagitis

Endoscopy is a frequent mode of investigation in patients in whom reflux esophagitis is suspected. This condition is present in 5 to 10% of all patients undergoing diagnostic EGD[1] and in 50 to 60% of patients thought to have gastroesophageal acid reflux disease (GERD).[1,39] According to endoscopic criteria, esophagitis can be classified into one of four levels:

Grade 1 (minimal esophagitis): Erythema of the distal esophagus with capillary dilation and, in some instances, friability of the mucosa.

Grade 2 (mild esophagitis): Loss of definition of the mucosal detail at the gastroesophageal junction with discrete erosions (Fig. 5–2). The erosions take on a deeper red hue than that of the surrounding mucosa and often extend distally to the region of the gastroesophageal junction. Pseudomembrane formation occasionally occurs.

Grade 3 (severe esophagitis): Ulcerations with granula-

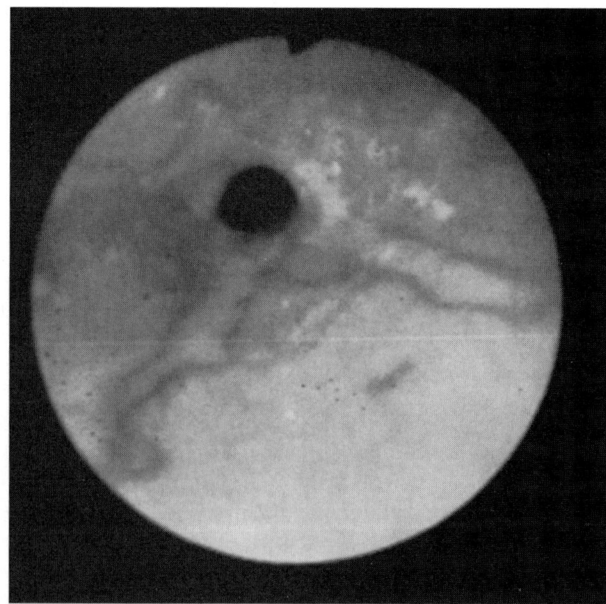

Figure 5–2. Grade II esophagitis, characterized by linear erosions and ulcerations.

tion tissue, as evidenced by either an inflammatory exudate or a pale ulcer bed (Fig. 5–3). There is also evidence of fibrosis within the wall of the esophagus, limiting distensibility during air insufflation.

Grade 4 (stricture): The presence of the findings of grade 3 esophagitis as well as a definite narrowing of the esophageal lumen (Fig. 5–4).

In addition to these typical findings of peptic esophagitis, unusual complications of esophageal inflammation include inflammatory pseudotumors of the esophagus, pseudopolyps, and mucosal bridging.[55]

The endoscopic criteria for the diagnosis of peptic esophagitis are not generally agreed on. Although several of the classification systems are quite similar, there is a disparity in the number of grades allowed, and the inclusion of erythema and stricture as criteria for esophagitis is not universally accepted. because endoscopic diagnosis of minimal esophagitis is frequently inaccurate, there is considerable difficulty in correlating the histologic findings obtained from endoscopic biopsies with the visual descriptions of the mucosa.[23] As a result, in the absence of frank ulceration, histologic evidence of esophagitis is frequently required to confirm the diagnosis.

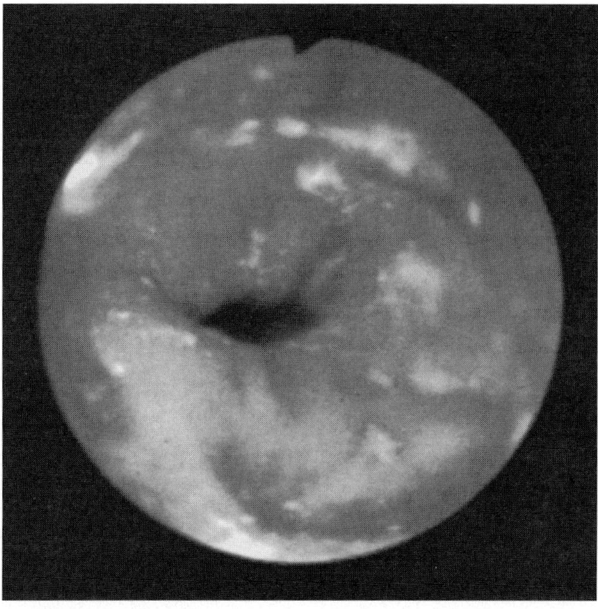

Figure 5–4. Grade IV esophagitis with severe inflammation and stricture formation.

Benign Strictures

Peptic strictures resulting from gastroesophageal acid reflux occur most often at or just above the squamocolumnar junction. In cases of severe reflux, the strictures may be long, allowing only a string of barium to pass from the upper esophagus to the stomach on contrast radiography. Other, less typical reflux strictures occur in patients with Barrett's esophagus, in whom the squamocolumnar junction is displaced orally. In such cases, the inflammatory stricture, although lying at or just above the squamocolumnar junction, is seen endoscopically and radiographically well above the esophageal hiatus, frequently at the level of the aortic arch.

Distinguishing benign reflux strictures from esophageal strictures with other causes, including malignancy, irradiation, and caustic ingestion, is not always straightforward. As always, a careful endoscopic approach including assessment of stricture length, location, vascularity, and friability is of key importance in achieving the correct diagnosis. Biopsy samples should generally be taken from the region of the stricture itself as well as above and below the stricture. A benign stricture can mask a carcinoma developing distally, particularly when it is associated with Barrett's esophagus.

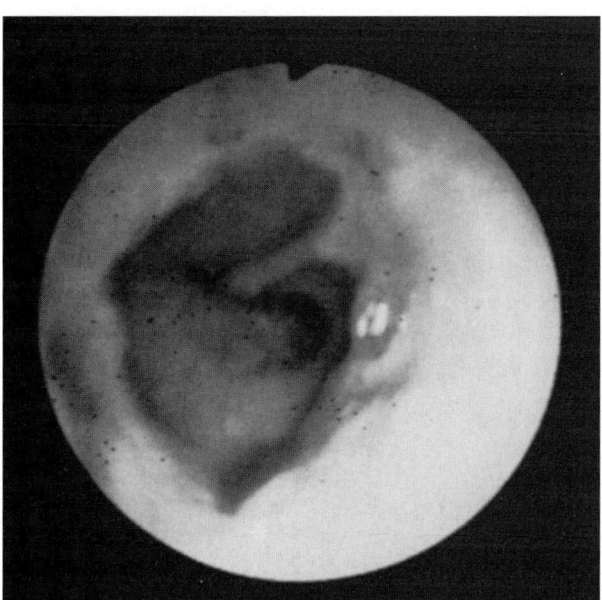

Figure 5–3. Grade III esophagitis, illustrating fibrosis within the esophageal wall, deep ulcerations, and pseudomembrane formation.

Lower Esophageal Ring

The lower esophageal ring (Schatzki's ring) was originally described in 1953 as a thin membrane of tissue near the gastroesophageal junction that was covered above by squamous epithelium and below by columnar (gastric) mucosa.[49] Endoscopically, such rings are visualized following air insufflation at the level of the distal esophagus. Although a hiatus hernia is frequently present, esophagitis is not common. Many of these rings measure more than 20 mm in maximum internal diameter and thus produce no symptoms.[40] When dysphagia is a presenting complaint, the rings may be disrupted by forceful passage of the endoscope through the remaining lumen. Rings smaller than 10 mm in internal diameter usually cannot be ruptured in this way, and dilation by another technique is normally required.[30] The endoscopic picture of such rings is so characteristic that a biopsy should not normally be required for confirmation of the diagnosis or to exclude other, more important pathologic entities.

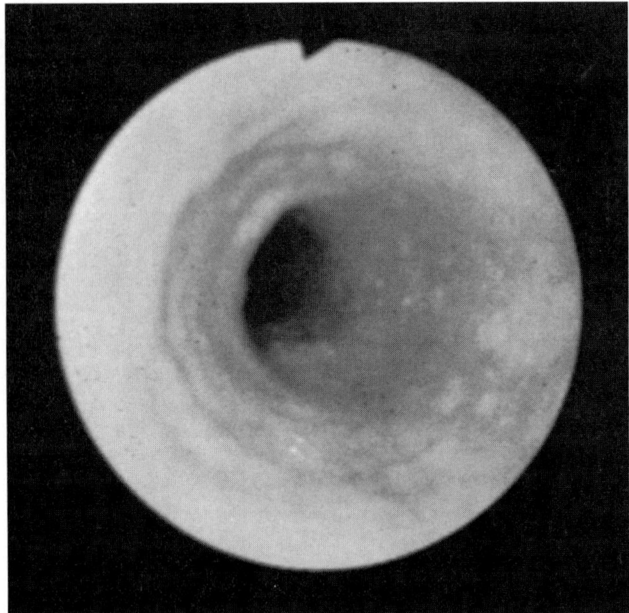

Figure 5–5. Early esophageal cancer, lying in the granular surface along the esophageal wall.

Malignant Tumors of the Esophagus

Early Diagnosis

In geographic areas in which esophageal cancer is endemic, early diagnosis by blind or endoscopically directed cytologic screening is frequently used for the early diagnosis of such cancers. These techniques also have been used in North America in high-risk populations with encouraging results. Early diagnosis is the primary method by which an improvement in survival statistics for esophageal cancer can be achieved.

Endoscopic diagnosis of dysplasia and early cancer of the esophagus is a great challenge for the endoscopist. Careful observation is necessary if the relatively minor abnormalities present in these stages are to be recognized. Early signs to look for include discoloration, subtle reddening, shallow mucosal depressions, an uneven or granular appearance of the mucous membrane, and plateau-like elevations (Fig. 5–5).[15,26,37,56]

In addition to endoscopically directed biopsies and brushings of all suspected regions of abnormality, systematic brushings and biopsies of other regions, particularly in the distal esophagus, are recommended for patients at high risk for esophageal cancer who are undergoing a screening examination. In early-stage cancers, the overall rate of positive endoscopic identification is approximately 93%, including 80% for endoscopic biopsy and 88% for directed brushing for cytology.[24]

Vital Staining

Vital stains can be used to great advantage in the identification of early lesions in the esophagus and in directing biopsies and brushings to appropriate areas.[28,35,38,56] Vital stains, including iodine (Lugol's solution), stain the normal esophageal squamous mucosa by turning the glycogen in the squamous cells black. Thus, normal esophageal mucosa appears dark gray-brown or black after iodine staining, whereas areas of carcinoma in situ or frankly invasive malignancy do not stain.[35] This method does not reliably detect dysplasia, which stains like normal mucosa about half the time.

Toluidine blue stains dysplastic and malignant mucosa an intense violet color. The method is not specific because areas of inflammation, peptic erosions, and ulcers also stain positively. Toluidine blue is taken up through widened intracellular bridges and has a strong affinity for cellular nuclei.[27] Overall, it is 85 to 90% accurate in staining squamous cancers of the esophagus.[14]

Rapidly growing tissues such as malignant tumors have an affinity for porphyrin. It is known that tumor cells take up and selectively retain hematoporphyrin derivatives. This knowledge has been used to provide an additional screening technique for esophageal cancer. It has theoretical value but has not yet been sufficiently refined to have achieved widespread clinical use. A hematoporphyrin derivative or protoporphyrin is injected intravenously, and endoscopy is performed after the substance has been eliminated from most normal tissues and selectively retained by tumor cells. These derivatives can be induced to fluoresce on exposure to blue-violet light in squamous carcinomas of the esophagus.

Diagnostic Techniques

When an area of obvious tumor is identified, careful biopsies and brushings are performed to achieve a diagnosis (Fig. 5–6). The accuracy of endoscopy in diagnosing such tumors is approximately 95%, although the accuracy of biopsy alone is only 83% and that of cytology alone is 85%, underscoring the usefulness of combining these modalities.[25,46] Diagnostic accuracy increases as more biopsies are taken, the optimal number being about four.[46]

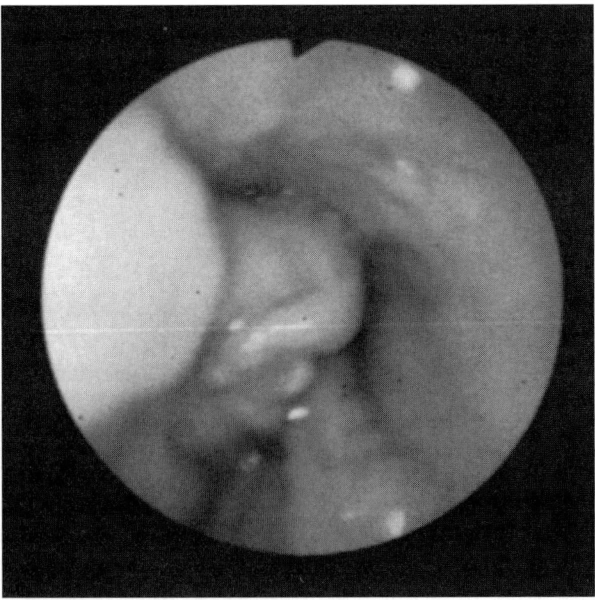

Figure 5–6. Squamous cell esophageal cancer with a large mass virtually occluding the distal lumen.

The gastroesophageal junction is a region in which it is particularly difficult to acquire adequate biopsies. In this area, brush cytology is significantly better than biopsy for the diagnosis of esophageal malignancy. Stenosing tumors are also more accurately diagnosed by brush cytology, because it is frequently difficult to direct the biopsy forceps to a desired location within the stenosis, particularly when the stenotic segment cannot be entered with the scope. When these measures fail to diagnose an area of suspected abnormality, biopsy through a rigid endoscope should be considered, because it has a diagnostic success rate approaching 100%.[46]

Other Esophageal Tumors

The most important esophageal tumor other than a primary malignancy of the esophagus or esophagogastric junction is the leiomyoma, a relatively rare lesion. In autopsy studies, it is present in 1 of slightly more than 1,000 cases, and certainly the clinical recognition of this benign lesion occurs even less often.[52] The tumor has no predilection to occur at any specific level within the esophagus. It is characteristically seen endoscopically as a mass bulging into the lumen of the esophagus and almost always is covered with normal mucosa. It is normally mobile, in contrast to invasive tumors, which appear fixed. Biopsies, when taken, have a very low yield in diagnosing these lesions. Because enucleation is a preferred mode for treating these tumors, it is generally recommended that endoscopic biopsy be avoided. This eliminates the risk of mucosal injury and the potential subsequent risk of perforation perioperatively. Multiple leiomyomas can exist and should be looked for.

Barrett's Esophagus

Barrett's esophagus is a premalignant condition requiring endoscopic or blind cytologic surveillance over time. It is important to recognize the presence of this epithelium during the initial endoscopic examination and to identify appropriately patients who are candidates for such surveillance.[21]

Barrett's esophagus appears endoscopically as a feathery red mucosa extending proximally from the region of the esophagogastric junction. It is diagnosed when a regular Z-line is identified 3 cm or more from the distal end of the lower esophageal sphincter or when tongues of columnar mucosa are found (Fig. 5–7). Frequently, the squamocolumnar junction in such patients is poorly visualized owing either to peptic esophagitis, which commonly involves the region of the mucosal junction and the squamous mucosa proximal to it, or stricturing in the same region.

The presence of a high benign stricture should alert one to the possible existence of Barrett's mucosa, and biopsies of the mucosa distal to the stricture are mandatory for diagnosis in such cases.[48] The Barrett's mucosa itself may be affected by typical shallow peptic ulcerations, or, less commonly, it may have deep ulcerations similar to those of true gastric ulcers. On occasion, these can penetrate into the mediastinum.[22]

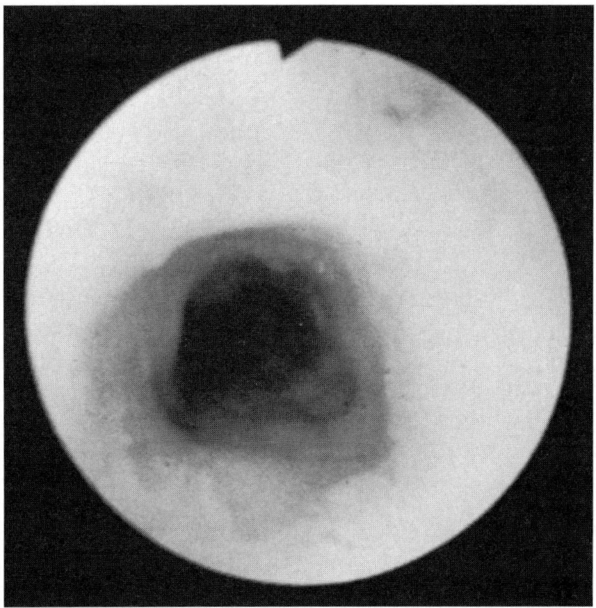

Figure 5–7. Barrett's esophagus with tongues of feathery red epithelium extending proximally toward the endoscope.

The overall sensitivity of visual endoscopic diagnosis of Barrett's esophagus ranges from 75 to 85%, and the specificity ranges from 85 to 90%.[21] As a result, histologic documentation of this entity is necessary. Biopsies are performed at 1-cm intervals beginning just below the lower esophageal sphincter and extending proximally well into the region of normal-appearing squamous mucosa. Biopsy of the normal squamous mucosa is important because squamous overgrowth of Barrett's epithelium has been reported. The accuracy of endoscopic detection of Barrett's esophagus can be improved by performing vital staining with toluidine blue, which serves as a positive stain for Barrett's esophagus. This technique raises the sensitivity of endoscopic detection of Barrett's esophagus to 95 to 100%.[13]

Esophageal Motor Disorders

Endoscopy is not the primary means of diagnosing esophageal motor disorders. One should rely on barium esophagograms and esophageal motility studies to document these problems. Endoscopy is performed when surgery is contemplated in a patient with a motility disorder or when other symptoms such as dysphagia are present.

Achalasia

Most patients with achalasia diagnosed radiographically or manometrically should undergo an initial endoscopic examination. There is an increased risk of esophageal carcinoma in these patients. In addition, there is an appreciable incidence of pseudoachalasia caused by tumors of the esophagogastric junction that cannot be identified reliably using the other two techniques. In patients with untreated achalasia, there is often a striking dilation of the body of the esophagus, frequently with retained food material. In such cases, it is usually wise to insert an Ewald tube for evacuation of the esophageal contents and then irrigate the esophagus until it is clean before attempting to perform endoscopy. This procedure not only improves the endoscopic view significantly but also minimizes the risk of aspiration during the procedure.

Diffuse Esophageal Spasm

In patients with diffuse esophageal spasm, endoscopy is normally recommended to rule out an obstructing lesion that may be causing dysphagia. The endoscopic picture shows concentric ring-like contractions throughout the distal two thirds of the esophageal body that correspond to the corkscrew appearance that is frequently seen radiographically. A similar appearance is sometimes evident in older patients undergoing endoscopy, corresponding to the condition of presbyesophagus.

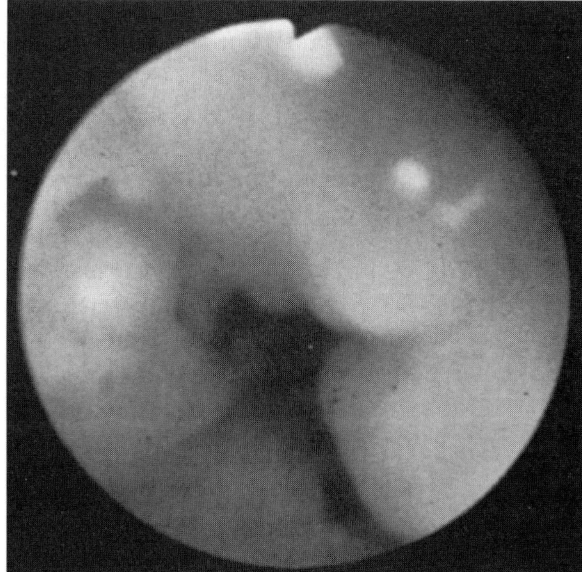

Figure 5–8. Esophageal varix with a polypoid appearance.

Scleroderma

Scleroderma causes a disorder of esophageal motility characterized by an absence of peristalsis in the distal two thirds of the esophagus and an absent lower esophageal high-pressure zone. As a result of intrinsically poor antireflux and distal esophageal clearance mechanisms, many patients with scleroderma involving the esophagus have significant reflux. The endoscopic appearance, therefore, is frequently one of severe reflux esophagitis associated with stricturing. Esophageal candidiasis is also common in this disorder.

Esophageal Varices

Esophageal varices are an important complication of cirrhosis and are frequently found in the absence of frank upper gastrointestinal bleeding. They appear as blue-gray columns with a slight elevation within the esophageal mucosa in their simplest form, or they may become serpentine or form very complex interconnected shapes within the esophageal wall. Their appearance is occasionally nodular (Fig. 5–8), and sometimes an unsuspecting endoscopist induces significant bleeding by performing an inappropriate biopsy.

It is useful to grade the size of varices for purposes of initial documentation and follow-up of treatment.[10,58] One technique is to compare the variceal width with the 5-mm opening of a standard cup biopsy forceps at a level 2 cm above the esophagogastric junction. Thus, grade I is a varix equal to one fourth of the forceps bite width, grade II to one half of the bite width, grade III to three quarters of the bite width, and grade IV to one or more bite widths.

Infectious Esophagitis

Esophagitis may arise as a result of a number of different infections, particularly the opportunistic type of infection that occurs in immunosuppressed patients. Typical symptoms and signs of infectious esophagitis include odynophagia, chest pain, fever, and bleeding. In patients suspected of having infectious esophagitis, additional preparation necessary before endoscopy includes sterilizing the endoscope and biopsy forceps and ensuring the availability of additional brushes for cytologic staining and cultures.

Candida species account for a significant percentage of cases of infectious esophagitis. Esophageal candidiasis is suspected with the presence of oral thrush or significant irregularity and occasional pseudodiverticulum formation in the esophageal wall on barium esophagogram. Its distribution does not typically correspond to that of peptic esophagitis because it may occur anywhere within the body of the esophagus in a discontinuous fashion. The endoscopic picture is variable and includes raised white plaques, ulceration, and stricture.[7] There is usually no accompanying exudate. Brushings are sent for culture and staining, and histologic examination of biopsies usually shows hyphae.

Viral esophagitis is most often due to cytomegalovirus and herpes simplex virus.[2,34,54] Viruses account for the greatest number of cases of infectious esophagitis among immunosuppressed patients. The endoscopic picture may include erosive esophagitis, bullae, or frank ulceration, occasionally of giant proportions. Diagnosis is made by taking brushings for cytology or biopsies for histology. Additional biopsy samples are sent in a special viral transport medium for culture, although viruses are identified in culture in only 40% of cases of viral esophagitis.

Caustic Injuries

Esophagoscopy is useful in the early assessment of the degree of severity of esophageal injury sustained following a caustic ingestion.[12,18,57,59] The presence or absence of burns of the lips and oropharynx are not reliable indicators of the existence or degree of esophageal injury. Flexible endoscopy is performed within 24 hours of injury, and an assessment of injury grade is assigned as follows: grade 1, erythema; grade 2, ulcerations and mild hemorrhage; and grade 3, multiple deep ulcerations or necrosis. The endoscope is advanced only until evidence of injury is seen. If only grade 1 injury is found, further cautious efforts to assess the degree of injury more distally may be of benefit because the most severe damage is sometimes at or near the gastroesophageal junction. Attempts to advance the scope through regions of grade 2 or grade 3 injury invite perforation.

Penetrating Trauma

Low- or high-velocity penetrating thoracic trauma results in infrequent but potentially lethal esophageal injuries.[31,45] Some advocate esophagoscopy as a primary diagnostic tool or as an adjunct to contrast esophagography in stable patients who are at risk from such injury. Endoscopy can be performed using a rigid or flexible scope, but in either case air insufflation is necessary to provide adequate views of all mucosal surfaces. The most difficult area to examine well is the cervical region, and this is unfortunately the most frequently injured site. Signs of penetrating esophageal trauma include bleeding, mucosal tears, or frank disruption with loss of luminal continuity. The false-positive rate for detecting a perforation on performing endoscopy for penetrating trauma approaches zero, whereas the false-negative rate for this indication is 10 to 20%.

Crohn's Disease of the Esophagus

Crohn's disease of the esophagus may appear as mild or ulcerative esophagitis in its early stages or as a stenosing esophagitis in its later stages.[32] These changes are limited predominantly to the distal esophagus but may extend more proximally in severe cases. Endoscopic recognition of Crohn's disease is possible only when the typical cobblestone pattern, similar to that seen in the colon, is present. In other cases, the endoscopic appearance is nonspecific, and the diagnosis is suspected only on the basis of histologic and radiographic findings, the history, and the physical examination.

ESOPHAGEAL ULTRASONOGRAPHY

Esophageal ultrasound became technically possible in the early 1980s with the introduction of modified ultrasound probes attached to endoscopes. Although the optics of current scopes are suboptimal, providing only side-viewing capabilities under normal circumstances, important intraesophageal and extraesophageal details within the neck, mediastinum, and upper abdomen can be examined by using this technology. Models of some scopes permit videoscopically directed needle aspiration for cytology and culture. Other scopes are capable of emitting two separate frequencies for differing depths of imaging and degrees of resolution.

Equipment

Esophageal ultrasound is performed using an endoscope measuring 12 mm in diameter with side-viewing capabilities and a modified tip that houses an ultrasound emitter-receiver. Most ultrasound endoscopes contain an instrument channel that permits directed biopsies. In addition, small (8.5-mm) ultrasound probes are available for evaluation of stenotic areas that will not permit passage of the larger standard ultrasound endoscopes. These scopes do not have viewing or biopsy capabilities, however.[8] The distal portion of the endoscope (excluding the ultrasound tip) is flexible and is directionally controlled by the operator.

The scope emits 7.5-, 10-, 12-, or 20-MHz signals, high-frequency sonic waves that are not used in most extracorporeal techniques and yield high-resolution sonographs with deep tissue penetration. Wide-angle pictures are provided by a 180-degree sectoral or a 360-degree radial view. A balloon tip capable of being filled with deaerated water provides the necessary contact with the esophageal wall to enhance sonographic evaluation. The scope is connected to a unit that processes and displays the sonograms for storage and evaluation.

Technique

Endoscopic ultrasound (EUS) is normally performed after formal endoscopic evaluation of the esophagus. The

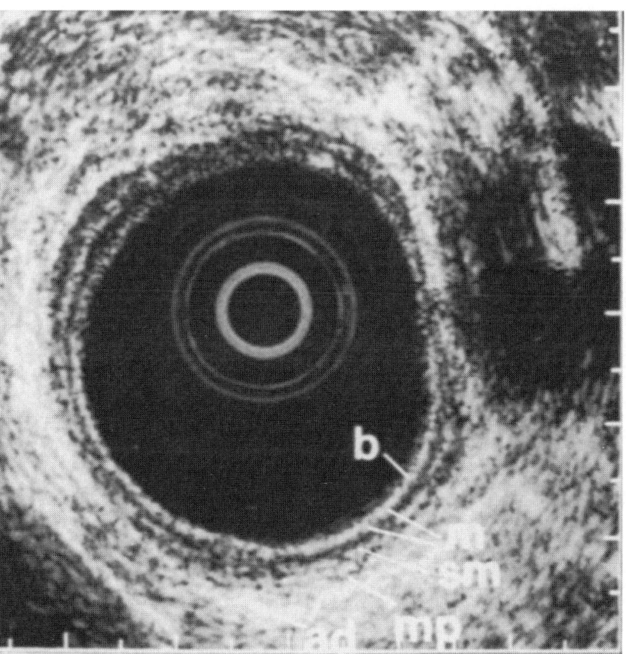

Figure 5–9. Normal esophageal sonograph showing five layers of the esophageal wall. (ad = adventitia, b = basement membrane [lamina propria], m = mucosa, mp = muscularis propria, sm = submucosa.) (From Tio, T.L., and Tytgat, G.N.J. [eds.]: Atlas of Transintestinal Ultrasonography. Aalsmeer, The Netherlands, Smith, Kline & French, 1986, p. 29, with permission.)

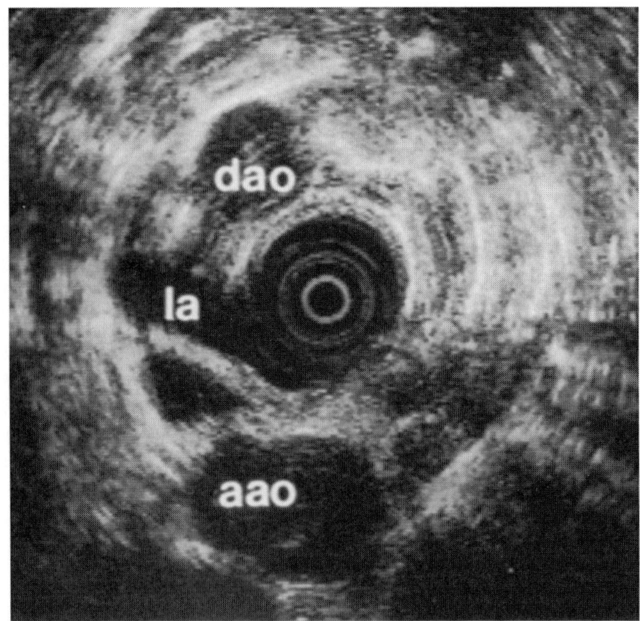

Figure 5–10. Midesophageal sonogram showing the ascending aorta (aao), left atrium (la), and descending aorta (dao). (From Tio, T.L., and Tytgat, G.N.J. [eds.]: Atlas of Transintestinal Ultrasonography. Aaslmeer, The Netherlands, Smith, Kline & French, 1986, p. 41, with permission.)

scope itself is inserted and advanced using a technique exactly like that used in normal endoscopy. All areas of the esophagus should be examined routinely, and recordings are made of regions of particular interest. In evaluating an esophageal carcinoma, it is recommended that recordings be made from multiple levels within the esophagus to assess concurrent mediastinal disease, particularly in the lymph nodes. In examining regions within

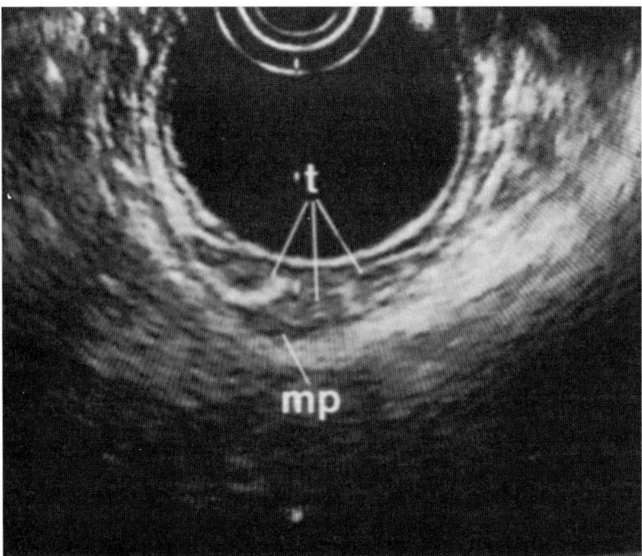

Figure 5–11. An early-stage tumor (t) is evident in this esophageal sonogram, demonstrating preservation of the muscularis propria (mp). (From Tio, T.L., and Tytgat, G.N.J. [eds.]: Atlas of Transintestinal Ultrasonography. Aalsmeer, The Netherlands, Smith, Kline & French, 1986, p. 99, with permission.)

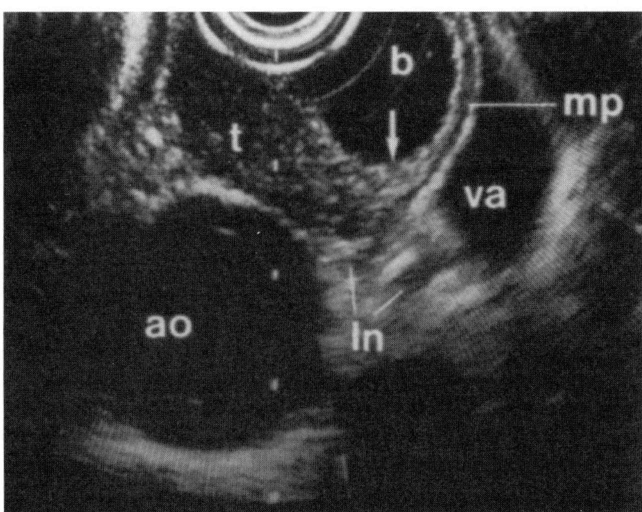

Figure 5–12. Esophageal sonogram in a patient with a large polypoid tumor (t) that extends transmurally. The ultrasound balloon (b) is eccentrically compressed. A portion of muscularis propria (mp) and a lymph node (ln) are visible. (ao = aorta, va = azygos vein.) (From Tio, T.L., and Tytgat, G.N.J. [eds.]: Atlas of Transintestinal Ultrasonography. Aalsmeer, The Netherlands, Smith, Kline, & French, 1986, p. 95, with permission.)

the stomach or duodenum, the various organs can be filled with deaerated water to transmit the sonographic signals. In this way, upper abdominal lymph nodes, particularly in the perigastric and celiac regions, can be visualized.

Staging Esophageal Malignancies

Endoscopic ultrasound has been used in Japan and northern Europe since the early 1980s for the purpose of staging upper gastrointestinal tract cancers. Five layers of normal esophageal wall are identified on the typical ultrasound image (Figs. 5-9 and 5-10). It is usually possible to identify a mass corresponding to an esophageal carcinoma and to correlate the depth of penetration of this mass with the impingement of the ultrasonographic abnormality on one or more of the layers of the esophagus (Fig. 5-11). In addition, lymph node metastases can be detected, even in the absence of lymph node enlargement, by noting one or more of the following abnormalities that are suspicious for malignancy within a node: (1) spherical shape, (2) a distinct border, and (3) heterogeneous echo spots within the nodes (Fig. 5-12).[11] Using these criteria, the depth of penetration of the primary tumor can be correctly assessed in up to 80 to 90% of cases, and involvement of identifiable mediastinal lymph nodes can be assessed with an accuracy of 70 to 80%.[3,29,43,44,60]

References

1. Akdamar, K., Ertan, A., Agrawal, N. M., et al.: Upper gastrointestinal endoscopy in normal asymptomatic volunteers. Gastrointest. Endosc., *32*:78, 1986.

2. Allen, J. I., Silvis, S. E., Sumner, H. W., et al.: Cytomegalic inclusion disease diagnosed endoscopically. Dig. Dis. Sci., *26:*133, 1981.
3. Altorki, N. K., Snady, H., and Skinner, D. B.: Endosonography for cancer of the esophagus and cardia: Is it worthwhile? Dis. Esophagus, *9:*198, 1996.
4. American Society for Gastrointestinal Endoscopy: Appropriate use of gastrointestinal endoscopy. Manchester, MA, 1992, p. 5.
5. American Society for Gastrointestinal Endoscopy: Antibiotic prophylaxis for gastrointestinal endoscopy. Gastrointest. Endosc., *42:*630, 1995.
6. Ancona, E., and Gayet, B.: Esophageal perforations. I: Etiology, diagnosis, localization and symptoms. *In* Siewert, J. R., and Hölscher, A. H. (eds.): Diseases of the Esophagus. Berlin, Springer-Verlag, 1988, p. 1327.
7. Bianchi Porro, G., Parente, F., and Cernuschi, M.: The diagnosis of esophageal candidiasis in patients with acquired immune deficiency syncrome: Is endoscopy always necessary? Am. J. Gastroenterol., *84:*143, 1989.
8. Binmoeller, K. F., Seifert, H., Seitz, U., et al.: Ultrasonic esophagoprobe for TNM staging of highly stenosing esophageal carcinoma. Gastrointest. Endosc., *41:*547, 1995.
9. Botoman, V. A., and Surawicz, C. M.: Bacteremia with gastrointestinal endoscopic procedures. Gastrointest. Endosc., *32:*342, 1986.
10. Cales, P., Zabotto, B., Meskens, C., et al.: Gastroesophageal endoscopic features in cirrhosis. Observer variability, interassociations, and relationship to hepatic dysfunction. Gastroenterology, *98:*156, 1990.
11. Catalano, M. F., Sivak, M. V., Jr., Rice, T., et al.: Endosonographic features predictive of lymph node metastasis. Gastrointest. Endosc., *40:*442, 1994.
12. Cello, J. P., Fogel, R. P., and Boland, R.: Liquid caustic ingestion. Arch. Intern. Med., *140:*501, 1980.
13. Chobanian, S. J., Cattau, E. L., Jr., Winters, C. A., Jr., et al.: In vivo staining with toluidine blue as an adjunct to the endoscopic detection of Barrett's esophagus. Gastrointest. Endosc., *33:*99, 1987.
14. Contini, S., Consigli, G. F., Di Lecce, F., et al.: Vital staining of oesophagus in patients with head and neck cancer: Still a worthwhile procedure. Ital. J. Gastroenterol., *23:*5, 1991.
15. Crespi, M., Grassi, A., Munoz, N., et al.: Endoscopic features of suspected precancerous lesions in high-risk areas for esophageal cancer. Endoscopy, *16:*85, 1984.
16. Dajani, A. S., Taubert, K. A., Wilson, W., et al.: Prevention of bacterial endocarditis. JAMA, *277:*1794, 1997.
17. Dark, D. S., Campbell, D. R., and Wesselius, L. J.: Arterial oxygen desaturation during gastrointestinal endoscopy. Am. J. Gastroenterol., *85:*1317, 1990.
18. Di Costanzo, J., Noirclerc, M., Jouglard, J., et al.: New therapeutic approach to corrosive burns of the upper gastrointestinal tract. Gut, *21:*370, 1980.
19. Diab, F. H., King, P. D., Barthel, J. S., and Marshall, J. B.: Efficacy and safety of combined meperidine and midazolam for EGD sedation compared with midazolam alone. Am. J. Gastroenterol., *91:*1120, 1996.
20. DiSario, J. A., Waring, J. P., Talbert, G., and Sanowski, R. A.: Monitoring of blood pressure and heart rate during routine endoscopy: A prospective, randomized, controlled study. Am. J. Gastroenterol., *86:*956, 1991.
21. Ferguson, M. K., Little, A. G., and Skinner, D. B.: Barrett's esophagus. *In* Tompkins, R. K. (ed.): Advances in Surgery, Vol. 21. Chicago, Year Book Medical Publishers, 1987, p. 127.
22. Ferguson, M. K., Little, A. G., and Skinner, D. B.: The clinical spectrum of benign penetrating Barrett's ulcers. *In* Siewert, J. R., and Hölscher, A. H. (eds.): Diseases of the Esophagus. Berlin, Springer-Verlag, 1988, p. 542.
23. Funch-Jensen, P., Kock, K., Christensen, L. A., et al.: Microscopic appearance of the esophageal mucosa in a consecutive series of patients submitted to upper endoscopy. Correlation with gastroesophageal reflux symptoms and macroscopic findings. Scand. J. Gastroenterol. *21:*65, 1986.
24. Guanrei, Y., He, H., Sungliang, Q., et al.: Endoscopic diagnosis of 115 cases of early esophageal carcinoma. Endoscopy, *14:*157, 1982.
25. Gupta, R. K., and Rogers, K. E.: Endoscopic cytology and biopsy in the diagnosis of gastroesophageal malignancy. Acta Cytol., *27:*17, 1983.
26. Hameeteman, W., den Hartog Jager, F. C. A., Tio, T. L., et al.: Early adenocarcinoma of the esophagus. *In* Siewert, J. R., and Hölscher, A. H. (eds.): Diseases of the Esophagus. Berlin, Springer-Verlag, 1988, p. 555.
27. Herlin, P., Marnay, J., Jacob, J. H., et al.: A study of the mechanism of the toluidine blue dye test. Endoscopy, *15:*4, 1983.
28. Hix, W. R., and Wilson, W. R.: Detection of occult carcinoma of the esophagus by toluidine blue staining in high risk patients. *In* Siewert, J. R., and Hölscher, A. H. (eds.): Diseases of the Esophagus. Berlin, Springer-Verlag, 1988, p. 118.
29. Holscher, A. H., Dittler, H. J., and Siewert, J. R.: Staging of squamous esophageal cancer: Accuracy and value. World J. Surg., *18:*312, 1994.
30. Jamieson, J., Hinder, R. A., DeMeester, T. R., et al.: Analysis of thirty-two patients with Schatzki's ring. Am. J. Surg., *158:*563, 1989.
31. Kelly, J. P., Webb, W. R., Moulder, P. V., et al.: Management of airway trauma. II: Combined injuries of the trachea and esophagus. Ann. Thorac. Surg., *43:*160, 1987.
32. Maffei, V. J., Zaatari, G. S., McGarity, W. C., et al.: Crohn's disease of the esophagus. J. Thorac. Cardiovasc. Surg., *94:*302, 1987.
33. Maroy, B., and Moullot, P.: Safety of upper gastrointestinal endoscopy with intravenous sedation by the endoscopist at office: 17,963 Examinations performed in a community center by two endoscopists over 17 years. J. Clin. Gastroenterol., *27:*368, 1998.
34. McBane, R. D., Gross, J. B., Jr.: Herpes esophagitis: Clinical syndrome, endoscopic appearance, and diagnosis in 23 patients. Gastrointest. Endosc. *37:*600, 1991.
35. Mori, M., Adachi, Y., Matsushima, T., et al.: Lugol staining pattern and histology of esophageal lesions. Am. J. Gastroenterol., *88:*701, 1993.
36. Nashef, S. A. M., and Pagliero, K. M.: Instrumental perforation of the esophagus in benign disease. Ann. Thorac. Surg., *44:*360, 1987.
37. Nishizawa, M., Okada, T., Hosoi, T., et al.: Detecting early esophageal cancers with special reference to the intraepithelial stage. Endoscopy, *16:*92, 1984.
38. Norberto, L., Cusumano, A., Bonavina, L., et al.: Endoscopic vital staining in the diagnosis of esophageal cancer. *In* Siewert, J. R., and Hölscher, A. H. (eds.): Diseases of the Esophagus. Berlin, Springer-Verlag, 1988, p. 135.
39. Olden, K., and Triadafilopoulos, G.: Failure of initial 24-hour esophageal pH monitoring to predict refractoriness and intractability in reflux esophagitis. Am. J. Gastroenterol., *86:*1142, 1991.
40. Ott, D. J., Kelley, T. F., Chen, M. Y., et al.: Use of a marshmallow bolus for evaluating lower esophageal mucosal rings. Am. J. Gastroenterol., *86:*817, 1991.
41. Quine, M. A., Bell, G. D., McCloy, R. F., et al.: Prospective audit of upper gastrointestinal endoscopy in two regions of England: Safety, staffing, and sedation methods. Gut, *36:*462, 1995.
42. Quine, M. A., Bell, G. D., McCloy, R. F., and Matthews, H. R.: Prospective audit of perforation rates following upper gastrointestinal endoscopy in two regions of England. Br. J. Surg., *82:*530, 1995.
43. Reed, C. E., Mishra, G., Sahai, A., et al.: Esophageal cancer staging: Improved accuracy by endoscopic ultrasound of celiac lymph nodes. Ann. Thorac. Surg., *67:*319, 1999.
44. Rice, T. W., Boyce, G. A., and Sivak, M. V.: Esophageal ultrasound and the preoperative staging of carcinoma of the esophagus. J. Thorac. Cardiovasc. Surg., *101:*536, 1991.
45. Richardson, J. D., Flint, L. M., Snow, N. J., et al.: Management of transmediastinal gunshot wounds. Surgery, *90:*671, 1981.
46. Ritchie, A. J., McGuigan, J., McManus, K., et al.: Diagnostic rigid and flexible oesophagoscopy in carcinoma of the oesophagus: A comparison. Thorax, *48:*115, 1993.
47. Sarr, M. G., Pemberton, J. H., and Payne, W. S.: Management of instrumental perforations of the esophagus. J. Thorac. Cardiovasc. Surg., *84:*211, 1982.
48. Savary, M., Ollyo, J. B., and Monnier, P.: Frequency and importance of endobrachyesophagus in reflux disease. *In* Siewert, J. R., and Hölscher, A. H. (eds.): Disease of the Esophagus. Berlin, Springer-Verlag, 1988, p. 529.
49. Schatzki, R., and Gray, J. E.: Dysphagia due to a diaphragm-like localized narrowing in the lower esophagus (lower esophageal ring). Am. J. Roentgenol., *70:*911, 1953.
50. Shamir, M., and Schuman, B. M.: Complications of fiberoptic endoscopy. Gastrointest. Endosc. *26:*86, 1980.
51. Shorvon, P. J., Eykyn, S. J., and Cotton, P. B.: Gastrointestinal instrumentation, bacteraemia, and endocarditis. Gut, *24:*1078, 1983.

52. Solomon, M. P., Rosenblum, H., and Rosato, F. E.: Leiomyoma of the esophagus. Ann. Surg., *199:*246, 1984.
53. Spach, D. H., Silverstein, F. E., and Stamm, W. E.: Transmission of infection by gastrointestinal endoscopy and bronchoscopy. Ann. Intern. Med., *118:*117, 1993.
54. St. Onge, G., and Bezahler, G. H.: Giant esophageal ulcer associated with cytomegalovirus. Gastroenterology, *83:*127, 1982.
55. Staples, D. C., Knodell, R. G., and Johnson, L. F.: Inflammatory pseudotumor of the esophagus. Gastrointest. Endosc., *24:*175, 1978.
56. Sugimachi, K., Kitamura, K., Baba, K., et al.: Endoscopic diagnosis of early carcinoma of the esophagus using Lugol's solution. Gastrointest. Endosc., *38:*657, 1992.
57. Symbas, P. N., Vlasis, S. E., Hatcher, C. R., Jr.: Esophagitis secondary to ingestion of caustic material. Ann. Thorac. Surg., *36:*73, 1983.
58. The Italian Liver Cirrhosis Project: Reliability of endoscopy in the assessment of variceal features. J. Hepatol., *4:*93, 1987.
59. Wiburg, F. A., Beukers, M. M., Bartelsman, J. F., et al.: Nasogastric intubation as sole treatment of caustic esophageal lesions. Ann. Otol. Rhinol. Laryngol., *94:*337, 1985.
60. Ziegler, K., Sanft, C., Zeitz, M., et al.: Evaluation of endosonography in TN staging of oesophageal cancer. Gut, *32:*16, 1991.

CHAPTER

6 Physiologic Diagnostic Studies

RODNEY J. MASON • TOM R. DEMEESTER

Clinical medicine has advanced through retrospective analysis, the relation of symptoms to anatomic or structural lesions, and the use of this relationship prospectively to diagnose disease. In time, biochemical or histologic abnormalities were identified as having a high probability of being caused by a disease process, such as alterations in metabolism, neoplasia, inflammation, and ischemia. Consequently, biochemical or histologic patterns are used to recognize and identify specific diseases in symptomatic patients. There are, however, abnormalities that cause symptoms in the absence of anatomic, histologic, or biochemical markers. For the most part, these are abnormalities of organ function that give rise to symptoms before the development of injury recognizable by structural, histologic, or biochemical changes.

Functional disorders of the esophagus are such an abnormality. They can exist for a period of time without causing morphologic changes while causing considerable symptoms. Typical symptoms of functional esophageal disorders are heartburn, regurgitation, and dysphagia. Ascribing these symptoms to a specific esophageal abnormality in the absence of structural or histologic findings and without further investigation can lead to an error in diagnosis. This is because a variety of gastric, duodenal, cardiac, and pulmonary disorders can cause symptomatology similar to esophageal abnormalities, making it difficult to differentiate and discriminate them from the latter. Further, functional esophageal disorders can present with atypical symptoms, such as chest pain, chronic cough, or shortness of breath, which lead the investigator to suspect abnormalities of the heart or lung. Complicating matters even more, functional esophageal disorders can also occur concomitantly with gastroduodenal, cardiac, and pulmonary disease. Consequently, objective methods are required to confirm the presence of a functional esophageal abnormality and to distinguish it from other conditions.

Even in the presence of histologic, endoscopic, or roentgenographic abnormalities that have classically supported a specific disease, the diagnosis may be incomplete without further investigation. This is because the underlying functional abnormality that led to the finding is not recognized. For example, esophagitis may be medication induced or secondary to gastroesophageal reflux disease (GERD). Increased esophageal exposure to gastric juice itself may be due to a mechanically defective lower esophageal sphincter, ineffective esophageal clearance function, or gastroduodenal disorders. A correct diagnosis of the abnormality and identification of the underlying cause is essential for the selection of the appropriate therapy and to avoid failure or recurrence. This requires a sound understanding of normal esophageal physiology and the functional abnormalities that may result in tissue injury if allowed to persist.[15,59]

PHYSIOLOGIC ASPECTS OF ESOPHAGEAL FUNCTION

The act of alimentation requires the passage of food and drink from the mouth into the stomach. One third of this distance consists of the mouth and hypopharynx, and two thirds consist of the esophagus. To comprehend the mechanics of alimentation, it is useful to visualize the gullet as a mechanical model in which the tongue and pharynx function as a piston pump with three valves, and the body of the esophagus and cardia function as a worm drive pump with a single valve. The three valves in the pharyngeal cylinder are the soft pallet, the epiglottis, and the cricopharyngeus. The valve of the esophageal pump is the lower esophageal sphincter. Failure of the valves or the pumps leads to abnormalities in swallowing—that is, difficulty in the propulsion of food from the mouth to the stomach or the regurgitation of gastric contents from the stomach into the pharynx.

Food is taken into the mouth in a variety of bite sizes, where it is broken up, mixed with saliva, and lubricated. Swallowing, once initiated, is entirely a reflex. When food is ready for swallowing, the tongue, acting like a piston, moves the bolus into the posterior oropharynx and forces it into the hypopharynx (Fig. 6–1). Concomitant with the posterior movement of the tongue, the soft palate is elevated, thereby closing the passage between the oropharynx and nasopharynx. This partitioning prevents pressure generated in the oropharynx from being dissipated through the nose. When the soft palate is paralyzed, as occurs after a cerebrovascular accident, the food is commonly regurgitated into the nasopharynx. During swallowing, the hyoid bone moves upward and anteriorly, elevating the larynx and opening the retrolaryngeal space. This brings the epiglottis under the tongue (Fig. 6–1). The backward tilt of the epiglottis covers the opening of the larynx to prevent aspiration. The entire pharyngeal part of swallowing occurs within 1.5 seconds.

The pressure in the hypopharynx rises abruptly during swallowing to reach at least 60 mmHg. A sizable pressure difference develops between the pharyngeal pressure and the less-than-atmospheric midesophageal or intrathoracic pressure (Fig. 6–2). This pressure gradient speeds the movement of food from the hypopharynx into the esoph-

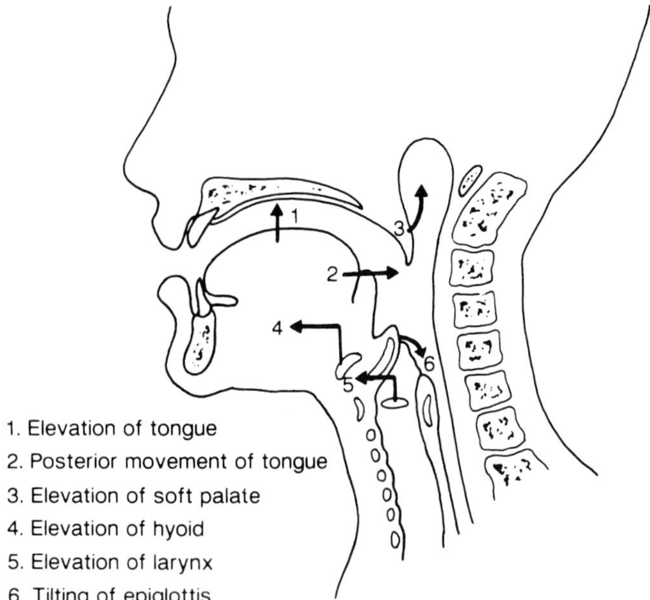

Figure 6–1. Sequence of events during the oropharyngeal phase of swallowing.

agus when the cricopharyngeus or upper esophageal sphincter relaxes and opens and the cervical esophagus is appropriately compliant. The bolus is propelled through the open sphincter by the piston-like action of the tongue and the peristaltic contractions of the posterior laryngeal constrictors and is sucked into the thoracic esophagus by the pressure differential. The compliance of the striated muscle of the cervical esophagus is crucial for this phase of swallowing, and its loss results in severe dysphagia. The upper esophageal sphincter closes within an additional 0.5 second, with the immediate closing pressure reaching approximately twice the resting level of 30 mmHg. This postrelaxation contraction continues down the esophagus as a peristaltic wave (Fig. 6–3). The high closing pressure and the initiation of the peristaltic wave prevent regurgitation of the bolus from the esophagus back into the pharynx. After the peristaltic wave has passed farther down the esophagus, the pressure in the upper, esophageal sphincter returns to its resting level (Fig. 6–3).

Swallowing can be started at will, or it can be reflexly elicited by the stimulation of areas in the mouth and pharynx, including the anterior and posterior tonsillar pillars or the posterior lateral walls of the hypopharynx. The afferent nerves of the pharynx are the glossopharyngeal nerve and the superior laryngeal branches of the vagus. Once aroused by stimuli entering via these nerves, the swallowing center in the medulla coordinates the complete act of swallowing by discharging impulses through the fifth, seventh, tenth, eleventh, and twelfth cranial nerves, as well as the motor neurons of Cl to C3. Discharges through these nerves occur in a rather specific pattern and last for approximately 0.5 second. Little is known about the organization of the swallowing center except that it can trigger swallowing after a variety of different inputs, but the response is always a rigidly ordered pattern of outflow. After a cerebrovascular accident, this coordinated outflow may be altered, causing mild abnormalities of swallowing. In more severe injury, swallowing can be grossly disrupted, leading to repetitive aspiration.

The striated muscles of the cricopharyngeus and the upper third of the esophagus are activated by efferent fibers distributed through the vagus nerve and its recurrent laryngeal branches. The integrity of innervation is required for the cricopharyngeus to relax in coordination with the pharyngeal contraction and resume its resting tone once a bolus has entered the upper esophagus. Concomitantly, the striated muscle of the cervical esophagus must have the compliance to dilate and to accept the swallowed bolus. Central nervous system damage from a variety of causes can interfere with the innervation of the larynx, cricopharyngeus, and upper esophagus. The resulting loss of muscle function and compliance can predispose the patient to aspiration or dysphagia.

The pharyngeal activity in swallowing initiates the esophageal phase. The body of the esophagus functions as a worm drive propulsive pump, due to the helical arrangement of its circular muscles, and is responsible

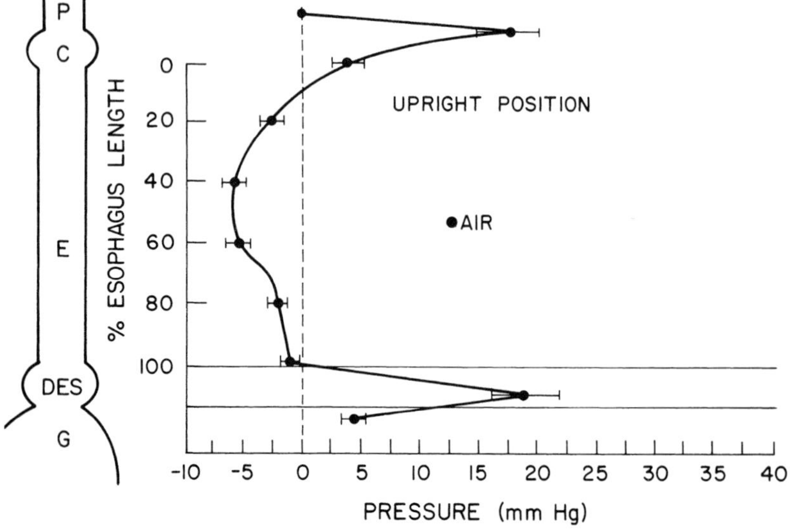

Figure 6–2. Resting pressure profile of the foregut showing the pressure differential between the atmospheric pharyngeal pressure (P), and the less than atmospheric midesophageal pressure (E), and the greater than atmospheric intragastric pressure (G), with the interposed high pressure zones of the cricopharyngeus (C) and distal esophageal sphincter (DES). The necessity for coordinated relaxation of the cricopharyngeus and DES in order to move a bolus into the stomach is apparent. Esophageal work occurs when a bolus is pushed across the pressure gradient from the midesophageal area (E) into the stomach (G). (From Waters, P.F., and DeMeester, T.R.: Foregut motor disorders and their surgical management. Med. Clin. North Am., *65*:1237, 1981, with permission.)

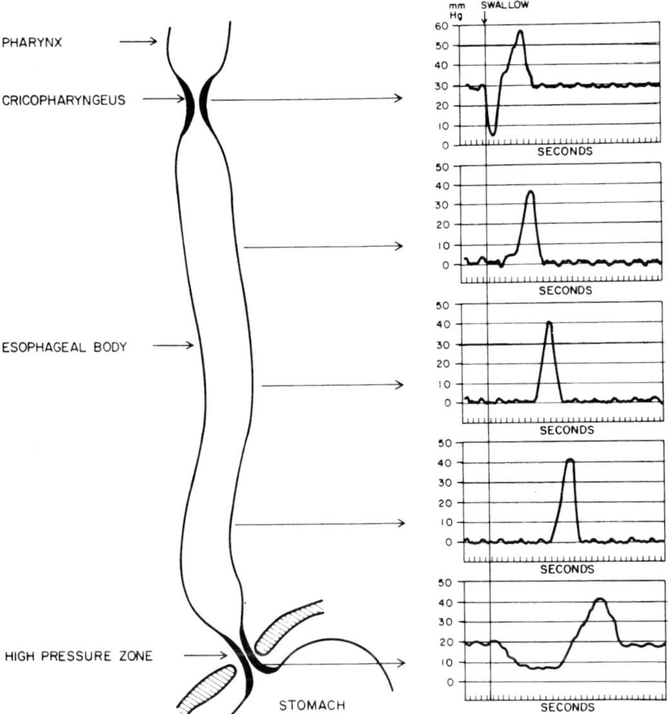

Figure 6–3. Intraluminal esophageal pressures in response to swallowing. (From Waters, P.F., and DeMeester, T.R.: Foregut motor disorders and their surgical management. Med. Clin. North Am., *65*:1238, 1981, with permission.)

for transmitting a bolus of food from the distal esophagus into the stomach. The esophageal phase of swallowing represents esophageal work done during alimentation, in that food is moved into the stomach from −6 mmHg intrathoracic pressure to an average of +6 mmHg of intra-abdominal pressure (i.e., a gradient of 12 mmHg [see Fig. 6–2]). Effective and coordinated smooth muscle function in the lower third of the esophagus is therefore important in pumping the food into the stomach. The peristaltic wave generates an occlusive pressure varying from 0.30 to 150 mmHg (see Fig. 6–3). The wave rises to a peak in 1 second, lasts at the peak for about 0.5 second, and then subsides in about 1.5 seconds. The entire course of the rise and fall of occlusive pressure may occupy one point in the esophagus for 3 to 5 seconds. The peak of a primary peristaltic contraction initiated by a swallow moves down the esophagus at 2 to 4 cm/sec and reaches the distal esophagus about 9 seconds after swallowing has been initiated (see Fig. 6–3). Consecutive swallows produce similar primary peristaltic waves, but when the act of swallowing is rapidly repeated, the esophagus remains relaxed and the peristaltic wave occurs only after the last movement of the pharynx. This phenomenon is referred to as *postdeglutitive inhibition*.

Progress of the wave down the esophagus is caused by sequential activation of its muscles initiated by efferent vagal nerve fibers that arise in the swallowing center. Continuity of the esophageal muscle is not necessary if the nerves remain intact. If the muscles but not the nerves are cut, the pressure wave begins distally below the cut, because it dies out at the proximal end above the cut. This allows a sleeve resection of the esophagus to be made without destroying its normal function. Afferent impulses from receptors within the esophageal wall are not essential for progress of the coordinated wave. However, afferent nerves do go to the swallowing center from the esophagus. If the esophagus is distended at any point, a contractual wave begins with a forceful closure of the upper esophageal sphincter and sweeps down the esophagus. This secondary contraction occurs without any movement of the mouth or pharynx. Secondary contractions can occur as an independent local reflex to clear the esophagus of material left behind after the passage of the primary wave but are less common than previously thought.

Despite the rather powerful occlusive pressure, the propulsive force of the esophagus is relatively feeble. If one attempts to swallow a bolus attached by a string to a counterweight, the maximum weight one can overcome is 5 to 10 g. Orderly contractions of the muscular wall and anchoring of the esophagus at its inferior end are necessary for efficient and aboral propulsion to occur. Loss of the inferior anchor, as occurs with a large hiatal hernia, can lead to inefficient propulsion.

The lower esophageal sphincter provides a pressure barrier between the esophagus and stomach and acts as the valve on the worm drive pump of the esophageal body. Although an anatomically distinct lower esophageal sphincter has been difficult to identify, microdissection studies show that in humans, the sphincter-like function of this segment is related to the architecture of the muscle fibers at the junction of the esophageal tube with the gastric pouch[42] (Fig. 6–4). The sphincter actively remains closed to prevent reflux of gastric contents into the esophagus and opens through relaxation that coincides with a pharyngeal swallow (see Fig. 6–3). The lower esophageal sphincter pressure returns to its resting level after the peristaltic wave has passed through the esophagus. Consequently, reflux of gastric juice that may occur through the open valve during a swallow is pumped back into the stomach. An important trigger for gastroesophageal reflux appears to be gastric distention, which results in a shortening of the lower esophageal sphincter as it is taken up into the fundus of the expanding stomach. The progressive shortening of the sphincter reaches a point where the pressure in the remaining length gives way and the sphincter opens, allowing reflux to occur. Loss of the sphincter barrier function also occurs if the pharyngeal swallow does not initiate a peristaltic contraction; then, the coincident relaxation of the lower, esophageal sphincter is unguarded, and reflux of gastric juice can occur. This appears to be the major cause of the so-called transient or spontaneous lower esophageal sphincter relaxations, thought by some to be a causative factor in GERD.[19] In dogs, a bilateral cervical parasympathetic blockade abolishes the relaxation of the lower esophageal sphincter that occurs with pharyngeal swallowing or distention of the esophagus.[49] This indicates that vagal function is important in maintaining the lower esophageal sphincter barrier function and in coordinating the relaxation of the lower esophageal sphincter with esophageal contraction.

The ability of the lower esophageal sphincter to pro-

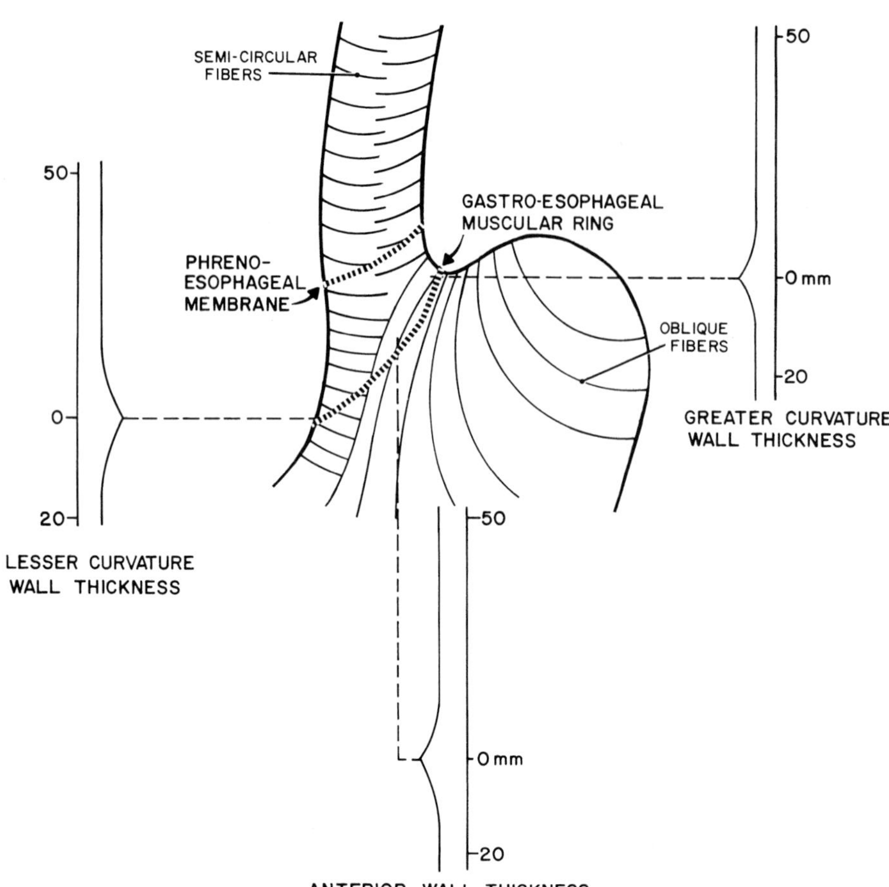

Figure 6–4. Schematic drawing showing wall thickness and orientation of fibers on microdissection of the cardia: At the junction of the esophageal tube with the gastric pouch, there is an oblique muscular ring composed of an increased muscle mass inside the inner muscular layer. On the lesser curve side of the cardia the muscle fibers of the inner layer are oriented transversely and form semicircular muscle clasps that insert into the submucosal connective tissues. On the greater curve side of the cardia, these muscle fibers form long oblique loops that run parallel to the lesser curve of the stomach and encircle the distal end of the cardia and gastric fundus. (From DeMeester, T.R., and Skinner, D.B.: Evaluation of esophageal function and disease. *In* Glenn, W.W.L. [ed.]: Thoracic and Cardiovascular Surgery, 4th ed. Norwalk, CT, Appleton-Century-Crofts, 1983, p. 461, with permission.)

tect the esophageal mucosa from excessive exposure to gastric juice depends on the resistance it imposes to the flow of gastric juice from an environment above atmospheric pressure, the stomach, into an environment below atmospheric pressure, the esophagus. Clinical and in vitro studies have shown that this resistance is due to the integrated mechanical effect of the sphincter pressure, overall length, and length exposed to the positive environmental pressure of the abdomen.[8,60,67]

PATHOPHYSIOLOGIC ASPECTS OF ESOPHAGEAL FUNCTION

In the normal situation, there is a coordinated interplay between the esophagus and its adjacent valves and compartments to propel food from the mouth to the stomach. Failure of the propulsive ability of a compartment hampers the forward movement of food and enhances regurgitation. Failure of the valve between two adjoining compartments results in exposure of the proximal compartment to the luminal contents of the distal compartment (i.e., gastroesophageal and esophagopharyngeal reflux).

Pharyngoesophageal Swallowing Disorders

Disorders of the pharyngoesophageal phase of swallowing result from a dyscoordination of the neuromuscular events involved in chewing, initiation of swallowing, and propulsion of the material from the oropharynx to the cervical esophagus. This results in dysphagia, nasal regurgitation, aspiration, and repetitive respiratory infections. The disorders can be categorized into one or a combination of the following: (1) inadequate oropharyngeal bolus transport, (2) inability to pressurize the pharynx, (3) inability to elevate the larynx and open the upper esophageal sphincter, (4) impaired cricopharyngeal muscle relaxation and pharyngeal contraction, and (5) decreased compliance of the pharyngoesophageal segment and cervical esophagus secondary to a restrictive myopathy.

The etiology of pharyngoesophageal swallowing disorders is usually an acquired disease that involves the central and peripheral nervous systems. Possible diseases and conditions include cerebrovascular accidents, brainstem tumors, poliomyelitis, multiple sclerosis, Parkinson's disease, pseudobulbar palsy, peripheral neuropathy, and operative damage to the cranial nerves involved in swallowing. Muscular diseases, such as radiation-induced myopathy, dermatomyositis, myotonic dystrophy, and myasthenia gravis, are less common. Occasionally, extrinsic compression through thyromegaly, cervical lymphadenopathy, or hyperostosis of the cervical spine can cause cervical dysphagia. It should be noted, however, that in our series, almost 40% of the patients had no discernible underlying disease process that could be identified.

The rapidity of the oropharyngeal phase of swallowing, the movement of the gullet, and the asymmetry

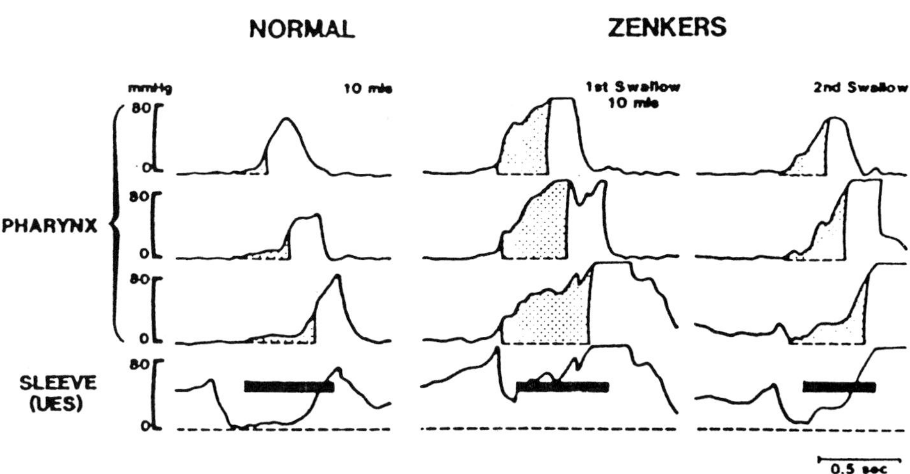

Figure 6–5. Manometric pharyngeal and upper esophageal sphincter (UES) tracing during a 10-ml swallow. In a patient with Zenker's diverticulum, there is a much higher intrabolus pressure wave *(stippled)* than in the normal control subject. Note that when the patient swallowed a second time to clear residual bolus from the pharynx, this lower volume bolus was associated with a lower but still abnormal intrabolus pressure and a shorter duration of UES opening on simultaneously performed videofluoroscopy *(bar)*. (From Cook, I.J., Gibb, M., Panagopoulos, V., et al.: Pharyngeal [Zenker's] diverticulum is a disorder of upper esophageal sphincter opening. Gastroenterology, *103*:1229, 1992, with permission.)

of the cricopharyngeus account for the difficulty in assessing abnormalities of esophagopharyngeal swallowing disorders with manometry. Videocineroentgenography is the most objective test to evaluate oropharyngeal bolus movement, pharyngeal contraction, cricopharyngeal relaxation, and the dynamics of airway protection during swallowing.[36] Careful analysis of videocineroentgenographic studies and manometry with specially designed catheter, ideally performed simultaneously, can identify the cause of pharyngoesophageal dysfunction in most situations.[45]

In patients with Zenker's diverticulum, it has been difficult to consistently demonstrate a motility abnormality of the pharyngeal phase of swallowing. The abnormality most apt to be present is a loss of compliance in the pharyngoesophageal segment manifested by an increased bolus pressure (Fig. 6–5).[13] Esophageal muscle biopsy results in patients with Zenker's diverticulum have shown histologic evidence of a restrictive myopathy correlating with decreased compliance of the upper esophagus on videocineradiographic and detailed manometric studies. These findings suggest that the diverticulum develops as a consequence of the repetitive stress of bolus transport through a noncompliant muscle of the pharyngoesophageal segment. Other roentgenographic manifestations of a noncompliant segment in the proximal esophagus are a cricopharyngeal bar or a more extended narrowing of the pharyngoesophageal segment. Dyscoordination of the sphincter relaxation with pharyngeal contraction together with impaired sphincter opening is another cause for the development of Zenker's diverticulum. This may not occur throughout the full length of the sphincter and can easily be missed on manometric assessment due to movement of the cricopharyngeus on swallowing. Failure of the cricopharyngeal muscle to relax on swallowing, the so-called cervical achalasia, and failure of an esophageal contraction to be initiated after a pharyngeal swallow have also been observed in patients with Zenker's diverticulum.[9]

Primary Motor Disorders of the Esophageal Body and Lower Esophageal Sphincter

Nonobstructive dysphagia (i.e., dysphagia in the absence of structural abnormalities) is the primary symptom of esophageal motor disorders. Its perception by the patient is a balance between the severity of the underlying cause that produces the difficulty and the patient's adjustment to that difficulty through the alteration in eating habits. Consequently, any complaint of dysphagia requires a detailed assessment of the patient's dietary history in addition to a clear understanding of the physiologic abnormalities that may cause the patient's symptoms.[59]

Abnormalities that occur in the worm drive pump of the esophageal body or the lower esophageal sphincter can give rise to a number of disorders in the esophageal phase of swallowing. These disorders are due to primary abnormalities in the esophagus or result from a more generalized neural, muscular, or systemic disease (Table 6–1). With the introduction of standard esophageal manometry, a number of primary esophageal motility disorders have been reclassified from nonspecific to separate disease entities; these include achalasia, diffuse esophageal spasm, the so-called nutcracker esophagus, and the hypertensive lower esophageal sphincter (Table 6–1).[65] The classification of these disorders usually is based on an analysis of the manometric recordings of 10 wet swallows performed in a laboratory setting (Table 6–2).[12]

The technique of ambulatory 24-hour monitoring of esophageal motor activity multiplies the number of esophageal contractions available for analysis and provides an opportunity to assess esophageal motor function

Table 6–1. Esophageal Motility Disorders

Primary
Achalasia, "vigorous" achalasia
Diffuse and segmental esophageal spasm
Nutcracker esophagus
Hypertensive lower esophageal sphincter
Nonspecific esophageal motility disorders
Secondary Esophageal Motility Disorders
Collagen vascular diseases: progressive systemic sclerosis, polymyositis and dermatomyositis, mixed connective tissue disease, systemic lupus erythematosus
Chronic idiopathic intestinal pseudo-obstruction
Neuromuscular diseases
Endocrine and metastatic disorders

Table 6–2. Manometric Characteristics of the Primary Esophageal Motility Disorders

Achalasia

Incomplete LES relaxation
Aperistalsis in the esophageal body
Elevated LES pressure
Increased intraesophageal baseline pressures relative to gastric baseline

Diffuse Esophageal Spasm

Simultaneous (nonperistaltic contractions) (>20% of wet swallows)
Repetitive and multipeaked contractions
Spontaneous contractions
Intermittent normal peristalsis
Contractions may be of increased amplitude and duration

Nutcracker Esophagus

Increased peristaltic amplitude in the distal esophagus (≥180 mmHg)
Increased mean duration of contractions (>7.0 seconds)
Normal peristaltic sequence

Hypertensive Lower Esophageal Sphincter

Elevated LES pressure
Normal LES relaxation
Normal peristalsis in the esophageal body

Nonspecific Esophageal Motility Disorders

Decreased or absent amplitude of esophageal peristalsis
Increased number of nonperistaltic or dropped contractions
Abnormal waveforms
Normal LES pressure and relaxation

LES = lower esophageal sphincter.

in a variety of physiological situations. This increases the accuracy and dependability of the measurement.[22] The application of ambulatory 24-hour esophageal motility monitoring has shown that there are marked differences in the classification of esophageal motor disorders between standard manometry and ambulatory motility monitoring (Fig. 6–6).[58] The degree of reclassification that occurs when analysis of esophageal motor function is conducted on the basis of ambulatory manometry indicates that the classic categories of esophageal motor disorders are inappropriate. This appears to be due to the intermittent expression of esophageal motor abnormalities that can be missed or overdiagnosed during the unphysiologic setting of standard manometry but are detected with a higher degree of reliability when motor activity is monitored over 24 hours under a variety of physiologic conditions. Based on these observations, esophageal motility disorders should be looked at as a spectrum of abnormalities that reflect various stages of deterioration of esophageal motor function rather than as separate entities.[59] This is supported by the observation that the severity of esophageal motor disorders can progress or regress during the natural course of the disease.

The symptom of dysphagia in patients without structural abnormalities of the esophagus can be caused by distal obstruction from a nonrelaxing lower esophageal sphincter or by disorganized contractions of the esophageal body. In patients with a nonrelaxing sphincter, the function of the esophageal body deteriorates secondarily to the distal obstruction and may recover if the obstruction is relieved early during the disease process. In patients with a primary motor disorder of the esophageal body, dysphagia appears to be due to an inability of the esophageal body to organize its motor activity into peristaltic contractions during meals. Ambulatory 24-hour monitoring of esophageal body function has shown that in normal asymptomatic volunteers, the prevalence of "effective contractions" (i.e., peristaltic contractions with sufficient amplitude to propel a bolus) increases with increasing states of consciousness (i.e., from sleep, to the upright position, and meal periods). This is probably due to a modulatory effect of the central nervous system on esophageal motor activity. Patients with nonobstructive dysphagia lack this ability to increase the prevalence of effective contractions with increasing states of consciousness.[52,57] Clinical studies using ambulatory esophageal motility have shown that the frequency of effective contractions increases during meal periods. Monitoring can be used to express the severity of esophageal body dysfunction on a linear scale. This can be related to the presence of nonobstructive dysphagia (Fig. 6–7), and it obviates the need for the current categories of esophageal motor disorders and permits an objective assessment of the

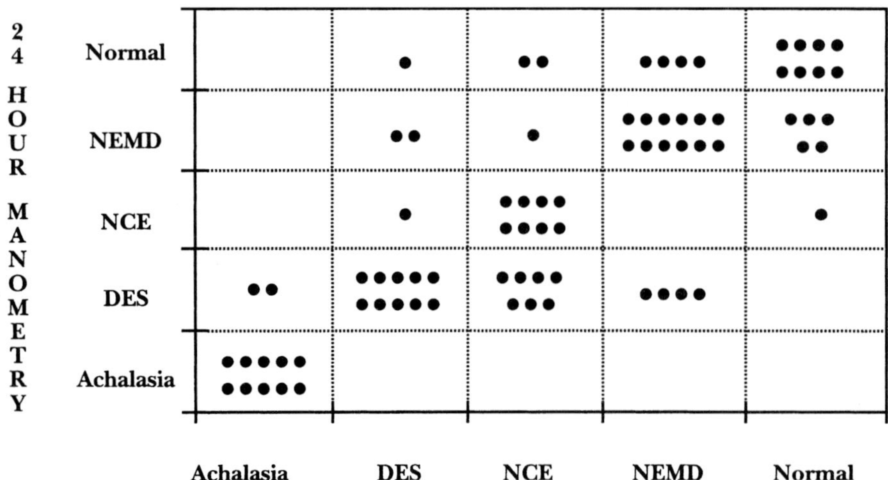

Figure 6–6. Classification of esophageal motor disorders in 108 patients with dysphagia or noncardiac chest pain according to the findings on standard or ambulatory 24-hour manometry. (DES, diffuse esophageal spasm; NCE, nutcracker esophagus; NEMD, nonspecific esophageal motor disorder.) (From Stein, H.J., DeMeester, T.R., Eypasch, E.P., and Klingman, R.P.: Ambulatory 24-hour esophageal manometry in the evaluation of esophageal motor disorders and noncardiac chest pain. Surgery, *110*:753, 1991, with permission.)

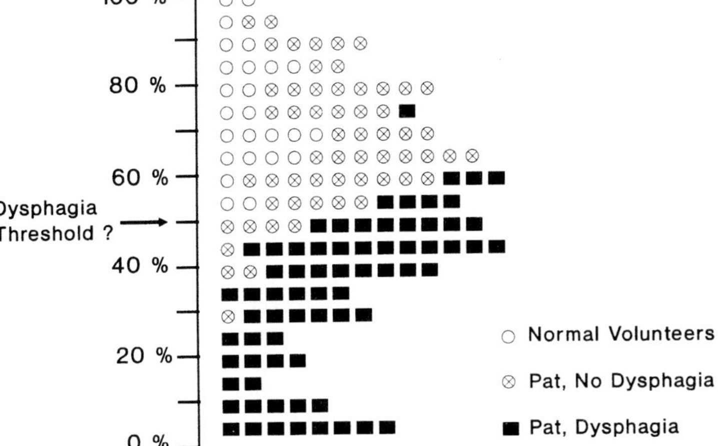

Figure 6–7. Prevalence of "effective contractions" during meal periods in normal volunteers, patients with nonobstructive dysphagia, and patients without dysphagia. Having less than 50% effective contractions during meals is associated with a high prevalence of nonobstructive dysphagia. Pat = patients.

effect of medical or surgical therapy on esophageal body function.[57]

Esophageal contractions of an abnormally high amplitude or long duration have been suggested to be responsible for chest pain in patients with esophageal motor disorders.[10] Ambulatory 24-hour motility monitoring in these patients has, however, shown that the amplitude and duration of esophageal contractions associated with chest pain episodes are similar to asymptomatic contractions, during the upright or supine recording. Esophageal chest pain episodes were preceded immediately by a markedly increased frequency of simultaneous and repetitive contractions (Fig. 6–8).[58] As in the heart, esophageal blood supply may be interrupted during bursts of disorganized muscular contractions. This may become crucial in situations where the resting blood flow to the esophagus is already compromised, as has been shown for the hypertrophic esophageal muscle in patients with esophageal motor disorders. A burst of disorganized motor activity in this situation may give rise to ischemic pain. Consequently, chest pain caused by a burst of uncoordinated esophageal motor activity under ischemic conditions has been called *esophageal claudication*.[58]

Roentgenographic abnormalities in motility disorders such as segmental spasms with compartmentalization of the esophagus or formation of a diverticulum are the anatomic results of disordered esophageal motor function. A detailed analysis will reveal that a motility disorder was usually present for years before the documentation of these roentgenographic findings. The development of a diverticulum may temporarily alleviate the symptom of initial dysphagia during eating and replace it with the symptom of postprandial regurgitation of undigested food. In those few patients with a diverticulum in whom an abnormality of esophageal body or lower esophageal sphincter function cannot be identified manometrically, a traction or congenital etiology for the diverticulum should be sought.

Secondary Esophageal Motor Disorders

Esophageal motility disorders may also result from more generalized neural, muscular, or systemic metabolic abnormalities. The esophagus is particularly affected by almost any of the collagen vascular disorders; the most common are progressive systemic sclerosis, mixed connective tissue disease, polymyositis, and dermatomyositis (see Table 6–1).[44,63,66] Eighty percent of patients with progressive systemic sclerosis have an esophageal motor abnormality. In most cases, the disease follows a prolonged course and usually affects only the smooth muscle

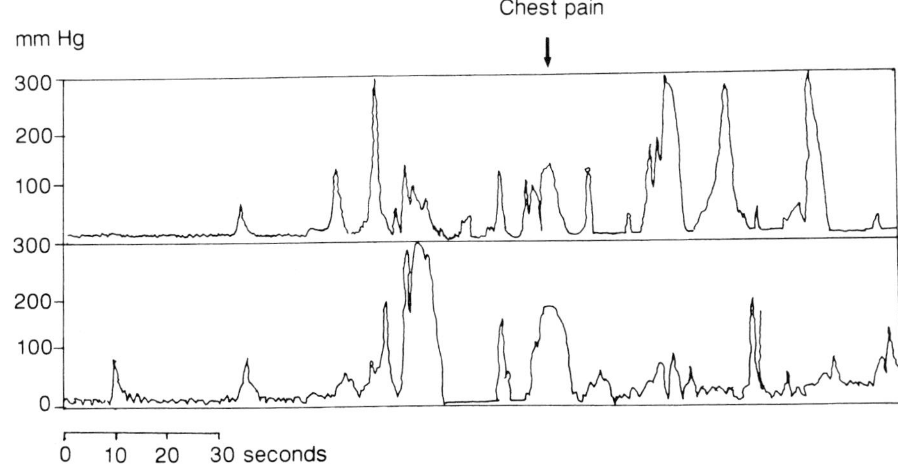

Figure 6–8. Ambulatory motility record of a patient with frequent episodes of noncardiac chest pain. Esophageal motor activity was recorded 10 cm *(top tracing)* and 5 cm *(bottom tracing)* above the lower esophageal sphincter. The patient experienced a spontaneous episode of severe chest pain associated with a high frequency of repetitive and simultaneous contractions in the distal esophagus. (From Stein, H.J., DeMeester, T.R. Eypasch E.P., and Klingman, R.P.: Ambulatory 24-hour esophageal manometry in the evaluation of esophageal motor disorders and noncardiac chest pain. Surgery, *110*:753, 1991, with permission.)

in the distal two thirds of the esophagus. Typical findings on esophageal manometry are normal peristalsis in the proximal striated esophagus, with weak or absent peristalsis in the distal smooth muscle portion. The lower esophageal sphincter pressure is progressively weakened as the disease advances, resulting in increased esophageal exposure to gastric juice due to a mechanically defective lower esophageal sphincter and poor clearance function of the esophageal body.[66]

In patients with polymyositis or dermatomyositis, the upper striated muscle portion is the major site of esophageal involvement, causing aspiration, nasopharyngeal regurgitation, and cervical dysphagia. Mixed connective tissue disease shows a mixture of the manometric findings of progressive systemic sclerosis and polymyositis.

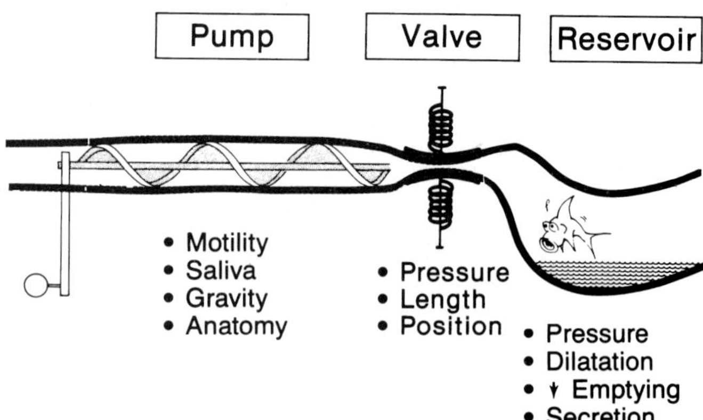

Figure 6–9. Mechanical model of the esophagus as a propulsive pump, the lower esophageal sphincter as a valve, and the stomach as a reservoir. Esophageal clearance of refluxed gastric juice is determined by the esophageal motor activity, salivation, gravity, and the presence of an anatomic alteration such as a hiatal hernia. The competency of the lower esophageal sphincter depends on its pressure, overall length, and length exposed to abdominal pressure. Gastric function abnormalities causing gastroesophageal reflux include increased intragastric pressure, gastric dilatation, decreased emptying rate, and increased gastric acid secretion. (From DeMeester, T.R., and Attwood, S.E.: Gastroesophageal reflux disease, hiatus hernia, achalasia of the esophagus and spontaneous rupture. *In* Schwartz, S.I., and Ellis, H. [eds.]: Maingot's Abdominal Operations, 9th ed. Norwalk, CT, Appleton & Lange, 1989, with permission.)

Gastroesophageal Reflux Disease

GERD is the most common foregut disorder in the Western world and accounts for approximately 75% of esophageal pathology. In about 50% of affected patients, it can lead to complications, such as esophagitis, stricture, ulceration, Barrett's esophagus, repetitive pulmonary aspiration, recurrent pneumonia, and progressive pulmonary fibrosis.[17] Despite its prevalence, GERD can be one of the most challenging diagnostic problems in benign esophageal disease, because symptoms or the finding of endoscopic or histologic esophageal mucosal injury are unreliable in indicating the presence of the disease. With the introduction of 24-hour esophageal pH monitoring, the basic pathophysiologic abnormality of GERD (i.e., increased esophageal exposure to gastric juice) has been quantified.[16,33] This has provided an opportunity to conceptualize the pathophysiology of a complicated disease process, stimulated a rational stepwise approach to determining the cause of increased esophageal exposure to gastric juice, and led to the design of specific therapy to correct the underlying abnormalities.

There are three known causes of increased esophageal exposure to gastric juice. The first is a mechanically defective lower esophageal sphincter. This cause accounts for about 60 to 70% of GERD and is due to inflammatory damage to the sphincter muscle.[67] The identification of this cause is important, because antireflux surgery is the only therapy designed to correct the abnormality. The other two causes are inefficient esophageal clearance of refluxed gastric juice and abnormalities of the gastric reservoir that result in transient loss of the sphincter barrier due to progressive shortening of the sphincter with gastric distention. Conceptually, these three main causes of gastroesophageal reflux can be thought of as abnormalities of a pump, a valve, or a reservoir (Fig. 6–9). The relative contributions of each of these components of the antireflux mechanism to increased esophageal exposure to gastric juice should be determined before the consideration of surgical therapy.

Failure of the lower esophageal sphincter can be caused by inadequate pressure, overall length, or intra-abdominal length (i.e., the portion of the sphincter exposed to the positive pressure environment of the abdomen on manometry). Failure of one or two of the components of the sphincter may be compensated for by the clearance of the esophageal body. Failure of all three sphincter components inevitably leads to increased esophageal exposure to gastric juice. The most common cause of a mechanically defective lower esophageal sphincter is inflammatory loss of myogenic function. This can result in a loss of sphincter pressure, overall length, abdominal length, or a combination. A normal sphincter pressure can be nullified by an inadequate abdominal length or an abnormally short overall length of the sphincter.[67] An adequate abdominal length of sphincter is important in preventing reflux caused by increases in intra-abdominal pressure. An adequate overall length is important in preventing reflux caused by gastric distention such as may occur with a meal.

The combined effects of sphincter pressure, overall length, and abdominal length can be determined by integrating the radial pressures exerted over the entire length of the sphincter. This can be done by calculating the volume of the three-dimensional sphincter pressure profile (i.e., the sphincter pressure vector volume).[7,60] The three-dimensional sphincter pressure profiles of a normal volunteer, a patient with Barrett's esophagus and a defective sphincter, and the same patient after Nissen fundoplication are shown in Figure 6–10.

A second cause of increased esophageal exposure to gastric juice is inefficient esophageal clearance of refluxed material.[27] By the failure to clear physiologic reflux, this can result in abnormal esophageal exposure to gastric juice in individuals who have a mechanically intact lower esophageal sphincter and normal gastric function. This situation is relatively rare, and ineffective clearance is more apt to be seen in association with a mechanically defective sphincter, where it augments the esophageal

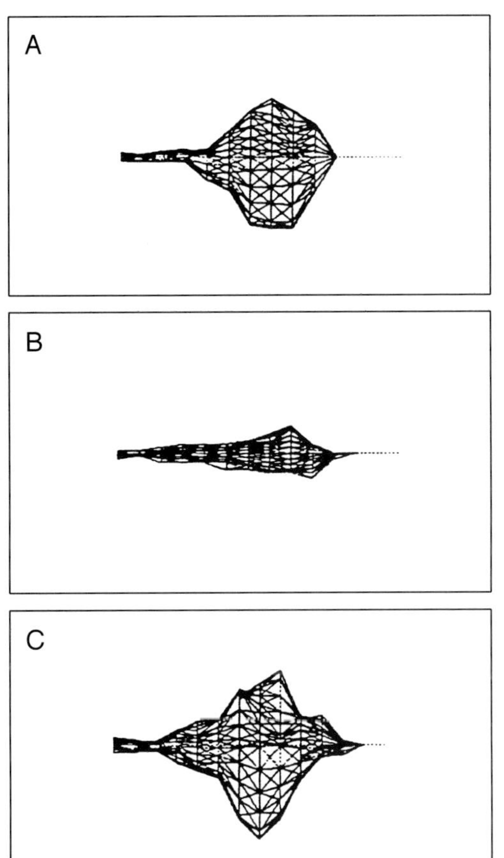

Figure 6–10. The three-dimensional lower esophageal sphincter pressure profile in a normal volunteer *(A)*, a patient with a mechanically defective sphincter *(B)*, and the same patient 1 year after Nissen fundoplication *(C)*. (From Stein, H.J., DeMeester, T.R., Naspetti, R., et al.: The three-dimensional lower esophageal sphincter pressure profile in gastroesophageal reflux disease. Ann. Surg., *214*:374, 1991, with permission.)

exposure to gastric juice by prolonging the duration of each reflux episode. The four factors important in esophageal clearance are gravity, esophageal motor activity, salivation, and anchoring of the distal esophagus in the abdomen. The bulk of refluxed gastric juice is cleared from the esophagus by a primary peristaltic wave initiated by a pharyngeal swallow. Secondary peristalsis initiated by either distention of the lower esophagus or a drop in the intraesophageal pH is less important. Combined videocineradiographic and manometric studies have shown that failure of esophageal clearance can be caused by nonperistaltic esophageal contraction waveform or contractions of low amplitude.[37] Salivation contributes to esophageal clearance by neutralizing the minute amount of acid that is left after a peristaltic wave. The presence of a hiatal hernia can also cause increased acid exposure by reducing the efficiency of esophageal contractions due to the loss of its distal anchor.

Gastric abnormalities that increase esophageal exposure to gastric juice include gastric dilatation, increased intragastric pressure, a persistent gastric reservoir, and increased gastric acid secretion.[17] The effect of gastric dilatation is to shorten the overall length of the lower esophageal sphincter, resulting in a decrease in the sphincter resistance to reflux. Increased intragastric pressures occur in patients with outlet obstruction due to scarred pylorus or duodenum, after vagotomy, or as a result of diabetic neuropathy. The persistence of the gastric reservoir results from delayed gastric emptying secondary to myogenic abnormalities as seen in patients with advanced diabetes, diffuse neuromuscular disorders, and postviral infections. Gastric hypersecretion can increase esophageal exposure to gastric juice by the physiologic reflux of the excessive volume of gastric juice of low pH that occurs in this condition.

The complications of gastroesophageal reflux result from the damage inflicted by gastric juice on the esophageal mucosa or the respiratory epithelium and the changes caused by their subsequent repair and fibrosis. Complications of GERD are classified as esophagitis, stricture, Barrett's esophagus, and pulmonary fibrosis secondary to repetitive aspiration, The presence of the complications of GERD is directly related to the prevalence of a mechanically defective sphincter (Fig. 6–11).[55] This indicates that a mechanically defective sphincter is the major factor in the development of complications of the disease.

The observation that complications of GERD do not always occur in patients with a defective sphincter and can occur in patients with a normal lower esophageal sphincter indicates that the composition of refluxed gastric juice is also an important factor in the pathogenesis of esophageal mucosal injury. Experimental studies have shown that 34% of GERD patients are identified on the basis of reflux of gastric juice with pH less than 4. Nine per cent are identified by the presence of bilirubin in refluxed duodenal juice, and 57% are identified on the basis of reflux of both gastric and duodenal juice; the latter situation causes the most injurious effects of refluxed gastric juice on the esophageal mucosa.[35] Clinical

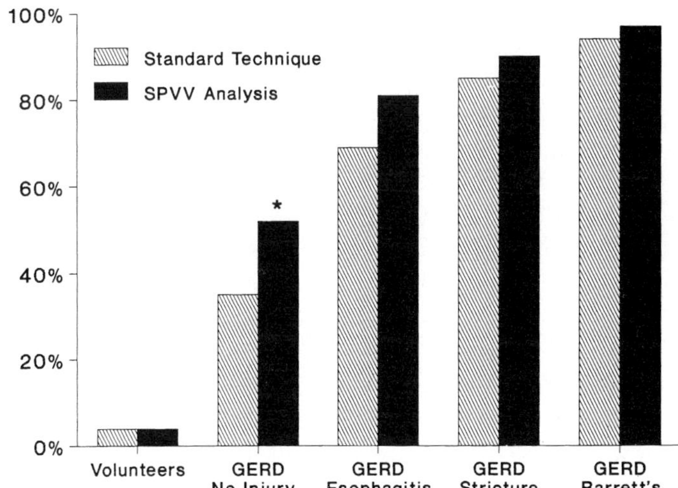

Figure 6–11. Prevalence of a mechanically defective sphincter in patients with increased esophageal exposure to gastric juice and no mucosal injury, esophagitis, stricture, and Barrett's esophagus using standard manometric techniques or analysis of the three-dimensional sphincter image (SPVV analysis). $P<.05$ versus standard technique. (From Stein, H.J., DeMeester, T.R., Naspetti, R., et al.: The three-dimensional lower esophageal sphincter pressure profile in gastroesophageal reflux disease. Ann. Surg., *214*:374, 1991, with permission.)

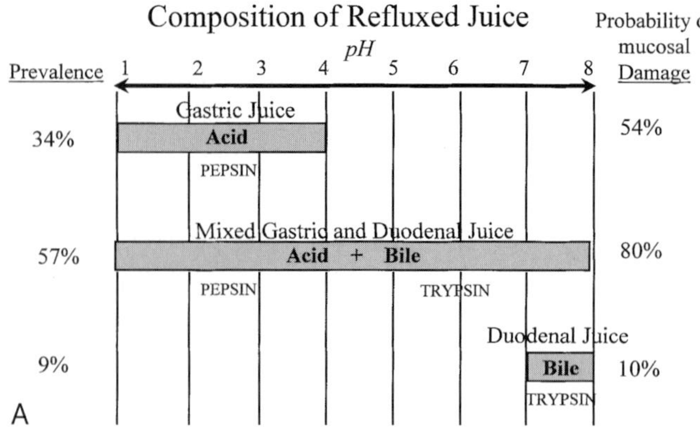

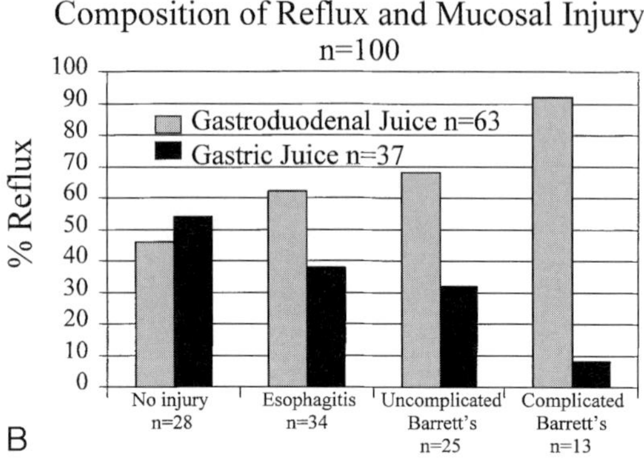

Figure 6–12. *A*, Prevalence of gastric acid reflux, gastroduodenal reflux, and duodenal reflux into the esophagus and the probability of mucosal injury based on the monitoring of 100 consecutive patients with gastroesophageal reflux disease defined by an increased esophageal exposure to acid and/or bilirubin. *B*, Prevalence of reflux of gastric acid juice or gastric acid and duodenal juice in 100 patients with various degrees of esophageal mucosal injury. (From Fein, M., Ireland, A.P., Ritter, M.P., et al.: Duodenogastric reflux potentiates the injurious effects of gastroesophageal reflux. J. Gastrointest Surg., *1*:27, 1997.)

studies confirmed this concept and showed that patients with increased esophageal exposure to gastric juice contaminated with alkaline duodenal contents have a higher prevalence and severity of complications than those who have only increased esophageal acid exposure (Fig. 6–12).[55] Complications of GERD are particularly frequent and severe in patients with a mechanically defective sphincter and the reflux of mixed gastroduodenal juice.

OBJECTIVE ASSESSMENT OF ESOPHAGEAL DISORDERS

A number of tests are available for the diagnosis of esophageal disease, but they vary greatly in reliability and appropriate application. The diagnostic tests may be divided into five broad groups: (1) tests to detect structural abnormalities of the esophagus, (2) tests to detect functional abnormalities of the esophagus, (3) tests to detect increased esophageal exposure to gastric and duodenal juice, (4) tests to provoke esophageal symptoms, and (5) tests of gastroduodenal function as they relate to esophageal disease.

Tests to Detect Structural Abnormalities of the Esophagus

The first diagnostic evaluation in patients with suspected esophageal disease should be a contrast roentgenographic examination of the esophagus with a full assessment of the stomach and duodenum followed by upper gastrointestinal endoscopy with biopsy. Effective roentgenographic evaluation of the esophagus is dependent on the use of a combination of different examining techniques. They are outlined in Chapter 4.

In any patient with dysphagia, endoscopy is indicated even in the face of a normal roentgenographic study. Regardless of the radiologist's interpretation of an abnormal finding, each structural abnormality of the esophagus should be confirmed visually and through a biopsy. Endoscopy and biopsy are also necessary to assess for the presence of complications of GERD (i.e., esophagitis, stricture, and Barrett's esophagus). Fiberoptic endoscopic examination of swallowing (FEES) is another valuable technique to assess pharyngeal sensitivity and swallowing. It provides a clear and direct view of the hypopharynx and larynx. Aspiration or the evidence of aspiration can be directly observed. It allows for the rapid clinical evaluation of patients in nursing homes, outpatient clinics, or intensive care units when videofluoroscopic examination is unavailable or unsuitable. It can evaluate vocal cord movement and the physical appearance of the pharyngeal and laryngeal structures.[41] The success of FEES has led to the development of transnasal and transoral diagnostic endoscopy in unsedated patients using narrow-diameter endoscopes (5.3 mm).[14]

The advance of endoscopic ultrasonography allows improved assessment of the esophageal wall. It is performed with a side-view endoscope with a radial scanning ultrasound probe mounted at its tip. Contact with the esophageal wall is accomplished with a water-filled balloon over the ultrasound probe. This provides a circular ultrasound cross section of the esophageal wall that can be visualized on an image processor. On the ultrasound image, the wall of the esophagus consists of five layers that correspond to the acoustic reflections and the interfaces between them. With this technique, thickening of the wall in the distal esophagus can easily be demonstrated in patients with achalasia and diffuse esophageal spasm. Fibrosis of the wall can be recognized in patients with scleroderma. Intramural tumors not seen on computed tomography or endoscopy can be detected and in some situations may be responsible for an observed motor disorder.[59]

Tests to Detect Functional Esophageal Abnormalities

Many patients with symptoms of an esophageal disorder do not show a structural abnormality on standard roentgenographic and endoscopic evaluation. In these situations, esophageal function tests are necessary to identify a functional disorder. The modern tests to evaluate esophageal function include stationary manometry of the pharyngoesophageal segment, esophageal body, and lower esophageal sphincter; ambulatory 24-hour esophageal motility monitoring; videocineroentgenography; and esophageal transit scintigraphy.

Stationary Esophageal Manometry

Stationary esophageal manometry is a widely used technique to examine the motor function of the esophagus and its sphincters. It is indicated whenever a motor abnormality of the esophagus is suspected on the basis of complaints of dysphagia, odynophagia, or noncardiac chest pain and when the barium swallow or endoscopy does not show a clear structural abnormality.[59] Esophageal manometry is particularly necessary to confirm the diagnosis of specific primary esophageal motility disorders (i.e., achalasia, diffuse esophageal spasm, nutcracker esophagus, and hypertensive lower esophageal sphincter).[65] It also identifies nonspecific esophageal motility abnormalities and esophageal motor disorders secondary to systemic disease, such as scleroderma, dermatomyositis, polymyositis, and mixed connective tissue disease. Stationary manometry is the most accurate method for assessing the function of the lower esophageal sphincter and has been the basis for the identification and classification of the motor disorders of the esophageal body.[12] In patients with disorders of the pharyngoesophageal phase of swallowing, manometry is complementary to and should ideally be performed simultaneously with videocineroentgenography.[11,38] In patients with GERD, manometry of the esophageal body can identify a mechanically defective lower esophageal sphincter as the cause of increased esophageal acid exposure and evaluate the adequacy of esophageal clearance function.[17]

Esophageal manometry is performed using electronic pressure-sensitive transducers located within a catheter or water-perfused catheters with lateral side holes attached to transducers outside the body. The catheter usually consists of a train of five or more pressure transducers or water-perfused tubes bonded together with lateral openings placed at 5-cm intervals from the tip and oriented radially around the circumference. A special catheter assembly consisting of four or eight lateral openings at the same level, oriented radially at 90 or 45 degrees to each other, is useful when constructing a three-dimensional image of the lower esophageal sphincter. Other specially designed catheters are used to assess the upper esophageal sphincter. When water-filled catheters are used, the rate of water infusion must be adjusted to obtain reliable and reproducible pressure tracings. This is best achieved by a low-compliance pneumohydraulic capillary infusion system.[1]

The manometric catheter is passed through the nose and esophagus and into the stomach, and the gastric pressure pattern is confirmed. The catheter is withdrawn across the cardia to identify the high-pressure zone of the lower esophageal sphincter. Although some advocate a steady, rapid withdrawal with the patient holding his or her breath, we have found that a stepwise withdrawal of the catheter at 0.5- or 1.0-cm intervals or a slow motorized pullback at a speed of 1 mm/sec for 60 seconds provides reproducible and more quantitative information and allows the patient to breathe normally during the procedure.[59,67] As the pressure-sensitive station is brought across the gastroesophageal junction, a rise in pressure

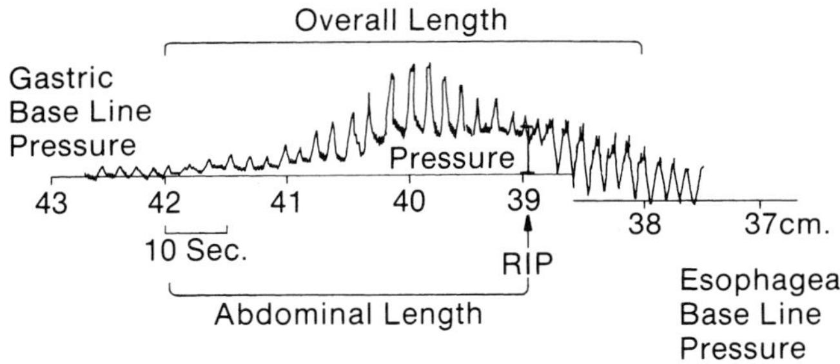

RIP = Respiratory Inversion Point

Figure 6–13. A sample manometric measurement of the lower esophageal sphincter. The distances are measured from the nares. (RIP, respiratory inversion point.) (From Zaninotto, G., DeMeester, T.R., Schwizer, W., et al.: The lower esophageal sphincter in health and disease. Am. J. Surg., *155*:105, 1988, with permission.)

off the gastric baseline identifies the beginning of the lower esophageal sphincter. The respiratory inversion point is identified when the positive excursions that occur with breathing in the abdominal cavity change to negative deflections in the thorax. The respiratory inversion point serves as a reference point at which the amplitude of lower esophageal sphincter pressure and the length of the sphincter exposed to abdominal pressure are measured. As the pressure-sensitive station is withdrawn into the body of the esophagus, the upper border of the lower esophageal sphincter is identified by the drop in pressure to the esophageal baseline. From these measurements, the resting pressure, abdominal length, and overall length of the sphincter are determined (Fig. 6–13). To account for the asymmetry of the sphincter, the pressure profile is repeated as each of the five radially oriented transducers is pulled through the sphincter and the values for sphincter pressure above gastric baseline, overall sphincter length, and abdominal length of the sphincter are averaged. Alternatively, if the pressure-sensitive stations are radially oriented at the same level on the catheters, a single pull-through is all that is necessary.

Table 6–3 shows the values for these parameters in 50 normal volunteers without subjective or objective evi-

Table 6–3. Normal Manometric Values of the Lower Esophageal Sphincter (n = 50)

		Percentile	
	Median	***2.5***	***97.5***
Pressure (mmHg)	13	5.8	27.7
Overall length (cm)	3.6	2.1	5.6
Abdominal length (cm)	2	0.9	4.7
	Mean	***Mean − 2 SD***	***Mean + 2 SD***
Pressure (mmHg)	13.8	4.6	23.0
Overall length (cm)	3.7	2.1	5.3
Abdominal length (cm)	2.2	0.6	3.8

From DeMeester, T.R., and Stein, H.J.: Gastroesophageal reflux disease. *In* Moody, F.G., Jones, R.S., Kelly, K.A., et al.: Surgical Treatment of Digestive Disease, 2nd ed. Chicago, Year Book Medical Publishers, 1989, p. 65, with permission.
SD = standard deviation.

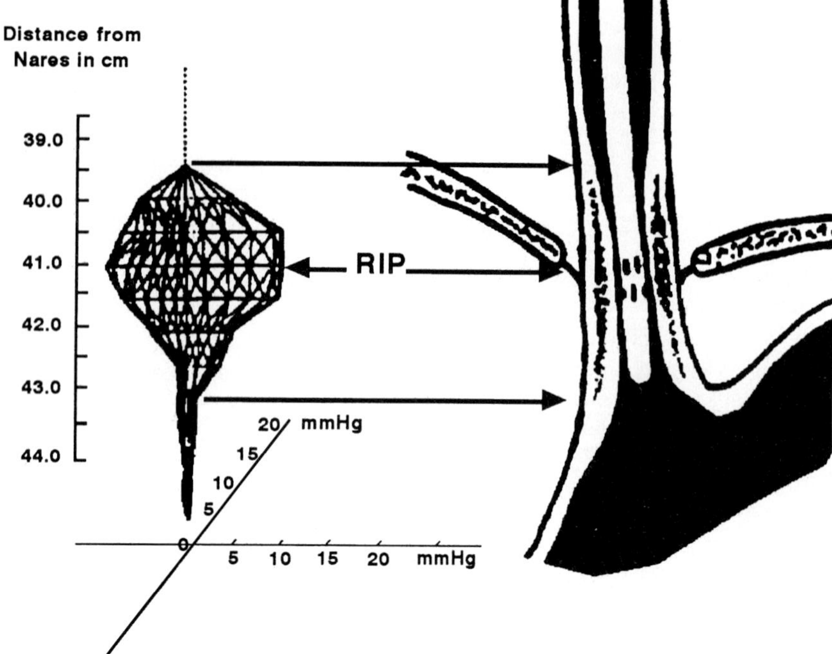

Figure 6–14. Computerized three-dimensional imaging of the lower esophageal sphincter; a catheter with four to eight radial side holes is withdrawn across the gastroesophageal junction. For each level of the pullback, the radially measured pressures are plotted around an axis representing gastric baseline pressure. (From Stein, H.J., DeMeester, T.R., Naspetti, R., et al.: The three-dimensional lower esophageal sphincter pressure profile in gastroesophageal reflux disease. Ann. Surg., *214*:374, 1991, with permission.)

dence of a foregut disorder. The level at which incompetence of the lower esophageal sphincter occurs was defined by comparing the frequency distribution of these values in the 50 healthy volunteers with the values for a population of similarly studied patients with symptoms of GERD.[67] The presence of increased esophageal exposure to gastric juice was documented by 24-hour esophageal pH monitoring. Based on these studies, a mechanically defective sphincter is identified by having one or more of the following characteristics: an average lower esophageal sphincter pressure of less than 6 mm Hg, an average length exposed to the positive pressure environment in the abdomen of 1 cm or less, and an average overall sphincter length of 2 cm or less. Compared with the normal volunteers, these values are below the 2.5 percentile for sphincter pressure, overall length, and the abdominal length.

If manometry of the lower esophageal sphincter is performed with four to eight radially oriented pressure transducers, a three-dimensional image of the sphincter can be constructed by plotting the pressures measured at each station of the pullback radially around an axis representing gastric baseline (Fig. 6–14).[7,60] For visual purposes, the three-dimensional reconstruction of the sphincter pressure image can be enhanced by applying a cubic curve-smoothing interpolation, which retains the original points while adding intermediate ones to give a smoother surface to the three-dimensional sphincter image and to improve its readability. Commercially available computer programs enable the creation of three-dimensional sphincter images that can be rotated on a computer screen. This allows inspection of the sphincter image for asymmetry (Fig. 6–15).

The volume circumscribed by the three-dimensional sphincter image integrates pressures exerted over the entire length and around the circumference of the sphincter into one value that represents sphincter resistance to reflux of gastric contents. This has been termed the *sphincter pressure vector volume*. The sphincter pressure vector volume can be calculated using standard trigonometric formulas. Validation studies and application of this

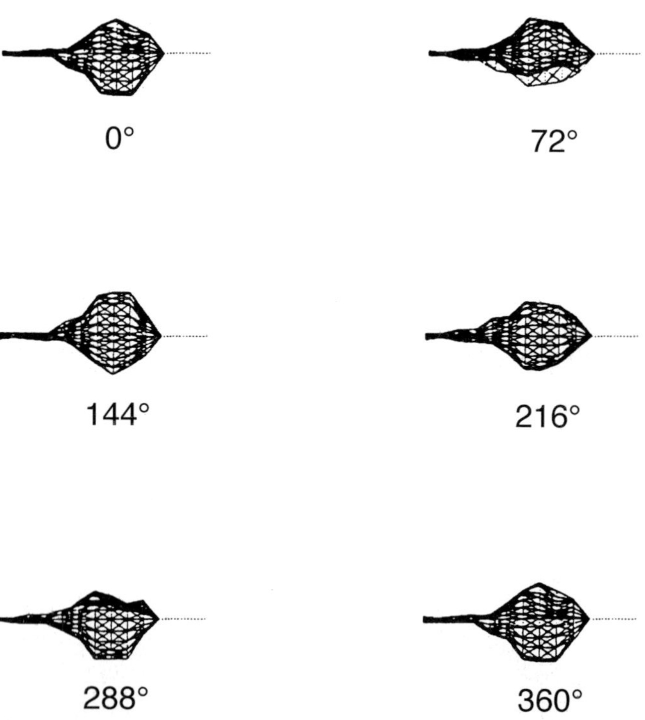

Figure 6–15. The three-dimensional sphincter pressure image of a normal volunteer shown from various angles. This is achieved by rotating the image around an axis representing gastric baseline. Note the marked asymmetry of the sphincter. (From Stein, H.J., DeMeester, T.R., Naspetti, R., et al.: The three-dimensional lower esophageal sphincter pressure profile in gastroesophageal reflux disease. Ann. Surg., *214*:374, 1991, with permission.)

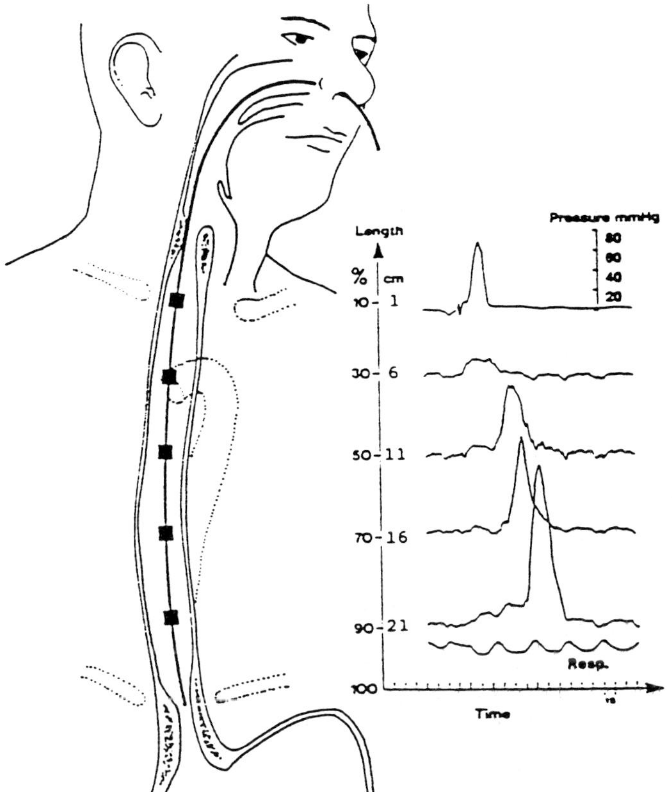

Figure 6–16. Schematic drawing showing the placement of the transducers for standard manometry and the pressure response throughout the esophageal body. (From Stein, H.J., DeMeester, T.R., and Hinder, R.A.: Outpatient physiologic testing and surgical management of foregut motility disorders. Curr. Probl. Surg., *29*:415, 1992, with permission.)

technique in a large number of patients with GERD have shown that calculation of the sphincter pressure vector volume is superior to standard techniques in assessing sphincter resistance to reflux of gastric juice (see Fig. 6–11).[60] This is particularly so in patients with increased esophageal acid exposure but no mucosal injury and in patients with borderline sphincter abnormalities.

To assess the relaxation and postrelaxation contraction of the lower esophageal sphincter, a pressure transducer is positioned within the high-pressure zone, with a distal transducer located in the stomach and the proximal transducer within the esophageal body. Ten wet swallows with 5 ml water are performed. The pressure of the lower esophageal sphincter should drop to the level of gastric pressure during each wet swallow. The function of the esophageal body is assessed with three to five pressure transducers located at various levels in the esophagus. To standardize the procedure, the most proximal pressure transducer is placed 1 cm below the well-defined cricopharyngeal sphincter, with the distal orifices trailing at 5-cm intervals over the entire length of the esophagus. With this method, a pressure response throughout the whole esophagus can be obtained on swallowing (Fig. 6–16). The response to 10 wet swallows with 5 ml room temperature water is recorded. Amplitude, duration, and morphology of contractions (i.e., number of peaks and repetitive activity) after each swallow are calculated at all recorded levels of the esophageal body. The delay between the esophageal contractions at the various levels of the esophagus is used to calculate the speed of wave propagation and to classify contractions as peristaltic, simultaneous, or not transmitted. Based on this information, motor disorders of the esophagus are identified and classified (see Table 6–2). Typical manometric tracings of a patient with nutcracker esophagus, diffuse esophageal spasm, and achalasia are shown in Figures 6–17 through 6–19. Display of a patient's values at the various levels of the esophagus against a background of normal values can make abnormalities more apparent[59] (Fig. 6–20).

Due to the rapidity of events during the pharyngeal phase of swallowing, manometry in patients with suspected cricopharyngeal dysfunction should be performed with specially designed catheters. Both water-perfused and electronic systems have been used. Some advocate that electronic pressure-sensitive transducers are superior because they have a much higher frequency response than water-perfused catheters and avoid the pharyngeal irritation that occurs with a water-perfused system.[11] The position, length, and pressure of the cricopharyngeal sphincter are assessed with a stationary pull-through technique. The manometry catheter is withdrawn in 0.5-cm intervals from the upper esophagus through the upper esophageal sphincter region into the pharynx. To ac-

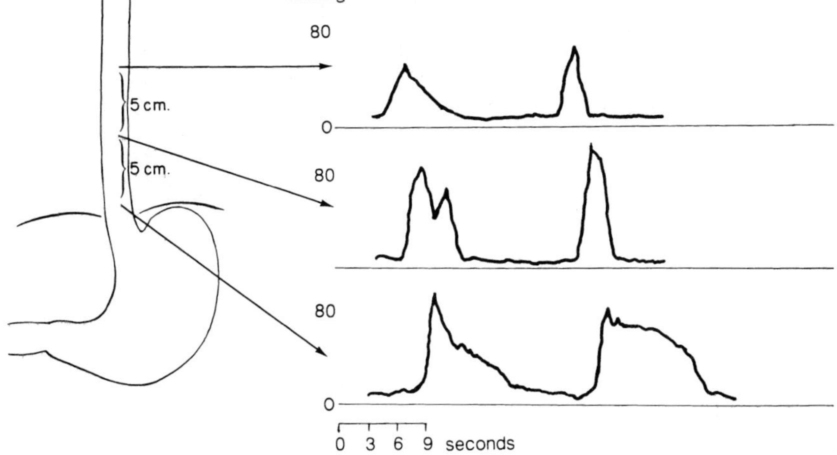

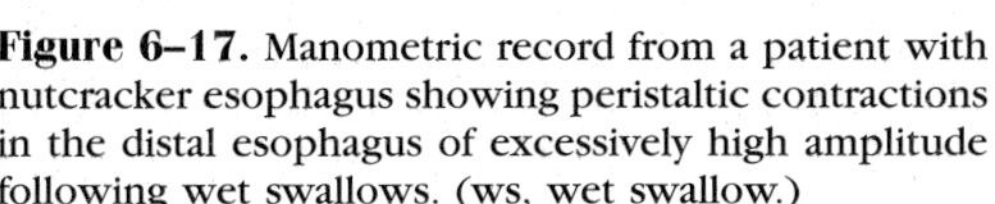

Figure 6–17. Manometric record from a patient with nutcracker esophagus showing peristaltic contractions in the distal esophagus of excessively high amplitude following wet swallows. (ws, wet swallow.)

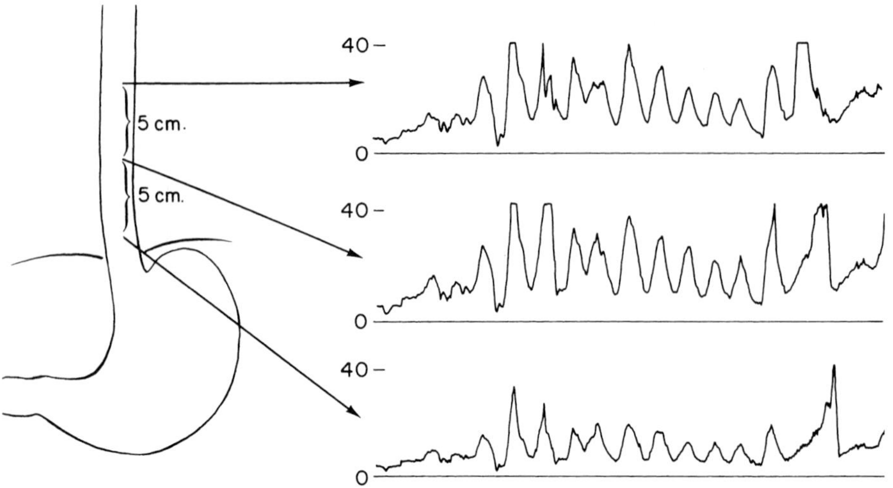

Figure 6–18. Manometric record from a patient with diffuse esophageal spasm showing repetitive, simultaneous contractions in the body of the esophagus over a length of 10 cm. (From Waters, P.F., and DeMeester, T.R.: Foregut motor disorders and their surgical management. Med. Clin. North Am., *65:*1248, 1981, with permission.)

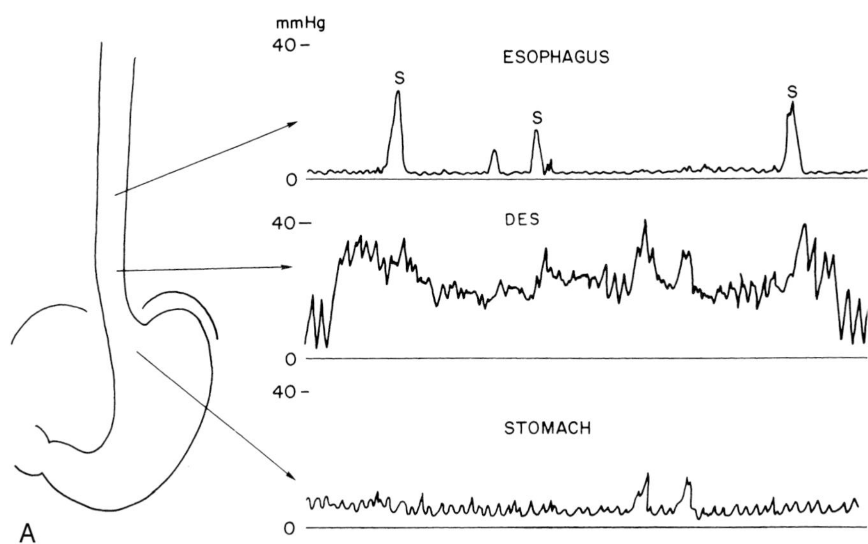

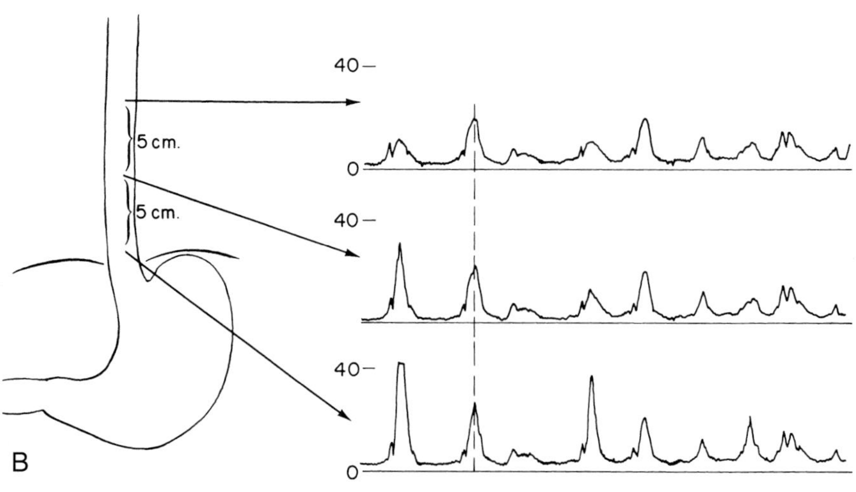

Figure 6–19. Manometric record from a patient with achalasia. *A*, failure of the distal esophageal sphincter (DES) to relax on swallows (S). *B*, aperistalsis in the body of the esophagus. Swallows are followed only by tertiary contractions. (From Waters, P.F., and DeMeester, T.R.: Foregut motor disorders and their surgical management. Med. Clin. North Am., *65:*1245, 1981, with permission.)

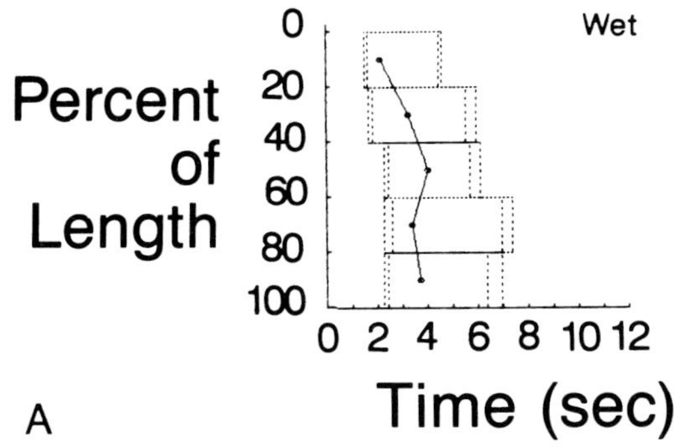

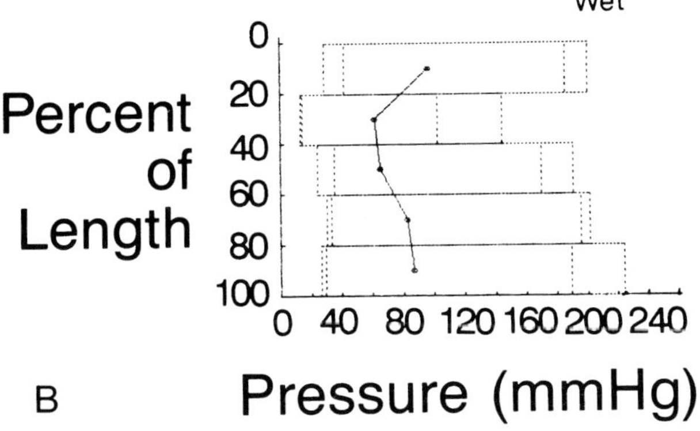

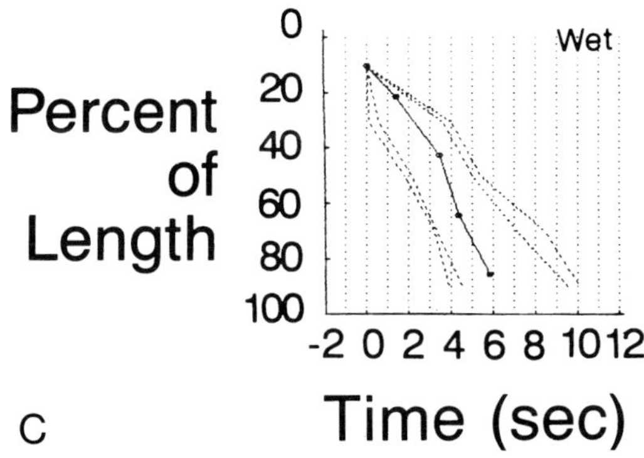

Figure 6–20. Graphic display of esophageal contraction characteristics at five levels of the esophagus (wet swallows). Patient values *(solid line)* are displayed against a background of normal values obtained in 60 asymptomatic volunteers *(broken lines:* fifth, tenth, ninetieth, and ninety-fifth percentiles). *A*, Duration of esophageal contractions. *B*, Amplitude of esophageal contractions. *C*, Wave progression.

count for the anatomic asymmetry of the upper esophageal sphincter (Fig. 6–21), five measurements with the pressure transducers oriented in various directions are made, and an average is calculated. A dedicated water-perfused catheter consisting of eight lateral ports located at 0.5-cm intervals is of special use to evaluate abnormalities of sphincter opening and to detect evidence of increased outflow resistance through the pharyngoesophageal segment. The opening of the upper esophageal sphincter is studied by placing one of the middle eight lateral pressure ports at the upper border of the cricopharyngeal sphincter while the other ports straddle the hypopharynx and upper esophagus (Fig. 6–22).[11] High-speed graphic recordings (50 mm/sec) are necessary to obtain an assessment of the coordination of cricopharyngeal relaxation with hypopharyngeal contraction. Carefully performed motility studies may demonstrate impaired sphincter opening, insufficient relaxation (Fig. 6–23) or premature contractions of the cricopharyngeus (Fig. 6–24), high sphincter pressure, or inadequate pharyngeal pressurization (Fig. 6–25). A decreased compliance of the upper esophageal sphincter caused by a restrictive myopathy can be recognized manometrically by the observation of a shoulder on the hypopharyngeal pressure wave (see Fig. 6–5). The size of this shoulder correlates directly with the degree of outflow obstruction. The sensitivity of manometry to detect abnormalities in pharyngoesophageal function is further increased by simultaneous videocineradiography.[13,38]

It should be remembered that all recorded manometric pressures are affected by variables such as age of the patient, posture, bolus characteristics, catheter diameter, swallowing frequency, and compliance of the perfusion system.[43] Because these parameters are not necessarily standardized, they must be controlled within an individual laboratory. Each laboratory should define normal values from volunteers who have no subjective or objective evidence of a foregut disorder; alternatively, one laboratory may adopt the normal values of another laboratory, provided identical procedures and equipment are used.

Ambulatory 24-Hour Esophageal Manometry

The intermittent and unpredictable occurrence of motor abnormalities and symptoms in patients with esophageal motility disorders limits the diagnostic value of stationary motility performed in a laboratory setting and consisting of 10 swallows over a short time period. The technique of ambulatory esophageal manometry was developed to overcome these shortcomings by monitoring esophageal motor activity over a prolonged period during a variety of physiologic activities and correlating esophageal motor abnormalities with spontaneously occurring symptoms.[22,32,48]

Due to the high sampling frequency required to evaluate esophageal motor activity, prolonged outpatient monitoring of esophageal motility became available only after the introduction of portable digital data recorders with large storage capacity. Today, ambulatory esophageal motility monitoring allows the evaluation of esophageal motor function based on more than 1,000 contractions recorded over an entire circadian cycle under a variety of physiologic conditions (i.e., upright activity, eating, and sleeping (Fig. 6–26). This provides a more than 100-fold larger database for the assessment of esophageal motor function than standard manometry.[57]

Ambulatory esophageal motility monitoring is usually performed using a catheter with three or more electronic pressure transducers placed in 5-cm intervals above the upper border of the manometrically determined lower esophageal sphincter (Fig. 6–27). The transducers are connected to a portable digital data recorder with sufficient memory to store pressure recordings from each channel over an entire circadian cycle. After placement

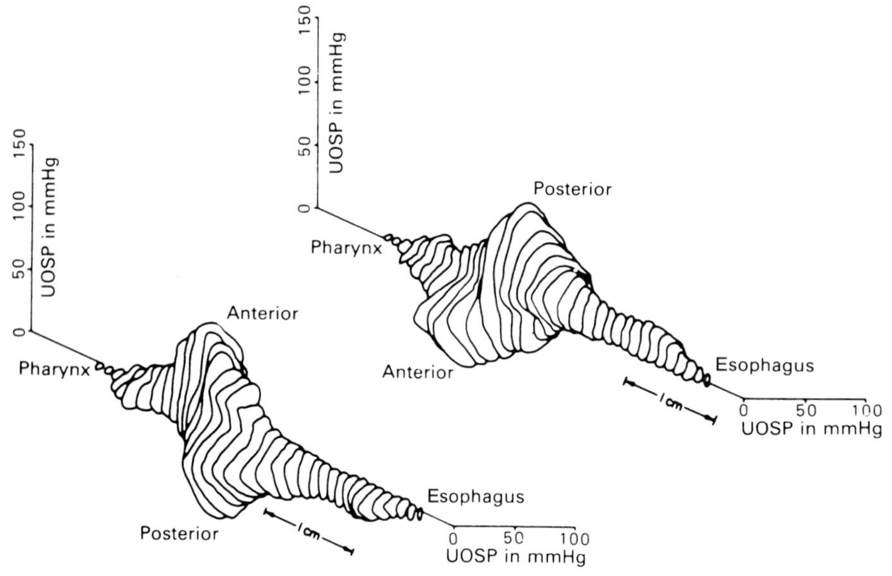

Figure 6–21. Three-dimensional pressure profile of the upper esophageal sphincter, illustrating the short axial zone of maximal pressure and the marked radial asymmetry. (UOSP, upper esophageal sphincter pressure.) (From Welch, R.W., et al.: Manometry of the normal upper esophageal sphincter and its alteration of laryngectomy. J. Clin. Invest, *63*:1039, 1979, with permission.)

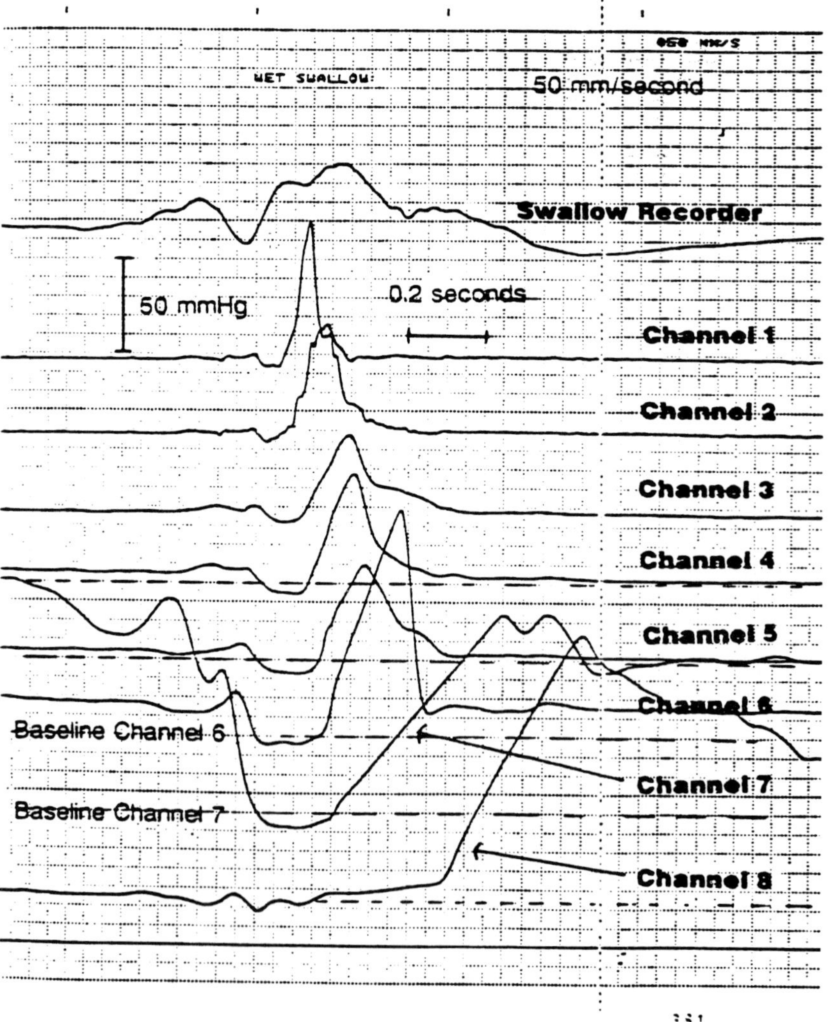

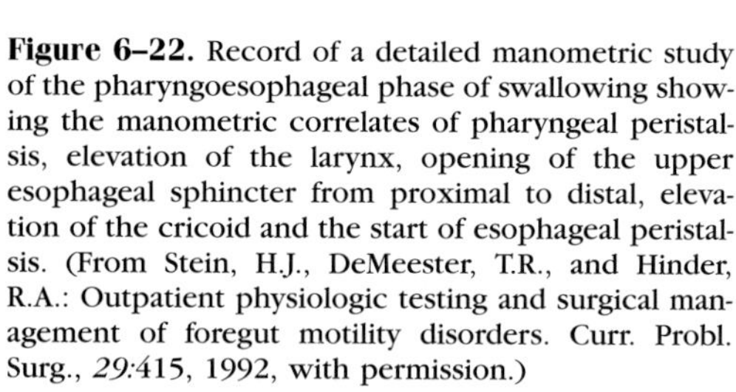

Figure 6–22. Record of a detailed manometric study of the pharyngoesophageal phase of swallowing showing the manometric correlates of pharyngeal peristalsis, elevation of the larynx, opening of the upper esophageal sphincter from proximal to distal, elevation of the cricoid and the start of esophageal peristalsis. (From Stein, H.J., DeMeester, T.R., and Hinder, R.A.: Outpatient physiologic testing and surgical management of foregut motility disorders. Curr. Probl. Surg., *29*:415, 1992, with permission.)

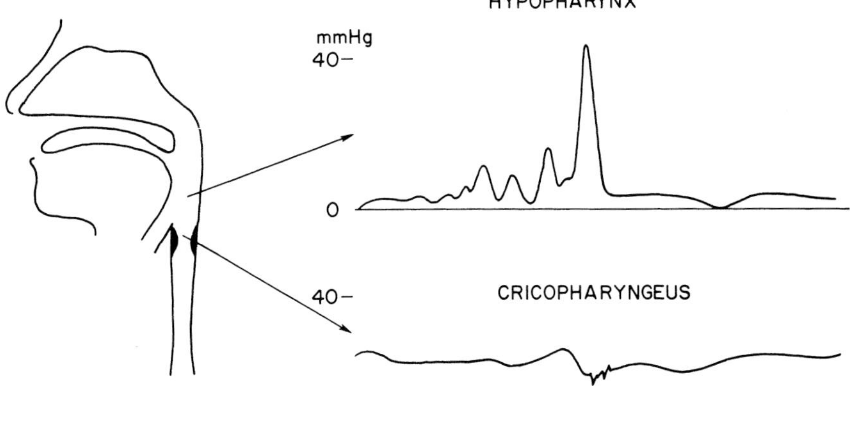

Figure 6–23. Manometric record showing absence of cricopharyngeal (upper esophageal) sphincter relaxation in response to pharyngeal contraction. (From Waters, P.F., and DeMeester, T.R.: Foregut motor disorders and their surgical management. Med. Clin. North Am., *65:*1259, 1981, with permission.)

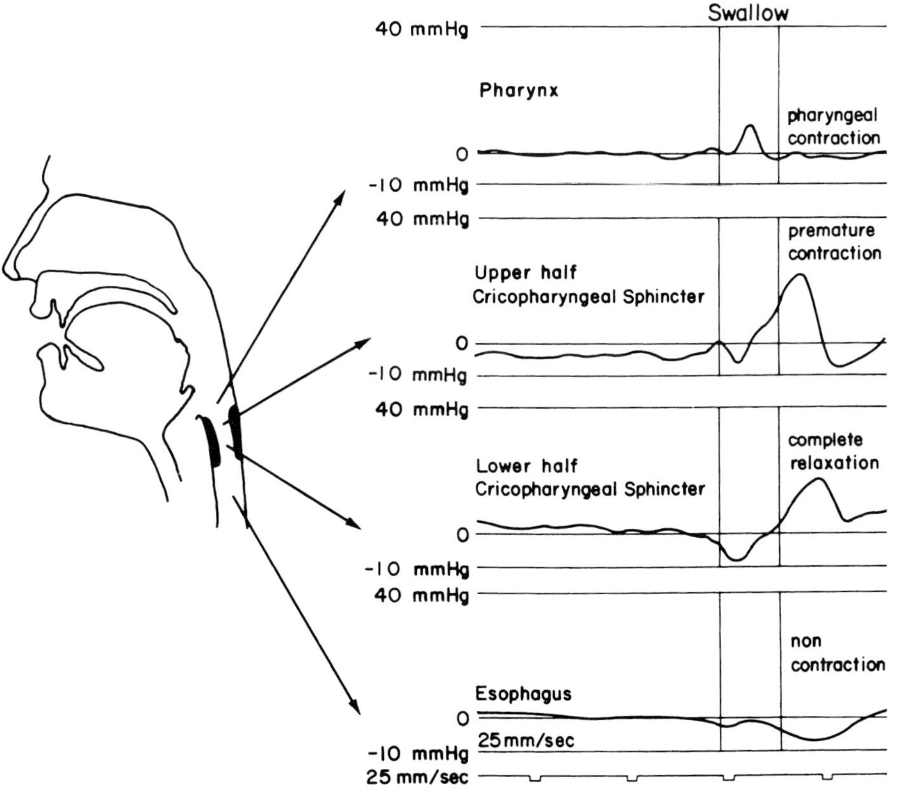

Figure 6–24. Manometric record showing premature contraction of the upper portion of the cricopharyngeal (upper esophageal) sphincter during pharyngeal contraction. No initiation of peristalsis is seen in the cervical esophagus. (From Waters, P.F., and DeMeester, T.R.: Foregut motor disorders and their surgical management. Med. Clin. North Am., *65:*1258, 1981, with permission.)

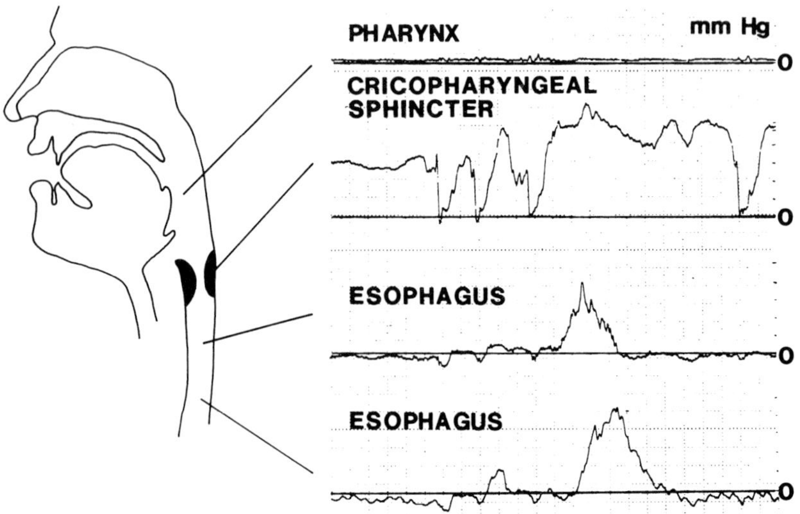

Figure 6–25. Manometric record showing absence of a pharyngeal pressure wave. Cricopharyngeal (upper esophageal) sphincter relaxation is normal and initiates cervical esophageal pressure waves. (From Bonavina, L., Khan, N.A., and DeMeester, T.R.: Pharyngoesophageal dysfunction. Arch. Surg., *20*:546, 1985, with permission.)

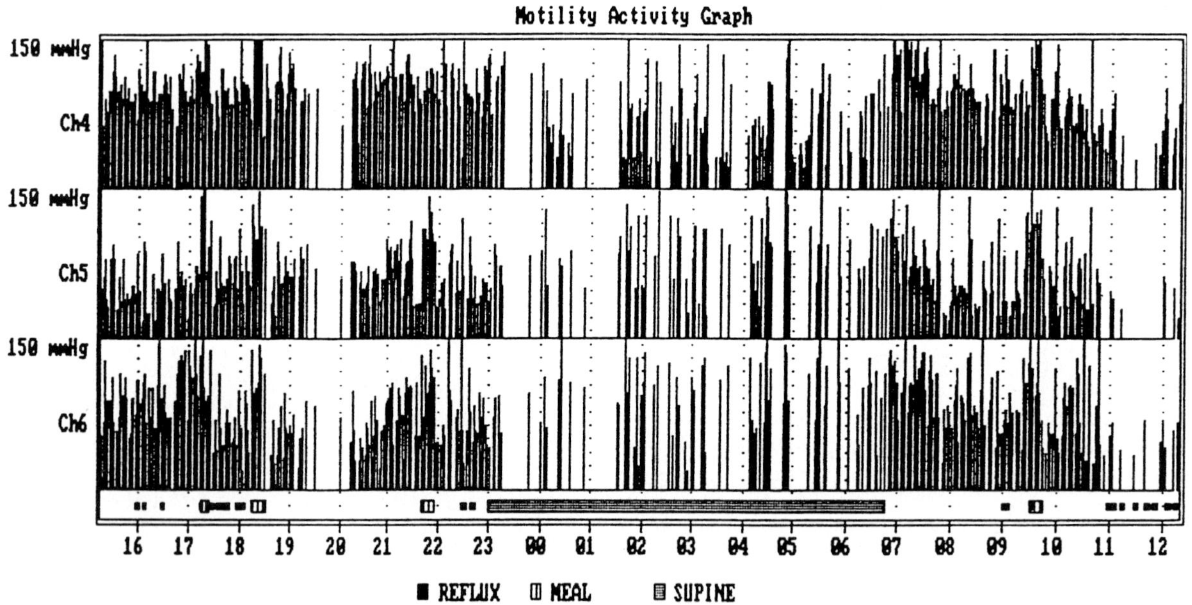

Figure 6–26. A condensed three-channel circadian esophageal motility tracing. Recording was started at 15:00 hours and terminated at 12:30 hours the next day. Time is shown on the X-axis. The three transducers were located 15 cm *(top tracing)*, 10 cm *(middle tracing)*, and 5 cm *(bottom tracing)* above the lower esophageal sphincter. Meal periods, the nighttime sleeping period, and reflux episodes are indicated at the bottom. Each recorded contraction is shown as a vertical line whose height reflects contraction amplitude. The circadian variability of esophageal motor activity can easily be recognized.

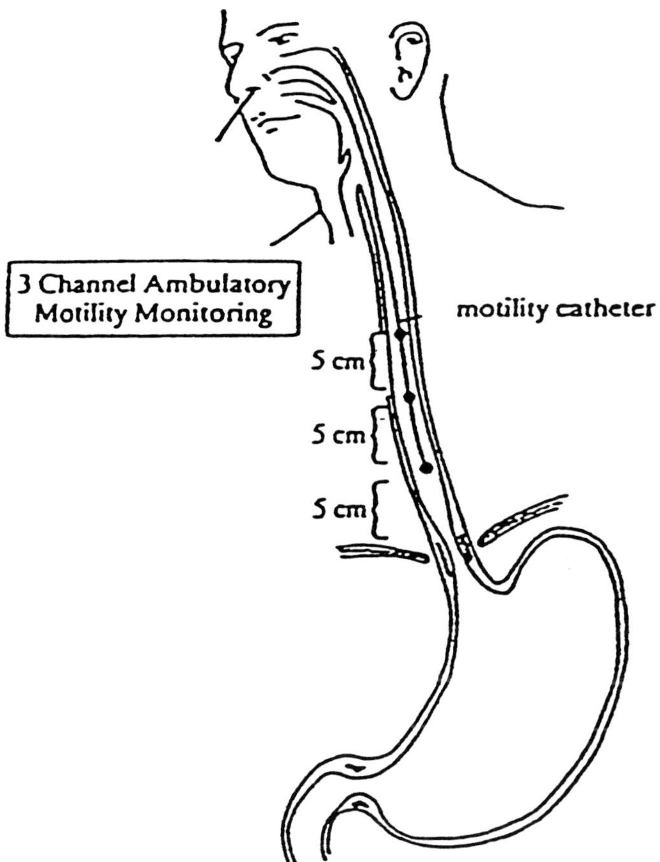

Figure 6–27. Placement of the electronic pressure transducers for ambulatory 24-hour esophageal motility monitoring. (From Stein, H.J., and DeMeester, T.R.: Indications, technique, and clinical use of ambulatory 24-hour esophageal motility monitoring in a surgical practice. Ann. Surg., *217*:128, 1993, with permission.)

of the transducers, the individuals are sent home and instructed to keep a diary for the next 24 hours, indicating when they retired for the night and awoke in the morning, when they ate their meals, and whenever a symptom occurred. The subjects are encouraged to perform normal daily activity during the study and to press an event marker when a spontaneous symptom occurs. After the 24-hour period, the subjects return to the laboratory where the pressure transducers are removed, and the data recorder is unloaded onto a personal computer. Data analysis is usually performed separately for the upright, supine, meal, and symptomatic periods with a computer program. This approach allows quantification of abnormal esophageal motor events and direct correlation of spontaneously occurring symptoms with motor abnormalities.

After its clinical introduction in 1985, ambulatory esophageal motility monitoring has been used primarily to identify esophageal motor abnormalities as the cause of noncardiac chest pain.[32,48] Recent studies in a larger number of unselected patients have uncovered that many patients do not experience these typical symptoms during the 24-hour monitoring period.[54,58] Even when a spontaneous episode of chest pain occurred during the monitored period, motor abnormalities associated with the symptoms were rare and gastroesophageal reflux was found to be a far more frequent cause of noncardiac chest pain than esophageal motor disorders. Consequently, ambulatory manometry in this situation should be performed simultaneously with esophageal pH monitoring and should be reserved for patients with daily symptoms.

Due to the enlarged database and the more physiologic conditions under which data are acquired, ambulatory manometry is superior to standard manometry in the evaluation of esophageal body function in patients with symptoms suggestive of a primary or secondary esophageal motor disorder.[57] The circadian motor pattern can be graphically displayed by showing the prevalence of peristaltic, simultaneous, and mixed contraction sequences (Fig. 6–28). The efficacy of esophageal motor activity can be shown graphically by plotting the prevalence of peristaltic contractions with sufficient amplitude to propel a bolus and clear refluxed gastric contents during the various monitoring periods (Fig. 6–29). Less than 50% of effective contractions during meals on ambulatory esophageal motility monitoring indicate the presence of a severe esophageal motor abnormality (see Fig. 6–7). Our experience with more than 300 ambulatory esophageal motility recordings in patients with esophageal motor disorder shows that this approach allows quantification of the severity of a motor disorder and objective assessment of the effects of medical or surgical therapy.[57]

Videocineroentgenography

High-speed cinerecording or videotaping of roentgenographic pharyngoesophageal contrast studies allows reevaluation of individual swallows through review of the study at various speeds. The study is very useful in the evaluation of the pharyngeal phase of swallowing. Observations that suggest oropharyngeal or cricopharyngeal dysfunction include misdirection of barium into the trachea or nasopharynx, prominence of the cricopharyngeal muscle (i.e., cricopharyngeal bar [Fig. 6–30]), a Zenker's diverticulum (Fig. 6–31), a narrow pharyngoesophageal segment, and stasis of the contrast medium in the valleculae or hypopharyngeal recesses (Fig. 6–32).[20] These findings are usually not specific but are common manifestations of neuromuscular disorders that affect the pharyngoesophageal area. Studies using liquid barium, barium-impregnated solids, or radiopaque pills greatly aid in the evaluation of normal and abnormal motility in the esophageal body. Loss of the normal stripping wave or segmentation of the barium column with the patient in the recumbent position can be correlates with reduced contraction amplitude or abnormal waveforms in the esophageal body on manometry (Fig. 6–33).[37,46] In addition, subtle structural abnormalities such as small diverticula, webs, and extrinsic impressions of the esophagus may be recognized only with motion-recording techniques.

Esophageal Transit Scintigraphy

Esophageal transit scintigraphy is another technique for the evaluation of esophageal function.[64] The esophageal

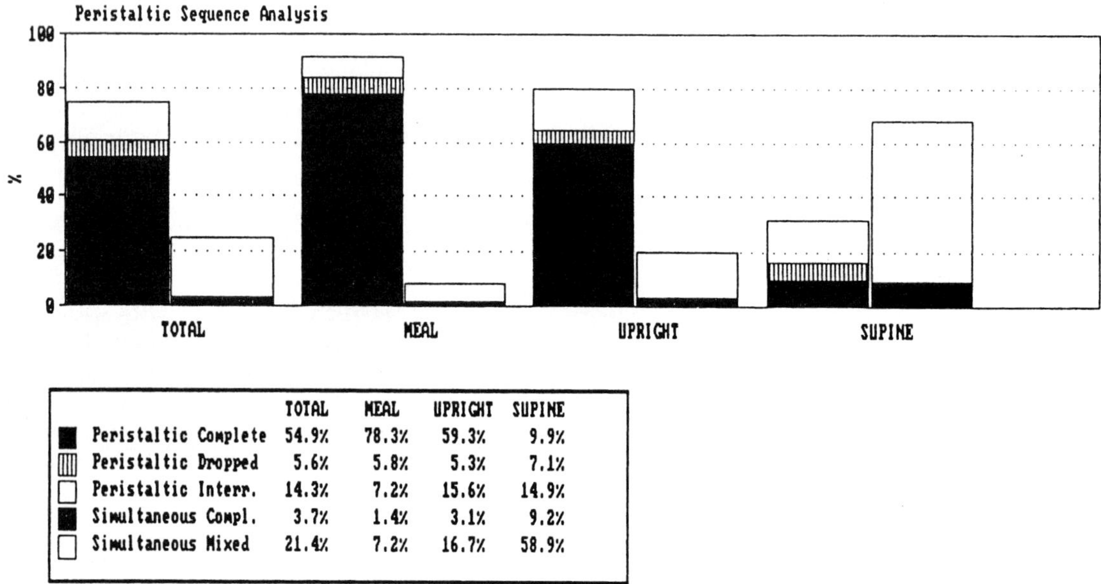

Figure 6–28. Peristaltic sequence analysis of the circadian esophageal motility record shown in Figure 6-26. The prevalence of peristaltic, simultaneous, and mixed contraction sequences during the various monitoring periods is shown.

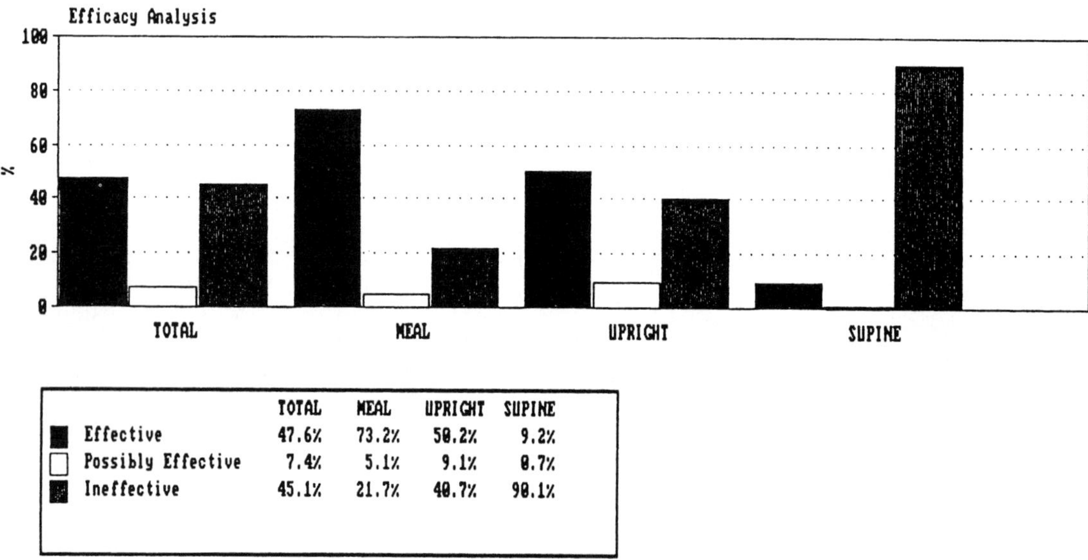

Figure 6–29. Efficacy analysis of the circadian esophageal motility record shown in Figure 6-26. The prevalence of efficient contractions (i.e., peristaltic contractions with sufficient amplitude to propel a bolus) during the various monitoring periods is shown.

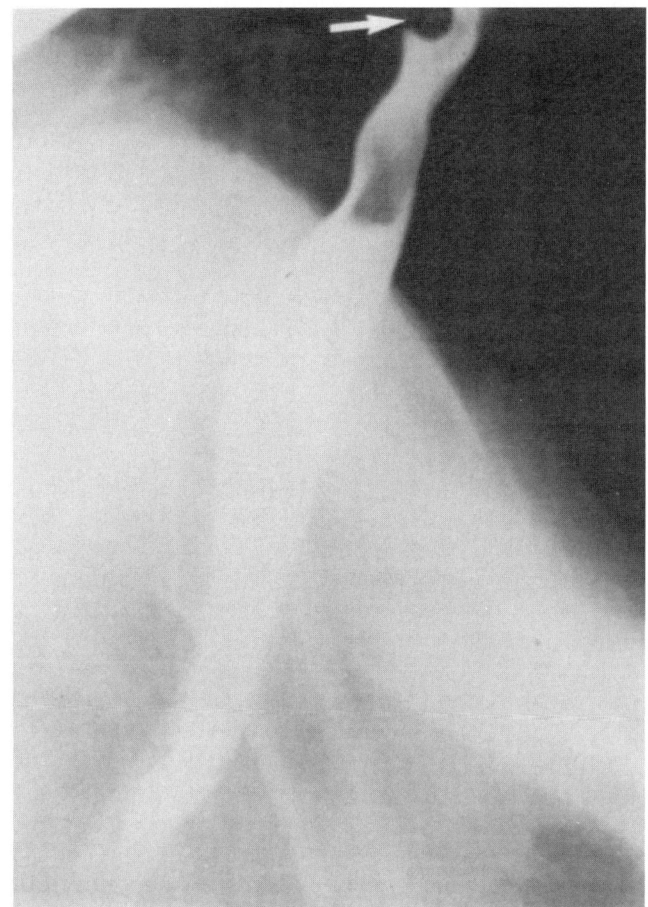

Figure 6–30. Barium contrast roentgenogram of pharyngeal swallowing activity showing a prominent cricopharyngeal indentation *(arrow)* in a patient who presented with dysphagia resulting from bulbar poliomyelitis. (From Bonavina, L., Khan, N.A., and DeMeester, T.R.: Pharyngoesophageal dysfunctions. Arch. Surg., *120:*543, 1985, with permission.)

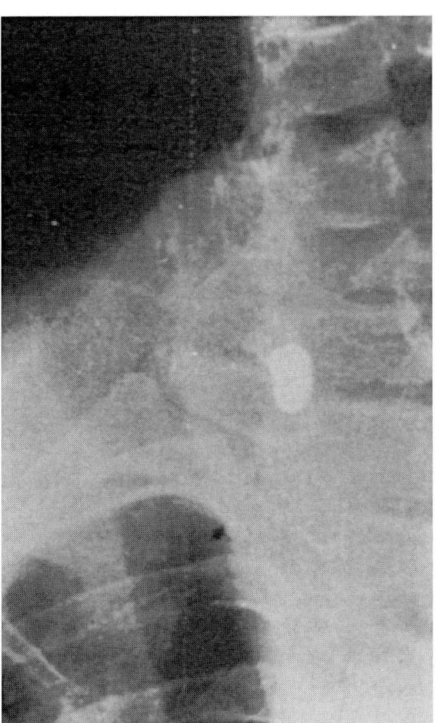

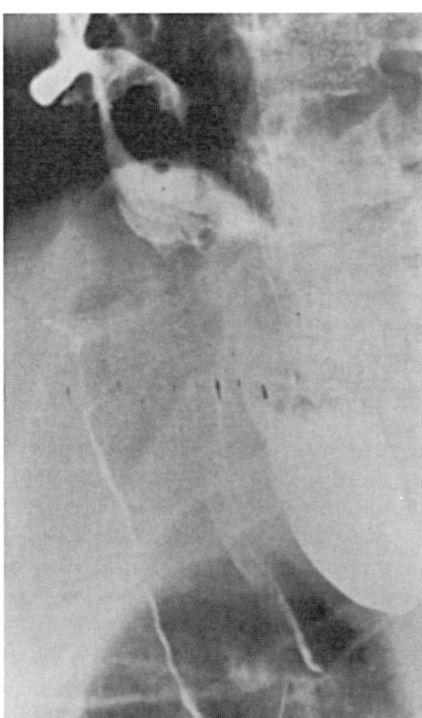

Figure 6–31. *Left*, Zenker's diverticulum, initially discovered 15 years ago and left untreated. *Right*, Note its marked enlargement and evidence of laryngeal inlet aspiration on recent esophagogram. (From Waters, P.F., and DeMeester, T.R.: Foregut motor disorders and their surgical management. Med. Clin. North Am., *65:*1257, 1981, with permission.)

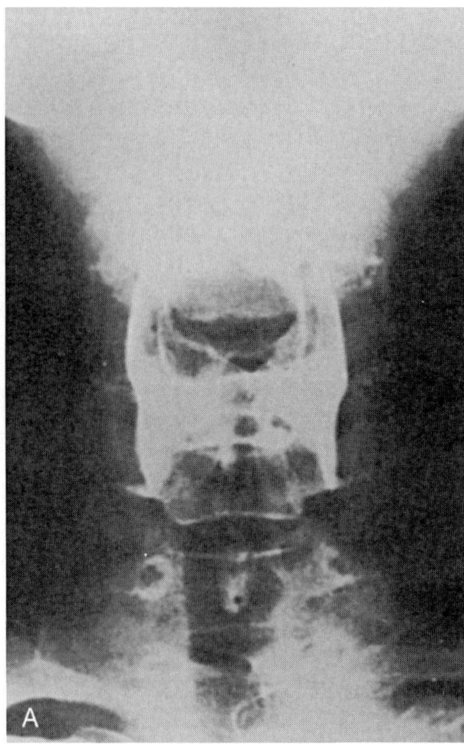

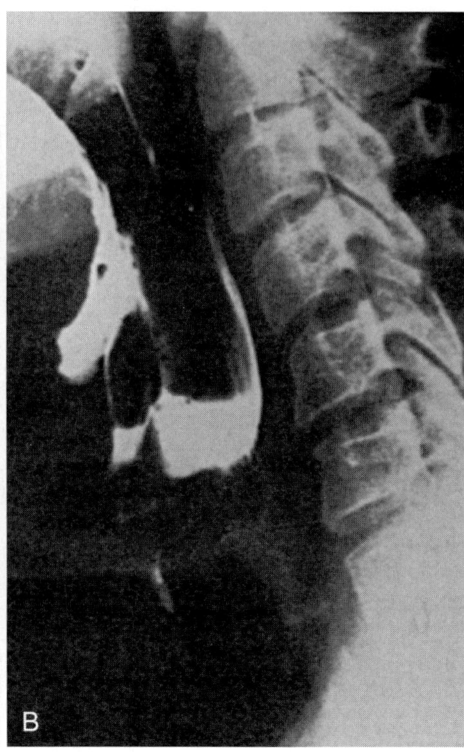

Figure 6–32. Esophagogram from a patient with cricopharyngeal achalasia. *A*, Anteroposterior film showing retention of the contrast medium at the level of the vallecula and piriform recesses, with no barium passing into the esophagus. *B*, Lateral film, taken opposite the C5–C6 vertebrae, showing posterior indentation of the cricopharyngeus, retention in the hypopharynx, and tracheal aspiration. (From Lafontaine, E.: Pharyngeal dysphagia. *In* DeMeester, T.R. and Matthews, H. [eds.]: International Trends in General Thoracic Surgery, Vol. 3, Benign Esophageal Disease. St. Louis, C.V. Mosby, 1987, p. 345, with permission.)

transit of a 10-ml water bolus containing sulfur colloid is recorded with a gamma camera. The transit time is measured separately in the proximal and distal esophagus. With this technique, delayed bolus transit can be shown in patients with a variety of esophageal motor disorders, including achalasia, scleroderma, diffuse esophageal spasm, nutcracker esophagus, and nonspecific motor disorders. It appears that transit scintigraphy is a reliable technique to quantify and document esophageal transit abnormalities.[51] However, the test lacks specificity, because it cannot define the precise nature of a swallowing abnormality. Its best use is to quantify the effect of an esophageal motor abnormality by measuring esophageal emptying time,

Tests to Detect Increased Esophageal Exposure to Gastric Juice

Before any rational therapy for GERD, the presence of increased esophageal exposure to gastric juice has to be confirmed objectively. Extensive clinical experience has shown that 24-hour esophageal pH monitoring has the highest sensitivity and specificity for the detection of acid GERD (Fig. 6–34). In patients in whom the refluxed gastric juice has a high probability of being contaminated with duodenal juice, combined gastric and esophageal pH monitoring or esophageal aspiration and direct analysis of the refluxed gastric juice may be helpful. The standard acid reflux test is useful in patients with previous gastric resection or achlorhydria or if the results of pH monitoring equivocate due to the prolonged action of antisecretory agents such as omeprazole. The diagnosis of gastroesophageal reflux by radiographic or scintigraphic methods lacks sensitivity.

24-Hour Esophageal pH Monitoring

The most direct method of measuring increased esophageal exposure to gastric juice is 24-hour monitoring of esophageal luminal pH with an indwelling pH probe placed 5 cm above the upper border of the lower esophageal sphincter. It quantifies the actual time the esophageal mucosa is exposed to acid gastric juice, measures the ability of the esophagus to clear refluxed acid, and correlates esophageal acid exposure to the patient's symptoms. A 24-hour monitoring period is necessary so that measurements are made over one complete circadian cycle.[18] This allows for assessment of the effect of physiologic activity such as eating or sleeping on the reflux of gastric juice into the esophagus (Fig. 6–35).

It is important to emphasize that 24-hour esophageal pH monitoring is not a test for reflux but rather a measurement of the esophageal exposure to gastric juice. The measurement is expressed in the time the esophageal pH is below a given threshold during the 24-hour period. This single assessment, although concise, does not reflect how the exposure has occurred; that is, did it occur in a few long episodes or several short episodes? Consequently, two other assessments are necessary: the frequency of the reflux episodes and their duration.

The units used to express esophageal exposure to gastric juice are (1) cumulative time the esophageal pH is below a chosen threshold (expressed as per cent of the total, upright, and supine monitored time), (2) frequency of reflux episodes below a chosen threshold (expressed as number of episodes per 24 hours), and (3) duration of the episodes (expressed as the number of episodes longer than 5 minutes per 24 hours and the time [in minutes] of the longest recorded episode).[18] Table 6–4 shows the normal values for these six compo-

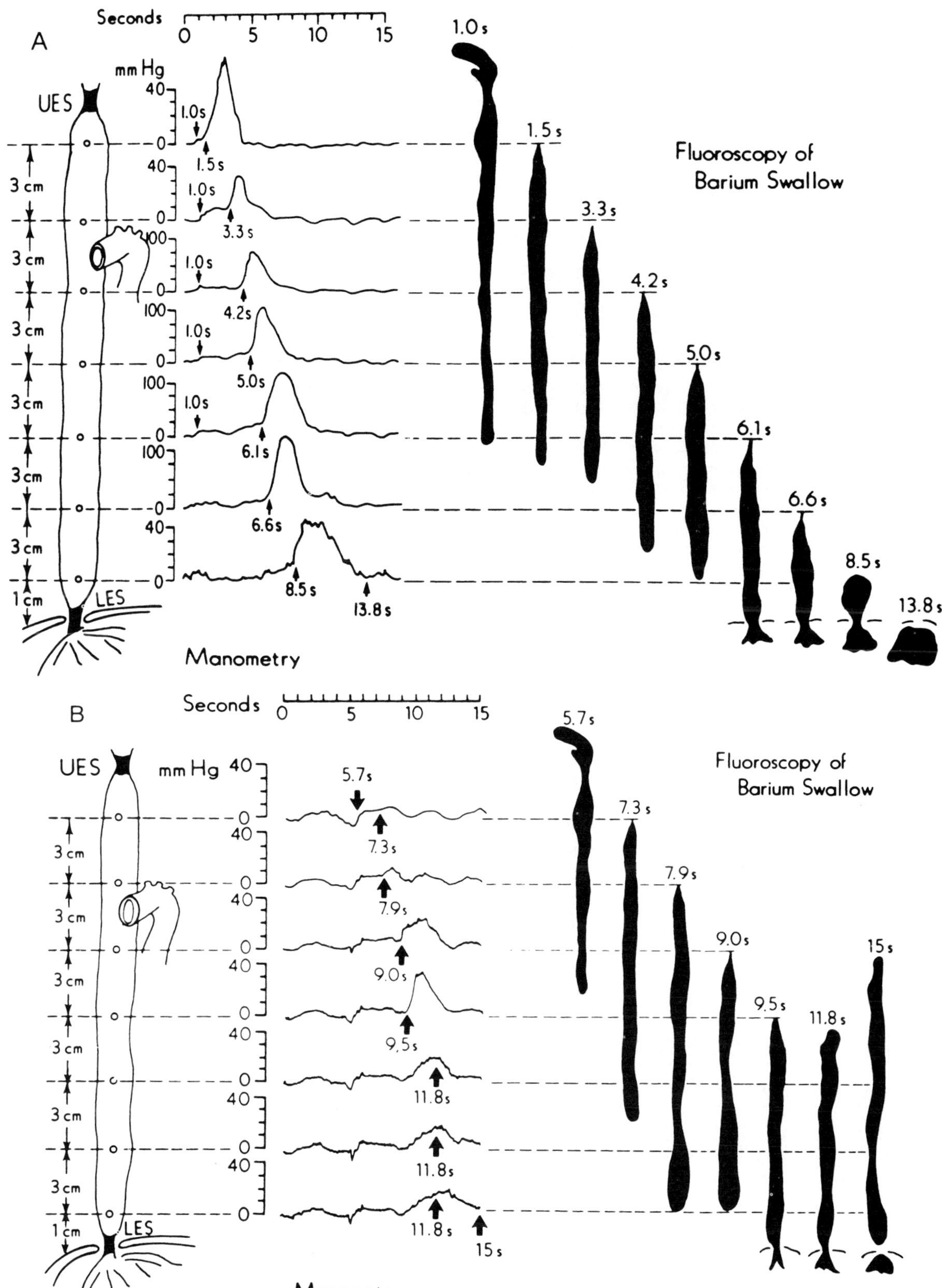

Figure 6–33. Correlation of manometry and the passage of a barium bolus. The tracings from the video images on the right depict the distribution of the barium bolus at the times indicated by arrows on the manometric record. *A*, Normal. *B*, Abnormal. In this example, minimal volume clearance occurs due to a failed peristaltic contraction. The peristaltic stripping wave progressed beyond the aortic arch to the middle of the esophagus and failed to propagate further, leaving most of the barium bolus in the distal esophagus. The manometric correlate of this event is shown on the *left*. The initial esophageal stripping action is associated with a feeble peristaltic contraction that progressed only as far as had the stripping wave. After the failure of the sequential peristaltic contraction, indicated by the 11.8-second mark, simultaneous waves were recorded from within the common cavity of the barium-distended esophagus. The simultaneous waves, recorded from the distal three recording sites, were of low amplitude and nearly identical waveform. After the termination of contractile activity (15 seconds) some barium was redistributed into the thoracic esophagus. This retrograde movement could be passive or, again, the result of the non-lumen-obliterating contraction of the distal esophageal segment. (From Kahrilas, P.J., Dodds, W.J., Hogan, W.J., et al.: Effect of peristaltic dysfunction on esophageal volume clearance. Gastroenterology, *94*:74, 1988, with permission.)

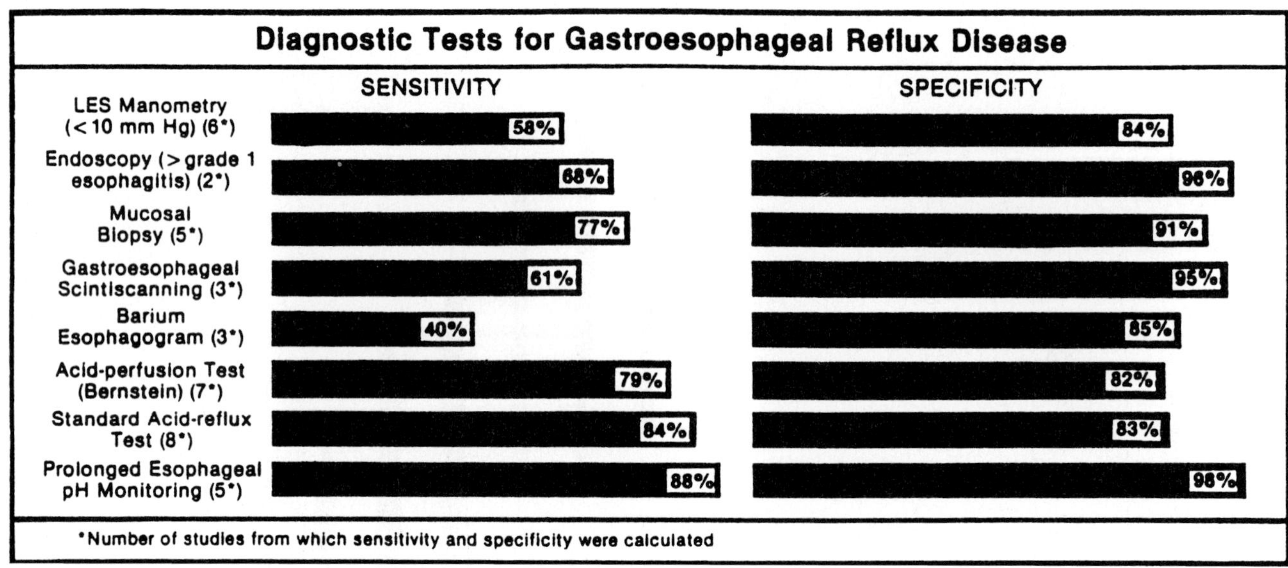

Figure 6–34. Sensitivity and specificity of diagnostic test for gastroesophageal reflux disease. (LES = lower esophageal sphincter.) (From DeMeester, T.R., and Stein, H.J.: Gastroesophageal reflux disease. *In* Moody, F.G., Jones, R.S., Kelly, K.A., et al. [eds.]: Surgical Treatment of Digestive Disease, 2nd ed. Chicago, Year Book Medical Publishers, 1989, p. 67, with permission.)

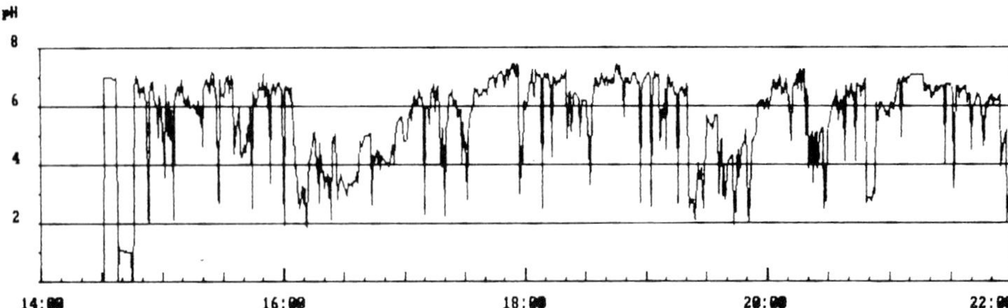

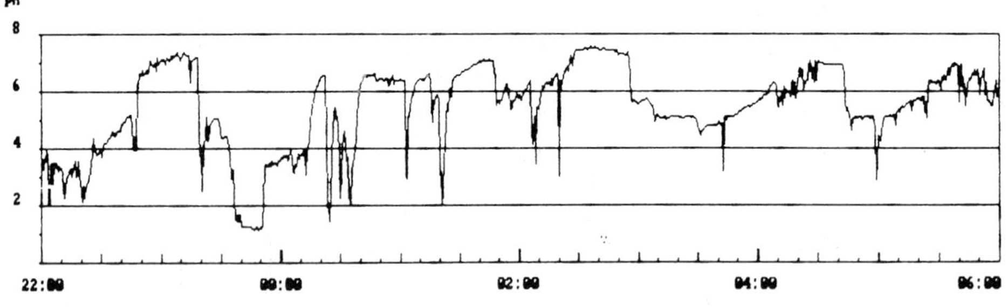

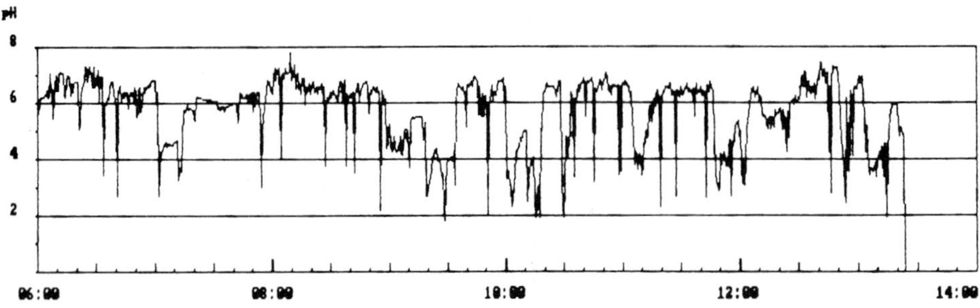

Figure 6–35. Display of a 24-hour esophageal pH monitoring study in a patient with increased esophageal acid exposure.

Table 6–4. Normal Values for Esophageal Exposure to pH <4 (n = 50)

Component	Mean	SD	95th Percentile
Total time	1.51	1.36	4.45
Upright time	2.34	2.34	8.42
Supine time	0.63	1.0	3.45
No. of episodes	19.00	12.76	46.90
No. >5 minutes	0.84	1.18	3.45
Longest episode	6.74	7.85	19.80

From DeMeester, T.R., and Stein, H.J.: Gastroesophageal reflux disease. *In* Moody, F.G., Jones, R.S., Kelly, K.A., et al. (eds.): Surgical Treatment of Digestive Disease, 2nd ed. Chicago, Year Book Medical Publishers, 1989, p. 65, with permission.

nents of the 24-hour record at each whole-number pH threshold derived from 50 asymptomatic control subjects. The upper limits of normal were established at the 95th percentile. Figure 6–36 shows the median and the 95th percentile of the normal values for each component (patient values are shown in black). If a symptomatic patient's values are outside the 95th percentile of normal subjects, he or she is considered abnormal for the component measured. Most centers use pH 4 as the threshold; with this threshold, there is a uniformity of normal values for the six components throughout the world.[21] This indicates that normal individuals have similar values for esophageal acid exposure despite nationality or dietary habits.

To combine the result of the six components into one expression of the overall esophageal acid exposure below a pH threshold, a pH score is calculated by using the standard deviation of the mean of each of the six components measured in the 50 normal subjects as a weighing factor.[34] By accepting an abstract zero level two standard deviations below the mean, the data measured in normal subjects can be treated as though they have a normal distribution. Thus, any measured patient value can be referenced to this zero point and in turn be awarded points based on whether it is below or above the normal mean value for that component. The equation used for the calculation illustrated in Figure 6–37 is

$$\text{Component score} = \text{patient value} - [\text{mean}/(\text{SD} + 1)]$$

This formula is used to score each of the six components of the 24-hour pH record obtained from the 50 normal subjects. The score for each component is added to obtain a composite score for each of the 50 normal subjects, and the upper level of a normal score is established at the 95th percentile. The upper limits of normal for the composite score for each whole number pH threshold are shown in Table 6–5. The median and 95th percentile for the composite score for each whole number pH threshold can also be expressed graphically (Fig. 6–38).

Relative operating characteristic curves confirmed that expression of the overall esophageal acid exposure using the composite score is superior to each individual component of the score in differentiating patients with and without GERD. The sensitivity, specificity, and predictive value of a positive and a negative test were all 96% when the composite score was used to express esophageal acid exposure.[31] Based on these studies and extensive clinical experience, 24-hour esophageal pH monitoring has emerged as the "gold standard" for the measurement of increased esophageal acid exposure.

In patients with symptoms of chronic cough, hoarseness, or aspiration, the placement of an additional pH electrode in the proximal esophagus or pharynx can be helpful. If reflux episodes reach the proximal esophagus or pharynx and a temporary relationship between these reflux episodes and the onset of the symptom can be documented, gastroesophageal reflux can be assumed to be the cause of the patient's complaint.[30]

24-Hour Ambulatory Detection of Esophageal Bilirubin Exposure

The potentially injurious ingredients of duodenal juice are bile acids and activated pancreatic enzymes, all of which can produce epithelial changes when incubated with strips of esophageal mucosa. Their presence in the esophagus can be proved conclusively only through aspiration over a prolonged period and assessment of the aspirated juice (Fig. 6–39). Ambulatory aspiration of esophageal contents is, however, cumbersome, requires a cooperative patient, and has largely been abandoned. A newer indirect method uses a special probe capable of detecting bilirubin in the refluxate.

The apparatus used to measure the presence of bilirubin consists of a portable opticoelectronic data logger, weighing 1200 g, that can be strapped to the patient's side and a fiberoptic probe, which can be passed transnasally and positioned anywhere in the lumen of the foregut (Bilitec 2000; Prodotec Srl, Florence, Italy; and Synectics Medical, Minneapolis, MN). The system allows for the spectrophotometric measurements of luminal bilirubin concentration.[4] The spectrophotometric probes are 3 mm in diameter and 140 cm in length and contain 30 plastic optical fibers, each 250 nm in diameter, bonded together and covered with biocompatible polyurethane.

Table 6–5. Normal Composite Score for Various pH Thresholds

pH Threshold	Upper Level of Normal Value (95th Percentile)
<1	14.2
<2	17.37
<3	14.10
<4	14.72
<5	15.76
<6	12.76
>7	14.90
>8	8.50

From DeMeester, T.R., and Stein, H.J.: Gastroesophageal reflux disease. *In* Moody, F.G., Jones, R.S., Kelly, K.A., et al. (eds.): Surgical Treatment of Digestive Disease, 2nd ed. Chicago, Year Book Medical Publishers, 1989, p. 65, with permission.

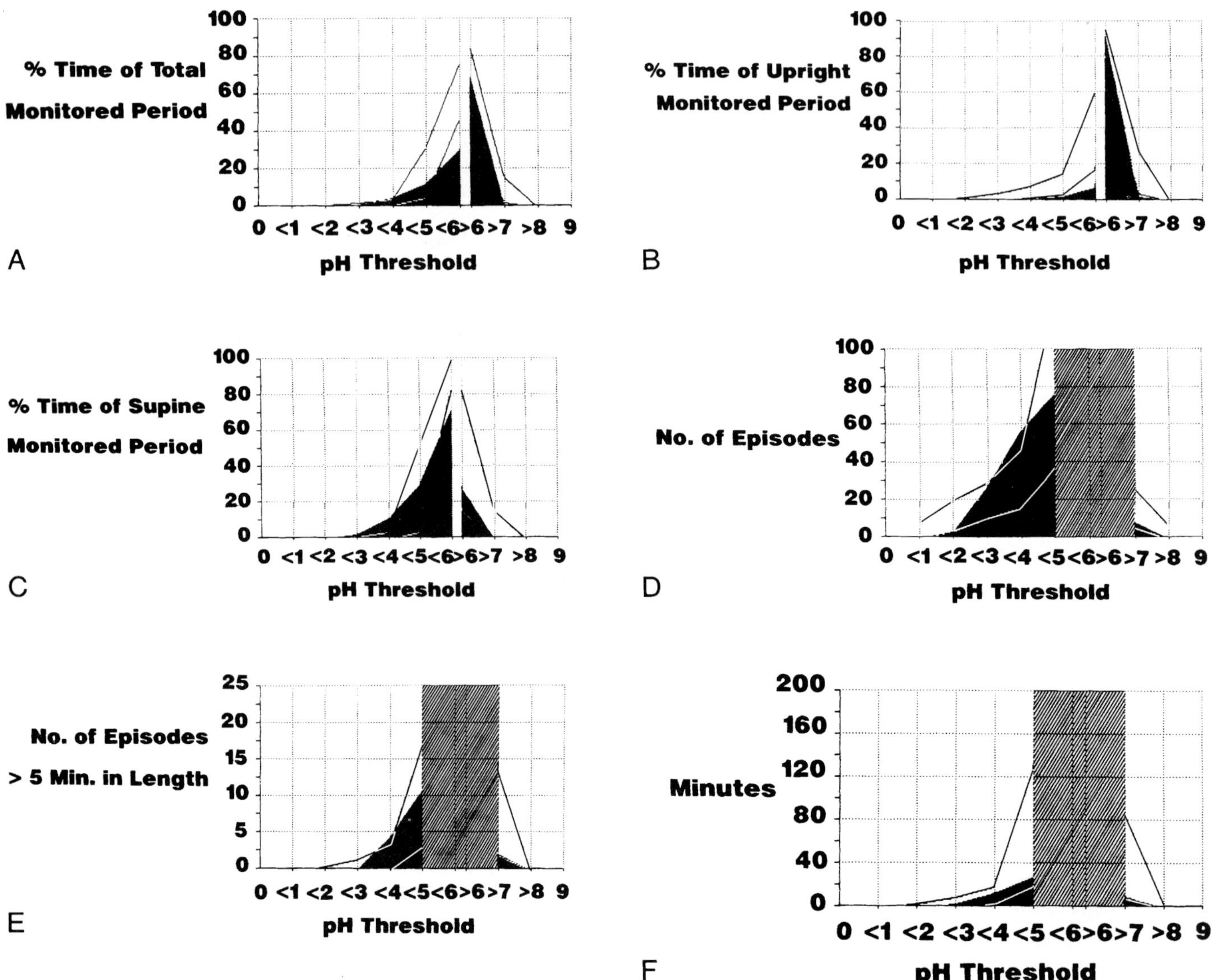

Figure 6–36. Graphic display of the median and ninety-fifth percentile levels in 50 normal individuals for pH thresholds above and below 6. The *black area* represents measurements made in the patient. The *lower line* shows the median and the upper line the ninety-fifth percentile value for the 50 normal subjects. When the *black area* exceeds the ninety-fifth percentile line for a given pH threshold, the patient has an abnormal value for the component measured. *A*, Percentage cumulative exposure for total time. *B*, Percentage cumulative exposure for upright time. *C*, Percentage cumulative exposure for supine time. *D*, Number of episodes. *E*, Number of episodes greater than 5 minutes in length. *F*, Length of longest episode. (From DeMeester, T.R., and Stein, H.J.: Gastroesophageal reflux disease. *In* Moody, F.G., Jones, R.S., Kelly, K.A., et al. [eds.]: Surgical Treatment of Digestive Disease, 2nd ed. Chicago, Year Book Medical Publishers, p. 67, 1989, with permission.)

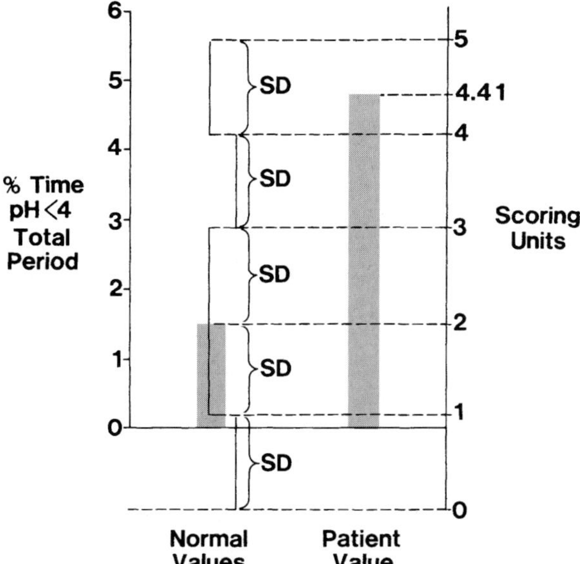

Figure 6–37. Concept of using the standard deviation as the scoring unit to score the component percentage time pH <4 for the total period. Note the establishment of an abstract zero point 2 standard deviations below the mean value for total-period acid exposure measured in normals. Theoretically, this allows scoring the measurement in patients as though the normal values were parametric. By this method, a patient who had a total acid exposure below pH 4 of 4.8% would have a score for this component of 4.41. (From DeMeester, T.R., and Stein, H.J.: Gastroesophageal reflux disease. *In* Moody, F.G., Jones, R.S., Kelly, K.A., et al. [eds.]: Surgical Treatment of Digestive Disease, 2nd ed. Chicago, Year Book Medical Publishers, p. 67, 1989, with permission.)

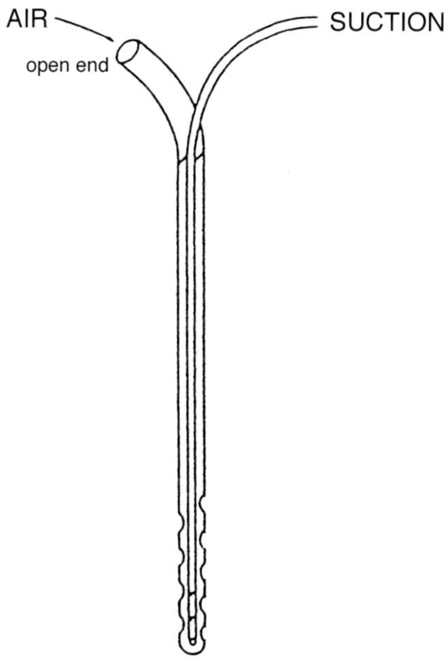

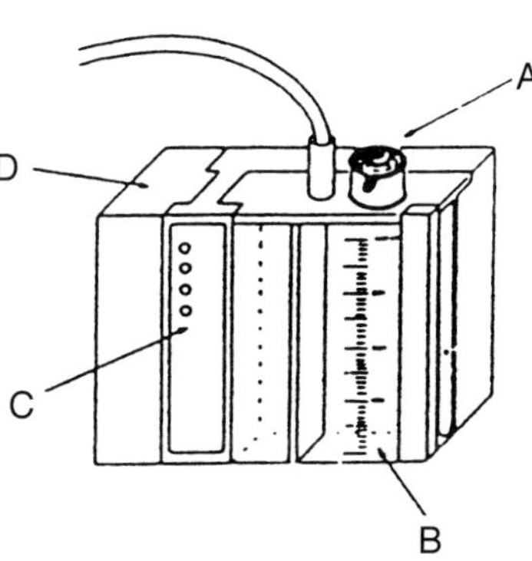

Figure 6–39. Catheter system *(top)* and portable vacuum pump *(bottom)* used for ambulatory esophageal reflux aspiration. *A*, Vacuum indicators. *B*, Replaceable container for aspirates. *C*, Control unit. *D*, Rechargeable battery. (From Stein, H.J., Feussner, H., Kaver, W., et al.: "Alkaline" gastroesophageal reflux: Assessment by ambulatory esophageal and pH monitoring. Am. J. Surg., *167*:163, 1994, with permission.)

Two plugs connect 50% of the optic fibers to the light-emitting diodes and 50% to the receiving photo diode. The tip of the probe contains a 2-mm space for sampling. Fluid and solids that have been processed in a blender can easily flow through the space, and their bilirubin concentration can be measured. The probes are flexible, durable, easy to sterilize, and reusable. The opticoelectronic unit acts simultaneously as a light signal generator, a data processor, and a data storage device. Further, the unit has two channels, allowing dual measurement with two probes if desired. The light source for each channel is provided by two light-emitting diodes that emit a 470-nm signal light (blue spectrum) and a 565-nm reference light (green spectrum). Reference and signal light-emitting diodes are stimulated alternately for a duration of 0.5 second. To avoid fluctuations in the source, the final 20 milliseconds of each pulse are used for signal processing. Optical signals reflected back from the probe are converted to electrical impulses by a photo diode. This electrical signal is then amplified and processed within the data logger. Absorbance readings are averaged every two cycles. The system is capable of recording 225 individual absorbance values per hour and allows up to 30 hours of continuous monitoring. In vitro and in vivo validation studies showed that spectrophotometry based on absorp-

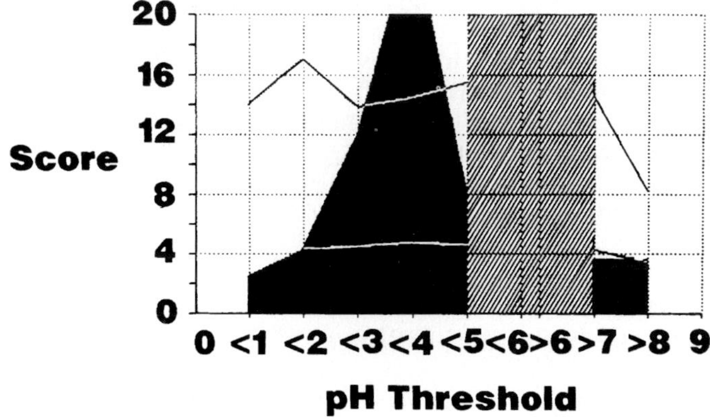

Figure 6–38. The composite score used to express the overall pH result. The *lower line* represents the median score and the *upper line* the ninety-fifth percentile of 50 normal subjects. The *black area* represents the composite score of the patient in Figure 6–34 with increased esophageal acid exposure measured at pH of <4. (From DeMeester, T.R., and Stein, H.J.: Gastroesophageal reflux disease. *In* Moody, F.G., Jones, R.S., Kelly, K.A., et al. [eds.]: Surgical Treatment of Digestive Disease, 2nd ed. Chicago, Year Book Medical Publishers, p. 67, 1989, with permission.)

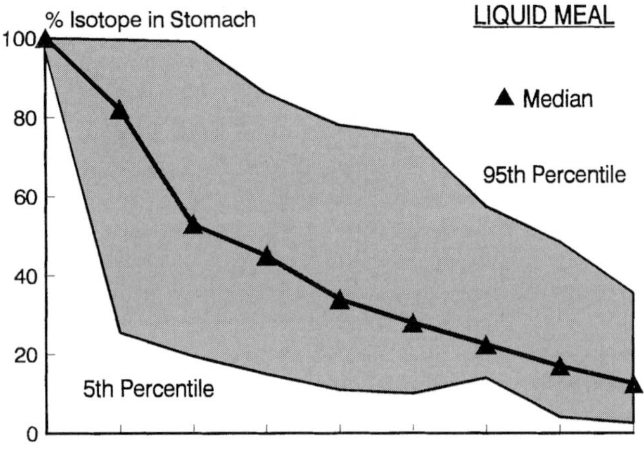

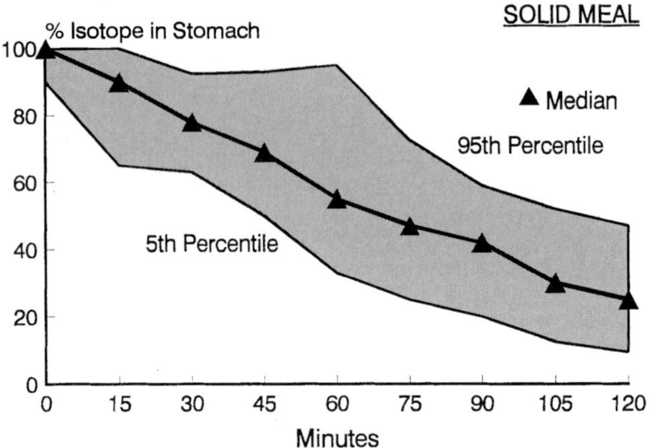

Figure 6–40. Gastric emptying of a liquid and solid meal. The *shaded area* and *line* represent the normal range and median in 20 volunteers. (From Stein, H.J., DeMeester, T.R., and Hinder, R.A.: Outpatient physiologic testing and surgical management of foregut motility disorders. Curr. Probl. Surg., *29*:415, 1992, with permission.)

tion at a wavelength of 453 nm is specific for bilirubin and that the absorbance spectrum is sufficient to detect bilirubin throughout human physiologic ranges. Further, the measurements are highly reproducible despite pH changes caused by environment or food intake. In addition, in a clinical study an absorbance threshold of 0.20 was found to be a reliable threshold to differentiate healthy subjects (Fig. 6–40) from reflux patients. Patients with Barrett's esophagus showed the highest individual values and a significantly higher exposure than controls when the esophageal pH was less than 4 or between 4 and 7, which are ranges in which pH monitoring cannot detect alkaline reflux (pH $>$ 7).[39]

Therefore, this test is a very useful and reliable complementary tool for esophageal pH monitoring in the investigation of patients with foregut symptoms. The combination of pH and bilirubin esophageal monitoring will further the understanding and care of patients with GERD.

Standard Acid Reflux Test

The development of powerful antisecretory agents such as proton pump inhibitors has, in some patients, created difficulty in the measurement of esophageal acid exposure. Many patients are placed on these medications before the study, altering normal physiology and thus complicating interpretation of ambulatory 24-hour esophageal pH monitoring. The acid-reducing effects of omeprazole have been noted to be present as long as 40 days after cessation of the drug. The standard acid reflux test (SART) can be used to provide information when it is suspected that the results of pH monitoring have been altered by medications or when patients do not tolerate a prolonged period without taking these medications.

The SART is performed after manometry by placing a pH electrode 5 cm above the upper border of the lower esophageal sphincter. The manometry catheter is advanced temporarily into the stomach, and 300 ml of 0.1N hydrochloric acid is infused. In children, the gastric acid load is reduced accordingly. The manometry catheter is flushed and then pulled back into the body of the esophagus. The pH of the esophagus is monitored 5 cm above the upper border of the sphincter while the patient rests quietly in the recumbent position and while performing four maneuvers: deep breathing, Valsalva, Mueller (inspiration against a closed glottis), and cough. These maneuvers are repeated in the right and left lateral decubitus position and with the head down 20 degrees, providing 16 possibilities for acid reflux to occur. A decrease in esophageal pH to less than 4 is considered evidence of reflux. At the beginning of the test, before the patient is placed in the recumbent position, the distal esophagus must have a pH greater than 4. In some patients, this necessitates standing erect and swallowing repeatedly to clear the esophagus of acid. Patients who cannot clear the esophagus in the erect position after 20 effective swallows monitored on a motility recording are considered to be abnormal in all positions and maneuvers. Among 90 healthy volunteers, only two individuals had more than two reflux episodes. Accordingly, one or two drops in pH during these challenges to the cardia are considered normal and three or more drops in pH are taken as evidence of a mechanical incompetence of the cardia. Patients with severe reflux may be unable to clear acid from the esophagus after reflux has been documented.[53]

When evaluated in a test population with an equal distribution of normal healthy subjects and patients with classic symptoms of GERD, the SART had a sensitivity of 59% and a specificity of 98%. This gave a positive predictive value of 96% and a negative predictive value of 75%, with an overall accuracy of 81%.[25]

Roentgenographic Detection of Gastroesophageal Reflux

The definition of roentgenographic gastroesophageal reflux varies depending on whether reflux is spontaneous or induced by various maneuvers. In only about 40% of patients with classic symptoms of GERD is spontaneous reflux observed by the radiologist (i.e., reflux of barium from the stomach into the esophagus with a patient in the upright position). In most patients who show this abnormality, the diagnosis of increased esophageal acid exposure can be confirmed by 24-hour, esophageal pH monitoring. Therefore, the roentgenographic demonstration of spontaneous regurgitation of barium into the esophagus in the upright position is a reliable indicator that reflux is present. Failure to see this does not, however, indicate the absence of disease.

Scintigraphic Detection of Gastroesophageal Reflux

A scintigraphic test for the detection of GERD was introduced in 1976 by Fisher and associates.[24] ^{99m}Tc sulfur colloid (100 Ci) is mixed with 300 ml physiologic saline and drunk by the patient or instilled into the stomach via a nasogastric tube. The patient is placed in the supine position, and abdominal pressure is augmented by an abdominal binder. Gastroesophageal reflux is identified and quantified with a gamma camera. A major disadvantage of the test is the short duration of the monitoring period and the unphysiologic means by which reflux is induced. Consequently, the sensitivity and specificity of this test for the diagnosis of GERD have been questioned.[28]

Tests to Provoke Esophageal Symptoms

The spontaneous occurrence of symptoms during a standard esophageal motility study is rare, especially in patients with noncardiac chest pain. Consequently, a number of provocative tests have been designed to identify the esophagus as the cause of these symptoms. Of these, intraesophageal acid perfusion (Bernstein test), edrophonium (Tensilon) test, and intraesophageal balloon distention are the most common. Common to all provocative tests is that they are dependent on the patient's perception and indirectly identify the esophagus as the cause of the symptoms. They do not definitely prove an esophageal cause of a spontaneously occurring symptom.

Acid Perfusion (Bernstein) Test

Since its introduction in 1958 by Bernstein and Baker,[6] the esophageal acid perfusion test has been widely used to determine whether a patient's symptoms can be reproduced by the infusion of acid into the esophagus. If positive, the test indicates that the esophagitis is sensitive to acid and increased esophageal exposure to acid is assumed. In the original technique, the distal esophagus is perfused with 0.1N HCl at a rate 6 to 8 ml/min with the patient sitting upright. Ideally, a placebo is also infused (i.e., acid is alternately perfused with physiologic saline without the patient knowing the identity of the perfusate). The patient is asked to report any symptom that develops during infusion. Consistent reproduction of the patient's usual symptoms only during acid perfusion and rapid abatement during saline perfusion indicates a positive test. The development of symptoms during both the saline test and the acid perfusion test or the development of symptoms foreign to the patient's usual experience represents an equivocal test. Failure to develop any symptoms during a 30-minute acid perfusion indicates a normal test.

Various investigators have reported that 34 to 100% of patients with typical symptoms of GERD have a positive acid perfusion test. Failure to include certain components of gastric juice (e.g., pepsin, bile, pancreatic enzymes, food) in the perfusate may account for some of the normal results. A false-negative result can also occur in patients who have an insensitive esophagus. False-positive results are seen in 15% of symptomatic subjects. Of concern is that symptomatic subjects whose pain is not due to reflux may have a similar incidence of false-positive tests, resulting in an erroneous diagnosis.

Edrophonium (Tensilon) Test

The edrophonium test has been introduced to identify chest pain of esophageal origin in patients in whom cardiac disease has been excluded.[5,50] The cholinesterase inhibitor edrophonium hydrochloride (Tensilon) is injected intravenously at a dose of 80 μ/kg. A syringe with 1 mg of the antidote atropine should always be at hand when performing the test. The test is ideally placebo controlled. A positive test is defined as replication of chest pain similar to the pain that the patient experiences spontaneously after edrophonium injection but not placebo injection. The test is positive in 20 to 30% of patients with noncardiac chest pain but not in asymptomatic volunteers.[50] In both normal volunteers and symptomatic patients, edrophonium causes a marked increase in amplitude and duration of esophageal contractions. Because reproduction of the patient's typical symptoms rather than a specific change in esophageal motility is considered the end point of the test, manometry does not have be performed. The disadvantages of the test are that its helpfulness is limited to only a small proportion of patients with chest pain, there is the risk of side effects, and it reproduces symptoms with an unphysiologic stimulus. The test should not be performed in patients with asthma, chronic obstructive airway disease, or cardiac arrhythmias. This test is rarely performed.

Esophageal Balloon Distention

Balloon distention of the esophagus was described in 1955 as a diagnostic test to distinguish esophageal from cardiac chest pain.[40] An inflatable balloon is positioned 10 cm above the lower esophageal sphincter and gradually inflated with air in 1-ml increments. Esophageal motility is simultaneously monitored. The test is considered positive when typical symptoms are reproduced with gradual distention of the balloon. Studies indicate that the procedure induces spastic esophageal motor activity and reproduces chest pain episodes in up to 50% of patients with noncardiac chest pain but not in volunteers.[3] Although the test has a greater diagnostic yield than drug provocative studies, it is relatively invasive and provides no information on spontaneously occurring symptoms.

Tests of Gastroduodenal Function as They Relate to Esophageal Disease

Esophageal disorders are frequently caused by abnormalities of gastroduodenal function. Abnormalities of the gastric reservoir or increased gastric acid secretion can be responsible for increased esophageal exposure to gastric juice. Reflux of gastric juice contaminated with duodenal contents (i.e., bile salts and pancreatic enzymes) is thought to have a role in the pathogenesis of esophagitis and complicated Barrett's esophagus.[59] Furthermore, functional disorders of the esophagus often are not confined to the esophagus alone but are associated with functional disorders of the rest of the foregut (i.e., stomach and duodenum). In any patient in whom a gastroduodenal disorder is suspected, it is essential to delineate the gastroduodenal anatomy to exclude structural abnormalities and a mechanical cause for the complaint before functional studies are performed.

The gastric secretory state has been classically assessed with gastric acid analysis. Gastric emptying and gastroduodenal motor function can be assessed with scintigraphic emptying studies, manometry, and electromyography. Cholescintigraphy is frequently used to assess the presence of excessive duodenogastric reflux. Twenty-four-hour gastric pH monitoring allows simultaneous evaluation of gastric acid secretion and an estimate of duodenogastric reflux and gastric emptying.

Gastric Acid Analysis

The gastric secretory state is usually evaluated by determination of the titratable acid in aspirated gastric juice. The test is performed after an overnight fast with the patient in a semirecumbent condition. The stomach is intubated, and the contents are completely aspirated. An aliquot of physiologic saline is instilled and immediately aspirated. Complete recovery of the instilled volume indicates correct position of the tube. Gastric acid is then aspirated every 5 minutes for 1 hour to assess basal acid secretion. Acid secretion is stimulated with pentagastrin or histamine, and aspiration is continued for an additional hour. The volume of the aspirated gastric juice is measured, and the hydrogen ion content is titrated.[59]

Interdigestive or basal gastric acid secretion is measured in the unstimulated state and varies between 0 and 5 mEq/hr in normal volunteers. The maximal secretory capacity of the stomach, which reflects the available parietal cell mass, is calculated after stimulation with pentagastrin or histamine and ranges between 10 and 15 mEq/hr in normal volunteers. Peak acid output, which is the two highest consecutive 15-minute acid values multiplied by 2, is another form of reporting the acid secretory potential of the stomach and avoids errors caused by isolated low acid values. Acid hypersecretors have a basal acid output of more than 5 mEq/hr and a maximum acid output (MAO) $>$30 mEq/hr.[59]

Recently, 24-hour gastric pH emptying pH monitoring has provided another measurement of gastric acid production. The cumulative frequency distribution of gastric pH value recorded every 4 to 6 seconds during a supine fasting period is plotted as the per cent of time the gastric pH was at various pH values. A patient with hypersecretion or achlorhydria is identified if their values fall above or below the normal range (Fig. 6–41).

Gastric Emptying Tests

Gastric emptying is best assessed with radionuclide-labeled meals. Emptying of solids and liquids can be evaluated simultaneously when both phases are marked with different tracers such as ^{99m}Tc or ^{111}In. Frequently used labeled solid and liquid meals include chicken liver, eggs, oatmeal, orange juice, or water. After ingestion of a labeled standard meal, anterior and posterior gamma camera images of the stomach area are obtained in 5- to 15-minute intervals for 1.5 to 2 hours. After correction for decay, the counts in the gastric area are plotted as a per cent of total counts at the start of imaging. Data can be shown as curves of emptying for liquid or solid against time with the 5th and 95th percentiles of normal values for comparison (see Fig. 6–40). A more simple technique of assessment is to derive the half-time, which is the time taken to empty 50% of the meal from the stomach.[59]

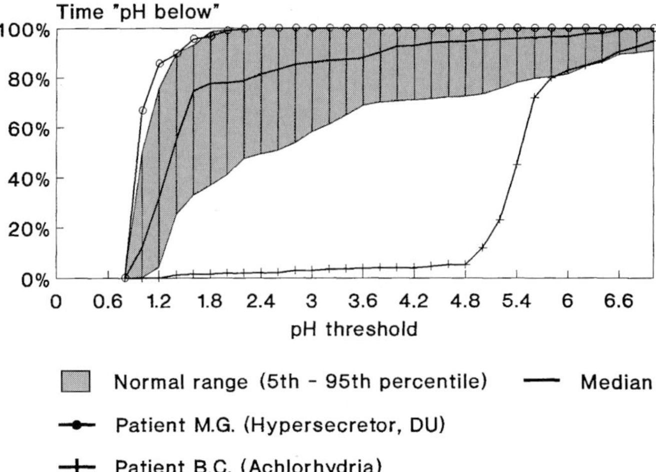

Figure 6–41. Cumulative frequency distribution of recorded gastric pH values during the supine period. The *shaded area* represents the fifth and ninety-fifth percentiles of 50 normal volunteers, the *solid line* shows the median. Patient M.G. has a marked "left shift" of his pH profile out of the normal range, suggesting gastric acid hypersecretion. Patient B.C. has a "right shift" of his pH profile, indicating hypochlorhydria. (From Stein, H.J., and DeMeester, T.R.: Integrated 24-hour ambulatory foregut monitoring in patients with complex foregut symptoms. Surg. Ann., *24*:161, 1992, with permission.)

A limitation of scintigraphic gastric emptying studies is that they fail to take into account rapid changes such as fast emptying in the first minutes after meal ingestion as seen after gastric resection. It is important to carry out testing with both a liquid and a solid meal, because some patients may show abnormalities of one and not the other and may be erroneously thought to have a normal rate of gastric emptying. The development of smaller, portable gamma counters and ultrasound imaging of the stomach offers new opportunities to study gastric emptying.

Cholescintigraphy

Scintigraphic hepatobiliary imaging is performed after the intravenous injection of ^{99m}Tc iminodiacetic acid derivatives such as disofenin (DISIDA). Gamma camera images of the upper abdomen that incorporate the gallbladder and stomach are obtained at 5-minute intervals for 60 minutes. Imaging is continued for an additional 30 minutes after stimulation of gallbladder contraction with the synthetic carboxyl-terminal octapeptide of cholecystoki-

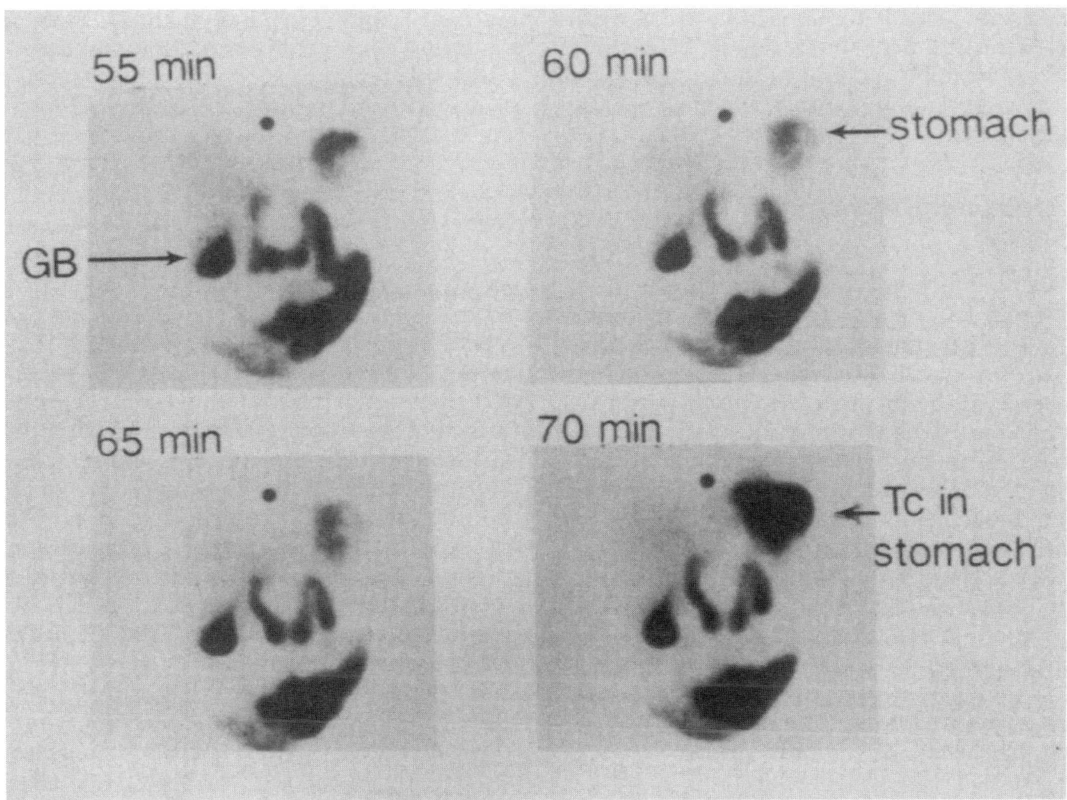

Figure 6–42. Cholescintigraphic scan showing duodenogastric reflux. Activity is seen in the location of the stomach 55, 60, and 65 minutes after injection of the radionuclide. The position of the stomach is confirmed at the end of the study by the oral administration of ^{99m}Tc pertechnetate shown in the final scan. (From Stein, H.J., Hinder, R.A., DeMeester, T.R., et al.: Clinical useof 24-hour gastric pH monitoring versus DISIDA scanning in the diagnosis of pathologic duodenogastric reflux. Arch. Surg., *125*:966, 1990, with permission.)

nin. Duodenogastric reflux is detected by an increase of radioactivity in the stomach area in the sequential images (Fig. 6–42). The clinical value of this test is limited due to its short duration and a false-positive rate of about 20% in normal volunteers. This is due to the inability of cholescintigraphy to differentiate physiologic from pathologic duodenogastric reflux.[62]

Additional Miscellaneous Tests

There are a number of other techniques and methods that have been and are being used to diagnose foregut abnormalities. These methods are, however, largely experimental and mainly conducted in the research or university setting. In many cases, the technology associated with the techniques is still too primitive and unrefined or the procedure is too cumbersome or user unfriendly to the patient. The methods and techniques used include the following:

1. The Barostat[2] measures tone in the proximal portion of the stomach.
2. Antroduodenal motility is used to evaluate pressure changes that occur in the stomach, pylorus, and duodenum after a meal.
3. Extrinsic cutaneous monitoring is conducted of small intestinal electrical activity.
4. Twenty-four-hour gastric pH monitoring is conducted.
5. Impendancometry allows for the measurement of bolus transport in hollow organs such as the esophagus.
6. Manovideofluorography is the simultaneous measurement of manometry and videofluoroscopy.

These techniques can all provide useful or additional information that may be of benefit to the patients. Their role in the routine evaluation of patients has yet to be determined.

Integrated Ambulatory Foregut Monitoring

The development of portable digital data recorders with large storage capacity now allows outpatient 24-hour monitoring of pharyngeal and esophageal motility simultaneous with esophageal and gastric pH.[56] Integrated evaluation of foregut motor and secretory function over an entire circadian cycle has thus become possible (Fig. 6–43*A* and *B*). Initial studies show that simultaneous outpatient monitoring of esophageal pH, gastric pH, and esophageal motor function with multiple pressure transducers and pH electrodes over 24 hours is tolerated with none or only minor discomfort in more than 95% of patients. In one study, integrated foregut monitoring established one or more functional or secretory abnormalities as the underlying cause of symptoms in 84% of the studied patients.[56] Gastroesophageal reflux, esophageal motor abnormalities, and prolonged postprandial alkalinization of the gastric pH suggestive of delayed gastric

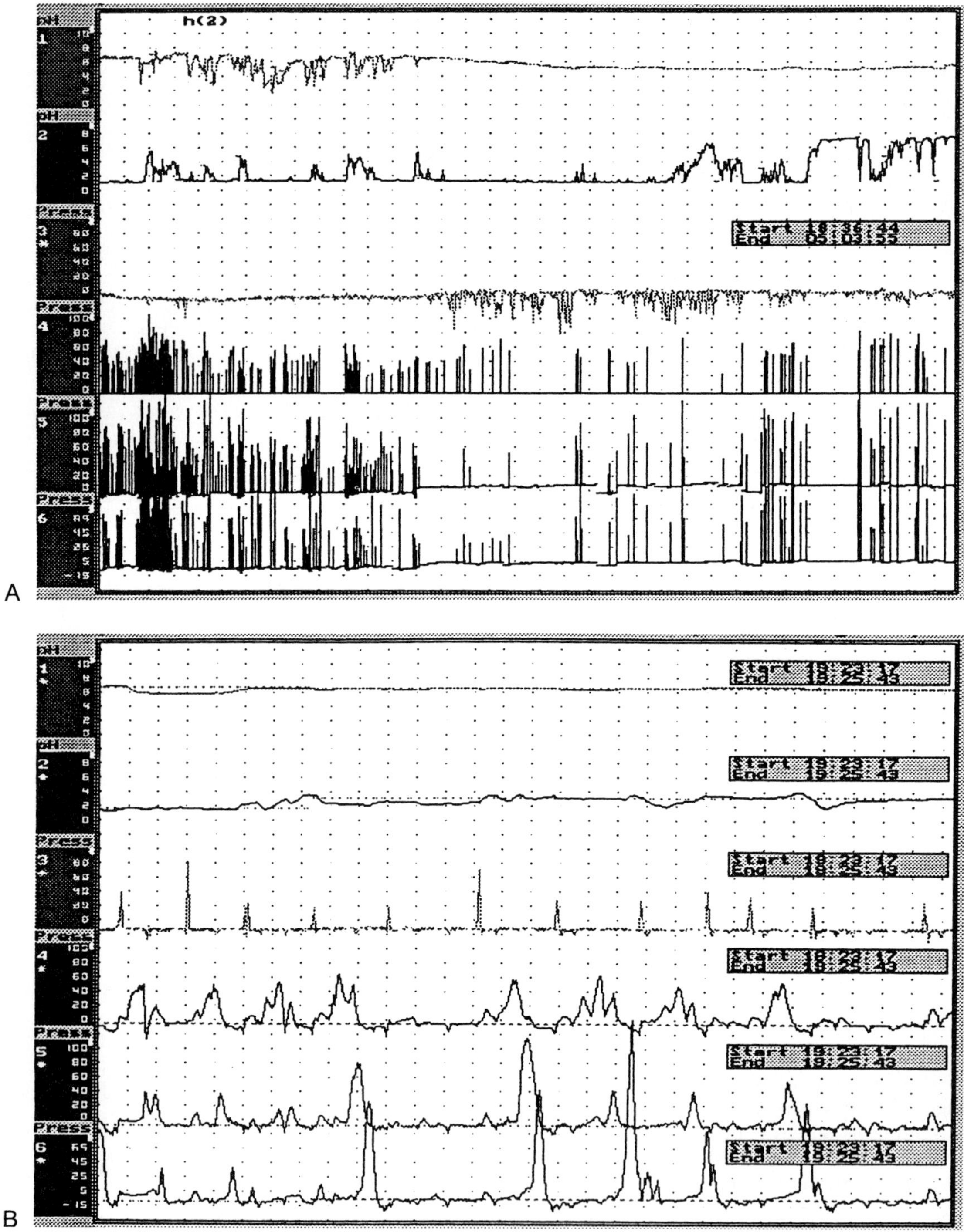

Figure 6–43. A representative tracing in a patient who had integrated foregut monitoring—that is, simultaneous monitoring of esophageal pH (first tracing from the top, 1); gastric pH (second tracing from the top, 2); pharyngeal pressure (third tracing from the top, 3); and pressures in the esophageal body 15, 10, and 5 cm above the lower esophageal sphincter (fourth, fifth, and sixth tracings from the top, 4 through 6) over an entire circadian cycle. *A*, Compressed data recorded between 18:36 and 05:00 hours the next morning. *B*, A 2-minute recording during dinner from 19:23 to 19:25 hours.

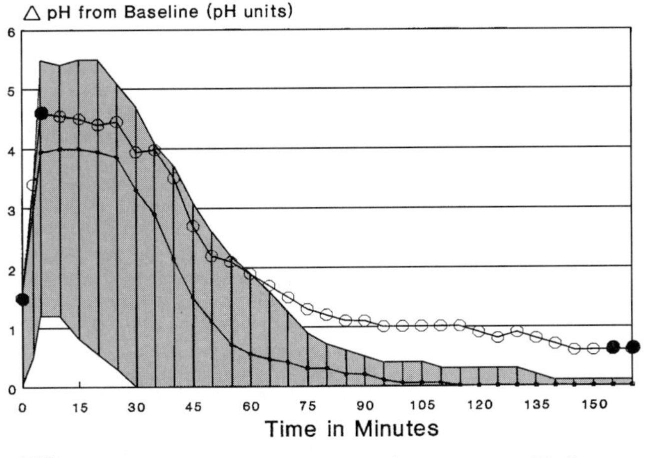

Figure 6–44. Postprandial alkalinization of the gastric pH measured as the change from baseline pH. The *shaded area* represents the fifth and ninety-fifth percentiles of 50 normal volunteers, the *solid line* shows the median. Patient J.B. showed a markedly prolonged postprandial alkalinization suggesting delayed gastric emptying. (From Stein, H.J., and DeMeester, T.R.: Integrated 24-hour ambulatory foregut monitoring in patients with complex foregut symptoms. Surg. Ann., *24:*161, 1992, with permission.)

emptying (Fig. 6–44), or a combination of these, were the most common diagnoses. This new technology represents the most physiologic way to assess foregut function and has potential to replace the series of individual laboratory tests that have been necessary to thoroughly evaluate patients with complex foregut disorders. Ambulatory integrated foregut monitoring and computerized evaluation of the recorded data put into the physician's hand the ability to evaluate foregut motor and secretory abnormalities within his or her office. This will place medical and surgical therapy of functional abnormalities of the foregut on a more scientific basis.[59]

References

1. Arndorfer, R.C., Stef, J.J., Dodds, W.J., et al.: Improved infusion system for intraluminal esophageal manometry. Gastroenterology, *73:*23, 1977.
2. Azpiroz, F., and Malagelada, J.R.: Gastric tone measured by an electronic barostat in health and postsurgical gastroparesis. Gastroenterology, *92:*934, 1987.
3. Barish, C.F., Castell, D.O., and Richter, J.E.: Graded esophageal balloon distention: A new provocation test for non-cardiac chest pain. Dig. Dis. Sci., *31:*1292, 1986.
4. Bechi, P., Pucciani, F., Baldini, F., et al.: Long-term ambulatory enterogastric reflux monitoring: Validation of a new fiberoptic technique. Dig. Dis. Sci., *38:*1297, 1993.
5. Benjamin, S.B., Richter, J.E., Cordova, C.M., et al.: Prospective manometric evaluation with pharmacologic provocation of patients with suspected esophageal motility dysfunction. Gastroenterology, *84:*893, 1983.
6. Bernstein, L.M., and Baker, C.A.: A clinical test for esophagitis. Gastroenterology, *34:*760, 1957.
7. Bombeck, C.T., Vaz, O., DeSalvo, J., et al.: Computerized axial manometry of the esophagus. Ann. Surg., *206:*465, 1987.
8. Bonavina, L., Evander, A., DeMeester, T.R., et al.: Length of the distal esophageal sphincter and competency of the cardia. Am. J. Surg., *151:*25, 1986.
9. Bonavina, L., Khan, N.A., and DeMeester, T.R.: Pharyngoesophageal dysfunctions: The role of cricopharyngeal myotomy. Arch. Surg., *120:*541, 1985.
10. Brand, D.L., Martin, D., and Pope, C.E.: Esophageal manometrics in patients with anginal type chest pain. Am. J. Dig. Dis., *23:*300, 1977.
11. Castell, D.A., Dalton, D.B., and Castell, D.O.: Pharyngeal and upper esophageal sphincter manometry in humans. Am. J. Physiol., *258:*173, 1990.
12. Castell, D.O., Richter, J.E., and Dalton, C.B. (eds.): Esophageal Motility Testing. New York, Elsevier, 1987.
13. Cook, I.J., Gibb, M., Panagopoulos, V., et al.: Pharyngeal (Zenker's) divertivulum is a disorder of upper esophageal opening. Gastroenterology, *103:*1229, 1992.
14. Craig, A., Hanlon, J., Dent, J., and Schoeman, M.: A comparison of transnasal and transoral endoscopy with small-diameter endoscopes in unsedated patients. Gastrointest. Endosc., *49:*292, 1999.
15. DeMeester, T.R.: Die chirurgische Perspektive der Funktionsdiagnostik. *In* Fuchs, K.H., and Hamelmann, H. (eds.): Gastrointestinale Funktionsdiagnostik in der Chirurgie. Berlin, Blackwell Wissenschaft, 1991, p. 3.
16. DeMeester, T.R., Johnson, L.F., Joseph, G.J., et al.: Patterns of gastroesophageal reflux in health and disease. Ann. Surg., *184:*459, 1976.
17. DeMeester, T.R., and Stein, H.J.: Gastroesophageal Reflux Disease. *In* Moody, F.G., Jones, R.S., Kelly, K.A., et al. (eds.): Surgical Treatment of Digestive Disease, 2nd ed. Chicago, Year Book Medical Publishers, 1989, p. 65.
18. DeMeester, T.R., Wang, C.I., Wernly, J.A., et al.: Technique, indications and clinical use of 24-hour esophageal pH monitoring. J. Thorac. Cardiovasc. Surg., *79:*656, 1980.
19. Dodds, W.J., Dent, J., Hogan, W.J., et al.: Mechanism of gastroesophageal reflux in patients with reflux esophagitis. N. Engl. J. Med., *307:*1547, 1982.
20. Ekberg, O., and Wahlgren, L.: Dysfunction of pharyngeal swallowing: A cineradiographic investigation in 854 dysphagial patients. Acta Radiol. Diagn., *26:*389, 1985.
21. Emde, C., Garner, A., and Blum, A.: Technical aspects of intraluminal pH-metry in man: Current status and recommendations. Gut, *23:*1177, 1987.
22. Eypasch, E.P., Stein, H.J., DeMeester, T.R., et al.: Ambulatory 24-hour esophageal motility monitoring: A new technique to define and clarify esophageal motor disorders. Am. J. Surg., *159:*144, 1990.
23. Fimmel C.J., Etienne, A., Cilluffo, T., et al.: Long-term ambulatory gastric pH monitoring: Validation of a new method and effect of H_2-antagonists. Gastroenterology, *88:*1842, 1985.
24. Fisher, R.S., Malmud, L.S., Roberts, G.S., et al.: Gastroesophageal (GE) scintiscanning to detect and quantitate GE reflux. Gastroenterology, *70:*301, 1976.
25. Fuchs, K.H., DeMeester, T.R., and Albertucci, M.: Specificity and sensitivity of objective diagnosis of gastroesophageal reflux disease. Surgery, *102:*575, 1987.
26. Fuchs, K.H., Hinder, R.A., DeMeester, T.R., et al.: Computerized identification of pathologic duodenogastric reflux using 24-hour gastric pH monitoring. Ann. Surg., *213:*13, 1991.
27. Helm, J.F., Riedel, D.R., Dodds, W.J., et al.: Determinants of esophageal acid clearance in normal subjects. Gastroenterology, *85:*607, 1983.
28. Hoffman, G.C., and Vansant, H.H.: The gastroesophageal scintiscan: Comparison of methods to demonstrate gastroesophageal reflux. Arch. Surg., *114:*727, 1979.
29. Houghton, L.A., Read, N.W., Heddle, R., et al.: Motor activity of the gastric antrum, pylorus, and duodenum under fasted conditions and after a liquid meal. Gastroenterology, *94:*1276, 1988.
30. Jacob, P., Kahrilas, P.J., and Herzon, G.: Proximal esophageal pH-metry in patients with "reflux laryngitis." Gastroenterology, *100:*305, 1991.
31. Jamieson, J.R., Stein, H.J., DeMeester, T.R., et al.: Ambulatory 24-hour esophageal pH monitoring: Normal values, optimal thresholds, specificity, sensitivity, and reproducibility. Am. J. Gastroenterol., *87:*1102, 1992.
32. Janssens, J., Vantrappen, G., and Chillibert, G.: 24-hour recording of esophageal pressure and pH in patients with non cardiac chest pain. Gastroenterology, *90:*1978, 1986.
33. Johnson, L.F., and DeMeester, T.R.: Twenty-four hour pH monitoring of the distal esophagus: A quantitative measure of gastroesophageal reflux. Am. J. Gastroenterol., *62:*325, 1974.

34. Johnson, L.F., and DeMeester, T.R.: Development of 24-hour intraesophageal pH monitoring composite scoring. J. Clin. Gastroenterol., *8:*52, 1986.
35. Johnson, L.F., and Harmon, J.W.: Experimental esophagitis in a rabbit model. J. Clin. Gastroenterol., *8*(Suppl.):26, 1986.
36. Kahrilas, P.J., Dodds, W.J., Dent, J., et al.: Upper esophageal sphincter function during deglutition. Gastroenterology, *95:*52, 1988.
37. Kahrilas, P.J., Dodds, W.J., and Hogan, W.J.: Effect of peristaltic dysfunction on esophageal volume clearance. Gastroenterology, *94:*73, 1988.
38. Kahrilas, P.J., Logemann, J.A., Shezhang, L., and Erfun, G.A.: Pharyngeal clearance during swallowing: A combined manometric and videofluoroscopic study. Gastroenterology, *103:*128, 1992.
39. Kauer, W.K.H., Burdiles, P., Ireland, A.P., et al.: Does duodenal juice reflux into the esophagus of patients with complicated GERD? Evaluation of a fiberoptic sensor for bilirubin. Am. J. Surg., *169:*98, 1995.
40. Kramer, P., and Hollander, W.: Comparison of experimental esophageal pain with clinical pain of angina pectoris and esophageal diseases. Gastroenterology, *29:*719, 1955.
41. Langmore, S.E., Schatz, K., and Olsen, N.: Fiberoptic endoscopic examination of swallowing safety: A new procedure. Dysphagia, *2:*216, 1988.
42. Lieberman-Meffert, D., Allgower, M., Schneid, P., and Blum, A.: Muscular equivalent of the esophageal sphincter. Gastroenterology, *76:*31, 1979.
43. Lydon, S.B., Dodds, W.J., Hogan, W.J., et al.: The effect of manometric assembly diameter on intraluminal esophageal pressure recording. Dig. Dis. Sci., *20:*968, 1975.
44. Marshall, J.B., Kretschmar, J.M., Gerhardt, D.C., et al.: Gastrointestinal manifestations of mixed connective tissue disease. Gastroenterology, *98:*1232, 1990.
45. Mason, R.J., Bremner, C.G., DeMeester, T.R., et al.: Pharyngeal swallowing disorders: Selection for and response to myotomy. Ann. Surg., *228:*598, 1998.
46. Massey, B.T., Doods, W.J., Hogan, W.J., et al.: Abnormal esophageal motility: An analysis of concurrent radiographic and manometric findings. Gastroenterology, *101:*344, 1991.
47. Mintchev, M.P., Kingma, Y.J., and Bowes, K.L.: Accuracy of cutaneous recordings of gastric electrical activity. Gastroenterology, *104:*1273, 1993.
48. Peters, L., Maas, L., Petty, D., et al.: Spontaneous non cardiac chest pain: Evaluation by 24-hour ambulatory esophageal motility and pH monitoring. Gastroenterology, *94:*878, 1988.
49. Price, L.M., El-Sharkawy, T.Y., Mui, H.Y., and Diamant, N.E.: Effects of bilateral cervical vagotomy on balloon-induced lower esophageal sphincter relaxation in the dog. Gastroenterology, *77:*324, 1979.
50. Richter, J.E., Hackshaw, B.T., and Wu, W.C.: Edrophonium: A useful provocative test for esophageal chest pain. Ann. Intern. Med., *103:*14, 1985.
51. Russell, C.O.H., Hill, L.D., Holmes, E.F., et al.: Radionuclide transit: A sensitive screening test for esophageal dysfunction. Gastroenterology, *80:*887, 1981.
52. Singh, S., Stein, H.J., DeMeester, T.R., and Hinder, R.A.: Nonobstructive dysphagia in gastroesophageal reflux disease—a study with combined ambulatory pH and motility monitoring. Am. J. Gastroenterol., *87:*562, 1992.
53. Skinner, D.B., and Booth, D.J.: Assessment of distal esophageal function in patients with hiatal hernia and gastroesophageal reflux. Ann. Surg., *172:*627, 1970.
54. Soffer, E.E., Scalabrini, P., and Wingate, D.L.: Spontaneous noncardiac chest pain: Value of ambulatory pH and motility monitoring. Dig. Dis. Sci., *34:*1656, 1989.
55. Stein, H.J., Barlow, A.P., DeMeester, T.R., and Hinder, R.A.: Complications of gastroesophageal reflux disease: Role of the lower esophageal sphincter, esophageal acid/alkaline exposure, and duodenogastric reflux. Ann. Surg., *216:*35, 1992.
56. Stein, H.J., and DeMeester, T.R.: Integrated 24-hour ambulatory foregut monitoring in patients with complex foregut symptoms. Surg. Ann., *24:*161, 1992.
57. Stein, H.J., and DeMeester, T.R.: Indications, technique, and clinical use of ambulatory 24-hour esophageal motility monitoring in a surgical practice. Ann. Surg., *217:*128, 1993.
58. Stein, H.J., DeMeester, T.R., Eypasch, E.P., and Klingman, R.P.: Ambulatory 24-hour esophageal manometry in the evaluation of esophageal motor disorders and noncardiac chest pain. Surgery, *110:*753, 1991.
59. Stein, H.J., DeMeester, T.R., and Hinder, R.A.: Outpatient physiologic testing and surgical management of foregut motility disorders. Curr. Probl. Surg., *29:*415, 1992.
60. Stein, H.J., DeMeester, T.R., Naspetti, R., et al.: The three-dimensional lower esophageal sphincter pressure profile in gastroesophageal reflux disease. Ann. Surg., *214:*374, 1991.
61. Stein, H.J., Feussner, H., Kauer, W., et al.: "Alkaline" gastroesophageal reflux: Assessment by ambulatory esophageal and pH monitoring. Am. J. Surg., *167:*163, 1994.
62. Stein, H.J., Hinder, R.A., DeMeester, T.R., et al.: Clinical use of 24-hour gastric pH monitoring vs. O-diisopropyl iminodiacetic acid (DISIDA) scanning in the diagnosis of pathologic duodenogastric reflux. Arch. Surg., *125:*966, 1990.
63. Steven, M.B., Hookman, P., Siegel, C.I., et al.: Aperistalsis of the esophagus in patients with connective-tissue disorders and Raynaud's phenomenon. N. Engl. J. Med., *270:*1218, 1964.
64. Tolin, R.D., Malmud, L.S., Reilley, J., and Fisher, R.S.: Esophageal scintigraphy to quantitate esophageal transit (quantitation of esophageal transit). Gastroenterology, *76:*1402, 1979.
65. Vantrappen, G., Janssens, J., Hellemans, J., and Coremans, G.: Achalasia, diffuse esophageal spasm, and related motility disorders. Gastroenterology, *76:*450, 1979.
66. Zamhost, B.J., Hirschberg, J., Ippoliti, A.F., et al.: Esophagitis in scleroderma: Prevalence and risk factors. Gastroenterology, *92:*421, 1987.
67. Zaninotto, G., DeMeester, T.R., Schwizer, W., et al.: The lower esophageal sphincter in health and disease. Am. J. Surg., *155:*104, 1988.

CHAPTER

7 Endoscopic Esophageal Ultrasonography

THOMAS W. RICE • GREGORY ZUCCARO, JR.

Endoscopic esophageal ultrasonography (EUS) has extended the endoscopic examination of the esophagus beyond the mucosa into the esophageal wall and periesophageal tissues. The diagnostic capabilities of surface ultrasound have been broadened by the endoscopic placement of ultrasound transducers adjacent to the gastrointestinal mucosa. These transducers, operating at relatively high frequencies, provide a detailed examination of the esophageal wall and surrounding tissues. EUS is the most significant advance in the diagnosis of esophageal disease since the introduction of flexible fiberoptic endoscopy. These intracorporeal examinations have proved beneficial in the diagnosis and treatment of both benign and malignant diseases of the esophagus and periesophageal tissues.

FUNDAMENTALS OF ULTRASONOGRAPHY

Sound waves are produced by the vibration of a source within a medium. The vibration produces cyclic compression and rarefaction (expansion) of the molecules in the medium, thus transmitting the sound wave through the medium. The number of cycles (compression and rarefaction) of a sound wave occurring in 1 second is the frequency and is measured in hertz (Hz). The frequency of sound waves audible to the human ear is between 20 and 20,000 Hz. Sound waves with frequencies higher than these (20,000 Hz) are ultrasound waves. The frequencies used in medical ultrasound imaging range from 1 million to 20 million Hz (1 to 20 MHz).

Ultrasound waves may be produced by the electrical excitation of a piezoelectric crystal. The application of a voltage across a crystal causes it to deform. Alternating electrical energy vibrates the crystal and produces sound waves. If a sound wave deforms a crystal, electrical energy is produced. It is this ability to convert electrical energy into sound energy and conversely to convert sound energy into electrical energy that allows these crystals to function as both transmitters and receivers (i.e., as *transducers*). These transducers are responsive to a limited range of frequencies; hence, more than one transducer may be required for an ultrasound examination.

The speed of a sound wave within a medium (tissue) is defined by the following relationship:

$$V = (K/p)^{1/2}$$

where V is the velocity of the sound wave, K is the bulk modulus of the tissue (a measure of stiffness), and p is the density of the tissue.

The resistance to passage of a wave through tissue is called the acoustic impedance (Z), which is defined by the following relationship:

$$Z = pV = (pK)^{1/2}$$

Sound waves travel best through dense or elastic tissues. Absorption of some of the energy of an ultrasound wave will occur as the wave passes through tissue. The amount of absorption is determined by tissue characteristics and the frequency of the sound wave. The higher the frequency, the greater the absorption.

The interactions that occur as a sound wave encounters different tissues are critical to the diagnostic capabilities of ultrasound. As a sound wave passes from one tissue to the next, a portion of the wave is transmitted into the new tissue and a portion is reflected. This reflected wave is received by the transducer and processed, providing the diagnostic information of ultrasound. The difference in acoustic impedance between the two tissues and the angle at which the sound wave enters the new medium (angle of incidence) determine the portion of the wave that is reflected and the portion that is transmitted. When there are similar acoustic impedances, most of the wave is transmitted. Soft tissues have excellent transmission qualities, and the density and velocity vary only by 12 to 14% among different soft tissues. Because the acoustic impedance is the product of velocity and density, the product of these small changes results in a 22% difference in the acoustic impedance between fat and muscle.[39] Useless bright echo images are obtained when an ultrasound wave encounters air or bone. Air is very compressible and has a low density, whereas bone, although dense, has a low compressibility and a high reflectivity. These properties account for the poor transmission of ultrasound waves from tissue to air or tissue to bone. The amount of reflected sound is also related to the angle of incidence; as the angle of incidence increases, less sound is reflected. In addition, sound waves are bent as they travel from one tissue to the next. This process is call *refraction*.

As a sound wave passes through tissue, a portion of its energy is lost; this process is called *attenuation*. Absorption, reflection, and refraction are major sources of energy loss. Some of the ultrasound wave is also lost by the process of scattering (diffusion). Scattering occurs when a sound wave encounters heterogeneous tissue. Tiny particles within tissue (such as fat in muscle) that are smaller than the ultrasound wavelength scatter the ultrasound wave. Attenuation increases as more tissues are encountered and as the wave travels farther from the source. Therefore, if the returning ultrasound wave is not processed, the same tissue would be imaged differently depending on its distance from the transducer. The intensity of the returning waves must be amplified (gain) to ensure that distant waves are correctly represented. Attenuation increases as ultrasound frequency increases.

Resolution is the ability to discriminate between different tissues with ultrasound waves. Depth or axial resolution is the ability to differentiate between two tissues along the path of the ultrasound wave. Lateral resolution is the ability to distinguish between adjacent tissues. Transducer characteristics and focusing determine resolution. Higher frequencies allow for better resolution but resultant decreased tissue penetration.

Pulse-echo technique is used in endoscopic ultrasonography. Ultrasound waves are emitted for a brief period, followed by a subsequent listening period during which the reflected ultrasound waves are received. The returning sound waves are displayed so that the brightness is proportional to the amplitude of the returning ultrasound waves. This is known as *B-mode ultrasonography.* Because the amplitude is presented in a range from white to gray to black, the display is also termed *gray-scale ultrasound.* Individual scans are shown at a rate at which the eye cannot detect single images (12/sec). This fast frame display is called *real-time ultrasound* and allows the ultrasonographer to study tissue temporally as well as spatially.

INSTRUMENTS AND TECHNIQUES

Because EUS provides an inadequate endoscopic inspection of the upper gastrointestinal tract, every ultrasound study should be preceded by a standard flexible endoscopic upper gastrointestinal examination. This provides precise location and mucosal definition (including biopsy) of the esophageal lesion and guides the ultrasound examination. Intravenous administration of a narcotic, such as meperidine, and a benzodiazepine, such as midazolam, usually provides adequate sedation. The ultrasound endoscope is generally passed blindly through the oropharynx and hypopharynx. Care must be taken because the distal tip containing the transducer is rigid. For complete examination, the endoscope must be passed beyond the esophagus and into the stomach.

The radial mechanical ultrasound endoscope (Fig. 7–1) is the principal instrument used for EUS. The ultrasound transducer is housed in the tip of the endoscope. It rotates at a speed of 7 revolutions per minute and produces a 360-degree sector scan perpendicular to the transducer tip. Because the transducer is adjacent to the tissues to be examined, higher frequencies than those used in extracorporeal ultrasound can be employed. In most models, two frequencies are available. One transducer images at 7.5 MHz and the other at 12 MHz. The 7.5-MHz transducer allows adequate study to a depth of 4 to 5 cm, whereas the 12-MHz transducer allows study to a depth of 1 to 2 cm. An acceptable acoustic interface between the transducer and the tissue being examined must be obtained to ensure good-quality ultrasound images. This is most commonly accomplished by covering the tip of the endoscope with a latex balloon, which can be filled with water to provide an excellent acoustic interface (see Fig. 7–1). A less commonly employed technique is the rapid insufflation of the esophageal lumen with water. This provides an excellent (but transient) acoustic interface without the tissue compression that can occur with the latex balloon. Located behind the transducer is the fiberoptic endoscope tip. This endoscope provides a limited field of view in a forward oblique direction. A 2-mm suction channel is oriented at this oblique angle.

The control section contains the deflection controls

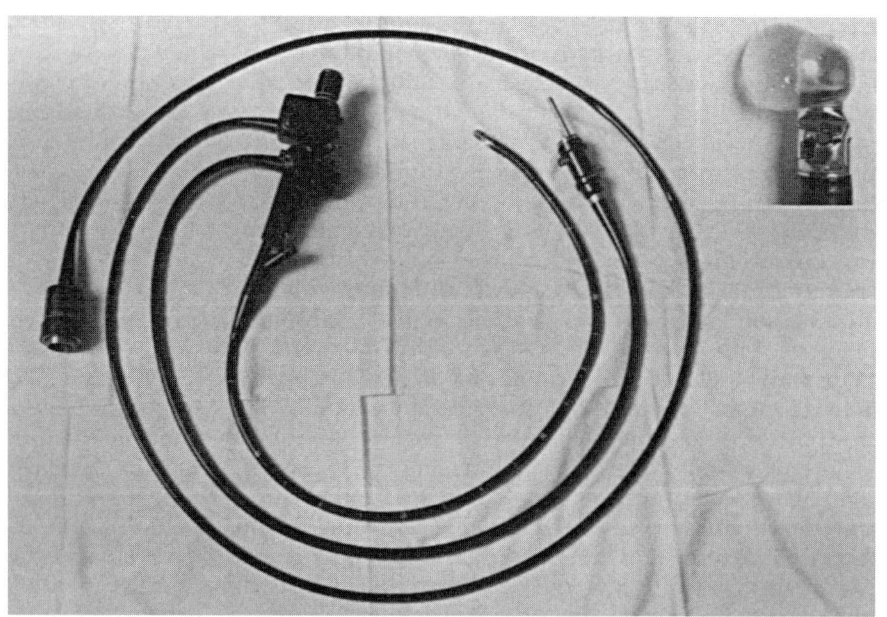

Figure 7–1. The Olympus GF-UM20 ultrasound endoscope. *Upper inset,* The distal tip of the ultrasound endoscope with the water-inflated contact balloon, which covers the ultrasound transducer. The forward oblique viewing endoscope and suction channel are proximal to the ultrasound transducer.

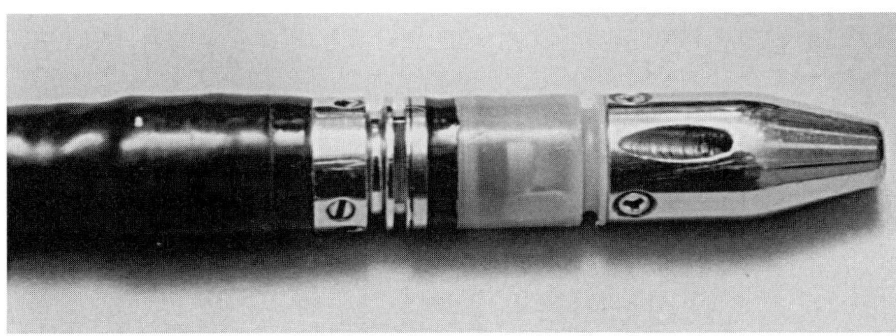

Figure 7–2. The radial mechanical blind probe. The tip is tapered, allowing for passage through tight strictures. The radial ultrasound transducer is positioned behind the tapered tip.

and air-water and suction valves similar to those on a standard endoscope (see Fig. 7-1). A water inflation-deflation system for the balloon is incorporated into the air-water and suction valve mechanisms. A DC motor and drive mechanism, which rotates the ultrasound transducer, are housed in the control section. Current ultrasound endoscopes are totally immersible.

The radial mechanical blind probe (Fig. 7-2) is available for the evaluation of esophageal strictures. This echoendoscope provides images similar to other larger-diameter radial mechanical echoendoscopes but has no endoscopic optical capabilities. Therefore, the instrument is less than 8 mm in diameter.

These instruments are used in conjunction with an image processor (Fig. 7-3). The controls of the image processor allow adjustment of gain, contrast, and sensitivity time control, which regulates the strength of the returning echo at different depths. On-screen calibration and labeling can be done with the image processor. The image may be displayed on a video monitor or stored in a computer, on videotape, or on Polaroid film. The image processor has been refined and miniaturized with successive generations of endoscopic ultrasound equipment. The current models are rack mounted and weigh about 80 lb.

The curvilinear electronic echoendoscope (Fig. 7-4), in contrast to the radial mechanical scanner, produces a field slightly more than 100 degrees in an oblique forward direction. It uses transducers with 5 and/or 7.5 MHz scanning frequencies, or both, allowing a 5 to 10 cm depth of penetration. This has several advantages: this system can provide color Doppler, and it allows direct visualization of cytology needles passed into and beyond the esophageal wall.

The availability of these two systems (radial mechanical and electronic linear) has increased the accuracy, but also the complexity, of EUS. For diagnostic purposes, the radial mechanical scanner is preferable because it allows a 360-degree view. Therefore, this echoendoscope system remains the "workhorse" of EUS. When a tissue sample for cytologic evaluation is required, however, the radial mechanical scanner does not allow safe directed passage of a needle into the esophageal wall or adjacent tissue. Therefore, a second instrument, the electronic linear echoendoscope, powered by a separate costly system, is employed for these purposes. It is possible to perform both diagnosis and fine-needle aspiration (FNA) with the electronic linear echoendoscope alone, but the limitation in viewing field requires significant torque on the insertion tube to image the esophageal wall and adjacent tissues in 360 degrees.

ULTRASOUND ANATOMY

The normal esophagus is usually viewed as five discrete layers by EUS (Fig. 7-5). These layers are seen as alternating hyperechoic (white) and hypoechoic (black) rings. Studies have demonstrated that the five layers seen by EUS correspond to the balloon-mucosa interface, the

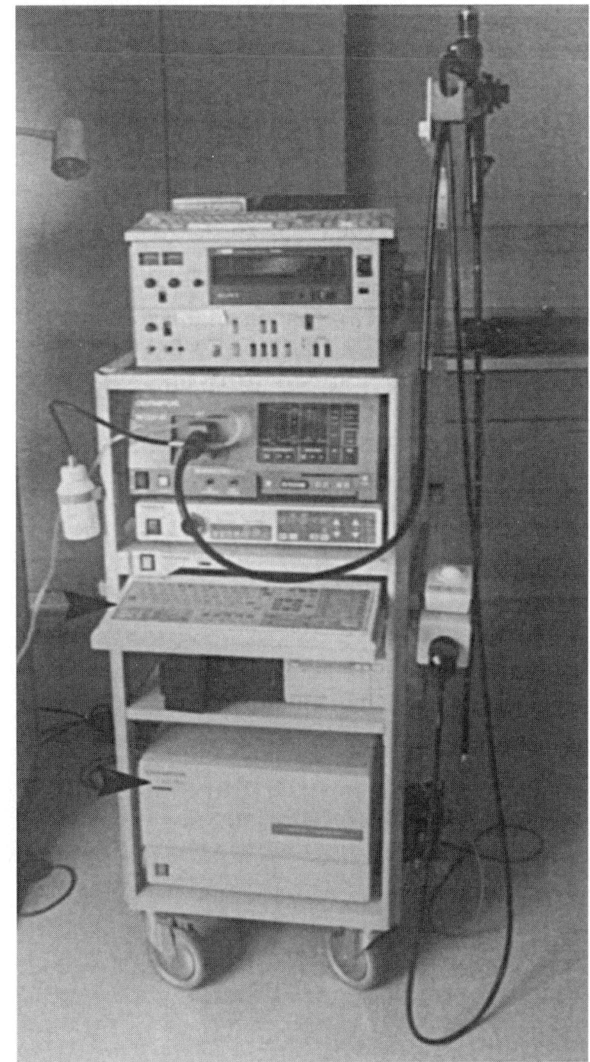

Figure 7–3. The Olympus EU-M20 image processor *(lower arrow)* is rack-mounted in a standard cart, which includes the other essential endoscopic equipment. The keyboard *(upper arrow)* can be used to measure and mark ultrasound findings.

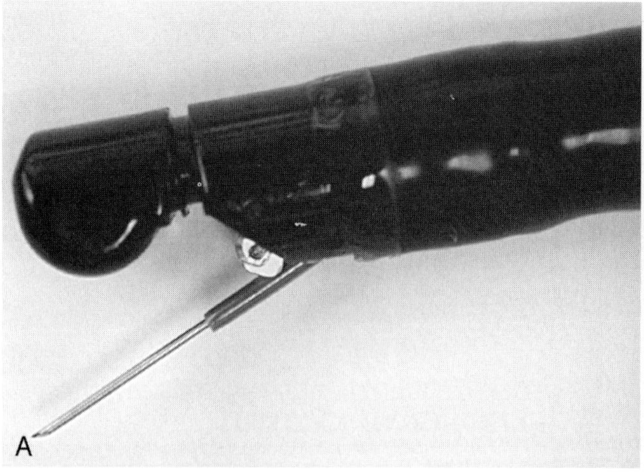

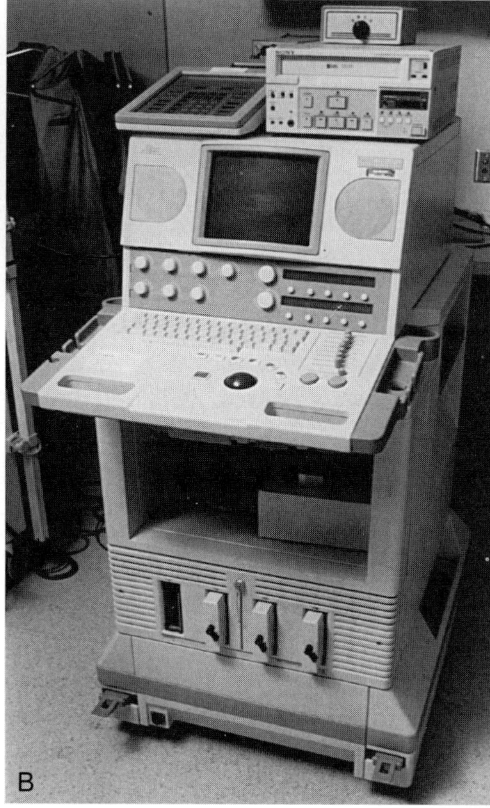

Figure 7–4. The curvilinear electronic endoscope *(A)* and image processor *(B)*. The optics and operating channel, through which a fine needle is passed, are positioned behind the linear ultrasound transducer. This echoendoscope requires a separate image processor.

mucosa deep to this interface, the submucosa and the acoustic interface between the submucosa and muscularis propria, the muscularis propria minus the acoustic interface between the submucosa and the muscularis propria, and the periesophageal tissue.[6,38] For clinical purposes, these layers represent the superficial mucosa, the deep mucosa, the submucosa, the muscularis propria, and the periesophageal tissue. In the upper esophagus, with overdistention of the examining balloon, or if the transducer is too close to the esophageal wall, only three layers of the esophageal wall may be apparent on the ultrasound image: the superficial mucosa, deep mucosa, and submucosa compose one hyperechoic layer. The thickness of each layer is about equal and does not repre-

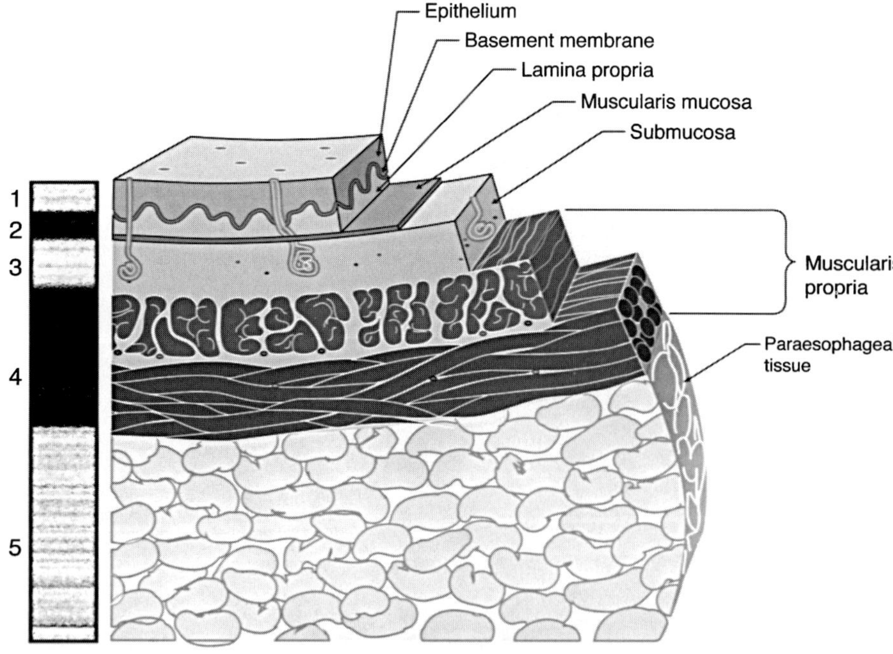

Figure 7–5. The esophageal wall is visualized as five alternating layers of differing echogenicity by esophageal ultrasound. The first layer, which is hyperechoic (white), represents the superficial mucosa (epithelium and lamina propria). The second layer, which is hypoechoic (black), represents the deep mucosa (muscularis mucosa). The third layer, which is hyperechoic (white), represents the submucosa. The fourth layer, which is black (hypoechoic), represents the muscularis propria. The fifth layer, which is hyperechoic (white) is the paraesophageal tissue.

sent the thickness of the tissue layer but instead represents the time it takes the ultrasound wave to traverse this layer.

ESOPHAGEAL CARCINOMA

The stage of an esophageal carcinoma, as defined by its anatomic extent, is the best predictor of outcome available for patients with esophageal carcinoma. Recent refinements in the staging of esophageal carcinoma have resulted in the present staging system, which is TNM based[20] (Table 7-1). The primary tumor (T) is defined only by the depth of invasion; EUS is ideally suited for this determination. T1 tumors are confined to the submucosa or more superficial esophageal layers. T2 tumors invade into but do not breach the muscularis propria. T3 tumors invade beyond the esophageal wall and into the paraesophageal tissue but do not invade adjacent structures. T4 tumors directly invade structures in the vicinity of the esophagus.

Regional lymph nodes (N) are characterized only by the presence or absence of metastases in lymph nodes in the area of the primary tumor. Regional lymph nodes are characterized by the presence (N1) or absence (N0) of metastases. Similarly, distant sites (M) are characterized by the presence (M1) or absence (M0) of metastases. The recent revision of the staging system for esophageal carcinoma subdivides distant metastatic carcinomas (M1) into M1a (distant, nonregional lymph node metastases) and M1b (other distant metastases).[20] M1a disease is further classified by tumor location; M1a tumors of the upper thoracic esophagus have metastasized to cervical nodes, and M1a tumors of the lower thoracic esophagus have metastasized to celiac lymph nodes. There is no M1a subdivision for midthoracic esophageal carcinomas because tumors in this location metastatic to nonregional lymph nodes have an equivalent prognosis as those metastatic to other distant sites. These TNM descriptors are grouped into stages with similar behavior and prognosis (see Table 7-1).

EUS may be used at two different periods in the course of esophageal carcinoma. The staging examination may be done before (clinical stage) or after (retreatment stage) treatment.

Table 7-1. TNM Staging of Esophageal Carcinomas

T: Primary Tumor

TX	Tumor cannot be assessed.
T0	No evidence of tumor
Tis	High-grade dysplasia
T1	Tumor invades the lamina propria, muscularis mucosa or submucosa. It does not breach the submucosa.
T2	Tumor invades into and not beyond the muscularis propria.
T3	Tumor invades the paraesophageal tissue, but does not invade adjacent structures.
T4	Tumor invades adjacent structures.

N: Regional Lymph Nodes

NX	Regional lymph nodes cannot be assessed.
N0	No regional lymph node metastases
N1	Regional lymph node metastases

M: Distant Metastasis

MX	Distant metastases cannot be assessed.
M1a	Upper thoracic esophagus metastatic to cervical lymph nodes Lower thoracic esophagus metastatic to celiac lymph nodes
M1b	Upper thoracic esophagus metastatic to other nonregional lymph nodes or other distant sites Midthoracic esophagus metastatic to either nonregional lymph nodes or other distant sites Lower thoracic esophagus metastatic to other nonregional lymph nodes or other distant sites

Stage Groupings

Stage 0	Tis	N0	M0
Stage I	T1	N0	M0
Stage IIA	T2	N0	M0
	T3	N0	M0
Stage IIB	T1	N1	M0
	T2	N1	M0
Stage III	T3	N1	M0
	T4	Any N	M0
Stage IVA	Any T	Any N	M1a
Stage IVB	Any T	Any N	M1b

Clinical Stage

The detailed images of the esophageal wall provided by EUS make it the most accurate modality available for determination of depth of tumor invasion (T) before treatment[7,14,28,67,71,79] (Figs. 7-6 to 7-8). The same definition of the esophageal wall is not offered by computed tomography (CT). The thickened esophageal wall, the principal CT finding in esophageal carcinoma, is not specific for esophageal carcinoma and lacks the definition required to distinguish T1, T2, and T3 tumors.[54]

In the differentiation of T3 from T4 tumors, EUS is superior to CT (Fig. 7-9). The evaluation of fat planes is used to define local invasion at CT examination. The obliteration or lack of fat planes is not sensitive in the prediction of local invasion, but the preservation of these planes is specific for the absence of T4 disease.[12,17,35,40,45,55,61,65] Compared with CT, EUS provides a more sensitive and reliable determination of vascular involvement.[25]

Experience with both examination technique and ultrasound interpretation is critical to determine depth of tumor invasion accurately. Seventy-five to 100 examinations are required before competence is obtained.[22,63] In a review of 21 series, the accuracy of EUS for T determination was 84%.[59] Accuracy is not constant and varies with T stage. In this meta-analysis, accuracy for T1 carcinomas was 83.5%, with 16.5% of tumors overstaged; accuracy for T2 was 73%, with 10% understaged and 17% overstaged; accuracy for T3 was 89%, with 5% understaged and 6% overstaged; and accuracy for T4 was 89%, with 11% understaged.[59] A review of the literature shows variation in accuracy with T stage: 75 to 82% for T1, 64 to 85% for T2, 89 to 94% for T3, and 88 to 100% for T4.[62]

Esophageal obstruction caused by a malignant high-grade stricture prohibits staging in 19 to 63% of examinations.[13,29,79] Failure to pass an ultrasound probe beyond a

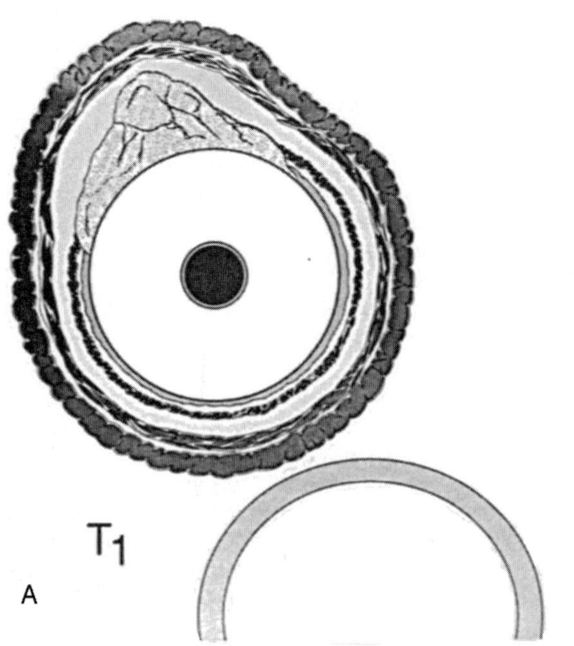

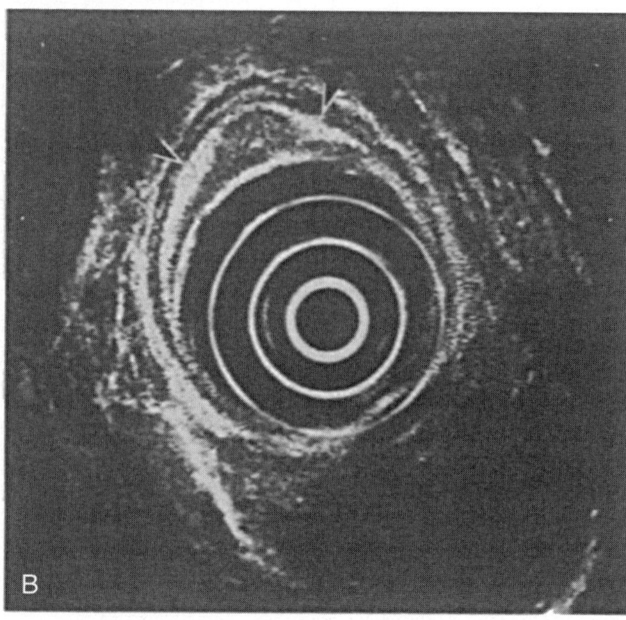

Figure 7-6. *A*, A T1 tumor invades but does not breach the submucosa. *B*, A T1 tumor as seen on esophageal ultrasound. The hypoechoic (black) tumor invades the hyperechoic (white) third ultrasound layer (submucosa) but does not breach the boundary between the third and fourth layers *(arrows)*. (From Rice, T.W., Boyce, G.A., Sivak, M.V., Jr., et al.: Esophageal ultrasound and the preoperative staging of carcinoma of the esophagus. J. Thorac. Cardiovasc. Surg., *101*:536, 1991, with permission.)

malignant stricture is an accurate predictor of advanced stage. More than 90% of these patients have stage III or IV disease.[69] Limited examination of the tumor above the stricture has variable accuracy but may be useful in staging if T3 or N1 disease is seen. Dilation of malignant strictures followed by EUS examination is associated with an increased incidence of perforation.[69] However, it allowed complete examination in 42% of patients with malignant strictures.[36] As an alternative to stricture dilation before EUS, the radial mechanical blind probe (see Fig. 7-3) may be passed with fluoroscopic guidance over a guidewire through most malignant strictures. If suspicious adenopathy is detected distal to the stricture, the endoscopist may consider dilation to facilitate passage of the curvilinear endoscope and allow FNA of the node. If no suspicious adenopathy is detected, the patient is not subjected to the risk of dilation. The problem of staging malignant strictures may be overcome by the use of

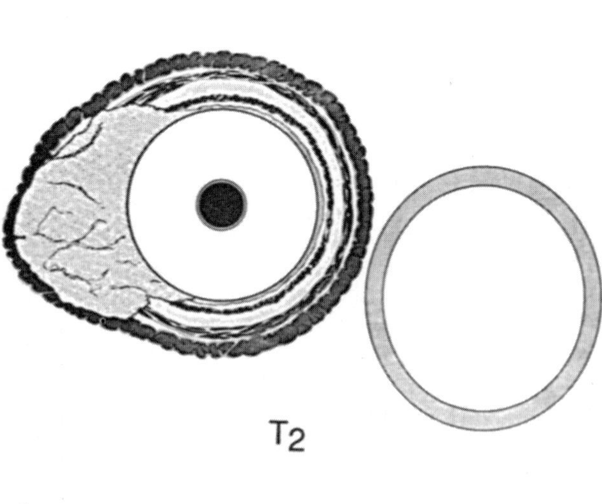

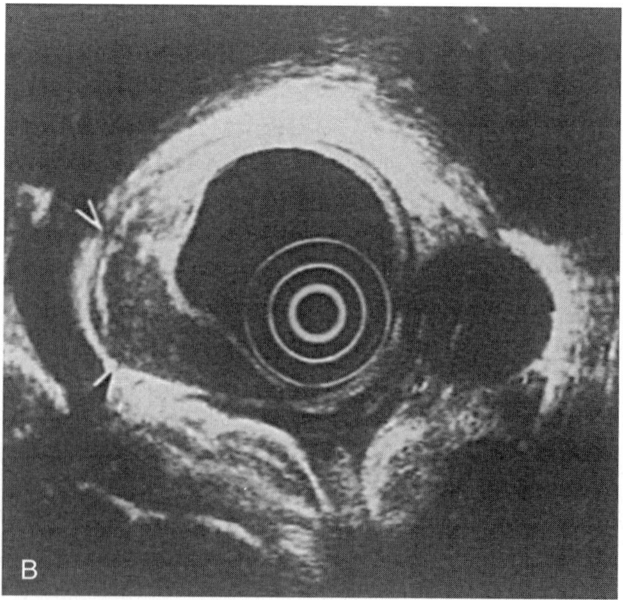

Figure 7-7. *A*, A T2 tumor invades but does not breach the muscularis propria. *B*, A T2 tumor as seen on esophageal ultrasound. The hypoechoic (black) tumor invades the hypoechoic (black) fourth ultrasound layer but does not breach the boundary between the forth and fifth layers *(arrows)*. (From Rice, T.W., Boyce, G.A., Sivak, M.V. Jr., et al.: Esophageal ultrasound and the preoperative staging of carcinoma of the esophagus. J. Thorac. Cardiovasc. Surg., *101*:536, 1991, with permission.)

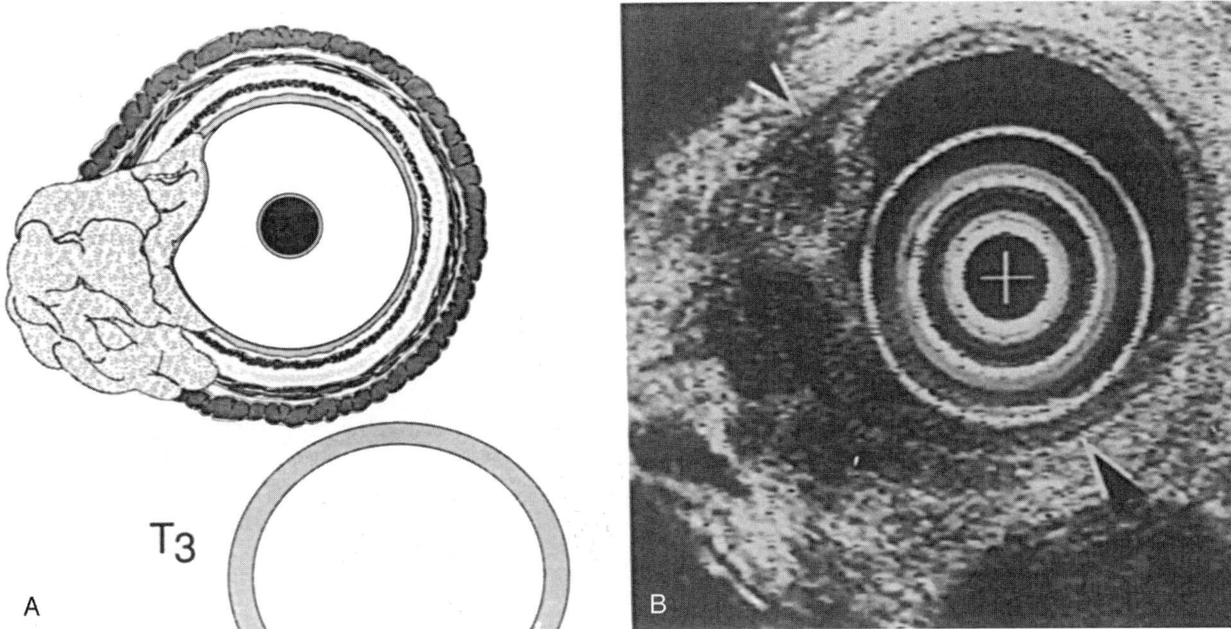

Figure 7–8. *A*, A T3 tumor invades the periesophageal tissue but does not involve adjacent structures. *B*, A T3 tumor as seen on esophageal ultrasound. The hypoechoic (black) tumor breaches the boundary between the fourth and fifth ultrasound layers *(arrows)* and invades the hyperechoic (white) fifth ultrasound layer (periesophageal tissue).

miniature ultrasound catheter probes. Passed through the biopsy channel of an esophagoscope and advanced through the stricture, these 20-MHz probes have accurately determined T stage in 85 to 90% of patients.[5,31,46,47] A limitation of these probes is their poor depth of penetration, such that lymph node status may not be accurately assessed.

Determination of N Status and Nonregional Lymph Node Status

In addition to size, EUS evaluates nodal shape, border, and internal echo characteristics in regional lymph node assessment (Fig. 7–10). Large (more than 1 cm), round, hypoechoic, nonhomogeneous, sharply bordered lymph

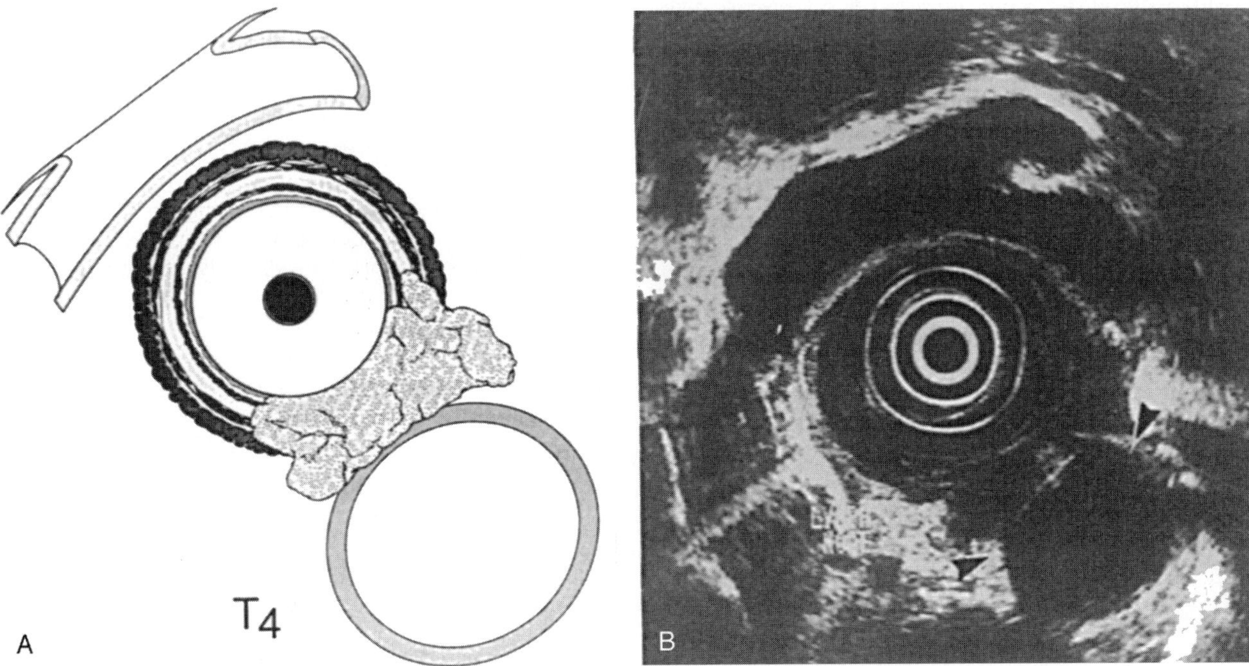

Figure 7–9. *A*, A T4 tumor invades the aorta. *B*, A T4 tumor as seen on esophageal ultrasound. The hypoechoic (black) tumor invades the aorta. The tumor breaches the boundary between the periesophageal tissue and the aorta *(arrows)*. (From Rice, T.W., Boyce, G.A., and Sivak, M.V., Jr.: Esophageal ultrasound and the preoperative staging of carcinoma of the esophagus. J. Thorac. Cardiovasc. Surg., *101*:536, 1991, with permission.)

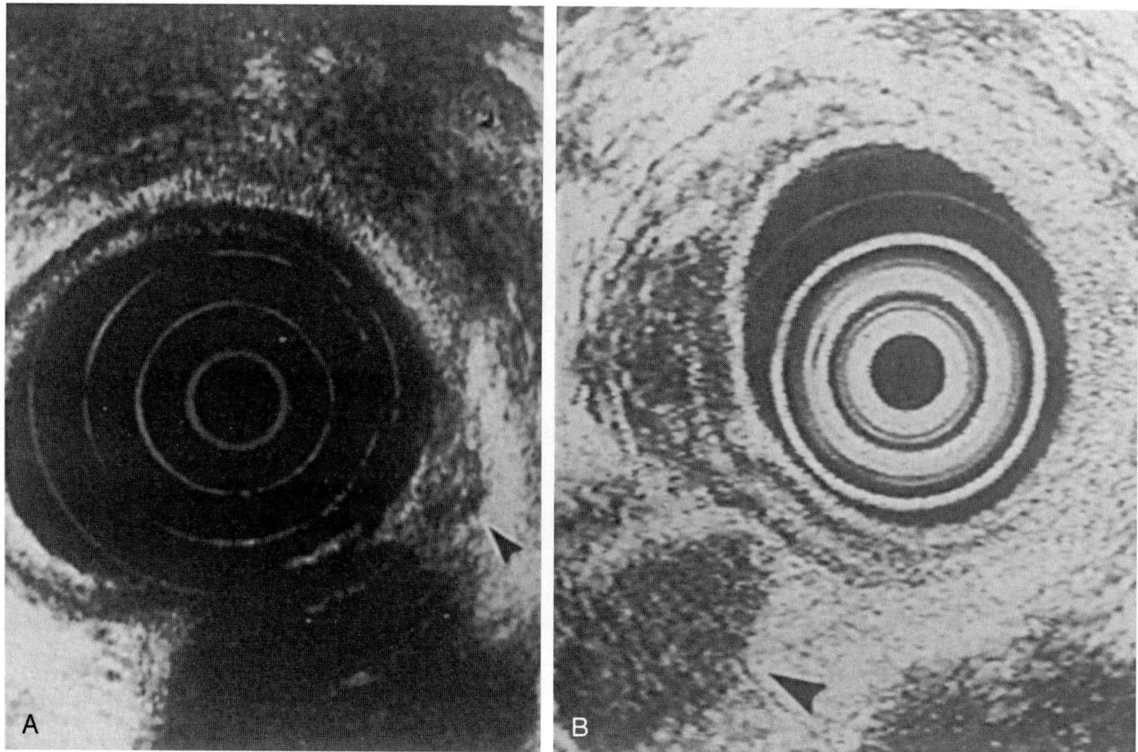

Figure 7-10. *A*, A N0 node *(arrow)* as seen on esophageal ultrasound (EUS). The node is 5 mm in diameter, has an ill-defined border, and a hyperechoic (white) internal structure. *B*, A N1 node *(arrow)* as seen on EUS. The large node, 12 mm in diameter, has a sharply demarcated border. The internal structure is hypoechoic (black) and is similar to that of the primary tumor. (From Rice, T.W., Boyce, G.A., and Sivak, M.V., Jr.: Esophageal ultrasound and the preoperative staging of carcinoma of the esophagus. J. Thorac. Cardiovasc. Surg., *101*:536, 1991, with permission.)

nodes are more likely malignant; small, oval or angular, hyperechoic, homogeneous lymph nodes with indistinct borders are more likely benign. In a retrospective review of 100 EUS examinations, the EUS determination of N stage was 89% sensitive, 75% specific, and 84% accurate.[9] The positive predictive value of EUS for N1 disease was 86%; the negative predictive value was 79%. A patient was 24 times more likely to have N1 disease if EUS detected regional lymph nodes. The single most sensitive predictor in detecting N1 was a hypoechoic internal echo pattern, followed by a sharp border, a round shape, and finally size greater than 1 cm. When all four factors are present, the accuracy of N1 detection is 80 to 100%.[4,9] Unfortunately, all four features are present in only 25% of N1 node.[4] In a meta-analysis of 21 series, the accuracy of EUS determination of N stage was 77%; for N0, 69%; and for N1, 89%.[59] The ability to use EUS to diagnose nodal metastases varies with location. It is better in the assessment of celiac nodes (accuracy, 95%; sensitivity, 83%; specificity, 98%; positive predictive value, 91%; negative predictive value, 97%) than in mediastinal nodes (accuracy, 73%; sensitivity, 79%; specificity, 63%; positive predictive value, 79%; and negative predictive value, 63%).[11]

Another predictor of N1 disease is close proximity of the regional node to the primary tumor. Comparison of the echo characteristic of the tumor and regional lymph nodes is useful for EUS lymph node evaluation. The relationship of T to N1 must be considered during EUS examinations. The incidence of N1 disease increases with deeper tumor invasion: for a patient with a poorly differentiated adenocarcinoma, the probability of N1 disease is 17% for T1 tumors, 55% for T2, 83% for T3, and 88% for T4.[58] In T3 and T4 carcinomas, an EUS assessment of N0 does not ensure absence of N1 disease.

Endosonography-directed fine-needle aspiration (EUS FNA) further refines clinical staging by adding tissue sampling to endosonography findings[73,74] (Fig. 7-11). In a multicenter study, 171 patients had EUS FNA of 192 lymph nodes.[75] The accuracy of EUS FNA in determination of lymph node status was as follows: sensitivity, 92%; specificity, 93%; positive predictive value, 100%; and negative predictive value, 86%. Two to three needle passes were made of each node. There was one nonfatal complication: an esophageal perforation at dilation of an esophageal stricture before EUS FNA. The combination of EUS and EUS FNA of celiac lymph nodes deemed positive by EUS had a sensitivity of 72%, a specificity of 97%, a positive predictive value of 95%, and a negative predictive value of 82%.[53] FNA confirmed positive EUS M1a disease in 88% of patients.

Determination of Non-nodal M1b Status

EUS has limited value in the screening for distant metastases (M1b). The distant organ must be in direct contact with the upper gastrointestinal tract for EUS to be useful (e.g., the left lateral segment of the liver and retroperitoneum are two such sites) (Fig. 7-12).

Retreatment Stage

After induction therapy, a subset of patients with esophageal cancer will be disease free. Because there are signifi-

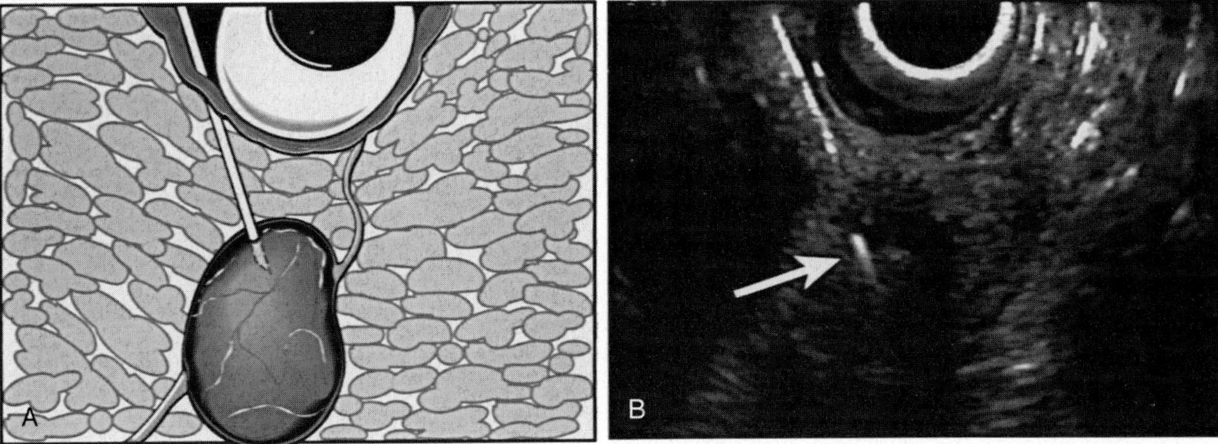

Figure 7–11. Esophageal ultrasound fine-needle aspiration of an N1 regional lymph node. *A*, An N1 regional lymph node undergoing FNA under curvilinear electronic endoscopic examination. *B*, Ultrasound image with needle *(arrow)* passed through the esophageal wall and into the N1 node.

cant morbidity and mortality associated with surgery for esophageal cancer, the ability to detect patients who have no residual cancer (T0 N0) after induction therapy is desirable. Esophageal ultrasonography has been applied in multiple clinical series for this purpose. Early series indicated that EUS was very accurate in determining T stage after chemotherapy. In these series, however, the presurgical therapy was largely ineffective in causing pathologic downstaging; therefore, EUS was accurate by merely indicating that no significant change had occurred.[1,30,60] In two earlier series in which radiation therapy was provided along with chemotherapy, accuracy of determination of T stage was again high (72 to 78%), but the prevalence of pathologic T0 disease was low or not reported.[16,24] Therefore, accuracy of T determination can again be attributed primarily to a lack of tumor response to chemoradiotherapy.

Later series incorporate more aggressive regimens of chemoradiotherapy, with higher rates of significant downstaging of tumor and pathologic T0, N0 disease. In these series, up to 31% of patients had pathologic T0, N0 disease after chemoradiotherapy.[80] EUS was poor at accurately determining T stage, with reported rates of 37 to 47%.[34,43,80] The most common mistake made in determining T stage was overstaging because EUS is unable to distinguish tumor from inflammation and fibrosis produced by chemoradiotherapy. Similar difficulties in distinguishing tumor from postchemoradiotherapy inflammation and fibrosis have also been reported with EUS staging of rectal cancers.[21]

EUS accuracy for N stage after chemoradiotherapy has been reported in only two clinical series. Both series show remarkably similar results, with reported accuracy of 64 to 71%.[43,80] The accuracy of N stage determination

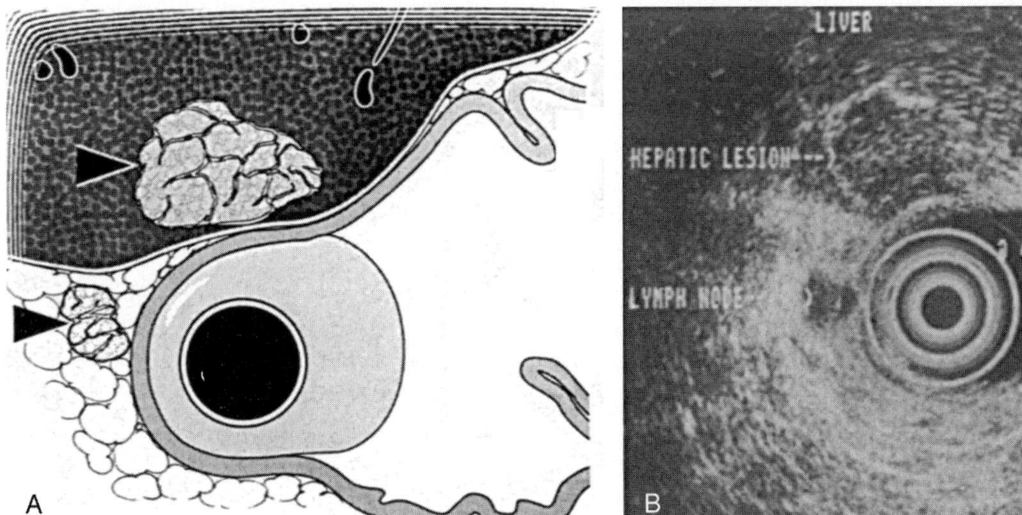

Figure 7–12. *A*, A hepatic metastasis *(upper arrow)* in the left lateral segment of the liver. The esophageal ultrasound probe is seen in the gastric cardia. *B*, A hepatic metastasis *(upper arrow)* as seen from the gastric cardia by esophageal ultrasound. The metastasis was imaged only by esophageal ultrasound. (From Rice, T.W., Boyce, G.A., Sivak, M.V., et al.: Esophageal carcinoma: Esophageal ultrasound assessment of preoperative chemotherapy. Ann. Thorac. Surg., 53:972, 1992, with permission.)

after chemoradiotherapy is lower than that of initial determination. This is because of an alteration in ultrasound appearance of nodes after chemoradiotherapy such that the established EUS criteria do not apply and because of residual foci of cancer within the nodes that are too small for detection by any modality other than pathologic analysis.

EUS has been useful in the diagnosis and restaging of patients with anastomotic recurrences that are not endoscopically visible.[10,44]

BENIGN ESOPHAGEAL DISEASES

The detailed examination of the esophageal wall provided by EUS has improved the diagnosis of benign esophageal tumors. EUS identification of intramural masses relies on both the layer from which the tumor arises (Table 7-2) and the ultrasound characteristics of the tumor. Homogeneous lesions that are anechoic, of intermediate echogenicity, or hyperechoic are almost exclusively benign.[37] A heterogeneous echo pattern may be seen in benign tumors, but this endosonographic finding, particularly in lesions greater than 3 to 4 cm in largest diameter, may be indicative of malignancy.

Cysts are echo free, rounded, and sometimes septated.[77] Lipomas are homogeneous, intensely hyperechoic lesions. Lipomas can often be recognized by endoscopy alone because they frequently have a yellow tint and are soft and pliable when probed. Granular cell tumors are typically found in the third ultrasound layer and may be hypoechoic or of intermediate echogenicity but generally are less hyperechoic than lipomas.[26,49,66] Unlike lipomas, granular cell tumors are firm to the touch and can be diagnosed by routine endoscopic biopsy. The most common benign esophageal tumors are smooth muscle tumors of the distal esophagus; in our practice, more than 70% of patients with benign intramural esophageal tumors referred for EUS have such smooth muscle tumors. Radiography reveals these lesions as smooth filling defects, endoscopy reveals normal overlying mucosa, and EUS displays hypoechoic tumors arising from the fourth ultrasound layer (muscularis propria) (Fig. 7-13). Because routine endoscopic biopsy specimens reveal only normal overlying squamous mucosa, EUS is the most helpful test in establishing the nature of the lesion. If a malignancy is suspected, FNA can be performed with EUS or endoscopic guidance.[8,74] This intervention is seldom necessary because the diagnosis can be established by EUS alone. EUS findings that suggest malignant degeneration are size larger than 4 cm, irregular borders, mixed internal echo pattern, or associated lymphadenopathy.[68]

Table 7-2. Endosonographic Classification of Esophageal Tumors

Endoscopic Ultrasound	Esophageal Tumor
First/second (mucosa/deep mucosa)	Fibrovascular polyp Retention cyst Squamous papilloma Tis esophageal cancer
Third (submucosa)	Lipoma Fibroma Neurofibroma Granular cell tumor T1 esophageal cancer
Fourth	Leiomyoma* T2 esophageal cancer

*Leiomyomas may also arise from the second ultrasound layer (muscularis mucosa), but these tumors arise much more commonly from the fourth ultrasound layer.

Esophageal varices have the typical appearance of blood vessels at EUS. They appear as tubular, round, or serpiginous echo-free structures. They may be visualized within the submucosal layer of the esophageal wall or in tissues adjacent to the esophagus (Fig. 7-14). These EUS patterns change after sclerosis.[76] Intravariceal sclerosis fills the varix with echogenic material, representing thrombus. Paravariceal injection leads to obliteration of the varix with hypoechoic extravariceal thickening.

The EUS findings in achalasia are controversial. Some authors have reported thickened esophageal wall in most patients examined.[3,15] However, this excessive thickening may be artifactual. In a dilated and convoluted esophagus, the ultrasound transducer may orient at an angle oblique to the esophageal wall, giving a false appearance of wall thickening.[19] The main role of EUS in achalasia is to exclude other mural abnormalities.[2,51,78]

EUS has not been helpful in the surveillance of patients with columnar-lined esophagus. The mucosal definition provided by EUS cannot differentiate dysplasia from intramucosal carcinoma.[18,72]

PARAESOPHAGEAL DISEASES

EUS has been used to examine mediastinal lymph nodes in patients with bronchogenic carcinoma.[22,41,42,52] In this setting, EUS has a reported positive predictive value of 77%, a negative predictive value of 93%, and an overall accuracy of 92%, using criteria similar to those used for regional lymph node evaluation in esophageal carcinoma.[42] However, anatomic constraints limit its usefulness for evaluation of lymph nodes in proximity to the airway. EUS-directed FNA provides cytologic differentiation between benign and malignant lymphadenopathy.[48] EUS-directed FNA has successfully diagnosed solid lesions of the mediastinum and lung.[23,32,33,50]

EUS has proved useful in the diagnosis of foregut cysts[56,70] (Fig. 7-15). These cysts are generally hypoechoic and located outside the esophageal wall. They may occasionally be found within the esophageal wall. If foregut cysts contain proteinaceous material, they may have a hyperechoic or an inhomogeneous (hyperechoic and hypoechoic) ultrasound appearance. Extrinsic esophageal compression may also be characterized with EUS.[64] However, examination of structures distant from the esophagus is best performed with transducers of lower frequencies. Transesophageal cardiac ultrasound provides better definition of these structures using probes with frequencies of 3 to 5 MHz.

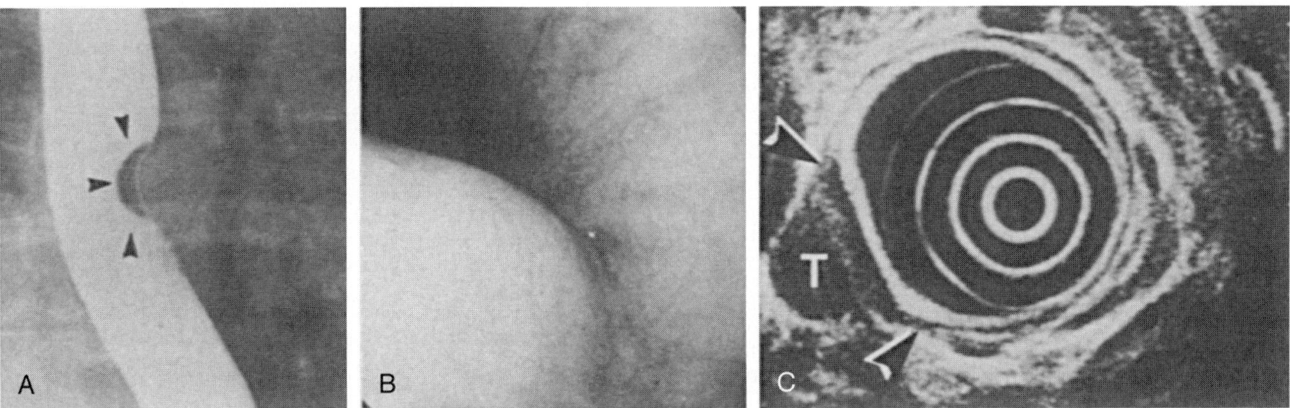

Figure 7–13. *A*, An esophageal leiomyoma. A barium esophagram shows an extraluminal mass *(arrows)*, with no mucosal involvement. *B*, The extraluminal mass at esophagoscopy. *C*, On esophageal ultrasound, a hypoechoic tumor (T) can be seen arising from the fourth ultrasound layer *(arrows)*. This intramural mass is confined to this layer with no invasion of adjacent layers.

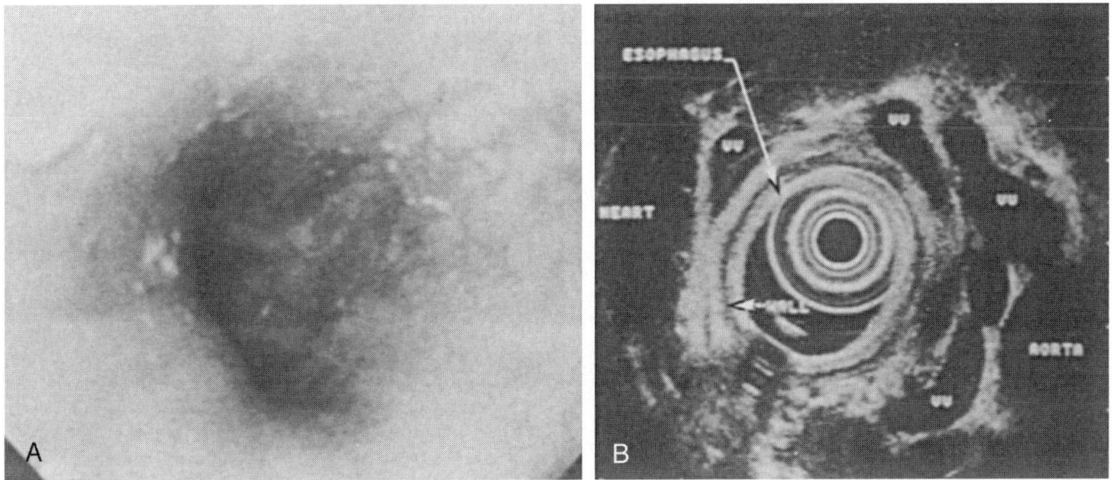

Figure 7–14. Paraesophageal varices. *A*, At endoscopy, small varices are not visible. *B*, On esophageal ultrasound, the varices (VV) are prominent anechoic, tubular, and rounded structures outside the esophageal wall.

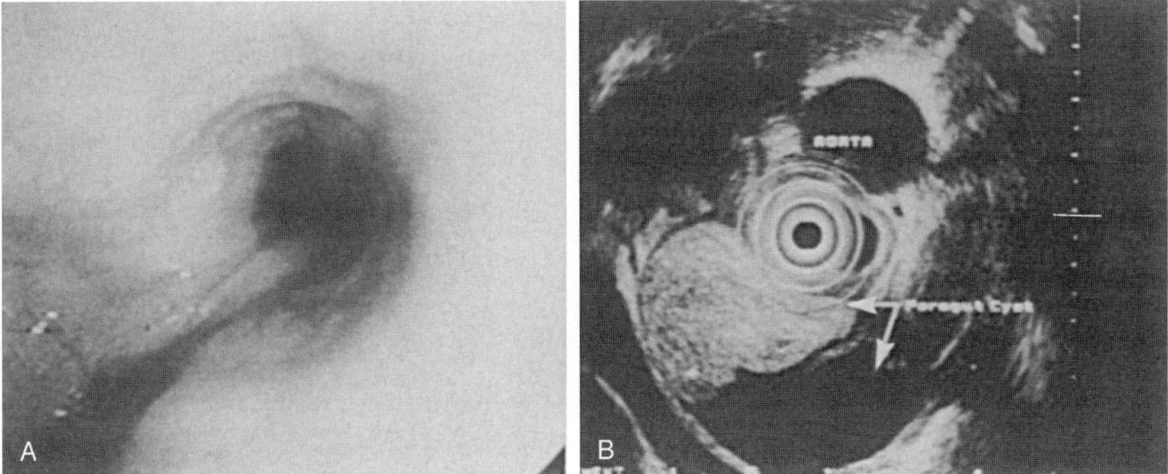

Figure 7–15. Foregut cyst. *A*, There is no extrinsic esophageal compression at esophagoscopy. *B*, On esophageal ultrasound, the cyst has two components, one anechoic (representing fluid) and the other hyperechoic (representing proteinaceous material). The cyst lies adjacent to the trachea and esophagus.

References

1. Adelstein, D.J., Rice, T.W., Boyce, G.A., et al.: Adenocarcinoma of the esophagus and gastroesophageal junction. Am. J. Clin. Oncol., *17:*14, 1994.
2. Barthet, M., Mambrini, P., Audibert, P., et al.: Relationships between endosonographic appearance and clinical or manometric features in patients with achalasia. Eur. J. Gastroenterol. Hepatol., *10:*559, 1998.
3. Bergami, G.L., Fruhwith, R., Di Mario, M., et al.: Contribution of ultrasonography in the diagnosis of achalasia. J. Pediatr. Gastroenterol. Nutr., *14:*92, 1992.
4. Bhutani, M.S., Hawes, R.H., and Hoffman, B.J.: A comparison of the accuracy of echo features during endoscopic ultrasound (EUS) and EUS-guided fine needle aspiration for diagnosis of malignant lymph node invasion. Gastrointest. Endosc., *45:*474, 1997.
5. Binmoeller, K.F., Seifert, H., Seitz, U., et al.: Ultrasonic esophagoprobe for TNM staging of highly stenosing esophageal carcinoma. Gastrointest. Endosc., *41:*547, 1995.
6. Bolondi, L., Casonova, P., Santi, V., et al.: The sonographic appearance of the normal gastric wall: An in vivo study. Ultrasound Med. Biol., *12:*991, 1986.
7. Botet, J.F., Lightdale, C.J., Zauber, A.G., et al.: Preoperative staging of esophageal cancer: Comparison of endoscopic US and dynamic CT. Radiology, *181:*419, 1991.
8. Caletti, G.C., Brocchi, E., Ferrari, A., et al.: Guillotine needle biopsy as a supplement to endosonography in the diagnosis of gastric submucosal tumors. Endoscopy, *23:*251, 1991.
9. Catalano, M.F., Sivak, M.V., Jr., Rice, T.W., et al.: Endosonographic features predictive of lymph node metastases. Gastrointest. Endosc., *40:*442, 1994.
10. Catalano, M.F., Sivak, M.V., Jr., Rice, T.W., et al.: Postoperative screening for anastomotic recurrence of esophageal carcinoma by endoscopic ultrasonography. Gastrointest. Endosc., *42:*540, 1995.
11. Catalano, M.F., Alcocer, E., Chak, A., et al.: Evaluation of metastatic celiac lymph nodes in patients with esophageal carcinoma: Accuracy of EUS. Gastrointest. Endosc., *50:*352, 1999.
12. Consigliere, D., Chua, C.L., Hui, F., et al.: Computed tomography for esophageal carcinoma: Its value to the surgeon. J. R. Coll. Surg. Edinb., *37:*113, 1992.
13. Dancygier, H., and Classen, M.: Endoscopic ultrasonography in esophageal diseases. Gastrointest. Endosc., *35:*220, 1989.
14. Date, H., Miyashita, M., Sasajima, K., et al.: Assessment of adventitial involvement of esophageal carcinoma by endoscopic ultrasonography. Surg. Endosc., *4:*195, 1990.
15. DeviEre, J., Dunham, F., Richaert, R., et al.: Endoscopic ultrasonography in achalasia. Gastroenterology, *96:*1210, 1989.
16. Dittler, H.J., Fink, U., Siewert, G.R.: Response to chemotherapy in esophageal cancer. Endoscopy, *26:*769, 1994.
17. Duignan, J.P., McEntee, G.P., O'Connell, D.J., et al.: The role of CT in the management of carcinoma of the esophagus and cardia. Ann. R. Coll. Surg. Engl., *69:*283, 1987.
18. Falk, G.W., Catalano, M.F., Sivak, M.V., Jr., et al.: Endosonography in the evaluation of patients with Barrett's esophagus and high-grade dysplasia. Gastrointest. Endosc., *40:*207, 1994.
19. Falk, G.W., Van Dam J., Sivak, M.V., et al.: Endoscopic ultrasonography (EUS) in achalasia. Gastrointest. Endosc., *37:*241, 1991.
20. Fleming, I.D., Cooper, J.S., Henson, D.E., et al. (eds): Digestive system: Esophagus. *In* AJCC Cancer Staging Manual, ed 5. Philadelphia, Lippincott-Raven, 1997, p. 65.
21. Fleshman, J.W., Myerson, R.J., Fry, R.D., et al.: Accuracy of transrectal ultrasound in predicting stage of rectal cancer before and after preoperative radiation therapy. Dis. Colon Rectum, *35:*823, 1992.
22. Fockens, P., van den Brande, J.H.M., van Dullemen, H.M., et al.: Endosonographic T-staging of esophageal carcinoma: A learning curve. Gastrointest. Endosc., *44:*58, 1996.
23. Fritscher-Ravens, A., Petrasch, S., Reinacher-Schick, A., et al.: Diagnostic value of endoscopic ultrasonography-guided fine-needle aspiration cytology of mediastinal masses in patients with intrapulmonary lesions and diagnostic bronchoscopy. Respiration, *66:*150, 1999.
24. Giovannini, M., Seitz, F.J., Thomas, P., et al.: Endoscopic ultrasonography for assessment of response to combined radiation therapy and chemotherapy in patients with esophageal cancer. Endoscopy, *29:*4, 1997.
25. Ginsberg, G.G., Al-Kawas, E.H., Nguyen, C.C., et al.: Endoscopic ultrasound evaluation of vascular involvement in esophageal cancer: A comparison with computed tomography. Gastrointest. Endosc., *39:*276, 1993.
26. Goldblum, J.R., Rice, T.W., Zuccaro, G. Jr., et al.: Granular cell tumors of the esophagus: A clinical and pathologic study of 13 cases. Ann. Thorac. Surg., *62:*860, 1996.
27. Gress, F.G., Savides, T.J., Sandler, A., et al.: Endoscopic ultrasonography, fine-needle aspiration biopsy guided by endoscopic ultrasonography, and computed tomography in the preoperative staging of non-small-cell lung cancer: a comparison study. Ann. Intern. Med., *127:*604, 1997.
28. Heintz, A., Höhne, U., Schweden, F., et al.: Preoperative detection of intrathoracic tumor spread of esophageal cancer: Endosonography versus computed tomography. Surg. Endosc., *5:*75, 1991.
29. Hordijk, M.L., Zander, H., van Blankenstein, M., et al.: Influence of tumor stenosis on the accuracy of endosonography in preoperative T staging of esophageal cancer. Endoscopy, *25:*171, 1993.
30. Hordijk, M.L., Kok, T.C., Wilson, J.H.P., et al.: Assessment of response of esophageal carcinoma to induction chemotherapy. Endoscopy, *25:*592, 1993.
31. Hunerbein, M., Ghadimi, B.M., Haensch, W., et al.: Transendoscopic ultrasound of esophageal and gastric cancer using miniaturized ultrasound catheter probes. Gastrointest. Endosc., *48:*371, 1998.
32. Hunerbein, M., Dohmoto, M., Haensch, W., et al.: Endosonography-guided biopsy of mediastinal and pancreatic tumors. Endoscopy, *30:*32, 1998.
33. Hunerbein, M., Ghadimi, B.M., Haensch, W., et al.: Transesophageal biopsy of mediastinal and pulmonary tumors by means of endoscopic ultrasound guidance. J. Thorac. Cardiovasc. Surg., *116:*554, 1998.
34. Isenberg, G., Chak, A., Canto, M.I., et a1.: Endoscopic ultrasound in restaging of esophageal cancer after neoadjuvant chemoradiation. Gastrointest. Endosc., *48:*158, 1998.
35. Kasbarian, M., Fuentes, P., Brichon, P.Y., et al.: Usefulness of computed tomography in assessing the extension of carcinoma of the esophagus and gastroesophageal junction. *In* Siewart, J.R., and Hölscher, A.H., (eds.): Diseases of the Esophagus. Berlin, Springer-Verlag, 1988, p. 185.
36. Kallemanis, G.E., Gupta, P.K., al-Kawas, F.H., et al.: Endoscopic ultrasound for staging esophageal cancer, with and without dilation, is clinically important and safe. Gastrointest. Endosc., *41:*540, 1995.
37. Kawamoto, K., Yamada, Y., Utsunomiya, T., et al.: Gastrointestinal submucosal tumors: Evaluation with endoscopic US. Radiology *205:*733, 1997.
38. Kimmey, M.B., Martin, R.W., Hagitt, R.C., et al.: Histologic correlates of gastrointestinal ultrasound images. Gastroenterology, *96:*433, 1989.
39. Kimmey, M.B., and Martin, R.W.: Fundamentals of endosonography. Gastrointest. Endosc. Clin. North Am., *2:*557, 1992.
40. Kirk, S.J., Moorehead, R.J., McIlrath, E., et al.: Does preoperative computed tomography scanning aid assessment of oesophageal carcinoma? Postgrad. Med. J., *66:*191, 1987.
41. Kobayashi, H., Danabara, T., Sugama, Y., et al: Observation of lymph nodes and great vessels in the mediastinum by endoscopic ultrasonography. Jpn. J. Med., *26:*253, 1987.
42. Kondo, D., Imaizumi, M., Abe, T., et al.: Endoscopic ultrasound examination for mediastinal lymph node metastases of lung cancer. Chest, *98:*586, 1990.
43. Laterza, E., deManzoni, G., Guglielmi, A., et al.: Endoscopic ultrasonography in the staging of esophageal carcinoma after preoperative radiotherapy and chemotherapy. Ann. Thorac. Surg., *67:*1466, 1999.
44. Lightdale, C.J., Botet, J.F., Kelson, D.P., et al.: Diagnosis of recurrent upper gastrointestinal cancer at the surgical anastomosis by endoscopic ultrasound. Gastrointest. Endosc., *35:*220, 1989.
45. Markland, C.G., Manhire, A., Davies, P., et al.: The role of computed tomography in assessing the operability of oesophageal carcinoma. Eur. J. Cardiothorac. Surg., *3:*33, 1989.
46. McLoughlin, R.F., Cooperberg, P.L., Mathieson, J.R., et al.: High resolution endoluminal ultrasonography in the staging of esophageal carcinoma. J. Ultrasound Med., *14:*725, 1995.
47. Menzel, J., Hoepffner, N., Nottberg, H., et al.: Preoperative staging of esophageal carcinoma: Miniprobe sonography versus conventional endoscopic ultrasound in a prospective histopathologically verified study. Endoscopy, *31:*329, 1999.

48. Mishra, G., Sahai, A.V., Penman, I.D., et al.: Endoscopic ultrasonography with fine-needle aspiration: An accurate and simple diagnostic modality for sarcoidosis. Endoscopy, *31*:377, 1999.
49. Palazzo, L., Landi, B., Cellier, C., et al.: Endosonographic features of esophageal granular cell tumors. Endoscopy, *29*:850, 1997.
50. Pedersen, B.H., Vilmann, P., Folke, K., et al.: Endoscopic ultrasonography and real-time guided fine-needle aspiration biopsy of solid lesions of the mediastinum suspected of malignancy. Chest, *110*:539, 1996.
51. Ponsot, P., Chaussade, S., Palazzo, L., et al.: Endoscopic ultrasonography in achalasia. Gastroenterology, *98*:253, 1990.
52. Potepan, P., Meroni, E., Spagnoli, I., et al.: Non-small cell lung cancer: Detection of mediastinal lymph node metastases by endoscopic ultrasound and CT. Eur. Radiol., *6*:19, 1996.
53. Reed, C.E., Misha, G., Sarai, A.V., et al.: Esophageal cancer staging: Improved accuracy by endoscopic ultrasound of celiac lymph nodes. Ann. Thorac. Surg., *67*:319, 1999.
54. Reinig, J.W., Stanley, J.H., Schabel, S.I.: CT evaluation of thickened esophageal walls. AJR *140*:941, 1983.
55. Rice, T.W., Boyce, G.A., Sivak, M.V., Jr., et al.: Esophageal ultrasound and the preoperative staging of carcinoma of the esophagus. J. Thorac. Cardiovasc. Surg., *101*:536, 1991.
56. Rice, T.W.: Benign cysts and neoplasms of the mediastinum. Semin. Thorac. Cardiovasc. Surg., *4*:25, 1992.
57. Rice, T.W., Boyce, G.A., Sivak, M.V., et al.: Esophageal carcinoma: Esophageal ultrasound assessment of preoperative chemotherapy. Ann. Thorac. Surg., *53*:972, 1992.
58. Rice, T.W., Zuccaro, G., Jr., Adelstein, D.J., et al.: Esophageal carcinoma: Depth of tumor invasion is predictive of regional lymph node status. Ann. Thorac. Surg., *65*:787, 1998.
59. Rösch, T.: Endosonographic staging of esophageal cancer: A review of literature results. Gastrointest. Endosc. Clin. North Am., *5*:537, 1995.
60. Roubein, L.D., DuBroe, R., David, C., et al.: Endoscopic ultrasonography in the quantitative assessment of response to chemotherapy in patients with adenocarcinoma of the esophagus and esophagogastric junction. Endoscopy, *25*:587, 1993.
61. Ruol, A., Rossi, M., Ruffatto, A., et al.: Reevaluation of computed tomography in preoperative staging of esophageal and cardial cancers: A prospective study. *In* Siewert, J.R., and Hölscher, A.H. (eds.): Diseases of the Esophagus. New York, Springer-Verlag, 1987, p. 194.
62. Saunders, H.S., Wolfman, N.T., and Ott, D.J.: Esophageal cancer: Radiologic staging. Radiol. Clin. North Am., *35*:281, 1997.
63. Schlick, T., Heintz, A., and Junginger, T.: The examiner's learning effect and its influence on the quality of endoscopic ultrasonography in carcinoma of the esophagus and gastric cardia. Surg. Endosc., *13*:894, 1999.
64. Silva, S.A., Kouzu, T., Ogino, Y., et al.: Endoscopic ultrasonography of oesophageal tumors and compressions. J. Clin. Ultrasound, *16*:149, 1988.
65. Söndenaa, K., Skaane, P., Nygaard, K., et al.: Value of computed tomography in preoperative evaluation of respectability and staging of oesophageal carcinoma. Eur. J. Surg., *158*:537, 1992.
66. Tada, S., Iida, M., Yao, T., et al.: Granular cell tumor of the esophagus: Endoscopic ultrasonography demonstration and endoscopic removal. Am. J. Gastroenterol., *85*:1507, 1990.
67. Tio, T.L., Cohen, P., Coene, P.P., et al.: Endosonography and computed tomography of esophageal carcinoma: Preoperative classification compared to the new (1987) TNM system. Gastroenterology, *96*:1478, 1989.
68. Tio, T.L., Tytgat, G.N., and den Hartog Jager, F.C.: Endoscopic ultrasonography for the evaluation of smooth muscle tumors in the upper gastrointestinal tract: An experience with 42 cases. Gastrointest. Endosc., *36*:342, 1990.
69. Van Dam, J., Rice, T.W., Catalano, M.F., et al.: High-grade malignant stricture is predictive of esophageal tumor stage: Risks of endosonographic evaluation. Cancer, *71*:2910, 1993.
70. Van Dam, J., Rice, T.W., Sivak, M.V., Jr., et al.: Endoscopic ultrasonography and endoscopically guided needle aspiration for the diagnosis of upper gastrointestinal tract foregut cysts. Am. J. Gastroenterol., *87*:762, 1992.
71. Vilgrain, V., Mompoint, D., Palazzo, L., et al.: Staging of esophageal carcinoma: Comparison of results with endoscopic sonography and CT. AJR *155*:277, 1990.
72. Waxman, I.: Endosonography in columnar-lined esophagus. Gastroenterol. Clin. North Am., *26*:607, 1997.
73. Wiersema, M.J., Hawes, R.H., Tao, L., et al.: Endoscopic ultrasound as an adjunct to fine needle aspiration cytology of the upper and lower gastrointestinal tracts. Gastrointest. Endosc., *38*:35, 1992.
74. Wiersema, M.J., Kochman, M.L., Chak, A., et al.: Real-time endoscopic ultrasound guided fine needle aspiration of a mediastinal node. Gastrointest. Endosc., *39*:429, 1993.
75. Wiersema, M.J., Vilmann, P., Giovannini M., et al.: Endosonography-guided fine-needle aspiration biopsy: Diagnostic accuracy and complication assessment. Gastroenterology, *112*:1087, 1997.
76. Yasuda, K., Cho, E., Nakajima, M., et al.: Diagnosis of submucosal lesions of the upper gastrointestinal tract by endoscopic ultrasonography. Gastrointest. Endosc., *36*:S17, 1990.
77. Yasuda, K., Nakajima, M., and Kawai, K.: Endoscopic ultrasonographic imaging of submucosal lesions of the upper gastrointestinal tract. Gastrointest. Endosc. Clin. North Am., *2*:615, 1992.
78. Ziegler, K., Sanft, C., Friedrich, M., et al.: Endosonographic appearance of the esophagus in achalasia. Endoscopy, *22*:1, 1990.
79. Ziegler, K., Sanft, C., Zeitz, M., et al.: Evaluation of endosonography in TN staging of oesophageal cancer. Gut, *32*:16, 1991.
80. Zuccaro, G., Jr., Rice, T.W., Goldblum, J.R., et al.: Endoscopic ultrasound cannot determine suitability for esophagectomy after aggressive chemoradiotherapy for esophageal cancer. Am. J. Gastroenterol., *94*:906, 1999.

CHAPTER

8 Esophageal Dilatation

TIMOTHY T. NOSTRANT • JOHN C. RABINE

Esophageal dilatation is the preferred treatment for dysphagia secondary to fixed narrowing of the esophagus. Although peptic acid-induced strictures of the esophagus are the most common indication for esophageal dilatation, malignant and medication-induced strictures are increasing in frequency as reasons for dilatation.[63] Other indications for esophageal dilatation are listed in Table 8-1. In addition to fixed narrowing of the esophagus, functional obstruction of the esophagus due to achalasia or other esophageal dysmotility syndromes is treated with pneumatic dilatation either as initial treatment or after failure of conservative medical treatment.[94]

Whereas all current dilating systems produce stricture dilatation either through stretching or fracture of fibrous scarring, there is minimal information about the actual effects with individual dilating systems.[63,71] Comparisons between dilating systems are usually anecdotal and frequently use historical rather than concurrent controls.[63,71] In addition, few prospective studies compare medical treatment (medications or dilatation) to surgery. The purpose of this chapter is to look at all past and current dilatation systems and put them into perspective relative to patient tolerance, ease of use, cost, cost-effectiveness compared with alternative treatment strategies, and available safety and efficacy data. Potential new longer term systems, such as wall stenting for both benign and malignant disease, are discussed.

Table 8-1. Indications for Esophageal Dilatation

Peptic Esophagitis
Chronic reflux esophagitis
Barrett's esophagus
Rings and Webs
Schatzki's rings
Congenital rings (upper and lower)
Plummer-Vinson syndrome
Caustic Injury
Lye ingestion
Acid ingestion
Pill-induced esophagitis
Iatrogenic Injury
Surgical anastomoses
Sclerotherapy
Nasogastric intubation
Radiation injury
Systemic Disease
Scleroderma
Crohn's disease
Sarcoidosis
Pemphigus
Bullous pemphigoid
Epidermolysis bullosa
Toxic epidermal necrolysis
Motility Disorders
Achalasia
Diffuse esophageal spasm
Nutcracker esophagus
Hypertensive lower esophageal sphincter
Nonspecific esophageal dysmotility
Infections
Candida
Herpesvirus
Cytomegalovirus
Human immunodeficiency virus

HISTORICAL PERSPECTIVE

The practice of esophageal dilatation began 4 centuries ago with the use of wax dilators for food impaction in the esophagus. Fabricus ab Acquadendente (1537-1619) was the first physician to use a blunt implement to push a foreign object from the esophagus into the stomach.[27] The original dilator "bougie" and the technique of "bougienage" received their names from the Algerian town of Bouginhay, which was the medieval capital of the wax candle trade.[27,54] Although wax bougies required pressure application for effect, passive therapy with an olive-shaped lead instrument was later developed. The first instance of achalasia dilation using a sponge-tipped whale bone was performed by Thomas Willis (1621-1675).[27,54] Minimal progress was made in esophageal dilatation for the next 2 centuries, until Sir Arthur Hurst developed the hollow dilator with a blunt end filled with mercury in 1915.[12,27,54] Mercury was used to give the dilator weight and employed gravity as an aid for dilatation, which was presumed at that time to be secondary to stricture stretching. Maloney refined the mercury dilator so that a tapered end would allow easier passage through tighter strictures with greater patient comfort.[12,27,54] Mercury bougienage was the only practical technique for esophageal dilatation until the late 1950s, when olive-shaped dilators on a solid metal shaft passed over a guidewire were developed for fluoroscopic dilatation of tight strictures (Eder-Puestow dilators).[91] Despite these advances, esophageal dilation was still used infrequently until the introduction of fiberoptic endoscopy in the 1960s and its widespread use in the diagnosis of upper gastrointestinal disorders over the next 3 decades.[90] Visualization of the stricture or narrowing allowed easier passage of the guidewires for olive dilatation, increasing the frequency of application of this technique.[90] After attaining adequate stricture dilatation, chronic mercury bougienage was then used to maintain esophageal patency. The introduction of hollow-core polyvinyl dilators (Savary-Gilliard, American) and balloon dilators using radiographic (Grunzig, Rigiflex) and endoscopic control (Rigiflex through-the-scope [TTS] system) in the mid 1980s has radically changed the approach to esophageal dilation and has substantially reduced the use of mercury dilators in most centers.[4,71]

TYPES OF DILATORS

Esophageal dilators can be divided into two basic groups: the push dilators (Fig. 8–1) and the balloon dilators (Fig. 8–2). The push dilators can be further subdivided into those that require guidewire passage and those that do not. Balloon dilators can be further classified as those requiring fluoroscopic placement and those that can be passed through the endoscope. Other types of dilators that have been advocated but are rarely used include tapered-tip endoscopes, mechanical dilators with monitoring for width and force of dilatation, and variably tapered plastic sheaths that fit over conventional pediatric or adult endoscopes.[60,63,66,71,94] Attaching a polyethylene balloon to a bronchoscope as a means of dilating tight strictures or placing a bolus of tape onto the distal shaft of the endoscope above the bending section each has been used as a cheaper alternative combining diagnosis and therapy in a single procedure.[60,66] The most commonly used systems today include mercury bougienage, Savary (American) polyvinyl dilators with guidewire, and balloon dilation using TTS instrumentation.[63,71,94]

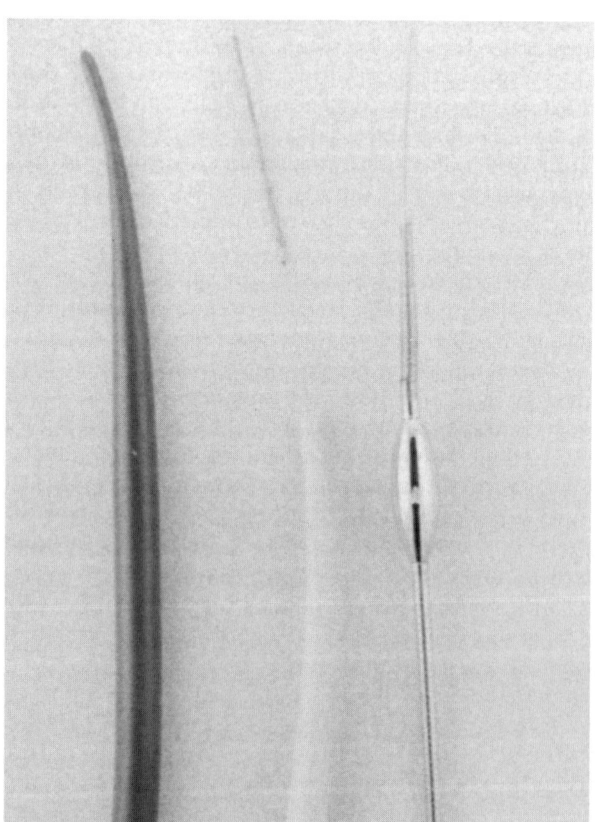

Figure 8–1. The push dilators: mercury dilator *(left)*; hollow polyvinyl dilator (American) with wire introducer in place *(middle)*; and Eder-Puestow dilator with flexible tip, olive dilator, and metal introducer *(right)*.

Mercury Bougienage

The most frequent form of esophageal dilatation is mercury bougienage (30 to 60% of all dilatations).[47] Mercury-filled dilators have several advantages over balloon and rigid over-the-wire dilators. Guidewires are not required and rare perforations secondary to the guidewire can be avoided. Bougies do not require fluoroscopy for passage in most cases and do not necessitate repeated endoscopy, which is required by the TTS balloon system. The major indications for mercury bougienage have been simple reflux strictures and congenital rings (Schatzki's ring) and webs.[29,45,47] Single passage of a large-caliber dilator (Nos. 48 to 60 French) is considered standard treatment of Schatzki's rings, with symptom-free intervals of more than 5 years in over 50% of patients followed for up to 75 months.[45] Similar long-term efficacy has been shown for simple reflux strictures with mean follow-up times of 50 months.[106] Details of how many patients with simple reflux strictures required use of olive or Savary dilators in addition to mercury dilators are scanty. Stoddard and Simms reported successful dilatation in 109 of 111 patients, with 92 having reflux strictures.[103] Of these patients, 102 required mercury dilators only. Dilatation efficacy appears to decrease if radiation-induced, malignant, or corrosive strictures are included, but overall success rates of 85% in all types of patients have been reported.[29,45,47,58,63,71,103,106] Strictures associated with Barrett's esophagus can be dilated with efficacy equal to that of simple reflux strictures.[47,71]

The role of mercury bougienage for tight strictures has not been fully clarified. Most authors suggest that strictures with diameters of less than 12 mm are not well suited to mercury bougienage.[4,47] Mercury dilators less than 30 French (10 mm) are very floppy and require fluoroscopy to confirm passage through the stricture. However, Kozarek was able to effectively dilate strictures with diameters down to 3 mm with mercury dilators alone and did not require fluoroscopy in most cases.[47,60]

Upper esophageal stricture dilatation with mercury dilators has not been systematically studied. Upper esophageal strictures most commonly occur after laryngectomy or are caused by radiation, malignancy, or postcorrosive injury.[47] Peptic strictures are rare except with Barrett's esophagus. Successful dilatation of upper esophageal strictures with mercury bougies occurred in only 55% of patients, but the success rate for patients with distal reflux strictures was 96.3%.[58,60] Most experts now agree that over-the-wire or balloon dilators are best for radiation-induced or malignant strictures, particularly if the strictures are tight, eccentric, or long (>2.5 cm) or have angulation and pseudodiverticula.[4,47,60,63,71]

Technique of Passage

Preprocedure barium examination and endoscopy should be done to confirm the diagnosis of esophageal stricture

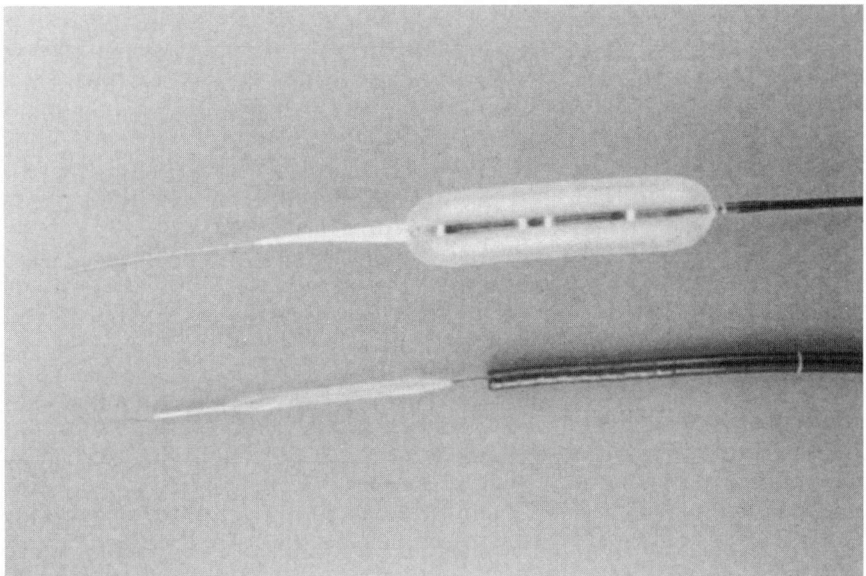

Figure 8–2. The balloon dilators: achalasia balloon dilator inflated with wire introducer in place *(top)* and through-the-scope (TTS) system passed through endoscope *(bottom)*.

and to rule out malignancy. The patient should fast for at least 6 to 8 hours prior to dilatation. Dilatation can be accomplished in the sitting or left lateral decubitus position.[47] Sedation prior to dilatation is still controversial but is frequently used to allay patient anxiety. Dilator selection should be based on the radiographic or endoscopically determined stricture diameter. Bougie sizes just below or at the level of stricture diameter should be used initially (1 mm = 3 French). Dilators should be cleaned with iodine solution just prior to use.[47,105] After pharyngeal anesthesia and lubrication, the dilator is passed over the forefinger and second finger into the posterior pharynx and the patient is asked to swallow. Both the passage and withdrawal of the dilators should be in one smooth motion. The first dilator to meet resistance is considered the first true dilatation. Maximal dilatation at a single session should be limited in most cases to no more than three dilator sizes above the first dilator to meet resistance (approximately a No. 9 French or 3 mm) to reduce the risk of perforation (the "rule of three").[61,105] Maximal dilatation should be accomplished in one to three sessions.[47,61,105]

The role of fluoroscopy with mercury bougienage is a current debate. Two studies have documented both a decreased success rate for stricture passage and a decreased operator accuracy for predicting success with blind bougienage.[8,114] McClave studied 43 patients with benign strictures in a randomized, controlled trial of 162 dilatations.[74] Successful dilatation rates for bougienage with and without fluoroscopy were 96% and 80%, respectively. There were more adverse events, such as tracheal intubation, without fluoroscopy. Most disturbing was the low rate of operator and patient perception of an adverse event (20%). Since not all units have fluoroscopy capabilities, only complicated strictures or resistant strictures should mandate fluoroscopic monitoring if mercury bougies are used.[47,63,74]

Redilatation rates after initial successful dilatation are varied. Some patients may not require redilatation for long periods. Up to 40% of patients may require only one dilatation.[41,87] Tight strictures may require short-interval redilation to ensure reasonable duration of response. Weekly dilatation until easy passage of a 44 French or larger dilator is accomplished is a common strategy.[47,63,71,91] Dilatation with up to a 60 French dilator for a Schatzki ring is preferable.[29,47] Neither the initial dilatation size nor the frequency of dilatation predicts ultimate response, and for most patients, recurrent dysphagia should be the signal for repeat dilatation.[41,47,63,71,87] Predictors for repeated dilatation are nonpeptic causes of strictures, fibrous strictures, more than two dilatation sessions, and maximal dilator size less than 44 French.[41,87,88]

Complications of mercury bougienage are infrequent and none are unique to this dilatation system. Complications of esophageal dilatation are discussed later. Mercury dilators have a manufacturer's shelf life of 2 to 4 years, after which they should be discarded.[20]

Eder-Puestow and Hollow Polyvinyl Dilators (Savary-Gilliard, American Endoscopy)

The Eder-Puestow dilation system was developed in 1951 as a means to dilate complicated strictures by using fluoroscopic guidewire placement of the metal olive dilator.[4,91] This system was the only practical means to dilate resistant or complicated strictures for 3 decades and was adapted for use with flexible endoscopes.[4,90,91] Hollow vinyl dilators were introduced in the mid 1980s and have almost completely replaced the Eder-Puestow system.[63,71,113]

There are two varieties of hollow polyvinyl dilators. The first version is known as the Savary-Gilliard (Wilson Cook) dilator and consists of semitransparent polyvinyl tubes with a 20-cm tapered tip and a central guidewire channel; a radiopaque band at the widest point of the dilator is difficult to see fluoroscopically. Impaction of the dilator on the tip of the guidewire is possible if the dilator is passed too far. Dilator sets are available in 70- and 100-cm lengths. Each set contains 16 dilators that range in size from 5 (15 French) to 20 mm (60 French), with 1-mm step-ups between dilators.[4,60,63,116]

The second variety (Bard, American Endoscopy) was an attempt to improve the Savary system. The dilators are impregnated with barium sulfate for easy fluoroscopic use. The guidewire system was improved for easier passage and longer life through a graduated spring device. The distal tapering was significantly shortened, and impaction and curling are much less frequent. American markings (tip of dilators to incisors) and European markings (maximal point of dilator to incisors) are aids in assessing stricture passage.[4,60]

Technique of Passage

Correct guidewire placement is the first crucial step. Routine endoscopy should be the standard first step for wire passage.[4,60] Pediatric endoscopes allow passage through all but the tightest strictures. The guidewire should be placed at least 20 to 25 cm beyond the lowest portion of the stricture. For practical purposes, wire placement in the antrum (≥60 cm) is most useful. The spring end should be parallel to the greater curvature of the stomach to decrease wire injury to the gastric wall. As the endoscope is withdrawn, the guidewire should be advanced an equal distance to prevent passage into the duodenum or inadvertent wire withdrawal above the stricture. Wire position is easily assessed by looking at the markings on the wire; each mark signifies 20 cm (i.e., 4-mark position = 80 cm from incisors). The distal wire end is sharp, and caution should be used or the sharp end hooded. As the dilator is passed over the wire, the endoscopic assistant should exert countertension but not actively pull on the wire. This technique facilitates passage through the cervical esophagus and decreases wire damage. After successful dilatation, the dilator is withdrawn and the wire advanced. Wire position should be within ±5 cm of the predilation distance before the next dilator is passed. The rule of three is even more important here than with mercury bougies, because resistance is more difficult to feel with the harder polyvinyl tubes.[4,60] Choice of dilator sizes is similar to that of mercury bougies. Dilators of size No. 48 French or larger will not pass through all types of mouthpieces, and only the largest mouthpieces should be used if the use of larger dilators is anticipated. Routine postprocedure esophagograms are not mandatory but are obtained immediately if there is any suspicion of perforation, as evidenced by back pain, persistent chest pain, fever, bloody emesis, or vomiting.

Complications

Complications unique to the Savary system include mucosal tearing and perforation induced by guidewires. The guidewire should be checked before each use, because a bent wire can serve as a lead point for esophageal perforation. Wire damage is more common with the Eder-Puestow system.[4,60] Correct placement and replacement during dilatation are crucial both for dilation effectiveness and for safety. If concerns occur, fluoroscopic confirmation may be necessary. Entrapment on the guidewire is caused by overzealous passage of the dilator. This should not occur if the markings are used to assess distance and further passage after the end hits a hard spot is avoided. Very hard resistance to passage is more commonly due to impending tip impaction than to stricture resistance.[4,60]

Eder-Puestow–Savary Comparisons

Head-to-head comparisons are few. Major complications are rare with both systems, although cervical esophageal trauma is more common with the Eder-Puestow system.[4,20,49,116] Speed of passage is slower with the Eder-Puestow system (5 minutes versus 2 minutes) and patient preference was highest with the Savary system. Dilatation effectiveness determined by the need to redilate, relief of dysphagia, postdilatation stricture size, return to baseline stricture size after dilatation, or time to redilation was equal with both techniques if initial stricture dilatation was identical.[4,49,116] Stricture dilation to 44 French or larger was more common with the Savary dilator in all forms of esophageal stricture.

Balloon Dilators

The development of polyethylene balloons for use in the gastrointestinal tract has allowed dilatation of previously inaccessible strictures in the colon, pancreas, biliary tree, and small intestine.[21,37,38,43,44,48,57,59,67,76,77,79,98] Their use in esophageal disease, although extensive, is still quite controversial given the highly effective systems already available.[21,62]

Esophageal graded polyethylene balloons range in size from 4 to 40 mm (12 to 120 French). The smaller sizes are relegated to the pancreaticobiliary tree and the larger French sizes to pneumatic dilatation in achalasia. The most commonly used sizes in esophageal stricture dilatation are 36, 45, and 54 French. Such balloons are affixed to 7 French semiflexible catheter shafts that range in size from 100 to 200 cm. The dilating balloon length ranges from 5.1 to 8.5 cm, with the longer balloons used for longer, straight strictures and the shorter ones used with angulated or short, tight strictures. Stepwise dilatation can be accomplished with a balloon dilator beginning in the proximal portion of the stricture and proceeding distally.[44,57,113] Newer dilating balloons, which allow dilatation across a range of sizes (12 to 15 mm and 15 to 18 mm) with a single disposable balloon, will reduce the need for passage of multiple dilating balloons.

Technique of Passage

Radiographic or TTS passage of dilating balloons is possible. The technique for passage is similar except that radiographic passage requires guidewire placement and endoscopic passage requires channel passage of the dilating balloon. Larger endoscopes with channel sizes larger than 3.2 mm are preferable and 4.2-cm channels are ideal.[59,60,63,67] Initial choice of balloon size should be 1 to 2 mm greater than a stricture diameter with both techniques. The balloon tip requires silicone for easy passage. The balloon should be fully deflated (with negative pressure maintained through stricture passage) and liberally lubricated. The dilating balloon should be passed completely through the stricture and the black catheter shaft seen at the top of the stricture. The balloon should be inflated fully and pulled up to the distal edge of the stricture. The balloon should then be deflated partially so it can be pulled back through the stricture and the midportion of the balloon placed in approximation to the tightest area of the stricture.[43,44] This technique decreases back-passage of the dilating balloon into the esophagus, which frequently happens when the balloon is suddenly inflated from complete deflation to maximal inflation. The balloon then is inflated slowly and repositioned to keep the midportion of the balloon in the stricture. Maximal dilating pressure varies inversely with balloon size and ranges between 30 and 45 lb/in^2 (2 to 3 atm) for 15- and 10-mm balloons, respectively. Either air or dilute contrast (10 to 25% diatrizoate [Hypaque]) can be used to inflate the balloon.[76] Dilute contrast allows better fluoroscopic imaging.[76] Maximal inflation should be maintained for 20 to 30 seconds and can be repeated two or three times.[60,76,77] Fluoroscopic obliteration of the stricture waist and endoscopic visualization of stricture dilatation are end-points of success.[76,77] Stricture dilatation with large balloon sizes can be performed in a similar manner at the same session. Stricture dilatation with balloons rarely gives a true diameter size (i.e., a successful 36 French dilatation does not equate to a 12-mm stricture diameter) and can be significantly less effective in dilating for stricture size enlargement than use of Savary or other push and guidewire systems.[59,62,63,67] Final dilatation size should depend on clinical necessity and may not be achievable at a single dilation session without significant risk for complication. After dilatation is finished, the balloon should again be deflated maximally and negative pressure maintained to allow easy withdrawal and minimize balloon damage. Balloon life expectancy is between one and ten uses per balloon.[60,63]

Indications and Contraindications

Dysphagia and food impaction are the major indications for esophageal dilatation. Weight loss is usually minimal because the patients have good appetites and do adapt their diets to prevent symptoms of food impaction.[15,21,71] Simply inquiring about the frequency of dysphagia may underestimate the severity of a stricture, because dietary changes can minimize symptoms.[15,21] If one uses a quantitative index for dysphagia with both a dysphagia and a diet scale as outlined by Cox, dilatation efficacy is more reliably evaluated.[21] This scale grades the severity of dysphagia on the basis of frequency of dysphagia and the types of food that cause symptoms. Symptoms will occur with water or mashed potatoes with only the most severe strictures, but meat stoppage may be seen in most strictures. History can also be helpful in eliminating precipitants of dysphagia such as nonsteroidal anti-inflammatory drugs (NSAIDs), quinidine, and doxycyline.

The major contraindication to esophageal dilatation is the lack of an informed patient who has participated in a frank discussion of alternative treatment strategies.[60,63] Uncooperative patients and patients with severe coagulopathy, active bleeding, acute severe abdominal symptoms, or a deeply ulcerated stenosis all have increased risk for complications and frequently have a poor response to dilatation. Inability to adequately predict a dilator's route during the dilatation process is a contraindication for blind passage.[60,63,71] Large pseudodiverticula, severe mucosal bridging, epiphrenic or Zenker's diverticula, severe stricture angulation, and a large hiatal hernia are relative contraindications to blind passage. Guidewire-directed dilatation may also be contraindicated when the guidewire length past the stricture is inadequate, such as after gastrectomy and gastroenterostomy. Severe baseline hypoxemia or hypercapnia or contraindications for endoscopy/sedation also frequently preclude safe esophageal dilatation, particularly with large dilators, which may cause tracheal compression.

Risk Factors and Complications

Potential complications from esophageal dilatation include both those from dilatation directly and those related to associated procedures such as endoscopy and mucosal biopsy. Bleeding risk is also increased above diagnostic endoscopy, although the margin appears small.[60,63] Recent trials report a risk of perforation of 0.2%, a risk of major bleeding of 0.07%, and a risk of death of 0.01%.[60,63,71] Minor complications of aspiration, chest pain, and postprocedure nausea and vomiting occurred in less than 0.2% of patients.[60,71] These rates compare favorably with the 0.4–0.6% risk of perforation reported in the 1976 American Society of Gastrointestinal Endoscopy survey.[100] Perforations in the cervical esophagus occurred predominantly with the Eder-Puestow dilators, and perforations in the thoracoabdominal esophagus occurred just above the stenosis and were seen with use of all dilator types.[60,63,71,100] Guidewire malposition or kinking and perforation in a large hiatal hernia seen with blind dilatation may be more common. Complications with the balloon system were thought to be fewer, because only radial forces would be applied to the stricture and the longitudinal forces applied by other systems were considered the major cause of perforation.[59,60] These theoretical arguments led to the suggestion that strictures could be dilated to full size in a single session with balloon dilators.[59,60] Initial reports of rapid dilatation using this technique showed rates of major complications as high as 2.1% and underscore the need for caution in dilating tight or angulated strictures.[59] Major risk factors for perforation included small stricture diameter, long stricture length, sharp angulation, and large hiatal hernia size.[59,60,63] The type of stricture dilated did not predict complication risk. A learning curve for endoscopists using new dilating systems may also be a component of complication risks. Controlled, randomized trials for different dilating systems such as mercury bougienage, Savary (American) guidewire dilatation, and balloon systems are not available at this time. Representative studies using different dilating systems are presented in Table 8–2.[21,35,41,46,73,81,87,116]

Table 8–2. Complication Rates of Esophageal Dilatation

Study	No. of Patients	Dilator Types	Complication Rate (%)
Ogilvie et al. (1980)	50	EP, C	2.0
Glick (1982)	76	MB, EP	1.3
Patterson et al. (1983)	154	MB, EP	3.8
Fellows et al. (1986)	100	C	2.0
Cox et al. (1988)	65	B, C, EP	0.0
Hands et al. (1989)	195	EP	3.6
Yamamoto et al. (1992)	123	EP, B	5.7
Marshall et al. (1996)	354	S	2.1

EP = Eder-Puestow, C = Celestin, MB = mercury bougienage, B = balloon dilators, S = Savary.

NATURAL HISTORY OF DILATED STRICTURES

Although stricture dilatation is widely used to treat all forms of benign esophageal strictures, the information on rate of stricture recurrence and long-term effectiveness of bougienage is limited. Patterson looked at 154 patients for time to redilatation and the percentage requiring redilatation.[87] Only 98 patients achieved initial dilatation to 40 French or greater and were followed for up to 48 months. Life-table analysis showed that the highest risk for redilatation was in the first year, and 48% of patients required redilatation in the first 12 months after initial successful dilatation. By the end of 4 years, 64% of patients required redilatation. After each redilatation session, approximately 40% of patients required no further dilatation. The perforation rate was not higher in the redilatation group. Initial severity of stricture, cause of stricture, presence of esophagitis, and initial extent of dilatation did not predict the need for repeat dilatation.[87] Glick also demonstrated a high rate of stricture recurrence and need for multiple dilatations.[41] Strictures recurred in 65% of 76 patients followed for a mean of 21.1 months after successful dilatation to 44 French. After two or more recurrences, the likelihood of repeat dilatation was 86 to 94% after each recurrence.[41,87] The interval for dilatations also decreased with each redilatation but was variable. However, after eight dilatation sessions, the frequency of dilatation was monthly. Agnew followed 58 patients with peptic strictures to define clinical predictors for frequent dilatations in the future.[2] Patients lacking pyrosis or having weight loss at presentation required more dilatations in the first year. Age, gender, and the presence of esophagitis or Barrett's esophagus did not correlate with the frequency of dilatation.[2] Despite the high number of dilatations, minimal morbidity and absent mortality underlined the safety and efficacy of dilatation for benign esophageal stricture.[41,87,88]

Penagini was the first to study the potential reasons behind the need for redilatation.[88] He showed that stricture size significantly increased from 7.0 ± 0.5 mm to 9.1 ± 0.5 mm after dilatation, but was back to baseline size by 12 weeks. Worsening symptoms followed this trend toward smaller size but were less severe than baseline symptoms prior to dilatation. The percentage of time pH was below 4 and the number of reflux episodes did not differ before or after dilatation, and acid-induced damage was not a factor in stricture recurrence in this study.[41,87,88]

The role of acid-reduction therapy after dilatation is still controversial. Until recently, clinicians aimed treatment at just mechanical stricture dilatation and gave little heed to coexistent esophagitis. In one of the earliest studies, Ferguson compared cimetidine, 400 mg four times a day, to placebo.[36] Esophagitis was improved with cimetidine but frequency of stricture dilatation did not differ between cimetidine and placebo. Similar findings were published by Starlinger et al.[102] Because standard H_2-receptor antagonists (H_2RA) are relatively weak acid reducers, more recent studies have centered on a proton pump inhibitor.[16,56,72] Koop and Arnold treated 31 patients with esophagitis resistant to H_2RA with omeprazole.[56] Patients were treated with omeprazole 40 mg/day until esophagitis disappeared and then were begun on maintenance treatment with 20 mg/day. Six patients had strictures, and none required redilatation after omeprazole treatment. Ching and co-workers demonstrated a need for redilatation after successful treatment with omeprazole in only 14% of patients during an 8-week follow-up period, but all patients with resistant esophagitis had redilatation during re-evaluation.[16] Recent studies using sequential endoscopic evaluation after treatment with omeprazole or twice-a-day H_2RA have shown an 80% redilatation frequency in patients with unhealed esophagitis, but only 25% of patients with healed esophagitis required redilatation.[72] These data emphasize the key role of esophagitis in stricture narrowing. Acid-reduction treatment in patients with strictures and acid reflux but no or minimal esophagitis awaits study.

The role of esophageal dilation for postsurgical or postirradiation strictures is less certain than that for peptic strictures. Dhir et al. followed 21 patients with proximal esophageal strictures after surgery or irradiation for head and neck cancer. Dilatation brought relief of dysphagia in 75% of patients, although technical success was achieved in 95%. Twenty per cent of patients required repeat dilation after a mean of 3 months, but the longest follow-up interval was only 36 weeks.[25]

Palliative dilatation for active esophageal cancers also has not been well studied. One prospective study of 15 patients with squamous cell carcinoma undergoing chemotherapy and radiation compared Savary system dilatation with dilatation and concomitant Nd:YAG laser use. The use of dilatation did not result in complications, and the addition of laser therapy did not improve symptoms.[5]

COMPARATIVE STUDIES WITH DILATING SYSTEMS

Randomized, controlled studies among mercury bougienage, Savary (Bard, American Endoscopy) guidewire dilators, and balloon systems are few. Retrospective comparisons between the Savary and Eder-Puestow systems show a lower rate of complications, easier use, and more patient comfort with the Savary system, but effectiveness was equal between the two systems with both initial and subsequent dilatations.[4,49] These facts are the major reasons that the Savary (Bard, American endoscopy) dilators have almost completely replaced the Eder-Puestow system.[60,63,113] Comparative studies between the Eder-Puestow and balloon dilating systems in both randomized and nonrandomized studies have shown either equal efficacy to or an advantage over the Eder-Puestow system.[21,116] Complication rates were equal to or slightly more with the Eder-Puestow system.[21,116] When balloon dilation is compared with serial Celestin and Eder-Puestow dilatation, patients undergoing bougie dilatation had better symptom control and required fewer future dilations.[22] There are few direct comparisons between the Savary (Bard, American Endoscopy) system and the balloon dilators.[98] The success rate was 96% or greater with both systems and redilatation frequency was equal.[98] The mean time interval to redilatation was longer (11 months versus 6 months) in patients treated with Savary dilators, although this was not statistically significant. Complication rates were equal between the two groups of 30 patients. Balloon dilators were used preferentially to dilate high, tortuous cervical and postoperative strictures, although Savary dilators were considered superior after a diameter of 10 mm was achieved. Ease of use and simplicity of equipment favored the Savary system. A more recent prospective study of 251 patients also demonstrated equal efficacy and safety between the Savary and balloon systems.[97] Another prospective randomized study comparing polyvinyl bougies with balloon dilators for peptic strictures has been performed with differing results. Thirty-four patients underwent dilation to a goal diameter of 45 French with the polyvinyl dilator and 15 mm with the balloon. After two years of follow-up, the bougie group required more sessions to achieve full dilation and had a higher rate of stricture recurrence.[95,96] Because mercury bougienage is considered standard treatment for routine esophageal strictures and other dilating systems routine for more complex strictures, there are no head-to-head comparisons between these systems. Representative noncontrolled studies are shown in Table 8–3.[21,35,41,46,81,87,116] On a final note, the overall rate of bacteremia and following dilation is approximately 20% and has been associated with the passage of multiple dilators.[80,117] This has led to the suggestion that balloon dilators (which can be passed through the endoscopy channel one time) may carry a lower risk of bacteremia, but this has not been critically studied to date.

Table 8–3. Dilatation Success

Study	Type of Dilatation	Maximal Dilator Used	Need for Redilatation (%)
Ogilvie et al. (1980)	EP, C	>45 French	60
Glick (1982)	MB, EP	≥44 French	65
Patterson et al. (1983)	MB, EP	>40 French	57
Fellows et al. (1986)	C	≥54 French	62
Cox et al. (1988)	B, C, EP	≥58 French	59
		20 mm	20
Hands et al. (1989)	EP	≥54 French	54
Yamamoto et al. (1992)	EP, B	≥45 French	35
		20 mm	

EP = Eder-Puestow, C = Celestin, MB = mercury bougienage, B = balloon dilators.

ACHALASIA

Achalasia of the esophagus is a degenerative neural disorder characterized by loss of ganglion cells within the myenteric plexus and reduction of nerve fibers in the esophageal wall.[1,92,94,108] Recent histochemical studies have demonstrated a decrease in both vasoactive intestinal polypeptide and nitrous oxide, which are known mediators of smooth muscle relaxation in many gastrointestinal sphincters in patients with achalasia.[1,94] Paradoxical esophageal contraction to known inhibitory peptides such as cholecystokinin (CCK) is consistent with inhibitory neuron loss in both the lower esophageal sphincter (LES) and smooth muscle portion of the esophageal body.[94]

Symptoms such as dysphagia and regurgitation are the hallmarks of achalasia. Dysphagia usually begins with solid foods, but liquid retention is also seen as the disease progresses. Postprandial retrosternal fullness with mild chest pain is common. Worsening of symptoms with meal progression or emotional stress is frequently described.[94] Regurgitation is present in 60 to 90% of patients, is nonbilious, and is frequently unprovoked.[94] Nocturnal regurgitation is a prelude to aspiration pneumonia. This regurgitation can be mistaken for an eating disorder, such as anorexia nervosa or bulimia in young women.[94]

Barium studies, endoscopy, and esophageal manometry are the standard diagnostic tests for achalasia. Barium studies reveal a dilated esophagus with tertiary contractions in the smooth muscle portion. The lower esophagus is constantly contracted, giving the characteristic "bird-beaking" appearance. Early in the course of the disease, barium studies are frequently normal and cannot be used to rule out achalasia at this stage.[83,94] Endoscopy is normal unless esophageal or gastric carcinoma is seen. Contraction of the LES can give a puckered appearance to the distal esophagus, and mild resistance can sometimes be felt as the endoscope passes into the stomach. *Candida* infection and mucosal ulcers can be seen secondary to stasis.[94] Evaluation of both sides of the LES and biopsy of any suspicious lesions must be done in all patients and particularly in those over the age of 50 years to rule out carcinoma.[94,108] Secondary achalasia can also be seen with distant tumors such as oat cell carcinoma, presumably on a neurohumoral basis.[94,108]

Esophageal manometry is necessary to establish the diagnosis. Four manometric features are characteristic of achalasia: (1) body aperistalsis, (2) incomplete or absent LES relaxation, (3) normal or elevated LES pressure, and (4) elevated intraesophageal pressure. Absence of body peristalsis and poor LES relaxation are mandatory for the diagnosis.[94,108]

Radionuclide studies are useful to determine the degree of impaired esophageal clearance and can be used to assess improvement following treatment.[50] Because poor esophageal emptying can be seen in other esophageal disorders including esophageal obstruction, the test must be considered supplemental to the diagnostic tests listed above.

TREATMENT OF ACHALASIA

Since the neural defect is not correctable, treatment aimed at increasing esophageal clearance is necessary. Pharmacotherapy aimed at decreasing LES pressure with agents such as calcium blocking agents or nitrates reduces LES pressure by only 30 to 40% and rarely works in the long term.[18,19,40,99] Recent trials showed an equal effect of nifedipine (20 mg) and balloon dilatation, but this requires substantiation.[18] Medical therapy should be reserved for those patients in whom dilatation or surgery is too risky or as a temporary therapy prior to definitive treatment.

Simple mercury or guidewire bougienage can be helpful initially but rarely works in the long term even with 58 or 60 French dilators.[70,71,94] Although some have advocated bougienage for recurrent symptoms after pneumatic dilatation, success rates are better with repeat pneumatic dilatation.[75] Recent studies in achalasia secondary to Chagas' disease have shown that LES pressure is decreased by 65% after pneumatic dilatation 1 year following treatment, while mercury bougienage reduced LES pressure by only 15% after a similar period.[93] Based on the poor response to bougienage, forceful dilatation has now become the standard technique for treating achalasia.[60,63,71]

Forceful dilatation to a diameter of 3 cm or greater (≥90 French) is necessary to tear esophageal smooth muscle and effect long-term results in achalasia patients.[94] Various forceful dilators including Mosher bags, the Starck metal dilator, the Brown-McHardy or Hurst-Tucker dilators, or hourglass-shaped bags (Rider-Moeller) attached to a semirigid metal post have all been replaced by the Rigiflex pneumatic balloon system.[94] Unique endoscopically placed balloon dilators (Witzel dilators) offer effective and safe treatment without the need for fluoroscopic control but are not available in the United States.[10,32]

Not only are there multiple dilators but the technique is not standardized.[9,10,17,23,24,32,34,39,52,68,82,84,101,109] Premedication should be used to allay anxiety, but consciousness should be maintained at all times. Initial dilator diameter is variable and ranges from 2.9 to 4.0 cm. Sequential use of dilators from 3.0 to 4.0 cm has been recommended by one group as a means of decreasing esophageal perforation while retaining excellent clinical results.[52] The maximal pressure needed and the duration of dilatation are not known. Pressures have ranged from 7 to 15 lb/in^2 (300 to 774 mmHg).[9,10,17,23,24,32,34,39,52,68,82,84,101,109] Dilatation duration has ranged from 20 seconds to 5 minutes with repeat dilatation done by several investigators.[9,10,17,23,24,32,34,39,52,68,82,84,101,109] Comparison trials are small, with almost equal efficacy and complications for all dilating systems.[9,10,17,23,24,32,34,39,52,68,74,82,84,101,109] A single-center report of Witzel and Rigiflex balloon dilatation for achalasia showed a slightly higher rate of perforation with the Witzel dilator (4-cm size) compared with sequential Rigiflex dilations (3.5- and 4.0-cm sizes), but the difference was not significant (5.2% versus 2.4%).[13] The Brown-McHardy dilator may be slightly more effective but is no longer commercially available.[101]

The procedure is usually done on an outpatient basis, although inpatient stay following the procedure may be necessary, particularly for elderly or infirm patients. The authors' unit uses both the Witzel dilator and the Rigiflex dilators. The Witzel dilator is our standard adult dilator, and the Rigiflex dilators are reserved for those patients who cannot be intubated or for children (3.0-cm balloon used). Both fluoroscopic and endoscopic guidance are used. Witzel dilatation is accomplished by passing the dilator over a standard adult gastroscope (29 French) and intubating the esophagus. The endoscope tip is passed into the antrum and the tip retroflexed. The distal end of the dilator is placed at the gastroesophageal junction and the distance noted. The scope is then passed until the midportion of the balloon straddles the gastroesophageal junction. The balloon is then inflated slowly with constant direct visualization and repositioning over 1 to 3 minutes until 300 mmHg is achieved or the patient has significant pain. The balloon is kept inflated for 3 minutes. The dilator is then deflated with negative pressure and withdrawn. The gastroesophageal junction should be examined for tears or perforation. Small amounts of blood may be present on the dilator at the end of the procedure. Repeat balloon inflation at the first treatment session is not used in the authors' center.

Fluoroscopic passage of the Rigiflex dilator or Brown-McHardy dilator is done in a similar manner with the patient in the sitting position. The balloon is passed until it is 40 to 50 cm from the incisors. The patient is then placed in the right anterior oblique position and the balloon passed until it straddles the diaphragm. The midportion of the balloon should straddle the waist of the narrowing. As dilatation progresses, the balloon tends to slip into the stomach and repositioning is necessary. Prevention of this tendency to ride up can be achieved by upward traction on the dilator. Pressure can vary from 9 to 15 lb/in^2 but should be increased until the waist of the narrowing is obliterated. High pressure can be maintained for 20 seconds to 1 minute and repeated.[39] Lower pressures should be needed to obliterate the waist on second dilatations if the first was successful. If high pressures are still necessary to achieve waist obliteration, then the initial procedure should be repeated. No more than two dilatations are recommended in a single session. Blood may be seen on the dilator, but its absence does not mean an unsuccessful dilatation.

The patient should be kept at least 4 hours following the procedure and radiologic studies obtained if there is any suspicion of perforation. Persistent chest pain, vomiting, hematemesis, back pain, tachycardia, or hypotension should mandate radiologic evaluation. Water-soluble contrast is used first and followed up with barium if no obvious leaks are seen. Intramural hematoma or localized small perforations can be handled medically in most situations, but the responsible surgeon should have the final say in most cases. Medical treatment includes bowel rest, broad-spectrum antibiotics, and total parenteral nutrition.[55,104] Progressive symptoms dictate surgical correction.

If dilatation has been successful and the patient is able to leave the unit, only clear liquids should be allowed on the first day.[9,10,32] Repeat evaluation the next day, preferably in person, is prudent. Diet can be progressed rapidly thereafter, and the patient usually notes improved swallowing even on the first day. Maximal improvement in swallowing may take several days to a week and mild chest pain may also be noted for a few days.[9,10,32] Increasing pain and fever are rare and mandate a full radiologic evaluation of the esophagus. True reflux after dilatation is uncommon and usually responds to a short course of standard H_2RAs.[9,10,32,94]

RESULTS OF PNEUMATIC DILATATION FOR ACHALASIA

Relief of dysphagia with pneumatic dilatation is variable, with a range between 32 and 98% and in most studies between 60 and 80%.[9,10,17,23,24,32,34,39,52,60,82,84,101,109] Studies that use standard clinic visit techniques have a tendency to overestimate success because of the patient's desire to please the doctor and by the patient's lack of knowledge of dietary changes, which minimize the patient's symptoms.[28,94] Predictive factors for immediate treatment efficacy include age, with younger patients (<40 years old) responding less well, and final diameter of the dilator used (≥3.6 cm responding best).[28] Sex, duration of symptoms, and investigation results did not predict treatment response. Long-term clinical response was best predicted by post-treatment LES pressure (≤10 to 30 mmHg predicted a good response); other long-term predictors of a good response have included age greater than 20 years, female gender, esophageal body diameter larger than 3 cm, and esophageal body pressure less than 15 mmHg.[3,28,89] The degree of pain with dilatation, the amount of blood on the dilator, insufflation pressures, and postprocedure esophageal emptying studies have not been shown to be predictive.[115] Some prospective studies using predetermined criteria for success and careful follow-up are less favorable to dilatation for long-term treatment. During the first few months after dilatation (one to four sessions), up to 80% of patients have an excellent subjective response.[28,89] However, using a structured interview and employing Kaplan-Meier plots, a single pneumatic dilatation resulted in a 1-year remission rate of 59% and a 5-year remission rate of only 26%.[28] However, repeat dilatations not only repeated the initial success but were followed by progressively longer remissions. Repeatedly dilated patients and nondilated or singly dilated patients fared equally well if surgery was chosen.[28,112] Thus, repeated dilatations are safe and effective and do not have to be limited in number if the patient prefers that option and has had initial success. Repeat pneumatic dilation in patients who have not had an initial successful dilatation has a low likelihood of success (<20%).[10,28,32]

Manometric changes following dilatation are common, with return of intermittent distal progressive peristalsis in 20% of patients after dilatation.[10,65,94,108] Lower esophageal sphincter pressure is immediately reduced after dilatation but tends to increase with time.[94,108] Relaxation of the LES does not return after dilatation, but the degree of relaxation (percentage of complete relaxation) does improve after treatment.[94,108] Bolus transit through the esophagus is still abnormal, although retention of radionuclide is decreased to 25% or less of baseline after successful dilatation.[50,83,94,108]

Immediate complications following pneumatic dilatation include chest pain, gastrointestinal bleeding, intramural hematoma, and esophageal perforation. Complication rates range from 1 to 16%, with perforation occurring in 4 to 6% (range, 1 to 13%).[9,10,17,23,24,32,34,39,52,68,82,84,94,101,109] Most perforations are small and localized and can be handled medically with antibiotics and hyperalimentation. Gastroesophageal reflux occurs in only 2% of patients after pneumatic dilatation because of residual pressure in the LES following dilation.[94,108]

COMPARISON STUDIES WITH SURGICAL MYOTOMY

Randomized, controlled trials comparing surgical myotomy and balloon dilatation for achalasia are few. One randomized, controlled trial compared 39 patients treated with balloon dilatation and 42 patients who underwent surgical myotomy.[23,24] Long-term results clearly showed in both the preliminary and follow-up studies that myotomy achieved a higher rate of a good long-term result, with 95% of patients having a good to excellent response, while only 65% of pneumatic dilatation patients had a similar response at 5 years.[23,24] Initial response was equal for the two groups, but only surgery maintained effectiveness over time. Post-treatment LES pressure was highly predictive of clinical response, with lesser degrees of LES pressure decrease in patients failing dilatation. A more recent study compared 20 pneumatic dilatation patients with 20 myotomy patients who had never undergone dilatation. At 4 to 6 months after the procedures, the dilatation group was more likely to have pyrosis and chest pain, although neither group had a greater propensity for developing esophagitis. The myotomy group had significantly lower LES pressures (7 versus 16 mmHg), although both interventions had similar clinical efficacy (symptom relief).[33]

Large comparison trials have given similar results.[82,84] Although mortality and morbidity are similar in the two groups of treated patients, long-term effectiveness is higher with surgery. Myotomy reduces LES pressure more dependably than pneumatic dilatation. The most significant complication of myotomy is symptomatic gastroesophageal reflux, with rates of 2 to 10% generally reported.[23,24,82,84] This reflux is frequently quite damaging because of poor acid clearance in a poorly motile or atonic esophagus. Peptic stricture, Barrett's esophagus, and severe dysphagia occur following myotomy.[23,24,82,84] Loose fundoplication has been advocated as prophylactic treatment to reduce postmyotomy acid reflux but can lead to severe dysphagia if esophageal motility is poor and LES pressure is too high.[23,24,92] Twenty-four-hour pH testing has demonstrated abnormal acid reflux in up to 28% of patients after myotomy, but most patients are asymptomatic.[23,24] Acid reflux scores after esophageal dilatation are much lower than scores after myotomy because of higher residual LES pressure following dilatation.[23,24] There have been no direct comparisons between endoscopic dilatation and laparoscopic Heller myotomy. This laparoscopic approach is 90% clinically effective, but prior dilatation has been associated with more complications after laparoscopic myotomy.[51,78,111] There are no compelling reasons to suspect that laparoscopic myotomy is less effective than the open technique, especially in comparison to endoscopic dilatation.

CHOICE OF TREATMENT

Controversy about whether surgical myotomy or pneumatic dilatation should be the initial treatment in patients with achalasia is still evident.[26,30,94,110] Although myotomy has a higher overall success rate, most patients do well following pneumatic dilatation and can be redilated with equal success if the initial response was good or excellent.[10,32,94,108] Cost-effectiveness studies have shown a 5.0 times greater cost for surgery initially and a 2.4 times increased cost when costs for treating failed patients after pneumatic dilation were factored in.[84,94] Only 12% of patients ultimately underwent myotomy over a 5-year follow-up period.[84] Clearly, patients with dilatation failures should have surgical myotomy, since redilatation is rarely successful.[10,32] Pneumatic dilatation should be considered a failure if two successive dilatation sessions produce minimal symptomatic improvement or rapidly recurring symptoms. Children and patients with a suspicion of secondary achalasia should have surgery as initial treatment.[83,94] Perforation risk with dilatation is significant but should not be a major consideration because of the reasonably low incidence and the fact that postperforation patients do equally as well with corrective surgery as those with initial surgical treatment.[10,32,94] Epiphrenic diverticula and a large hiatal hernia are still considered relative contraindications because of higher perforation rates.[94,108]

Recent innovations in achalasia treatment were based on the fact that excitatory neural input through acetylcholine release is unopposed by inhibitory input at the LES in patients with achalasia, thereby preventing LES relaxation. This excitatory input can be blocked with botulinum toxin injection into the LES (usually 80 to 100 units total divided among four or five injections). Initial studies demonstrated excellent but short-lived clinical and manometric improvement when botulinum toxin was compared to placebo.[7,85] Recent randomized, comparative trials between botulinum toxin injection and pneumatic dilatation have demonstrated a superior response with pneumatic dilation, with more patients clinically responding (70% versus 22%), a greater effect on LES pressure, less barium retention, and less need for retreatment in the first 12 months.[107] The role of botulinum toxin may be relegated to patients with high-risk medical conditions, the elderly, and potential salvage treatment after failed myotomy or pneumatic dilatation.[6,42,86]

FUTURE DIRECTIONS IN ESOPHAGEAL DILATATION

More permanent prosthetic devices such as wall stents are still in their infancy.[64] Difficulty in placement, higher complication rates, and an unknown longevity make these devices less attractive for long-term treatment of benign strictures of the esophagus.[64] Technical advances in dilators, such as ones that detect a fall in wall tension or resistance as tissue is dilated, may reduce complications.[63,64,94]

Although dilatation remains the major nonsurgical treatment choice for mechanical and functional esophageal obstruction, only continued comparison to other alternative modalities will allow proper placement of esophageal dilatation in the physician's treatment armamentarium.

References

1. Aggestrup, S., Uddman, R., Sundler, F., et al.: Lack of vasoactive intestinal polypeptide nerves in esophageal achalasia. Gastroenterology, *84*:924, 1983.
2. Agnew, S. R., Pandya, S. P., Reynolds, R. P., et al.: Predictors for frequent esophageal dilations of benign peptic strictures. Dig. Dis. Sci., *41*:931, 1996.
3. Alonso, P., Gonzalez-Conde, B., Macenlle, R., et al.: Achalasia: The usefulness of manometry for evaluation of treatment. Dig. Dis. Sci., *44*:536, 1999.
4. Anand, B. S.: Eder-Puestow and Savary dilators. Hepatogastroenterology, *39*:494, 1992.
5. Anand, B. S., Saeed, Z. A., Michaletz, P. A., et al.: A randomized comparison of dilation alone versus dilation plus laser in patients receiving chemotherapy and external beam radiation for esophageal carcinoma. Dig. Dis. Sci., *43*:2255, 1998.
6. Annese, V., Basciani, M., Lombardi, G., et al.: Perendoscopic injection of botulinum toxin is effective in achalasia after failure of myotomy or pneumatic dilation. Gastrointest. Endosc., *44*:461, 1996.
7. Annese, V., Basciani, M., Perri, F., et al.: Controlled trial of botulinum toxin injection versus placebo and pneumatic dilation in achalasia. Gastroenterology, *111*:1418, 1996.
8. Bailey, A. D., and Goldner, F.: Can clinicians accurately assess esophageal dilation without fluoroscopy? Gastrointest. Endosc., *34*:373, 1990.
9. Barkin, J. S., Guelrud, M., Reiner, D. K., et al.: Forceful balloon dilation: An outpatient procedure for achalasia. Gastrointest. Endosc., *36*:123, 1990.
10. Barnett, J. L., Eisenman, R., Nostrant, T. T., and Elta, G. H.: Witzel pneumatic dilation for achalasia: Safety and long-term efficacy. Gastrointest. Endosc., *36*:482, 1990.
11. Becker, B. S., and Burakoff, R.: The effect of verapamil on the lower esophageal sphincter pressure in normal subjects and in achalasia. Am. J. Gastroenterol., *78*:773, 1983.
12. Bolstad, D. S.: The management of strictures of the esophagus. Ann. Otol. Rhinol. Laryngol., *75*:1019, 1966.
13. Borotto, E., Guadric, M., and Samama, J.: Risk factors of oesophageal perforation during pneumatic dilatation for achalasia. Gut, *39*:9, 1996.
14. Botulinum toxin. Lancet, *340*:1508, 1992.
15. Castell, D. O., and Donner, M. W.: Evaluation of dysphagia: A careful history is crucial. Dysphagia, *2*:65, 1987.

16. Ching, C. K., Shaheen, M. Z., and Homes, G. K. T.: Is omeprazole more effective in the treatment of reflux esophagitis with associated peptic stricture? Gastroenterology, *98:*A30, 1990.
17. Clagett, O. T.: Achalasia: Dilation or myotomy? J. Thorac. Cardiovasc. Surg. *53:*757, 1967.
18. Coccia, G., Bortolotti, M., Michetti, P., and Dodero, M.: Prospective clinical and manometric study comparing pneumatic dilatation and sublingual nifedipine in the treatment of oesophageal achalasia. Gut, *32:*604, 1991.
19. Coccia, G., Bortolotti, M., Michetti, P., and Dodero, M.: Return of esophageal peristalsis after nifedipine therapy in patients with idiopathic esophageal achalasia. Am. J. Gastroenterol., *87:*1705, 1992.
20. Cox, J. G. C., Dakkak, M., Buckton, G. K., and Bennett, J. R.: Dilators for esophageal stricture—a description of a new bougie and a comparison of current instruments. Gastrointest. Endosc., *35:*551, 1989.
21. Cox, J. G., Winter, R. K., Maslin, S. C., et al.: Balloon or bougie for dilatation of benign oesophageal stricture? An interim report of a randomised controlled trial. Gut, *29:*1741, 1988.
22. Cox, J. G., Winter, R. K., Maslin, S. C., et al.: Balloon or bougie for dilation of benign esophageal strictures? Dig. Dis. Sci., *39:*776, 1994.
23. Csendes, A., Braghetto, I., Henriquez, A., and Cortes, C.: Late results of a prospective randomized study comparing forceful dilatation and oesophagomyotomy in patients with achalasia. Gut, *30:*299, 1989.
24. Csendes, A., Velasco, N., Braghetto, I., and Henriquez, A.: A prospective randomized study comparing forceful dilatation and esophagomyotomy in patients with achalasia of the esophagus. Gastroenterology, *80:*789, 1981.
25. Dhir, V., Swaroop, S., Mohandas, K. M., et al.: Dilation of proximal esophageal strictures following therapy for head and neck cancer: Experience with Savary Gilliard dilators. J. Surg. Oncol., *63:*187, 1996.
26. Donahue, P. E., Schlesinger, P. K., Bombeck, C. T., et al.: Achalasia of the esophagus. Ann. Surg., *203:*505, 1986.
27. Earlam, R., and Cunha-Melo, J. R.: Benign esophageal strictures: Historical and technical aspects of dilation. Br. J. Surg., *68:*829, 1981.
28. Echardt, V. F., Aignherr, C., and Bernhard, G.: Predictors of outcome in patients with achalasia treated by pneumatic dilation. Gastroenterology, *103:*1732, 1992.
29. Eckardt, V. F., Kanzler, G., and Willems, D.: Single dilation of symptomatic Schatzki rings. A prospective evaluation of its effectiveness. Dig. Dis. Sci., *37:*577, 1992.
30. Ellis, H. F.: Treatment of achalasia: A continuing controversy. Ann. Thorac. Surg., *45:*447, 1988.
31. Ellis, H. F., Crozier, R. E., and Watkins, E., Jr.: Operation for esophageal achalasia. J. Thorac. Cardiovasc. Surg., *88:*344, 1984.
32. Elta, G. H., Nostrant, T. T., and Wilson, J. A.: Treatment of achalasia with the Witzel pneumatic dilator. Gastrointest. Endosc., *33:*101, 1987.
33. Felix, V. N., Cecconello, I., Zilberstein, B., et al.: Achalasia: A prospective study comparing the results of dilatation and myotomy. Hepatogastroenterology, *45:*97, 1998.
34. Fellows, I. W., Ogilvie, A. L., and Atkinson, M.: Pneumatic dilatation in achalasia. Gut, *24:*1020, 1983.
35. Fellows, I. W., Raina, S., and Holmes, G. K. T.: Celestin dilatation of benign esophageal strictures: A review of 100 patients. Am. J. Gastroenterol., *81:*1052, 1986.
36. Ferguson, R., Dronfield, M. W., and Atkinson, M.: Cimetidine in treatment of reflux esophagitis with peptic stricture. BMJ, *2:*472, 1979.
37. Fregonese, D., DiFalco, G., and DiToma, F.: Balloon dilatation of anastomotic intestinal stenoses: Long-term results. Endoscopy, *22:*249, 1990.
38. Frimberger, E.: Endoscopic treatment of benign esophageal stricture. Endoscopy, *15:*199, 1983.
39. Gelfand, M. D., and Kozarek, R. A.: An experience with polyethylene balloons for pneumatic dilation in achalasia. Am. J. Gastroenterol., *84:*924, 1989.
40. Gelfond, M., Rozen, R., and Gilat, T.: Isosorbide dinitrate and nifedipine treatment of achalasia: A clinical, manometric and radionuclide evaluation. Gastroenterology, *83:*963, 1982.
41. Glick, M. E.: Clinical course of esophageal stricture managed by bougienage. Dig. Dis. Sci. *27:*884, 1982.
42. Gordon, J. M., and Eaker, E. Y.: Prospective study of esophageal botulinum toxin injection in high-risk achalasia patients. Am. J. Gastroenterol., *92:*1812, 1997.
43. Graham, D. Y., and Smith, J. L.: Balloon dilatation of benign and malignant esophageal strictures. Gastrointest. Endosc., *31:*171, 1985.
44. Graham, D. Y., Tabibian, N., Schwartz, J. T., and Smith, J. L.: Evaluation of the effectiveness of through-the-scope balloons as dilators of benign and malignant gastrointestinal strictures. Gastrointest. Endosc., *33:*432, 1987.
45. Groskreutz, J. L., and Kim, C. H.: Schatzki's ring: Long-term results following dilation. Gastrointest. Endosc., *36:*479, 1990.
46. Hands, L. J., Papauramidis, J., Bishop, H., et al.: The natural history of peptic oesophageal strictures treated by dilatation and antireflux therapy alone. Ann. R. Coll. Surg. Engl., *71:*306, 1989.
47. Harrison, M. E., and Sanowski, R. A.: Mercury bougie dilation of benign esophageal strictures. Hepatogastroenterology, *39:*497, 1992.
48. Hegedüs, V., and Poulsen, P. E.: Balloon dilatation of alimentary tract strictures. Acta Radiol. Diagn., *27:*681, 1986.
49. Hine, K. R., Hawkey, C. J., Atkinson, M., and Holmes, G. K. T.: Comparison of the Eder-Puestow and Celestin techniques for dilating benign oesophageal strictures. Gut, *25:*1100, 1984.
50. Holloway, R. H., Krosin, G., Lange, R. C., et al.: Radionuclide esophageal emptying of a solid meal to quantitate results of therapy in achalasia. Gastroenterology, *84:*771, 1983.
51. Hunter, J. G., Trus, T. L., Branum, G. D., et al.: Laparoscopic Heller myotomy and fundoplication for achalasia. Ann. Surg., *225:*655, 1997.
52. Kadakia, S. C., and Wong, R. K. H.: Graded pneumatic dilation using Rigiflex achalasia dilators in patients with primary esophageal achalasia. Am. J. Gastroenterol., *88:*34, 1993.
53. Katz, P. O., Gilbert, J., and Castell, D. O.: Pneumatic dilatation is effective long-term treatment for achalasia. Dig. Dis. Sci., *43:*1973, 1998.
54. Kelly, H. D. R.: Origins of oesophagology. Proc. R. Soc. Med., *62:*781, 1969.
55. Kim-Deobald, J., and Kozarek, R. A.: Esophageal perforation: An 8-year review of a multispecialty clinic's experience. Am. J. Gastroenterol., *87:*1112, 1992.
56. Koop, H., and Arnold, R.: Long-term maintenance treatment of reflux esophagitis with omeprazole: Prospective study in patients with H_2 blocker resistant esophagitis. Dig. Dis. Sci., *36:*552, 1991.
57. Kozarek, R. A.: Endoscopic Gruntzig balloon dilation of gastrointestinal stenoses. J. Clin. Gastroenterol., *6:*401, 1984.
58. Kozarek, R. A.: Proximal strictures of the esophagus. J. Clin. Gastroenterol., *6:*505, 1984.
59. Kozarek, R. A.: Hydrostatic balloon dilation of gastrointestinal stenoses: A national survey. Gastrointest. Endosc., *32:*15, 1986.
60. Kozarek, R. A.: Esophageal dilation and prostheses. Endosc. Rev., *4:*9, 1987.
61. Kozarek, R. A.: Complications of reflux esophagitis and their medical management. Gastroenterol. Clin. North Am., *19:*713, 1990.
62. Kozarek, R. A.: Dilation therapy for gastric outlet obstruction. Are balloons a bust? (Editorial). J. Clin. Gastroenterol., *17:*2, 1993.
63. Kozarek, R. A.: Gastrointestinal dilation. *In* Yamada, T. (ed.): Textbook of Gastroenterology. New York, J.B. Lippincott, 1991, p. 2587.
64. Kozarek, R. A., Ball, T. J., and Patterson, D. J.: Metallic self-expanding stent application in the upper gastrointestinal tract: Caveats and concerns. Gastrointest. Endosc., *38:*1, 1992.
65. Lamet, M., Fleshler, B., and Achkar, E.: Return of peristalsis in achalasia after pneumatic dilatation. Am. J. Gastroenterol., *80:*602, 1985.
66. Lehman, G. A., and O'Connor, K. W.: Endoscopic tape dilator—a simple and inexpensive method to dilate upper gastrointestinal strictures. J. Clin. Gastroenterol., *7:*208, 1985.
67. Lindor, K. D., Ott, B. J., and Hughes, R. W., Jr.: Balloon dilatation of upper digestive tract strictures. Gastroenterology, *89:*545, 1985.
68. Lishman, A. H., and Dellipiani, A. W.: Management of achalasia of the cardia by forced pneumatic dilation. Gut, *23:*541, 1982.
69. Little, A. G., Soriano, A., Ferguson, M. K., et al.: Surgical treatment

of achalasia: Results with esophagomyotomy and Belsey repair. Ann. Thorac. Surg., *45:*489, 1988.
70. Mandelstam, P., Block, C., Newell, L., and Dillon, M.: The role of bougienage in the management of achalasia—the need for reappraisal. Gastrointest. Endosc., *28:*169, 1982.
71. Marks, R. D., and Richter, J. E.: Peptic strictures of the esophagus. Am. J. Gastroenterol., *88:*1160, 1993.
72. Marks, R., Richter, J. C., Koehler, R., et al.: Does medical therapy improve dysphagia in patients with peptic strictures and esophagitis? Gastroenterology, *102:*A118, 1992.
73. Marshall, J. B., Afridi, S. A., King, P. D., et al.: Esophageal dilation with polyvinyl dilators over a marked guidewire: Practice and safety at one center over a 5-year period. Am. J. Gastroenterol., *91:*1503, 1996.
74. McClave, S. A., Wright, R. A., and Brady, P. G.: Prospective randomized study of Maloney esophageal dilation—blinded versus fluoroscopic guidance. Gastrointest. Endosc., *36:*272, 1990.
75. McJunkin, B., McMillan, W. O., Duncan, H. E., et al.: Assessment of dilation methods in achalasia: Large diameter mercury bougienage followed by pneumatic dilation as needed. Gastrointest. Endosc., *37:*18, 1991.
76. McLean, G. K., Cooper, G. S., Hartz, W. H., et al.: Radiologically guided balloon dilation of gastrointestinal strictures (part I). Radiology, *165:*35, 1987.
77. McLean, G. K., Cooper, G. S., Hartz, W. H., et al.: Radiologically guided balloon dilation of gastrointestinal strictures (part II). Radiology, *165:*41, 1987.
78. Morino, M., Rebecchi, F., Festa, V., et al.: Preoperative pneumatic dilatation represents a risk factor for laparoscopic Heller myotomy. Surg. Endosc., *11:*359, 1997.
79. Myer, C. M., Ball, W. S., and Bisset, G. S., III: Balloon dilatation of esophageal strictures in children. Arch. Otolaryngol. Head Neck Surg., *117:*529, 1991.
80. Nelson, D. B., Sanderson, S. J., and Azar, M. M.: Bacteremia with esophageal dilation. Gastrointest. Endosc., *48:*563, 1998.
81. Ogilvie, A. L., Fergusion, R., and Atkinson, M.: Outlook with conservative treatment of peptic esophageal stricture. Gut, *20:*23, 1980.
82. Okike, N., Payne, W. S., Neufeld, D. M., et al.: Esophagomyotomy versus forceful dilation for achalasia of the esophagus: Results in 899 patients. Ann. Thorac. Surg., *28:*119, 1979.
83. Ott, D. J., Richter, J. E., Wu, W. C., et al.: Radiographic evaluation of esophagus immediately after pneumatic dilatation for achalasia. Dig. Dis. Sci., *32:*962, 1987.
84. Parkman, H. P., Reynolds, J. C., Ouyang, A., et al.: Pneumatic dilatation or esophagomyotomy treatment for idiopathic achalasia: Clinical outcomes and cost analysis. Dig. Dis. Sci., *38:*75, 1993.
85. Pasricha, P. J., Ravich, W. J., Hendrix, T. R., et al.: Intrasphincteric botulinum toxin for the treatment of achalasia. N. Engl. J. Med., *332:*774, 1995.
86. Pasricha, P. J., Ravich, W. J., and Kalloo, A. N.: Botulinum toxin for achalasia. Lancet, *341:*244, 1993.
87. Patterson, D. J., Graham, D. Y., Smith, J. L., et al.: Natural history of benign esophageal stricture treated by dilatation. Gastroenterology, *85:*346, 1983.
88. Penagini, R., Dabbagh, M. A., Misiewicz, J. J., et al.: Effect of dilatation of peptic esophageal strictures on gastroesophageal reflux, dysphagia, and stricture diameter. Dig. Dis. Sci., *33:*389, 1988.
89. Ponce, J., Garrigues, V., Pertejo, V., et al.: Individual prediction of response to pneumatic dilation in patients with achalasia. Dig. Dis. Sci., *41:*2135, 1996.
90. Price, J. D., Stanciu, C., and Bennett, J. R.: A safer method of dilating oesophageal strictures. Lancet, *1:*1141, 1974.
91. Puestow, K. L.: Conservative treatment of stenosing diseases of the esophagus. Postgrad. Med. *18:*6, 1955.
92. Qualman, S. J., Haupt, H. M., Yang, P., and Hamilton, S. R.: Esophageal Lewy bodies associated with ganglion cell loss in achalasia: Similarity to Parkinson's disease. Gastroenterology, *87:*848, 1984.
93. Raizman, R. E., DeRezende, J. M., and Neva, F. A.: A clinical trial with pre- and post-treatment manometry comparing pneumatic dilation with bougienage for treatment of Chagas' megaesophagus. Am. J. Gastroenterol., *74:*405, 1980.
94. Richter, J. E.: Motility disorders of the esophagus. *In* Yamada, T. (ed.): Textbook of Gastroenterology. New York, J.B. Lippincott, 1991, p. 1083.
95. Saeed, Z. A., Ramirez, F. C., Hepps, K. S., et al.: An objective end point for dilation improves outcome of peptic esophageal strictures: A prospective randomized trial. Gastrointest. Endosc., *45:*354, 1997.
96. Saeed, Z. A., Winchester, C. B., Ferro, P. S., et al.: Prospective randomized comparison of polyvinyl bougies and through-the-scope balloons for dilation of peptic strictures of the esophagus. Gastrointest. Endosc., *41:*159, 1995.
97. Scolapio, J. S., Pasha, T. M., Gostout, C. J., et al.: A randomized prospective study comparing rigid to balloon dilators for benign esophageal strictures and rings. Gastrointest. Endosc., *50:*13, 1999.
98. Shemesh, E., and Czerniak, A.: Comparison between Savary-Gilliard and balloon dilatation of benign esophageal strictures. World J. Surg., *14:*518, 1990.
99. Short, T. P., and Thomas, E.: An overview of the role of calcium antagonists in the treatment of achalasia and diffuse oesophageal spasm. Drugs, *43:*177, 1992.
100. Silvis, S. E., Nebel, O., Rogers, G., et al.: Endoscopic complications: Results of the 1974 American Society for Gastrointestinal Endoscopy survey. JAMA, *235:*928, 1976.
101. Stark, G. A., Castell, D. O., Richter, J. E., and Wu, W. C.: Prospective randomized comparison of Brown-McHardy and microvasive balloon dilators in treatment of achalasia. Am. J. Gastroenterol., *85:*1322, 1990.
102. Starlinger, M., Appel, W. H., Schemper, M., and Schiessel, R.: Long-term treatment of peptic esophageal stenosis with dilatation and cimetidine: Factors influencing clinical result. Eur. Surg. Res., *17:*207, 1985.
103. Stoddard, C. J., and Simms, J. M.: Dilation of benign oesophageal strictures in the outpatient department. Br. J. Surg., *7:*752, 1984.
104. Swedlund, A., Traube, M., Siskind, B. N., and McCallum, R. W.: Nonsurgical management of esophageal perforation from pneumatic dilatation in achalasia. Dig. Dis. Sci., *34:*379, 1989.
105. Tulman, A. B., and Boyce, H. W.: Complications of esophageal dilation and guidelines for their prevention. Gastrointest. Endosc., *27:*229, 1981.
106. Tytgat, G. N. J.: Dilation therapy of benign esophageal stenoses. World J. Surg., *13:*142, 1989.
107. Vaezi, M. F., Richter, J. E., Wilcox, C. M., et al.: Botulinum toxin versus pneumatic dilatation in the treatment of achalasia: A randomized trial. Gut, *44:*231, 1999.
108. VanTrappen, G., and Hellemans, J.: Treatment of achalasia and related motor disorders. Gastroenterology, *79:*144, 1980.
109. VanTrappen, G., Hellemans, J., Deloof, W., et al.: Treatment of achalasia with pneumatic dilatations. Gut, *12:*268, 1971.
110. VanTrappen, G., and Janssens, J.: To dilate or to operate? That is the question. Gut, *24:*1013, 1983.
111. Vogt, D., Curet, M., Pitcher, D., et al.: Successful treatment of esophageal achalasia with laparoscopic Heller myotomy and Toupet fundoplication. Am. J. Surg., *174:*709, 1997.
112. Vreden, S. G. S., and Yap, S. H.: Pneumatic dilation for the treatment of achalasia. Neth. J. Med., *36:*228, 1990.
113. Webb, W. A.: Esophageal dilation: Personal experience with current instruments and techniques. Am. J. Gastroenterol., *83:*471, 1988.
114. Wesdorp, K., Bartelsman, J. F., den Hartog Jager, F. C., et al.: Results of conservative treatment of benign esophageal strictures: A follow-up study of 100 patients. Gastroenterology, *82:*487, 1982.
115. Wong, R. K., and Maydonovitch, C.: Utility of parameters measured during pneumatic dilation as predictors of successful dilation. Am. J. Gastroenterol., *91:*1126, 1996.
116. Yamamoto, H., Hughes, R. W., Schroeder, K. W., et al.: Treatment of benign esophageal stricture by Eder-Puestow or balloon dilators: A comparison between randomized and prospective nonrandomized trials. Mayo Clin. Proc., *67:*228, 1992.
117. Zuccaro, G., Richter, J. E., Rice, T. W., et al.: Viridans streptococcal bacteremia after esophageal stricture dilation. Gastrointest. Endosc., *48:*568, 1998.

VOLUME

I

Operative Approaches: The Hill Repair, The Belsey Mark IV Procedure, The Nissen Fundoplication, The Collis-Nissen Operation, and Barrett's Esophagus

CHAPTER

9 Overview: Hiatal Hernia, Gastroesophageal Reflux, and Their Complications

CLEMENT A. HIEBERT

GASTROESOPHAGEAL REFLUX: PERSPECTIVES ON THE HISTORY OF AN IDEA

Ideas become fossilized in names. For the first half of the twentieth century, surgeons were mesmerized by the idea that something called a hernia, which looked like a hernia and caused pain in the area of the affliction, should be managed like a hernia. Nissen,[36] protégé of the renowned Ferdinand Sauerbruch, recalled that his mentor at the turn of the century was so seduced by the implication of the diagnosis that he would actually section the hiatal rim of an ordinary sliding hiatal hernia to release the supposedly throttled stomach. For more than five decades, textbooks of surgery relegated hiatal hernia to chapters dealing with scrotal, umbilical, and other coelomic ruptures. Thoracic and abdominal surgeons, who had yet to learn about gastroesophageal reflux, knew threatened turf when they saw it and jousted over the advantages of pushing or pulling on their migrant quarry. Regardless of from which side of the diaphragmatic fence they argued, however, the surgical prescription was a rupture remedy: release and reposition the incarcerated stomach. Tether it so it would stay put, and narrow the hiatal escape route just in case.

The beginning of the end of this traditional and altogether too anatomic thinking was signaled by Allison[2] in his classic paper that illuminated the sliding hiatal hernia as a *physiologic* disorder of wrong-way traffic at the gastroesophageal junction. The anatomic culprit was a bad valve, and the burning symptoms were the lament of an esophagus awash with gastric ferments.

Allison's description of a typical patient cannot be improved on:

> A woman of 59 years of age complains that for six years she has suffered from intense burning pain behind the lower part of the sternum, which rises up toward, or even into, the neck. The pain may spread into the jaw, the ear, or the hard palate, or radiate through to the back between [the] shoulder blades or down the arm. It comes on especially when she exerts herself stooping forward, as in washing the floor, bending over the washtub, poking the fire, or fastening her shoes. It wakes her in the middle of the night, especially if she is sleeping on her back or her right side, and she seeks relief from what she describes as an agonizing pain by sitting upright and taking a few sips of water, milk, or alkaline mixture. She says that her throat usually feels dry and burning. When she swallows she may be conscious of the passage of food down the gullet, it may cause a feeling of soreness, and may sometimes lodge toward the lower end of the sternum, causing pain which is immediately relieved as the bolus passes into the stomach. If she bends forward after a meal, food or sour fluid rises into her throat and has to be swallowed again. Her husband says that for belching she takes the first prize. Four years ago, she was thought to have cholecystitis, but removal of either a normal or abnormal gallbladder did not cure her. Roentgenography of her stomach and duodenum shows no evidence of ulcer. She has tried all of the advertised stomach medicines with only temporary relief and has finally been told that "the nerves of her stomach have been upset by the change of life."

Allison thought that the normal valve mechanism at the gastroesophageal junction depended on the muscular arch formed by the right crus of the diaphragm, an attractive symmetric arrangement with the puborectalis sling around the anorectal junction at the other end of the alimentary tract. In each case, angulation of the passageway plus a pinchcock action of the adjacent pelvic or thoracic diaphragm achieved continence. Allison's remedy for the incontinent gastroesophageal junction was to reunite the stretched-out posterior fibers of the right crus with loose sutures and to shorten and reattach the splayed phrenoesophageal ligament to the undersurface of the diaphragm. Whether the phrenoesophageal membrane lacked substance or the sutures between it and the diaphragm put radial stress on the lower esophageal sphincter is moot. Results were less than satisfactory, and the Allison repair fell on hard times.

Given the disappointment of a promising operation that did not weather well, interest in Allison's observations might have petered out if it had not been for two separate and simultaneous fresh streams of activity, the first in the operating theaters of Frenchay Hospital, Bristol, and the Kantonsspital of the University of Basel and the second in the Gastrointestinal Laboratories of the Mayo Clinic and the Boston University, School of Medicine. In the first case, Belsey[5,7] and Nissen[35] independently put the final touches on operations that effectively discouraged reflux and also stood up to use. In the second case, Code[12] and Ingelfinger[25] proved with manometry the existence of a physiologic lower esophageal sphincter and, in so doing, put the imprimatur of scientific respectability on the antireflux goal of surgeons. From these two dissimilar streams of endeavor have flowed virtually all of our modern concepts of esophageal transport. Protégés of Belsey and Nissen carried their ideas and techniques to America, whereas followers of Code and Ingelfinger supplied the tools and critical judgment for a whole generation of manometrists who now look over the surgeon's shoulder.

At the time that Belsey and Nissen were working on their antireflux operations, there was great controversy over exactly what constituted the barrier to reflux. The Allison concept of a diaphragmatic pinchcock mechanism has already been noted. Other hypotheses included an acute angle of entry of the esophagus into the stomach, creating a flap valve, a mucosal rosette (bung), and the "liver tunnel." An eye of faith was required to appreciate most of these, but, after all, that sphinx of a sphincter,[26] the lower esophageal sphincter, remains something of a mystery, too. The cherished hope that simply measuring the lower esophageal sphincter would sort out candidates for antireflux surgery has not worked out. In a similar vein, it would be nice to relate that operative design followed laboratory revelation. This was not the case. Belsey's Mark IV operation was the product of astute observation, trial and error, failure, and frustration in the settings of the operating room and follow-up clinic.

Both the Belsey and Nissen operations had already proved their worth by the time manometry laboratories were prepared to certify them. Belsey had long before recognized that the normal locus of the gastroesophageal junction was several centimeters below the hiatus and had set his operative goal accordingly. For good measure, he added a crescentic overlay of stomach both to serve as a sphincter and to affix a length of intra-abdominal esophagus. Belsey waited 7 years before he was sufficiently satisfied with the durability of his operation to publish the results.[7,19] He called the procedure the Mark IV operation to remind surgeons that, although this might not be his last thought on the subject, neither was it his first!

Nissen's fundoplication was serendipitous,[36] a discovery illustrative of Pasteur's dictum that chance favors the prepared mind. In 1937, he was faced with an insecure esophagogastric anastomosis following a resection for a benign esophageal ulcer and decided to dunk it into the gastric wall "as is done with the feeding tube in Witzel's method of gastrostomy." The patient was lost to follow-up, but 16 years later a relative informed Nissen of the patient's good health; on further inquiry, Nissen learned that there were no reflux symptoms. Two years after this, he treated a woman with reflux without hiatal hernia and resurrected the fundoplication technique that had been effective 18 years before in the quite different setting of an esophagogastric anastomosis. This was the first "Nissen repair." Rossetti and Hell[45] modified the Nissen repair to include only the anterior stomach wall in the wrap. The idea was to reduce dissection in the vicinity of the vagal nerves.

A third contributor to operative design in the modern era was Hill, who made the fresh and interesting observation that in a "normal" cadaver, the gastroesophageal junction is primarily tethered *posteriorly.*[22] He claimed that this fibroelastic posterior shackle is loosened in a sliding hernia. Hill's operation relies on sutures placed from the upper lesser curvature of the stomach to the posterior parietes or, more anatomically, between the median arcuate ligament and the anterior and posterior phrenoesophageal fascial bundles. An alleged feature of his operation is its applicability to patients with grade IV esophagitis and stricture. Hill has answered skeptics with meticulous preoperative, intraoperative, and postoperative manometric data.

Each of these three major accepted methods of repair emphasizes redeployment of the gastroesophageal junction so that the lower esophageal sphincter resides entirely within the abdomen. In addition, the Belsey and Nissen repairs bolster the natural intrinsic sphincter with a fold of stomach, 270 degrees in the Belsey procedure and 360 degrees in the Nissen operation. In contrast, Hill argues that the natural valve includes an oblique entry of the esophagus into the stomach that is accentuated and strengthened by the anchoring sutures of the repair. Technical details of each of these three operations are described in subsequent sections of this chapter.

INCIDENCE AND IMPORTANCE OF THE HIATAL HERNIA PROBLEM

Although its exact prevalence in the normal population remains unknown, it is certain that hiatal hernia is the most common abnormality, reported on barium studies of the upper gastrointestinal tract. Women are more likely to be afflicted than men, the highest incidence occurring in the fifth and sixth decades of life. Skinner[49] estimates that routine gastrointestinal series show hiatal hernia in 10% of the population, with 5% of this group having pathologic reflux. If these figures are correct, significant gastroesophageal reflux disease is present in more than 1 million Americans. To be sure, one may take issue with the fact that the radiologic examinations were presumably requested for upper gastrointestinal symptoms and that the reported frequency, therefore, is unnaturally high. Identification of the stomach above the hiatus, moreover, depends both on the technique used by the radiologist and the sensitivity of his or her interpretation. When maneuvers such as abdominal compression are used, the incidence of hiatal hernia has been recorded in as many as 54.6% of patients.[52] Similarly, if encouraged and looked for, reflux has been found in more than 60% of another large group of patients, all ostensibly without symptoms.[34] As if to confound the skeptical clinician further, one of five patients with proven symptomatic reflux has no radiologically demonstrable hiatal hernia.[49] This case exists when the esophagus joins the stomach like the neck of an inverted funnel. It is an important concept and merits some reflection (Fig. 9-1).

INCOMPETENCE OF THE LOWER ESOPHAGEAL SPHINCTER WITHOUT HIATAL HERNIA

Reference has already been made to Nissen's first fundoplication for reflux in a patient with reflux but no

THE SPECTRUM OF THE HIATAL HERNIA/REFLUX PROBLEM

	Patulous Cardia	Sliding Hiatal Hernia	Early Incarceration (rolling phase)	End Stage Incarceration
Schematic	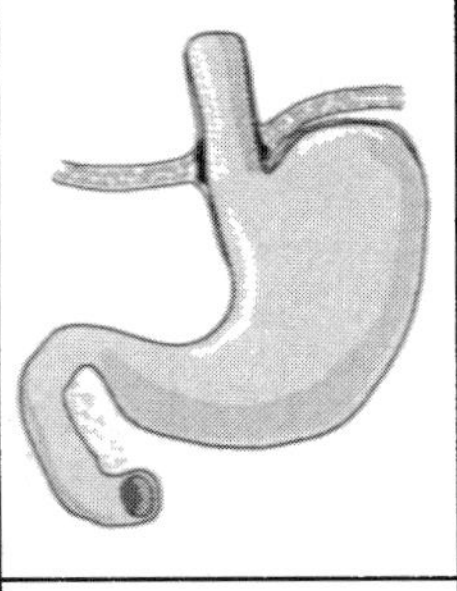	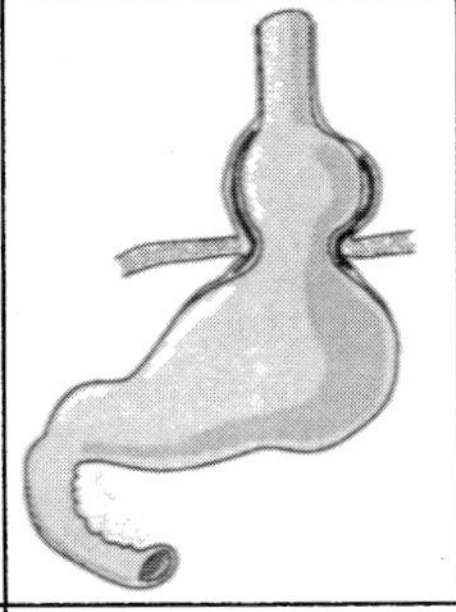	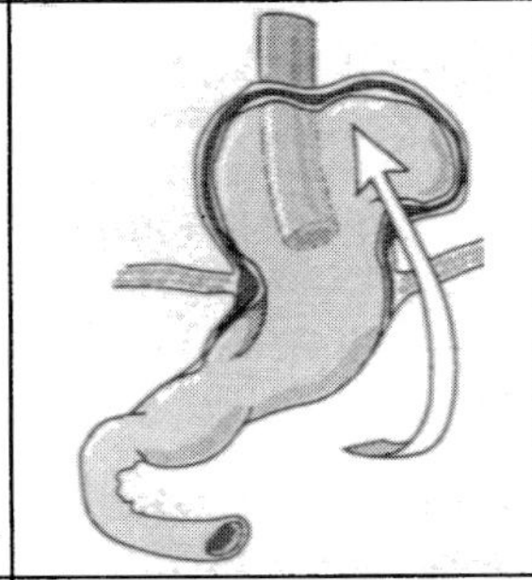	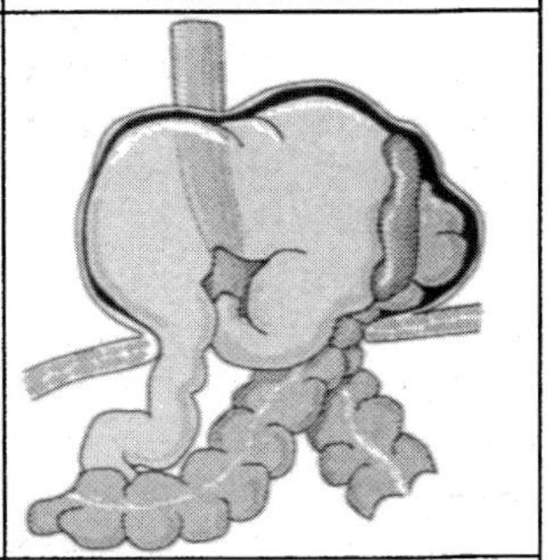
Radiologic Picture	GE junction widened but undisplaced	GE junction above diaphragm	GE junction near hiatus. A third or more of stomach in chest.	GE junction near hiatus. Most of stomach in chest. (spleen and colon may also migrate)
Dominant Symptoms	Posturally aggravated • heartburn / regurgitation • epigastric / substernal pain		• Early satiety, fullness, post prandial pain • Variable reflux symptoms.	Symptoms may be meager - then catastrophic complications!
Complications	Esophagitis, stricture, bleeding, aspiration		• Ulceration of stomach • Chronic bleeding	• Acute obstruction • Strangulation • Ulceration and acute hemorrhage • Perforation, aspiration
Indications for Operation	• Failed medical therapy • Presence of complications		Presence of a third or more of stomach above diaphragm with or without symptoms	Presence of a massive incarcerated hernia

Figure 9–1. The surgeon must understand the variably deranged physiology as well as the anatomic consequences of slack tethers and a wide hiatus.

hernia. The first published report of the Mark IV operation in North America, in fact, was made by Hiebert and Belsey,[19] who presented 71 patients with isolated gastroesophageal reflux culled from a group of 640 patients with hiatal hernia repairs that were done at Frenchay Hospital between 1951 and 1959. At that time, radiologists were wont to belittle the "clinical significance" of a small hiatal hernia, even though, as it turns out, reflux symptoms tend to be worse when the thoracic reservoir is small. Belsey shelved roentgenograms in favor of direct interpretation of the afflicted esophagus by means of rigid esophagoscopy with the patient awake. He argued convincingly that what mattered was a gaping and incompetent cardia rather than the presence or absence of a hernia. Symptoms of this isolated defect of the hiatal valve mechanism were identical to those characteristic of a sliding hiatal hernia. Endoscopy showed loss of vertical movements of the lower esophagus with respiration consistent with a slack phrenoesophageal membrane. The cardia opened during inspiration, and through the opening, a tide of gastric fluid rose and fell with each breath. The existence of reflux through a widened but undisplaced gastroesophageal junction has subsequently been validated by modern manometry and pH testing.[13] The reflux in this condition may be serious and chronically disabling, and knowledge of it may not only spare patients from a diagnosis of anxiety neurosis but also allow them the same advantages of modern therapy that would be expended if there were a visible rupture to validate the incompetent sphincter. The results of surgery are as dramatic and durable as those of surgery designed to repair a sliding hiatal hernia.[20]

HIATAL HERNIA IN INFANTS AND CHILDREN

As in adults, gastroesophageal reflux is a more suitable term than hiatal hernia in infants and children because it directs attention to the physiologic disorder rather than the incidental anatomic anomaly. The trouble is, of course, that reflux is ubiquitous in infants. The problem is to sort out Shakespeare's[48] "infant mewling and puking in his mother's arms" from the child headed for lifelong swallowing and aspiration problems because of virulent gastroesophageal reflux.

The pathognomonic symptom of *uncomplicated* chalasia or sliding hiatal hernia in infancy is regurgitation.

This form of regurgitation begins a few days after birth when feedings are increased and tends to be effortless but occasionally is projectile. Compared with the regurgitation of normal infants, which is usually confined to the first 2 hours after feeding, reflux through an incompetent cardia tends to last longer.[32] Bile seldom appears in the vomitus, but there may be streaks of blood.

Although pulmonary problems, dehydration, failure to thrive, esophagitis, stricture, bleeding, and anemia are frequently listed as the classic symptoms of gastroesophageal reflux in infants, they are, in fact, complications of that reflux. *Pulmonary complications* include apnea, choking, chronic cough, wheezing, and pneumonia. The diagnosis of gastroesophageal reflux should therefore be considered in all cases of recurrent respiratory problems that are otherwise not explained. The recovery of fat-laden macrophages by bronchoscopy is said to be confirming evidence that food has been inhaled.

Esophagitis in infancy may be severe and rapid in onset.[7] Belsey reports the development of an inflammatory *stricture* in as short a period as 6 weeks. Why all infants do not suffer the same fate is a mystery. Reflux episodes can be documented in duration and severity with prolonged pH testing.[10,30,31] Cleansing peristaltic waves can be identified by manometry, but the ability of the epithelial lining of the infant gullet to stifle digestion is not measurable. Esophagitis may lead to stricture, chronic bleeding, and failure to thrive. The babies are small, thin, and malnourished. Up to 70% of them are below the fifteenth percentile in weight, and 88% are below the fiftieth percentile.[28] The child may be loathsome to the parents.

Associated diseases and major congenital anomalies are frequently seen.

Diagnosis

The serious nature of an infant's rumination is usually not appreciated until one or more of the mentioned complications have supervened. A barium study demonstrates reverse flow through a patulous cardia, but a hernia may be hard to define unless it is large. Because an obstruction at the pylorus or beyond can exacerbate cardial incompetency in 20% of cases,[44] it is useful to perform a technetium sulfur colloid scintiscan as well as a barium study. Both tests can be useful in defining the status of the upper and lower ends of the stomach. Seibert and colleagues[47] found that the scintiscan had a specificity of 93% and a sensitivity of 79% compared with the barium study figures of 21 and 86%, respectively, in the detection of reflux. *Twenty-four-hour pH testing* can be done in infancy and is the most accurate reflux detection technique available. The duration and frequency of episodes of esophageal pH measuring less than 4.0 form the basis of a scoring system of severity (pH testing is discussed in Chapter 2).

Esophagoscopy is the sine qua non for assessing esophagitis. Clinical or radiologic clues may prove elusive, but endoscopy and biopsy can be used to identify early esophagitis, allowing definitive treatment to begin. The most serious consequences of gastroesophageal reflux in infants and children are those stemming from neglected esophagitis, particularly aspiration and malnourishment.

Treatment

Feedings thickened with cereal, positioning of the infant in the prone position with the head end of the body elevated 30 degrees, antacids, H_2 blockers, and occasionally metoclopramide are the salient features of medical management. Improvement is the rule, and about two thirds of afflicted children stop vomiting with treatment. When followed to adulthood, 90% of unoperated subjects are said to remain free from symptoms if esophagitis is absent from the start.[3] Jewett and Waterston[28] reported that 80 (13%) of 602 babies and children with hiatal hernia required an operation; one third were operated on after medical treatment failed, and the remainder had surgery for esophagitis as determined by roentgenography or esophagoscopy. Failure of medical treatment is indicated by continued inhalation of feedings, pneumonia, inanition, bleeding, or increased esophagitis.[29] Medical treatment of large hernias in children is futile.

Surgery consists of restoring competency to the cardia, usually by performing either a Belsey or a loose Nissen wrap. The latter procedure has been very popular. When stenosing esophagitis has supervened, a resection and short-segment colon interposition, which is described by Waterston[56] and Belsey,[6] is the treatment of choice. Lesser grades of esophagitis deserve a full trial of medical treatment.

ASSESSMENT OF GASTROESOPHAGEAL REFLUX

History

The most pathognomonic clue is a history of postprandial posturally aggravated symptoms of substernal burning (Fig. 9-2). Dysphagia without weight loss is present in about half of patients, and about the same number have chronic regurgitation or effortless vomiting.[19]

Radiography

Radiography can be used to define coexisting foregut anatomy, identify a hiatal hernia, determine its type, and, on occasion, display gastroesophageal reflux. Failure to identify reflux on radiography in no way excludes the diagnosis. Occasionally, a barium study taken when the patient has a full stomach is helpful in eliciting reflux that has failed to show itself during fasting.[33]

Endoscopy

Endoscopy is as indispensable in the evaluation of the esophagus as colonoscopy is in the study of large bowel disease. It is the only way to identify an early stage of

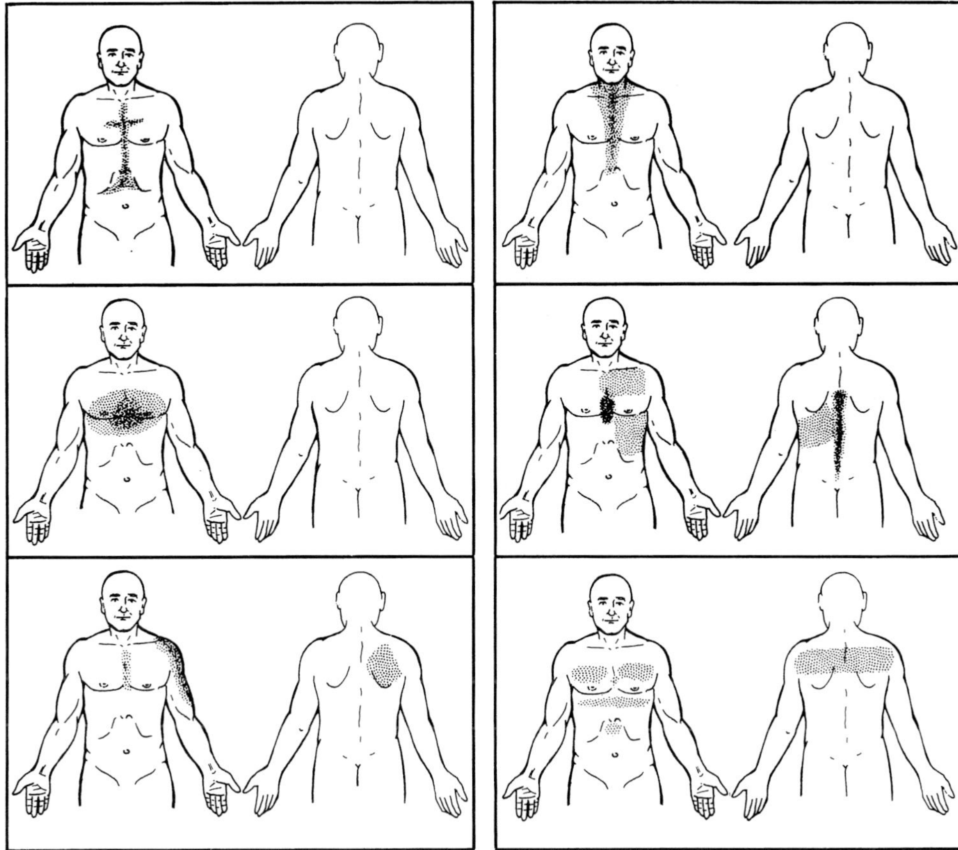

Figure 9–2. Pain patterns. The location of the discomfort from gastroesophageal reflux varies. Patients themselves shaded in the original sketches.

esophagitis as well as a curable malignancy. A more extended examination provides direct evidence that the stomach, pylorus, and duodenum are not part of the problem.

Manometry

Manometry may be most useful in defining disorders of propulsion, such as scleroderma, achalasia, or diffuse spasm. Knowledge of a weakly propulsive esophagus may help the surgeon decide how much of a reflux barrier to construct.

Acid Perfusion Test

An acid perfusion test, performed by instilling 0.1 N hydrochloric acid (HCl)[9] into the lower gullet through a fine catheter, may reproduce the symptoms that are troublesome to the patient, but the test must be conducted with a placebo perfusion of water.

Xylocaine Test

A simple office maneuver, the reverse of the acid perfusion test, consists of asking the patient with substernal pain to swallow 15 ml of 0.5% viscous lidocaine hydrochloride (Xylocaine). Abolishment of the distress is a positive result but does not necessarily indicate that the ulceration or inflammation is in the esophagus.

24-Hour pH Study

A 24-hour esophageal pH study can be used to test the frequency and duration of reflux episodes as the patient goes about his or her daily activities. The patient notes the times of symptoms, and this record is then related to the pH recording.

Acid Reflux Test

Measurement of esophageal pH after instillation of 200 ml of 0.1 N HCl in the stomach is the most sensitive test for reflux but lacks specificity; normal patients also experience reflux episodes.

By no means are all of these tests necessary in every patient with a suspected gastroesophageal reflux problem. When symptoms elude definition by conventional barium studies and endoscopy, or when there is suspicion of a motility problem, additional tests are performed.

MEDICAL MANAGEMENT OF GASTROESOPHAGEAL REFLUX

A rational approach toward medical treatment of gastroesophageal reflux aims to (1) decrease gastric acidity, (2) enhance mechanical factors that favor one-way traffic through the foregut, and (3) boost esophageal mucosal resistance.[54]

An estimated 60 million adult Americans have heartburn at least once a month, and 60% of those afflicted choose over-the-counter medication rather than a visit to the physician.[50] Most of those who do seek medical advice respond to inexpensive measures such as a diet that is low in fat, highly soluble carbohydrates, and caffeine. Chocolate, alcohol, and tobacco are notorious stokers of the reflux furnace. Elevating the head of the bed by 6 inches may discourage retrograde flow of gastric contents during sleep, but such advice is easier to prescribe than to follow.

When lifestyle changes and simple antacids fail to relieve symptoms, pharmacologic manipulation of the secretion, concentration, and transport of gastric acid is an option. Sucralfate or prostaglandin analogues may help to shield the esophageal mucosa, and H_2-receptor antagonists such as cimetidine, ranitidine, famotidine, and nizatidine often reduce acidity to a tolerable level. By far the most efficacious remedy for refractory gastroesophageal reflux is the proton pump inhibitor, omeprazole.[14,17,24] Conventional doses of H_2-receptor antagonists are said to leave 30 to 50% of patients unrelieved, as compared with omeprazole, which induces healing of esophagitis in 90% of patients so treated.[17] *The trouble is that these medications are expensive, and treatment over the span of a lifetime—at least one that is measured in decades—may be far more costly than an operation.* A second concern is the inability of drugs to prevent aspiration of gastric contents, whatever the pH. Cooper and Jeejeebhoy observe that symptoms of aerophagia are best handled by metoclopramide and a diet low in fat and high in fiber.[15]

ESOPHAGITIS

"Symptoms of esophagitis" is a phrase commonly heard in discussions by clinicians of patients with symptoms of gastroesophageal reflux. It is an erroneous phrase because esophagitis is a pathologic entity, not a clinical hunch. Indeed, some patients with severe, posturally aggravated discomfort have reflux but no esophagitis, and some patients with fiery, ulcerated, and even stenosing esophagitis deny having any symptoms. Like the disparity of complaints among individuals with acute sunburn, it may be a matter of pain threshold.

The development of esophagitis depends on the duration, frequency, volume, and virulence of the refluxed material; the effectiveness of the clearing waves of peristalsis; and the resilience of the afflicted esophageal cells. When the corrosive tide of gastric or intestinal fermentation overcomes the capacity of the mucosal cells to regenerate, ulcerative esophagitis exists. If unchecked, it may eventually involve the full circumference and thickness of the esophageal wall. The final stage is a stricture, which typically is conical, 1 or 2 cm in length, and localized to the gastroesophageal junction. Longer strictures are more commonly associated with Barrett's epithelium or prolonged recumbency.

The role of radiology in diagnosis is limited. By the time esophagitis has advanced to such a point that it can be recognized on barium examination, a stricture is on the way. It is the esophagoscope to which the surgeon must turn for early diagnosis.

Esophagitis is a determination made by the pathologist, but the endoscopist, as the purveyor of tissue, can easily distinguish the more severe forms of the condition. Skinner and Belsey[7] have proposed four grades of esophagitis:

1. Mucosal hyperemia and edema
2. Superficial mucosal ulceration with an overlay of gray fibrin membrane
3. Deeper ulcerations with submucosal fibrosis and muscular shortening of the esophagus
4. Organic stenosis with panmural fibrosis and associated enlargement of the mediastinal lymph nodes

Owing to the shortening and stiffening of the esophagus that occur with grades III and IV esophagitis, reduction of a hiatal hernia is frequently impossible without a concomitant lengthening procedure. Resection and colon interposition are ordinarily reserved for the special cases of iatrogenic perforation above a stricture, a Barrett's esophagus with a bleeding or penetrating ulcer, severe dysplasia, and stricture at a young age.

The spectrum of visible changes that occur with esophagitis varies from one observer to the other according to Thompson,[53] who suggests that the color of the squamous mucosa has less to do with inflammation than the thickness of the squamous layer, the density of submucosal capillaries, and the eye of the beholder. Ismail-Beigi and associates[27] described the histologic criteria for early esophagitis. Hyperplasia of the basal cell layer and thinning of the squamous layer were cited as evidence of faster turnover of basal cells in proportion to the chemical injury. The authors believe that these criteria are a more sensitive index of mild reversible disease.

Compared with the more diffuse inflammatory changes just described, the histologic findings in the pseudostricture of the Schatzki type[46] consist of a submucosal annular inflammation at the junction of the stomach and esophageal mucosa. There is always a small hiatal hernia, and there may be reflux symptoms. Most Schatzki's rings require no treatment unless they are accompanied by significant symptoms or are small (less than 12 mm) and associated with dysphagia.[40]

The most important factor in the treatment of benign peptic strictures is prevention. It is unfortunate that the symptoms of an early stricture are often mild and may escape the concerned attention of both patient and physician. A surgeon dealing with esophageal reflux and stricture should be familiar with both rigid and flexible esophagoscopy. The rigid instrument serves as a lightweight probe that enables the operator to gauge the firmness of the obstruction and sometimes to elicit an indication from the awake patient that the afflicted area has been touched. Graded tapered bougies up to about No. 26 French can be passed without buckling through the instrument. For very tight strictures, balloon-tipped catheters passed through the side port of a flexible scope can be very useful for the initial dilatation. Finally, Maloney or Savary dilators passed through the mouth allow satisfactory treatment of virtually all patients in the older age group. Frequency of treatments varies from monthly to yearly. The physician should let the symptoms be the guide. The onset of dysphagia in response to well-chewed food should coincide with the scheduled endoscopic session. The intervals for each patient turn out to be rather constant. Surgery for reflux-induced stricture is discussed in a subsequent section of this chapter.

ASPIRATION SECONDARY TO GASTROESOPHAGEAL REFLUX

The clinical picture of gastroesophageal reflux ranges from unexplained bouts of hoarseness or paroxysms of coughing with meals to repeated severe pulmonary infections accompanied by fever, chest pain, and hemoptysis. Chronic nocturnal cough that disappears on sitting up and is otherwise unexplained points to the esophagus, as does the association of heartburn and cough. A patient who has repeated episodes of pneumonia, especially pneumonia that presents in the same lobe or segments, should be asked what sleeping position is favored. Aspiration may be associated with lung abscess, chronic bronchiectasis, or bronchitis. In each circumstance, awareness by the physician of the possible relationship between respiratory complaints and occult gastroesophageal reflux is of the essence. History taking provides the physician with the clues, but verification of the hypothesis generally awaits a demonstration of disordered anatomy at the gastroesophageal junction or the foregut. When other causes of the respiratory complaints have been eliminated and the presence of gastroesophageal reflux has been verified, antireflux treatment may be associated with a dramatic improvement in the airway problem.

A patient with gastroesophageal reflux is especially vulnerable during induction of anesthesia, when an unheralded gush of gastric contents may flood the pharynx and then the lungs. The result can be catastrophic, indeed lethal.

BARRETT'S ESOPHAGUS

No other aspect of esophageal anatomy and pathology has occasioned more debate among surgeons, endoscopists, pathologists, gastroenterologists, physiologists, and philosophers than the curious condition of Barrett's esophagus. What else can one say about an organ that is an esophagus on the outside and a stomach (or intestine) on the inside? Despite much study, the riddle of Barrett's esophagus remains. Do the little islands or tongues of columnar epithelium proximal to the endoscopically visualized gastroesophageal junction represent the same condition as the long mucous cylinder described by Barrett?[4] Where does the real esophagus end and the stomach begin—at the meeting place of the columnar and squamous epithelium, at the locus of the lower esophageal sphincter, or at the hiatal junction? And what is the pedigree of the columnar cells—metaplasia of squamous epithelium or migration of gastric mucosa? Is esophagitis the companion or the precursor of the condition? What are the risks of malignant change? How can one speak confidently about treatment when the nature of the ailment is so uncertain?

Surgeons are for the most part left to cope alone with managing disorders associated with (but not necessarily caused by) Barrett's esophagus. They include the following:

1. Pure gastroesophageal reflux with or without hiatal hernia. If the reflux is severely symptomatic and medicines and diet are ineffective, an antireflux operation is indicated.
2. Esophagitis with superficial ulcerations usually located at or above the squamocolumnar junction. This condition must be treated. A medical trial is usual and appropriate before the patient is offered an operation to correct reflux.
3. Stricture. Strictures require stretching and antireflux measures. If the patient is otherwise well, an operation should be considered, the choice depending on the severity and duration of the problem. Extirpation and correction are the options. If the surgeon elects the former, the anastomosis should be placed high in the chest or in the neck, both to get rid of the abnormal gullet and to prevent new reflux problems associated with a low anastomosis. If the esophagus has been shortened by inflammation, a Collis lengthening procedure with a Belsey or Nissen wrap as devised by Pearson and Henderson[41] and modified by Henderson[18] should be done. The partial fundoplication procedure provides less obstruction to the passage of food, but the full wrap may offer more reflux protection.
4. An acute, penetrating, sharply circumscribed defect in the columnar epithelium that resembles a gastric ulcer both in appearance and behavior. A Barrett's ulcer has clear-cut edges, is usually posterior, and tends to lie longitudinally. Painful swallowing rather than reflux may dominate the clinical picture in the early stages; back pain is an ominous signal of deeper penetration. Perforation into the mediastinum, pleural space, airway, or pericardium is possible. Acute hemorrhage is a second recognized complication and may be life-threatening. Barrett's ulcers bleed, whereas reflux ulcers weep. Barrett's ulcers, like esophagitis, may occasionally respond to medical treatment but usually do not. Resection may be life-saving.
5. Malignant potential. Although antireflux surgery may be associated with regression of Barrett's epithelium, it is not an effective means of preventing malignant degeneration.[51] In the selected group of patients seen by a surgeon, about 10% of patients with Barrett's epithelium have an associated adenocarcinoma. Compared with the high *prevalence* seen in a surgeon's practice, the *incidence* of esophageal adenocarcinoma in a cancer-free patient population with Barrett's esophagus is 1 case per 441 patient-years of follow-up.[11] It is not surprising, therefore, that the actuarial survival of patients with Barrett's esophagus without cancer, compared with citizens living in the same region of the country, shows that longevity is uninfluenced by a diagnosis of Barrett's epithelium.

MASSIVE INCARCERATED (PARAESOPHAGEAL) HERNIA

The so-called paraesophageal hernia refers to massive herniation of the gastric body in front of a gastroesophageal junction that supposedly remains anchored at or just below the hiatus. Pearson and colleagues[42] considered the pure paraesophageal hernia a rare sighting and argued convincingly that a massive adult hernia is virtually always the end stage of a sliding hernia. Support for this thesis comes from manometric definition of the level of the lower sphincter, endoscopic measurements, and operative records showing the location of the esophagogastric junction in 56 patients. It seems too much to expect for doctors, who can't decide whether to spell foregut with an "O" or an "E," that "paraesophageal" will yield to exact nomenclature overnight. All the same, the observations are convincing, and "massive incarceration" it is.

A surgeon encounters fewer than five of these patients for every 100 patients with a sliding hiatal hernia he or she sees. In contrast to the sliding hernia of the cardia, a massive hernia is a classic coelomic rupture, incarcerated and triggered for bleeding, obstruction, or strangulation and perforation. Because of its relative rarity and because, ironically, the modern doctor is now attuned to equating the syndrome of hiatal hernia with reflux, detailed understanding of the paraesophageal hiatal hernia has lagged behind knowledge of the smaller but more common sliding variety.

Surgical Anatomy

The gastroesophageal junction of a massive incarcerated hernia is bound at or near the hiatus by various mesenteric tethers, the anterior ones to the diaphragm, liver, and spleen having yielded, whereas the major attachment to the posterior parietes has held firm. Given a wide or yielding hiatus, the mobile greater curvature of the stomach body can prolapse anterior to the gastroesophageal junction into the posterior mediastinum. This movement is achieved, as noted by Allison in 1951,[2] by a rolling of the body of the stomach along its long axis. The greater curvature winds up at the apex of the sac, and what was originally the anterior aspect of the stomach faces posteriorly. Because the greater curvature of the stomach has close connections with the transverse colon, the latter may join the migration along with the omentum and later the spleen. The expanding sac displaces the lower lobes of the lung, particularly on the right side. The processes of sliding and rolling may be simultaneous events, and many of these hernias are mixtures of the sliding and parahiatal varieties.[16,42]

The literature contains sporadic references to the condition of *parahiatal* herniation, in which penetration of the diaphragm through a separate opening occurs. If this condition exists at all, it is very rare. Except as a consequence of trauma, I have never knowingly encountered it.

Clinical Observations

A massive incarcerated hernia seldom occurs before middle age and is most common in patients 70 years of age and older. It is an unsettling fact that such herniation occurs at a time in life when chronic vague aches are deemed natural. All too frequently, the symptoms of a massive incarcerated hernia are neither severe enough to take the patient to the doctor early nor specific enough to generate a concerned response when the patient does go. The complaints of an uncomplicated massive incarcerated hernia include breathlessness with meals, early satiety, a sense of fullness, queasiness, or mild dysphagia. A careful history may reveal that symptoms of gastroesophageal reflux have been gradually exchanged over the years for obstructive ones. This finding can be an ominous clue that a sliding hernia has become a large rupture. (It must also be noted that disappearing symptoms of gastroesophageal reflux may also presage the development of a tumor at the gastroesophageal junction.) Up to 85% of patients have a remote history of reflux symptoms. Finally, acute respiratory embarrassment, aspiration, bleeding, or acute gastritis may be the first clue to a massive incarcerated hernia in 30 to 40% of patients. Allen and associates at the Mayo Clinic,[1] in a study of 147 patients with intrathoracic stomach, conclude that obstructive symptoms are especially ominous and recommended elective repair. Belsey and Skinner[7] described a group of 21 asymptomatic and untreated patients, of whom 6 died from catastrophic complications.

Diagnosis

An air-fluid level in the lateral radiograph of the chest associated with the previously noted postprandial symptoms makes the diagnosis. A radiocontrast study in the patient without obstruction can differentiate between a true hernia and diaphragmatic paralysis or eventration. If the patient's condition is satisfactory, flexible endoscopy can rule out other causes of dysphagia and can assess the presence or absence of esophagitis. Esophagitis suggests adding an antireflux maneuver to the surgery.

Treatment

The presence of a massive incarcerated hernia is in itself an indication for repair, given the life-threatening complications that can develop so swiftly even in a patient who has been symptom free for many years. Exceptions to this caveat are patients with generalized atherosclerotic complications, advanced pulmonary disease, or terminal decrepitude. The prospects for a full recovery from an elective herniorrhaphy are excellent compared with a 50% or higher operative risk when the operation is done under emergency circumstances.[43]

Standard textbook descriptions of the anatomy of paraesophageal hernias have been clouded by grouping these hernias with *parahiatal* hernias, supposedly because a slip of diaphragmatic muscle intervenes between the hernia and the esophageal hiatus. The hypothesis is attrac-

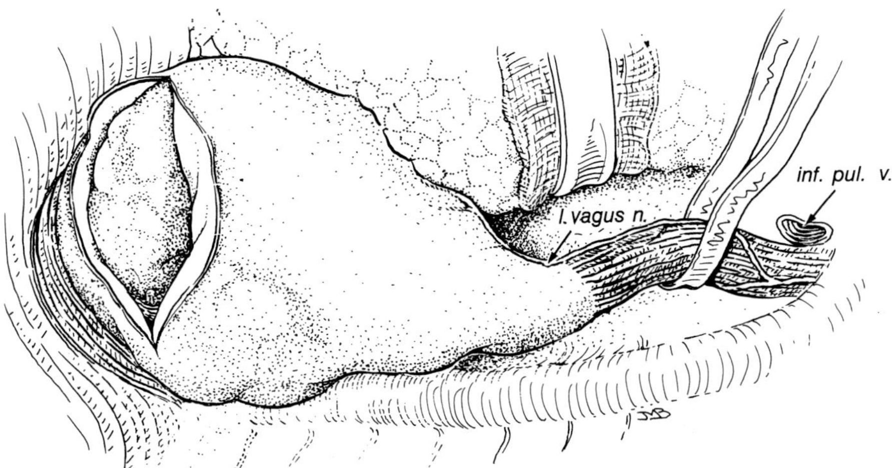

Figure 9–3. Transthoracic approach to paraesophageal hiatal hernia—first step. The esophagus is encircled and cleared to the inferior pulmonary vein, after which the sac is opened close to the diaphragm.

tive, but there are probably more drawings of the concept than there are instances of it.

Similarly, the pure paraesophageal hernia (with the gastroesophageal junction fixed at or below the hiatus) is rare. In the usual case, both sliding and rolling components are present. Because of this and because reflux has been documented in as many as 60% of patients with massive incarcerated hiatal hernias,[54] we have generally added an antireflux step to the operation. Ellis and associates[16,58] argue that this is unnecessary except when the lower esophageal sphincter has been proved slack on manometric testing. In the emergency setting, at least, it is not reasonable to roust a manometry laboratory technician out of bed merely to vindicate omission of a few plicating sutures.

Should the hernia be approached through the abdomen or the chest? The school of thought to which I belong favors a transthoracic approach through the sixth or seventh interspace (Figs. 9–3 through 9–5). Mobilization of the esophagus is begun well above the sac to avoid injury to the vagus nerves. The nerves can be traced downward as one dissects away the hernia sac and mobilizes the lower esophagus and cardia.

The purpose of these maneuvers is to gain length and allow the stomach to be restored to the abdomen without tension. When the gastroesophageal junction reaches comfortably below the hiatus without tension, a standard antireflux operation is performed. I prefer the Belsey Mark IV operation. The point is that one must not merely convert an asymptomatic paraesophageal hernia into an iatrogenic symptomatic sliding hernia. Owing to its long-standing position in the chest, the gastroesophageal junction does not always drop down with ease, and occasionally the Pearson modification of Collis' lengthening procedure is necessary.[38]

Closure of the hiatus and large defects where the crus is thin may be more easily accomplished anterior to the esophagus, but it is preferable in the transthoracic approach to rejoin the two halves of the right crus posteriorly with six or more 2-0 nonabsorbable sutures. The sutures should not be drawn tight lest they strangulate the intervening tissue. At the completion of this operation, the gastroesophageal junction may be displaced somewhat more anteriorly than it is when the defect is small.

Massive incarcerated hernias may also be repaired

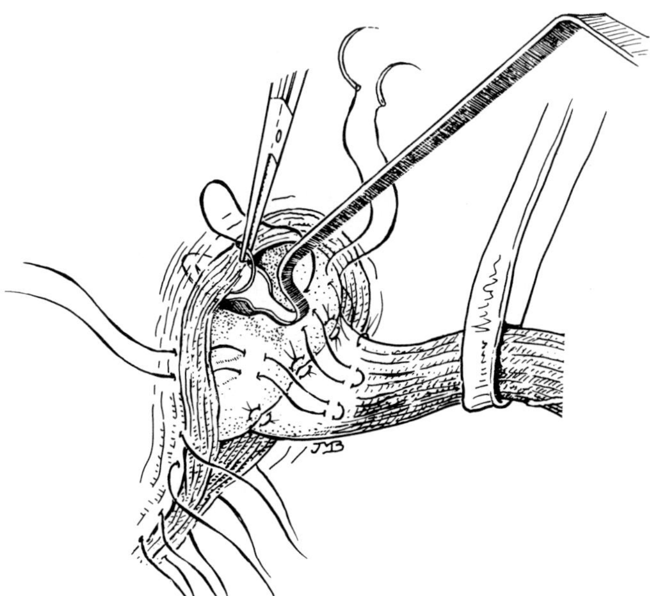

Figure 9–4. Transthoracic approach—second step. An antireflux operation, in this case the Belsey Mark IV, is performed.

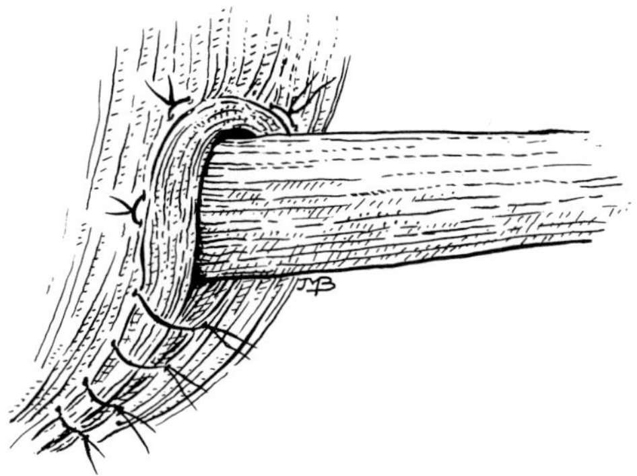

Figure 9–5. Transthoracic repair completed. The transcrural sutures are placed posteriorly. On occasion, anterior sutures may be required as well if the defect is huge.

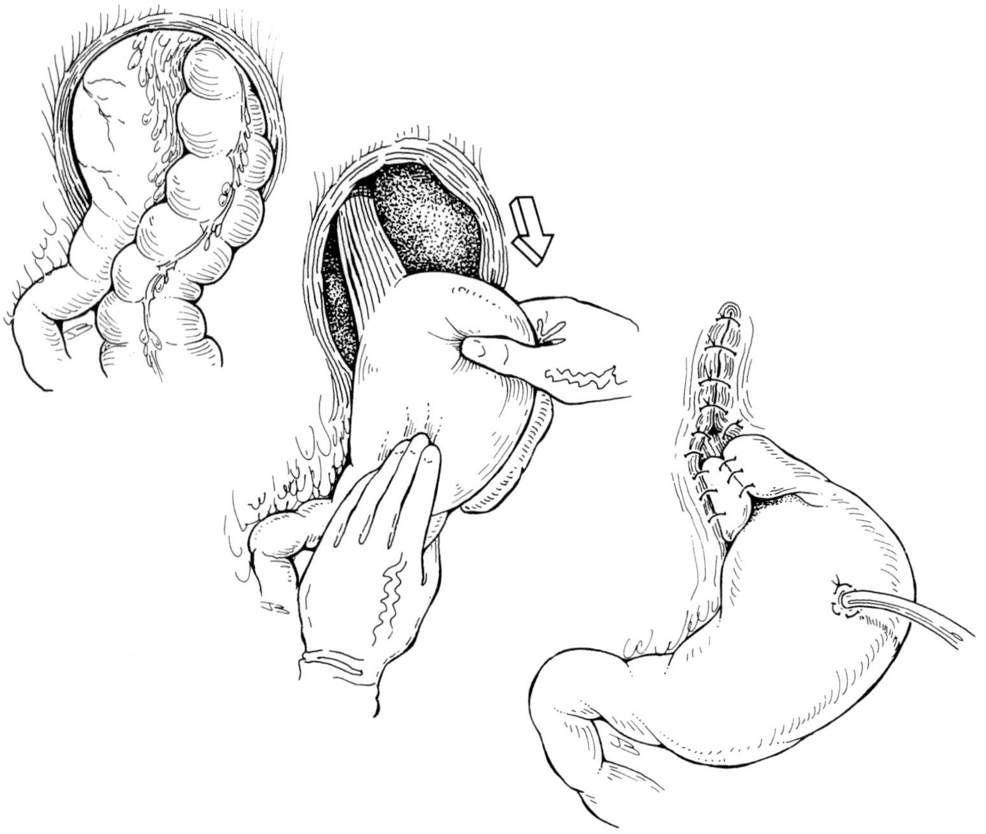

Figure 9–6. Abdominal approach to paraesophageal hiatal hernia. Gentle reduction, closure of the hiatus (either anteriorly or posteriorly), an antireflux maneuver, and fixation of the stomach both at the hiatus and at the gastrostomy site are the essential operative components.

through the abdominal route (Fig. 9-6). Through an upper midline incision, the left lobe of the liver is released, and the stomach is reduced manually. If nasogastric decompression has been inadequate, great care must be taken to avoid squeezing gastric contents into the esophagus or, even worse, disrupting the tense gastric wall. On occasion, it may be necessary to incise the hiatal rim or to remove the gastric contents with a trocar.

The sac is excised close to the diaphragmatic margin, taking care to avoid the vagus nerves. When the defect is large and the crura are thin, closure of the hiatus may be more easily accomplished anterior to the esophagus. Mattress sutures with Teflon felt bolsters almost always succeed in bringing the diaphragmatic margins together. As in the thoracic approach, care must be exercised not to tie these sutures so tightly that the intervening tissue is devitalized.

After the stomach has been reduced, it should be fixed in an untwisted position and tethered either by fundoplicating sutures that include the hiatus or gastropexy sutures as recommended by Hill. Although an antireflux maneuver is theoretically mandatory only for patients who have documented incompetence of the lower esophageal sphincter, these data may not be available. We generally place the necessary sutures to avert this complication. Finally, a Witzel gastrostomy provides a point of additional fixation and also serves as a vent during the first postoperative week.

When strangulation or perforation exists, the gangrenous stomach is better removed through the transthoracic route. Resection of nonviable tissue and control of infection are primary considerations, whereas reestablishment of esophagogastric continuity is a secondary concern. Some patients are simply too sick to tolerate a one-stage operation. In those circumstances when the area of necrosis is large, Orringer[39] recommends that the distal esophagus should not be closed and left in the potentially infected field of the lower mediastinum but rather that the entire thoracic esophagus be mobilized into the neck through the thoracic incision. After this step, the mediastinum is irrigated and drained, and the thoracotomy is closed. The patient is subsequently repositioned so that a feeding jejunostomy can be inserted through a limited abdominal incision. An oblique left cervical incision paralleling the anterior border of the sternocleidomastoid muscle allows the previously mobilized thoracic esophagus to be delivered out of the wound. Next, Orringer recommends making a subcutaneous tunnel on the anterior chest wall into which the esophagus is passed and terminated with a low presternal stoma. Such a stoma is ostensibly more easily cared for than a cervical esophagostomy. Once the patient has recovered from the insult of the operation and the associated infection, restoration of alimentary continuity can then be undertaken with a substernal intestinal conduit. Although I have had no experience with Orringer's operation, it is clear that it represents yet one more alternative to stage III construction by one of the more traditional approaches.

SUMMARY

1. Massive incarcerated hernias, in contrast to the small and far more common sliding variety, are potentially

lethal and should ordinarily be repaired once they are diagnosed regardless of the presence or absence of symptoms.

2. Pure paraesophageal hiatal hernias are rare, and in most cases, there are both sliding and rolling components of the anatomic problem. The physiologic consequences of this situation result in gastroesophageal reflux, symptoms of gastric obstruction, or both.

3. An operation should ideally deal with both components of the problem (i.e., control of reflux and reduction and fixation of the stomach in its normal intra-abdominal location).

4. Many patients have relative esophageal shortening that requires a lengthening Collis gastroplasty to achieve a tension-free and reflux-free reconstruction of the gastroesophageal junction.

RECURRENCES

Orringer and colleagues[37] analyzed the operative results of 892 patients operated on at Frenchay Hospital by the *Mark IV technique* between 1955 and 1965 and established long-term recurrence rates for patients who were followed for from 3 to 15 years. Among the 883 survivors of surgery, the overall rate of recurrence of the problem was 11%. There were differences for procedures done by the consultant (5.9%) and by the house staff (14.6%). When grade IV esophagitis was present, 45% of the operations failed. The recurrence rate for children was 20%.

Hill and associates[23] described 25 patients with failed *Nissen operations*. All of the patients had either recurrent hernias with reflux symptoms or dysphagia; 15 had a motility disorder. The most common operative finding was lack of a suitably snug wrap. Disruption of the fundoplication resulting from sutures pulling out had occurred in 6 patients. Obstruction at the level of the wraparound due to intussusception or because the original fold was too snug constituted a third category of failure. Maher and colleagues[34] looked at recurrences after 65 Hill repairs done during a 6-year period. The average follow-up was 15.6 months. Twenty-three per cent of patients developed radiographically recurrent hiatal hernia, although the incidence of recurrent esophagitis was only 9%. Two patients had postoperative strictures. Preoperative risks of a poor result after a Hill repair were the presence of Barrett's epithelium, ulcer, or stricture (100%), or alkaline esophagitis (33%).

It is clear from the foregoing that a recurrence of symptoms is the end result of an operation designed by, named for, or done by a colleague. Then there is the subject of "modified repairs" masquerading under the original eponym. I submit that most operations for hiatal hernia are tailored not only to the patient's anatomy but also to the operator's knowledge and technical skill. This conclusion raises the nice question of whether an operation with the multiple geometric variables of a hiatal hernia repair can ever be learned from a book.

Reoperation for recurrent herniations can be extremely tedious and involves dismantling the previous repair and completely freeing up the anatomy. In so doing, the vagus nerves are likely to be traumatized, further diminishing the likelihood of a satisfactory outcome. Belsey[8] advocates that a second repair be done by the most experienced surgeon on the team. If a third operation is necessary, Belsey's advice is to do a short-segment left colon interposition.

Recurrent hernia is a plague for both patient and surgeon. In a small community, a single disgruntled patient can make antacids a lot easier to swallow. We must select our patients carefully and operate skillfully.

FOLLOW-UP

Good results with gastroesophageal reflux surgery depend on (1) proper selection of patients, (2) a meticulous operation, (3) optimal postoperative care, and (4) scrutiny of results. Scrutiny of results requires the continual and long process of fine tuning the operative technique based on the outcome seen in one's patients. This requires careful postoperative notes as well as proper questions in the follow-up clinic.

What constitutes a good result? The immediate goal of the surgeon is to eliminate gastroesophageal reflux while preserving other functions of the esophagus. These functions include (1) the agreeable passage of masticated food to the stomach, (2) prevention of aspiration, (3) provision of a barrier for one-way flow at the gastroesophageal junction, (4) provision for venting of gastric gas, and (5) the capacity for vomiting.

In questioning patients in the clinic, it is important to ask about all of these matters as well as about the inadvertent introduction of new problems such as a painful incision, bloating, flatulence, or dysphagia. Reflux cure is not the same as a good result. A string looped around the gastroesophageal junction will, after all, cure reflux.

Results may also be defined by radiography, endoscopy, and manometry. The patient may have an excellent clinical result but have a recurrence on a barium swallow. By the same token, severe symptoms may occur even though the barium study shows neither recurrent hernia nor residual reflux. The question arises: If manometry is required to assess the situation preoperatively, should it not also be used in defining success postoperatively? Costs and inconvenience to patients are obviously factors that militate against excessive testing.

Long-term follow-up must be defined as a minimum of 5 years, or, better still, 10 years before statements are made about the efficacy of any new operation. We have discovered recurrences as long as 20 years from the original operation[21] (Fig. 9-7). In addition to recurrences, undesirable complaints with regard to swallowing, belching, and so on may develop remote from the immediate operative period.

Finally, what about the overall success of the operation? Would the patient, knowing what he or she does at the time of questioning, go through the procedure again? No laboratory test can substitute for diligent questioning. As Belsey has so often noted, a "satisfied customer" is the best indication of a good result.

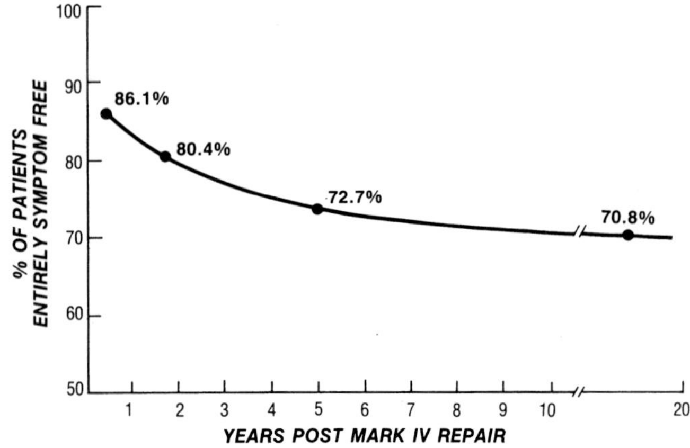

Figure 9–7. Long-term follow-up of operative patients. The population of entirely symptom-free patients declines even into the second decade. (From Hiebert, C.A., and O'Mara, C.S.: The Belsey operation for hiatal hernia: A 20-year experience. Am. J. Surg., *137*:532, 1979, with permission.)

References

1. Allen, M.S., Trastek, V.F., Deschamps, C., and Pairolero, P.C.: Intrathoracic stomach. J. Thorac. Cardiovasc. Surg., *105*:253, 1993.
2. Allison, P.R.: Reflux esophagitis, sliding hiatus hernia and the anatomy of repair. Surg. Gynecol. Obstet., *92*:419, 1951.
3. Astley, R., Carre, M.A., and Langmead-Smith, R.: A 20-year prospective follow-up of childhood hiatal hernia. Br. J. Radiol., *40*:400, 1977.
4. Barrett, N.R.: Chronic peptic ulcer of the oesophagus and "oesophagitis." Br. J. Surg., *38*:175, 1950.
5. Belsey, R.: Diaphragmatic hernia. *In* Modern Trends in Gastroenterology. London, Butterworth, 1952, p. 134.
6. Belsey, R.: Reconstruction of the esophagus with left colon. J. Thorac. Cardiovasc. Surg., *49*:33, 1965.
7. Belsey, R., and Skinner, D.B.: Surgical management of esophageal reflux and hiatus hernia: Long-term results with 1,030 patients. J. Thorac. Cardiovasc. Surg., *53*:33, 1967.
8. Belsey, R.: Surgical treatment of hiatus hernia and reflux esophagitis: Introduction. World J. Surg., *1*:421, 1977.
9. Bernstein, L.M., and Baker, L.A.: A clinical test for esophagitis. Gastroenterology, *34*:760, 1958.
10. Boix-Ochoa, J., LaFuente, J.M., and Gil-Vernet, J.M.: Twenty-four hour pH monitoring in gastroesophageal reflux. J. Pediatr. Surg., *15*:74, 1980.
11. Cameron, A.J., Ott, B.J., and Spencer, P.W.: The incidence of adenocarcinoma in columnar-lined (Barrett's) esophagus. N. Engl. J. Med., *313*:857, 1985.
12. Code, C.F., Creamer, B., Schlegel, J.F., et al.: An Atlas of Esophageal Motility in Health and Disease. Springfield, IL, Charles C Thomas, 1958.
13. Cohen, S., and Harris, L.D.: Does hiatus hernia affect competence of the gastroesophageal sphincter? N. Engl. J. Med., *284*:1053, 1971.
14. Collen, M.J., and Strong, R.M.: Comparison of omeprazole and ranitidine in treatment of refractory gastroesophageal reflux disease in patients with gastric acid hypersecretion. Dig. Dis. Sci., *37*(6):897, 1992.
15. Cooper, J.D., and Jeejeebhoy, K.N.: Gastroesophageal reflux: Medical and surgical management. Ann. Thorac. Surg., *31*:577, 1981.
16. Ellis, F.H., Crozier, R.E., and Shea, J.A.: Paraesophageal hiatus hernia Arch. Surg., *121*:416, 1986.
17. Fiorucci, S., Santucci, L., and Morelli, A.: Effect of omeprazole and high doses of ranitidine on gastric acidity and gastroesophageal reflux in patients with moderate-severe esophagitis. Am. J. Gastroenterol., *85*(11):1458, 1990.
18. Henderson, R.D.: Reflux control following gastroplasty. Ann. Thorac. Surg., *24*:206, 1977.
19. Hiebert, C.A., and Belsey, R.B.: Incompetency of gastric cardia without radiologic evidence of hiatus hernia. J. Thorac. Cardiovasc. Surg., *42*:352, 1961.
20. Hiebert, C.A.: The recognition and management of gastroesophageal reflux without hiatal hernia. World J. Surg., *1*:445, 1977.
21. Hiebert, C.A., and O'Mara, C.S.: The Belsey operation for hiatal hernia: A twenty-year experience. Am. J. Surg., *137*:532, 1979.
22. Hill, L.D.: An effective operation for hiatal hernia: An eight-year appraisal. Ann. Surg., *166*:681, 1967.
23. Hill, L.D., Ilves, R., Stevenson, J.K., et al.: Reoperation for disruption and recurrence after Nissen fundoplication. Arch. Surg., *114*:542, 1979.
24. Hixson, L.J., Kelley, C.L., Jones, W.N., and Tuohy, C.D.: Current trends in the pharmacotherapy for gastroesophageal reflux disease. Arch. Intern. Med., *152*(*4*):717, 1992.
25. Ingelfinger, F.J., Kramer, P., and Sanchez, G.C.: Gastroesophageal vestibule, its normal function and its role in cardiospasm and gastroesophageal reflux. Am. J. Med. Sci., *228*:417, 1954.
26. Ingelfinger, F.J.: the sphincter that is a sphinx. N. Engl. J. Med., *284*:1095, 1971.
27. Ismail-Beigi, F., Horton, P.F., and Pope, C.E.: Histological consequences of gastroesophageal reflux in man. Gastroenterology, *58*:163, 1970.
28. Jewett, T.C., Jr., and Waterston, D.J.: Surgical management of hiatal hernia in children. J. Pediatr. Surg., *10*:757, 1975.
29. Johnson, D.G.: Current thinking on the role of surgery in gastroesophageal reflux. Pediatr. Clin. North Am., *32*:1165, 1985.
30. Johnson, L.F., and DeMeester, T.R.: Twenty-four hour pH monitoring of the distal esophagus: A quantitative measure of gastroesophageal reflux. Am. J. Gastroenterol., *62*:325, 1974.
31. Jolley, S.G., Johnson, D.G., and Herbst, J.J.: An assessment of gastroesophageal reflux in children by extended pH monitoring of the distal esophagus. Surgery, *84*:16, 1978.
32. Jolley, S.G., Herbst, J.J., Johnson, D.G., et al.: Patterns of postcibal gastroesophageal reflux in symptomatic infants. Am. J. Surg., *138*:946, 1979.
33. Maglinte, D.D.T., Schultheis, T.E., Kroll, K.L., et al.: Survey of the esophagus during the upper gastrointestinal examination in 500 patients. Radiology, *147*:65, 1983.
34. Maher, J.W., Hollenbeck, M.D., and Woodward, E.R.: An analysis of recurrent esophagitis following posterior gastropexy. Ann. Surg., *187*:227, 1978.
35. Nissen, R.: Eine einfache Operation zur Beeinflussung der Refluxoesophagitis. Schweiz. Med. Wochenschr., *86*:590, 1956.
36. Nissen, R.: Reminiscences: Reflux esophagitis and hiatal hernia. Rev. Surg., *27*:307, 1970.
37. Orringer, M.B., Belsey, R.H.R., and Skinner, D.B.: Long-term results of the Mark IV operation for hiatal hernia and analyses of recurrences and their treatment. J. Thorac. Cardiovasc. Surg., *63*:25, 1972.
38. Orringer, M.B., and Sloan, H.: Combined Collis-Nissen reconstruction of the esophagogastric junction. Ann. Thorac. Surg., *25*:16, 1978.
39. Orringer, M.B.: Symptomatic paraesophageal hernia. *In* Fischer, J.E. (ed.): Common Problems in Gastrointestinal Surgery. Chicago, Year Book Medical Publishers, 1989, p. 37.
40. Ottinger, L.W., and Wilkins, E.W.: Late results with Schatzki rings undergoing destruction of the ring and hiatus herniorrhaphy. Am. J. Surg., *139*:591, 1980.
41. Pearson, F.G., and Henderson, R.D.: Long-term follow-up of peptic strictures managed by dilatation, modified Collis gastroplasty, and Belsey hiatus hernia repair. Surgery, *80*:396, 1976.
42. Pearson, F.G., Cooper, J.D., Ilves, R., et al.: Massive hiatal hernia with incarceration: A report of 53 cases. Ann. Thorac. Surg., *35*:45, 1983.
43. Postlethwait, R.W.: Surgery of the Esophagus, 2nd ed. Norwalk, CT, Appleton-Century-Crofts, 1986, p. 257.
44. Randolph, J.: Discussion. *In* Jewett, T.C., Jr., and Waterston, D.J.: Surgical management of hiatal hernia in children. J. Pediatr. Surg., *10*:757, 1975.
45. Rossetti, M., and Hell, K.: Fundoplication for the treatment of gastroesophageal reflux in hiatal hernia. World J. Surg., *1*:439, 1977.
46. Schatzki, R., and Gary, J.E.: Dysphagia due to a diaphragm-like localized narrowing in the lower oesophagus ("lower oesophageal ring"). AJR, *70*:911, 1953.
47. Seibert, J.J., Byrne, W.J., Euler, A.R., et al.: Gastroesophageal reflux–the acid test: Scintigraphy of the pH probe? AJR, *140*:1087, 1983.

48. Shakespeare, W.: As You Like It, Act II, scene vii, 1599.
49. Skinner, D.B.: Esophageal hiatal hernia. *In* Sabiston, D.C., and Spencer, F.C. (eds.): Gibbons's Surgery of the Chest, 4th ed., Vol. 2. Philadelphia, W.B. Saunders, 1983, p. 773.
50. Sontag, S.J.: The medical management of reflux esophagitis: Role of antacids and acid inhibition. Gastroenterol. Clin. North Am., *19*(3):683, 1990.
51. Spechler, J.S., and Goyal, R.K.: Barrett's esophagus. N. Engl. J. Med., *315*:362, 1986.
52. Stilson, W.L., Sanders, I., Gardiner, G.A., et al.: Hiatal hernia and gastroesophageal reflux: A clinicoradiological analysis of more than 1,000 cases. Radiology, *93*:1323, 1969.
53. Thompson, H.: Symposium on gastroesophageal reflux and its complications: The spectrum of pathological change. Gut, *14*:237, 1972.
54. Vantrappen, G., and Janssens, J.: Pathophysiology and treatment of gastro-oesophageal reflux disease. Scand. J. Gastroenterol. Suppl., *165*:7, 1989.
55. Walther, B., DeMeester, T.R., LaFontaine, E., et al.: Effect of paraesophageal hernia on sphincter function and its implication on surgical therapy. Am. J. Surg., *147*:111, 1984.
56. Waterston, D.J.: Colonic replacement of esophagus (intrathoracic). Surg. Clin. North Am., *44*:1441, 196.
57. Williamson, W.A., Ellis, F.H., Streitz, J.M., Jr., and Shahian, D.M.: Paraesophageal hiatal hernia: Is an antireflux procedure necessary? Ann. Thorac. Surg., *56*:447, 1993.

CHAPTER

10 The Hill Repair*

RALPH W. AYE • LUCIUS D. HILL • STEFAN J. M. KRAEMER

Gastroesophageal reflux disease (GERD) with its complications of heartburn, esophagitis, and pneumonitis is the most common abnormality of the upper gastrointestinal tract.[1] Despite the high incidence of GERD, the pathophysiology of this disorder has been poorly understood until recently. Basically, gastroesophageal reflux occurs when the antireflux barrier fails. To understand the disorder as well as the principles of surgical correction, it is essential to understand the components of the antireflux barrier (ARB).

The antireflux barrier consists of the gastroesophageal valve (GEV), the lower esophageal sphincter (LES), the diaphragm, posterior fixation of the gastroesophageal junction (GEJ), and esophageal clearance. In 1956, Fyke and associates[2] produced manometric evidence for a lower esophageal sphincter. All attention was then focused on the LES as the sole barrier to reflux. The GEV—which had been described 100 years earlier and noted by Allison, Barrett, Johnstone, and many others—was ignored. With the advent of the fiberoptic scope and the ability to view the GEJ with the retroflexed scope, it became clear that the GEV is an important component of the ARB.

In our cadaver dissections, it was noted that with the stomach left in situ, a barrier to the flow of water from the stomach to the esophagus could be demonstrated. Because there is no sphincter pressure in a cadaver, it was concluded that the GEV represented the barrier. We then viewed the valve with the retroflexed endoscope and demonstrated it in the normal subject. The musculomucosal fold created by the angle of entry of the esophagus into the stomach extends 3-4 cm along the lesser curve. This fold adheres to the scope through all phases of respiration; opens only with swallowing, belching, and vomiting; and closes promptly. These valves were scored as grade I GEV (Fig. 10-1). A valve that is only slightly less well defined and opens occasionally was graded as grade II GEV (Fig. 10-2). The grade III valve opens frequently, remains open for varying periods of time, is poorly defined, and is usually associated with a hiatal hernia (Fig. 10-3). The grade IV valve shows no musculomucosal fold. The esophageal orifice is wide open, and it is invariably accompanied by a hiatal hernia (Fig. 10-4).

It is noteworthy that in 32 patients with or without a history of reflux, the GEV was graded by gastroenterologists blinded to the clinical status of the patient. No patient with a grade I or II GEV showed reflux, whereas all patients with a grade III or IV valve showed reflux.

*Supported by: The Ryan Hill Research Foundation, The Norcliffe Foundation, and John and Ruth Braun.

These studies show clearly that the GEV is an important component of the ARB. The role of surgery, therefore, is to reestablish a normal grade I, 180-degree valve in a patient who has lost the valve and is therefore suffering from reflux.

We have previously published these findings regarding the valve.[3] The GEV had not been previously mentioned in any anatomy book. The editors of *Gray's Anatomy*[4] asked for more information about the valve, which we sent to them, and they now include two pages regarding the GEV. The valve has also been confirmed by Contractor and his group[5] at the King Fahad Hospital in Saudi Arabia. Peters and DeMeester's group[6] at the University of Southern California has published a paper confirming the grading of the valve. With such wide confirmation, it is time for both gastroenterologists and surgeons to recognize the importance of the valve from both the clinical and the surgical standpoints.

In addition to re-creating the valve, calibrating the LES is important and can be done with intraoperative measurement of the sphincter pressure. The relationship of the LES to the valve is shown in Figure 10-5. This computer-generated view shows that the sphincter resides inside the valve and aids the valve in discriminating among gas, liquids, and solids. It also does the discriminatory work, and the valve does the heavy work, to prevent reflux. Increased intragastric pressure serves to close the valve against the lesser curve.

Posterior fixation of the GEJ is essential. This is lost when a patient develops a hiatal hernia and the GEJ ascends into the posterior mediastinum. The esophagus can no longer generate the propulsive waves that are necessary for esophageal clearance, because the esophagus no longer has a fulcrum from which to work. One should recall that the entire gastrointestinal tract, including the hollow as well as the solid viscera in humans and most vertebrate animals, is suspended by the dorsal mesentery to the posterior body wall. The esophagus is no exception to the rule. Extensive cadaver dissections demonstrate that the esophagus is primarily fixed posteriorly by a dense plate of fibroareolar tissue that extends from the median arcuate ligament all the way to the aortic arch. The posterior attachment of the GEJ by the dorsal mesentery to the preaortic fascia is vital to the integrity of the entire barrier to reflux. It has been demonstrated in the cadaver that when the posterior attachment is divided the GEJ slides into the chest and the effect of the GEV is lost. This is also demonstrated with the retroflexed endoscope in humans. As the GEJ ascends into the posterior mediastinum, the valve is lost and

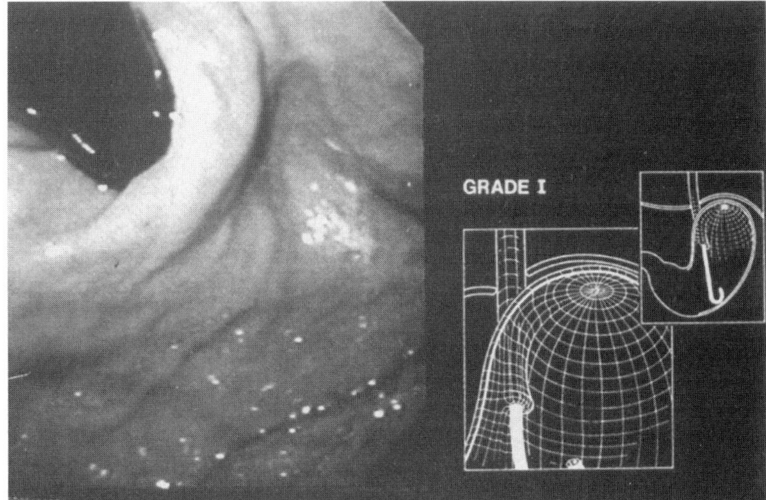

Figure 10–1. Grade I flap valve. Note the ridge of tissue, which is closely approximated to the shaft of the retroflexed endoscope. It extends 3 to 4 cm along the lesser curve.

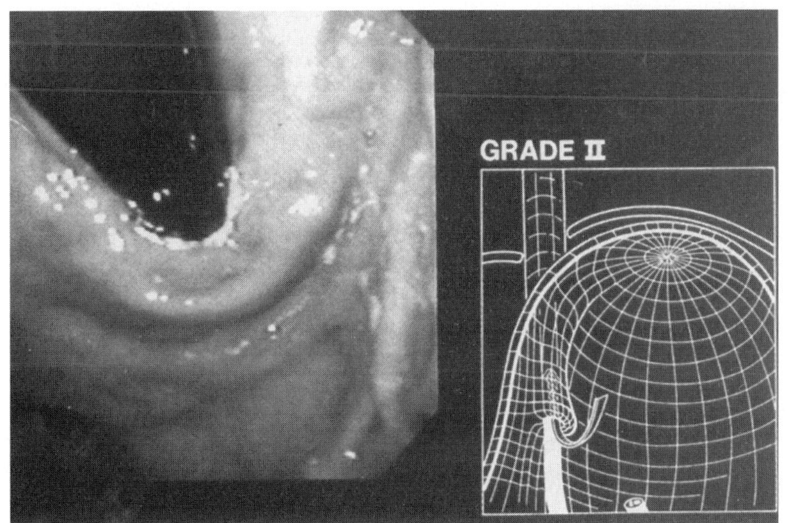

Figure 10–2. Grade II flap valve. The ridge is slightly less well defined than in grade I, and it opens rarely with respiration and closes promptly.

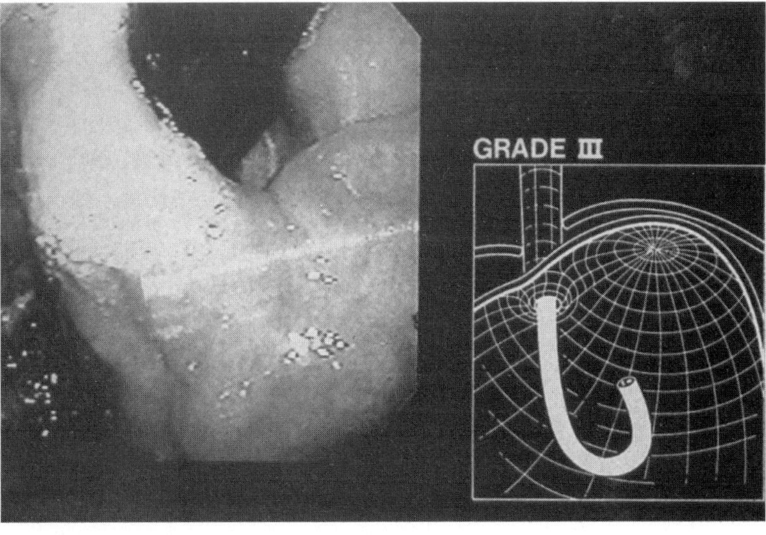

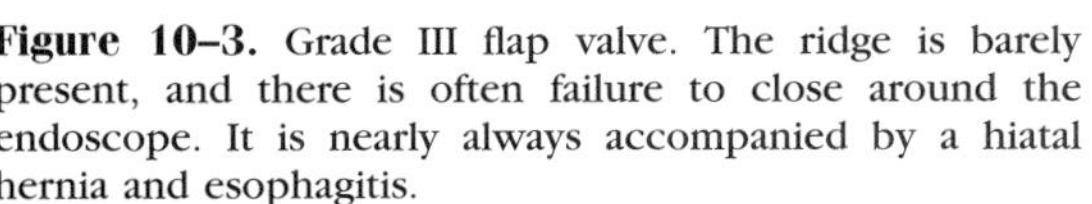

Figure 10–3. Grade III flap valve. The ridge is barely present, and there is often failure to close around the endoscope. It is nearly always accompanied by a hiatal hernia and esophagitis.

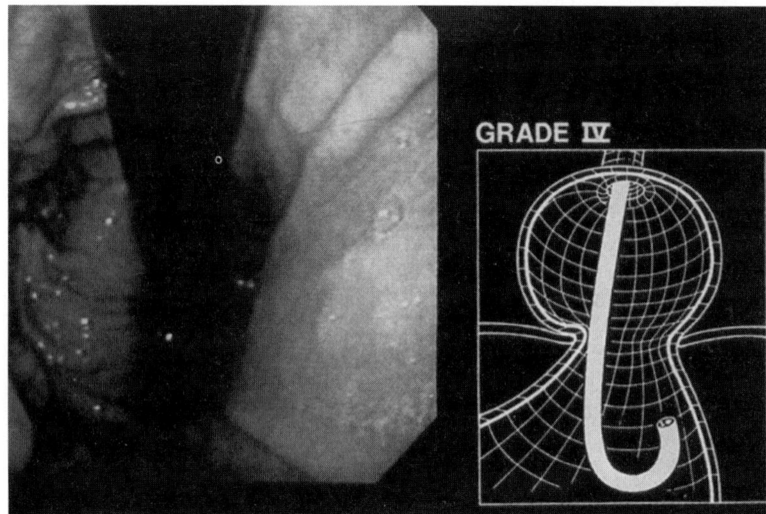

Figure 10–4. Grade IV flap valve. There is no muscular ridge at all. The gastroesophageal area stays open all the time, and squamous epithelium can often be seen from the retroflexed position. A hiatal hernia is always present, as is esophagitis.

the sphincter is distracted. Reattachment of the GEJ is therefore important for restoration of esophageal function.

Closure of the enlarged diaphragmatic opening is important to prevent recurrence of the hiatal hernia. The diaphragm should be closed loosely about the esophagus so that at least one finger can be placed alongside the esophagus with a nasogastric tube in the lumen. Fixation of the cardia to the rim of the diaphragm is also important to accentuate the valve and to close the opening into the posterior mediastinum to prevent herniation of the cardia into the posterior mediastinum.

To summarize, the goals of surgery are:

1. Restoration of the GEV
2. Calibration of the LES to the proper range
3. Posterior fixation of the GEJ to restore esophageal peristalsis and clearance
4. Reduction of the hiatal hernia
5. Closure of the diaphragm

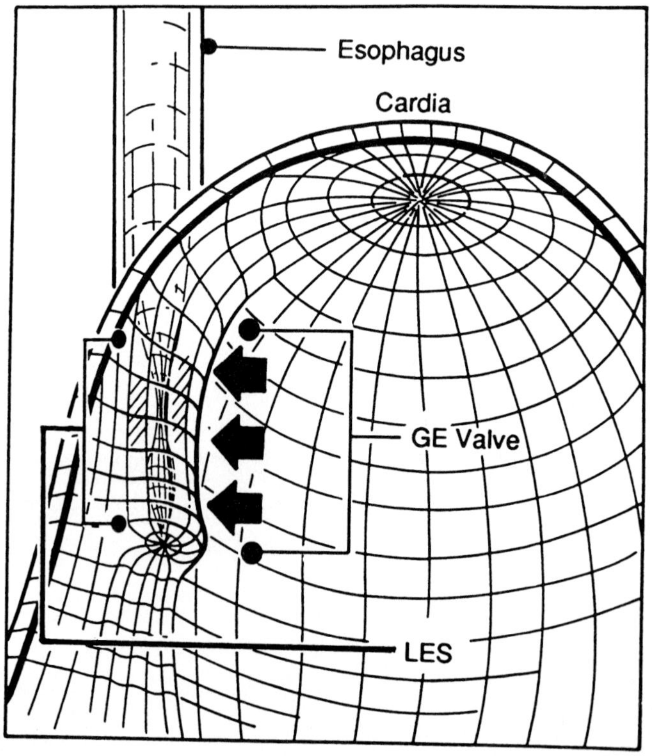

Figure 10–5. The relationship of the lower esophageal sphincter (LES) to the gastroesophageal valve (GE Valve). The sphincter resides inside the valve; aids the valve in discriminating among gas, liquid, and solids; and helps prevent reflux. The arrows are pressure vectors demonstrating that increased intragastric pressure closes the valve.

INDICATIONS FOR SURGERY

Because the symptoms of esophagitis, including heartburn and dysphagia, are so common, it is important that the indications for surgery remain strict. The important indications for surgery are as follows:

Intractability. The most common indication for surgery is failure to respond to medical management, or intractability. Medical management should be carried out by a gastroenterologist or internist interested in gastrointestinal disorders. If the patient fails a medical management program under the guidance of a competent physician who specializes in gastrointestinal disorders, he or she should be considered for surgery.

Esophagitis. The features of esophagitis have been clearly outlined by Brand and others.[9] The symptoms may vary from edema and erythema of the mucosa accompanied by spasm to severe forms of ulcerative esophagitis with stricture.

Stricture and Ulceration. Approximately 14% of patients in our series have undergone surgery for stricture; 2.5% have had discrete ulceration with or without stricture. The presence of a stricture usually indicates that refractory esophagitis has been allowed to proceed too long. Bleeding from ulcers is usually slow and may produce a chronic anemia. Perforations have been reported, and we have seen perforations into the mediastinum and even into the pericardium. These complications are rare but indicate that large hiatal hernias can contribute to a variety of problems. In addition to peptic ulceration, large hernias may produce pressure on the heart and lungs and create chest discomfort as well as limit cardiorespiratory reserve.

Bleeding. Bleeding from the esophagus is usually chronic and low grade, producing persistent anemia. Rarely, a tear in the esophagus from severe reflux or penetrating ulceration with submucosal bleeding may lead to acute, serious bleeding. Approximately 10% of the patients in our series had chronic anemia.

Respiratory Complications. Larrain and Pope[7] reported on an excellent survey of the pulmonary complications of gastroesophageal reflux. These complications are often overlooked by physicians. A number of patients in our series have been under long-term treatment for what was considered to be asthma. On careful questioning, it was learned that the so-called asthma occurred when the patient was lying down or followed episodes of reflux. In these individuals, surgery is rewarding because it not only relieves the symptoms of reflux but also eliminates the symptoms related to aspiration or overflow into the tracheobronchial tree.

Large Hernias. In a small group of patients with sliding hiatal hernia, surgery is required because the hernia is large enough to produce pressure symptoms in the chest with cardiorespiratory embarrassment. In these individuals, episodes of incarceration may cause pain so severe that it is interpreted as a myocardial infarction. In patients with large hernias, in addition to pressure symptoms, trauma to the stomach occurs at the point where the diaphragm impinges on the displaced viscus and can lead to what is termed a callous ulceration of the gastric mucosa, which may bleed either chronically or acutely. In our experience, large hernias—even those that result with the entire stomach in the chest—have done well with surgery.

Barrett's Esophagus. Patients with documented Barrett's esophagus who have progressive and increasing dysplastic changes in the Barrett's epithelium while on intensive medical management are candidates for operative reflux control. Studies by Reid and associates[8] using flow cytometry to correlate genomic instability (diploidy/aneuploidy) have provided additional data to identify patients with Barrett's epithelium who are at increased risk for developing esophageal cancer. Esophageal reflux is currently the primary factor investigated in the evolution of Barrett's epithelium. Patients who have had successful antireflux surgery have been shown to have regression of Barrett's esophagus after control of reflux. Patients with severe dysplasia should be evaluated by a pathologist experienced with Barrett's esophagus. If severe dysplasia is present, the patient may well have carcinoma in situ and is a candidate for resection of the Barrett's epithelium.

Upright Reflux. In a study involving two large medical institutions, Swedish Medical Center and Virginia Mason Medical Center, it was found that upright reflux is as common as supine reflux. Upright reflux in this study was defined as refluxing primarily in the upright position. The three categories of reflux are supine, upright, and combined (in which the patient refluxes in both the supine and upright positions). Some reports have suggested that patients with upright reflux do poorly with surgery and that surgery should be withheld in some instances. We have operated on a large number of patients with upright reflux and find that they do as well as patients with combined or with supine reflux.

PREOPERATIVE EVALUATION

Preoperative evaluation of the symptoms of GERD should identify the presence and severity of reflux and its potential complications and exclude or document coexistent problems. Upper gastrointestinal radiographs, although the most common initial examination, are somewhat insensitive to reflux. Radiographs, however, demonstrate stenosis and show its level and length of extension, ulceration, and the type of hiatal hernia that is present. Other, more objective tests include esophageal manometry with pH studies. These tests are important to establish the level of acid in the stomach, the volume of acid that is refluxing into the esophagus, and the pressure of the LES. These studies can be used postoperatively to evaluate the success of the operation. In our laboratory, a sphincter pressure of less than 10 mmHg raises the question of sphincter incompetence. A sphincter pressure in the range of 30 mmHg or more raises the possibility of a hypertensive sphincter or so-called super squeeze. In addition, esophageal manometry can demonstrate the motility of the esophagus and the presence of high-pressure, simultaneous waves, which should raise a suspicion of diffuse spasm.

Twenty-four-hour pH monitoring not only gives an indication of the extent of reflux, but also is important in that it identifies those patients who reflux in the upright position.

Preoperative endoscopy, with or without biopsy, provides valuable information regarding the presence of esophagitis, ulceration, and Barrett's esophagus and serves to exclude carcinoma.

Radionuclide studies are an additional valuable test for the detection of reflux, especially in patients who cannot tolerate or who refuse intubation for the pH and manometric studies. Our laboratory demonstrated very clearly that radionuclide studies not only can demonstrate reflux but also can help separate early achalasia from diffuse spasm as well as other motility disorders. They can also serve to detect delayed gastric emptying.

TECHNIQUE

The Hill repair is being done both with the conventional open technique and with the laparoscopic method.

Open Technique

The conventional open technique is accomplished through an upper abdominal midline incision. The abdomen is thoroughly explored. The pylorus in particular is examined carefully for any evidence of pyloric stenosis that might impede gastric emptying. The triangular ligament of the left lobe of the liver is divided so that the left lobe can be retracted to the patient's right. This exposes the esophageal hiatus with its covering phrenoesophageal membrane. An upper hand retractor with two blades is placed to facilitate exposure of the upper abdomen. The phrenoesophageal membrane is then divided on the diaphragm (Fig. 10-6), keeping as much of the fibroareolar tissue that makes up the phrenoesophageal bundles as possible with the GEJ. These bundles normally hold the GEJ in place in the diaphragm and will be used to anchor the GEJ to the preaortic fascia. The lesser omentum is divided, and the esophageal hiatus is exposed. The esophagus is gently diverted to the patient's left and the attachment of the cardia to the diaphragm is divided. We are usually able to accomplish the repair without dividing the short gastric vessels, which is rarely required. This dissection must be done with care to avoid damaging the spleen. Division of the phrenogastric and superior portions of the gastrosplenic ligament mobilizes the upper part of the gastric fundus. The fundus can then be rotated so that the posterior part of the stomach can be visualized. This allows the GEJ to be retracted downward and the hiatal hernia to be reduced. The bundles of tissue that constitute the anterior and posterior attachments of the GEJ to the diaphragm—the anterior and posterior phrenoesophageal bundles—can then be displayed. By retracting these caudally, an intra-abdominal segment of the esophagus becomes visible. The anterior and posterior vagus nerves are visualized and kept in view to avoid damaging them.

Preoperative endoscopy should rule out pyloric stenosis or duodenal ulcer. It is imperative to relieve any gastric outlet obstruction to obtain a good result from an antireflux procedure. On the other hand, to add a vagotomy to the routine hiatal hernia reduction is unwise. In our experience, this has led to complications of vagotomy without benefit to the patient.

Dissection of the celiac axis has been a deterrent to performing this operation in the opinion of other surgeons. If it is difficult to locate the median arcuate ligament (MAL) or the surgeon is not familiar with this area, a safer alternative procedure is recommended. By retracting the esophagus to the patient's left, the surgeon can expose the esophageal hiatus. The fibroareolar tissue overlying the aorta and the esophageal hiatus can simply be divided by dissection, thereby exposing the aorta. A finger is then passed gently beneath the preaortic fascia down to the celiac artery, and the preaortic fascia can be lifted off the aorta. The fascia can be grasped with a Babcock clamp and sutures placed through the preaortic fascia. This is a much simpler and safer approach than dissecting out the celiac artery. This technique was described by Vansant,[11] and we use it quite frequently. In passing the finger behind the fascia, care must be taken not to damage short branches that pass from the aorta to the crura. By staying in the midline, these branches are avoided. We find that this approach is preferable, and we now rarely dissect out the median arcuate ligament.

The crura of the esophageal hiatus are loosely approximated behind the esophagus with nonabsorbable sutures. The crura are closed so that a finger can be placed alongside the esophagus to ensure that the closure is not too tight.

The stomach is then rotated to expose the anterior and posterior phrenoesophageal bundles. The bundles are grasped with Babcock clamps well above the left gastric artery, taking care not to traumatize the vagal nerves. Strong, nonabsorbable sutures are used for the repair. Sutures are taken through the anterior and poste-

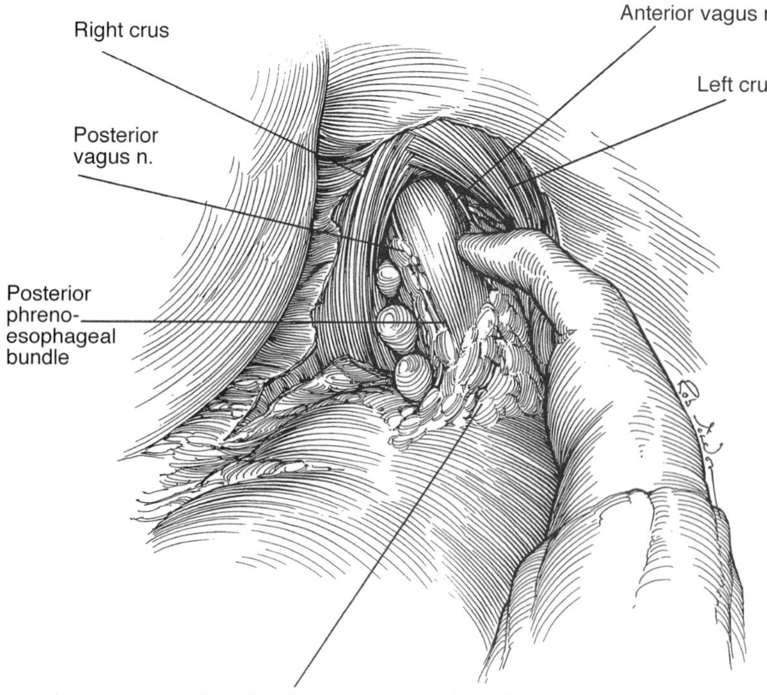

Figure 10-6. The phrenoesophageal bundles are taken close to the diaphragm so that they can be used in the repair.

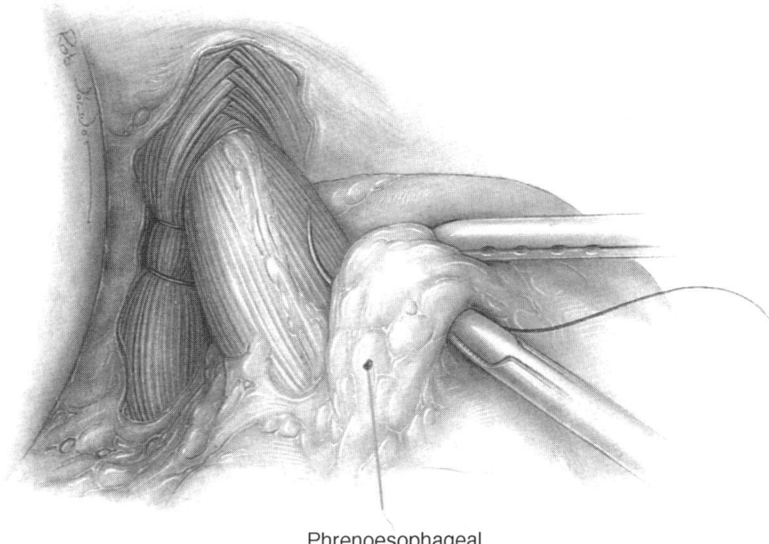

Figure 10–7. Sutures are taken through the anterior and posterior phrenoesophageal bundles.

rior phrenoesophageal bundles (Fig. 10–7). These are then passed through the preaortic fascia, which is lifted well off the aorta with a Babcock clamp. Usually, four sutures are placed in the anterior and posterior phrenoesophageal bundles and are carried through the preaortic fascia (Fig. 10–8). These sutures are placed with the vagus nerves in full view to avoid damaging them. A single knot is placed in the top two sutures, which are then clamped with long hemostats (Fig. 10–9). Measurement of the barrier pressure is then obtained by passing the side hole of the modified nasogastric tube attached to a monitor through the GEJ. If the pressure is above 45

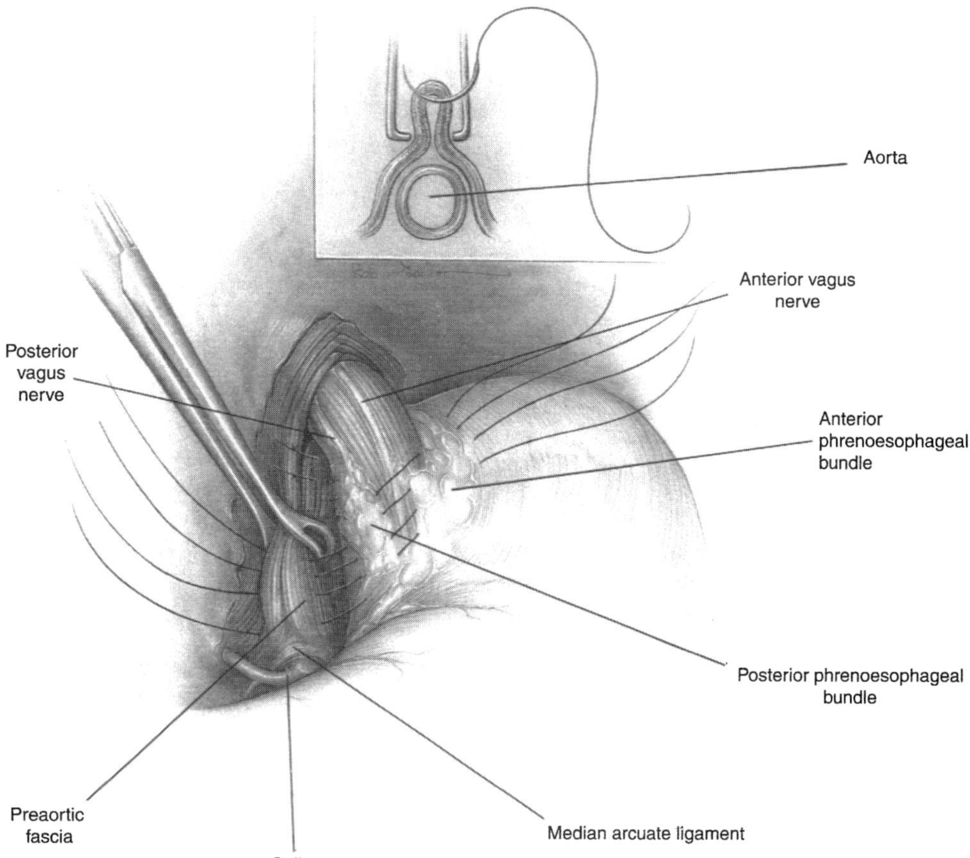

Figure 10–8. Four sutures are placed in the anterior and posterior phrenoesophageal bundles and carried through the preaortic fascia.

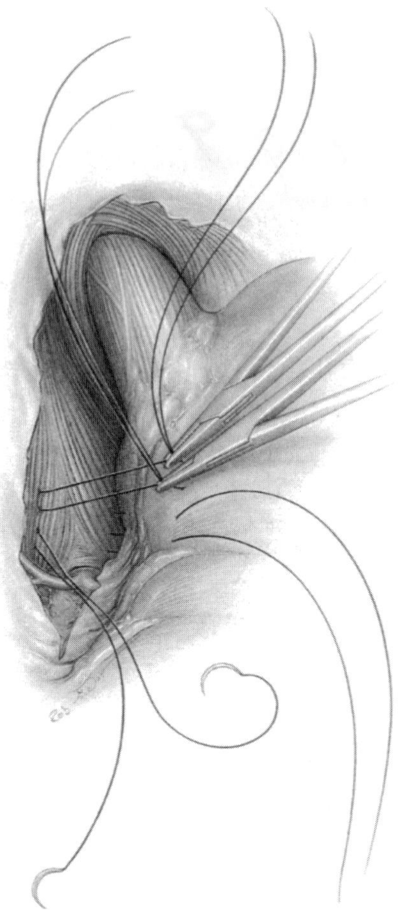

Figure 10–9. A single knot is placed in the top two sutures, which are then clamped with two long hemostats.

mmHg, the sutures are loosened. If it is below 25 mmHg, the sutures are tightened, depending on the problem at hand. After the proper pressure is obtained, all four sutures are tied (Fig. 10–10).

In the open repair, the valve and crura of the esophagus can be palpated and a final pressure measurement is taken. The barrier is usually 3 to 4 cm long. Additional cardiodiaphragmatic sutures are taken. The final appearance of the repair is shown in Figure 10–11. In addition to restoring the sphincter, the GEV is accentuated and can be readily palpated through the wall of the stomach. The valve measures from 3 to 4 cm along the lesser curve and is important in the prevention of reflux. In patients who have had previous operations with scarring and destruction of the GEJ, the valve may be destroyed or inadequate. In these cases, a gastrostomy is performed and the valve is secured with sutures in the anterior and posterior edges of the valve, thereby lengthening the valve to 3 to 4 cm. Attempts to calibrate the cardia with a bougie are unsatisfactory. It is impossible to determine whether the wrap around the bougie is too tight or too loose.

Intraoperative Manometry

In 1977, our group first reported the use of a simplified method to measure the pressure in the antireflux barrier during surgery.[10] This measurement is obtained by simply modifying the nasogastric tube that is routinely used in these patients. The tip of the smaller Silastic sump portion of the tube is sealed at the end, and a 1-mm side hole is cut 12 cm from the tip of the tube. This small Silastic tube is attached to a strain gauge and to a manometer that produces a digital reading. If a manometer is not available, the pressure tube can simply be attached to the central venous pressure (CVP) line that the anesthesiologist has available. The side hole is passed across the GEJ at operation and a baseline pressure is obtained prior to repair. As the side hole passes through the junction, both a tracing and a digital readout are obtained. After the repair, if the pressure is higher than 40 mmHg, the sutures that have been placed are loosened. If the pressure is below 20 mmHg, the sutures are tightened. This process is continued until a pressure of between 25 and 40 mmHg is obtained. The side hole must be pulled at a steady, slow rate through the barrier. If it is pulled through too rapidly, a peak pressure will be missed. It should be emphasized that sophisticated equipment is not needed for pressure measurements. The CVP line available in the operating room can be monitored by the anesthesiologist and yields an accurate pressure.

In the repair of recurrent hernias, there is no doubt that intraoperative pressure measurement could help in avoiding some of the disastrous complications of the Nissen procedure that occur when the wrap is either too loose or too tight. Intraoperative manometry is very simple and does not require sophisticated equipment. The pressure lines used by anesthesiologists—for example, the CVP transducer, which is available in every operating room—can be used to monitor the sphincter pressure. It has been stated that measuring the pressure with the

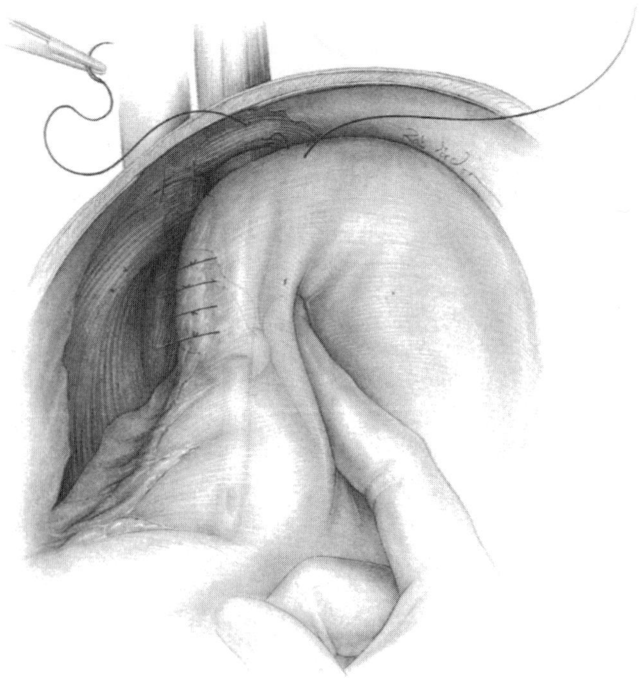

Figure 10–10. All four sutures are tied, and a final pressure measurement is taken.

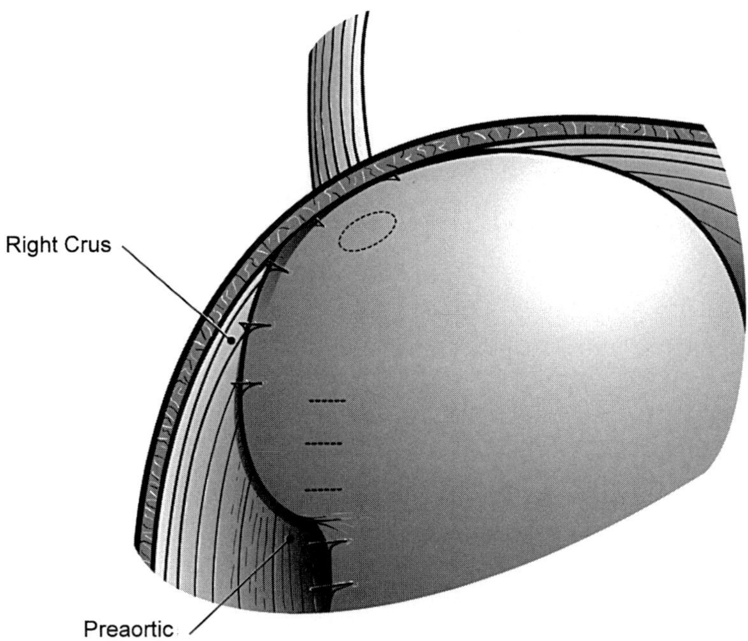

Figure 10–11. The cardiodiaphragmatic sutures complete the repair.

patient under anesthesia is not valid because of the effect of anesthesia. It should be kept in mind that relaxation of sphincters and incontinence occur only in the fourth plane of anesthesia. We have checked the pressures both with and without the use of anesthesia, and the anesthesia has no effect on the sphincter pressure. We measure the sphincter pressure before surgery and after surgery, but it is far more important to measure it during surgery than at any other time.

Further efforts to simplify intraoperative manometrics and to make the technique more readily available are under way. The present technique is safe and simple and requires only a few minutes to obtain valuable information. It is our opinion that in a major antireflux operation that is so dependent on the construction of an adequate barrier, intraoperative assessment of the barrier should become a standard part of any technique that is used.

Laparoscopic Technique

The laparoscopic technique is basically the same as the open technique except that an abdominal incision is not made, pneumoperitoneum is used, and the instruments are designed for working through trocars. The operation is performed through two 10-mm ports and three or four 5-mm ports.

Pneumoperitoneum is established. A 30-degree 5-mm laparoscope (forward oblique) connected to a video camera is used. Trocars and retractors are introduced under direct vision. This can be seen in Figure 10–12, which shows the placement of trocars. The phrenoesophageal membrane is incised close to its diaphragmatic origin over the esophageal hiatus, thereby retaining the phrenoesophageal bundles on the stomach. These bundles of tissue represent the aggregate of fibroareolar tissue that normally holds the GEJ in the diaphragm. They represent a strong aggregate of tissue suitable for holding the GEJ to the preaortic fascia. The diaphragm and the preaortic fascia are exposed, and the crura are then closed loosely about the esophagus. Four sutures are then placed through the anterior and posterior phrenoesophageal bundles and carried through the preaortic fascia (see Fig. 10–8). The top two sutures, which set the tension for the LES, are then tied with a single throw in the knot (see Fig. 10–9). A pressure measurement of the LES is obtained by using a modified nasogastric tube as previously described. The side hole is passed across the GEJ and a pressure is obtained. If the pressure is too high, around 40 mmHg, the sutures are loosened. If the pressure is too low, around 10 to 15 mmHg, the suture is

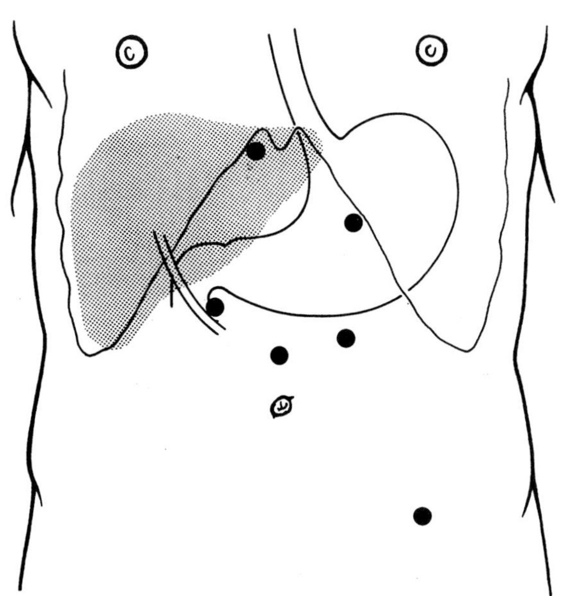

Figure 10–12. Trocar placement.

tightened to bring the pressure into the correct range. This ensures that the pressure is not so high that the patient will have dysphagia.

When the correct pressure is obtained, all the sutures are tied (see Fig. 10–10). Four to five additional sutures are then taken from the fundus of the stomach to the rim of the diaphragm (see Fig. 10–11). These sutures close the opening of the esophageal hiatus to prevent recurrent herniation and serve to accentuate the GEV.

RESULTS

The report by Brand et al. indicated that antireflux operations last only 2 to 3 years and then fail.[9] The series reported here, including the Seattle experience with 2,390 antireflux surgeries and a 91% rate of good to excellent results over 33 years, refutes that opinion. This represents the largest series with the longest follow-up reported. Good results with antireflux operations often reflect only control of reflux. The incidence of dysphagia and fistula formation must be included in the evaluation of these operations.

In our experience with more than 400 redo operations—which were primarily for failed Nissen procedures—dysphagia, slipped wrap, and fistulas are as common as recurrent reflux. These serious complications are rare to nonexistent with the Hill procedure.

The Hill procedure can be performed in other institutions as indicated by a multi-institution study. This multi-institution study includes Massachusetts General Hospital, University of Virginia, University of Kansas, and Queens University as well as Seattle. It is noteworthy that the good to excellent results in these institutions were consistent, varying between 90 and 92% over 10 years.

The Hill procedure can be performed for a wide array of patients and results in low mortality and morbidity. There has been only one mortality in the last 700 cases of primary repairs. The mortality rate is higher for redo operations, indicating that the best time to correct reflux is during the first operation.

DISCUSSION

It is important to point out that the Hill repair is not a fundoplication. The phrenoesophageal bundles are imbricated, and there is no wrap of the stomach around the lower esophagus. This operation very often is erroneously described as partial fundoplication or a wrap. There is no intention on the part of the authors of this procedure to do a blind wraparound of the stomach but rather a careful calibration of the antireflux barrier, restoration of the GEV, and posterior fixation of the GEJ. There is no wrap to slip. The basic differences between the gastroesophageal restoration repair and the Nissen repair are as follows:

1. The Hill procedure depends on augmentation of intrinsic pressure and its special features. By placing tension on the collar-sling musculature, the repair automatically restores the GEV, which has been shown to be important in the prevention of reflux. The Nissen repair, on the other hand, depends on extrinsic pressure of the wrap around the lower esophagus with indirect pressure on the lower esophagus.

2. The Hill procedure anchors the GEJ posteriorly to its normal primary attachment, the preaortic fascia. The Nissen repair is allowed to float freely and the GEJ is not anchored. The unanchored esophagus has no fulcrum from which to operate and almost always develops a dysmotility, because the esophagus cannot generate propulsive waves.

3. In the Hill procedure, no sutures into the esophagus are used because the esophagus has no serosa and no strength. The Nissen procedure employs esophageal sutures to hold the wrap in place. The weakness of these sutures accounts for the frequency of the slipped Nissen. If these sutures are taken deeply, there is a risk of fistula formation from the esophagus.

4. In the Hill procedure, intraoperative pressure measurement is used to calibrate the barrier created at operation, giving an objective assessment of the competence of the reflux barrier. This should be done in all repairs, including the Hill, the Belsey, and the Nissen. In the Nissen procedure, the surgeon relies on either a bougie or a finger placed up into the esophageal lumen. We have seen a number of patients in whom a large bougie was used only to find that as soon as the bougie was removed, the wrap, which was made too tight, simply closed down or that the wrap was made loosely and remained open after removal of the bougie.

We have been interested in determining whether technologic and other advances have had an impact on outcome. We analyzed 200 cases before the use of intraoperative manometrics and 200 cases following the use of intraoperative manometrics. The results of premanometric cases show an 89% rate of good to excellent results. Analysis of 200 recent cases performed with the use of newer technology showed a 94.6% good to excellent result over 5 years. Therefore, the statistics do indicate that the addition of newer technology has improved results.

Our observations on the GEV reported here have improved our understanding of reflux disease and have improved the management of these patients.

The Hill repair is technically feasible laparoscopically, providing a safe and effective definitive antireflux repair.

In conclusion, antireflux surgery designed to restore normal anatomy and function gives long-lasting, good results with freedom from reflux, dysphagia, and serious complications and with low mortality and morbidity.

Acknowledgments

We wish to acknowledge the help of Hope Dumais, Bette Glass, and Wm. Dudson Bacon.

References

1. Hill, L.D., Aye, R.W., and Ramel, S.: Antireflux surgery. A surgeon's look. Gastroenterol. Clin. North Am., *19*:745, 1990.

2. Fyke, R.E., Code, C.F., and Schlegel J.F.: The GE sphincter in healthy human beings. Gastroenterologia, *86:*135, 1956.
3. Hill, L.D., Kozarek, R.A., Kraemer, S.J.M., et al.: The gastroesophageal flap valve: In vitro and in vivo observations. Gastrointest. Endosc., *44*, No. 5, 1996.
4. Gray's Anatomy, The anatomical basis of medicine and surgery. Alimentary system. Edinburgh, Churchill Livingstone, 1995, p. 1757.
5. Contractor, Q.Q., Akhtar, S.S. and Contractor, T.Q.: Endoscopic and gastroesophageal flap valve. J. Clin. Gastroenterol., *28:*233, 1999.
6. Oberg, S., Peters, J.H., DeMeester, T.R., et al.: Endoscopic grading of the gastroesophageal valve in patients with symptoms of gastroesophageal reflux disease. Surg. Endosc., *13:*1184, 1999.
7. Larrain, A., and Pope, C.E.: Respiratory complications of gastroesophageal reflux. *In* Hill, L.D., Kozarek, R., McCallum, R., et al. (eds): The Esophagus: Medical and Surgical Management. Philadelphia, W.B. Saunders, 1988, p. 70.
8. Reid, B.J., Haggitt, R.C., and Rubin, C.E.: Barrett's esophagus and esophageal adenocarcinoma. *In* The Esophagus: Medical and Surgical Management, Philadelphia, W.B. Saunders, 1988, p. 157.
9. Brand, D.L., Eastwood, I.R., Martin, D., et al: Esophageal symptoms, manometry, and histology before and after antireflux surgery: A long-term follow-up study. Gastroenterology, *76:*1393, 1979.
10. Hill, L.D: Intraoperative measurement of lower esophageal sphincter pressure. J. Thorac. Cardiovasc. Surg., *75:*378, 1978.
11. Vansant, J.H., Baker, J.W., and Ross, D.G.: Modification of the Hill technique for repair of hiatal hernia. Surg. Gynecol. Obstet., *143:*637, 1976.

CHAPTER

11 The Belsey Mark IV Antireflux Procedure

RONALD BELSEY

The designation Mark IV was coined to indicate that the final technique emerged as the result of a series of clinical trials of various techniques intended to restore a competent valvular mechanism to the cardia. The fourth and final variant was applied initially in 1952 and has been used routinely since that time without modification.[12,15] At that time, the functional activity of the normal reflux-controlling mechanism, as well as its failure, could be assessed only on clinical, radiologic, and endoscopic evidence. The pH probe was still experimental, and esophageal manometry was not yet available. It is salutary to reflect that the four surgical antireflux techniques that have survived to the present day—the Nissen fundoplication,[11] the Hill gastropexy,[6] the Collis gastroplasty,[4] and the Mark IV procedure—were all developed before the appearance of the spate of investigative techniques for assessing esophageal function, normal and abnormal, currently practiced in the esophageal laboratory. The available evidence, mainly endoscopic, and data gleaned from postoperative studies suggested that restoration of a 4- to 5-cm segment of lower esophagus to the high-pressure infradiaphragmatic zone is an essential element in reestablishing control of reflux. The development of the Mark IV antireflux procedure was conceived on this assumption. Earlier surgical trials—the Mark I, II, and III versions—revealed problems in permanent maintenance of an adequate intra-abdominal segment as revealed by long-term postoperative follow-up. Throughout the development phase, technical simplicity was a constant target to facilitate communication of the technique to the average surgical resident in training. It has not been found necessary to introduce any significant modifications into the original technique. Annual modifications cast doubt on the conceptual basis of any surgical technique.

The lower esophageal sphincter, or, more accurately, the "high-pressure zone," may have a role in preventing reflux when it is situated in the normal anatomic position, but once divorced from the hiatus and the normal insertion of the phrenoesophageal membrane, the so-called sphincter frequently fails to resist the negative intrathoracic pressure and the gastroesophageal gradient. The principle of restoring a 4- to 5-cm segment of lower esophagus to the high-pressure infradiaphragmatic region was based on the difficulty of determining the extent of the hypothetical "sphincter." This principle was supported by observations derived from long-term postoperative follow-up. DeMeester and colleagues[5] have more recently devised an experimental model that confirms the principle of the Mark IV procedure and the necessity for a 4-cm intra-abdominal segment to establish 90 to 100% competence at the gastroesophageal junction.

TECHNIQUE OF THE MARK IV REPAIR

Specific Preoperative Preparation

When the patient has esophagitis of grade I or II, has been following routine medical treatment, and has no pulmonary complications, surgical correction can proceed without delay. In cases complicated by more severe esophagitis of grade III or IV with dysphagia, an intensive preoperative course of medical therapy can influence the operative outcome significantly. A history of aspiration pneumonitis or signs indicative of resulting lung damage call for an intensive course of thoracic physiotherapy to reduce the risk of postoperative complications.

A reflux-induced stricture consists of three components: first, transmural fibrosis due to collagen deposition[14]; second, chronic inflammatory edema and hyperemia associated with the more superficial mucosal ulceration (extensive nonspecific periesophageal lymphadenitis may also be present); and third, muscle spasm in response to the acute inflammatory element. The second and third factors may contribute significantly to the radiologic and endoscopic appearance of a stricture and are reversible. An intensive course of preoperative medical therapy can reduce the edema and spasm and convert a situation in which resection and reconstruction appear inevitable to a simpler therapeutic problem for which an antireflux procedure, augmented by dilatation when necessary, will prove adequate.

Anesthesia

Double-lumen tracheal intubation is not necessary. A completely atelectatic lung on the side of the thoracotomy is mobile and flaccid and difficult to displace with retractors. A partially inflated lung is easier to control.

Position on the Table

The Mark IV antireflux procedure is performed through a left sixth interspace thoracotomy with the patient in the full right lateral position. The patient's spine is maintained in a true horizontal position. The use of a mechanical bridge to open up the thoracotomy incision may cause persistent postoperative back pain and should be avoided.

Thoracotomy Technique

Access is achieved through an oblique posterolateral thoracotomy incision over the sixth left interspace.[3] The latissimus dorsi and serratus anterior muscles are divided as low as possible or dissected from their costal origins to maintain maximum function. The intercostal tissues are dissected from the upper border of the seventh rib, and the left pleura is entered through the periosteal bed of this rib. The intercostal incision is carried forward to the costal margin. Posteriorly, the sacrospinalis is retracted laterally, and 1 cm of the posterior end of the seventh rib is resected subperiosteally beneath the muscle, which will stabilize the cut ends of the seventh rib when it is restored to its normal position during wound closure. The seventh intercostal bundle is ligated and divided before the ribs are retracted to prevent traction injuries to the posterior nerve roots. Most post-thoracotomy discomfort arises in the cord or posterior roots rather than in the lateral chest wall. In children, it is not necessary to divide a rib. The sixth and seventh ribs should be separated gently and only enough to achieve manual access to the hiatus. Aggressive distraction by a mechanical rib spreader such as the Finochietto spreader, will inevitably increase postoperative discomfort. Adequate exposure is essential, especially when the procedure is performed by residents in training. A longer incision causes less postoperative discomfort than a restricted incision involving aggressive rib distraction and the possible resulting rib fracture.

The technique of closure is equally important. The sixth and seventh ribs should be restored to their normal relationship by loosely tied pericostal sutures. Tight approximation of these ribs causes pain. Airtight closure of the intercostal incision is unnecessary with correctly placed catheter drainage of the pleura, and no surgical emphysema will result. The chest wall is repaired in three layers using continuous monofilament stainless-steel wire suture material, which causes no tissue reaction and does not retard healing or create stitch sinuses if superficial wound infection occurs. The thoracotomy technique has been described in some detail because attention to these points reduces or eliminates postoperative discomfort.

Extended Left Thoracotomy

When access to the upper abdomen is necessary to permit treatment of additional pathologic conditions such as cholecystitis or peptic ulceration of the stomach or duodenum, the incision is extended forward and downward to the margin of the rectus sheath; the costal margin is then divided at the anterior extremity of the sixth interspace, and the oblique muscles are divided for 1 to 2 inches. The diaphragm is then separated from its costal origin anteriorly for a distance of about 15 cm, leaving a 1-cm fringe on the chest wall for subsequent reattachment, and retracted cephalad with its nerve supply intact. Excellent exposure of the upper abdomen is thus achieved. During closure, a short segment of the costal margin can be resected to prevent any unsightly overlap of the cut ends, but these ends should not be wired together because a painful chondritis may ensue, necessitating later resection of the inflamed cartilage. The costal margin rapidly stabilizes, without the use of sutures in the cartilage.

Mobilization of the Esophagus

The mediastinal pleura is incised vertically from the diaphragm to the aorta (Fig. 11–1). The lower esophagus is mobilized from the mediastinum in the plane adjacent to the surrounding anatomic structures. This technique minimizes the risk of damage to the vagus nerves during mobilization. Great care is taken to avoid opening the right pleura to prevent the unseen accumulation of blood in the right pleural cavity. Mobilization involves division of the "middle esophageal artery," a constant vessel running from the descending aorta to the midpoint of the infra-aortic segment of the esophagus. Failure to divide this vessel results in inadequate immobilization, which is one cause of failure of the Mark IV technique in the hands of the less experienced surgeon. Care is taken to avoid trauma to the vagi. The left vagus is clearly visible during the demobilization; contact with the right vagus

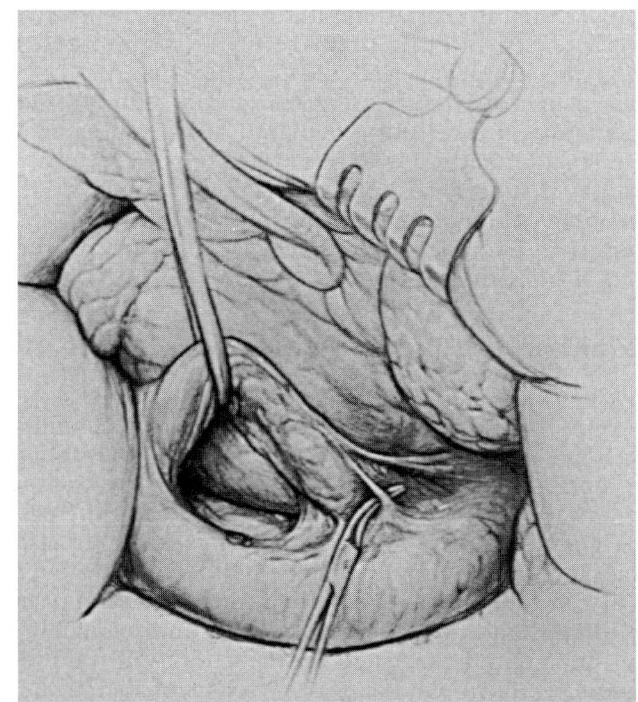

Figure 11–1. Through a left sixth interspace posterolateral thoracotomy, the esophagus is mobilized up to the region of the aortic arch. The middle esophageal artery and the esophageal branches of the bronchial arteries are divided. (From Belsey, R.: Hiatal herniorrhaphy. *In* Malt, R. [ed.]: Surgical Techniques Illustrated. Philadelphia, W.B. Saunders, 1985, with permission.)

can be maintained by palpation on the deeper surface of the organ during the mobilization. Division of the inferior bronchial artery and its esophageal branch may also be necessary to achieve adequate mobilization. After the proximal mobilization to the region of the aortic arch or to the point where the vagus nerves run from the lung roots to the esophagus, the dissection is carried caudad. The vagus nerves are left in place on the esophagus. Posteriorly, the dissection is carried down to the right crus of the diaphragm. Adequate mobilization of the esophagus and cardia is the single most important step in the Mark IV technique and can be achieved only by the thoracotomy route.

Mobilization of the Cardia

Mobilization of the cardia is commenced anteriorly by dividing the pleural reflection transversely as it passes from the muscular ring of the hiatus to the mediastinum (Fig. 11-2). Upward traction on the esophagus by an encircling tape places tension on the phrenoesophageal membrane, revealing its insertion into the muscular wall of the esophagus. The membrane is divided transversely at right angles to the long axis of the esophagus. The next plane to be entered, the extraperitoneal plane, is identified by the appearance of extraperitoneal fat. Transverse incision of this fatty layer and further upper traction will enable the peritoneum to be divided transversely around the anterior aspect of the cardia. Division of the peritoneal reflection and endoabdominal fascia is continued laterally until the short gastric vessels appear. Division of the upper one or two vessels may be necessary. On the lateral aspect of the cardia, division of the peritoneal reflection and endoabdominal fascia is continued medially until the left lobe of the liver appears. The cardia is firmly bound to the posterior abdominal wall by a thick band of tissue, a condensation of the upper limit of the gastrohepatic omentum. This band contains an important vessel known as Belsey's artery. Accidental division of the band results in troublesome hemorrhage. To identify this vessel, an index finger is passed downward and medially into the greater sac of the peritoneal cavity to identify the gastrohepatic omentum. The finger then passes posteriorly through the gastrohepatic omentum, which offers little resistance, at a point between the palpable left gastric artery and Belsey's artery in the upper thickened band of the omentum, into the lesser sac, and then upward and laterally behind the cardia. The peritoneum of the lesser sac can be divided by the exploring finger in the space between the two halves of the right crus. The band can now be divided between clamps, and a double ligature is placed around the proximal end for greater security. Division of the band and its contained vessel results in a dramatic improvement in the mobilization of the cardia.

Another common error is to attempt to identify Belsey's artery from above. Downward dissection along the posterior aspect of the cardia causes the surgeon to enter the plane deep to the visceral peritoneum on the posterior aspect of the stomach, possibly resulting in perforation of that organ.

Removal of the Fat Pad

After mobilization of the cardia has been completed, the fundus of the stomach is drawn up into the thorax through the hiatus (Fig. 11-3). The next step is removal of the fat pad in front of the cardia and all fibrofatty tissue from the anterior aspect of the esophagus. The two vagus nerves are mobilized from the muscle layer in continuity and allowed to drop back posteriorly behind the esophagus. Inadvertent damage to both vagus nerves during mobilization, which can occur when the local anatomy has been disorganized by previous surgical attempts to control reflux, makes it advisable to extend the thoracotomy anteriorly, separate the diaphragm from its

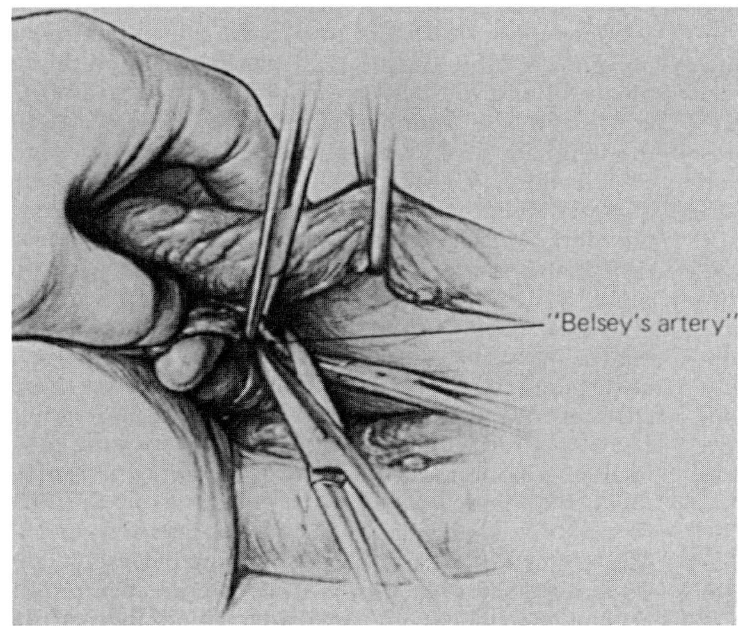

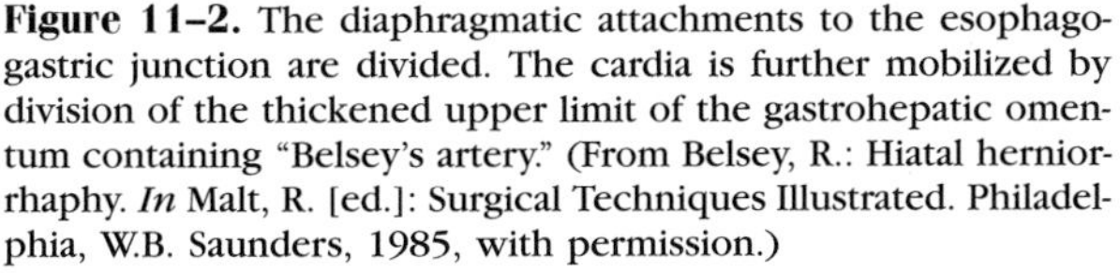
Figure 11–2. The diaphragmatic attachments to the esophagogastric junction are divided. The cardia is further mobilized by division of the thickened upper limit of the gastrohepatic omentum containing "Belsey's artery." (From Belsey, R.: Hiatal herniorrhaphy. *In* Malt, R. [ed.]: Surgical Techniques Illustrated. Philadelphia, W.B. Saunders, 1985, with permission.)

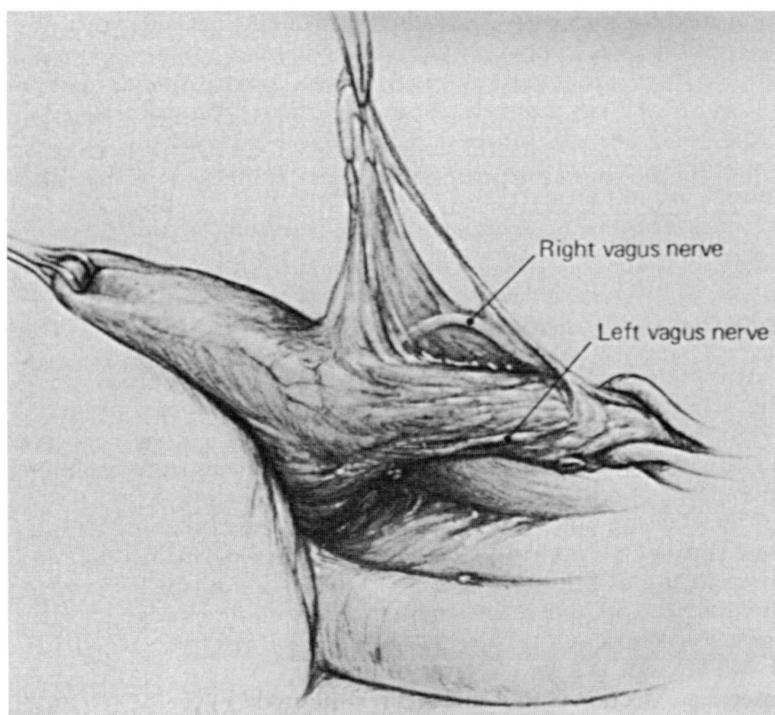

Figure 11–3. The fat pad is excised from the anterior aspect of the cardia and lower esophagus. The vagus nerves are mobilized in continuity and displaced posteriorly for protection. (From Belsey, R.: Hiatal herniorrhaphy. *In* Malt, R. [ed.]: Surgical Techniques Illustrated. Philadelphia, W.B. Saunders, 1985, with permission.)

origin on the chest wall, and perform a pyloromyotomy to prevent gastric stasis.

Preparation of the Posterior Buttress

After mobilization of the esophagus and cardia has been completed, the posterior buttress can be prepared (Fig. 11–4). The posterior buttress is created by approximating the two halves of the right crus. Failure to maintain this buttress permits posterior recurrence. Narrowing of the hiatus as such has no significant role in controlling reflux in the context of this technique.

With forward traction applied on the central tendon of the diaphragm near its medial margin by a powerful tissue forceps, the tendinous core of the inner limb of the right crus is tensed into greater prominence as an easily palpable dense band of tissue. The tension on the central tendon also elevates the inner limb of the right crus off the inferior vena cava. Starting posteriorly near the aorta, strong interrupted sutures of 0 linen thread or silk, preferably on atraumatic needles, are passed through the tense tendinous core of the inner limb and through the superficial margin of the outer limb, including the firmly adherent overlying pleura. A common mistake is to pass these stitches through the weak intercrural muscle fibers, which will not hold sutures. Two or three additional sutures are placed progressively anteriorly at 1-cm intervals. An average Mark IV repair requires three such sutures, but in cases of a grossly dilated hiatus, up to six sutures may be necessary. These sutures are left in place and tied later when the fundoplication has been completed and restored to the abdomen.

240-Degree Fundoplication

With the fundus drawn up into the thorax through the hiatus, the 240-degree fundoplication is now created (Fig. 11–5). A 2-0 linen or silk suture on a fine curved atraumatic needle is passed vertically through the seromuscular layer of the stomach about 2 cm below the esophagogastric junction, at the level of the original but now

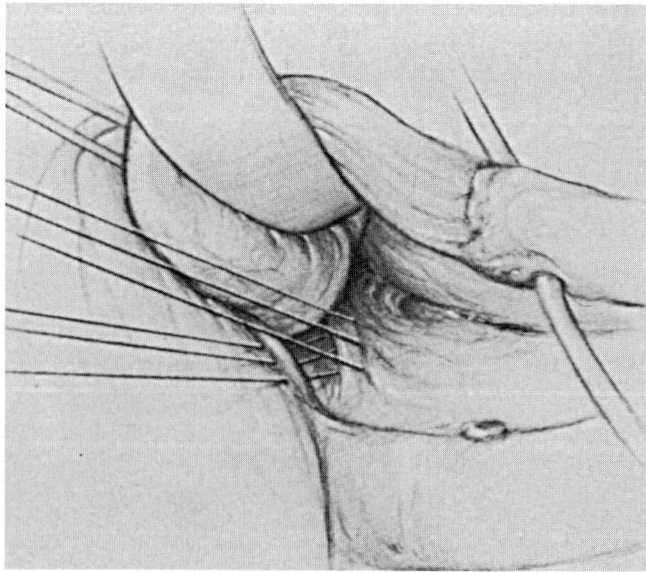

Figure 11–4. Preparation of the posterior buttress. Stout interrupted sutures are passed through the two limbs of the right crus. Three to six sutures may be required, depending on the size of the hiatus. These sutures are tied at a later stage. (From Belsey, R.: Hiatal herniorrhaphy. *In* Malt, R. [ed.]: Surgical Techniques Illustrated. Philadelphia, W.B. Saunders, 1985, with permission.)

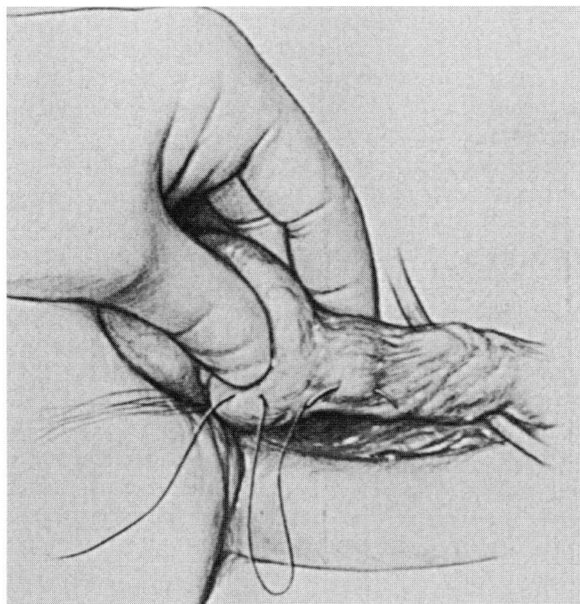

Figure 11–5. Commencement of the fundoplication. An atraumatic nonabsorbable suture is passed vertically through the seromuscular layer of the stomach and the muscular layer of the esophagus. The mucosae must not be perforated. (From Belsey, R.: Hiatal herniorrhaphy. *In* Malt, R. [ed.]: Surgical Techniques Illustrated. Philadelphia, W.B. Saunders, 1985, with permission,)

divided peritoneal reflection, and then vertically through the muscle layer of the esophagus 2 cm above the junction and well lateral to the midline of the esophagus. The suture is then reversed (Fig. 11-6) and passed down through the muscle layer of the esophagus in the opposite direction 3 to 4 mm nearer the middle line of the esophagus to include an adequate bite of esophageal muscle and then through the seromuscular layer of the stomach 1 cm medial to the original point of entry of the stitch (Fig. 11-7). This stitch must not perforate either the gastric or the esophageal mucosa. The thickness of the muscle layer of the esophagus and the admissible depth of this suture can be assessed by palpation, provided no nasogastric tube remains in the lumen of the esophagus. Any tube inserted preoperatively should be removed at this stage. When the wall is thickened by fibrosis resulting from chronic esophagitis, a deeper bite and a more secure grip on the wall of the esophagus can be taken. Protection of the mucosa is enhanced by upward displacement of the esophagogastric junction manually, thus shortening the organ and bunching up the muscle layer off the underlying mucosa. Three mattress sutures are placed in the first row of the fundoplication. The second suture is placed in the midline and the third medially near the right vagus. The ends of these sutures are shortened independently to prevent a loop of the suture material sawing through the brittle esophageal muscle and tied very gently to achieve tissue apposition without tissue strangulation. The placement of these sutures is such that when tied they achieve a 240-degree fundic wrap around the lower 2 cm of esophagus (Fig. 11-8).

The three mattress sutures in the second row are first passed through the diaphragm at the point where the central tendon fuses with the muscular ring of the hiatus (Fig. 11-9). With the help of a spoon retractor inserted through the hiatus to protect the abdominal viscera, the suture is passed from above downward through the diaphragm into the bowl of the spoon and then up and out through the hiatus. Further passage of this suture through the wall of the stomach and the muscle layer of the esophagus follows the same pattern as that outlined in

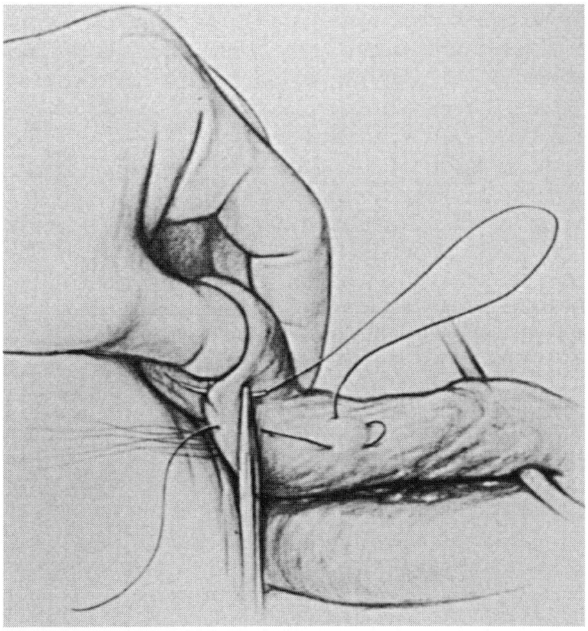

Figure 11–6. The mattress suture is reversed. Note the relative size of the bites of the esophageal muscle and gastric wall. (From Belsey, R.: Hiatal herniorrhaphy. *In* Malt, R. [ed.]: Surgical Techniques Illustrated. Philadelphia, W.B. Saunders, 1985, with permission.)

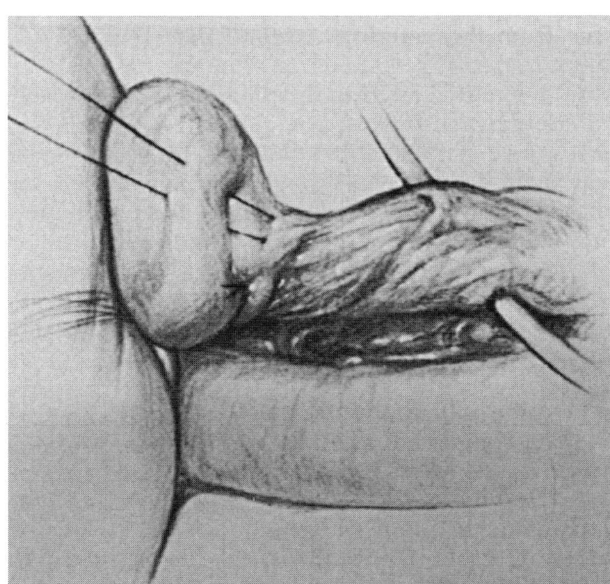

Figure 11–7. The first fundoplicating suture is tied. The second or midline suture is in place. (From Belsey, R.: Hiatal herniorrhaphy. *In* Malt, R. [ed.]: Surgical Techniques Illustrated. Philadelphia, W.B. Saunders, 1985, with permission.)

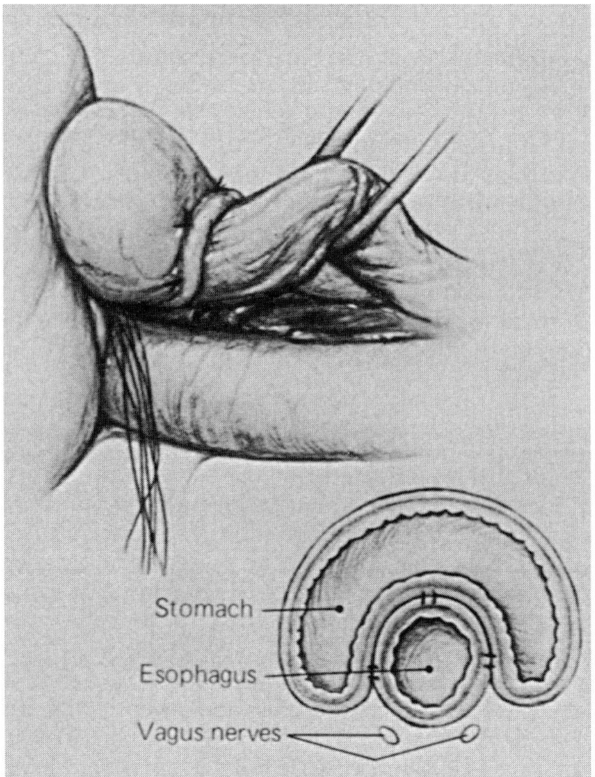

Figure 11–8. The first fundoplicating layer is completed, embracing 240 degrees of the esophageal circumference. The vagus nerves are protected by repositioning them posteriorly. (From Belsey, R.: Hiatal herniorrhaphy. *In* Malt, R. [ed.]: Surgical Techniques Illustrated. Philadelphia, W.B. Saunders, 1985, with permission.)

the first row but it is placed 2 cm lower in the stomach and 2 cm higher on the esophagus. When reversed, this suture includes a 5-mm strip of esophageal muscle. The suture is passed through the seromuscular layer of the stomach at the same level as the original point of entry. Again with the help of the spoon retractor, the suture is finally passed down through the hiatus and up through the edge of the central tendon of the diaphragm 1 cm medial to the original point of entry (Fig. 11–10). Three sutures are placed in the second row in locations corresponding to those in the first row to embrace 240 degrees of the circumference of the hiatus and the esophagus. They are not tied until after the hernia has been reduced. Larger rather than smaller bites of the muscle wall ensure a more lasting hold on this layer and discourage any recurrence. Correct placement of these fundoplication sutures is critical to the success of the operative technique. The use of Teflon pledgets to buttress the sutures in the esophageal muscle layer has been suggested but is unnecessary, provided the mattress sutures creating the fundoplication are correctly placed and tied with restraint sufficient to achieve tissue apposition only (Fig. 11–11).

Reduction of the Reconstructed Cardia

The reconstructed cardia is returned to the abdomen through the hiatus and tucked forward below the diaphragm manually rather than by exerting traction on the second row of fundoplicating sutures. If adequate mobilization of the esophagus and cardia has been achieved, the fundoplication should lie below the hiatus without tension and with no tendency to retract back into the thorax. Any tendency toward upward prolapse suggests inadequate mobilization of the esophagus or acquired shortening of the organ secondary to chronic fibrosing esophagitis. In the latter situation, a physiologic repair may not be possible, and a modified Collis gastroplasty or resection of the ulcerated segment and replacement by an isoperistaltic segment of left colon or

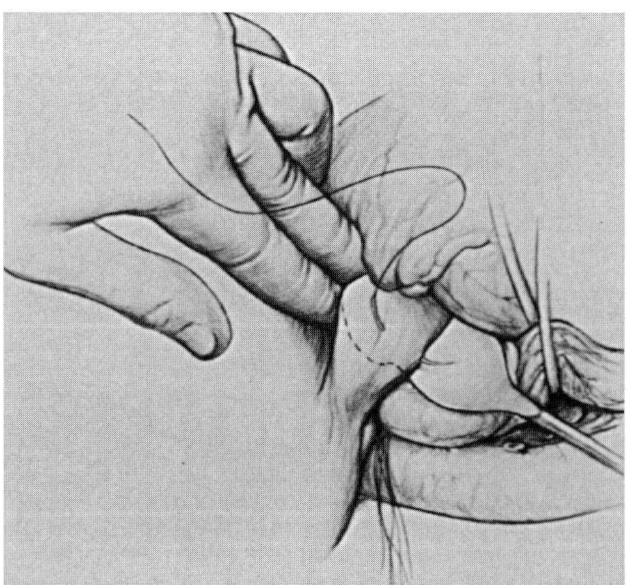

Figure 11–9. Commencement of the second fundoplicating layer using the spoon retractor. (From Belsey, R.: Hiatal herniorrhaphy. *In* Malt, R. [ed.]: Surgical Techniques Illustrated. Philadelphia, W.B. Saunders, 1985, with permission.)

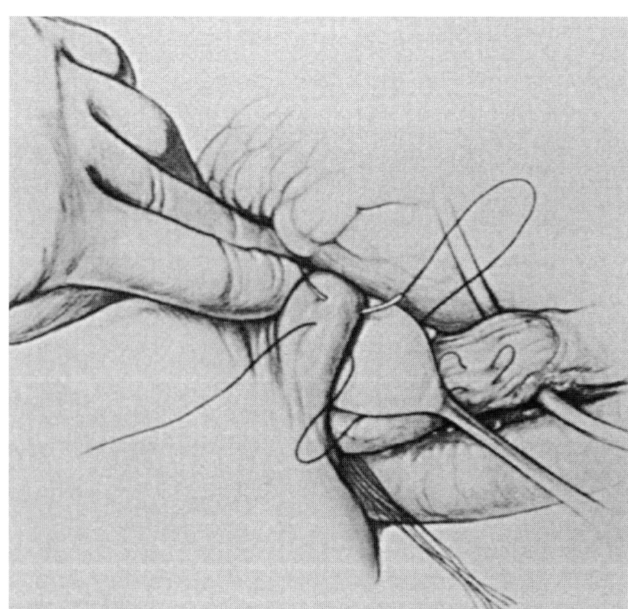

Figure 11–10. The mattress suture includes adequate bites of stomach and esophageal muscle as in the first layer; it is reversed and finally passed up through the central tendon of the diaphragm. (From Belsey, R.: Hiatal herniorrhaphy. *In* Malt, R. [ed.]: Surgical Techniques Illustrated. Philadelphia, W.B. Saunders, 1985, with permission.)

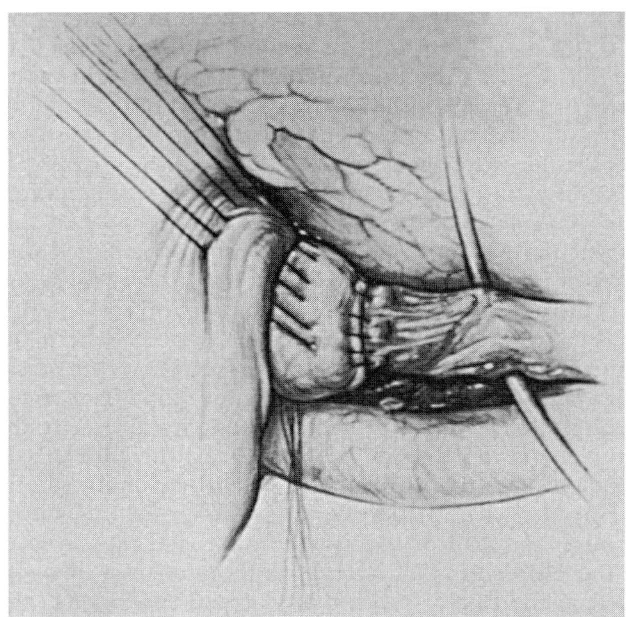

Figure 11–11. The three mattress sutures of the second layer are in position before manual reduction of the hernia. (From Belsey, R.: Hiatal herniorrhaphy. *In* Malt, R. [ed.]: Surgical Techniques Illustrated. Philadelphia, W.B. Saunders, 1985, with permission.)

jejunum may be necessary. If in doubt, a repair under moderate tension may succeed in view of the firmer grip obtainable on the fibrosed and thickened muscle layer. In the presence of grade III or grade IV chronic fibrosing esophagitis, the patient should be prepared before the operation for a resection and interposition procedure when it is indicated.

After the hernia has been reduced, the second fundoplicating row of sutures is now gently pulled up independently, again to avoid damage to the esophageal muscle and to "snuggle" the reconstructed cardia up against the undersurface of the diaphragm (Fig. 11–12). Sutures in the second row are again tied very gently. When the technique is performed correctly, there should be 4 cm of the sphincter zone of the lower esophagus, partially embraced by the fundic wrap, in the high-pressure region below the diaphragm and a further 1 cm surrounded by the muscle ring of the hiatus and the two limbs of the approximated right crus.

Creating the Posterior Buttress

The posterior buttressing sutures passed earlier through the two limbs of the right crus are now tied from behind forward to approximate the two limbs. The first throw of the final suture knot is tied, and the resulting size of the hiatus is assessed for adequacy by digital exploration (Fig. 11–13). If there is no constriction of the esophagus, the knot is completed. When the buttress has been completed, it should be possible to pass an index finger easily through the triangular hiatus posterior to the esophagus. If the finger cannot be passed easily, the final approximating suture should be cut out. It is better to leave the hiatus too loose than too tight because mechanical constriction of the lower esophagus plays no part in the control of reflux in this procedure (Fig. 11–14).

Closure

The mediastinal pleura is not repaired because residual collections of blood or serum are easier to drain from the pleural cavity than from the mediastinum. A single intercostal catheter is inserted into the midaxillary line and positioned with the tip high in the pleural cavity in the paravertebral gutter. No nasogastric tube need be inserted routinely because the 240-degree fundoplication does not cause the gas-bloat syndrome. Should intubation

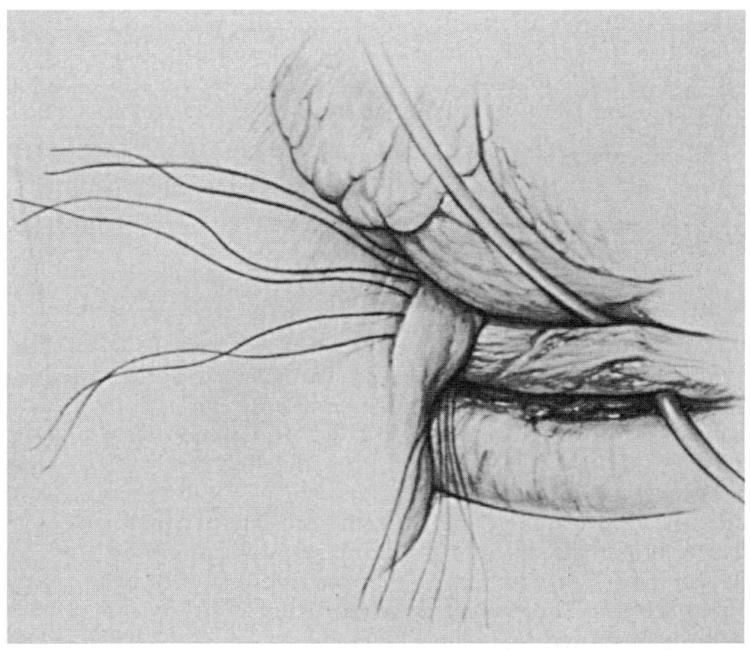

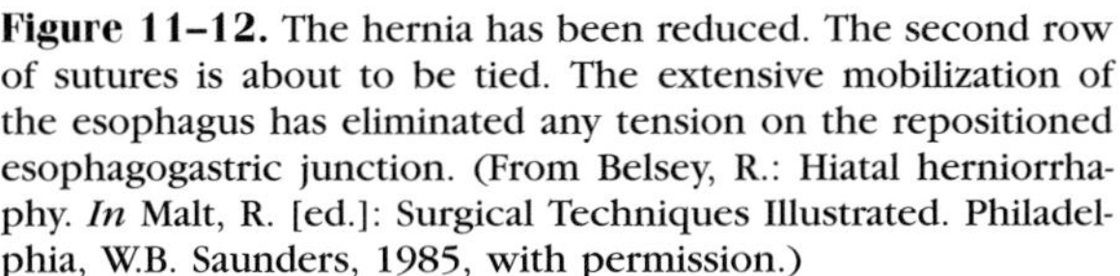

Figure 11–12. The hernia has been reduced. The second row of sutures is about to be tied. The extensive mobilization of the esophagus has eliminated any tension on the repositioned esophagogastric junction. (From Belsey, R.: Hiatal herniorrhaphy. *In* Malt, R. [ed.]: Surgical Techniques Illustrated. Philadelphia, W.B. Saunders, 1985, with permission.)

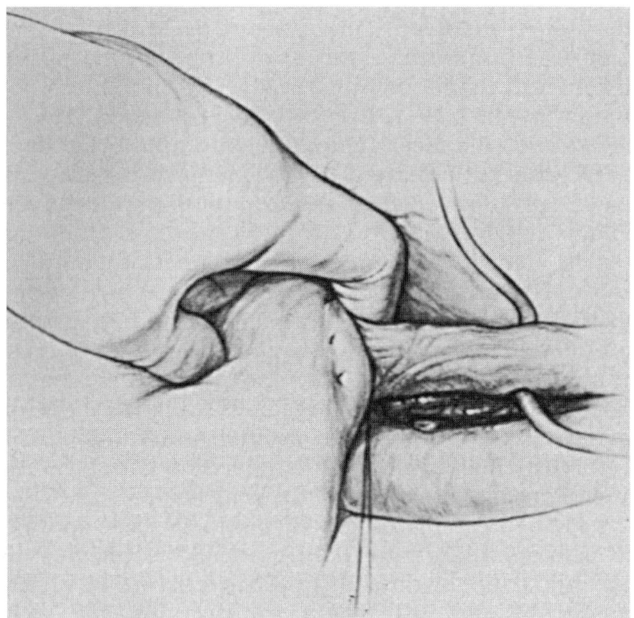

Figure 11–13. The second row has been tied. The posterior buttress sutures are tied from behind forward. Before the last stitch is completed, the absence of constriction at the hiatus is confirmed by digital exploration. (From Belsey, R.: Hiatal herniorrhaphy. *In* Malt, R. [ed.]: Surgical Techniques Illustrated. Philadelphia, W.B. Saunders, 1985, with permission.)

be necessary later for a specific indication, the tube can be passed easily through the reconstructed cardia without risk.

The thoracotomy incision is closed, paying due attention to those steps in the technique designed to minimize post-thoracotomy pain. To recapitulate, these steps are as follows:

1. A high thoracotomy incision is made, never lower than the sixth interspace.
2. If the posterior end of the seventh rib is divided and 1 cm resected, the seventh neurovascular bundle must be ligated and divided before the rib spreader is inserted to prevent traction injury to the posterior nerve roots.
3. Aggressive separation of the ribs must be avoided; manual separation sufficient only to permit the entry of one hand is maintained by simple spreaders incorporating no mechanical assistance.
4. During closure, the sixth and seventh ribs are restored to their original relationship with pericostal sutures to prevent subsequent lung herniation; close approximation of the ribs is a common cause of postoperative pain.
5. Sutures are avoided in the sensitive intercostal tissues; with correct placement of the drainage catheter, no chest wall emphysema will occur.
6. A catheter inserted in the midaxillary line causes less discomfort than one placed posteriorly. The intercostal catheter is attached to an underwater seal in the operating room to encourage rapid re-expansion of the lung.

POSTOPERATIVE CARE

A chest radiograph is taken in the recovery room to ascertain that the intercostal catheter is correctly positioned, that the lung is re-expanding, and that no fluid is accumulating in either pleural cavity. Thoracic physiotherapy is recommended as soon as the patient regains consciousness. It is important to explain to the patient that although coughing will hurt during the first few postoperative days, it will not cause any harm. Patients frequently suppress the cough mechanism voluntarily for fear of bursting sutures or promoting complications. Sedation is kept to a minimum to avoid depression of the cough reflex. The patient is warned that if he or she fails to cough and maintain a clear airway, he or she will require physical therapy.

Broad-spectrum antibiotic therapy is maintained for the first 5 postoperative days. The intercostal catheter may be removed at the end of 48 hours or when drainage of serum falls below 200 cm^3 in a 24-hour period. Sips of clear fluid are permitted on the first postoperative day. The patient is rapidly restored to a semisolid diet. Ice cream is readily accepted by the patient after esophageal surgery. A significant advantage of the thoracic route for antireflux surgery is the avoidance of any trauma to the small intestine and the rapid return of normal peristalsis.

Ambulation is commenced on the evening of the oper-

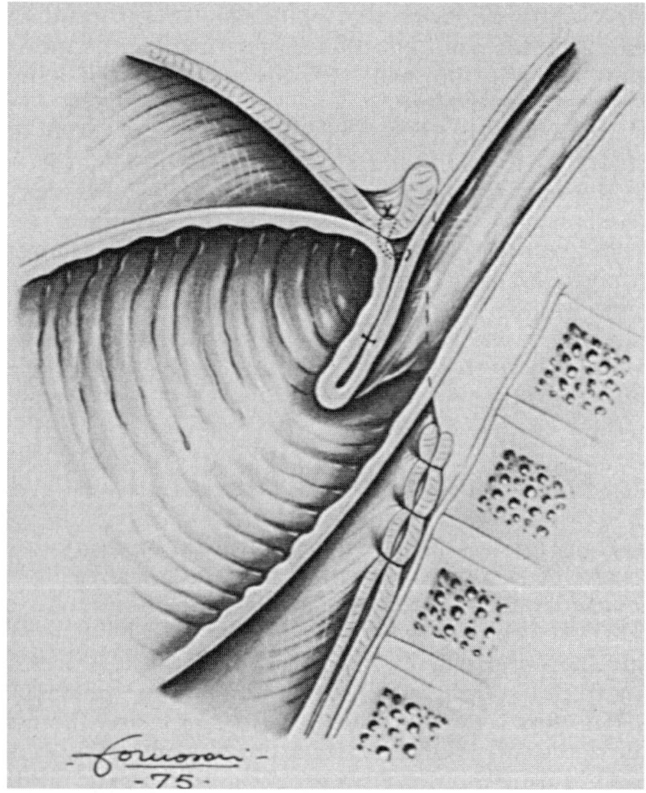

Figure 11–14. Diagrammatic representation of the principle of the Mark IV repair. Note the posterior buttress and the absence of any constriction at the hiatus. (From Stipa, S.: Hiatal herniorrhaphy. *In* Malt, R. [ed.]: Surgical Techniques Illustrated. Philadelphia, W.B. Saunders, 1985, with permission.)

ation or the following morning. While in bed, the patient's legs are kept raised to maintain venous drainage. If esophagitis was present before the operation, antacids are prescribed for the first postoperative month. A postoperative barium swallow is performed to determine whether the procedure was correctly performed, to exclude any suture problems in the repair, and to form a basis for comparison in subsequent barium studies.

POSTOPERATIVE COMPLICATIONS

There are few specific postoperative complications of the Mark IV procedure other than those normally associated with a transthoracic operation. Segmental or lobar atelectasis may occur in the immediate postoperative period, particularly in the right lower lobe, resulting from the frequent presence of aspiration pneumonitis in this segment. Response to aggressive thoracic physiotherapy is prompt. Mild transient dysphagia may occur during the first week owing to tissue edema in the reconstructed cardia. Persistent dysphagia indicates an error in surgical technique, probably too-aggressive narrowing of the hiatus. The gas-bloat syndrome does not occur after the 240-degree fundoplication.

Inadvertent mucosal perforation during mobilization of the cardia when previous surgery has disorganized the local anatomy can be corrected at operation. The closure is buttressed by the fundoplication. Small diverticula in the region of the repair, revealed in the postoperative barium study, call for no treatment in the symptom-free patient. Failure to secure Belsey's artery may result in intraperitoneal hemorrhage; this complication can be prevented. Small bowel ileus is avoided by the protection from trauma afforded by access to the upper abdomen through the extended left thoracotomy incision. Postthoracotomy discomfort has already been discussed and can largely be prevented.

The only late complication observed has been recurrent reflux caused by errors in technique. The dramatic late complications that have been reported after abdominal total fundoplication have not been encountered with the Mark IV technique.[7,8,10]

ADVANTAGES OF THE THORACIC APPROACH

1. The essential mobilization of the esophagus and cardia demanded by the Mark IV technique is possible only by using the thoracic route.

2. Adequate access to the upper abdomen to allow attention to be paid to coexistent upper abdominal pathologic lesions is afforded by the extended left thoracotomy incision described earlier.

3. For correction of recurrent reflux, particularly after multiple prior surgical adventures, the thoracic approach is now considered mandatory.[9] Disorganization of the local anatomy warrants adequate exposure of the mediastinum to permit mobilization of the esophagus and cardia. Intra-abdominal adhesions can be separated under direct vision by extending the incision into the upper abdomen. Doubt about the integrity of the vagi is an indication for a pyloromyotomy, possibly through the same incision. After complete mobilization, a Mark IV repair can be performed. Disorganization of the local anatomy by multiple prior operations, when complicated by chronic fibrosing ulcerative esophagitis, may prohibit any attempt to perform a physiologic repair. Resection of the destroyed segment and replacement by an isoperistaltic segment of jejunum or colon[1] is indicated in such cases. Maintenance of an 8- to 10-cm segment of the transplant in the high-pressure infradiaphragmatic zone constitutes an effective reflux-controlling mechanism that is adequate to prevent any further esophagitis. The patient should be fully prepared for the possibility of an interposition procedure before the operation. The final decision about the therapeutic program can be made at operation.

4. The same philosophy dictates a thoracic approach in patients with grade III or grade IV esophagitis with an undilatable or difficult to dilate stricture in whom a modified Collis gastroplasty[13] or resection and reconstruction may be necessary.

5. The Mark IV procedure is an effective antireflux adjunct to a long myotomy performed for achalasia or diffuse esophageal spasm. The 240-degree fundoplication does not cause dysphagia in cases of esophageal neuromotor dysfunction.[2]

6. The transthoracic Mark IV technique is preferable in patients with type II (paraesophageal) hernia, in whom adhesions between the intrathoracic stomach and surrounding mediastinal structures may render mobilization by the abdominal route hazardous. The presence of this abnormality since birth may result in defects in esophageal development and congenital shortening, requiring extensive mobilization to permit reduction of the hernia. Simple reduction may convert a type II hernia into a type I hernia and may precipitate reflux that was not present previously. It is essential to supplement reduction by an antireflux procedure; the Mark IV technique has been satisfactory in this situation. Gross congenital shortening may call for a modified Collis gastroplasty, a further indication for a thoracic approach.

7. The transthoracic Mark IV technique has proved satisfactory in the management of chronic reflux resistant to medical treatment in infants and children. In this age group, severe irreversible stenosis is frequently observed at the time of the initial diagnosis. The thoracic approach offers a wider spectrum of therapeutic options, including resection and reconstruction when indicated.

Results of the Belsey Mark IV Operation

Long-term results of reflux control after the Mark IV hiatal hernia repair were determined in 892 patients operated on between 1955 and 1965.[12] Follow-up was complete in 86%, and 94% of patients were followed for more than 3 years. The operative mortality rate was 1%, and the overall recurrence rate was 11%. In patients followed for 3 to 10 years, the recurrence rate was 12%, and in patients followed more than 10 years, it was 14.7%. About 84% of patients had either excellent or good results from operation at their last follow-up evaluation. Most recurrences occurred within 5 years of the initial operation.

A satisfactory result after the Mark IV repair is clearly related to the experience of the operating surgeon. Recurrence rates for the consultant (Belsey) and house staff were 5.9 and 14.6%, respectively. The type of hiatal hernia present and the degree of esophagitis in the absence of stricture did not significantly influence the results. However, when the Mark IV repair was performed in patients with severe esophagitis and stricture, there was a 45% failure rate (9 of 20 patients). The recurrence rate in children (20%) was twice that in adults.

Of the 98 patients with unsatisfactory surgical results, 32 were treated medically, and 45 required reoperation. Twenty-one patients with recurrence required no treatment. Twenty-four of 33 patients who had a second Mark IV repair and 8 of 9 patients who underwent resection and either colonic interposition or esophagogastrostomy had good or excellent results, an overall success rate of 76%.

References

1. Belsey, R.: Reconstruction of the esophagus with left colon. J. Thorac. Cardiovasc. Surg., *49:*33, 1966.
2. Belsey, R.: Functional diseases of the esophagus. J. Thorac. Cardiovasc. Surg., *52:*164, 1966.
3. Belsey, R.: Hiatal herniorrhaphy. *In* Malt, R. (ed.): Surgical Techniques Illustrated. Philadelphia, W.B. Saunders, 1985, p. 29.
4. Collis, J.: An operation for hiatus hernia with short esophagus. J. Thorac. Cardiovasc. Surg., *34:*768, 1957.
5. DeMeester, T., Wernly, J., Bryant, G., et al.: Clinical and in vitro analysis of determinants of gastroesophageal competence. Am. J. Surg., *137:*39, 1979.
6. Hill, L.: An effective operation for hiatal hernia: An 8 year appraisal. Ann. Surg., *166:*681, 1967.
7. Hill, L., Ilves, R., Stevenson, J., et al.: Reoperation for disruption and recurrence after Nissen fundoplication. Arch. Surg., *114*(4): 542, 1979.
8. Leonardi, H., Crozierre, R., and Ellis, F.: Reoperation for complications of Nissen fundoplication. J. Thorac. Cardiovasc. Surg., *81:*50, 1981.
9. Little, A., Ferguson, M., and Skinner, D.: Reoperation for failed antireflux operations. J. Thorac. Cardiovasc. Surg., *91:*511, 1986.
10. Mansour, K., Burton, H., Miller, J., et al.: Complications of intrathoracic Nissen wrap. Ann. Thorac. Surg., *32:*173, 1981.
11. Nissen, R.: Gastropexy and fundoplication in the surgical treatment of hiatal hernia. Am. J. Dig. Dis., *6:*954, 1961.
12. Orringer, M., Skinner, D.B., and Belsey, R.: Long-term results of the Mark IV operation for hiatal hernia and analyses of recurrences and their treatment. J. Thorac. Cardiovasc. Surg., *63:*25, 1972.
13. Pearson, F., Cooper, J., and Nelems, J.: Gastroplasty and fundoplication in the management of complex reflux problems. J. Thorac. Cardiovasc. Surg., *76:*665, 1978.
14. Sandry, R.: Pathology of reflux esophagitis. *In* Skinner, D., Belsey, R., Hendrix, T., et al. (eds.): Gastroesophageal Reflux and Hiatal Hernia. Boston, Little, Brown, 1972.
15. Skinner, D.B., and Belsey, R.: Surgical management of esophageal reflux and hiatus hernia: Long-term results with 1030 patients. J. Thorac. Cardiovasc. Surg., *53:*33, 1967.

CHAPTER

12 The Nissen Fundoplication: Operative Technique and Clinical Experience

HIRAM C. POLK, JR. • MARK A. WILSON

The discovery of the existence and pathophysiology of gastroesophageal reflux disease (GERD) proceeded in a sequential and orderly manner. Unfortunately, as a result of Allison's widely read and appreciated article,[1] excessive emphasis was placed on the existence of a hiatal hernia, and insufficient emphasis was placed on the true underlying process of abnormal acid reflux. Not surprisingly, a large number of patients, often without significant acid reflux or esophagitis, underwent either transabdominal or transthoracic repair of hiatal hernias. Often the operations failed either anatomically or symptomatically because relatively few of the patients had symptoms that were related to the anatomic abnormalities described radiographically and discovered at operation. Many individuals in Western societies who are of middle or older age will have radiographically demonstrable hiatal hernias. Often, occasional heartburn may be present, but comparatively few patients have symptomatic reflux esophagitis.

The re-emergence of reflux esophagitis as the primary indication for surgery dates to the 1970s and represents an important component of the current understanding of GERD. Acid reflux accounts for about 75% of esophageal pathology in Western societies and seems to be increasing in frequency.[2] Forty per cent of adult Americans report heartburn at least monthly,[3] and at least 7% have daily symptoms.[4,5] Symptomatic patients are often managed well without surgery, provided they are willing to comply with a sequence of simple lifestyle and medicinal measures. Approximately one third of persons with reflux symptoms require daily medical therapy,[3] although many patients frequently self-medicate with over-the-counter preparations, especially H_2-receptor antagonists. Interestingly, patients with symptomatic GERD have a markedly impaired quality of life that is comparable to that of patients with better recognized chronic illnesses, such as congestive heart failure and refractory angina pectoris.[5]

The primary underlying pathologic process that accounts for reflux symptoms and complications is increased esophageal exposure to gastric acid. Mechanical defects of the lower esophageal sphincter are the most common cause of GERD and are present in at least 70% of patients.[6] Overly frequent relaxation of the sphincter has also been implicated in an additional subset of patients with normal sphincter pressures. Less frequently, inefficient esophageal clearance of refluxed gastric juice and certain gastric abnormalities may be contributory. Esophageal motor defects or inadequate intra-abdominal fixation of the esophagus due to a large hiatal hernia may also result in impaired esophageal clearance. Gastric abnormalities of excessive acid secretion, delayed emptying due to anatomic obstruction or paresis, or increased gastric pressure may augment physiologic reflux. Delineation of these factors is important because antireflux surgery corrects only lower esophageal sphincter defects and is more likely to induce dysphagia or gastric distention in the case of substantial esophageal motor or gastric abnormalities.[7]

DIAGNOSIS

The diagnosis of GERD is often obvious owing to typical symptoms of heartburn and regurgitation. Heartburn usually responds rapidly to medical therapy and may recur after the discontinuation of medications or other measures. A minority of patients present with primary complaints due to complications of reflux disease, such as fibrotic stricture, and sequelae of regurgitation, such as nocturnal choking, coughing, and globus. The atypical symptoms of reflux disease include chest pain, wheezing, chronic cough, hoarseness, and pharyngeal discomfort. All of these symptoms overlap substantially with other common medical conditions, and often the role of gastric juice reflux in the genesis of these complaints is not obvious. The elusiveness of this relationship is evidenced by the absence of heartburn in more than 50% of patients with posterior laryngitis due to reflux.[8] Reflux should be sought if atypical symptoms are unexplained or refractory to appropriate therapies for coexistent conditions. The diagnosis of either idiopathic pulmonary fibrosis or bronchiectasis should prompt an investigation for possible reflux because of the recent recognition that these diseases are commonly associated with reflux disease.[9]

Although reflux is typically diagnosed clinically or suspected radiographically, confirmation before the consideration of operative intervention is crucial. In the past, this was frequently demonstrated by the presence of esophagitis endoscopically or histologically. Because of the nearly ubiquitous availability and the use of both over-the-counter and prescription medications, many pa-

Table 12–1. Diseases Associated With Reflux Esophagitis

Disease	Association, %
Cholelithiasis	26
Duodenal ulcer	15
Gastric ulcer	5
Surgical colonic disease	2
Angina pectoris	3
Nocturnal asthma	2
No other disorder	70

tients may not have esophagitis at the time of initial endoscopy. For patients with normal results of esophagoscopy or atypical symptoms, 24-hour pH monitoring without medical therapy can confirm pathologic reflux. The cost-effectiveness of this relatively costly procedure must be ultimately proved, especially for surgeons who are highly cost accountable. Unequivocally abnormal reflux is typically considered to occur during more than 7% of the 24-hour period,[10] whereas 4 to 7% is abnormal when there is good correlation with symptoms. The coexistence of other diseases, such as cholelithiasis, peptic ulcer disease, or dyspepsia, should also be carefully considered, because they are relatively common (Table 12–1). Even for patients with documented reflux, other coexistent processes, such as coronary artery disease, bronchospasm, or chronic sinusitis, may contribute to the symptom complex. The cause and effect of reflux in these presentations may be difficult to discriminate. Therapy with high doses of proton pump inhibitors may facilitate the diagnostic process in certain patients.

THERAPY OPTIONS

The goals of therapy are to control symptoms, to resolve esophagitis, and to manage or prevent complications. Lifestyle modifications (Table 12–2) should be emphasized to all patients and are requisite to other medical therapies or surgical intervention. We believe that expensive medications, such as proton pump inhibitors, generally should not be initiated until the efficacy of this simple six-point plan is determined. Studies that compared medical and surgical therapy of symptomatic GERD have often suggested similar outcomes, although some indicate superior results for operative repair.[11] Discussions of these issues continue and have been further stimulated by the acceptance of proton pump inhibitors for long-term maintenance therapy and the widespread adaptation of minimally invasive surgical techniques for operative therapy. Many factors must be considered when therapies are compared; these include the efficacy of symptom resolution or the development of new symptoms, the need for ongoing therapy, the control of disease progression, overall cost, and patient satisfaction. At present, no one study has comprehensively addressed these issues. Open Nissen fundoplication controls reflux symptoms in more than 90% of patients at 10 years after surgery.[7] The traditional indication for operative therapy has been failure of medical management with reflux complications or persistent symptoms. The patient who requires chronic therapy with proton pump inhibitors for disease control is also appropriately considered for surgery, especially if he or she is of a young age. Despite the increasing acceptance of the laparoscopic approach for surgery, the appropriate indications for surgery should not be altered.

Table 12–2. Non-operative Management of Gastroesophageal Reflux

Elevation of the head of the bed
No liquids after 8:00 P.M.
Abstinence from tobacco, alcohol, and chocolate
Antacid mints
Gaviscon
Elimination of tight garments
Weight loss, if possible
Omeprazole (Prilosec), as prescribed

PREOPERATIVE EVALUATION

The goal of preoperative evaluation is to confirm the presence of GERD and to select the best treatment option for each individual based on clinical presentation and gastroesophageal function.[12] Upper gastrointestinal endoscopy should be performed on all surgical candidates to assess for reflux complications and is best performed by the operating surgeon or an endoscopist with substantial experience in esophagoscopy and reflux disease. If possible, erosive esophagitis should be healed before surgery to reduce periesophageal inflammation. If Barrett's esophagus is present, thorough biopsies of the abnormal epitheliums are required, and the presence of dysplasia or adenocarcinoma requires specific further evaluation. Upper endoscopy can also be used to evaluate the size and type of hiatal hernia. The identification of a large (>5 cm) sliding hernia, a paraesophageal hernia, or esophageal scarring is important. These findings may indicate the presence of esophageal shortening, which would dictate a different operative approach. Strictures of the gastroesophageal junction should be dilated preoperatively to prevent postoperative dysphagia. A contrast esophagram is routinely performed and should be repeated if not performed within several weeks before surgery. We have frequently found that the disease process or esophageal anatomy has changed during the time from more remote contrast studies.

The role of esophageal manometry has been controversial. We have tended to reserve manometry for patients in whom abnormal motor function of the esophagus is suspected based on symptoms or radiographic or endoscopic findings. However, some studies claim that routine preoperative esophageal manometry can alter decision making in about 14% of patients.[12] It is unclear whether routine manometry is cost-effective to identify the small number of patients with esophageal motor defects that are not evidenced by an otherwise careful preoperative evaluation. Moreover, in our opinion, ambulatory pH monitoring is not necessary in all patients. Endoscopic evidence of erosive esophagitis is sufficient to substantiate significant reflux disease. Patients without reflux complications and those with atypical reflux symptoms should undergo pH monitoring to confirm the presence of pathologic reflux. Gastric emptying studies are selectively performed for patients at risk for gastroparesis, such as those with diabetes or those with significant nausea, vomiting, bloating, or postprandial fullness.

INCISIONAL PREFERENCE

For many years, much comment has been made as to whether operations should be performed through a transabdominal or transthoracic incision. The focus has shifted to an appropriate selection of patients for minimally invasive surgical procedures. Too frequently, it has been the technical skill and preference of the surgeon rather than the needs of the patient that have dictated the operative approach. In the majority of patients, careful and objective study provides clear-cut indications of which route is better.[13] The majority of procedures may be appropriately performed via a transabdominal approach. The true danger is the inadvisable transabdominal operation in a patient in whom there is substantial esophageal shortening. In this circumstance, it is difficult to perform adequate mobilization to obtain sufficient intraabdominal esophageal length for a tension-free fundoplication. This has been our most common indication for recommending a thoracic approach. Transabdominal Collis gastroplasty for esophageal shortening is also feasible in certain cases.

Laparoscopic fundoplication has become the preferred operative approach for surgical therapy of reflux disease at an increasing number of centers. We reiterate that the indications for surgery should not be altered because of the availability of a minimally invasive technique. There are no specific contraindications for laparoscopic fundoplication beyond open procedures, but several factors merit consideration. The most important decisions relate to whether surgery is warranted and to what procedure is most likely to provide the best outcome for the individual patient. The selection of a traditional open versus a laparoscopic approach is dependent on the surgeon's skill and training, the patient's disease process, and the patient's understanding of surgical options, including relative advantages and disadvantages of the approaches. Laparoscopic antireflux procedures are technically demanding and require advanced suturing skills and two-handed dissection abilities. Further, the learning curve for these procedures is longer and requires more cases than for laparoscopic cholecystectomy. Relative contraindications to a laparoscopic approach include previous upper abdominal surgery, morbid obesity, hepatomegaly, esophageal shortening, and massive hiatal hernia. These conditions do not preclude laparoscopic repair but are more likely to result in conversion to open procedures or in poor outcome unless the operating surgeon is highly experienced.

OPEN OPERATIVE TECHNIQUE

The principles of successful surgery for reflux disease are entirely predicated on the creation of a valvular mechanism that will control the reflux of gastric acid into the lower esophagus. There should be a requisite emphasis on the correction of associated hiatal hernias because maintenance of the esophogagastric junction below the diaphragm greatly enhances the physiologic effects on the lower esophageal sphincter mechanisms. The transabdominal operation is best performed through an upper midline incision. Xiphoid excision may be of benefit in an occasional patient. Thorough exploration of the abdomen is performed, and the decision to address associated diseases is confirmed. Attention is then turned to the esophageal hiatus. The first maneuver is to mobilize the left lobe of the liver, to fold it upon itself, and to retract it to the patient's right with a Harrington retractor. A transverse incision of the anterior peritoneum over the gastroesophageal junction is made and converted into an inverted U. This is extended to the first short gastric vessels laterally and to the ascending branch of the left gastric artery medially (Fig. 12–1). The operator's fingers may then be directed around the esophagus. Digital palpation should allow for identification of the diaphragmatic crura and the posterior vagus nerve. Both vagus nerves are included in the esophageal mobilization, and the structures are controlled with a Penrose drain. If substantial periesophageal inflammation persists, caution must be exercised to remain particularly wide of the esophagus to decrease the possibility of iatrogenic perforation. Palpation of the nasogastric tube or a No. 40 French Maloney bougie may facilitate the identification of the bounds of the esophagus. Esophageal mobilization is completed, usually via blunt dissection, and permits visualization of the diaphragmatic crura. We believe that crural repair is an essential part of the operation.

At this point, it is helpful to recognize the unique role of the bare area of the stomach to understand why a hiatal hernia is usually a true sliding hernia (Fig. 12–2). The posterior gastric fundus is a retroperitoneal structure and usually is easily mobilized from the pancreas and other retroperitoneal tissues. This blunt dissection is relatively easily accomplished by working from the right side of the esophagus and along the lesser curvature above

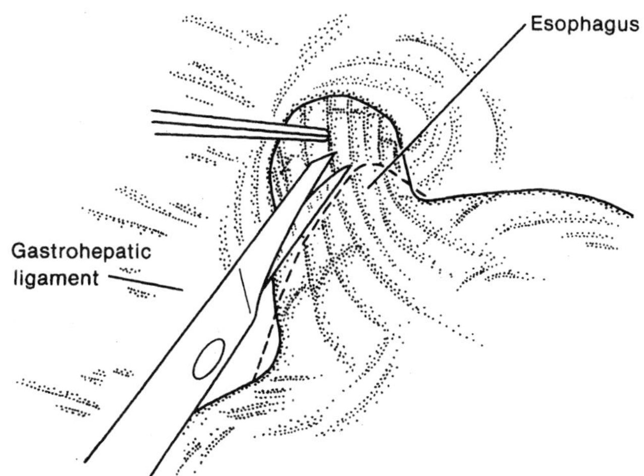

Figure 12–1. Nissen fundoplication. After the liver is mobilized and retracted, a transverse incision of the anterior peritoneum is made over the gastroesophageal junction and is converted into an inverted U.

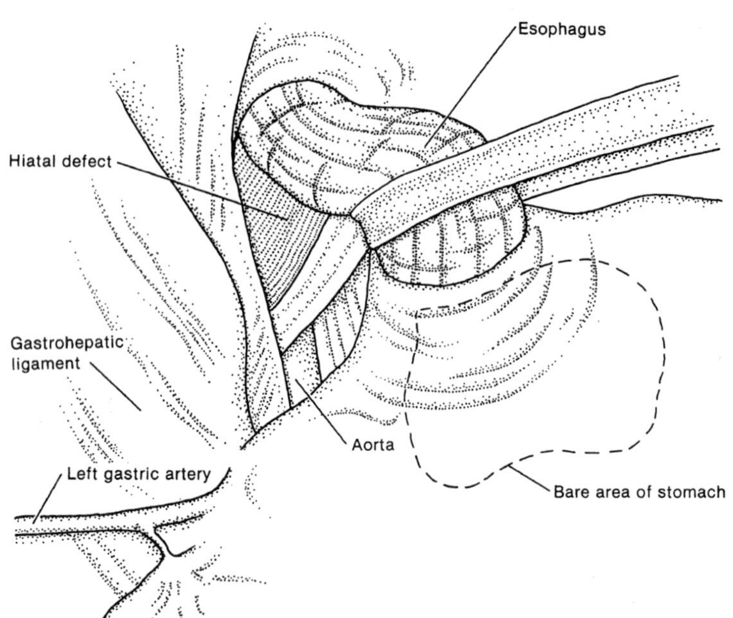

Figure 12–2. Unique role of the bare area of the stomach.

the insertion of the left gastric artery. A detailed anatomic study of fresh cadavers demonstrated the importance of this step in appropriate gastric mobilization.[14] At the same time, division of the short gastric vessels is not uniformly necessary for successful surgery and is important for fundic mobilization in a minority of patients. Posterior mobilization of the fundus at the bare area of the stomach is of greater importance than lateral mobilization of the greater curvature. On completion of these measures, crural repair is performed.

If a surgeon is experienced with operations for hiatal hernia, it is not always necessary to insert a bougie to prevent inadvertent narrowing of the esophagus. On the other hand, a surgeon without substantial experience or one who performs the operations less frequently should introduce a Maloney bougie to avoid constricting sutures about the esophagus. The crural repair is accomplished with interrupted 0 silk sutures by taking fairly wide bites of the muscular substance of the crura (Fig. 12–3). We try to tighten the crura to allow the tip of the operator's index finger to be introduced alongside the esophagus when the dilator has been removed (Fig. 12–4). When this has been accomplished, the posterior gastric fundus is mobilized to the medial side of the esophagus and is grasped with Babcock clamps to provide the full fundoplication as described by Nissen (Fig. 12–5).[15] It is important to use the posterior portion of the gastric fundus for the wrap. Use of the anterior stomach as described by Rosetti may result in lateral traction on the esophagus and is probably associated with a higher postoperative rate of dysphagia. The use of adequate posterior gastric mobilization avoids these difficulties. Recent literature has tended to recommend a shorter length of wrap, between 1.5 and 2.5 cm. We have continued to believe that a 3- to 4-cm wrap that is loosely constructed with an adequately mobilized gastric fundus is desirable. The actual repair is constructed with three or four sutures of 2–0 silk with partial-thickness bites of the esophagus. We no longer routinely suture the wrap or esophagus to the diaphragm but do secure the plication to the insertion of the esophagus along the lesser curvature of the stomach with the lowest suture. This maneuver acts to prevent the so-called slipped Nissen, which is uncommon unless the left gastric artery has been transected for mobilization. On completion of the wrap, the operator should be able to pass at least two fingers underneath the wrap and alongside the bougie and the esophagus (Fig. 12–6). Suction drains are occasionally used for reoperations, for extremely difficult procedures, and whenever gastrotomy or esophagotomy complicates a procedure.

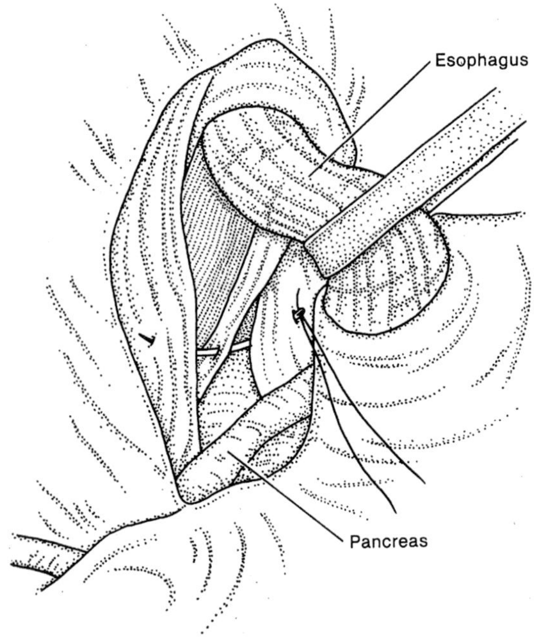

Figure 12–3. Crural repair during Nissen fundoplication.

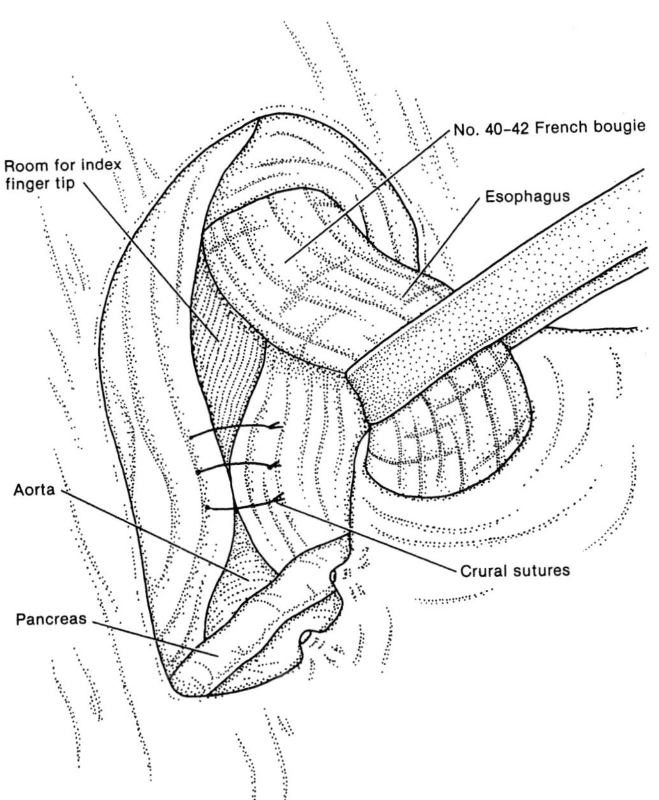

Figure 12–4. Tightening of crural suture sufficient to allow room for index finger alongside the esophagus when the dilator has been removed.

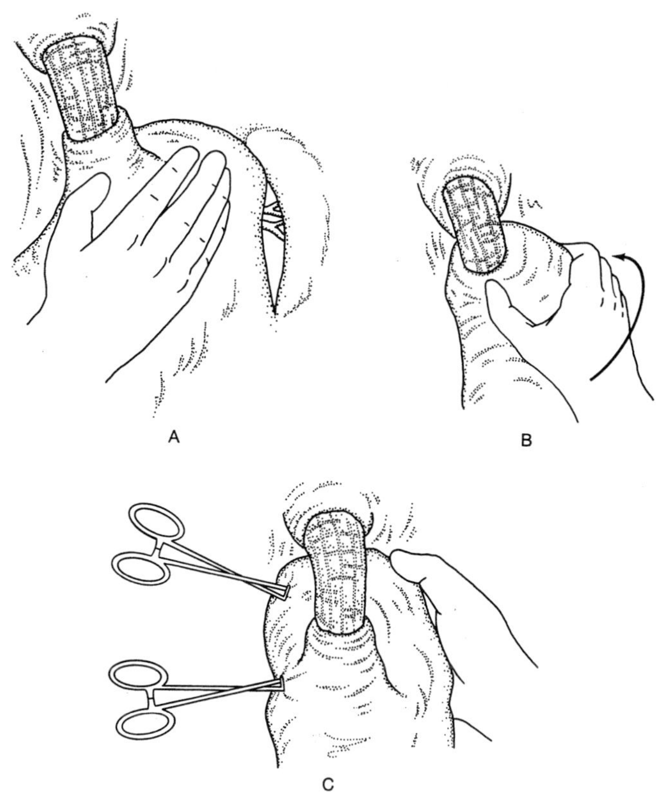

Figure 12–5. Mobilization of posterior gastric fundus to medial side of esophagus and grasping with Babcock clamps to provide full Nissen fundoplication.

The thoracic procedure is exactly the same operation but conducted in a different order. This is one of the reasons that we believe the Nissen fundoplication to be the procedure of choice for both thoracic and abdominal approaches.[16,17] We perform this operation through the subperiosteally resected bed of the fifth or sixth rib. Although some surgical inconvenience of the higher thoracotomy incision is experienced, there may be a lower incidence of intercostal neuralgia than with a lower thoracotomy. The posterior mediastinal pleura is incised after mobilization of the inferior pulmonary ligament. The esophagus is surrounded, and the hernia sac is opened circumferentially. This technique of dissection leaves a rim of phrenoesophageal ligament, hernia sac, and peritoneum attached to the esophagus. Blunt dissection is usually sufficient to mobilize the crura, which fall sharply posteriorly and away from the surgeon. After accentuation of the hernia and construction of the fundoplication, the wrap is reduced into the abdomen. The crura are then closed behind the plication, with care taken to obtain sufficient bites. Thus, the crural closure and fundoplication are performed in the reverse of what is done in the transabdominal operation.

We rarely use partial posterior fundoplication as described by Toupet[18]—typically when esophageal motor dysfunction exists. Hiatal closure and fundic mobilization are performed as described earlier. The posterior portion of the plication is secured to the posterior portions of the right and left crura with individual sutures after standard

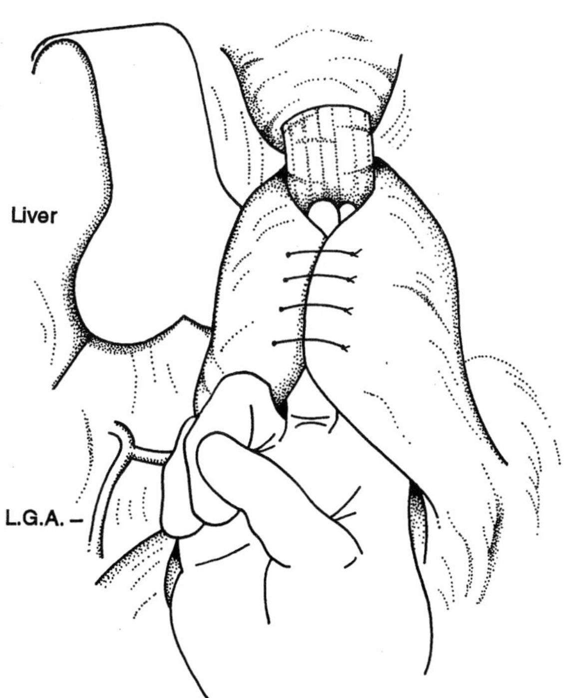

Figure 12–6. Completion of wrapping of gastric fundus, after which the operator should be able to pass two fingers under the wrapped portion and along the bougie and the esophagus. L.G.A. = left gastric artery.

closure of the crura. In this respect, our repair differs from the original description, in which a separate hiatal closure was not performed. The anterosuperior portion of the gastric fundus is secured on both the right and left sides to the crura anteriorly. Two or three interrupted 2-0 nonabsorbable sutures are used to approximate the fundus to the esophagus on either side to create a posterior 270-degree plication.

LAPAROSCOPIC OPERATIVE TECHNIQUE

The principles of laparoscopic antireflux procedures should adhere closely to those for the open operation. The techniques for dissection vary from those of open procedures due to inherent differences of the approaches. Patients are placed in a modified Lloyd-Davis position, and pneumatic compression devices are applied to the lower extremities. An initial trochar is inserted in the midline or just to the left of the midline about 15 cm from the xiphoid, and a 15-mmHg carbon dioxide pneumoperitoneum is established. An additional four trochars are inserted subcostally (two right and two left) in the upper abdominal quadrants. An angled 30- or 45-degree laparoscope is critical for adequate visualization of the hiatus. The left lobe of the liver is retracted anteriorly, but unlike in the open procedure, the triangular ligament is not divided. The initial dissection begins with one of two techniques. Our preference has been to divide the gastrohepatic ligament anterior to the caudate lobe of the liver to allow identification of the right diaphragmatic crus. Care must be taken to inspect for and avoid a replaced left hepatic artery. The hepatic branch of the vagus nerve should also be identified and preserved, if possible. The peritoneum overlying the anterior esophagus is then incised, and the epiphrenic fat pad is mobilized interiorly from the gastroesophageal junction. Alternatively, the dissection may begin to the anterior left side of the esophagus with incision of the peritoneal reflection and reflection of the fat pad. Isolation of the esophagus is best performed by initially dissecting the right crus to develop a space between the crus and the esophagus. It is safest to dissect the crus, instead of dissecting the esophagus as in open operation. Early identification of the vagus nerves is important, and the posterior nerve is usually left in its natural position with the esophagus and is included in the fundoplication.

After identification of the posterior decussation of the crura, initial dissection along the left crus is performed. As the dissection in this region proceeds further posteriorly, it becomes difficult to visualize the phrenogastric attachments and to mobilize the bare area of the stomach from the retroperitoneum. Because of the importance of adequate fundic mobility to allow a tension-free wrap, this posterior mobilization should not be compromised. Unlike the open procedure, this mobilization cannot be fully performed from the lesser curvature approach. In our experience, the posterior dissection almost always requires ligation and division of the short gastric vessels to permit exposure of the posterior gastric wall for mobilization. Short gastric vessels may be hemoclipped and cut, or they can be coagulated with bipolar devices or the harmonic scalpel ultrasonic scissors. This posterior dissection is thus performed from the left side instead of the right side, as in the open technique. As the higher short gastric vessels are encountered, traction on the posterior body of the stomach inferiorly and to the right facilitates exposure. After complete dissection of the left crus, the right crus is further dissected and the retroesophageal space is completed. This region should always be directly visualized to lessen the likelihood of iatrogenic perforation. The nasogastric tube and esophageal stethoscope should be withdrawn into the proximal esophagus to further minimize the risk of perforation during dissection. The esophagus is encircled with a Penrose drain that is used to retract the esophagus interiorly and to the left. Circumferential esophageal dissection above the hiatus is completed to mobilize a minimum of 3 cm of tension-free esophagus into the abdomen.

Posterior crural approximation is performed with interrupted size 0 nonabsorbable sutures that are tied intracorporeally. The hiatal closure is sized by the insertion of a bougie per orum. It is critical that the individual who inserts the bougie observes its passage on the video monitor to lessen the possibility of perforation. After partial withdrawal of the dilator, the posterosuperior portion of the fundus is passed posteriorly through the retroesophageal window under direct vision. The wrap should remain in place without being grasped. The dilator is readvanced, and the wrap is completed. Sutures are placed from the left fundus through a partial thickness of the anterior esophagus and into the wrapped stomach. Usually, three 2-0 nonabsorbable sutures are placed with each including a portion of the esophageal wall. The tension of extracorporeal knots is difficult to appreciate, and in this location, sutures may tear through the esophagus. Intracorporeal knot tying allows the most precise determination of adequate tension and a lesser degree of tissue trauma. The wrap is inspected to ensure a loosely constructed fundoplication, and the dilator is removed. Suturing of the wrap to the diaphragm has been espoused by some to lessen intrathoracic migration, but we have not routinely included these sutures.

RESULTS AND COMPLICATIONS

The results of the abdominal and thoracic operations have been similar. They have comparable failure rates, although there is a slightly higher incidence of recurrent hernia after the thoracic operation. It is fair to remember that most patients undergoing the throracic approach have been selected for that operation as a result of significant esophageal shortening. By any grading of disease, these patients have more advanced esophagitis. Overall, we believe that the operations are similar with regard to outcome. The results of our open procedures are presented in Table 12-3; these data confirm that antireflux surgery is not a placebo and that esophagitis resolves postoperatively. In some patients, several months are required for resolution,[19] possibly related to distal esophageal stasis rather than to continued reflux. In every case,

Table 12–3. Clinical Results of Fundoplication

Clinical Result		%
Excellent	Asymptomatic	85
Good	Improved but occasionally symptomatic	11
Failed	Persisting or progressive heartburn or dysphagia	4
Reoperation needed	For symptomatic failure	1
Death	In hospital	0.5

there has been resolution of microscopic esophagitis, and this remains true during extended follow-up, exceeding 20 years in several patients. These results are comparable to those reported by others experienced with antireflux procedures.[7,20] Improvement in atypical symptoms of hoarseness or pulmonary complaints often occurs more slowly during a period of up to one year.

Reports of laparoscopic fundoplication were initially limited by small patient numbers and very short follow-up. More recent reports with larger patient numbers suggest that laparoscopic antireflux procedures can be performed by experienced surgeons with outcomes comparable to the open operation.[21] The recurrence of reflux at 3 to 4 years after surgery parallels rates observed for open fundoplication. As outlined earlier, there are features of the laparoscopic procedure that differ from those of the open operation and that require specific recognition by the operator. Complications are therefore more frequent during the learning curve of the laparoscopic approach. Delayed recognition of iatrogenic perforation in several patients who were referred to us has resulted in substantial morbidity rates. Based on our geographic referral patterns, we believe that the incidence of fundoplication "slippage" is higher for operators' early laparoscopic procedures than for the open operation. This may be the result of difficulty in assessing the size of tissue bites laparoscopically, anatomic problems in wrap construction, or faulty suturing technique.

Complications may be considered based on occurrence during surgery, early after surgery, or late after surgery. In general, complications are of a similar type for both open and laparoscopic procedures, although the incidence varies with the technique and with operator experience. The mortality rate is less than 1% in most series of open antireflux procedures and is less frequent in laparoscopic operations. Bleeding may occur from an aberrant left hepatic artery in the gastrohepatic ligament, the left gastric artery, short gastric vessels, or the spleen. Open procedures have a 1 to 4% occurrence of splenectomy, whereas this is rarer with laparoscopic procedures. Perforation of the esophagus or stomach occurs in 1 to 3% of operations, regardless of whether they were performed laparoscopically or open. Perforation is most likely to occur during a surgeon's early experience, with obese patients, with patients with large hiatal hernias or severe periesophagitis, and with reoperative procedures. Inadvertent technical problems with creation of the fundoplication are probably more common with laparoscopic procedures, because there is a tendency to grasp the anterior stomach too close to the lesser curvature or too far distally. Resulting distortion of the proximal stomach may result in failure to control reflux or in the onset of dysphagia. Pneumothorax occurs infrequently with laparoscopic fundoplication procedures. Inadvertent vagal nerve injury may cause or worsen preexisting diarrhea and may contribute to postprandial symptoms of bloating and nausea.

Gas bloat has been variably reported with open fundoplications, but it generally is reported to occur in 5 to 15% of laparoscopic patients. Conversely, as many as half of patients may have difficulty vomiting after surgery regardless of an open or a minimally invasive approach. Intragastric trapping of swallowed air due to difficulty belching is the probable primary cause of gas bloat, but unrecognized preoperative gastric dysmotility and vagal injury may also contribute. These symptoms are self-limited in many patients but may be troublesome and difficult to treat for others. Dietary modifications and prokinetic agents may be beneficial. Dysphagia probably is the most common occurrence in the early postoperative period, with an incidence reported between 0 and 99% depending on the care with which patients are questioned. In most cases, dysphagia gradually improves without specific therapy except for the patient remaining on a liquid or soft diet. Cold foods or drinks tend to accentuate dysphagia. Persistent difficulties after the first 4 weeks may require dilatation,[22] but long-term dysphagia persists in only about 1% of patients. Inadequate fundic mobilization is more often an issue in the genesis of dysphagia than in a wrap that is too tight per se. Severe dysphagia in the early postoperative period mandates barium esophagography. Total or near-total obstruction at the fundoplication should be treated with reoperation, because endoscopic dilatation is not of benefit in this setting. Intraoperative assessment for fundic mobility is important, and endoscopic examination may facilitate evaluation of the wrap after reconstruction.

Recurrent reflux may be due to disruption of the wrap, to slippage of a previously adequate wrap, or to incorrect wrap construction. Reflux recurs in 1 to 5% of patients at 1 year after surgery. Long-term follow-up with open fundoplication demonstrates a 4 to 10% recurrence rate at 10 years, and follow-up at 4 years after laparoscopic repair suggests an incidence of about 3%. Slippage often presents with recurrent reflux symptoms, with or without dysphagia, and has a higher incidence in patients with esophageal shortening. Patients at a high risk of "slippage" are those with large hiatal hernias (>6 cm), impaired esophageal motility, or severe esophagitis with stricture. Extensive mediastinal mobilization of the esophagus may allow a sufficient intra-abdominal length to be obtained, but other cases may require a lengthening procedure, such as a Collis gastroplasty. Although Collis gastroplasty has been performed laparoscopically,[23] this substantially increases procedural difficulty, and collected long-term outcomes are not yet available.

SPECIAL CONSIDERATIONS

Much has been written about the role of surgery in the treatment of patients with Barrett's esophagus. The specific criteria that are required for the diagnosis of Barrett's esophagus continue to be discussed. It is clear that there is a spectrum of Barrett's esophagus that ranges from microscopic intestinalization of the esophageal mucosa in the absence of endoscopic abnormalities to larger and longer lesions that are overt. It is now generally accepted that columnar change of the esophageal mucosa is the result of abnormal gastroesphageal reflux. Many patients will have had chronic symptoms of reflux, but up to 40% will have few, if any, symptoms.[24] Once dysplasia occurs, there is unlikely to be a reversal to nondysplastic epithelium,[25,26] although low-grade dysplasia is often difficult to discriminate from an inflammatory component. Antireflux procedures will resolve reflux symptoms[27] and probably prevent extension of mucosal changes. However, there is a lesser likelihood that columnar mucosa will regress, and the effect on malignant transformation has not been clearly established.[28] The increased risk of adenocarcinoma in patients with Barrett's esophagus must be recognized so that surveillance can be performed.

Esophageal shortening is not common, but it must be recognized and prepared for before surgery.[29] Patients with large hiatal hernias, strictures, or severe Barrett's esophagus with submucosal fibrosis are at an increased risk of esophageal shortening. A review of upper gastrointestinal radiographs by an experienced surgeon will typically identify the patient with shortening or at substantial risk. Mediastinal mobilization is the first approach and is more readily accomplished via a transthoracic approach than via the open transabdominal route. However, laparoscopy provides excellent visualization of the lower esophagus for several centimeters above the hiatus, often permitting safe dissection to the level of the inferior pulmonary ligament. When mobilization is inadequate to provide sufficient intra-abdominal esophageal length, it is of paramount importance to not construct the Nissen wrap under tension. A lengthening procedure, typically a Collis gastroplasty, should be performed instead, followed by fundoplication around the neoesophagus.

Paraesophageal hernia is an issue for patients undergoing initial surgery as well as those who have had previous antireflux procedures. These hernias are especially treacherous in the elderly. Primary repair of these hernias or those with a mixed sliding and paraesophageal component has been performed laparoscopically with good results.[30] These laparoscopic procedures are often more difficult than standard antireflux procedures and require flexibility in the operative approach, often with initial dissection to the left of the esophagus. Regardless of whether the repair is performed open or laparoscopically, primary suture repair is typically feasible. Prosthetic mesh is used for repair only when the tissue quality is judged to be truly inadequate. The addition of a fundoplication to crural repair for pure paraesophageal hernias (type II) has been controversial. We believe that the majority of patients do have evidence of reflux,[31] and we typically include a fundoplication in the procedure.

Paraesophageal herniation may occur at any time during the postoperative course and appears to be more frequent after laparoscopic antireflux surgery.[32] Contributory factors probably include inadequate hiatal closure, technical difficulties with suturing of the crura, and increased intra-abdominal pressure from early postoperative emesis or inordinate physical activity. Efforts to prevent occurrence of paraesophageal herniation should include mandatory hiatal closure, attention to adequate delineation of the hiatal anatomy, appropriate suturing during laparoscopic repairs, and prevention of postoperative emesis by gastric decompression and/or antiemetics. Patients who are identified as having paraesophageal hernias in the early postoperative period should undergo reoperation for correction and not be observed.

CONCLUSION

Nissen fundoplication is a proved and effective long-term therapy for GERD. Appropriate patient selection and attention to surgical technique are keys to obtaining satisfactory results. The minimally invasive approach appears to provide results comparable to those of open fundoplication, but long-term results continue to be assessed.

References

1. Allison, P.R.: Reflux esophagitis, sliding hiatal hernia, and the anatomy of repair. Surg. Gynecol. Obstet., *92:*419, 1951.
2. DeMeester, T.R., and Stein, H.J.: Surgical treatment of gastroesophageal reflux disease. *In:* Castell, D.O. (ed.). *The Esophagus.* Boston, Little, Brown, 1992, pp. 579–625.
3. Gallup Survey on Heartburn Across America. Princeton, NJ, The Gallup Organization, March 28, 1988.
4. Spechler, S.J.: Epidemiology and natural history of gastro-esophageal reflux disease. Digestion, *51:*24, 1992.
5. Dimenas, E., Glise, H., Hallerback, B., et al.: Quality of life in patients with upper gastrointestinal symptoms: an improved evaluation of treatment regimens? Scand. J. Gastroenterol., *28:*681, 1992.
6. Stein, H.J., DeMeester, T.R., and Perry, R.P.: The three-dimensional lower esophageal sphincter pressure profile in gastroesophageal reflux disease: Effect of antireflux procedures. Ann. Surg., *216:*35, 1992.
7. DeMeester, T.R., Bonavina, L., and Albertucci, M.: Nissen fundoplication for gastroesophageal reflux disease: Evaluation of primary repair in 100 consecutive patients. Ann. Surg., *204:*9, 1986.
8. Koufman, J.A.: The otolaryngologic manifestations of gastroesophageal reflux disease (GERD): A clinical investigation of 225 patients using ambulatory 24-hour monitoring and an experimental investigation of the role of acid and pepsin in the development of laryngeal injury. Laryngoscopy, *101:*1, 1991.
9. El-Serag, H.B., and Sonnenberg, A.: Comorbid occurrence of laryngeal or pulmonary disease with esophagitis in United States military veterans. Gastroenterology, *113:*755, 1997.
10. Jamieson, G.G., and Duranceau, A.C.: The investigation and classification of reflux disease. *In:* Jamieson, G.G. (ed.): Surgery of the Esophagus. London, Churchill-Livingstone, 1988, pp. 201–211.
11. Spechler, S.J., and the Department of Veterans Affairs Gastroesophageal Reflux Disease Study Group: Comparison of medical and surgical therapy for complicated gastroesophageal reflux disease in veterans. N. Engl. J. Med., *326:*786, 1992.
12. Waring, J.P., Hunter, J.G., Oddsdottir, M., et al.: The preoperative evaluation of patients considered for laparoscopic antireflux surgery. Am. J. Gastroenterol., *90:*35, 1995.
13. Polk, H.C., Jr., and Zeppa, R.: Fundoplication for complicated hiatal hernia. Ann. Thorac. Surg., *7:*202, 1969.
14. Wald, H., and Polk, H.C., Jr.: Anatomical variations in hiatal and upper gastric areas and their relationship to difficulties experienced in operations for reflux esophagitis. Ann. Surg., *197:*389, 1983.
15. Nissen, V.R.: Eine einfache Operation zur beeinflussurgder Refluxoesophagitis. Schweiz. Med. Wochenschr., *86:*1, 1956.

16. Polk, H.C., Jr.: An approach to reflux esophagitis complicating sliding hiatal hernia. *In* Schwartz, S.I. (ed.): Modern Techniques in Surgery. New York, Futura, 1980, p. 1.
17. DeMeester, T.R., Johnson, L.F., and Kent, A.H.: Evaluation of current operations for the prevention of gastroesophageal reflux. Ann. Surg., *180:*511, 1974.
18. Toupet, A.: Technique d'oesophago-gastroplastie avec phreenogastropexie appliquée dans la cure radicale des hernies hiatales et comme complement de l'opération de Heller dans les cardiospasmes. Acad. Chir., *11:*394, 1863.
19. Richardson, J.D., Larson, G.M., Richardson, R.L., et al.: Properly conducted fundoplication reverses histologic evidence of esophagitis. Ann. Surg., *197:*763, 1983.
20. Dunnington, G.L., and DeMeester, T.R.: Outcome effect of adherence to operative principles of Nissen fundoplication by multiple surgeons: The Department of Veterans Affairs Gastroesophageal Reflux Disease Study Group. Am. J. Surg., *166:*654, 1993.
21. McKernan, J.B., and Champion, J.K.: Minimally invasive antireflux surgery. Am. J.Surg., *175:*271, 1998.
22. Wo, J.M., Trus, T.L., Richardson, W.S., et al.: Evaluation and management of postfundoplication dysphagia. Am. J. Gastroenterol. *91:*2318, 1996.
23. Johnson, A.B., Oddsdottir, M., and Hunter, J.G.: Laparoscopic Collis gastroplasty and Nissen fundoplication: A new technique for the management of esophageal foreshortening. Surg. Endosc., *12:*1055, 1998.
24. Gruppo Operativo per lo Studio delle Precancerosi dell'Esfago (GOSPE). Barrett's esophagus: Epidemiological and clinical results of a multicentre survey. Int. J. Cancer, *48:*364, 1991.
25. Levine, D.S.: Barrett's esophagus. Sci. Am. Sci. Med., *1:*16, 1994.
26. Haggitt, R.C.: Barrett's esophagus, dysplasia, and adenocarcinoma. Hum. Pathol., *25:*982, 1994.
27. Farrell, T.M., Smith, C.D., Metreveli, R.E., et al.: Fundoplication provides effective and durable symptom relief in patients with Barrett's esophagus. Am. J. Surg., *178:*18, 1999.
28. Williamson, W.A., Ellis, F.H., Gibb, S.P., et al.: Effect of antireflux surgery on Barrett's mucosa. Am. Thorac. Surg., *49:*537, 1990.
29. Gastal, O.L., Hagen, J.A., Peters, J.H., et al.: Short esophagus: Analysis of predictors and clinical implications. Arch. Surg., *134:*633, 1999.
30. Perdikis G., Hunter, J.G., Filipi, C.J., et al. Laparoscopic paraesophageal hernia repair. Arch Surg., *132:*586, 1997.
31. Fuller, C.B., Hagen, J.A., DeMeester, T.R., et al.: The role of fundoplication in the treatment of type II paraesophageal hernia. J.Thorac. Cardiovasc. Surg., *111:*655, 1996.
32. Watson D.I., Jamieson, G.G., Devitt, P.G., et al.: Paraoesophageal hiatus hernia: An important complication of laparoscopic fundoplication. Br. J. Surg., *82:*521, 1995.

CHAPTER

13

Reflux Stricture and Short Esophagus

MARK B. ORRINGER

Esophageal reflux strictures result from the inflammatory reaction that is induced in the esophagus by exposure to regurgitated gastric contents, both acid and alkaline.[8,112] Why only some patients with gastroesophageal reflux develop strictures is unknown, but patients with reflux strictures tend to be older with a longer history of reflux and to have more reduced lower esophageal sphincter pressure and abnormal esophageal motility compared with reflux patients without strictures.[56] Gastroesophageal reflux occurs independently of the presence of a hiatal hernia, and incompetence of the lower esophageal sphincter, not the size of the hernia, is the critical pathologic lesion. As a result of the esophageal epithelial burn caused by exposure to gastric contents, ulceration, submucosal edema, and inflammatory cellular infiltration occur. The inflammation may involve the muscular layers of the esophageal wall as well as periesophageal soft tissues. Surrounding mediastinal edema and lymphadenopathy are not uncommon. With healing, various degrees of fibrosis occur. Acute reflux esophagitis tends to be cyclic, and, with time, progressive mural fibrous infiltration occurs, initially in the submucosa but ultimately involving the muscle and periesophageal tissues. Contraction of collagen within the esophageal scar produces both circumferential narrowing, which reduces the size of the lumen, and esophageal shortening of various degree. This process of true shortening of the distance between the esophageal introitus and the esophagogastric junction occurs in a fashion similar to that seen with contracture that follows a caustic esophageal injury.

Considerable controversy regarding the term *short esophagus* has existed for nearly 40 years. Barrett[6] acknowledged Albers as being the first to describe peptic ulceration of the esophagus. Tileston[124] reported 44 patients with ulcerative reflux esophagitis and also described associated esophageal stenosis.[124] As the term reflux esophagitis was popularized as a distinct clinical entity by Allison[2] and Barrett,[6] the occurrence of columnar epithelium distal to the stenosis in many of these patients began to be recognized. Although he was a pioneer in his efforts to define reflux esophagitis, Barrett unfortunately concluded that any portion of the swallowing passage that is lined by columnar epithelium is stomach.[6] Thus the term *short esophagus* was coined, because the columnar-lined lower esophagus distal to the stricture was regarded as stomach. The erroneous notion was born that reflux strictures always occur at the anatomic esophagogastric junction, and intestinal interpositions were performed to replace the "missing" esophageal segment.

With time, it became apparent that the columnar-lined lower esophagus is an *acquired* lesion that results from reflux esophagitis.[3,71,72] With the development of techniques of esophageal manometry came the observation that in patients with a columnar-lined lower esophagus, there is a definite though weak lower esophageal sphincter mechanism at the *anatomic* esophagogastric junction, well below the squamocolumnar *epithelial* junction. As a result, some investigators have disputed the very existence of a short esophagus and argue that the esophagogastric junction can always be reduced below the diaphragmatic hiatus for an antireflux operation.[47,57] This is clearly *not* the viewpoint of most esophageal surgeons, who recognize that fibrous contracture may occur in the esophagus just as it does at other sites in the body in response to a burn. In fact, it has becoming increasingly apparent that acquired esophageal shortening in response to gastroesophageal reflux may occur even in patients who do not have fibrosis or stricture formation. Clinical experience has repeatedly identified patients undergoing transthoracic hiatal hernia repairs for gastroesophageal reflux without stricture formation in whom it is difficult to reduce the esophagogastric junction below the diaphragm without tension. It appears, therefore, that the term *short esophagus* does not necessarily imply that a stricture is present and may also be applied appropriately in patients who at the time of hiatal hernia repair are found to have an unacceptable degree of stretch on the distal esophagus once the esophagogastric junction is reduced below the diaphragm. Because the majority of antireflux operations are performed transabdominally, assessment of tension on the distal esophagus at the completion of the repair is seldom possible; therefore, the frequency with which esophageal shortening occurs is grossly underestimated. The presence of a reflux stricture or a short esophagus in a patient undergoing an antireflux operation may have direct implications on the type of surgical procedure performed and will be the subject of this chapter.

ANATOMIC VARIATION AND EVALUATION

Esophageal reflux strictures tend to be one of three general varieties. Most reflux strictures are only 1 to 2 cm in

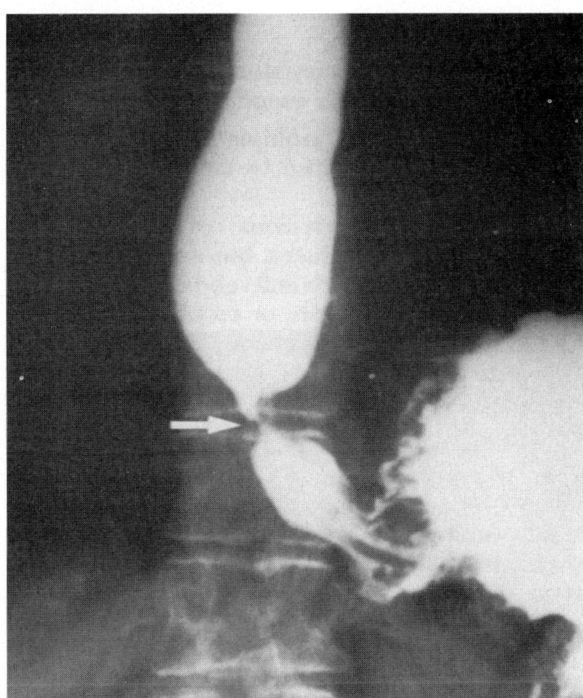

Figure 13–1. Barium esophagograms demonstrating the most frequent type of esophageal reflux stricture: a short, less than 2-cm stenosis *(arrow)* occurring at the esophagogastric junction just proximal to a sliding hiatal hernia. (From Orringer, M.B.: Short esophagus and peptic stricture. *In* Sabiston, D.C., Jr., and Spencer, F.C. [eds.]: Surgery of the Chest, 6th ed. Philadelphia, W.B. Saunders, 1995, p. 1059, with permission.)

length and are localized to the anatomic esophagogastric junction (Fig. 13-1). Less frequently, lengthy strictures involving the distal half or third of the esophagus occur, particularly following nasogastric intubation in critically ill patients who are supine for many days, after protracted vomiting, or in association with gastric outlet obstruction (Fig. 13-2). The third variety is the short stricture that occurs in the mid or upper thoracic esophagus at the squamocolumnar epithelial junction in a patient with Barrett's esophagus (Figs. 13-3 and 13-4). The presence

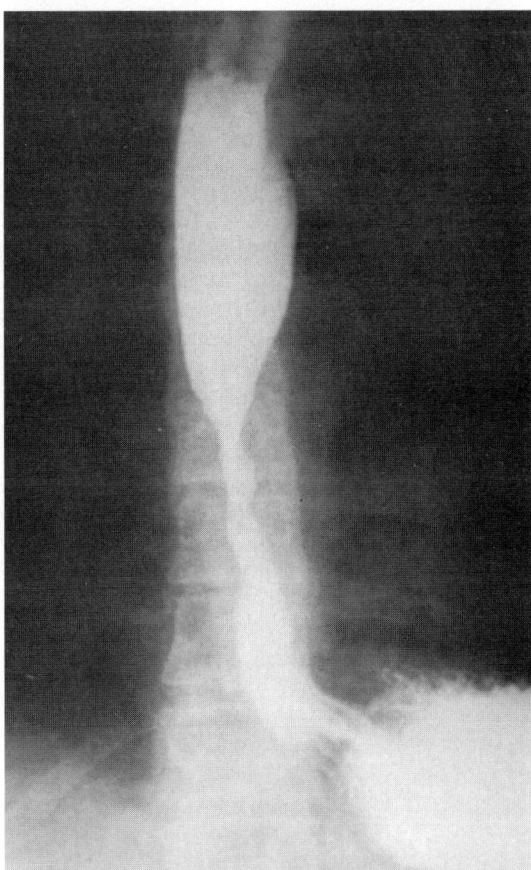

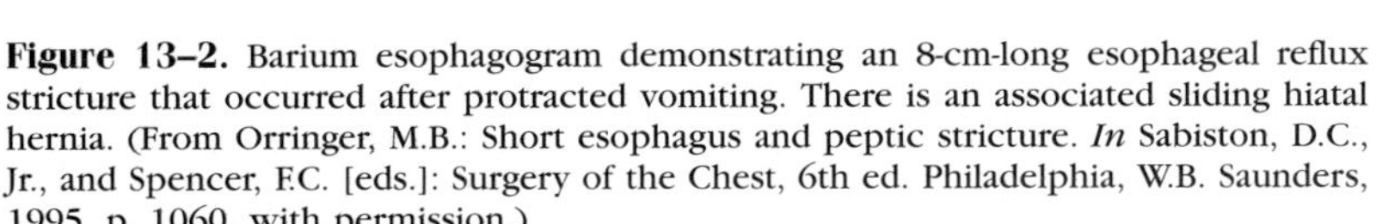

Figure 13–2. Barium esophagogram demonstrating an 8-cm-long esophageal reflux stricture that occurred after protracted vomiting. There is an associated sliding hiatal hernia. (From Orringer, M.B.: Short esophagus and peptic stricture. *In* Sabiston, D.C., Jr., and Spencer, F.C. [eds.]: Surgery of the Chest, 6th ed. Philadelphia, W.B. Saunders, 1995, p. 1060, with permission.)

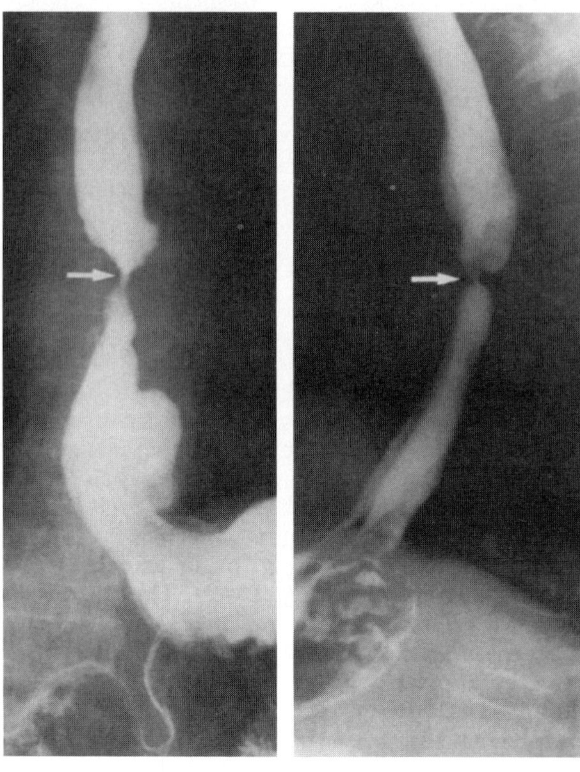

Figure 13–3. Posteroanterior *(left)* and lateral *(right)* views from an esophagogram demonstrating a short midesophageal stricture *(arrows)* in a patient with chronic reflux symptoms and dysphagia. This "high" stricture suggested a Barrett's esophagus. At endoscopy, there was normal squamous epithelium down to the squamocolumnar epithelial junction, which was located at the site of the stricture. The esophagus distal to the stenosis was lined by columnar epithelium. A small sliding hiatal hernia is present.

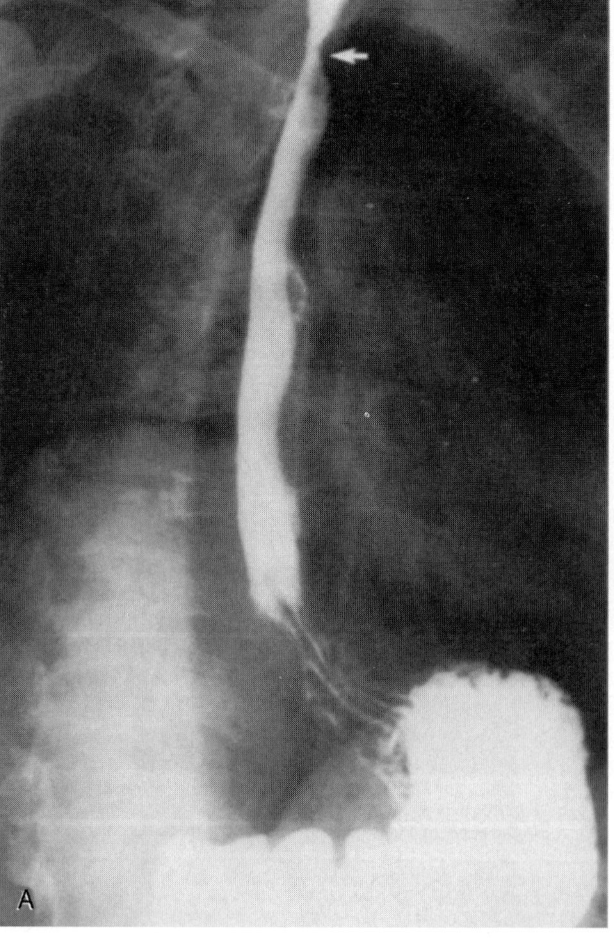

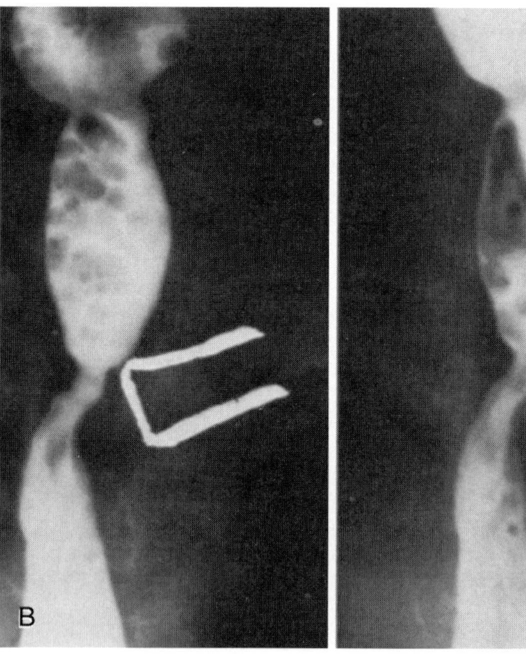

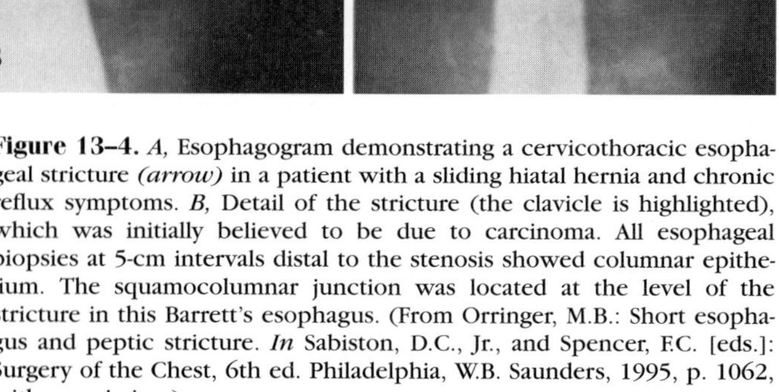

Figure 13–4. *A,* Esophagogram demonstrating a cervicothoracic esophageal stricture *(arrow)* in a patient with a sliding hiatal hernia and chronic reflux symptoms. *B,* Detail of the stricture (the clavicle is highlighted), which was initially believed to be due to carcinoma. All esophageal biopsies at 5-cm intervals distal to the stenosis showed columnar epithelium. The squamocolumnar junction was located at the level of the stricture in this Barrett's esophagus. (From Orringer, M.B.: Short esophagus and peptic stricture. *In* Sabiston, D.C., Jr., and Spencer, F.C. [eds.]: Surgery of the Chest, 6th ed. Philadelphia, W.B. Saunders, 1995, p. 1062, with permission.)

of a benign mid or upper esophageal stricture in a patient with gastroesophageal reflux should always alert the physician to the possibility of Barrett's esophagus, because the stricture occurs characteristically at the squamocolumnar epithelial junction, and the esophagus distal to the stricture is lined by columnar epithelium. A sliding hiatal hernia is usually but not always present.

The presence of an esophageal reflux stricture is typically diagnosed by means of a barium esophagogram obtained in a patient who has dysphagia or reflux symptoms. Although it would obviously be desirable to treat gastroesophageal reflux before mural fibrosis occurs, early diagnosis of reflux esophagitis is hampered by the curious nature of this disease. First, a notoriously poor correlation between the patient's symptoms and the degree of esophagitis present prevents the physician from relying on the patient's complaints alone as being the most important indicator of the need for endoscopy. Thus, some young patients with severe reflux symptoms may have no or minimal endoscopic evidence of esophagitis, whereas some older patients who have never had enough reflux symptoms to seek medical attention in the past present with dysphagia due to established reflux strictures. Second, the barium esophagogram, one of the most readily available studies for evaluation of the esophagus, fails to detect esophagitis consistently and reliably before mural fibrosis occurs, and the degree of esophageal narrowing indicated by the barium esophagogram provides no real information about the likelihood of being able to dilate the stricture successfully. The narrowing seen on a barium esophagogram in a patient with a reflux stricture has two components: (1) the edema and cellular inflammatory reaction of acute reflux esophagitis, and (2) varying degrees of fibrosis that have resulted from previous reflux episodes. The ease with which progressively larger esophageal dilators can be passed through the radiographic narrowing (i.e., the "hardness" of the stricture) cannot be predicted from the barium swallow.

A variety of classifications of esophageal reflux strictures have been proposed. Esophagitis is an endoscopic diagnosis, and several well-established classifications of reflux esophagitis may be applied to strictures. In the endoscopic grading of reflux esophagitis proposed by Skinner and Belsey,[115] four grades of esophagitis are recognized:

Grade I: Distal esophageal mucosal erythema (which may obscure the esophagogastric squamocolumnar epithelial junction).

Grade II: Mucosal erythema with superficial ulceration, typically linear and vertical and with an overlying fibrinous membranous exudate that is easily wiped away, leaving a bleeding surface (which is often misinterpreted as "scope trauma" by the inexperienced endoscopist).

Grade III: Mucosal erythema with superficial ulceration and associated mural fibrosis—a dilatable "early" stricture.

Grade IV: Extensive ulceration and fibrous luminal stenosis, which may represent irreversible panmural fibrosis.

In the Savary-Monnier clarification,[77] there are five grades of reflux esophagitis:

Grade 1: Single or multiple erosions (may be erythematous or covered by exudate) *on a single mucosal fold.*

Grade 2: Multiple erosions covering *several mucosal folds* (may be confluent, but not circumferential).

Grade 3: Multiple circumferential erosions.

Grade 4: Ulcer, stenosis, or esophageal shortening.

Grade 5: Barrett's epithelium: columnar mucosa reepithelialization in the form of an island, strip, or circumferential.

Regardless of which endoscopic grading system is used, such objectivity in describing the pathologic changes seen endoscopically is preferable to the traditional distinctions of "mild," "moderate," or "severe" esophagitis, which have inherent wide variation and observer variability. It is important to emphasize, particularly to physicians who do not frequently treat patients with reflux esophagitis, that the radiologic report of a mild esophageal reflux stricture does *not* imply that the process has been diagnosed at a sufficiently early stage that conservative therapy is likely to be successful. A mild radiographic stricture is an *advanced* stage of esophagitis, and institution of appropriate therapy is long overdue.

In addition to the endoscopic grading of esophagitis, there is a need to classify reflux strictures according to the degree of resistance encountered during attempts at dilation. The "hardness" of a reflux stricture—that is, the degree of fibrosis present—has direct implications on the likelihood of successful treatment with conservative measures. The severity of a stricture can be classified on the basis of the degree of resistance encountered during dilation. A *mild* stricture is defined as one in which minimal resistance is encountered as progressively larger dilators are passed through the stenosis. *Moderate* strictures require some, but not excessive, forceful dilation. *Severe* strictures require forceful dilation and are associated inevitably with marked periesophageal inflammation and mural thickening of the esophagus. The determination of the severity of a reflux stricture may not be possible until at operation the anesthetist passes progressively larger esophageal dilators by mouth with the mobilized esophagus supported by the surgeon's hand.

TREATMENT

Endoscopic Assessment

Two critical questions must be answered about every newly diagnosed esophageal stricture: (1) Is the stricture benign or malignant, and (2) if benign, can it be dilated? The relative technologic explosion in the variety of available flexible fiberoptic esophagogastroscopes and instrumentation possible through them has resulted in this instrument becoming the most common means of assessing the esophageal lumen and stenoses visually. Rigid esophagoscopy still has its place in the esophageal surgeon's armamentarium because it provides larger and more meaningful biopsy specimens with which to assess changes of reflux esophagitis,[70] but its use is now restricted to the patient in whom passage of the flexible instrument is not possible, and general anesthesia is required. Endoscopic assessment of any esophageal stricture requires adequate patient sedation and anesthesia, because this is an uncomfortable procedure that mandates the surgeon's complete concentration on the endoscopic field, not on a moving, struggling patient.

Adequate esophageal biopsies and brushings for cytologic evaluation of the stricture should be performed in the initial endoscopic assessment of the stricture, as the combination of esophageal biopsy and brushings establishes the diagnosis of carcinoma in more than 95% of patients with a malignant stricture. If there is no evidence of neoplasm with either of these studies, there is a high likelihood that the esophageal stenosis is benign. After the biopsy, dilation of the stenosis is performed. The standard adult flexible esophagoscope is the size of a No. 32 French esophageal dilator, and a mild stricture can be dilated directly by advancing the instrument through it. After this, passage of progressively larger Hurst-Maloney tapered dilators is performed beginning with a No. 32 French size and advancing to at least a No. 46 French size, but preferably larger depending on the resistance encountered. Virtually every reflux stricture that can be dilated by mouth to a No. 40 French size bougie can be dilated later intraoperatively to the 54 to 60 French range (see later section, "Surgical Treatment"). Patients with intractable esophagitis or dysphagia who are likely candidates for antireflux surgery, therefore, need not undergo dilation much beyond a No. 40 French size preoperatively unless relatively little resistance is encountered to passage of the bougies. Those for whom periodic dilations and an antireflux medical regimen are thought to be the preferred treatment of the reflux stricture must undergo dilation to at least a No. 46 French size to restore comfortable swallowing.

With a more severe stricture, it is dangerous to advance either a rigid or the flexible esophagoscope through it at the initial assessment. In the past, prior to the availability of the Savary-Gilliard dilating system,[69] patients had hard strictures dilated under general anesthesia through a rigid esophagoscope with gum-tipped bougies passed under direct vision through the stenosis (Fig. 13-5). Most standard rigid esophagoscopes accommodate up to a No. 26 French bougie in this manner. After reaching this size, the esophagoscope is removed and the dilation is continued blindly by passing Hurst-Maloney, mercury-filled, tapered rubber dilators through the patient's mouth. With particularly dense hard strictures, such blind passage of dilators is not performed because curling of the dilator within the esophagus proximal to the stricture may result in a perforation (Fig. 13-6). Fluoroscopic guidance may be a useful adjunct for safer passage of Maloney dilators in those with more severe esophageal strictures.[125] Several alternative methods of dilation are available in such cases, and the surgeon should be familiar with a variety of methods of dilation.

When performing the initial endoscopic evaluation of a high-grade, hard stricture through a rigid esophagoscope, rather than attempting to pass dilators blindly through the stenosis, the standard rigid esophagoscope through which the stricture has been dilated to a No. 26

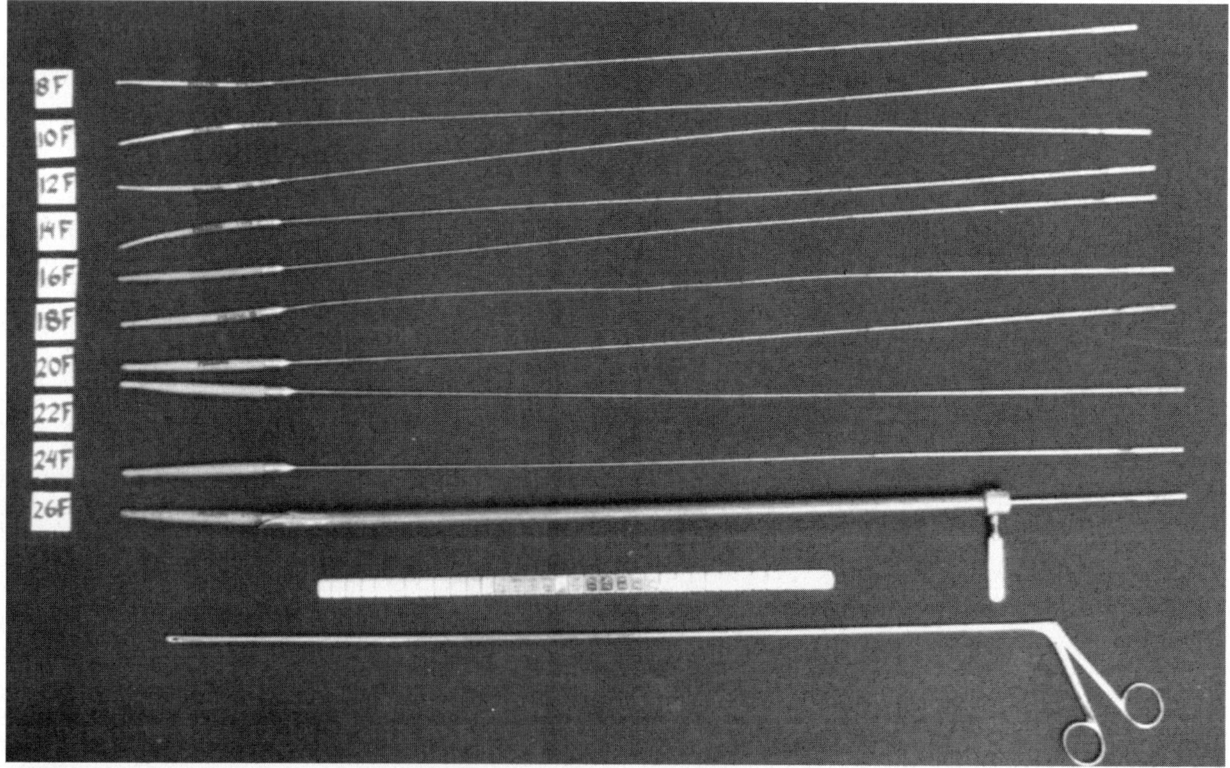

Figure 13-5. Equipment needed for the initial evaluation of an esophageal reflux stricture: a ruler for precise localization of the pathology (in centimeters from the incisor teeth); a biopsy forceps (and cytology brush, not shown) to exclude carcinoma with biopsies and brushings of the stricture; and gum-tipped Jackson dilators, manipulated gently through the stricture, to assess the length and pliability of the obstruction. The No. 26 French dilator is the largest size that passes through the standard 45-cm rigid esophagoscope.

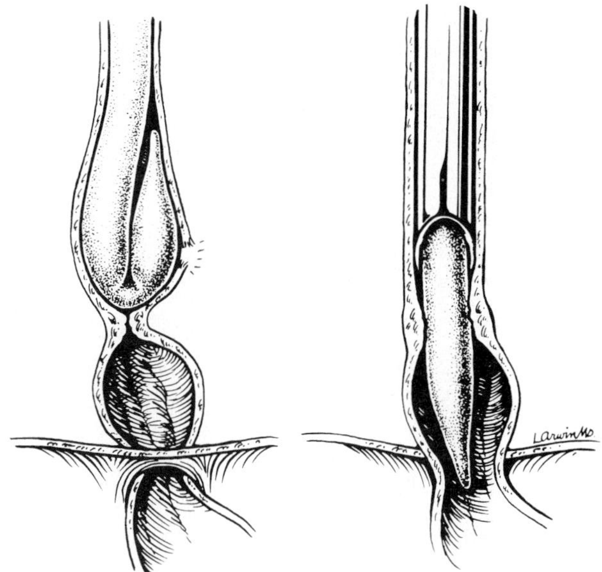

Figure 13–6. *Left,* Esophageal perforation due to "curling" of an esophageal dilator passed blindly in an attempt to dilate a tight stricture. *Right,* A special-order large, rigid esophagoscope (see also Fig. 13–7) accommodates up to a No. 50 French dilator and permits dilation of the stricture under direct vision. (From Orringer, M.B.: Complications of esophageal surgery and trauma. *In* Greenfield, L.J. [ed.]: Complications in Surgery and Trauma, 2nd ed. Philadelphia, J.B. Lippincott, 1990, p. 310, with permission.)

French bougie under direct vision is removed and replaced with a special-order, 45-cm-long rigid esophagoscope (Pilling Company), which accommodates up to a No. 50 French bougie (Fig. 13–7). This esophagoscope is nearly the size of a sigmoidoscope, and the greatest morbidity risk associated with its use involves its insertion through the upper esophageal sphincter, where considerable experience is required to prevent a perforation. However, once this esophagoscope is introduced into the esophagus and advanced to the level of the stricture, dilation *under direct vision* can be performed using progressively larger dilators, beginning with a No. 28 French and proceeding to a No. 50 French size.

The above techniques of dilation using the rigid eso-

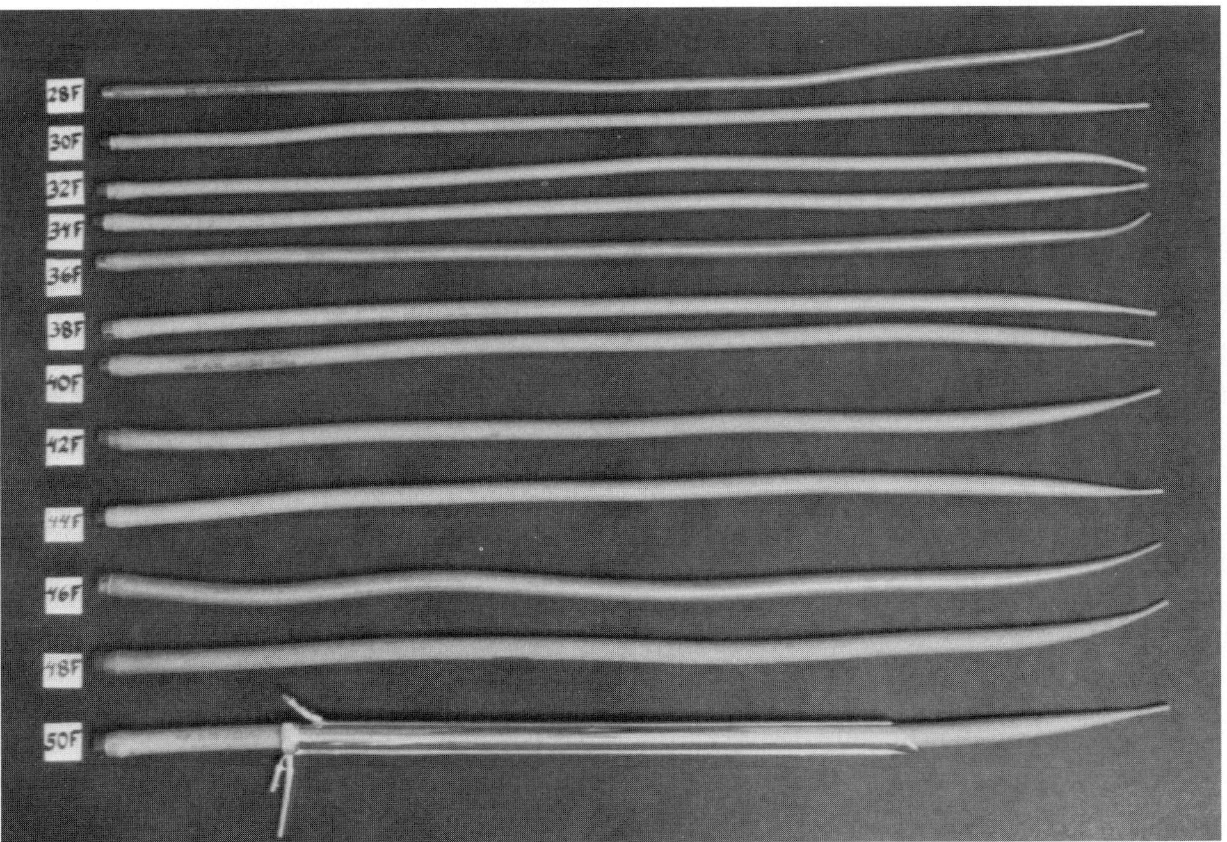

Figure 13–7. Tapered Maloney esophageal dilators and the special-order Pilling 45-cm esophagoscope, which will accommodate a No. 50 French dilator, used to dilate dense, severe reflux strictures under direct vision.

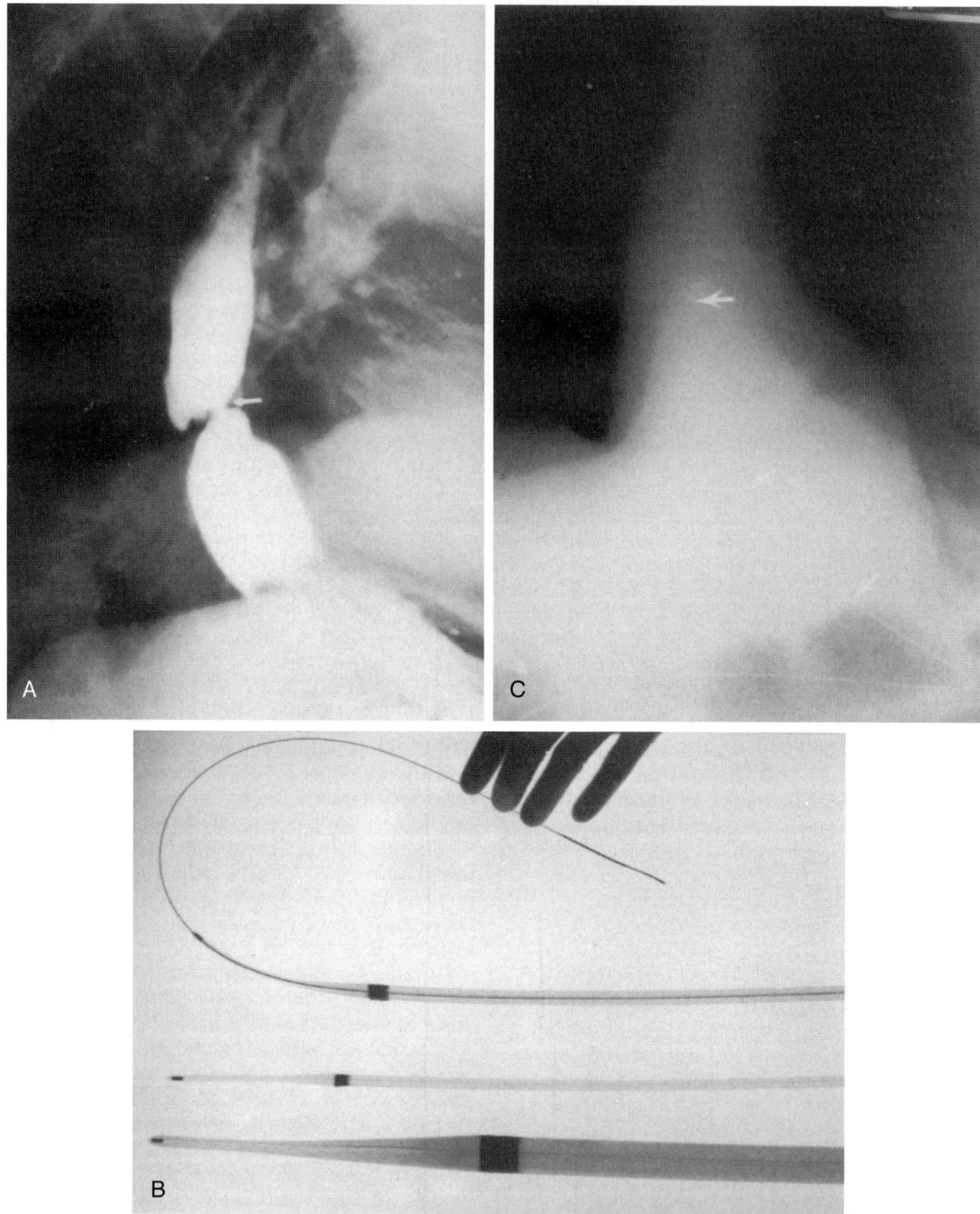

Figure 13–8. Esophagogram showing *(A)* eccentric complex reflux stricture *(small arrow)* at esophagogastric junction proximal to a large sliding hiatal hernia. Because of the diverticulum-like configuration of the lumen in the region of the stricture, blind passage of a Maloney bougie was thought to be unsafe. *B,* Several sizes of the polyvinyl Savary-Gilliard dilators with a guidewire passed through the upper dilator. *C,* Radiographic confirmation of the proper course of the endoscopically placed Savary guidewire *(arrows)* through the esophageal stenosis and into the stomach (same patient as shown in *A*). Progressively larger Savary dilators up to a No. 54 French were passed over the wire and through the stricture. Blind passage of Maloney dilators on an outpatient basis was then achieved without difficulty. (From Orringer, M.B.: Short esophagus and reflux stricture. *In* Sabiston, D.C., Jr., and Spencer, F.C. [eds.]: Surgery of the Chest, 6th ed. Philadelphia, W.B. Saunders, 1995, p. 1066, with permission.)

phagoscope have all but been replaced by availability of the Savary-Gilliard dilating system (Fig. 13–8). When the flexible esophagoscope cannot be manipulated through the stenosis to achieve dilation, the Savary guidewire passed through the esophagoscope is insinuated through the stricture and into the stomach. After removing the esophagoscope, progressively larger tapered polyvinyl Savary dilators are passed over the guidewire until there is an adequate lumen to permit endoscopic assessment with biopsies and cytologic brushings. Alternatively, balloon dilation over a guidewire or under endoscopic guidance has been shown to provide effective treatment of reflux strictures.[107]

Several rules of thumb have been developed regarding the extent to which a reflux stricture can be dilated at the initial assessment. Passage of the dilators until blood is seen on the bougie, advancing only two or three sizes a dilating session once resistance is encountered, and so forth have been described.[23] In my experience, there is little evidence that such protracted dilation carries any less risk of perforation than controlled careful dilation under direct vision at a single sitting. In more than 20 years of treating patients with esophageal strictures, I have carried out rigid endoscopy, biopsy, and brushing of reflux strictures with dilation to the maximum allowable size (as determined by the degree of resistance encountered) as described earlier. Once it has been established that the stricture can be dilated to the 46 to 50 French range, a decision to try either conservative management with periodic bougienage and a medical antireflux regimen or antireflux surgery must be made.

Non-operative Management

Because an esophageal reflux stricture represents an advanced stage of esophagitis, it is tempting for the surgeon to adopt the view that operative therapy is long overdue in such patients. However, as indicated earlier, reflux symptoms often correlate poorly with the degree of esophagitis that is present. At least one quarter of the patients we treat for peptic strictures have had no or insignificant pyrosis or regurgitation before the onset of dysphagia from their esophageal stenoses. These patients have remained relatively asymptomatic as their esophageal inflammation has progressed through the initial pathologic and endoscopic stages of reflux esophagitis. Because dysphagia is their only significant symptom, if adequate dilatation of the stricture can be achieved, the patient may be quite satisfied. Many readily accept an outpatient esophageal dilatation several times a year as a relatively minor price to pay for comfortable swallowing. It seems unwise to inflict the potential adverse effects of antireflux surgery on such a patient. In fact, some authors have used dilatation alone, without an antireflux regimen, as treatment for reflux strictures and have reported success rates of approximately 65%.[17,33,91] More recent data, however, demonstrate the value of healing coexistent esophagitis. The use of the proton pump inhibitor omeprazole after endoscopic dilatation is more effective than treatment with the H_2-receptor antagonist ranitidine: healing of esophagitis is better, the need for subsequent dilatations is less; dysphagia is better relieved, and it is more cost effective.[54,63,64]

The decision in favor of operative intervention, therefore, must take into consideration the patient's associated reflux symptoms, if any. In the patient with a dilatable reflux stricture and no or little associated acute mucosal ulceration and friability, after the initial dilation to at least a No. 46 to 50 French range, a return visit for an outpatient dilatation is scheduled for 2 weeks later. At this time, without sedation or anesthesia, a No. 40 or 42 French dilator is passed to give patients confidence that they can in fact swallow a dilator, and then one or two additional dilators are passed to maintain a No. 46 to 50 French caliber lumen. If no resistance is encountered with the passage of any of these dilators, patients are instructed in a medical antireflux regimen, including omeprazole, and is scheduled for a repeat outpatient dilatation procedure in 3 months. But they are given specific instructions to return earlier if recurrent dysphagia warrants dilatation before this time. If resistance to the passage of Nos. 46 to 50 French dilators is encountered, the treatment is repeated in 2 weeks, and the interval between dilatations is gradually increased, again letting the onset of dysphagia serve as the patient's barometer of the need for another treatment.

Considering the pathophysiology of a reflux stricture, as indicated earlier, dilatation therapy alone is not adequate treatment. A strict antireflux medical regimen including the use of omeprazole should be carefully reviewed with the patient, and the need for compliance should be emphasized. True elevation of the head of the bed at night (not simply propping up on several pillows), regular use of antacids after meals and at bedtime, and refraining from eating for several hours before retiring at night remain the mainstay of medical therapy. A variety of pharmacologic interventions are now included in the armamentarium against gastroesophageal reflux.[102] Addition of an H_2-receptor–blocking medication (e.g., cimetidine[7,11,36] or ranitidine[35,48]), particularly at bedtime, may be helpful. It must be remembered, however, that these drugs, which decrease gastric acid and pepsin production, are also associated with a low but definite incidence of complications: hepatic and renal injury, gynecomastia, impotence, diarrhea, lethargy, and occasionally bone marrow suppression. Metoclopramide has been used for the treatment of gastroesophageal reflux because it increases distal esophageal sphincter tone, increases gastric emptying, and relaxes the pyloric sphincter.[8,34,39,99] However, neurologic side effects of this drug may occur. Domperidone, a peripherally acting dopamine antagonist, has also been used for the medical control of reflux symptoms.[13,127] This drug may improve reflux symptoms by increasing the rate of gastric emptying. Its incidence of associated adverse effects—dry mouth, skin rash, headaches, and diarrhea—seems low. Sucralfate (aluminum sucrose sulfate) is currently being used as a cytoprotective agent in patients with esophagitis because it forms a viscous fluid that binds protein exudate in areas of ulceration and inflammation.[78]

The proton-pump inhibitors, e.g., omeprazole, are the newest drugs in the medical armamentarium against acid reflux disease.[60] Initial concern in the United States about continuous omeprazole therapy was generated by the initial laboratory trials that showed an increased incidence of small bowel tumors in rats receiving high doses of the drug. This phenomenon has not been duplicated in any other species of laboratory animal or in humans, and in Europe omeprazole has been used continuously for years in patients with gastroesophageal reflux disease without an increased incidence of neoplasia. Omeprazole is a potent acid inhibitor, and its efficacy in treating reflux esophagitis is well documented.[53] Not every patient can tolerate omeprazole, however, and some patients who have an initial excellent response to the drug experience a "breakthrough" phenomenon in which reflux symptoms return despite the medication. During the 1990s, there also were several reports of the use of steroids injected endoscopically into the stricture to increase the effectiveness of dilatation therapy.[52,58,137] Regardless of the specifics of therapy, the combination of an antireflux medical regimen and dilatation for reflux strictures has been reported to be successful in 75 to 88% of patients so treated.[16,75,104,132,135] Such data must of course be scrutinized carefully, analyzing the types of strictures treated (i.e., mild, moderate, or severe), the method of treatment, and the criteria of success or failure of therapy.

Some argue that the presence of a Barrett's esophagus per se is an indication for antireflux surgery to prevent the subsequent development of carcinoma.[113] It appears, however, that the presence of *atypia* in the Barrett's epithelium, not simply the metaplastic epithelium alone, is the major risk factor associated with the subsequent development of adenocarcinoma.[4] The incidence of malignant degeneration of Barrett's epithelium in which no epithelial dysplasia is evident on biopsy is probably in the range of 1 to 2%.[19] Consequently, the patient who presents with a reflux stricture associated with a Barrett's esophagus *without* endoscopic ulceration or histologic evidence of atypia on biopsy may be treated quite effectively with intermittent dilations, a medical antireflux regimen, and endoscopic surveillance at 1- or 2-year intervals to exclude the development of neoplastic changes.

In deciding on medical versus surgical therapy for an esophageal reflux stricture, an honest appraisal of the patient's response to dilatation and medical therapy is needed. Although some patients have never had noticeable reflux symptoms before the onset of dysphagia from their reflux strictures and are well managed with periodic dilatations and an antireflux medical program, others have experienced chronic severe reflux symptoms that have gradually subsided as dysphagia occurs. Once the stenosis is dilated and the dysphagia is relieved, gastroesophageal reflux recurs, and reflux symptoms again become troublesome for the patient. In this situation, relief of the esophageal obstruction alone does not adequately control the patient's symptoms from esophagitis. As indicated earlier, one point of view, most often articulated by gastroenterologic colleagues, is that esophageal bougienage in combination with antireflux medical therapy is the treatment of choice for virtually all patients with reflux strictures. They point to the poor operative results with long-term reflux control in patients with strictures treated with standard hiatal hernia repairs (e.g., the Belsey, Nissen, or Hill operations) or the technical difficulty of operations used for esophageal resection and reconstruction in these patients. However, more modern surgical advances have altered the traditional operative approach to reflux strictures. There is clearly a small but definite population of patients with reflux strictures who because of intractable reflux symptoms or dysphagia despite aggressive medical therapy are candidates for surgical intervention for control of their gastroesophageal reflux.

Surgical Treatment

Esophagus-Sparing Procedures

The current surgical treatment of esophageal reflux strictures has evolved gradually since reflux esophagitis as a distinct pathologic entity was recognized in the early 1950s. Initially, such strictures were often considered to represent an irreversible fibrous reaction and were treated with operations of considerable magnitude. These included distal esophageal resection with esophagogastrostomy[9,28]; jejunal interposition[2,3,5,67]; colonic interposition[10,38,73,76]; the reversed gastric tube[38]; plastic operations on the distal esophageal stricture[121,122,136]; and resection of the stricture with esophagogastrostomy in combination with antrectomy, vagotomy, and Roux-en-Y gastroenterostomy.[29,92]

Hayward first suggested that most reflux strictures could be treated successfully with operative dilatation in combination with an antireflux operation.[37] Hill was the first in the United States to advocate this approach.[47] However, the presence of a peptic stricture with its inevitable esophageal shortening adversely affects long-term reflux control after standard antireflux operations. In a large retrospective review of the results of the Belsey Mark IV operation, it was reported that the incidence of recurrent reflux or hernia in patients with strictures or severe esophagitis at the time of their operation was 45% compared with an 11% incidence of recurrent reflux or hernia in those without esophagitis or stricture.[85] Based on these data, Belsey advocated distal esophagectomy and reconstruction with colon rather than a standard hiatal hernia repair in patients with a stricture with significant esophagitis and shortening. Similarly, Donnelly and associates reported a 75% incidence of recurrent reflux when the Belsey repair was carried out in patients with reflux strictures.[27] Mural inflammation, esophagitis, and esophageal shortening, which are characteristic of peptic esophageal strictures, prevent the *tension-free* reduction of the 3 to 5 cm of distal esophagus below the diaphragm that is the prerequisite for the Belsey repair and also require that the fundoplication sutures be placed between the stomach and the inflamed distal esophagus. Such repairs, done under tension and requiring sutures in an inflamed and abnormal esophageal wall, do not "hold," and therefore recurrence is more common. All three of the most popular standard antireflux operations—the Belsey[116] and Nissen[74] fundoplications and the Hill posterior gastropexy[45,46]—advocate an intra-abdominal location of the gastroesophageal junction and sutures in the distal esophageal or periesophageal tissues. Therefore, the long-term success of any of these procedures *must* be jeopardized in the presence of mural inflammation or esophageal shortening (see Figs. 26-5 and 26-6 in Chap. 26, Complications of Esophageal Surgery). One advantage of the transthoracic approach for reflux control in patients with an esophageal reflux stricture is the capability it provides to mobilize the shortened esophagus superiorly, if necessary, to the level of the aortic arch, to facilitate a reduction of the esophagogastric junction below the diaphragm.[59,85] An alternative maneuver that is aimed at providing additional esophageal length in the presence of shortening is the performance of a circular myotomy just below the level of the aortic arch. This approach has been used in combination with a standard Belsey repair with good results in patients with reflux strictures.[1] The need for such maneuvers, however, is an acknowledgment of the surgeon's concern about the degree of tension on the repair and suggests to the author that an alternative operation is needed.

Despite the rather obvious undesirability of attempting to "drag" the esophagogastric junction of a shortened esophagus below the diaphragm, treatment of reflux strictures with a combination of dilatation and a standard antireflux procedure, either a Hill posterior gastropexy[66] or a Nissen fundoplication,[23] has become common. The majority of these latter operations have been performed transabdominally, and therefore the ability to assess the degree of tension on the distal esophagus when the repair is completed is less than ideal. Attempting to pull-down a shortened esophagus from an abdominal approach may produce elongation of the proximal stomach that is then inappropriately identified as the distal esophagus and wrapped by the fundoplication. The resultant "slipped Nissen" seen on subsequent barium esophagograms is more a function of an improperly performed initial operation than disruption of the repair. On the other hand, a properly performed fundoplication that encircles the distal esophagus, which has been reduced beneath the diaphragm under tension, is subject to dehiscence and slippage (Fig. 13-9). To circumvent the problem of trying to maintain the fundoplication below the diaphragm in a patient with esophageal shortening, some have advocated leaving the fundoplication within the thorax and have documented reflux control with this approach.[55,68,98,109,110] This approach, however, creates an iatrogenic paraesophageal hiatal hernia with its potential for mechanical complications of strangulation, perforation, ulceration, and bleeding, each of which has been reported following intrathoracic fundoplication.[18,62,106] The Thal fundic path operation was initially utilized in patients with reflux strictures[122] and was subsequently applied to a number of problems involving the esophagogastric junction (hiatal hernia with reflux esophagitis, achalasia, and perforation)[121] under the mistaken notion that it would prevent gastroesophageal reflux. It soon became apparent that the addition of a Nissen fundoplication to the Thal operation was required for reflux control[49,61,123,136] (Fig. 13-10). Although conceptually relatively simple, there are two major disadvantages to this approach: first, reliance on the healing of the diseased, intentionally opened esophagus to which the gastric fundus is sutured, and second, the need for an intrathoracic fundoplication with the complications of paraesophageal herniation as described earlier (see Fig. 26-19 in Chap. 26, Complications of Esophageal Surgery). Suture-line leak and problems related to the paraesophageal hernia have been reported.[100,105,119] Although effective reflux control can be achieved whether the fundoplication is intra-abdominal or intrathoracic, there are obvious advantages when the reconstructed esophagogastric junction is intra-abdominal in location.

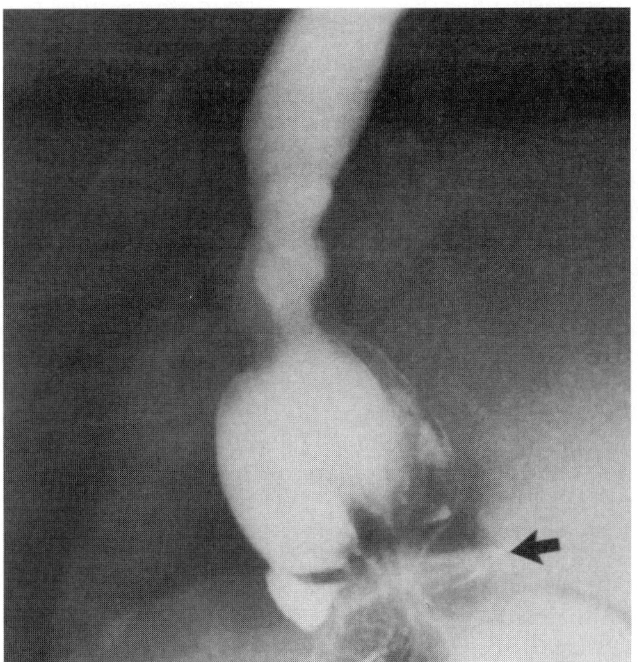

Figure 13-9. Esophagogram demonstrating a "slipped Nissen" fundoplication in an obese woman with esophageal shortening due to reflux esophagitis. She had undergone an antireflux operation 9 months earlier. After initial control of reflux symptoms, regurgitation, pyrosis, and obstructive symptoms began. The stomach has "telescoped" through the fundoplication, the horizontal folds of which *(arrow)* can still be seen below the diaphragm. There is a recurrent hiatal hernia, and intermittent obstruction occurs when food is lodged at the point of gastric constriction by the fundoplication.

Combined Collis-Belsey Procedure. In 1971, Pearson and associates reported excellent reflux control in patients with strictures treated with the combination of the esophagus-lengthening Collis gastroplasty[21,22] and the Belsey repair.[97] Resolution of the distal esophageal stricture followed control of gastroesophageal reflux and permitted comfortable swallowing. The rationale for this approach followed logically the conclusions of the long-term Belsey study[85]: it should be possible to minimize recurrent reflux in a patient undergoing an antireflux operation if additional distal esophageal length is available, thereby minimizing tension on the repair and avoiding the need to suture to the diseased esophagus. The combined Collis-Belsey operation is a transthoracic procedure performed through the sixth intercostal space (Fig. 13-11). After mobilizing the distal esophagus, the gastric fundus is delivered into the chest through the diaphragmatic hiatus without the routine use of a diaphragmatic counterincision. This involves routine ligation and division of several short gastric vessels along the high greater curvature of the stomach. With the surgeon's hand supporting the esophagogastric junction and strictured lower esophagus to reduce the risk of disruption, progressively larger Hurst-Maloney tapered dilators, up to the range of a No. 56 to 58 French, are passed by the anesthetist per os. It may be necessary to apply considerable force to the dilator to achieve satisfactory intraoperative dilation of the stricture. With a No. 56 or 58 French dilator displaced against the lesser curvature of the stomach and the fundus retracted upward, the GIA stapler is applied to the stomach adjacent to the dilator and parallel

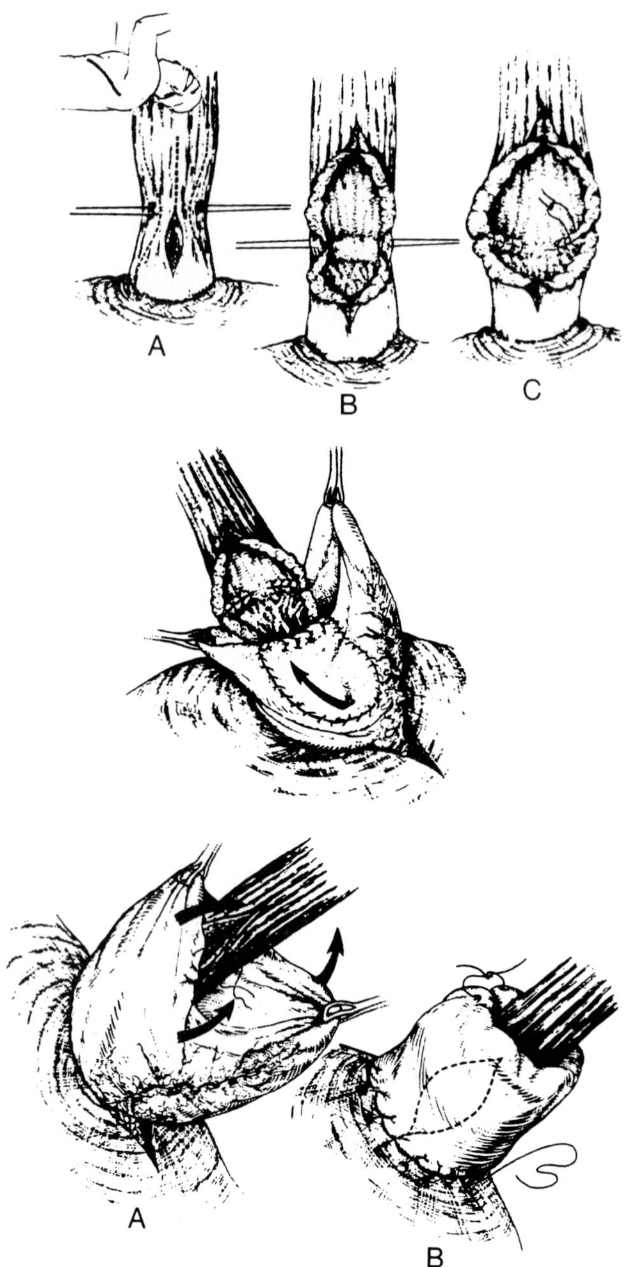

Figure 13–10. Combined Thal fundic patch operation and Nissen fundoplication for esophageal reflux stricture. *Top panel: A,* Longitudinal incision of the stricture. *B,* Opened stricture. *C,* Transverse closure of the incision, which widens the area of stenosis but shortens the esophagus. *Middle,* A split-thickness skin graft has been sutured to the gastric fundus to provide epithelial continuity within the esophagus. *Bottom panel: A,* The fundic path is sutured into the esophageal defect. *B,* A fundoplication is completed for reflux control. (From Thomas, H.F., Clarke, J.M., Rayl, J.E., et al.: Results of the combined fundic patch-fundoplication operation in the treatment of reflux esophagitis with stricture. Surg. Gynecol. Obstet., *135:*241, 1972, by permission of *Surgery, Gynecology and Obstetrics.*)

to the lesser curvature. Use of the GIA stapler for construction of the gastroplasty tube keeps the operation closed.[86] Advancement of the knife assembly creates a 5-cm-long gastric tube extension of the functional esophagus. On rare occasions, it may be necessary to apply the stapler a second time to gain an additional 2 to 3 cm of esophageal length. The staple suture line is oversewn, the dilator is removed, and the standard posterior crural sutures (No. 1 silk) are placed but left untied.

After intraoperative dilation of the stricture and construction of the gastroplasty tube, a standard Belsey repair around the new distal esophagus (i.e., the gastroplasty tube) was recommended by Pearson and associates[97] (Fig. 13–12*C*). After placing and tying the two rows of three horizontal mattress sutures each and securing the stomach below the diaphragm, the posterior crural sutures are tied, resulting in a tension-free segment of intra-abdominal "esophagus" compressed by the partial fundoplication (Fig. 13–12*C*). In contrast to the standard Belsey Mark IV operation, the combined Collis-Belsey procedure involves suturing to a resilient healthy gastroplasty tube rather than to the inflamed distal esophagus. The additional esophageal length gained by construction of the gastroplasty tube avoids the need to pull the esophagogastric junction below the diaphragm under tension. Pearson and Henderson.[93,96] reported excellent relief of dysphagia and reflux symptoms in 25 of 33 patients with reflux strictures treated with the Collis-Belsey procedure and followed for 5 to 12 years.

Collis-Nissen Procedure. Although reports of the results of the combined Collis-Belsey procedure were initially favorable,[87,95,126] data began to emerge showing unsatisfactory long-term reflux control as assessed with the intraesophageal pH electrode. Orringer and Sloan[89] suggested that there was an inadequate amount of remaining gastric fundus to perform a functioning 240-degree Belsey fundoplication after construction of the gastroplasty tube (Fig. 13–13). They demonstrated with postoperative esophageal pH studies that even after construction of a 3- to 7-cm intra-abdominal segment of functional distal esophagus with the Collis procedure, if there were an inadequate Belsey fundoplication, reflux control might not be achieved. To improve reflux control after performance of the Collis gastroplasty, Henderson and Marryatt[41,42] and Orringer and associates[84,88] described use of a 360-degree Nissen-type fundoplication. An uncut gastroplasty combined with a total fundoplication was described by Bingham[12] and Demos et al.[24,26] and used in patients with reflux strictures. The cut Collis-gastroplasty combined with a 360-degree fundoplication has become the author's preferred approach in patients with dilatable reflux strictures that are amenable to an antireflux operation. Patients in whom initial endoscopic assessment has indicated that the stricture is benign and can be dilated with a No. 40 French bougie will most likely have stenoses that can be dilated to the No. 56 French or so range at the time of a Collis-Nissen repair. If, on the other hand, passage of a No. 40 French dilator is not possible, the surgeon must be prepared for an esophageal resection and reconstruction, the exact type and approach depending upon the surgeon's preference and experience. In patients with strictures that are too tight to accommodate a No. 40 French bougie, the colon is prepared preoperatively if there has been previous gastric surgery in the event that an esophagectomy is required. This is also done in patients with recurrent reflux esophagitis after prior failed hernia repairs, because repeat mobilization of the upper stomach may

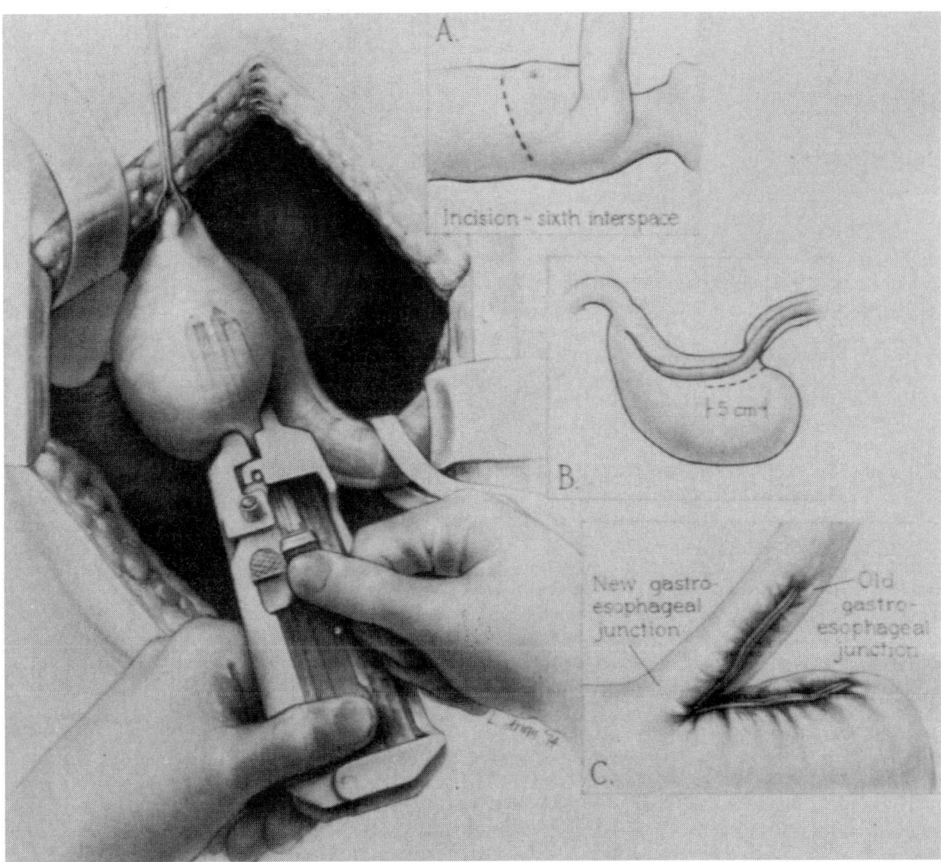

Figure 13–11. Construction of the Collis gastroplasty tube using the GIA surgical stapler. *A,* Sixth left interspace incision used. *B,* The No. 54 or 56 French dilator inserted through the stricture is displaced against the lesser curvature of the stomach. The *dotted line* indicates the site of application of the stapler. The main illustration shows the advancement of the knife assembly. *C,* The new functional distal esophagus is a 5-cm tube of healthy stomach. (From Orringer, M.B., and Sloan, H.: An improved technique for the combined Collis-Belsey approach to dilatable esophageal strictures. J. Thorac. Cardiovasc. Surg., *68:*298, 1974, with permission.)

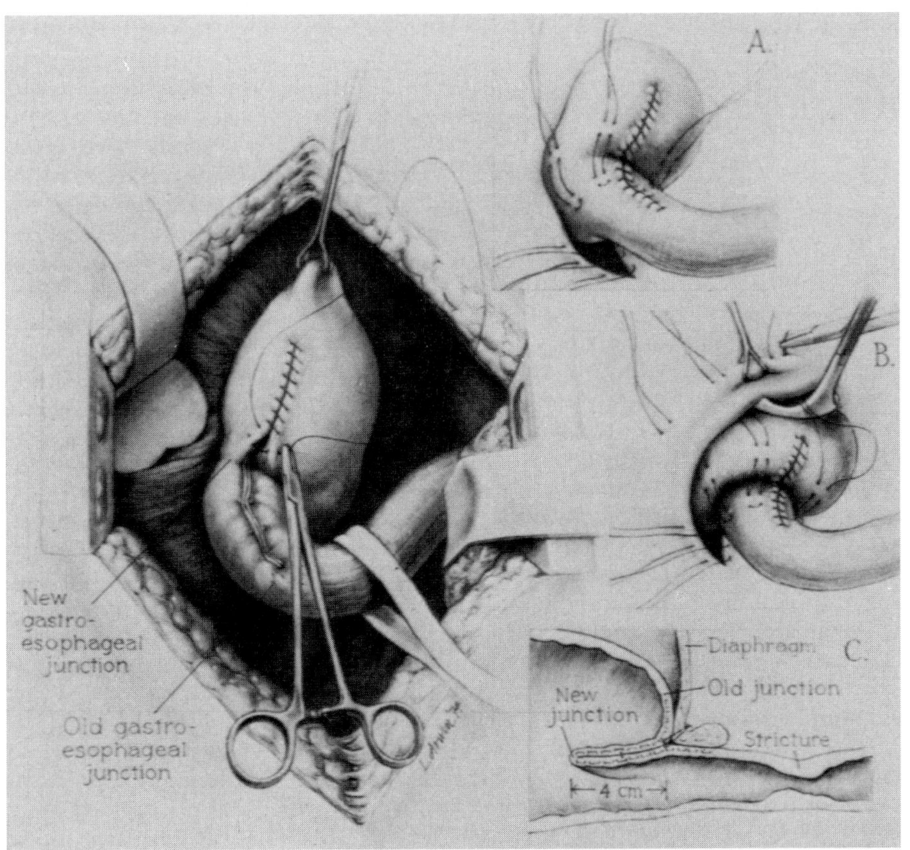

Figure 13–12. Belsey reconstruction of the esophagogastric junction after construction of the Collis gastroplasty tube. *Main illustration,* Oversewing the staple suture line. *A,* Placement of the first row of three mattress sutures between the new distal "esophagus" and the gastric fundus. The posterior crural sutures have been placed but are left untied at this point. *B,* Placement of the second row of mattress sutures through the diaphragm, gastric fundus, and distal esophagus 2 cm proximal to the first row. *C,* The completed repair reduced beneath the diaphragm shows a 4-cm intra-abdominal distal esophageal segment (the gastroplasty tube) partially compressed by the Belsey fundoplication. The posterior crural sutures have been tied. (From Orringer, M.B., and Sloan, H.: An improved technique for the combined Collis-Belsey approach to dilatable esophageal stricture. J. Thorac. Cardiovasc. Surg., *68:*298, 1974, with permission.)

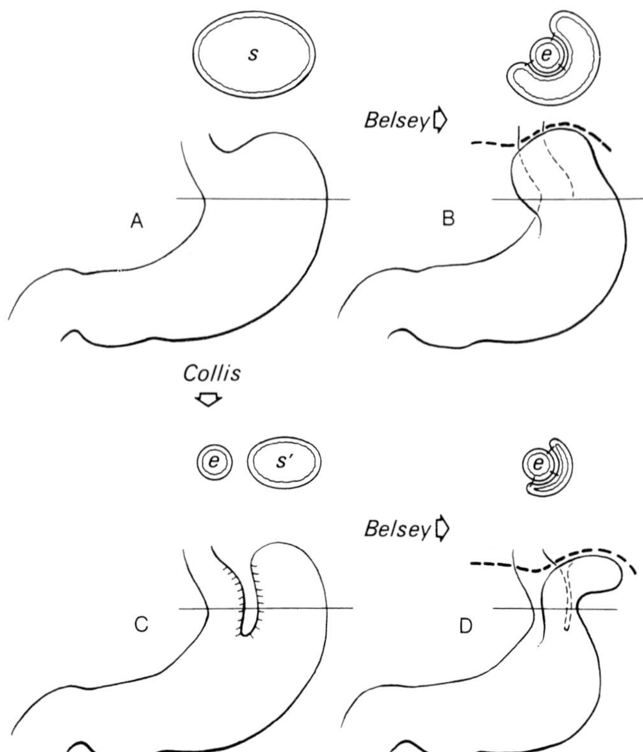

Figure 13–13. Decreased amount of gastric fundus available for Belsey repair after Collis procedure. *A,* Cross section through the gastric fundus in the plane indicated shows the area of stomach *(s)* available for the standard Belsey Mark IV repair with a 240-degree gastric wrap as shown in *B. C,* Construction of the Collis gastroplasty tube *(e)* results in a smaller area of stomach *(s')* available for the Belsey repair. *D,* Only a limited 180-degree fundoplication is possible after the Collis procedure, and the elongated, narrowed gastric fundus is angulated beneath the diaphragm *(dotted line)* as the second row of sutures of the Belsey repair are tied. (From Orringer, M.B., and Sloan, H.: Complications and failings of the combined Collis-Belsey operation. J. Thorac. Cardiovasc. Surg., *74:*726, 1977, with permission.)

leave a gastric fundus of questionable viability and one that is not suited for the safe construction of a Collis gastroplasty tube.

In the combined Collis-Nissen operation, five or six short gastric vessels are routinely divided as the gastric fundus and greater curvature of the stomach are delivered into the chest through the diaphragm hiatus. Careful ligation of these vessels without undue tension is required to avoid injury to the spleen and unrecognized intra-abdominal hemorrhage. Adhesions from earlier operations at the hiatus may necessitate a diaphragmatic counterincision for exposure. When necessary, a 5- to 10-cm peripheral diaphragmatic counterincision is made 4 to 5 cm from the diaphragmatic attachment to the costal arch. Whenever possible, division of the costal arch is avoided to minimize postoperative incisional pain and problems with chest wall instability.

The reflux stricture is supported by the surgeon and dilated per os to the 56 or 58 French range, and the gastroplasty tube is constructed. One application of the GIA stapler with the resulting 5-cm additional esophageal length is almost always adequate (see Fig. 13–11). In initial reports,[84,88] strictures were dilated intraoperatively to the No. 54 to 60 French range, the gastroplasty tube was constructed over these bougies, and these large dilators were removed and replaced with a No. 46 French bougie around which the fundoplication was performed. A 5- to 6-cm fundoplication was constructed incorporating the proximal 3 to 4 cm of stomach and the distal 3 to 4 cm of gastroplasty tube (Figs. 13–14 and 13–15). Currently, in order to avoid narrowing of the "neoesophagus," thereby producing postoperative dysphagia, construction of the gastroplasty and the fundoplication have been performed with either a No. 54 French dilator (in women) or a No. 56 French dilator (in men) within the esophagus.[118] Furthermore, the fundoplication is limited to 3 cm in length and is performed only around the gastroplasty tube, not the proximal stomach (Fig. 13–16). The fundoplication is fashioned with four interrupted seromuscular 2-0 silk sutures placed 1 cm apart, with each suture passing through the gastric fundus, then the gastroplasty tube, and finally through the gastric fundus again. These sutures are tied with the No. 54 or 56 French dilator within the gastroplasty tube, and the silk suture line is then oversewn with a 4-0 running polypropylene Lembert seromuscular stitch. This is done prophylactically to prevent a fundoplication suture leak. After reducing the fundoplication beneath the diaphragm, the posterior crural sutures are tied to narrow the hiatus until it admits one finger comfortably alongside the esophagus, which now contains no dilator. Silver clip markers are placed at the apex of the gastroplasty tube (the new esophagogastric junction) before beginning the fundoplication and at the edges of the diaphragmatic hiatus after reduction of the fundoplication into the abdomen. The distance between these two sets of silver markers on postoperative roentgenograms indicates the intra-abdominal segment of functional esophagus wrapped by the fundoplication (Fig. 13–17).

Results of Collis-Nissen Procedure. As indicated previously, the severity of each stricture is graded intraoperatively depending on the degree of resistance encountered as the dilator is passed through it: A *mild* stricture is easily dilated with minimal resistance; a *moderate* stricture requires some, but not excessive, forceful dilation; and a *severe* stricture requires vigorous forceful dilation. Although the severity of the stricture (i.e., the ease with which it can be dilated) cannot be predicted by its appearance radiographically or endoscopically, almost every reflux stricture can be dilated intraoperatively with the esophagus supported by the surgeon's hand as the dilator is passed. Occasionally, antegrade dilation as described earlier is not possible, and it may be necessary to resort to retrograde passage of Hegar dilators through a high gastrotomy.[40,44] This has been necessary in only one of the author's patients.

Stirling and Orringer[118] reported the results of intraoperative dilation and the combined Collis gastroplasty-Nissen fundoplication procedure in 64 patients (average age of 51 years) with esophageal reflux strictures. In the same period of time, 30 patients (average age of 59 years) with reflux strictures and dysphagia but *without* significant reflux symptoms were treated successfully with intermittent outpatient esophageal dilations and a strict antireflux medical regimen. Esophageal resections

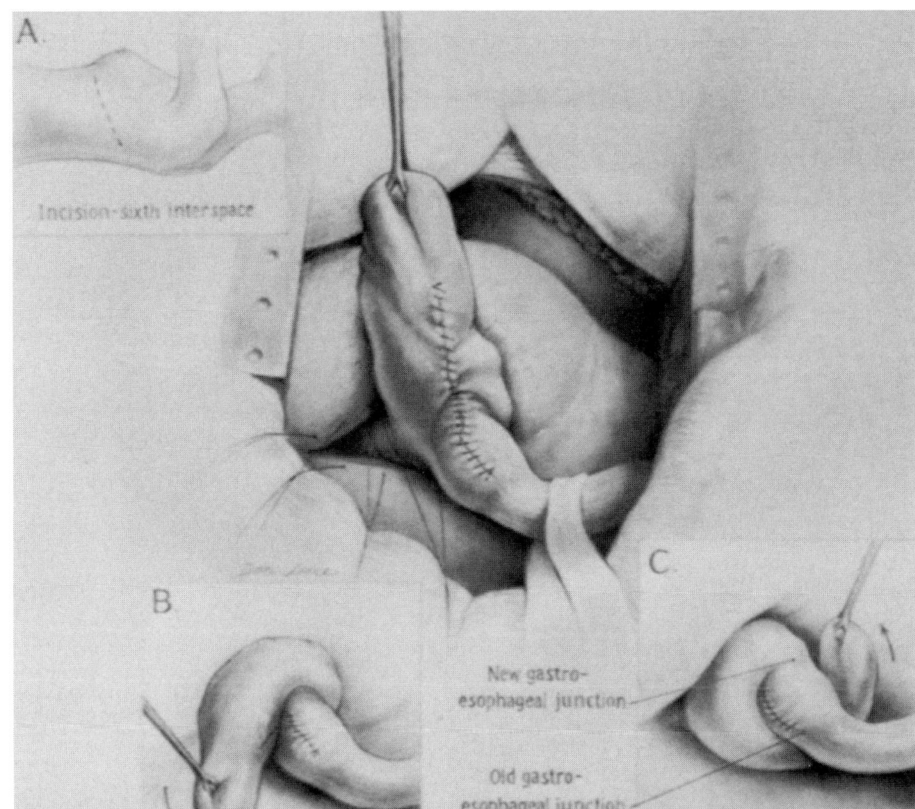

Figure 13–14. Construction of a 360-degree fundoplication after the Collis procedure. *Main illustration,* Elongated narrow gastric fundus remaining after the Collis procedure. The posterior crural sutures have been placed but not tied. *A,* The sixth left interspace incision used for the operation. *B* and *C,* Wrapping the gastric fundus behind the gastroplasty tube and adjacent upper stomach. (From Orringer, M.B., and Sloan, H.: Combined Collis-Nissen reconstruction of the esophagogastric junction. Ann. Thorac. Surg., *25:*16, 1978, with permission.)

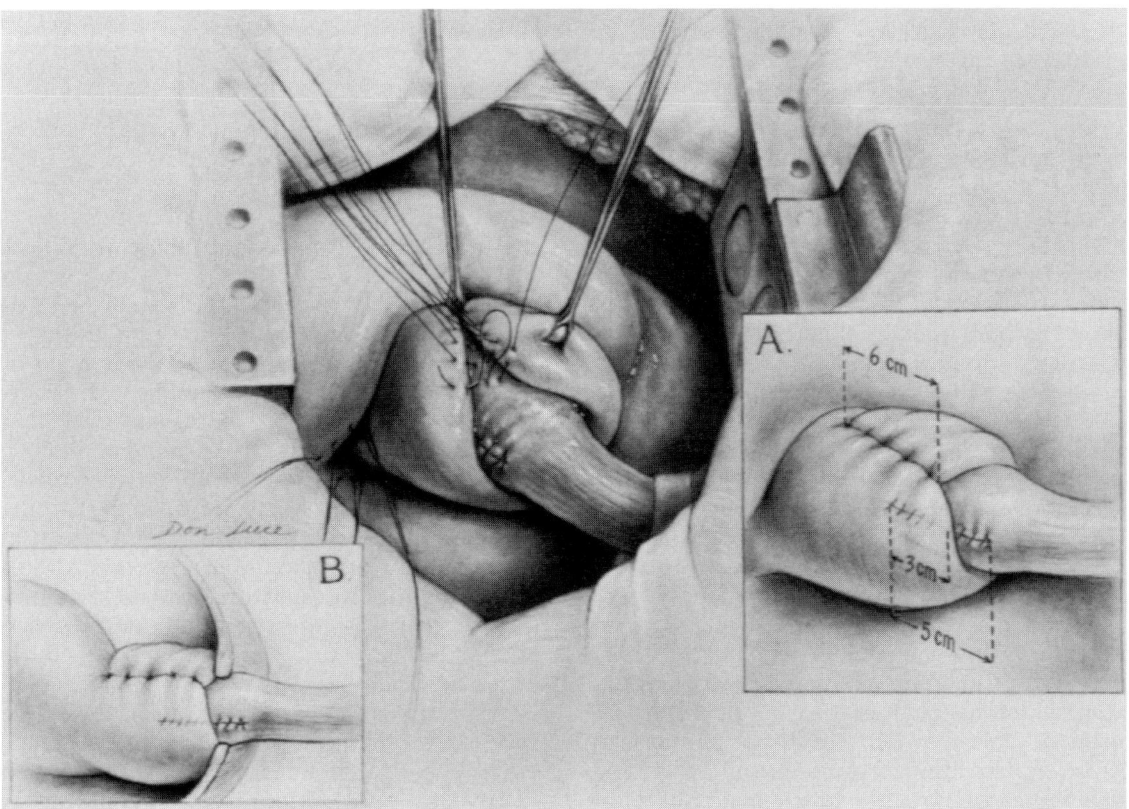

Figure 13–15. Construction of a 360-degree fundoplication around a Collis gastroplasty tube. *Main illustration,* Seromuscular sutures being placed between the gastric fundus, the gastroplasty tube, and gastric fundus again. As originally described, the initial three sutures incorporated the proximal stomach, and the remaining three sutures incorporated the gastroplasty tube. *A,* When the fundoplication sutures are tied, the wrap includes 3 cm of gastroplasty tube and 3 cm of proximal stomach. *B,* The fundoplication reduced beneath the diaphragm without tension. The posterior crural sutures are tied. (From Orringer, M.B., and Sloan, H.: Combined Collis-Nissen reconstruction of the esophagogastric junction. Ann. Thorac. Surg., *25:*16, 1978, with permission.)

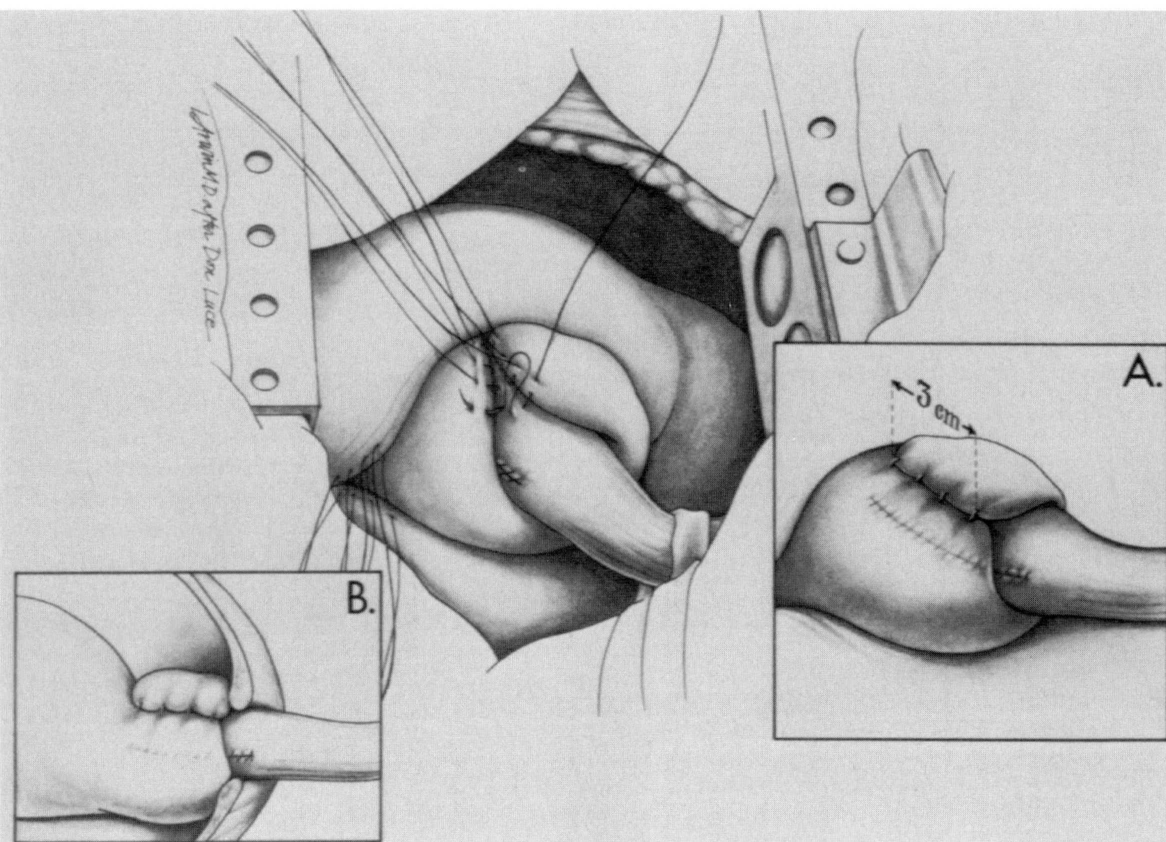

Figure 13-16. Currently advocated 3-cm long fundoplication after Collis gastroplasty. Four seromuscular 2-0 silk sutures placed 1 cm apart *(main illustration)* result in a 3-cm-long fundoplication around the gastroplasty tube *(A)*, not the proximal stomach. *B,* The fundoplication reduced beneath the diaphragm. (From Stirling, M.C., and Orringer, M.B.: The combined Collis-Nissen operation for esophageal reflux strictures. Ann. Thorac. Surg., *45:*148, 1988, with permission.)

were performed in 17 other patients with reflux strictures, 14 of whom had associated esophageal pathology (megaesophagus of achalasia, severe dysplasia in Barrett's epithelium, caustic stricture, or inability to perform a redo fundoplication because of previous antireflux repairs) and three because of inability to dilate the stricture or because the stricture was disrupted during attempted dilation. These authors found that more than 95% of esophageal reflux strictures could be dilated to a size compatible with comfortable swallowing (at least to No. 46 French, but generally No. 54 or 56 French). There was one postoperative death (1.6% mortality rate) from a pulmonary embolus 2 weeks after surgery among their 64 patients undergoing the Collis-Nissen operation. Two patients (3%) experienced esophageal leaks, which healed after drainage. Four patients were lost to follow-up, and the remaining 59 patients were followed an average of 43 months. At the time of latest follow-up, symptomatic reflux was eliminated or mild in 88% of this group, 8% required an antireflux medical regimen to control reflux symptoms, and 4% had poorly controlled reflux symptoms (Table 13-1). In this report, the severity of the stricture preoperatively did not significantly influence the likelihood of unsatisfactory subjective reflux control postoperatively. These patients were followed with routine preoperative and periodic postoperative esophageal manometry and standard acid reflux testing with the intraesophageal pH electrode (Table 13-2). Using such objective testing, good reflux control was documented with the standard acid reflux test in 47 (94%) of 50 patients studied after 1 year, but 10 (34%) of 29 patients studied 2 to 5 years postoperatively had abnormal reflux. However, seven of these ten objective failures of reflux control at 2 to 5 years had no symptoms of reflux. The increase in distal esophageal high-pressure zone pressure and length achieved with the Collis-Nissen operation (see Table 13-2) was maintained over time. It is important to note that patients with severe strictures were significantly ($P < 0.05$) more likely to develop recurrent abnormal reflux as documented with the pH probe at 2- to 5-year follow-up than patients with less severe strictures. It was postulated that the need for repeated frequent dilations in patients with more severe panmural fibrosis may ultimately disrupt the fundoplication, thus predisposing the patient to recurrent gastroesophageal reflux. In 81% of their patients, dysphagia was satisfactorily relieved (no dysphagia or mild dysphagia not requiring dilation) (see Table 13-1). Seven (12%) required occasional dilations for treatment of their dysphagia, and four (7%) required regular dilations. The severity of the stricture has a direct bearing on the need for early postoperative dilations, 50% of those with mild strictures requiring at least one postoperative dilation compared with 73% of those with moderate strictures and 100% of those with severe strictures. However, of the 38 patients (64%) who required postoperative dilations, 27 (72%) required

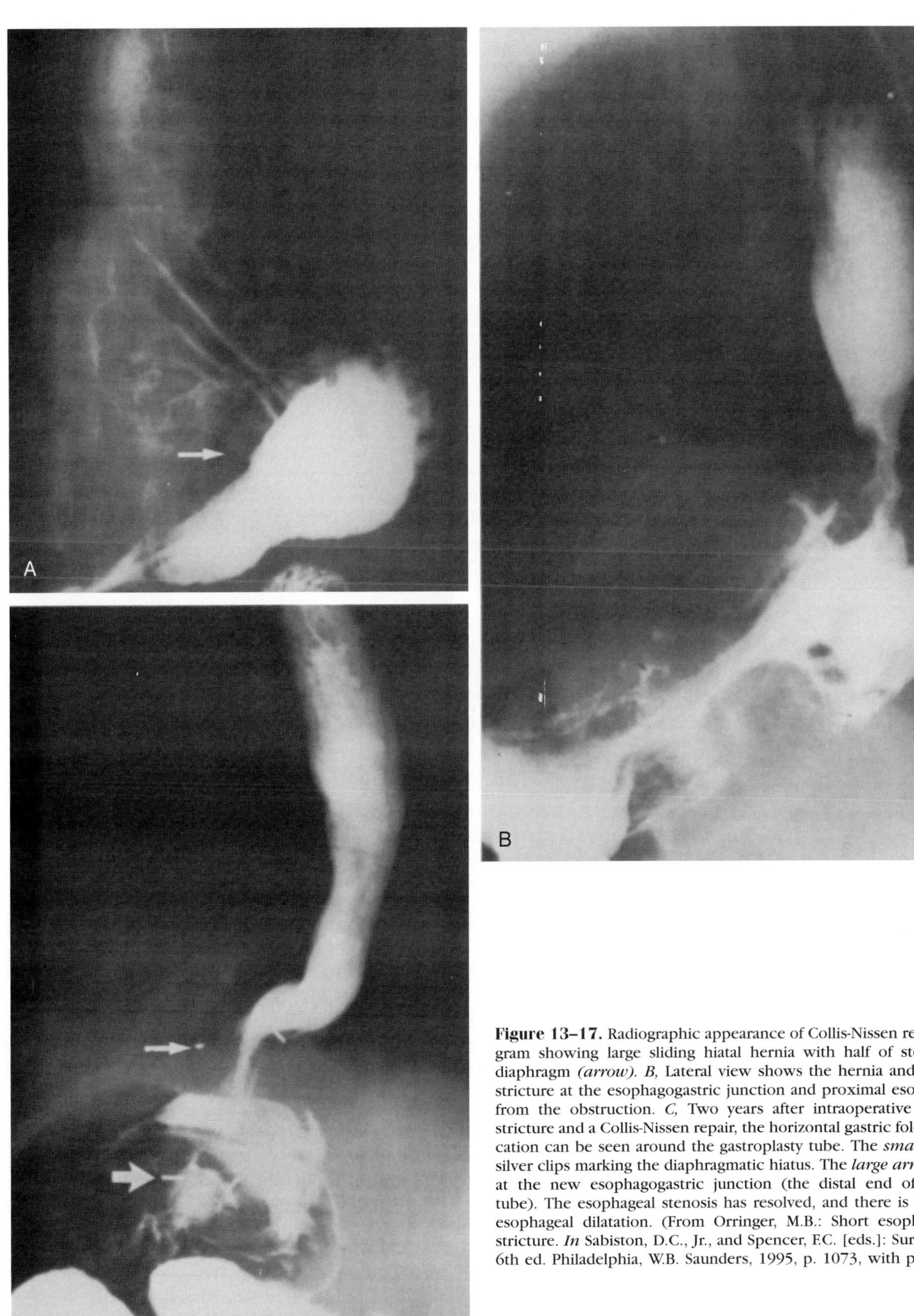

Figure 13–17. Radiographic appearance of Collis-Nissen repair. *A,* Esophagogram showing large sliding hiatal hernia with half of stomach above the diaphragm *(arrow). B,* Lateral view shows the hernia and associated reflux stricture at the esophagogastric junction and proximal esophageal dilatation from the obstruction. *C,* Two years after intraoperative dilatation of the stricture and a Collis-Nissen repair, the horizontal gastric folds of the fundoplication can be seen around the gastroplasty tube. The *small arrow* indicates silver clips marking the diaphragmatic hiatus. The *large arrow* indicates clips at the new esophagogastric junction (the distal end of the gastroplasty tube). The esophageal stenosis has resolved, and there is now no proximal esophageal dilatation. (From Orringer, M.B.: Short esophagus and peptic stricture. *In* Sabiston, D.C., Jr., and Spencer, F.C. [eds.]: Surgery of the Chest, 6th ed. Philadelphia, W.B. Saunders, 1995, p. 1073, with permission.)

Table 13–1. Subjective Results of Collis-Nissen Operation for Esophageal Reflux Strictures (59 Patients)

	Mild Stricture* (*n* = 34)			Moderate Stricture* (*n* = 15)			Severe Stricture* (*n* = 10)			Total (*n* = 59)			
	No.	*%*		*No.*	*%*		*No.*	*%*		*No.*		*%*	
Reflux†													
None	28	82	91	12	80	87	8	80	80	48	52	81	88
Mild	3	9		1	7		0	0		4		7	
Moderate	2	6		2	13		1	10		5		4	
Severe	1	3		0	0		1	10		2		4	
Dysphagia‡													
None	26	76	85	9	60	73	7	70	80	42	48	70	81
Mild	3	9		2	13		1	10		6		10	
Moderate	3	9		3	20		1	10		7		12	
Severe	2	6		1	7		1	10		4		7	
Clinical status§													
Excellent	24	70	82	6	40	67	7	70	70	37	45	63	77
Good	4	12		4	27		0			8		14	
Fair	5	15		3	20		1	10		9		15	
Poor	1	3		2	13		2	20		5		8	

From Stirling, M.C., and Orringer, M.B.: The combined Collis-Nissen operation for esophageal reflux strictures. Ann. Thorac. Surg., *45*:148, 1988, with permission.
*Stricture: Mild = easily dilated; moderate = requiring some force to dilate; severe = requiring very forceful dilation.
†Reflux: Mild = requires no treatment; moderate = controlled by medical therapy; severe = uncontrolled by medication or need for reoperation.
‡Dysphagia: Mild = requires no dilation; moderate = requires occasional dilation; severe = requires regular dilations or reoperation.
§Clinical status: Excellent = asymptomatic; good = minimal reflux symptoms or mild dysphagia requiring no treatment; fair = symptoms controlled by medication or dilation; poor = symptoms severe or reoperation required.

early dilation only (within the first 6 postoperative months) to achieve resolution of their dysphagia. When comparing the overall degree of preoperative and postoperative dysphagia in these patients, dysphagia was found to be improved postoperatively in 49 (83%), unchanged in seven (12%), and more severe in three (5%).

The overall *subjective* clinical status of the patients reported by Stirling and Orringer included an evaluation of both reflux symptoms *and* dysphagia (see Table 13–1). Excellent results (no symptoms) were thus achieved in 37 patients (63%), good results (mild symptoms not requiring treatment) in eight (14%), fair results (reflux symptoms *or* dysphagia controlled by medical therapy or dilation) in nine (15%), and poor results (severe uncontrolled symptoms) in five (8%). Therefore, the Collis-Nissen operation was successful (no symptoms or mild symptoms not requiring treatment) in 77% of these patients.

Five variables that might influence the overall clinical outcome after the Collis-Nissen operation were analyzed (Table 13–3). Patients with scleroderma, severe preoperative dysphagia, follow-up greater than 48 months, or more severe strictures were less likely to obtain a good clinical result than their counterparts, but these differences were not statistically significant. However, patients who had a stricture *and* a previously failed antireflux operation were significantly ($P < 0.05$) less likely to have a good result than those with no prior operation. Four patients in this group required reoperation. One patient who had a mild stricture developed a paraesophageal hernia 3 years after the Collis-Nissen repair and despite reoperation had only a fair result. Two patients were treated with a transhiatal esophagectomy without thoracotomy for recurrent reflux esophagitis, and results were good. One patient with a severe stricture before the initial Collis-Nissen repair underwent a pyloromyotomy and revision of the fundoplication for recurrent reflux esophagitis 4 years later with subsequent good results. Patients with esophageal reflux strictures who are being treated with an antireflux procedure should be informed preoperatively that subsequent postoperative dilations may be required. In any patient who complains of dysphagia following the Collis-Nissen repair, outpatient esophageal dilations are used liberally. In addition, in patients with moderate or severe strictures requiring forceful intraoperative dilatation, a No. 50 French Maloney dilator is passed at the bedside before discharge from the hospital. If resistance is encountered as this dilator is passed, outpatient dilations are performed at 2-week intervals until resistance is no longer encountered. If no resistance is encountered as the dilator is passed 1 week after operation, subsequent dilations are carried out only if dysphagia recurs.

It is a sobering but mandatory exercise to apply statistical methods to the results of antireflux surgery as just described. Although the combined Collis-Nissen operation combined with intraoperative dilatation has successfully controlled both reflux symptoms and dysphagia in 77% of the author's patients with reflux strictures, a 23% failure rate still leaves much to be desired. Although it is now apparent that most reflux strictures can be dilated intraoperatively, it is clear that not every patient whose stricture is dilated will experience a good long-term result from an antireflux operation, persistent dysphagia due to established panmural fibrosis being the limiting factor. Thus, additional long-term data analysis is needed to predict in advance those patients with dilatable strictures who will do well with a Collis-Nissen repair and those in whom esophageal resection is a better option. A 24% risk of recurrence was previously reported in patients

Table 13–2. Objective Results of Collis-Nissen Operation for Esophageal Reflux Strictures

	Mild Stricture*		
Esophageal Functional Tests	***Preoperative* (n = *36*)**	***1 yr* (n = *27*)**	***2–5 yr* (n = *17*)**
Acid reflux test			
Normal (0–1+)	2 (5%)	26 (96%)	12 (71%)
Abnormal (2–3+)	34 (95%)	1 (4%)	5 (29%)
Distal HPZ‡			
Pressure (mmHg)	3.5 ± 3.9	11.6 ± 3.5	10.8 ± 3.4
Length (cm)	1.4 ± 1.6	4.4 ± 1.1	3.8 ± 1.1
	Moderate Stricture*		
	***Preoperative* (n = *16*)**	***1 yr* (n = *13*)**	***2–5 yr* (n = *5*)**
Acid reflux test			
Normal (0–1+)	2 (12%)	12 (92%)	5 (100%)
Abnormal (2–3+)	14 (88%)	1 (8%)	0
Distal HPZ			
Pressure (mmHg)	1.4 ± 3.0	11.3 ± 3.8	11.2 ± 4.6
Length (cm)	0.7 ± 1.5	3.8 ± 1.1	4.0 ± 1.2
	Severe Stricture*		
	***Preoperative* (n = *9*)**	***1 yr* (n = *10*)**	***2–5 yr* (n = *7*)**
Acid reflux test			
Normal (0–1+)	1 (11%)	9 (90%)	2 (28%)†
Abnormal (2–3+)	8 (89%)	1 (10%)	5 (72%)
Distal HPZ			
Pressure (mmHg)	6.4 ± 4.5	10.8 ± 2.7	7.9 ± 3.7†
Length (cm)	2.1 ± 1.7	4.1 ± 1.5	3.3 ± 1.6
	Total		
	***Preoperative* (n = *61*)**	***1 yr* (n = *50*)**	***2–5 yr* (n = *29*)**
Acid reflux test			
Normal (0–1+)	5 (8%)	47 (94%)	19 (66%)
Abnormal (2–3+)	56 (92%)	3 (6%)	10 (34%)
Distal HPZ			
Pressure (mmHg)	3.4 ± 4.1	11.4 ± 3.4	10.2 ± 3.8
Length (cm)	1.3 ± 1.6	4.2 ± 1.2	3.7 ± 1.2

From Stirling, M.C., and Orringer, M.B.: The combined Collis-Nissen operation for esophageal reflux strictures. Ann. Thorac. Surg., *45*:148, 1988, with permission.

*Stricture: Mild, easily dilated; moderate, requiring some force to dilate; severe, requiring very forceful dilation.

†$P < 0.05$ compared with mild and moderate strictures at 2 to 5 years.

‡HPZ, distal esophageal high-pressure zone. HPZ pressure and length data are reported as mean ± standard deviation.

undergoing redo antireflux operations.[106] Patients who have esophageal reflux strictures *and* a history of a failed previous repair have an even higher risk of recurrence (50%), and this has been documented in other reports as well.[66] On the basis of this information, we now believe that esophageal resection and reconstruction is a more reliable option in patients with reflux strictures and a history of antireflux surgery, those with associated underlying esophageal disease (e.g., megaesophagus, scleroderma, caustic stricture), and those in whom disruption of the stricture occurs during attempted intraoperative dilation.

Excellent results with the combined Collis gastroplasty-fundoplication procedures for the treatment of reflux strictures have been reported by others.[15,20] Pearson and associates[94] reported the results obtained in 430 patients undergoing a modified Collis gastroplasty and partial fundoplication for complex reflux problems, including 138 with short esophagus and peptic stricture or gross ulcerative esophagitis. With excellent long-term follow-up, 93% of these 215 latter patients had a good result (asymptomatic or minor symptoms not requiring treatment), 4% had a fair result (improved, but symptoms or endoscopic findings that required either medication or dilatation), and 3% had a poor result (unimproved or worse).

Resection

As indicated earlier, there are situations in which a patient with an esophageal reflux stricture is best treated with esophageal resection. The ideal approach and the organ with which to replace the esophagus remain controversial issues. The author believes that distal esophagectomy with an intrathoracic esophagogastric anastomosis is a *poor* operation for the patient with reflux esophagitis with or without a stricture. Resection of the lower esophageal sphincter and creation of a hiatal hernia with a portion of the stomach above and a portion below the diaphragm explain the reported incidence of reflux esophagitis in the residual esophagus in 20 to 40% of patients undergoing an intrathoracic esophagogastric anastomosis.[114] Although a variety of operative techniques have been developed with the intent of preventing gastroesophageal reflux after an intrathoracic esophagogastric anastomosis,[14,25,76,129] none has proved to be consistently reliable or gained widespread acceptance. This is an unacceptable option in patients with benign disease and results only in recurrent esophageal stenosis due to reflux esophagitis. Distal esophagectomy and reconstruction with either a jejunal[101] or short-segment colonic interposition[10] are excellent options in patients with reflux strictures requiring resection. Both of these operations, however, are of considerable magnitude and are technically demanding. If an anastomotic stricture develops, dilatation of an esophagojejunal or esophagocolonic anastomosis is dangerous.

During the 1980s and 1990s, *total* thoracic esophagectomy with a cervical esophagogastric anastomosis became a preferred approach in patients requiring esophageal resection and reconstruction for both benign and malignant disease.[79,80,83] Even in patients with distal esophageal pathology, the author chooses to remove the entire thoracic esophagus and place the anastomosis in the neck to avoid the potential for mediastinitis from an anastomotic leak. The stomach is positioned in the posterior mediastinum in the original esophageal bed, and an end-to-side cervical esophagogastric anastomosis is constructed several centimeters from the apex of the gastric fundus, which is suspended from the prevertebral fascia. Clinically significant gastroesophageal reflux is extremely uncommon after a properly performed cervical esophagogastric anastomosis. Thus, thoracic esophagectomy with a cervical esophagogastric anastomosis has become an excellent option in patients with recurrent

Table 13–3. Effect of Variables on Clinical Outcome (59 Patients)

Variable	Satisfactory Results*		Unsatisfactory Results*	
	No. of Patients	***%***	***No. of Patients***	***%***
Scleroderma (n = 11)	6	55	5	45
No scleroderma (n = 48)	39	81	9	19
Mild-moderate preoperative dysphagia† (n = 38)	31	82	7	18
Severe preoperative dysphagia† (n = 21)	14	67	7	33
Follow-up <48 mo (n = 25)	16	64	9	36
Follow-up >48 mo (n = 34)	29	85	5	15
Mild stricture‡ (n = 34)	28	82	6	18
Moderate-severe stricture‡ (n = 25)	17	68	8	32
Prior reflux operation (n = 10)	5	50§	5	50§
No prior reflux operation (n = 49)	40	82	9	18

From Stirling, M.C., and Orringer, M.B.: The combined Collis-Nissen operation for esophageal reflux strictures. Ann. Thorac. Surg., *45*:148, 1988, with permission.

*Clinical results: Satisfactory, no symptoms or mild symptoms not requiring treatment; unsatisfactory, significant symptoms requiring treatment with antacids or dilation.

†Preoperative dysphagia: Mild, no dilations; moderate, requiring occasional dilations; severe, requiring regular dilations.

‡Stricture: Mild, easily dilated; moderate, requiring some force to dilate; severe, requiring very forceful dilation.

§$P < 0.05$ prior reflux operations compared with no prior reflux operations.

reflux esophagitis after multiple prior failed antireflux operations because symptomatic reflux is generally eliminated with this procedure. However, the need for a periodic postoperative cervical esophagogastric anastomotic dilatation due to stricture formation at this site negates the effectiveness of an operation being performed to relieve dysphagia. A cervical esophagogastric anastomotic leak after transhiatal esophagectomy is a predictor of subsequent difficulty; nearly half of such leaks result in an anastomotic stricture once healing of the fistula is complete. Dilation of a cervical esophagogastric anastomosis is far safer than dilatation of an intrathoracic esophagocolic or esophagojejunal anastomosis. Attention to the details of construction of the cervical esophagogastrostomy reduces the need for postoperative dilations and provides long-term comfortable swallowing as well as relief of the majority of reflux symptoms in these patients.[90] In their 1993 review of the long-term functional results of esophageal substitution with stomach for benign esophageal disease, the author and associates reported that less than 10% of their patients undergoing transhiatal esophagectomy and a cervical esophagogastric anastomosis had troublesome nocturnal regurgitation.[83] More recently, this experience has been corroborated in the largest reported experience with transhiatal esophagectomy and a cervical esophagogastric anastomosis.[82] Of the 1085 esophagectomies performed, 285 (26%) were for benign disease, and of these, 42 were for reflux strictures. Clinically significant reflux symptoms occurred in less than 10%, and only one patient has had pulmonary complications resulting from aspiration (see Chap. 25, Transhiatal Esophagectomy Without Thoracotomy). The need for postoperative anastomotic dilatation had been common after transhiatal esophagectomy and a cervical esophagogastric anastomosis. Focus on minimization of trauma to the mobilized stomach and use of a side-to-side stapled cervical esophagogastric anastomotic technique have dramatically reduced the incidence of anastomotic leak as well as the need for subsequent dilatations.[81]

One final method of indirect resectional therapy for esophagitis with stricture is partial gastrectomy with Roux-en-Y biliary diversion. The earliest report of resolution of benign esophageal stenosis following partial gastrectomy for peptic ulcer disease was made by Wangensteen and Levin.[128] The importance of bile in refluxed gastric contents in the development of severe esophagitis was then recognized both clinically and experimentally.[31,32,108,111] After this, several surgeons began to treat reflux strictures by partial gastrectomy and Roux-loop gastrojejunostomy.[120,134] Others advocated antrectomy and Roux diversion in conjunction with resection for the stricture.[50,92,133] A randomized trial comparing the efficacy of a Nissen fundoplication with antrectomy, vagotomy, and Roux diversion for severe esophagitis, generally with stricture, was reported by Washer and associates.[131] The results were not significantly different. And although good results from Roux diversion have been reported,[43,130] failures of this treatment have also been documented.[65]

The author has no personal experience with this method of treating esophagitis but nonetheless has difficulty accepting this approach to reflux disease. It is difficult to rationalize leaving in place the inflamed, scarred, strictured esophagus, which may contain Barrett's epithelium with its premalignant potential, while sacrificing the healthy stomach, probably the best organ with which to replace the esophagus. If dilation therapy with an antireflux operation, preferably a Collis-Nissen or Collis-Belsey procedure, cannot control the reflux esophagitis and stricture, resection of the *esophagus* and replacement with a gastric interposition and a cervical esophagogastric anastomosis, if possible, seems much more direct and conceptually appealing than sacrificing a portion of an otherwise normal stomach.

References

1. Allen, S.M., and Matthews, H.R.: Circular myotomy and Belsey repair for acquaired shortening of the oesophagus. Eur. J. Cardiothorac. Surg., 7:645, 1993.

2. Allison, P.R.: Peptic ulcer of oesophagus. Thorax, *3:*20, 1948.
3. Allison, P.R., Johnston, A.S., and Royce, G.B.: Short esophagus with simple peptic ulceration. J. Thorac. Surg., *12:*432, 1943.
4. Appleman, H.D., Kalish, R.J., Clancy, P.E., et al.: Distinguishing features of adenocarcinoma in Barrett's esophagus and in the gastric cardia. *In* Spechler, S.J., and Goyal, R.K. (eds.): Barrett's Esophagus: Pathophysiology, Diagnosis, and Management. New York, Elsevier, 1985, p. 167.
5. Barnes, W.A., and Redo, S.F.: Evaluation of esophagojejunostomy in the treatment of lesions at the esophagogastric junction. Ann. Surg., *146:*224, 1957.
6. Barrett, N.R.: Chronic peptic ulcer of the oesophagus and "oesophagitis." Br. J. Surg., *38:*175, 1950.
7. Behar, J., Brand, D.Z., Brown, F.C., et al.: Cimetidine in the treatment of symptomatic gastroesophageal reflux. Gastroenterology, *74:*441, 1978.
8. Behar, J., and Ramsby, G.: Gastric emptying and antral motility in reflux esophagitis: Effect of oral metoclopramide. Gastroenterology, *74:*253, 1978.
9. Belsey, R.: Diaphragmatic hernia. *In* Jones, F.A. (ed.): Modern Trends in Gastroenterology. New York, Hoeber, 1952, p. 128.
10. Belsey, R.H.: Reconstruction of the esophagus with left colon. J. Thorac. Cardiovasc. Surg., *49:*33, 1965.
11. Bennett, J.R., Martin, H.D., and Buckton, G.: Cimetidine in reflux oesophagitis. Digestion, *26:*166, 1983.
12. Bingham, J.A.W.: Evolution and early results of constructing an antireflux valve in the stomach. Proc. R. Soc. Med., *67:*4, 1974.
13. Blackwell, J.N., Heading, R.C., and Fetter, M.R.: Effect of domperidone on lower esophageal sphincter pressure and gastroesophageal reflux in patients with peptic oesophagitis: Progress with domperidone. R. Soc. Med. (Int. Cong. Symp. Series), *36:*57, 1981.
14. Bombeck, C.T., Coelho, R.G., and Nyhus, L.M.: Prevention of gastroesophageal reflux after resection of the lower esophagus. Surg. Gynecol. Obstet., *130:*1035, 1970.
15. Bonavino, L., Fontebasso, V., Bardini, R., et al.: Surgical treatment of reflux stricture of the oesophagus. Br. J. Surg., *80:*317, 1993.
16. Bremner, C.G.: Combined technique of esophageal endoscopy, dilatation and biopsy using the Celestin system of dilatation. *In* Demeester, T.R., and Skinner, D.B. (eds.): Esophageal Disorders: Pathophysiology and Therapy. New York, Raven Press, 1985, p. 501.
17. Buchin, P.J., and Spiro, H.M.: Therapy of esophageal stricture: A review of 84 patients. J. Clin. Gastroenterol., *3:*121, 1981.
18. Burnett, H.F., Read, R.C., Morris, W.B., et al.: Management of complications of fundoplication and Barrett's esophagus. Surgery, *82:*521, 1977.
19. Cameron, A.J., Ott, B.J., and Payne, W.S.: The incidence of adenocarcinoma in columnar-lined (Barrett's) esophagus. N. Engl. J. Med., *313:*857, 1985.
20. Chen, L., Nastros, D., Hu, C., et al.: Results of the Collis-Nissen gastroplasty in patients with Barrett's esophagus. Ann. Thorac. Surg., *68:*1014, 1999.
21. Collis, J.L.: An operation for hiatus hernia with short esophagus. Thorax, *12:*181, 1957.
22. Collis, J.L.: Gastroplasty. Thorax, *16:*197, 1961.
23. Condon, R.E.: Intraoperative dilation and fundoplication for benign peptic oesophageal stricture. *In* Jamieson, G.G. (ed.): Surgery of the Oesophagus. Edinburgh, Churchill Livingstone, 1988, p. 341.
24. Demos, N.J.: Stapled, uncut gastroplasty for hiatal hernia: 12-year follow-up. Ann. Thorac. Surg., *38:*393, 1984.
25. Demos, N.J., and Biele, R.M.: Intercostal pedicle method for control of postresection esophagitis. J. Thorac. Cardiovasc. Surg., *80:*679, 1980.
26. Demos, N.J., Smith, N., and Williams, D.: A new gastroplasty for strictured short esophagus. N.Y. State J. Med., *75:*57, 1975.
27. Donnelly, R.J., Deverall, P.B., and Watson, D.A.: Hiatus hernia with and without stricture: Experience with the Belsey Mark IV repair. Ann. Thorac. Surg., *16:*301, 1973.
28. Dunlop, E.E.: Problems in the treatment of reflux esophagitis. Gastroenterology, *86:*287, 1956.
29. Ellis, F.H., Jr., Anderson, H.A., and Clagett, O.T.: Treatment of short esophagus with stricture by esophagogastrectomy and antral excision. Ann. Surg., *148:*526, 1958.
30. Ellis, F.H., Jr., and Gibb, S.P.: Esophageal reconstruction for complex benign esophageal disease. J. Thorac. Cardiovasc. Surg., *99:*192, 1990.
31. Gillison, E.W., Capper, W.M., Airth, G.R., et al.: Hiatus hernia and heartburn. Gut, *10:*609, 1969.
32. Gillison, E.W., and Nyhus, L.M.: Bile reflux, gastric secretion and heartburn. Br. J. Surg., *58:*864, 1971.
33. Glick, M.E.: Clinical course of esophageal stricture managed by bougienage. Dig. Dis. Sci., *27:*884, 1982.
34. Goldstein, F., Thornton, J.J., Abramson, J., et al.: Bile reflux gastritis and esophagitis in patients without prior gastric surgery, with pilot study of the therapeutic effects of metoclopramide. Am. J. Gastroenterol., *76:*407, 1981.
35. Goy, J.A., Maynard, J.H., McNaughton, W.M., et al.: Ranitidine and placebo in the treatment of reflux oesophagitis: A double-blind randomized trial. Med. J. Aust., *2:*558, 1980.
36. Greaney, M.G., and Invin, T.T.: Cimetidine for treatment of symptomatic gastroesophageal reflux. Br. J. Clin. Pract., *35:*21, 1981.
37. Hayward, J.: The treatment of fibrous stricture of the esophagus associated with hiatus hernias. Thorax, *16:*45, 1961.
38. Heimlich, H.J.: Peptic esophagitis with stricture treated by reconstruction of the esophagus with a reversed gastric tube. Surg. Gynecol. Obstet., *114:*673, 1962.
39. Heitman, P., and Muller, N.: The effect of metoclopramide on the gastroesophageal junctional zone and the distal esophagus in man. Scand. J. Gastroenterol., *5:*621, 1970.
40. Henderson, R.D.: Benign strictures of the esophagus. *In* Shields, T.W. (ed.): General Thoracic Surgery. Philadelphia, Lea & Febiger, 1989, p. 1012.
41. Henderson, R.D.: Reflux control following gastroplasty. Ann. Thorac. Surg., *24:*206, 1977.
42. Henderson, R.D., and Marryatt, G.V.: Total fundoplication gastroplasty (Nissen gastroplasty): Five-year review. Ann. Thorac. Surg., *39:*74, 1985.
43. Herrington, J.L., and Mody, B.: Total duodenal diversion for treatment of reflux esophagitis uncontrolled by repeated antireflux procedures. Ann. Surg., *183:*636, 1976.
44. Herrington, J.L., Jr., Wright, R.S., Edwards, W.H., et al.: Conservative surgical treatment of reflux esophagitis and esophageal stricture. Ann. Surg., *181:*552, 1975.
45. Hill, L.D.: An effective operation for hiatal hernia: An eight year appraisal. Ann. Surg., *166:*681, 1967.
46. Hill, L.D.: Intraoperative manometry of lower esophageal sphincter pressures. J. Thorac. Cardiovasc. Surg., *75:*378, 1978.
47. Hill, L.D., Gelfand, M., and Bauermeister, D.: Simplified management of reflux esophagitis with stricture. Ann. Surg., *172:*638, 1970.
48. Hine, K.R., Holmes, G.K., Melikian, V., et al.: Ranitidine in reflux oesophagitis. A double-blind placebo controlled study. Digestion, *29:*119, 1984.
49. Hollenbeck, J.I., and Woodward, E.R.: Treatment of peptic esophageal stricture with combined fundic patch fundoplication. Ann. Surg., *182:*472, 1975.
50. Holt, C.J., and Large, A.M.: Surgical management of reflux esophagitis. Ann. Surg., *153:*555, 1961.
51. Ismail-Beigi, F., Horton, P.F., and Pope, C.E.: Histologic consequences of gastroesophageal reflux in man. Gastroenterology, *58:*163, 1970.
52. Kirsch, M., Blue, M., DeSai, R.K., et al.: Intralesional steroid injections for peptic esophageal strictures. Gastrointest. Endosc., *37:*180, 1991.
53. Klinkenberg-Knol, E.C., Festen, H.P., Jansen, J.B., et al.: Long-term treatment with omeprazole for refractory reflux esophagitis: Efficacy and safety. Ann. Intern. Med., *121:*161, 1994.
54. Kozarek, R.A.: Hydrostatic balloon dilation of gastrointestinal stenosis: a national survey. Gastrointest. Endosc., *32:*15, 1986.
55. Krupp, S., and Rosetti, M.: Surgical treatment of hiatal hernia by fundoplication and gastropexy (Nissen repair). Ann. Surg., *164:*927, 1966.
56. Kuo, W.H., and Kalloo, A.N.: Reflux strictures of the esophagus. Gastrointest. Endosc. Clin. North Am., *8:*273, 1998.
57. Lam, C.R., and Gahagan, T.H.: Special comment: The myth of the short esophagus. *In* Nyphus, L.M., and Harkins, H.N. (eds.): Hernia. Philadelphia, J.B. Lippincott, 1964, p. 450.
58. Lee, M., Kubik, C.M., Polhemus, C.D., et al.: Preliminary experience with endoscopic intralesional steroid injection for refractory

upper gastrointestinal strictures. Gastrointest. Endosc., *41*:598, 1995.
59. Little, A.G., Naunheim, K.S., Ferguson, M.K., et al.: Surgical management of esophageal strictures. Ann. Thorac. Surg., *45*:144, 1988.
60. Lundell, L.: Acid suppression in the long-term treatment of peptic stricture and Barrett's esophagus. Digestion, *51*(1):49, 1992.
61. Maher, J.W., Hocking, M.P., and Woodward, E.R.: Long-term follow-up of the combined fundic patch fundoplication for treatment of longitudinal peptic strictures of the esophagus. Ann. Surg., *194*:64, 1981.
62. Mansour, K., Burton, H., Miller, J., et al.: Complications of intrathoracic Nissen fundoplication. Ann. Thorac. Surg., *32*:173, 1981.
63. Marks, R.D., Richter, J.E., Rizzo, J., et al.: Omeprazole versus H_2-receptor antagonist in treating patients with peptic strictures and esophagitis. Gastroenterology, *106*:907, 1994.
64. Marks, R.D., and Richter, J.E.: Peptic strictures of the esophagus. Am. J. Gastroenterol., *88*:1160, 1993.
65. Matikainen, M.: Antrectomy, Roux-en-Y reconstruction and vagotomy for recurrent reflux esophagitis. Acta Chir. Scand., *150*:643, 1984.
66. Mercer, C.D., and Hill, L.D.: Surgical management of peptic esophageal stricture. J. Thorac. Cardiovasc. Surg., *91*:371, 1986.
67. Merendino, K.A., and Dillard, D.H.: The concept of sphincter substitution by an interposed jejunal segment for anatomic and physiologic abnormalities at the esophagogastric junction. Ann. Surg., *142*:486, 1955.
68. Moghissi, I.: Intrathoracic fundoplication for reflux stricture associated with short esophagus. Thorax, *38*:36, 1983.
69. Monnier, P., Hsieh, V., and Savary, M.: Endoscopic treatment of esophageal stenosis using Savary-Gilliard bougies: Technical innovations. Acta Endosc., *15*:119, 1985.
70. Monnier, P., and Savary, M.: Contribution of endoscopy to gastroesophageal reflux disease. Scand. J. Gastroenterol., *19*:26, 1984.
71. Mossberg, S.M.: The columnar lined esophagus (Barrett's syndrome): An acquired condition? Gastroenterology, *50*:671, 1966.
72. Naef, A.P., Savary, M., and Ozello, L.: Columnar-lined lower esophagus: An acquired lesion with malignant predisposition. J. Thorac. Cardiovasc. Surg., *70*:826, 1975.
73. Neville, W.E., and Clowes, G.H.A., Jr.: Surgical treatment of the complications resulting from cardioesophageal incompetence. Dis. Chest, *43*:572, 1963.
74. Nissen, R.: Gastropexy and "fundoplication" in surgical treatment of hiatal hernia. Am. J. Dig. Dis., *6*:954, 1961.
75. Ogilvie, A.L., Ferguson, R., and Atkinson, M.: Outlook with conservative treatment of peptic oesophageal stricture. Gut, *21*:23, 1980.
76. Okada, N., Kuriyama, T., Urmenoto, H., et al.: Esophageal surgery: A procedure for posterior invagination esophagogastrostomy in one stage without positional change. Ann. Surg., *179*:27, 1974.
77. Ollyo, J.B., Ch. Fontolliet, E., and Brossard, F.L.: Savary's new endoscopic classification of reflux oesophagitis. Gullet, *22*:307, 1992.
78. Orlando, R.C.: Effect of sucralfate on the esophageal epithelium. Curr. Concepts Gastroenterol., *6*:34, 1984.
79. Orringer, M.B.: Transhiatal esophagectomy for benign disease. J. Thorac. Cardiovasc. Surg., *90*:649, 1985.
80. Orringer, M.B.: Transhiatal esophagectomy without thoracotomy for carcinoma of the thoracic esophagus. Ann. Surg., *200*:282, 1984.
81. Orringer, M.B., Marshall, B., and Iannettoni, M.D.: Eliminating the cervical esophagogastric anastomotic leak with a side-to-side stapled anastomosis. J. Thorac. Cardiovasc. Surg., *119*:277, 2000.
82. Orringer, M.B., Marshall, B., and Iannettoni, M.D.: Transhiatal esophagectomy: Clinical experience and refinements. Ann. Surg., *230*:392, 1999.
83. Orringer, M.B., Marshall, B., and Stirling, M.C.: Transhiatal esophagectomy for benign and malignant disease. J. Thorac. Cardiovasc. Surg., *105*:265, 1993.
84. Orringer, M.B., and Orringer, J.S.: The combined Collis-Nissen operation: Early assessment of reflux control. Ann. Thorac. Surg., *33*:534, 1982.
85. Orringer, M.B., Skinner, D.B., and Belsey, R.H.: Long-term results of the Mark IV operation for hiatal hernia and analyses of recurrences and their treatment. J. Thorac. Cardiovasc. Surg., *63*:25, 1972.
86. Orringer, M.B., and Sloan, H.: An improved technique for the combined Collis-Belsey approach to dilatable esophageal strictures. J. Thorac. Cardiovasc. Surg., *68*:298, 1974.
87. Orringer, M.B., and Sloan, H.: Collis-Belsey reconstruction of the esophagogastric junction. J. Thorac. Cardiovasc. Surg., *71*:295, 1976.
88. Orringer, M.B., and Sloan, H.: Combined Collis-Nissen reconstruction of the esophagogastric junction. Ann. Thorac. Surg., *25*:16, 1978.
89. Orringer, M.B., and Sloan, H.: Complications and failings of the combined Collis-Belsey operation. J. Thorac. Cardiovasc. Surg., *74*:726, 1977.
90. Orringer, M.B., and Stirling, M.C.: Cervical esophagogastric anastomosis for benign disease: Functional results. J. Thorac. Cardiovasc. Surg., *96*:887, 1988.
91. Patterson, D.J., Graham, D.Y., Smith, J.L., et al.: Natural history of benign esophageal stricture treated by dilation. Gastroenterology, *85*:346, 1983.
92. Payne, W.S.: Surgical treatment of reflux esophagitis and stricture associated with permanent incompetence of the cardia. Mayo Clin. Proc., *45*:553, 1970.
93. Pearson, F.G.: Surgical management of acquired short esophagus with dilatable peptic stricture. World J. Surg., *1*:463, 1977.
94. Pearson, F.G., Cooper, J., Patterson, G., et al.: Gastroplasty and fundoplication for complex reflux problems. Ann. Surg., *206*:473, 1987.
95. Pearson, F.G., and Henderson, R.D.: Experimental and clinical studies of gastroplasty in the management of acquired short esophagus. Surg. Gynecol. Obstet., *136*:737, 1973.
96. Pearson, F.G., and Henderson, R.D.: Long-term follow-up of peptic strictures managed by dilatation, modified Collis gastroplasty, and Belsey hiatus hernia repair. Surgery, *80*:396, 1976.
97. Pearson, F.G., Langer, B., and Henderson, R.D.: Gastroplasty and Belsey hiatal hernia repair. J. Thorac. Cardiovasc. Surg., *61*:50, 1971.
98. Pennell, T.: Supradiaphragmatic correction of esophageal reflux strictures. Ann. Surg., *193*:655, 1981.
99. Perkel, M.S., Moore, C., Hersh, T., et al.: Metoclopramide therapy in patients with delayed gastric emptying. Dig. Dis. Sci., *24*:662, 1979.
100. Polk, H.C., Jr.: Fundoplication for reflux esophagitis: Misadventures with the operation of choice. Ann. Surg., *183*:645, 1976.
101. Polk, H.C., Jr.: Jejunal interposition for reflux esophagitis and esophageal stricture unresponsive to valvuloplasty. World J. Surg., *4*:731, 1980.
102. Pope, C.E., II.: Acid reflux disorders. N. Engl. J. Med., *331*:656, 1994.
103. Popov, V.I.: Reconstruction of the esophagus in cases of stricture. Arch. Surg., *82*:226, 1961.
104. Rago, E., Boesby, S., and Spencer, J.: Results of Eder-Puestow dilatation in the management of esophageal peptic structures. Am. J. Gastroenterol., *78*:6, 1983.
105. Richardson, J.D., Larson, G.M., and Polk, H.C., Jr.: Intrathoracic fundoplication for shortened esophagus: A treacherous solution to a challenging problem. Am. J. Surg., *143*:29, 1982.
106. Rossman, F., Brantigan, C.O., and Sawyer, R.B.: Obstructive complications of the Nissen fundoplication. Am. J. Surg., *138*:860, 1979.
107. Saeed, Z.A., Ramirez, F.C., Hepps, K.S., et al.: An objective end point for dilation improves outcomes of peptic esophageal strictures: A prospective randomized trial. Gastrointest. Endosc., *45*:354, 1997.
108. Safaie-Shirazi, S., DenBesten, L., and Zike, W.L.: Effects of bile salts on the ionic permeability of the esophageal mucosa and their role in the production of esophagitis. Gastroenterology, *68*:728, 1975.
109. Safaie-Shirazi, S., Sike, W.L., Anuras, S., et al.: Nissen fundoplication without crural repair. Arch. Surg., *108*:424, 1974.
110. Safaie-Shirazi, S., Zike, W.L., and Masson, E.E.: Esophageal strictures secondary to reflux esophagitis. Arch. Surg., *110*:629, 1975.
111. Salo, J.A., and Kivilaakso, E.: Role of bile salts and trypsin in the pathogenesis of experimental alkaline esophagitis. Surgery, *98*:525, 1983.
112. Sandry, R.J.: Pathology of reflux esophagitis. *In* Skinner, D.B., Belsey, R.H., Hendrix, T.R., et al. (eds.): Gastroesophageal Reflux and Hiatal Hernia. Boston, Little, Brown, 1972, p. 43.
113. Skinner, D.B.: The columnar-lined esophagus and adenocarcinoma (Editorial). Ann. Thorac. Surg., *40*:321, 1985.

114. Skinner, D.B., and Belsey, R.H.: Reconstruction with stomach. *In* Skinner, D.B., and Belsey, R.H.: Management of Esophageal Disease. Philadelphia, W.B. Saunders, 1988, p. 228.
115. Skinner, D.B., and Belsey, R.H.: Surgical management of esophageal reflux and hiatus hernia. J. Thorac. Cardiovasc. Surg., *53:*33, 1967.
116. Skinner, D.B., and Belsey, R.H.: Surgical management of esophageal reflux and hiatus hernia and long term results with 1,030 patients. J. Thorac. Cardiovasc. Surg., *53:*33, 1967.
117. Stirling, M.C., and Orringer, M.B.: Surgical treatment of the failed antireflux operation. J. Thorac. Cardiovasc. Surg., *92:*667, 1986.
118. Stirling, M.C., and Orringer, M.B.: The combined Collis-Nissen operation for esophageal reflux strictures. Ann. Thorac. Surg., *45:*148, 1988.
119. Strug, B.S., Jordan, P.H., Jr., and Jordan, G.L., Jr.: Surgical management of benign esophageal strictures. Surg. Gynecol. Obstet., *138:*74, 1974.
120. Tanner, N.C., and Westerholm, P.: Partial gastrectomy in the treatment of esophageal stricture after hiatal hernia. Am. J. Surg., *115:*449, 1968.
121. Thal, A.P.: A unified approach to surgical problems of the esophagogastric junction. Ann. Surg., *168:*542, 1968.
122. Thal, A.P., Hatafuko, T., and Kurtzman, R.: New operation for distal esophageal stricture. Arch. Surg., *90:*464, 1965.
123. Thomas, H.F., Clarke, J.M., Rayl, J.E., et al.: Results of the combined fundic patch fundoplication operation in the treatment of reflux esophagitis with stricture. Surg. Gynecol. Obstet., *135:*241, 1972.
124. Tileston, W.: Peptic ulcer of the oesophagus. Am. J. Med. Sci., *132:*240, 1906.
125. Tucker, L.E.: The importance of fluoroscopic guidance for Maloney dilation. Am. J. Gastroenterol., *87:*1709, 1992.
126. Urschel, H.C., Razzuk, M.A., Wood, R.E., et al.: An improved surgical technique for the complicated hiatal hernia with gastroesophageal reflux. Ann. Thorac. Surg., *15:*443, 1973.
127. Valenzuela, J.E.: Effects of domperidone on the symptoms of reflux oesophagitis: Progress with domperidone. R. Soc. Med. (Int. Cong. Symp. Series), *36:*51, 1981.
128. Wangensteen, O.H., and Levin, N.L.: Gastric resection for esophagitis and stricture of acid-peptic origin. Surg. Gynecol. Obstet., *88:*560, 1949.
129. Wara, P., Oster, M.J., Funch-Jensen, P., et al.: A long-term follow-up of patients resected for benign esophageal stricture using the ink-well esophagogastrectomy. Ann. Surg., *190:*214, 1981.
130. Washer, G.F., Gear, M.W.L., Dowling, B.L., et al.: Duodenal diversion with vagotomy and antrectomy for severe or recurrent reflux esophagitis and stricture: An alternative to operation at the hiatus. Ann. R. Coll. Surg., *68:*222, 1986.
131. Washer, G.F., Gear, M.W.L., Dowling, B.L., et al.: Randomized prospective trial of Roux-en-Y duodenal diversion versus fundoplication for severe reflux oesophagitis. Br. J. Surg., *71:*181, 1984.
132. Watson, A.: The role of antireflux surgery combined with fiberoptic endoscopic dilatation in peptic esophageal strictures. Am. J. Surg., *148:*346, 1984.
133. Weaver, A.W., Large, A.M., and Walt, A.J.: Surgical management of severe reflux esophagitis. Am. J. Surg., *119:*15, 1970.
134. Wells, C., and Johnston, J.H., Hiatus hernia: Surgical relief of reflux oesophagitis. Lancet, *268:*937, 1955.
135. Wesdorp, I.C., Bartelsman, J.F., denHartog Jager, F.C., et al.: Results of conservative treatment of benign esophageal strictures: A follow-up study of 100 patients. Gastroenterology, *82:*487, 1982.
136. Woodward, E.R.: Sliding esophageal hiatal hernia and reflux peptic esophagitis. Mayo Clin. Proc., *50:*523, 1975.
137. Zein, N.N., Gresetn, J.M., and Perrault, J.: Endoscopic intralesional steroid injection in the management of refractory esophageal strictures. Gastrointest. Endosc., *41:*598, 1995.

CHAPTER

14 Barrett's Esophagus: Morphologic Considerations

BARBARA J. MCKENNA • HENRY D. APPELMAN

NORMAL ESOPHAGEAL MUCOSA AND SUBMUCOSA

The normal esophageal mucosa comprises two discrete layers. Moist, stratified squamous epithelium on the surface covers a lamina propria composed of loose, fibrous tissue that contains scattered lymphoid cells but very few other inflammatory cells (Fig. 14-1). This layer in turn lies on a thick muscularis mucosae composed of prominent smooth muscle bundles. Beneath this muscle layer is the submucosa, another loose, fibrovascular connective tissue region, in which are embedded clusters of mucus-producing submucosal glands. From these submucosal glands, ducts penetrate the muscularis mucosae, lamina propria, and stratified squamous epithelium to empty onto the surface.

DEFINITION OF BARRETT'S MUCOSA

Barrett's mucosa is a postreflux metaplasia involving the lower esophagus in continuity with the proximal stomach in which columnar epithelium replaces the normal squamous epithelium[2,21,39] (Fig. 14-2). Barrett's mucosa is believed to be the result of destruction of the distal esophageal squamous epithelium owing to contact with irritant gastric or gastroduodenal contents. Instead of healing with squamous re-epithelialization, the surface of the injured area is replaced by columnar epithelium, possibly arising from ducts of submucosal glands, the gastric cardiac mucosa, or some other source. A length of distal esophagus covered by columnar mucosa is then established that persists indefinitely.[4]

DISTRIBUTION

Grossly, in Barrett's mucosa the squamocolumnar junction, seen as the junction of the white squamous mucosa and the pink or red columnar mucosa, is displaced proximally. The displacement is often in the form of tongue-like extensions, especially when the Barrett's segment is short. Longer segments of Barrett's mucosa are likely to have circumferential involvement of the distal esophagus. The proximal margin of columnar mucosa is commonly irregular and patches of squamous mucosa, known as squamous islands, may be trapped within the columnar mucosa. Occasional erosions and ulcers are found, especially near the junction between the Barrett's mucosa and the squamous mucosa[36] (Fig. 14-3).

At one time, the definition of Barrett's required involvement of at least 2 or 3 cm of the distal esophagus. Because the normal endoscopic squamocolumnar junction (Z-line) often has an irregular, sawtooth, or undulating configuration that may span a length of distal esophagus up to 2 cm long, shorter segments of columnar mucosa were not designated as Barrett's. Even without this irregular squamocolumnar junction, it is now recognized that cardiac mucosa may extend into the lower 2 cm of the esophagus circumferentially. However, more recently, short segments of Barrett's esophagus, involving 1 to 3 cm of the distal esophagus, have been recognized and are not uncommon. These segments usually consist of the upward extension of tongues of columnar mucosa above the Z-line that show intestinalized epithelium on biopsy, as described later.

Not all columnar mucosa in the esophagus is Barrett's mucosa. Commonly, small velvety pink or red patches, referred to as inlet patches, are located at the level of the cricoid cartilage, far from the normal gastroesophageal junction. They consist of gastric-body or antral-type mucosa and are thought to be developmental aberrations. Inlet patches have nothing to do with reflux and do not imply a need for follow-up or surveillance. They are generally recognized readily by a trained endoscopist (Fig. 14-4).[15] All the changes that affect the stomach, including *Helicobacter pylori* gastritis and atrophic gastritis, can affect the mucosa in the inlet patch.

EPITHELIAL TYPES IN BARRETT'S ESOPHAGUS

At one time, histologic descriptions of Barrett's esophagus identified three types of mucosa, two of which had gastric-type glands and the third of which contained intestinal-type cells. The finding of any of these in the appropriate setting (i.e., located more than 3 cm above the gastroesophageal junction) was considered equivalent to a diagnosis of Barrett's esophagus.[23] Only one of these types, the one in which intestinal-type goblet cells are found, currently is considered the fully diagnostic type, although the other mucosal types may also be present.[11]

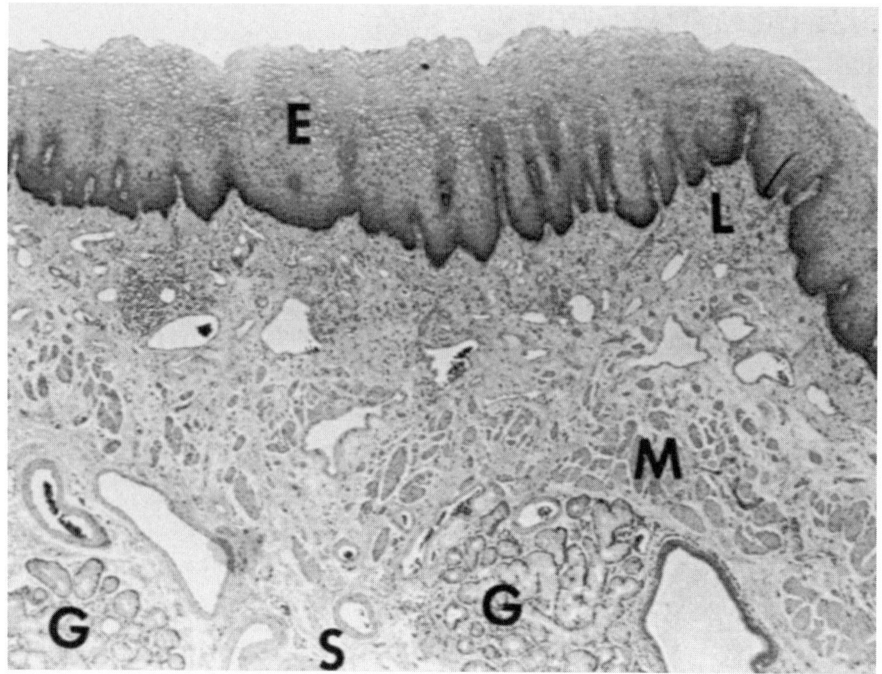

Figure 14–1. Normal esophageal mucosa with its two components of squamous epithelium *(E)* and lamina propria *(L)*. At the base of the mucosa is the muscularis mucosae *(M)*, and submucosa *(S)* with mucous glands *(G)*. (Hematoxylin and eosin, ×33.)

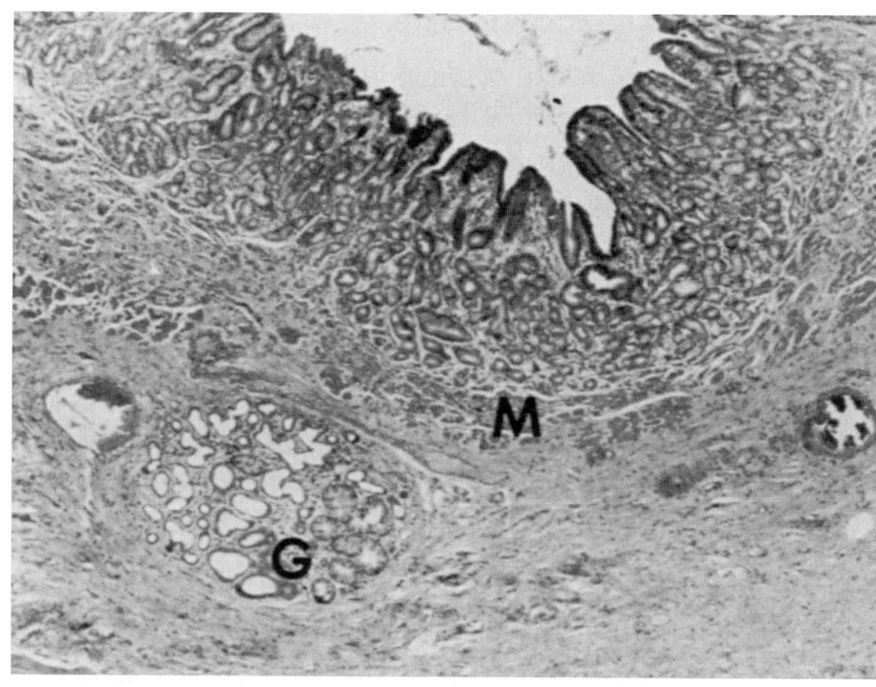

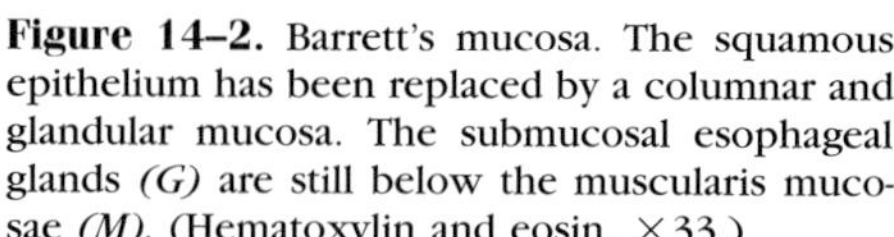
Figure 14–2. Barrett's mucosa. The squamous epithelium has been replaced by a columnar and glandular mucosa. The submucosal esophageal glands *(G)* are still below the muscularis mucosae *(M)*. (Hematoxylin and eosin, ×33.)

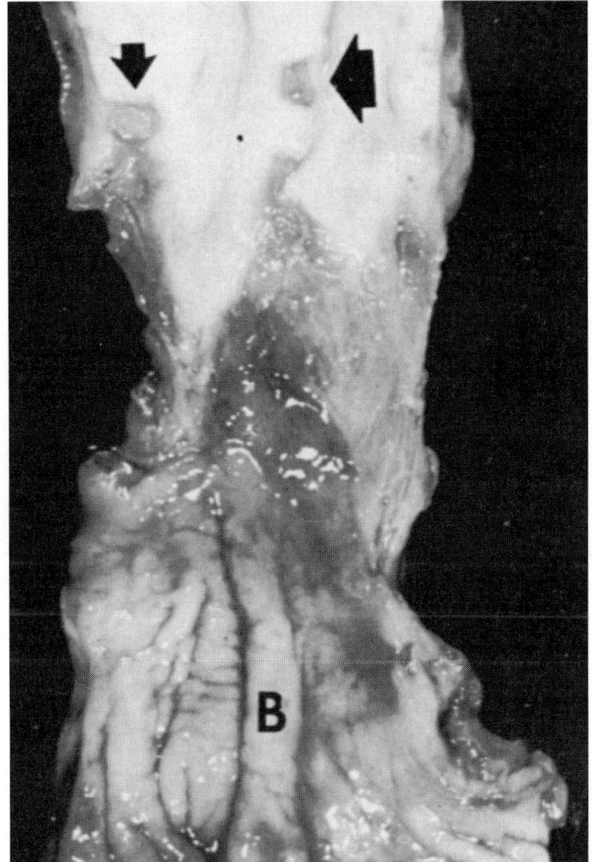

Figure 14–3. Gross picture of Barrett's mucosa *(B)* at the bottom, which resembles gastric mucosa. The squamous esophageal mucosa above is white, and there is an ulcer at the junction. Note the islands of Barrett's mucosa within the squamous epithelium *(arrows)*.

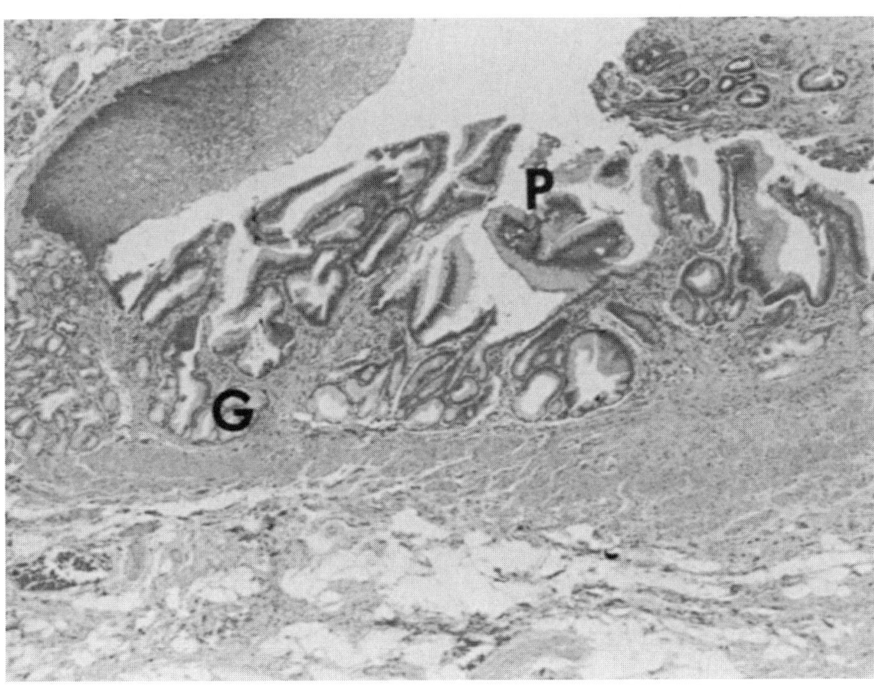

Figure 14–4. An inlet patch: ectopic gastric mucosa in the cervical esophagus has both pits *(P)* and glands *(G)*. (Hematoxylin and eosin, ×33.)

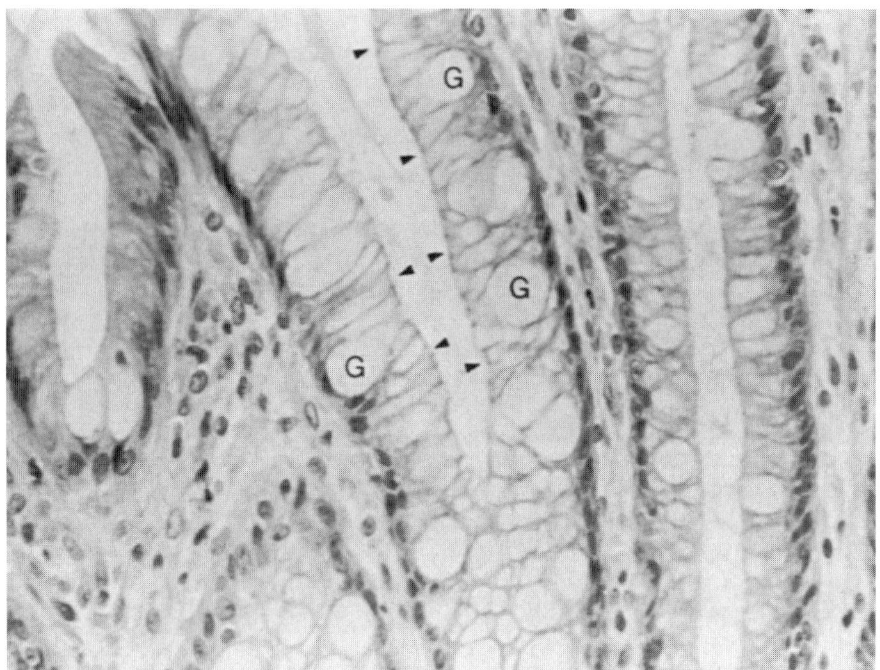

Figure 14–5. Incomplete intestinal metaplasia in the specialized Barrett's mucosa has goblet cells *(G)* among gastric-type surface cells or intermediate cells *(arrows)*. (Hematoxylin and eosin, ×330.)

The diagnostic type of mucosa has been called the specialized or distinctive type. Its defining feature is the presence of intestinal-type goblet cells. These cells occur on the surface and line pit- or crypt-type structures, where they are dispersed among epithelial cells resembling gastric foveolar cells that are sometimes referred to as intermediate cells (Fig. 14–5). This epithelium has also been designated "incomplete intestinal metaplasia" because only the goblet-cell component of intestinal epithelium is present, and not the other components such as Paneth cells and absorptive cells. Much less frequently, complete intestinal metaplasia occurs in which stretches of epithelium containing goblet cells, absorptive cells, Paneth cells, and even endocrine cells of the intestinal type are found (Fig. 14–6). The surface contour is generally flat to undulating or, less commonly, has a villous configuration (Figs. 14–7 and 14–8). A scant glandular compartment is usually composed of discrete nests of mucus-secreting glands, although fundic glandular epithelium may also be present (see Figs. 14–7 and 14–8).

The other types of mucosa that have been described in Barrett's esophagus are not diagnostic because they do not contain goblet cells. The first of these is a modified fundic or body-type mucosa in which there are clusters

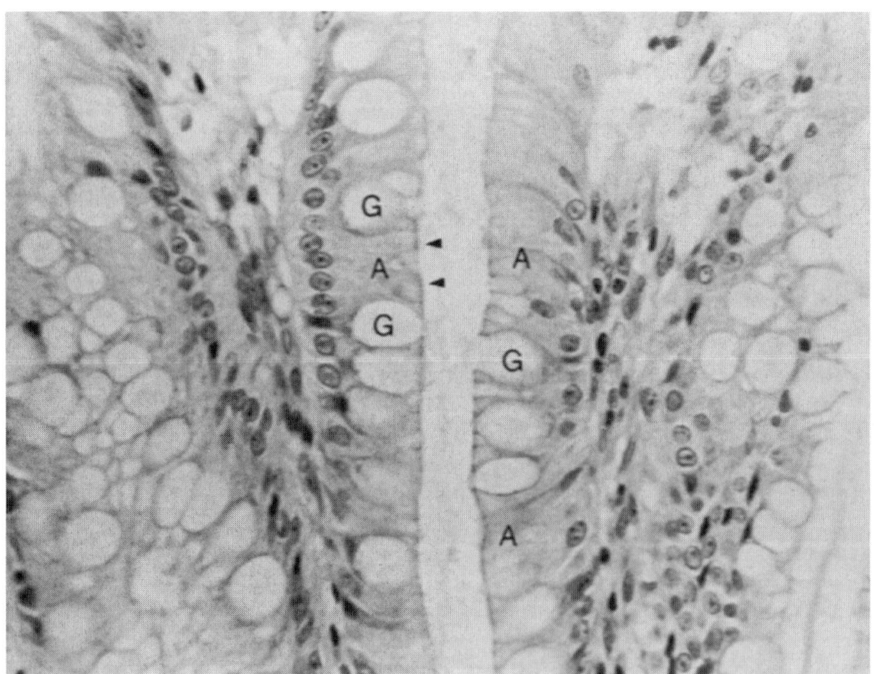

Figure 14–6. Complete intestinal metaplasia in Barrett's mucosa has goblet cells *(G)*, absorptive cells *(A)*, and a brush border on the luminal surface *(arrows)*. (Hematoxylin and eosin, ×330.)

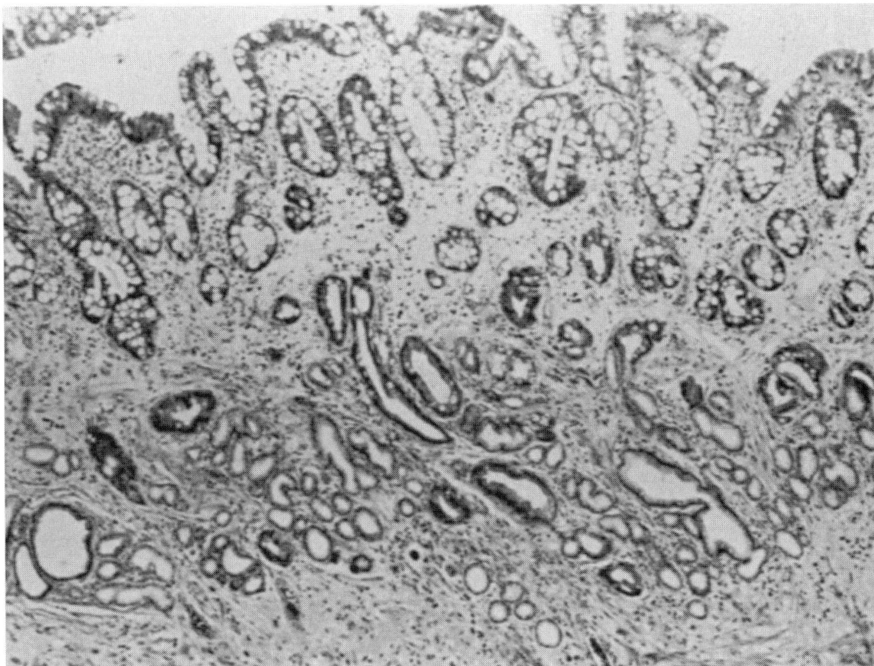

Figure 14–7. Flat Barrett's mucosa with intestinal metaplasia on the surface and clusters of cardiac-type mucous glands at the base. (Hematoxylin and eosin, ×53.)

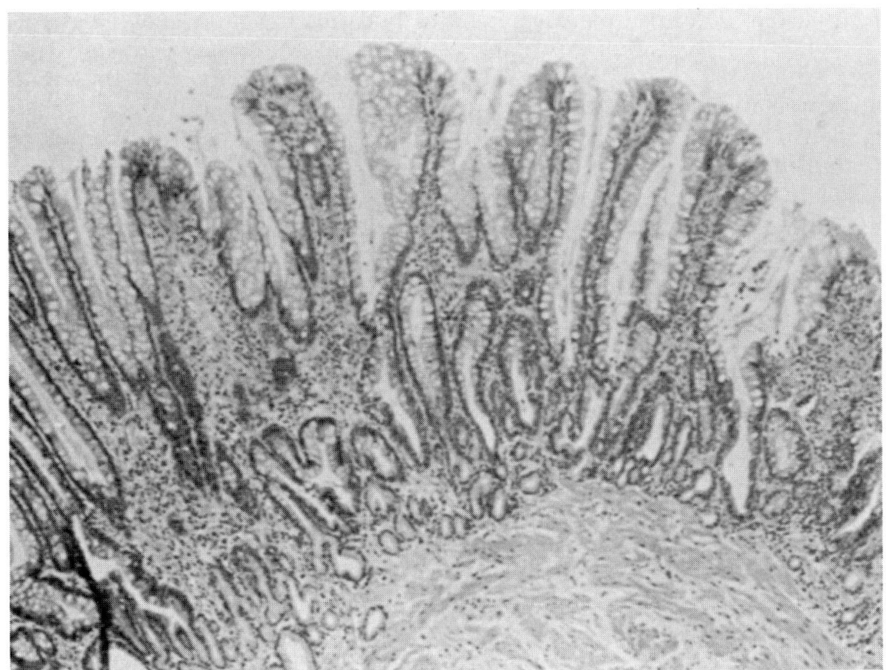

Figure 14–8. This Barrett's mucosa has a villiform surface. (Hematoxylin and eosin, ×53.)

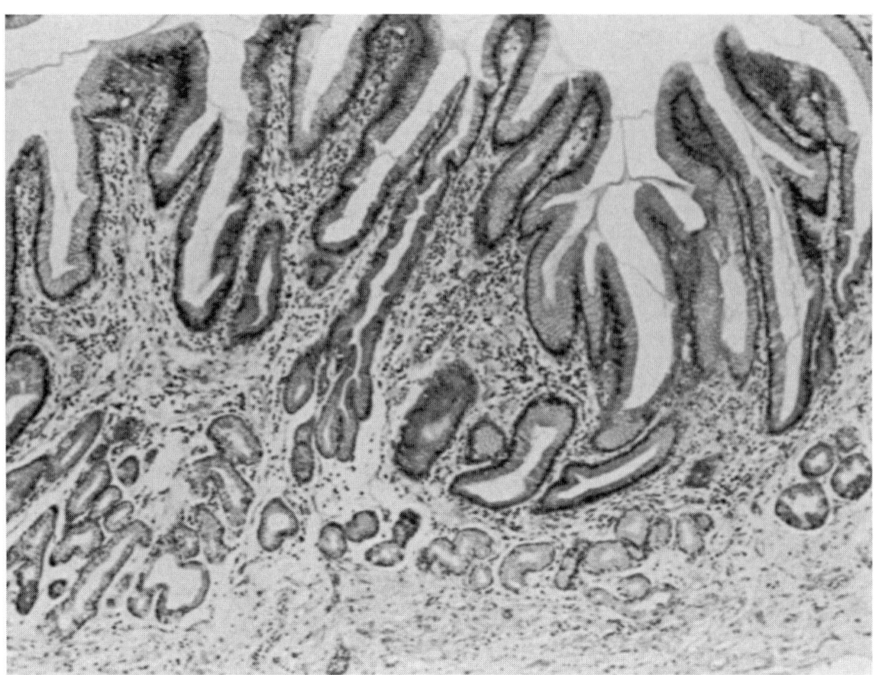

Figure 14–9. Cardiac-type mucosa has pits and clusters of mucous glands at the base but no goblet cells. (Hematoxylin and eosin, ×53.)

of glands containing parietal cells and chief cells that are identical to those found in gastric body mucosa. However, the volume of the glandular compartment is less than that in the normal gastric body, whereas the pit compartment is proportionately larger. The other mucosal type has been designated as junctional mucosa. This mucosa resembles gastric cardiac mucosa, except that the glandular compartment is often relatively atrophic (Fig. 14–9).[14,15,32,39]

Partial healing of Barrett's mucosa with replacement of the surface columnar epithelium by squamous epithelium also occurs and is referred to as pseudoregression. There is often residual columnar epithelium, including intestinalized tubules and glands, beneath the squamous surface in such areas. This process may be the source of some of the squamous islands observed grossly (Fig. 14–10). Pseudoregression may result from acid suppression or from laser or photodynamic ablation. We do not know whether the risk for dysplasia and carcinoma for the Barrett's mucosa covered by squamous epithelium is the same as that for the other Barrett's mucosae.

MUCIN HISTOCHEMISTRY

Different types of epithelial mucin exist in the specialized or distinctive mucosa of Barrett's esophagus, in both the gastric-type surface cells and the goblet cells. The three histochemical staining reactions used to separate the types of mucin are[16,18]:

1. The periodic acid–Schiff (PAS) technique, which stains many types of mucin, including neutral mucin, such as occur in gastric surface epithelium, cardiac mucosal glands, antral mucosal glands, and Brunner's glands in the duodenum. With this technique, neutral mucin is stained red or magenta.

2. The Alcian blue (AB) technique, which, at a pH of 2.5, stains all acid mucopolysaccharides blue. The goblet cells throughout the entire gastrointestinal tract stain with this technique.

3. The high iron diamine (HID) technique, which is a specific histochemical stain for sulfated acid mucopolysaccharides; they stain dark purple or brownish. This technique stains normal colonic goblet cells, which have a high content of sulfated acid mucopolysaccharides; small intestinal goblet cell mucin does not stain, however, because it is not sulfated.

These stains may be used in combination. For example, when PAS and AB are combined at pH 2.5, PAS stains only neutral mucin, whereas AB stains only acidic mucin. Some cells occasionally stain purplish when this combination is used, indicating that they contain both neutral and acid mucin.

The combination of AB and HID separates acid mucins into those that are sulfated and those that are not. Using this combination, the sulfated mucins stain dark purple or brownish with HID, whereas the nonsulfated mucins, almost all of which are sialomucins, stain blue with AB. Some cells may contain both sulfated and nonsulfated mucins, producing a dirty grayish-blue cast.

Using these combination techniques, it is possible to identify three types of intestinal metaplasia in Barrett's mucosa. They are identical to the three types that occur in gastric mucosa in atrophic gastritis.[6,16,18] *Complete intestinal metaplasia* consists of stretches of epithelium that have all the characteristics of small intestinal epithelium, with goblet cells, absorptive cells, Paneth cells, and even endocrine cells (Fig. 14–11). There are no interspersed cells of the gastric surface type. The goblet cells stain only with AB when the PAS-AB and HID-AB combinations are used, indicating that they contain only sialomucins, and not sulfated or neutral mucins. This complete type of intestinal metaplasia has been designated as type I.

Figure 14–10. Pseudoregression in Barrett's mucosa has squamous epithelium on top of and partly replacing the intestinalized tubules. (Hematoxylin and eosin, ×83.)

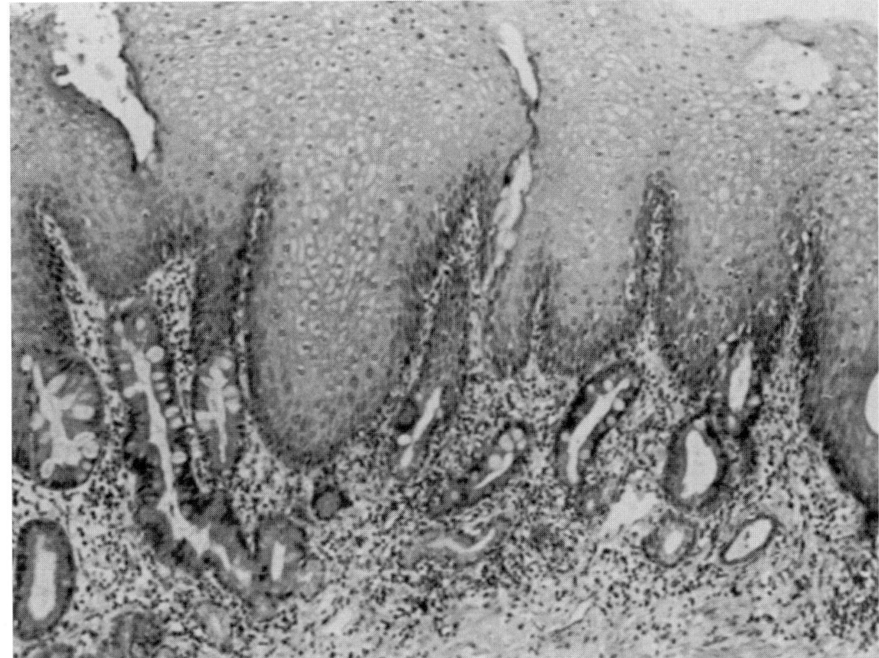

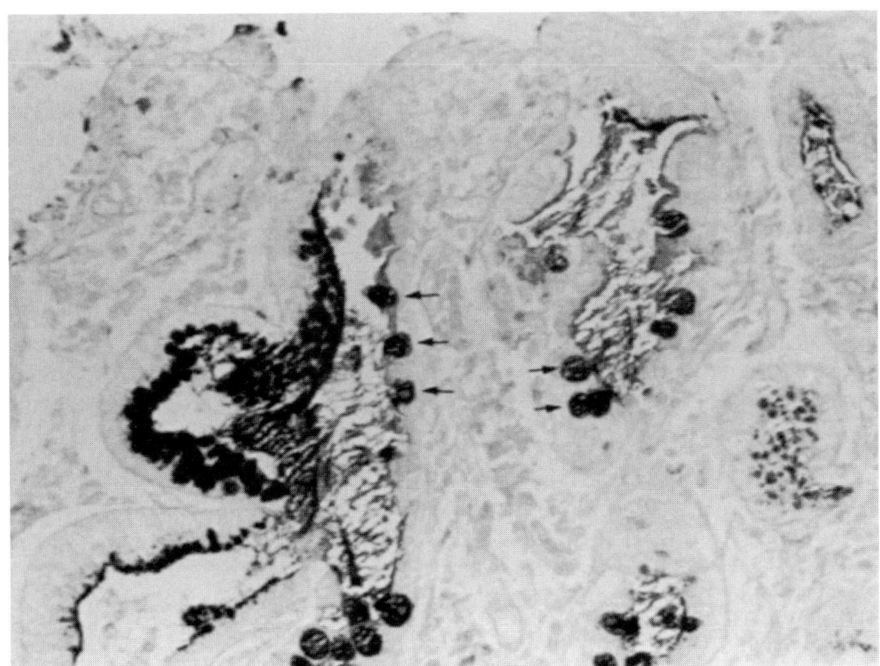

Figure 14–11. Complete intestinal metaplasia. The goblet cells *(arrows)* are dark, as is the glycocalyx, the mucous coat on the cell surfaces. The tubule at the far left has complete intestinal metaplasia on its right side and residual pit epithelium on the left with uniform apical dark-staining mucous droplets. (Alcian blue/PAS, ×132.)

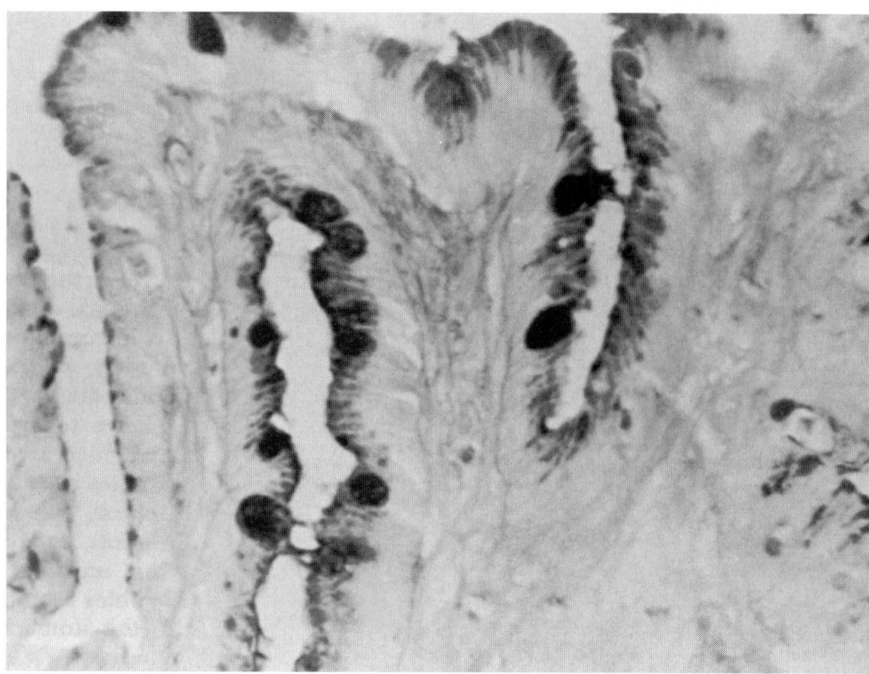

Figure 14–12. Incomplete intestinal metaplasia has goblet cells *(dark blobs)* mixed with the paler apical mucous vacuoles in the surrounding intermediate cells. (Alcian blue/PAS, ×330.)

There are two types of *incomplete intestinal metaplasia*, which are incomplete in that they contain intestinal-type goblet cells in a field of gastric-type surface cells that are sometimes also called intermediate cells (Fig. 14–12).[6] The difference between the two types relates to whether some intermediate cells contain sulfated mucins. The presence of sulfated mucins in the goblet cells is not important. In both types, the goblet cells contain either sulfated mucins or sialomucins, or both. In the first type, the intermediate cells or gastric-type surface cells contain either neutral mucins or sialomucins, but no sulfated mucins are present. This form of intestinal metaplasia has been designated as type II.[6,16] In the second type of incomplete intestinal metaplasia, some of the intermediate or gastric-type surface cells contain sulfated mucins. They also may contain neutral mucins or sialomucins. This type of metaplasia has been designated as type III.[6,16]

The significance of these different types of intestinal metaplasia lies in their association with dysplasia and carcinoma and whether they can serve as markers of neoplastic risk. This issue is discussed in detail later, in the "Barrett's Mucosa and Carcinoma" section.

DIAGNOSIS OF BARRETT'S ESOPHAGUS BY BIOPSY

The only reason to make a diagnosis of Barrett's mucosa with a biopsy is to identify a patient who has a significant risk for developing esophageal adenocarcinoma and so is a candidate for endoscopic surveillance. The biopsy diagnosis of Barrett's mucosa depends on the identification of specialized columnar epithelium—that containing goblet cells—in a biopsy from an area in the esophagus that is endoscopically suggestive of Barrett's mucosa. The finding of goblet cells is not sufficient alone, because as many as 20% of adults who undergo upper endoscopy have goblet cells in biopsies of the gastric cardia.[9,13,38] Therefore, the diagnosis of Barrett's depends on close correlation between the endoscopic findings and the histologic appearance. It is important to be sure that the biopsy sample is definitely taken from within the tubular esophagus, and it may be important to know the exact site of the biopsy in relation to the position of the lower esophageal sphincter. This may be difficult because often the endoscopist is not certain where this sphincter is. The diagnosis is made easier if this mucosa is found in biopsies from tongues of pink mucosa extending proximally from the normal squamocolumnar junction or Z-line into the lower esophagus, especially if these tongues appear to be more than merely exaggerations of the normal Z-line. In cases in which the precise relationship to the lower esophageal sphincter is not clear, there may be confirmation that the biopsy comes from the tubular esophagus, such as an esophageal submucosal gland duct penetrating the columnar mucosa. When any gastric-type mucosa without goblet cells is present in the biopsy, then the diagnosis of Barrett's mucosa cannot be made. It is generally not necessary to employ special histochemical stains for mucins to be able to identify goblet cells, because they have a characteristic appearance on routine hematoxylin and eosin (H&E) stained slides. Table 14–1 gives guidelines for diagnosing biopsies taken from columnar mucosa in the lower esophagus and proximal stomach.

A biopsy with squamous metaplasia on the surface and underlying Barrett's mucosa containing goblet cells—the "pseudoregression" described earlier—is also diagnostic when there is appropriate endoscopic correlation.

BARRETT'S MUCOSA AND CARCINOMA

The development of adenocarcinoma is a well-recognized complication of Barrett's esophagus.[2,34,36] These carcinomas occur in either short-segment or long-segment Bar-

Table 14–1. The Diagnosis of Barrett's Mucosa

Histologic and Endoscopic Features	Diagnosis
Columnar epithelium with goblet cells	
more than 2 cm in the distal esophagus	Barrett's mucosa, long segment
less than 2 cm in distal esophagus	Barrett's mucosa, short segment
Columnar epithelium with goblet cells at the gastroesophageal junction	Goblet cells at the cardia
Cardiac or body-type gastric mucosa without goblet cells from lower esophagus	No Barrett's mucosa; either cardia or hiatal hernia

rett's mucosa. To be identified as a Barrett's carcinoma, the tumor must occur within a field of Barrett's mucosa.[5,33] Precursor epithelial changes known as dysplasia often are found somewhere adjacent to the carcinoma. Grossly, these tumors often are ulcerated, with heaped-up or nodular edges (Fig. 14–13). Other gross appearances, such as polypoid, plaque-like, or diffusely infiltrating lesions, also occur. From a histologic standpoint, these tumors are adenocarcinomas of variable differentiation that are identical to those found in the stomach, and especially in the cardia (Figs. 14–14, 14–15, and 14–16).[8,12,17] This is understandable because Barrett's carcinomas and gastric-body and antral carcinomas in most cases arise from similar incompletely intestinalized epithelium. It is not known whether this is true of gastric cardiac carcinomas.

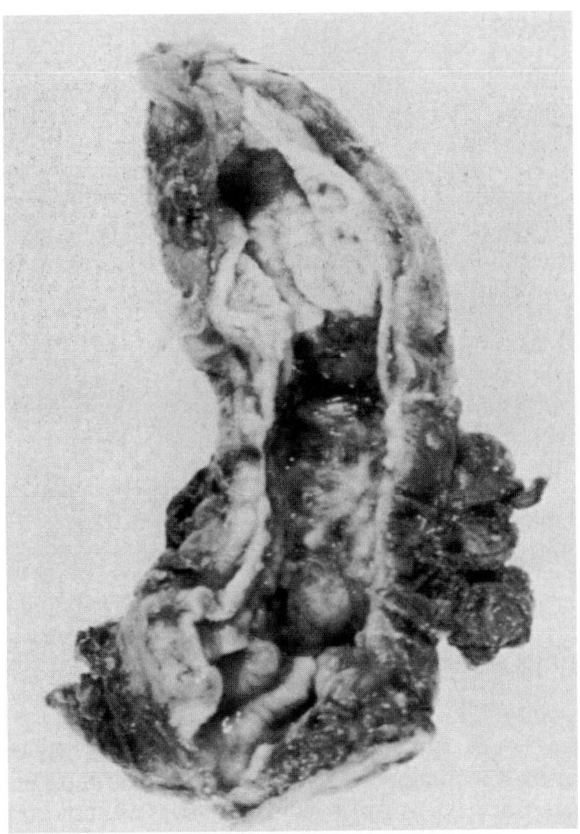

Figure 14–13. This carcinoma in a Barrett's mucosa has a mixture of nodular and ulcerated features and is confined to the tubular esophagus.

Determining the magnitude of the risk of carcinoma in Barrett's mucosa has been elusive. Most studies agree that most Barrett's carcinomas are found at presentation; that is, the cancer and the Barrett's mucosa are discovered at the same time. In a study from the Mayo Clinic published in 1985,[2] 20 cancers were found within a group of 122 patients with Barrett's mucosa. In 18 of these 20 cases, both the carcinoma and the Barrett's mucosa were found at the initial examination. Only 2 of the remaining 104 patients had developed carcinoma on follow-up, an incidence of one tumor per 441 patient-years of follow-up. In a similar study in Boston published in 1984,[35] 8 of 10 carcinomas were detected among 113 patients with Barrett's mucosa at initial evaluation. Two cancers had developed in the remaining 105 patients at the time of follow-up, an incidence of one cancer per 175 patient-years of follow-up. A study in England places the incidence at one cancer per 56 patient-years of follow-up.[30] Thus, although there may be some geographic or population differences in the estimation of incidence, in all these studies the risk of esophageal carcinoma in people with Barrett's mucosa is at least 20 to 50 times the risk for esophageal squamous cancer in the general population.[37]

Yet, even with the data indicating increased risk for adenocarcinoma, we currently do not know whether every patient with Barrett's mucosa should undergo surveillance, nor do we know the true prevalence of Barrett's esophagus in the population. Barrett's mucosa is a postreflux event, and heartburn is the characteristic symptom of reflux, but heartburn is an extraordinarily common symptom. If we were to perform esophagoscopy on every patient with heartburn and take multiple-level biopsies from the esophagus, we would be able to identify the symptomatic population with Barrett's mucosa. In one such study, it was found that Barrett's mucosa occurs commonly in patients with long-standing symptomatic reflux.[41] However, many patients with Barrett's mucosa do not have typical symptoms and may even be asymptomatic.[2,3] They would not be identified in any such study. It is believed that, were they to be identified, the population of patients with Barrett's carcinoma in the United States alone would be too huge for surveillance purposes.[41] It must be remembered that any surveillance study must have a low cost:benefit ratio, indicating that the cost is relatively small considering the benefits that accrue. It would be ideal, then, to identify a specific subset of high-risk patients that constitutes a more manageable group for cancer surveillance. So far, we have not been able to identify this high-risk group based on clinical features.

Because it is the specialized mucosa that seems to be the bed for carcinomas, recent studies have focused on the different types of intestinal metaplasia and their use in defining a high-risk population. It has been suggested that type III incomplete intestinal metaplasia with sulfated acid mucins in the intermediate or gastric-type surface cells helps in identifying esophagi at high risk.[16,24] In general, this type of metaplasia appears to have a high

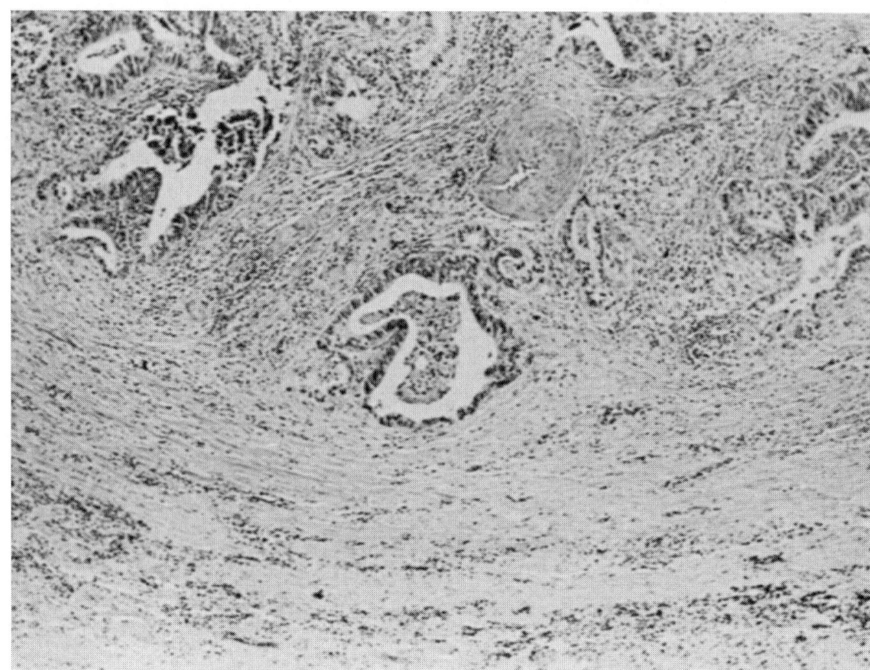

Figure 14–14. Well-differentiated Barrett's carcinoma forms clearly defined tubular structures. (Hematoxylin and eosin, ×33.)

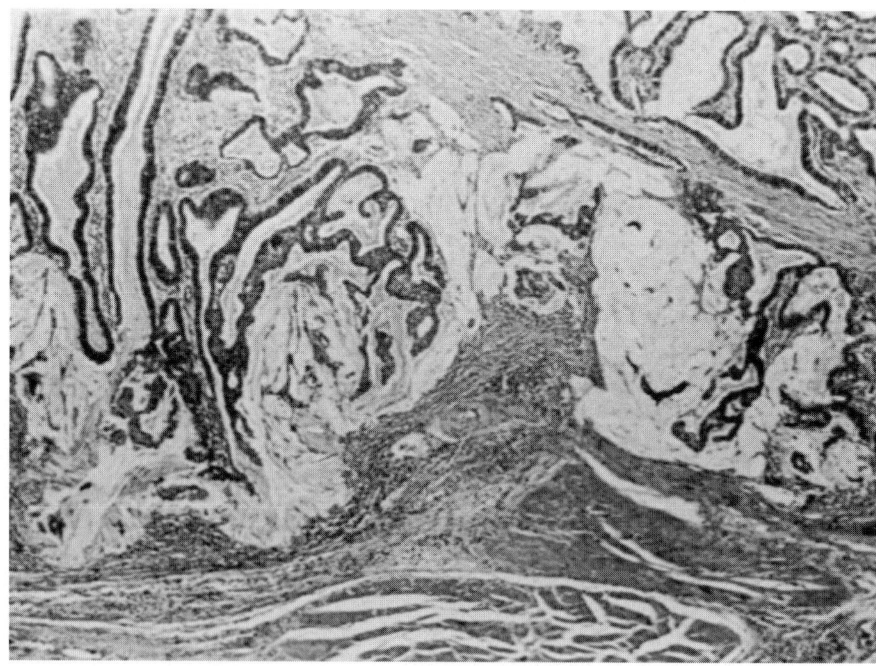

Figure 14–15. Mucinous Barrett's carcinoma has columns of carcinoma surrounded by large pools of mucin. (Hematoxylin and eosin, ×33.)

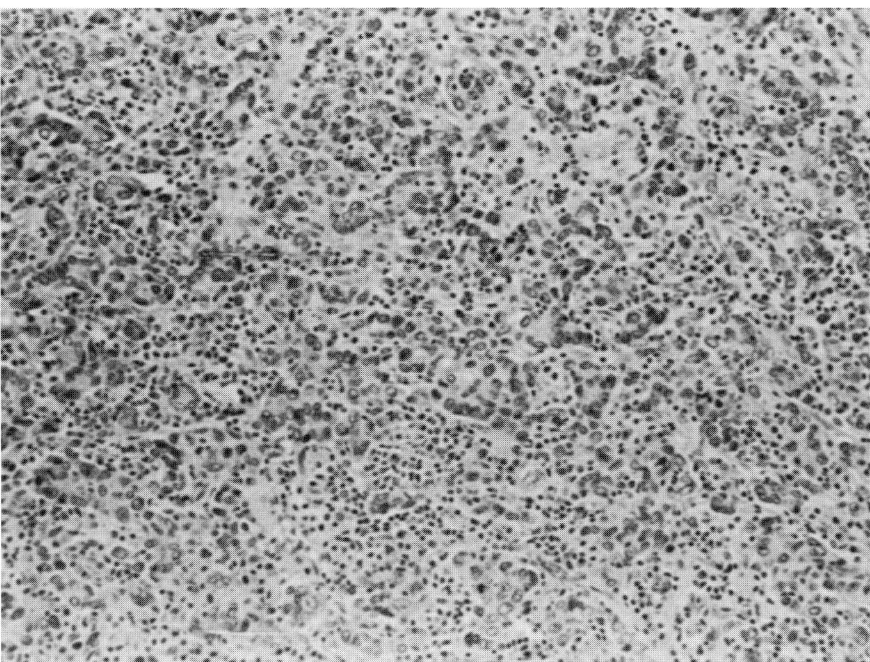

Figure 14–16. Anaplastic carcinoma has strands of carcinoma cells that do not form tubules. (Hematoxylin and eosin, ×132.)

association with carcinoma, but it also occurs often in patients with Barrett's mucosa without carcinoma or carcinoma precursors.[32] Furthermore, when it does occur, it may exist in a very patchy fashion and biopsy specimens may easily miss the patches. Therefore, identification of a high-risk group based on identification of sulfated mucins in the intermediate cells results in both too many false-negatives and too many false-positives to be useful.

The longer the segment of Barrett's mucosa, the greater is the risk of carcinoma. One study from England suggests that patients with long-segment Barrett's have a greater risk of developing dysplasia and carcinoma than those with short-segment Barrett's.[14] Another study, from the United States, suggests that the amount of surface area of esophagus that contains Barrett's mucosa is related to the amount of dysplastic mucosa, but the amount of dysplasia is not related to the risk of carcinoma.[20] This may be true, but we do not know the exact cancer risk per centimeter of Barrett's mucosa.[26,31]

To date, then, we have not identified a high-risk group of patients with Barrett's mucosa, based on either clinical or histologic criteria, who are more in need of surveillance for the development of carcinoma or its precursors than are other individuals. This failure has resulted in considerable conflict. In some centers, it is believed that Barrett's mucosa is too prevalent for its presence alone to constitute an indication for surveillance. In other institutions, Barrett's mucosa, once it has been identified, is a lesion that requires surveillance.

The goal of a surveillance program is to identify patients who may be treated for neoplastic complications at a curative stage. Because the development of adenocarcinoma in Barrett's mucosa is known to be preceded by the morphologically identifiable histologic changes designated as low-grade and high-grade dysplasia, one goal of surveillance of these patients is to find these preinvasive lesions as markers of patients at risk for developing invasive carcinoma and to treat them early with the goal of cure. Another goal is to identify carcinomas when they are minimally invasive and treat them at this early stage.

The histologic appearances and terminology that have been adopted for preinvasive neoplastic lesions in Barrett's mucosa are the same as those that are used for colitic dysplasia.[28] The term dysplasia is reserved for epithelium that is considered to be unequivocally neoplastic. Such epithelium has an increase in nuclear size relative to cytoplasmic volume, nuclear hyperchromatism, increased numbers of mitoses, stratification of nuclei and cells, decreased cytoplasmic maturation with less mucus production, and, sometimes, nuclear pleomorphism. With this definition, anything that occurs in Barrett's mucosa that resembles adenomatous or dysplastic epithelium as seen in the stomach, duodenum, or colon becomes part of the Barrett's dysplasia spectrum. If we apply the definitions for low-grade and high-grade dysplasia that are used for colitic dysplasia, then low-grade dysplasia includes those forms of neoplastic epithelium that more closely resemble normal epithelium, generally those with basal nuclei and lesser degrees of nuclear and cytoplasmic abnormality (Fig. 14–17). High-grade dysplasia includes neoplastic epithelium with more nuclear stratification, greater nuclear abnormalities, less cytoplasmic maturation, and, often, more disordered architecture; thus, this tissue resembles adenomas with higher grades of dysplasia and even epithelium that resembles that of adenocarcinoma (Figs. 14–18 and 14–19).

In the classification of the epithelial changes that occur in patients with ulcerative colitis, not only are low-grade and high-grade dysplasias defined, but also there is a group of epithelial alterations that are not clearly either dysplastic or regenerative. These epithelia are designated as "indefinite for dysplasia."[28] In Barrett's mucosa, the epithelia that are highly dysplastic are usually easily iden-

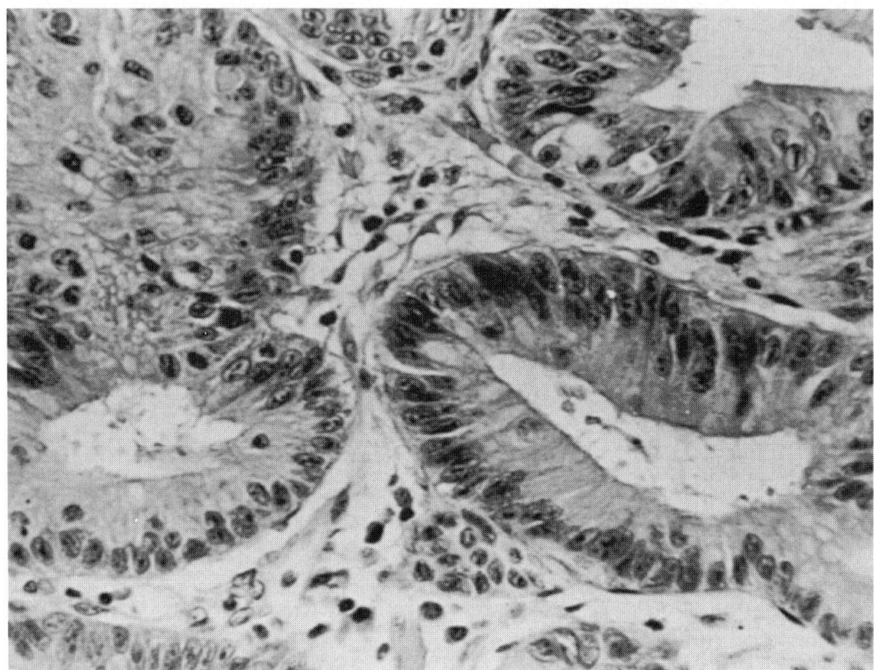

Figure 14–17. Low-grade dysplasia in Barrett's mucosa. These tubules have crowded cells, increased nuclear size, and nuclear stratification limited to the basal half of the cells. (Hematoxylin and eosin, ×330.)

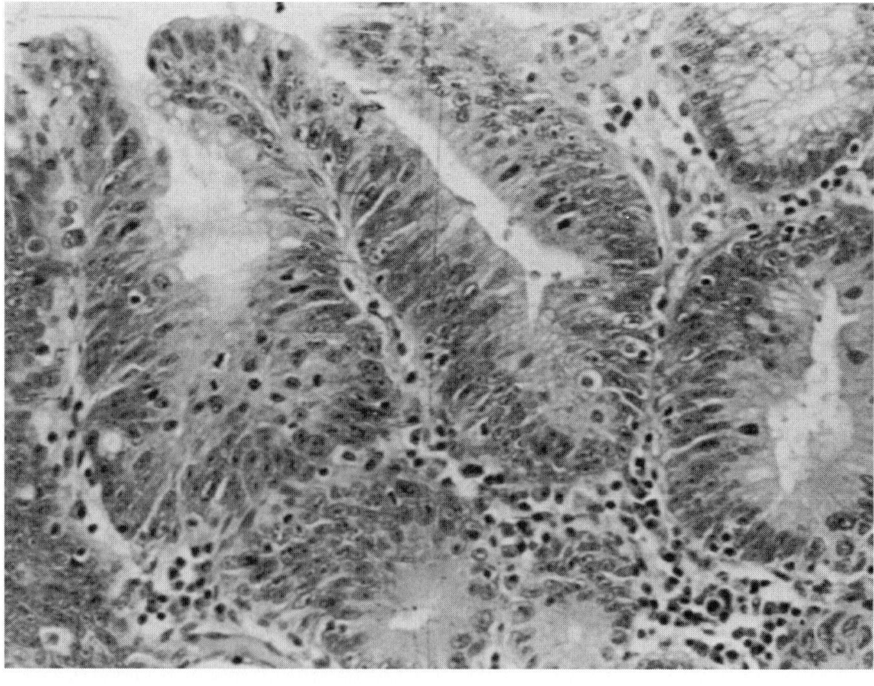

Figure 14–18. High-grade Barrett's dysplasia. This mucosa has cells even more crowded than those in Figure 14–17, with nuclear stratification extending to the luminal surface. (Hematoxylin and eosin, ×208.)

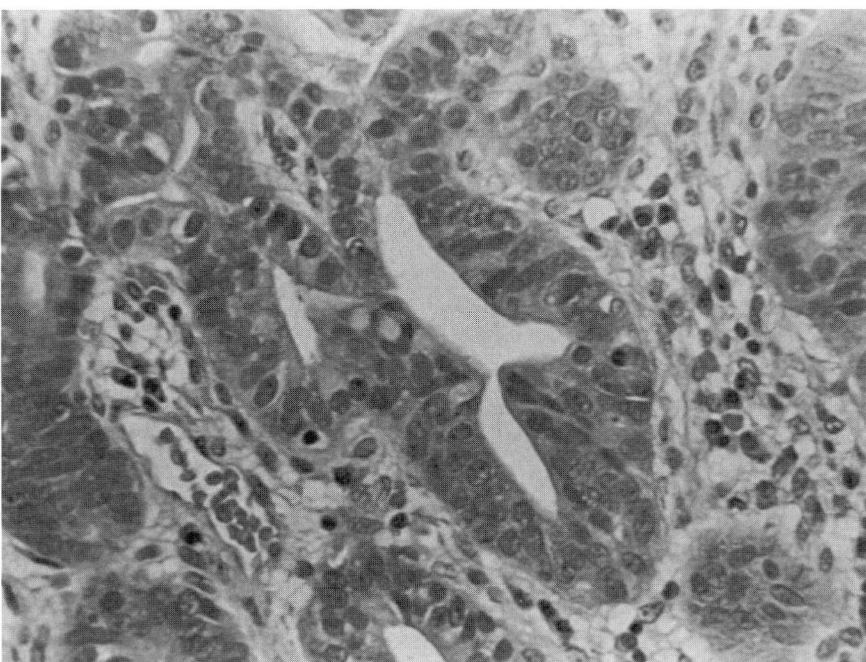

Figure 14–19. Another example of high-grade Barrett's dysplasia. In this complex branching tubule, the nuclei are large, have lost all polarity, and appear at all levels of the cells. (Hematoxylin and eosin, ×330.)

tified. The low-grade dysplastic changes are more difficult to define. According to a group of expert pathologists, the problem of separating low-grade dysplasia from atypical regenerative epithelium is even greater in patients with Barrett's mucosa than in those with colitic mucosa.[25] Many Barrett's mucosae contain regenerative epithelium, presumably as a result of ongoing injury. Because the histologic features of regenerative epithelium may sometimes approach the degree of abnormality present in dysplastic epithelium, especially in low-grade dysplasia, these two are not always definitively separable. The category of "indefinite for dysplasia" is used to identify epithelium in which this separation is not possible (Table 14–2). In some centers, epithelia that are indefinite for dysplasia as well as for low-grade dysplasia are considered together as a single group because the management implications are the same.

Every surveillance program must have some end-point. Obviously, the identification of invasive adenocarcinoma in patients with Barrett's mucosa is a clear indication for esophagectomy and is the end-point used by some. However, in many centers the end-point that has been established is the finding of high-grade dysplasia, because it seems to be a marker of high risk for concurrent carcinoma. Several studies report that when high-grade dysplasia is discovered, the likelihood of a concurrent invasive carcinoma is about 30%.[12] However, in other studies, high-grade dysplasia is followed with more frequent endoscopic examinations, and some high-grade dysplasias are treated with different types of ablation.[19] In these centers, the indication for resection is carcinoma invading the lamina propria. Thus, the indications for resection vary from center to center, and no consensus exists on the appropriate end-point.

Table 14–2. Epithelial Changes in Barrett's Esophagus

Designation	Recommended Management
Negative (no dysplasia)	Ignore? Continue surveillance?
Indefinite (cannot tell if dysplasia is present)	Follow-up with shorter interval
Positive (dysplasia)	
Low-grade	Follow-up with shorter interval
High-grade	Follow-up with very short interval? Resection?
Intramucosal carcinoma (invasion of lamina propria)	Resection

Complicating the situation is the lack of well-defined standards for surveillance. For instance, no standards dictate how often a patient should have esophagoscopy and biopsy, or how many biopsy samples should be taken, or at which sites they should be taken. Some pathologists believe that examination of brush cytologic specimens, in addition to biopsy specimens, increases diagnostic yield.[7] Dysplasia and low-stage carcinomas can be found in flat, innocuous-appearing mucosa as well as in abnormal-appearing mucosa, so there are often no endoscopic markers of where to perform a biopsy.[27] One recommendation is to take four-quadrant biopsy samples at 2-cm increments along flat mucosa as well as of all endoscopic lesions.[27] Likewise, the proper approach to take when high-grade dysplasia is found in a biopsy is not clear-cut. For instance, should a pathologist who is expert in the field review every diagnosis of high-grade dysplasia? Some authors believe this should be done.[27,36] Does a diagnosis of high-grade dysplasia constitute an indication for esophagectomy? Should the follow-up period, whatever it may be, be shortened and rebiopsy and possibly brush cytology undertaken if esophagectomy is not performed? Furthermore, what constitutes a shortened follow-up interval? What should be done for patients with low-grade dysplasia? Does this lesion require a shorter period of follow-up? Some low-grade dysplasias evolve into high-grade lesions. Which ones will, and how long will this evolution take? At the moment, these questions have not been answered, the data are still inconclusive, and it is possible that anything that is done for these patients may be performed on the basis of a best estimate and on the clinical status of the individual.[27]

To summarize, we know that many people in the general population suffer from chronic heartburn. In this population, and even in the population without heartburn, short-segment Barrett's mucosa appears to be common. We have not identified a set of clinical or histologic features that defines a high-risk clinical group within the population with Barrett's mucosa that requires cancer surveillance. Finally, once surveillance programs are undertaken, we are not absolutely certain what courses of action will be dictated by the biopsy changes that are found. In some centers, the finding of clear-cut, confirmed, high-grade columnar dysplasia is an indication for resection, because of the high risk of unsuspected, concurrent invasive adenocarcinoma. In other centers, the indication for resection is invasive carcinoma.

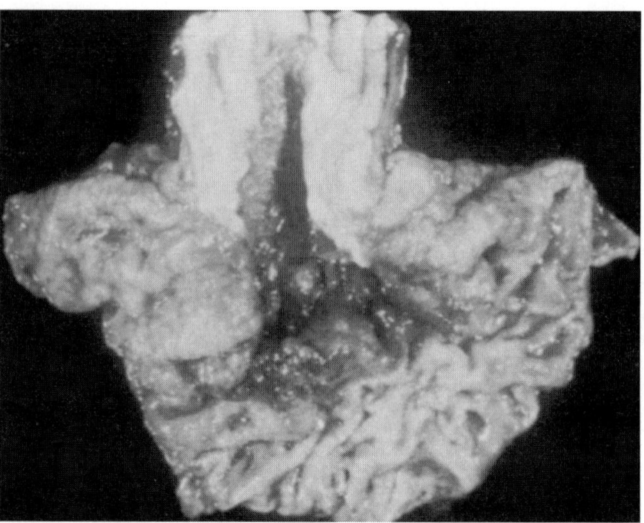

Figure 14–21. This cardiac carcinoma is mainly ulcerating. The large part of the ulcer is below the junction, but there is an extension into the totally squamous-lined distalmost esophagus.

RELATIONSHIP BETWEEN BARRETT'S CARCINOMA AND OTHER ADENOCARCINOMAS OCCURRING ABOUT THE CARDIOESOPHAGEAL JUNCTION

Barrett's carcinoma is only one form of adenocarcinoma that occurs close to the cardioesophageal junction. Identical carcinomas occur on the gastric side within the cardiac mucosa; they are called cardiac carcinomas (Figs. 14–20 and 14–21).[17,39,40] To complicate matters, there is a group of carcinomas that span and obliterate the junction, do not have any clear-cut Barrett's mucosa around them, and do not have any dysplasia on either the gastric side or the esophageal side (Fig. 14–22). These carcinomas constitute a group of junctional carcinomas of uncertain origin. In our experience, more than 90% of the carcinomas that occur in this region can be separated into either the Barrett's or the cardiac type, with less than 10% classified as junctional carcinomas of uncertain origin.[1]

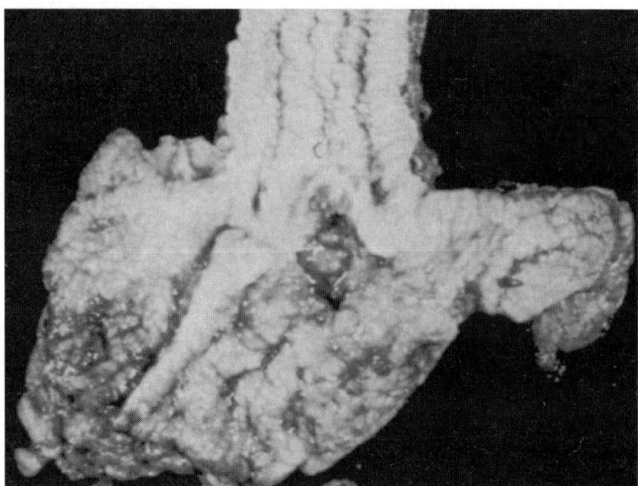

Figure 14–20. Cardiac carcinomas such as this one arise immediately below the cardioesophageal junction. This tumor has a central ulcer with nodular, somewhat radiating folds below.

Carcinomas that arise in the gastric cardia are slightly more difficult to define than those arising in Barrett's mucosa, mainly because the cardiac mucosa itself is such a small region, and its extent is quite unpredictable. In general, the cardiac region comprises the 1 to 2 cm surrounding the opening of the esophagus, immediately below the cardioesophageal junction. It has a columnar mucosa almost identical to that found in the distal stomach with a superficial pit compartment and a deep glandular compartment composed of clusters of neutral mucin-secreting glands. A carcinoma can be identified as a cardiac carcinoma if it arises immediately below the esophagogastric junction, lies predominantly within that region, and replaces all or most of the cardiac mucosa while sparing the distal stomach. It is ideal to find dysplasia in the cardiac mucosa at only the edges. However, when these carcinomas are found, they tend to be at a high stage and large; as a result, because the area of cardiac mucosa itself is so small, there may be no residual cardiac mucosa in which to identify dysplasia. Thus, although it is common to find dysplasia in Barrett's mucosa at the edges of Barrett's carcinomas, the identification of cardiac dysplasia at the edges of cardiac carcinomas is unusual, occurring in only about 10% of cases.[17] The precursor of cardiac carcinoma is not known. It has been suggested that intestinal metaplasia in the cardia is a precursor, but there is little evidence to support this. As mentioned earlier, goblet cells at the gastric cardia are common.

Grossly, cardiac carcinomas have a tendency to be ulcerating with heaped-up edges, and this complex commonly surrounds the opening of the esophagus (see Fig. 14–20). Occasionally, these carcinomas extend across the cardioesophageal junction and into the distal squamous-lined part of the tubular esophagus (see Fig. 14–21).

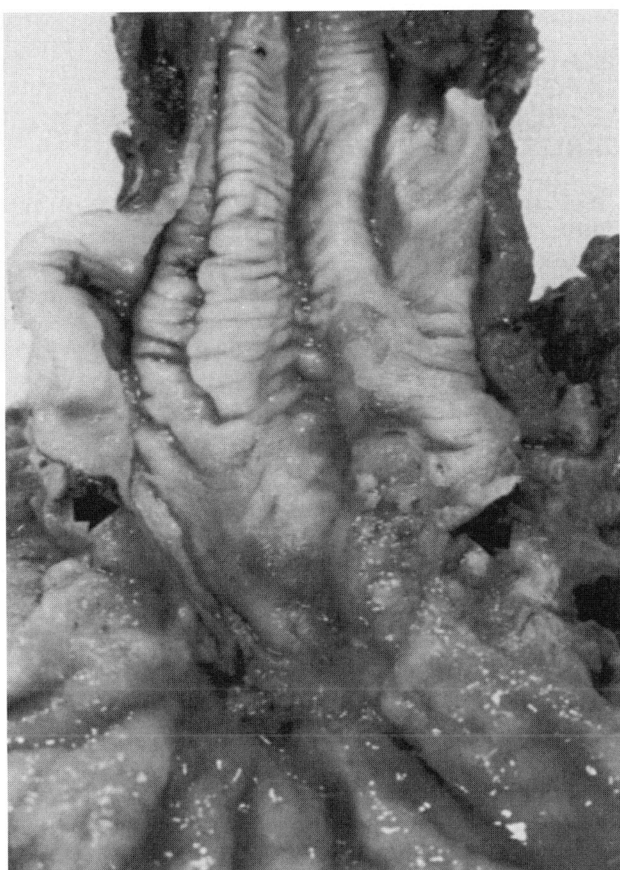

Figure 14–22. This carcinoma crosses the cardioesophageal junction *(arrows)* and has almost equal components on both sides. It is impossible to tell whether it arose in the cardia or in a Barrett's mucosa.

As mentioned earlier, from the standpoint of gross and microscopic features, there are no significant differences between Barrett's and cardiac carcinomas.

Epidemiologic factors associated with cardiac carcinomas vary from one study to the next, perhaps because of geographic and/or definitional differences. Like patients with Barrett's carcinoma, those with cardiac carcinoma are likely to be white males, but it is not clear whether cardiac carcinomas are a consequence of reflux or whether other factors are more important. In some studies, cardiac carcinomas have a stronger association with alcohol use and/or smoking than do Barrett's carcinomas,[1,17,29] but in other studies this is not the case.[10,22,39,40] In contrast, Barrett's carcinomas tend to occur in patients who have precursors of Barrett's mucosa, including hiatal hernias, and almost half the patients in one series neither smoked nor drank.[1] Many of the discrepancies in these findings may relate to the criteria used, in that the criteria for designating a carcinoma near the cardioesophageal junction as either cardiac or esophageal in origin were not the same from one study to the next. In addition, other factors, perhaps environmental ones, may contribute to the differences in epidemiologic associations.

References

1. Appelman, H.D., Kalish, R.J., Clancy, P.E., et al.: Distinguishing features of adenocarcinoma in Barrett's esophagus and in the gastric cardia. *In* Spechler, S.J., and Goyal, R.K. (eds.): Barrett's Esophagus: Pathophysiology, Diagnosis, and Management. New York, Elsevier, 1985, p. 167.
2. Cameron, A.J., Ott, B.J., and Payne, W.S.: The incidence of adenocarcinoma in columnar-lined (Barrett's) esophagus. N. Engl. J. Med., *313*:857, 1985.
3. Cameron, A.J., Zinmeister, A.R., Ballard, D.J., and Carney, J.A.: Prevalence of columnar-lined (Barrett's) esophagus. Gastroenterology, *99*:918, 1990.
4. Cameron, A.J., and Lomboy, C.T.: Barrett's esophagus: Age, prevalence, and extent of columnar epithelium. Gastroenterology, *103*:1241, 1992.
5. Clark, G.W., Ireland, A.P., Peters, J.H., et al.: Short-segment Barrett's esophagus: A prevalent complication of gastroesophageal reflux disease with malignant potential. J. Gastrointest. Surg., *1*:113, 1997.
6. Filipe, M.I., Potet, F., Bogomoletz, W.V., et al.: Incomplete sulphomucin-secreting intestinal metaplasia for gastric cancer: Preliminary data from a prospective study from three centres. Gut, *26*:1319, 1985.
7. Geisinger, K.R., Teot, L.A., and Richter, J.E.: A comparative cytopathologic and histologic study of atypia, dysplasia, and adenocarcinoma in Barrett's esophagus. Cancer *69*:8, 1992.
8. Gillen, P., Keeling, P., and Hennessy, T.P.J: Barrett's esophagus: Risk factors for malignancy (Abstract). Gut, *28*:A1379, 1987.
9. Goldblum, J.R., Vicari, J.J., Falk, G.W., et al.: Inflammation and intestinal metaplasia of the gastric cardia: The role of gastroesophageal reflux and *H. pylori*. Gastroenterology, *114*:633, 1998.
10. Gray, J.R., Coldman, A.J., and MacDonald, W.C.: Cigarette and alcohol use in patients with adenocarcinoma of the gastric cardia or lower esophagus. Cancer, *69*:2227, 1992.
11. Haggitt, R.C.: Barrett's esophagus, dysplasia, and adenocarcinoma. Hum. Pathol., *25*:982, 1994.
12. Hamilton, S.R., and Smith, R.R.L.: The relationship between columnar epithelial dysplasias and invasive adenocarcinoma arising in Barrett's esophagus. Am. J. Clin. Pathol., *87*:301, 1987.
13. Hirota, W.K., Loughney, T.M., Lazas, D.J., et al.: Specialized intestinal metaplasia, dysplasia and cancer of the esophagus and esophagogastric junction: Prevalence and clinical data. Gastroenterology, *116*:277, 1999.
14. Iftikhar, S.Y., James, P.D., Steele, R.J.C., et al.: Length of Barrett's oesophagus: An important factor in the development of dysplasia and adenocarcinoma. Gut, *33*:1155, 1992.
15. Jabbari, M., Goresky, C.A., Lough, J., et al.: The inlet patch: Heterotopic gastric mucosa in the upper esophagus. Gastroenterology, *89*:352, 1985.
16. Jass, J.R.: Mucin histochemistry of the columnar epithelium of the oesophagus: A retrospective study. J. Clin. Pathol., *34*:866, 1981.
17. Kalish, R.J., Clancy, P.E., Orringer, M.B., et al.: Clinical epidemiologic and morphologic comparison between adenocarcinomas arising in Barrett's esophageal mucosa and in the gastric cardia. Gastroenterology, *86*:461, 1984.
18. Lee, R.G.: Mucins in Barrett's esophagus: A histochemical study. Am. J. Clin. Pathol., *81*:500, 1984.
19. Levine, D.S., Haggitt, R.C., Blount, P.L., et al.: An endoscopic biopsy protocol can differentiate high-grade dysplasia from early adenocarcinoma in Barrett's esophagus. Gastroenterology, *105*:40, 1993.
20. McArdle, J.E., Lewin, K.J., Randzil, G., and Weinstein, W.: Distribution of dysplasia and early invasive carcinoma in Barrett's esophagus. Hum. Pathol., *23*:479, 1992.
21. Naef, A.P., Savary, M., and Ozzello, L.: Columnar-lined lower esophagus: An acquired lesion with malignant predisposition. J. Thorac. Cardiovasc. Surg., *70*:826, 1975.
22. Palli, D., Bianchi, S., Decarli, A., et al.: A case-control study of cancers of the gastric cardia in Italy. Br. J. Cancer, *65*:263, 1992.
23. Paull, A., Trier, J.S., Dalton, M.D., et al.: The histologic spectrum of Barrett's esophagus. N. Engl. J. Med., *295*:476, 1976.
24. Peuchmaur, M., Potet, F., and Goldfain, D.: Mucin histochemistry of the columnar epithelium of the oesophagus (Barrett's oesophagus): A prospective biopsy study. J. Clin. Pathol., *37*:607, 1984.
25. Reid, B.J., Haggitt, R.C., Rubin, C.E., et al.: Criteria for dysplasia in Barrett's esophagus: A cooperative consensus study (Abstract). Gastroenterology, *88*:1552, 1985.
26. Reid, B.J., and Rubin, C.E.: When is the columnar-lined esophagus premalignant? (Abstract). Gastroenterology, *88*:1552, 1985.
27. Reid, B.J., Weinstein, W.M., Lewin, K.J., et al.: Endoscopic biopsy

can detect high-grade dysplasia or early adenocarcinoma in Barrett's esophagus without grossly recognizable neoplastic lesions. Gastroenterology, *94:*81, 1988.
28. Riddell, R.H., Goldman, H., Ransohoff, D.F., et al.: Dysplasia in inflammatory bowel disease: Standardized classification with provisional clinical applications. Hum. Pathol., *14:*931, 1983.
29. Rios-Castellanos, E., Sitas, F., Sheperd, N.A., and Jewell, D.P.: Changing pattern of gastric cancer in Oxfordshire. Gut, *33:*1312, 1992.
30. Robertson, C.S., Mayberry, J.F., James, P.D., et al.: Value of endoscopic surveillance in the early detection of malignant changes in Barrett's oesophagus (Abstract). Gut, *28:*A1379, 1987.
31. Rosenberg, J.C., Budev, H., Edwards, R.C., et al.: Analysis of adenocarcinoma in Barrett's esophagus utilizing a staging system. Cancer, *55:*1353, 1985.
32. Rothery, G.A., Patterson, J.E., Stoddard, C.J., et al.: Histological and histochemical changes in the columnar lined (Barrett's) oesophagus. Gut, *27:*1062, 1986.
33. Schnell, T.G., Sontag, S.J., and Chejfec, G.: Adenocarcinomas arising in tongues of short segments of Barrett's esophagus. Dig. Dis. Sci., *37:*137, 1992.
34. Smith, R.R.L., Hamilton, S.R., Boitnott, J.K., et al.: The spectrum of carcinoma arising in Barrett's esophagus: A clinicopathologic study of 26 patients. Am. J. Surg. Pathol., *8:*563, 1984.
35. Spechler, S.J., Robbins, A.H., Rubins, H.B., et al.: Adenocarcinomas and Barrett's esophagus: An overrated risk? Gastroenterology, *87:*927, 1984.
36. Spechler, S.J., and Goyal, R.K.: Barrett's esophagus. N. Engl. J. Med., *315:*362, 1986.
37. Spechler, S.J.: Endoscopic surveillance for patients with Barrett's esophagus: Does the cancer risk justify the practice? (Editorial). Ann. Intern. Med., *106:*902, 1987.
38. Spechler, S.J., Zeroogian, J.M., Antonioli, D.A., et al.: Prevalence of metaplasia at the gastro-oesophageal junction. Lancet, *344:*1533, 1994.
39. Thompson, J.J., Zinsser, K.R., and Enterline, H.T.: Barrett's metaplasia and adenocarcinoma of the esophagus and gastroesophageal junction. Hum. Pathol., *14:*42, 1983.
40. Wang, H.H., Antonioli, D.A., and Goldman, H.: Comparative features of esophageal and gastric adenocarcinomas: Recent changes in type and frequency. Hum. Pathol., *17:*482, 1986.
41. Winters, C. Jr., Spurling, T.J., Chobanian, S.J., et al.: Barrett's esophagus: A prevalent occult complication of gastroesophageal reflux disease. Gastroenterology, *92:*118, 1987.

CHAPTER

15 Barrett's Esophagus: Surgical Implications

VICTOR F. TRASTEK

In 1906, Tileston reported on peptic ulcerations arising in the lower esophagus lined by columnar epithelium.[38] In 1950, Barrett (Fig. 15-1), at the Brompton Hospital in London, described a condition characterized by a columnar epithelium-lined tube extending below the squamocolumnar junction in patients with hiatal hernia and reflux. Barrett postulated initially that this tube was an attenuated segment of stomach drawn into the chest by a shortened esophagus. Subsequently, Allison and Johnstone[1] suggested that the condition described by Barrett was indeed a columnar epithelium-lined lower esophagus with cephalad displacement of the squamocolumnar junction above the anatomic esophagogastric junction. During the ensuing decades, a clearer picture of the genesis, morphology, complications, and implications of Barrett's esophagus has become evident. Today, Barrett's ulcer, Barrett's stricture, and Barrett's carcinoma have all been well described and suggest that this process with its associated secondary complications may best be described as Barrett's disease.[6,16,24,27]

The initial explanation of this condition was that the aberrant mucosa was entirely congenital, but the frequent association of Barrett's esophagus with hiatal hernia, hypotensive lower esophageal sphincter, and symptomatic reflux with a positive acid reflux test result has overwhelmingly suggested that the condition is an acquired process that is a consequence of chronic gastroesophageal and duodenal content reflux.[3,9,17] Findings constituting further evidence of an acquired and reflux-initiated condition are peptic ulceration within the columnar epithelium-lined segment (Barrett's ulcer), frequent development of an inflammatory stenosis at the displaced squamocolumnar junction, and esophagitis in the squamous epithelium just above the squamocolumnar junction. Indeed, cephalad migration of the squamocolumnar junction has been frequently observed, and antireflux procedures have been routinely noted to arrest progression and resolve stenosis, inflammation, and ulceration. Also against the theory of congenital causation is the fact that usually the cervical or high thoracic esophagus of the developing fetus is the last area of columnar epithelium to be replaced by squamous epithelium. Finally, the production of Barrett's esophagus in laboratory animals has added validity to the hypothesis that the condition is acquired and reflux induced.[5]

Although it remains unclear which patients will develop Barrett's esophagus and in whom it will progress to adenocarcinoma, it does appear that there may be an inherited predisposition for this process. Families with multiple members over more than one generation who have Barrett's esophagus and adenocarcinoma have been reported.[11,17]

The nature of Barrett's metaplasia of the lower esophagus has been the subject of considerable scrutiny and of pivotal interest since it became evident that this epithelium could be the origin of the adenocarcinoma of the esophagus. How it develops, whether as a "creeping" or sloughing process, is unclear.[8] Work done by Gillen suggests that the epithelium arises from multipotential stem cells located in submucosal esophageal glands.[12] Three types of columnar epithelial metaplasia have been defined: (1) specialized villiform type, resembling intestinal mucosa; (2) junctional cardial epithelium with mucus-secreting cells free of chief and parietal cells; and (3)

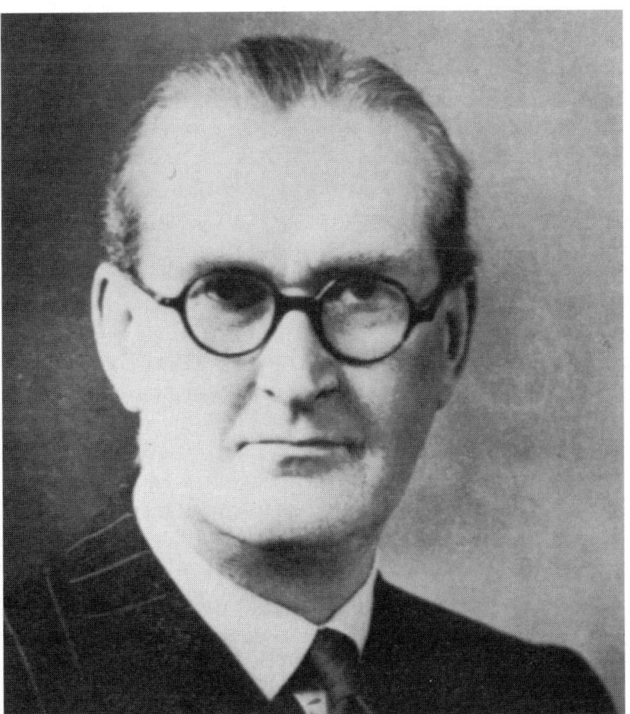

Figure 15-1. Norman Rupert Barrett (1903-1979) was the first to draw attention to the phenomenon of the columnar epithelium-lined lower esophagus, which bears his name and is still a clinical enigma. (From Payne, W.S.: Norman Rupert Barrett, C.B.E., F.R.C.S., M.Chir. [1903-1979]. Cardiopulm. Med., *18*:8, 1979, by permission of the American College of Chest Physicians.)

Table 15–1. Results of Studies of the Incidence of Esophageal Cancer in Patients With Barrett's Esophagus*

Study Findings	Study Center: *Boston VA Hospital*†	*Mayo Clinic*‡	*Lahey Clinic*§
Patients (total no.)	115	122	108
Prevalence of esophageal cancer (%)	7	15	22
Cancer-free patients followed up (no.)	105	104	41
Mean (range) length of follow-up (yr)	3.3 (0.1–20)	8.5 (3 to >15)	4 (1–11)
Patients in whom cancer developed during follow-up (no.)	2	2	2
Length of follow-up before cancer development in each patient (yr)	5.3 and 8	6 and 10	3.5 and 4.3
Incidence of esophageal cancer (cases/person-years)	1/175	1/441	1/81
Estimated increased risk above that in general population	40-fold	30-fold	Not available

*From Spechler, S.J., and Goyal, R.K.: Barrett's esophagus. N. Engl. J. Med., *315*:362, 1986, by permission of the *New England Journal of Medicine.*
†From Spechler, S.J., Robbins, A.H., Rubins, H.B., et al.: Adenocarcinoma and Barrett's esophagus: An overrated risk? Gastroenterology, *87*:927, 1984.
‡From Cameron, A.J., Ott, B.J., and Payne, W.S.: The incidence of adenocarcinoma in columnar-lined (Barrett's) esophagus. N. Engl. J. Med., *313*:857, 1985.
§From Sprung, D.J., Ellis, F.H., Jr., and Gibb, S.P.: Incidence of adenocarcinoma in Barrett's esophagus (Abstract). Am. J. Gastroenterol., *79*:817, 1984.

gastric-fundic type with chief and parietal cells.[23] Currently, specialized intestinal metaplasia is the only form at risk for progression to dysplasia and subsequent adenocarcinoma.[7] Biopsy proof of this form is required to confirm the diagnosis of Barrett's esophagus, whether it is of the long-segment (≥ 3 cm) or the short-segment (< 3 cm) variety.[30]

BARRETT'S ESOPHAGUS: A PREMALIGNANT CONDITION?

In 1952, Morson and Belcher[21] were the first to call attention to the development of adenocarcinoma in the columnar epithelium-lined lower esophagus of Barrett. As both Barrett's esophagus and its association with cancer have become more widely recognized, the prevalence of both conditions, either singly or in combination, has increased.

Making this increase even more striking is the finding that there appears to be a marked underestimation of the true prevalence of Barrett's esophagus in the general population. A clinical autopsy review by Cameron and associates[10] demonstrated that the estimated age- and sex-specific prevalence of Barrett's esophagus based on autopsy findings was 376 in a population of 100,000, approximately 16 times more than what had been clinically diagnosed in the same geographic area. The incidence of the development of Barrett's esophagus in patients with gastroesophageal reflux is not well documented. Lomboy and colleagues[19] reported seven patients with reflux esophagitis who developed Barrett's metaplasia over a mean interval of 1.6 years. Also, Schnell and coworkers[31] followed 725 patients whose initial biopsy showed no evidence of Barrett's esophagus; 8% later developed Barrett's metaplasia.

The reported prevalence of adenocarcinoma in the columnar epithelium-lined lower esophagus has varied widely, from 6.6% to 46%.[9,14,15,22,29,33] Although such data have alerted us to a propensity for the development of malignant disease in Barrett's esophagus, such data cannot be used to assess the risk of cancer developing later in a patient with benign Barrett's esophagus.

The report of Hawe and coworkers[15] in 1973 was the first study that attempted to address this problem. Among 85 patients diagnosed in a 20-year period as having benign Barrett's esophagus, retrospective follow-up showed that cancer of Barrett's esophagus developed in only two. More stringent incidence studies were provided by three subsequent reports (Table 15–1).[9,36,37] Along with this is the finding that the incidence of adenocarcinoma of the esophagus and esophagogastric junction seems to be rising not only in the United States but also in western Europe[25] (Fig. 15–2). Obviously, all of these studies have shortcomings, because it is not known how long patients had had Barrett's esophagus before diagnosis and entry into the study, nor is it certain that the diagnostic criteria for entry were not overly selective. In any event, longer-term follow-up of larger numbers of patients is required to place this problem in better perspective. For the present, at least, it is reassuring to note that the survival of patients with benign Barrett's esophagus is roughly similar to that of an age- and sex-adjusted general population (Fig. 15–3).

BARRETT'S ESOPHAGUS WITH CANCER

At the Mayo Clinic between 1970 and 1985, 62 patients underwent resection for invasive adenocarcinoma of the

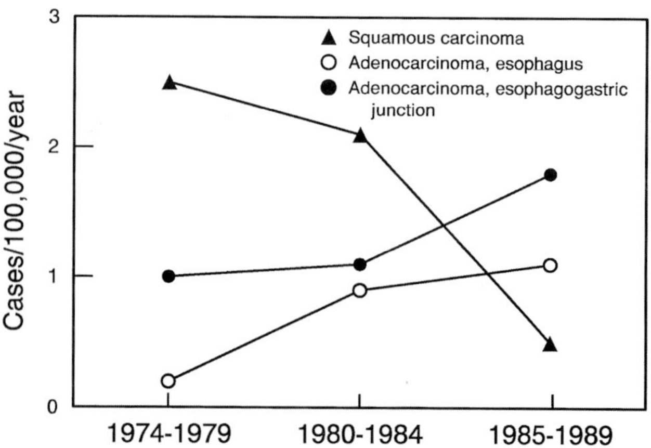

Figure 15–2. Incidence of squamous carcinoma, esophageal adenocarcinoma, and adenocarcinoma of the esophagogastric junction during three discrete periods.

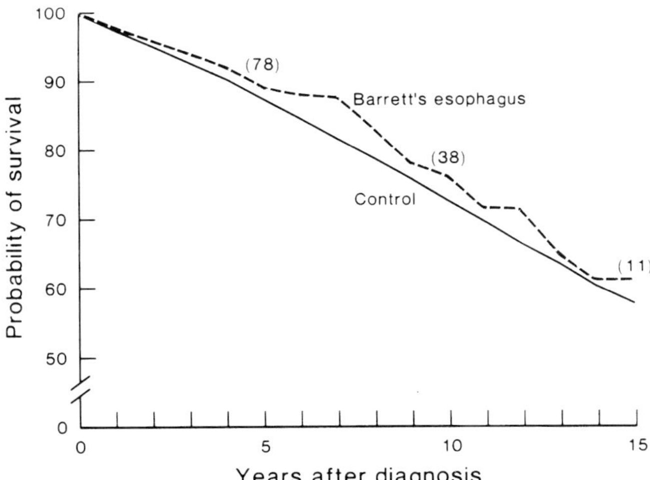

Figure 15–3. Comparison of age- and sex-adjusted survival rates for 104 patients with Barrett's esophagus and a control population. The numbers in parentheses indicate patients still at risk. (From Cameron, A.J., Ott, B.J., and Payne, W.S.: The incidence of adenocarcinoma in columnar-lined [Barrett's] esophagus. N. Engl. J. Med., *313*:857, 1985. Reprinted by permission of the New England Journal of Medicine.)

Table 15–2. Location of Squamocolumnar Junction in Barrett's Esophagus and Site of Adenocarcinoma Arising in the Columnar Epithelium in 62 Patients

Level of Involved Esophagus	No. of Patients: *Highest Level of Barrett's Esophagus*	No. of Patients: *Highest Location of Carcinoma**
Upper third (to 24 cm)	2	1
Middle third (24–32 cm)	32	12
Lower third (32 cm–GE junction†)	28	49

From Payne, W.S., McAfee, M.K., Trastek, V.F., et al.: Adenocarcinoma of the columnar epithelial-lined lower esophagus of Barrett. *In* Delarue, M.C., Wilkins, E.W., Jr., and Wong, J. (eds.): International Trends in General Thoracic Surgery, Vol. 4. St. Louis, C. V. Mosby, 1988, p. 256, by permission of the publisher.

*Eight of the 62 resected specimens had multicentric malignant lesions, and these were often diffuse and confluent.

†GE = gastroesophageal.

esophagus associated with Barrett's esophagus (Table 15–2). The ages of these patients ranged from 36 to 84 years (median, 60 years); 59 of the 62 were men. During this same period, one additional patient with just atypia (dysplasia) and three additional patients with carcinoma in situ also underwent resection, but they were excluded from the 62 patients above and the following staging-survival analysis.[2] Twelve (19%) of the 62 patients had stage I disease ($T_1N_0M_0$), and only one of these died of recurrent disease, with a mean follow-up of 41 months. Thirteen patients (21%) had stage II disease ($T_2N_0M_0$); six died, and seven (54%) were alive without evidence of disease. Thirty-seven patients had stage III disease ($T_{1-3}N_1M_0$). In this group, there were four operative deaths; at follow-up, four of the remaining 33 patients were living, but 2 of these had known recurrences (10.8% survival). All four patients with atypia or in situ cancer were living and well at follow-up 1 to 5 years after resection.

On pathologic examination, 35 of 62 resected specimens showed high-grade dysplasia or carcinoma in situ in otherwise benign columnar epithelium adjacent to the invasive cancer. There did not appear to be any consistently predominant type of residual benign Barrett's columnar epithelium associated with neoplasm. Eight of the 62 resected specimens had multicentric malignant foci within Barrett's epithelium (Fig. 15–4). A solitary focus of malignancy, which was more common, was frequently found at the squamocolumnar epithelial juncture (Fig. 15–5).

Of special interest was the observation that five patients underwent resection of the esophagus during this period entirely on the basis of the results of biopsy of the columnar epithelium-lined lower esophagus, which showed only high-grade dysplasia in four patients and carcinoma in situ in one patient. In all five, this was the only histologic finding of concern. In one patient, however, the esophageal radiograph suggested malignancy. In three of these five cases, an obvious invasive cancer was defined in the surgical specimen. Others have commented on the occurrence of the epithelial atypia and its association with cancer in patients with Barrett's esophagus,[13,14,18,28,33-35] but our early experience has led us to use this occurrence as an indication for resection, even in the absence of clinically apparent biopsy-proven invasive malignant disease.

We subsequently reported on 19 patients who had

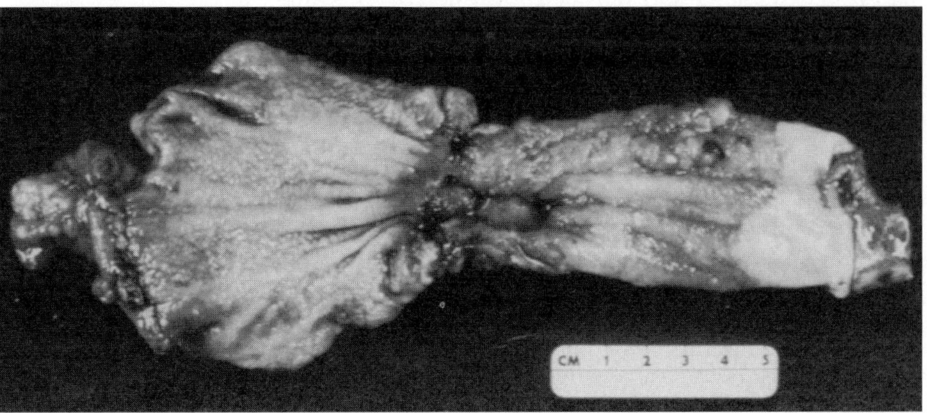

Figure 15–4. Thoracic esophagus and lesser curvature of stomach show multicentric (two) foci of invasive carcinoma in Barrett's esophagus. Progressive dysphagia to solids developed in the patient, a 59-year-old man with an anatomic sliding esophageal hiatal hernia who did not have a history of gastroesophageal reflux symptoms or alcohol or tobacco abuse. Subsequent radiography and endoscopy defined columnar epithelium-lined lower esophagus with squamocolumnar junction just above the aortic arch and more distal invasive cancer near the esophagogastric junction. Not until the specimen was opened was the second, higher-invasive cancer appreciated.

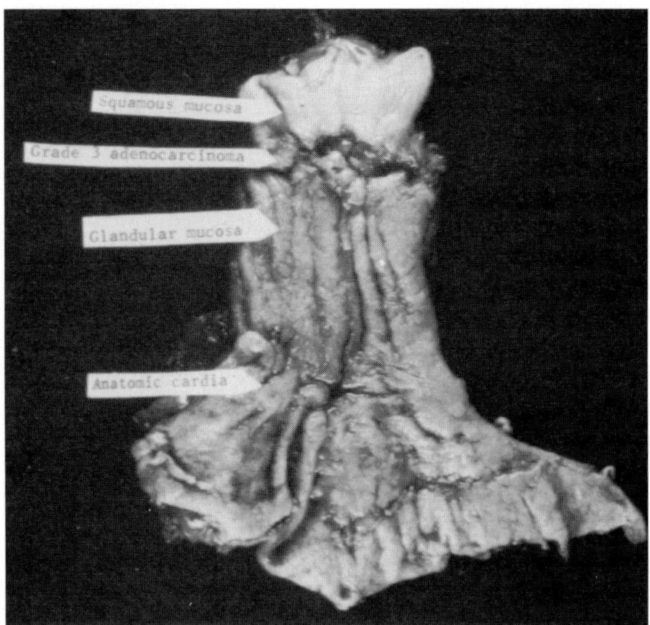

Figure 15–5. Adenocarcinoma developing at the site of the cephalad-displaced (5 cm) squamocolumnar junction. (From Hawe, A., Payne, W.S., Weiland, L.H., et al.: Adenocarcinoma in the columnar epithelial lined lower [Barrett] oesophagus. Thorax, *28*:511, 1973, with permission.)

only high-grade dysplasia on preoperative endoscopic biopsy. Eighteen patients underwent resection without operative death, and nine patients (50%) had invasive carcinoma. Follow-up at 35 months showed recurrent carcinoma in two patients, with an overall 5-year survival rate of 66.7%.[21] After this report, we had the opportunity to observe another 19 patients, and when we combined the groups, we had 38 patients with 36 resections, 15 of whom had invasive carcinoma (41.7%).[39] The overall 5-year survival rate was the same, and there continued to be no operative deaths. When looking at these two groups, it was clear that significant abnormalities (nodules, stenosis, or ulcers) found at the time of endoscopy were significant. Of the 23 patients with abnormal endoscopic appearance, 22 had resection and 13 were found to have invasive disease (61.9%). Of the 15 patients with normal-appearing Barrett's mucosa without abnormality, 14 had resection, and 1 was found to have invasive disease. The role of further observation in patients with high-grade dysplasia and normal-appearing Barrett's mucosa is open to controversy, and we await the long-term results of those following such patients. Until then, our surgical group still considers biopsy-proven high-grade dysplasia an indication for resection (Table 15–3).

Although little evidence exists to suggest that antireflux procedures reverse atypia or indeed the progression of Barrett's epithelium, one could question whether all patients with benign Barrett's esophagus with positive acid-reflux test results, regardless of symptoms or complications, should have an antireflux procedure performed.[6,14,22] Skinner[32] suggested this approach and that an effective antireflux procedure might prevent subsequent malignancy. In McDonald's series of 113 patients with Barrett's esophagus who underwent an antireflux procedure, 3 patients (2.7%) were found to develop adenocarcinoma after repair. Of interest, although follow-up was a median of 6.5 years and up to 18.2 years, all three of the adenocarcinomas were noted early, at 13, 25, and 39 months.[20] It is unclear whether repair in any way protected against the development of later carcinomas. Because only surgical repair completely eliminates reflux, the benefit of early intervention must be considered, even if the patient is asymptomatic. We now give strong consideration to laparoscopic repair in these patients. Although still under evaluation, the ability to ablate the residual mucosa may reinforce the ability to reduce the risk of carcinoma.

Surveillance for patients with apparently benign Barrett's esophagus is recommended. Obviously, such patients have an increased risk of development of adenocarcinoma, but the anticipated detection rate is low enough to frustrate patient compliance with frequent examinations. Brush or balloon cytology for early detection may prove to be a more acceptable alternative for the patient, but its ability to detect occult cancer in Barrett's esophagus or epithelial atypia (dysplasia) has not been fully exploited or defined. For the present, we recommend surveillance endoscopy with large "four-quadrant" biopsies every 2 cm of Barrett's mucosa and thorough biopsy of any abnormal areas (see Table 15–3).

FUTURE

Little did Norman Barrett and the many others who contributed along the way realize the importance of their observations concerning the columnar epithelium-lined esophagus. Certainly, this is one of the most exciting areas in general thoracic surgery. Progress in the knowledge and treatment of Barrett's disease, particularly as it applies to those who may progress to adenocarcinoma, is important. Better understanding of the pathophysiology of the development of metaplasia and progression to invasive cancer is clearly the first step. Ultimately, early intervention may be the best hope to improve survival in these patients. This has been suggested by the results of resection in patients with high-grade dysplasia alone. The ability to differentiate those patients who have high-risk mucosa by analysis of endoscopic biopsy would be very helpful. The use of biologic markers, such as oncogenes, tumor suppressor genes, flow cytometry, and the like,

Table 15–3. Epithelial Changes in Barrett's Esophagus

Designation	Implication
Negative (no dysplasia)	Continue surveillance—at least biyearly.
Indefinite (cannot tell if dysplasia is present)	Repeat biopsy.
Positive (dysplasia)	
Low grade	Continue surveillance—every 6 months.
High grade	Resection
Intramucosal carcinoma (invasion of lamina propria)	Resection

may provide information on which patients need immediate resection and which ones can be observed closely. Surveillance of patients who are found to have Barrett's disease needs to continue. Last, one must consider the opportunity to intervene with the Barrett's disease at an earlier point in time. Prophylactic antireflux procedure in those patients with known Barrett's disease would allow for elimination of both acid- and duodenal-content reflux. Coupling this with complete ablation of the Barrett's mucosa might lead to a reduction in the risk of developing invasive carcinoma. The answers to these important questions will come only from the combined teamwork of the surgeon, gastroenterologist, pathologist, and basic scientist.

References

1. Allison, P.R., and Johnstone, A.S.: The oesophagus lined with gastric mucous membrane. Thorax, *8:*87, 1953.
2. American Joint Committee on Cancer: Manual for Staging of Cancer, 2nd ed. Philadelphia, J.B. Lippincott, 1983, p. 61.
3. Attwood, S.E.A., DeMeester, T.R., Bremner C., et al.: Alkaline gastroesophageal reflux: Implications in the development of complications in Barrett's columnar-lined esophagus. Surgery, *106:*764, 1989.
4. Blot, W.J., Devesa, S.S., Kneller, R.W., et al.: Rising incidence of adenocarcinoma of the esophagus and gastric cardia. JAMA, *265:*1287, 1991.
5. Bremner, C.G., Lynch, V.P., and Ellis, F.H., Jr.: Barrett's esophagus: Congenital or acquired? An experimental study of esophageal mucosal regeneration in the dog. Surgery, *68:*209, 1970.
6. Burgess, J.N., Payne, W.S., Andersen, H.A., et al.: Barrett esophagus: The columnar-epithelial-lined lower esophagus. Mayo Clin. Proc., *46:*728, 1971.
7. Cameron, A.J., Lombay, T.C., and Carpenter, H.A.: Adenocarcinoma of the esophagogastric junction in Barrett's esophagus. Gastroenterology, *109:*1541, 1995.
8. Cameron, A.J., and Lombay, T.C.: Barrett's esophagus: Age, prevalence, and extent of columnar epithelium. Gastroenterology, *103:*1241, 1992.
9. Cameron, A.J., Ott, B.J., and Payne, W.S.: The incidence of adenocarcinoma in columnar-lined (Barrett's) esophagus. N. Engl. J. Med., *313:*857, 1985.
10. Cameron, A.J., Zinsmeister, A.R., Ballard, D.J., et al.: Prevalence of columnar-lined (Barrett's) esophagus: Comparison of population-based clinical and autopsy findings. Gastroenterology, *99:*918, 1990.
11. Crabb, D.W., Berk, M.A., Hall, T.R., et al.: Familial gastroesophageal reflux in the development of Barrett's esophagus. Ann. Intern. Med., *103:*52, 1985.
12. Gillen, P., Keeling, P., Byrne, P.J., et al.: Experimental columnar metaplasia in the canine oesophagus. Br. J. Surg., *75:*113, 1988.
13. Haggitt, R.C., Tryzelaar, J., Ellis, F.H., et al.: Adenocarcinoma complicating columnar epithelium-lined (Barrett's) esophagus. Am. J. Clin. Pathol., *70:*1, 1978.
14. Harle, I.A., Finley, R.J., Belsheim, M., et al.: Management of adenocarcinoma in a columnar-lined esophagus. Ann. Thorac. Surg., *40:*330, 1985.
15. Hawe, A., Payne, W.S., Weiland, L.H., et al.: Adenocarcinoma in the columnar epithelial lined lower (Barrett) oesophagus. Thorax, *28:*511, 1973.
16. Heitmann, P., Strauszer, T., Sapunar, J., et al.: Lower esophagus lined with columnar epithelium: Morphological and physiological correlation. Gastroenterology, *53:*611, 1967.
17. Jochem, V.J., Fuerst, P.A., and Fronkes, J.: Familial Barrett's esophagus associated with adenocarcinoma. Gastroenterology, *102:*1400, 1992.
18. Levine, M.S., Caroline, D., Thompson, J.J., et al.: Adenocarcinoma of the esophagus: Relationship to Barrett mucosa. Radiology, *150:*305, 1984.
19. Lomboy, C.T., Cameron, A.J., and Carpenter, H.A.: Development of Barrett's esophagus: How long does it take? (Abstract). Am. J. Gastroenterol., *86:*1298, 1991.
20. McDonald, M.L., Trastek, V.F., Allen, M.S., et al.: Barrett's esophagus: Does an anti-reflux procedure reduce the need for endoscopic surveillance? J. Thorac. Cardiovasc. Surg., *111:*1135, 1994.
21. Morson, B.C., and Belcher, J.R.: Adenocarcinoma of the oesophagus and ectopic gastric mucosa. Br. J. Cancer, *6:*127, 1952.
22. Naef, A.P., Savary, M., and Ozzello, L.: Columnar-lined lower esophagus: An acquired lesion with malignant predisposition; report on 140 cases of Barrett's esophagus with 12 adenocarcinomas. J. Thorac. Cardiovasc. Surg., *70:*826, 1975.
23. Paull, A., Trier, J.S., Dalton, M.D., et al.: The histologic spectrum of Barrett's esophagus. N. Engl. J. Med., *295:*476, 1976.
24. Pedersen, S.A., Hage, E., Nielsen, P.A., et al.: Barrett's syndrome: Morphological and physiological characteristics. Scand. J. Thorac. Cardiovasc. Surg., *6:*191, 1972.
25. Pera, M., Cameron, A.J., Trastek, V.F., et al.: Increasing incidence of adenocarcinoma of the esophagus and esophagogastric junction. Gastroenterology, *104:*510, 1993.
26. Pera, M., Trastek, V.F., Carpenter, H.A., et al.: Barrett's esophagus with high-grade dysplasia: An indication for esophagectomy? Ann. Thorac. Surg., *54:*199, 1992.
27. Pera, M., Trastek, V.F., Pairolero, P.C., et al.: Barrett's disease: Pathophysiology of metaplasia and adenocarcinoma. Ann. Thorac. Surg., *56:*1191, 1993.
28. Poleynard, G.D., Marty, A.T., Birnbaum, W.B., et al.: Adenocarcinoma in the columnar-lined (Barrett) esophagus: Case report and review of the literature. Arch. Surg., *112:*997, 1977.
29. Radigan, L.R., Glover, J.L., Shipley, F.E., et al.: Barrett esophagus. Arch. Surg., *112:*486, 1977.
30. Schnell, T., Sontag, S., and Schejfec, G.: Adenocarcinoma arising in tongues or short segments of Barrett's esophagus. Dig. Dis. Sci., *37:*137, 1992.
31. Schnell, T., Sontag, S., Chejfec, G., et al.: An attempt to define the incidence of development of Barrett's esophagus (BE). Gastroenterology, *106:*A175, 1994.
32. Skinner, D.B.: The columnar-lined esophagus and adenocarcinoma (Editorial). Ann. Thorac. Surg., *40:*321, 1985.
33. Skinner, D.B., Walther, B.C., Riddell, R.H., et al.: Barrett's esophagus: Comparison of benign and malignant cases. Ann. Surg., *198:*554, 1983.
34. Smith, J.L., Jr.: Pathology of adenocarcinoma of the esophagus and gastroesophageal region, and "Barrett's esophagus" as a predisposing condition. *In* Stroehlein, J.R., and Romsdahl, M.M. (eds.): Gastrointestinal Cancer. New York, Raven Press, 1981, p. 125.
35. Smith, R.R.L., Hamilton, S.R., Boitnott, J.K., et al.: Spectrum of carcinoma arising in Barrett esophagus: A clinicopathologic study of twenty-five patients (Abstract). Lab. Invest., *46:*78A, 1982.
36. Spechler, S.J., Robbins, A.H., Rubins, H.B., et al.: Adenocarcinoma and Barrett's esophagus: An overrated risk? Gastroenterology, *87:*927, 1984.
37. Sprung, D.J., Ellis, F.H., Jr., and Gibb, S.P.: Incidence of adenocarcinoma in Barrett's esophagus (Abstract). Am. J. Gastroenterol., *79:*817, 1984.
38. Tileston, W.: Peptic ulcer of the esophagus. Am. J. Med. Sci., *132:*240, 1906.
39. Trastek, V.F., Pera, M., Pairolero, P.C., et al.: High-grade dysplasia in Barrett's esophagus: Role of surveillance and resection. Paper presented at the 19th Annual Meeting of the Western Thoracic Surgical Association, June 23–26, 1993, Carlsbad, CA.

VOLUME

I

Esophageal Motor (Functional) Disorders and Esophageal Diverticula

CHAPTER

16 Functional Disorders of the Esophagus

ALEX G. LITTLE

The function of the esophagus is to transport saliva and food from the mouth to the stomach. To function effectively, there must be an appropriately timed and forceful relaxation or contraction of the upper and lower esophageal sphincters, and the esophageal body must peristalse normally. An understanding of normal function (see Chap. 1, Anatomy and Embryology, and Chap. 2, Physiology) is crucial to the surgeon who is attempting to correct or improve a condition of dysfunction. In addition, it is necessary to recognize that the esophageal function is dependent on integration within and coordination with both the oropharyngeal aspects of swallowing and the gastroduodenal secretory and clearance functions. Not only must each swallowed bolus successfully transit the esophageal body, but also two additional biologic functions must be met: guiding food and air into the appropriate organs, despite their sharing of a common chamber (the pharynx), and protecting the esophagus from the damaging reflux of gastric contents. Like other portions of the gastrointestinal tract, the esophagus is part of a continuous digestive organ, and an awareness of the continuous nature of this system is important to understanding function and dysfunction.

When the esophagus dysfunctions, an individual experiences one or a combination of a limited number of symptoms. The most common symptom is *dysphagia,* or difficulty swallowing. When dealing with any patient with swallowing difficulty, it is important for the clinician to try to distinguish between whether this represents difficulty in clearing a food bolus from the mouth—oropharyngeal dysphagia—or is a problem of esophageal transit—so-called esophageal dysphagia. It is not always possible to make this distinction clinically, but it is helpful to attempt to do so because this will guide investigations and focus them predominantly on oropharyngeal function or on esophageal function.

Another symptom that the patient may experience is a *cough,* which presumably is secondary to aspiration. Aspiration can occur as a consequence of a dysfunctional oropharyngeal phase of swallowing, so that saliva or food is diverted into the larynx rather than the esophagus. Alternatively, there may be regurgitation from the esophagus into the pharynx with subsequent aspiration, especially during sleep.

Finally, the patient may experience *chest pain* as a consequence of esophageal dysfunction. This chest pain may be caused directly by the esophagus, even if mechanisms are unclear, or may be owing to acid reflux from the stomach. This final symptom of heartburn is, of course, secondary to gastroesophageal reflux, which is extensively described in Chapter 9.

Esophageal dysfunction can be thought of in terms of both anatomy and etiology. This chapter attempts to combine these perspectives and discusses sequentially disorders of the upper esophageal sphincter (UES), disorders of the esophageal body, and disorders of the lower esophageal sphincter (LES). Obviously, there is overlap, because some processes cause dysfunction of more than one of these anatomic segments. Finally, esophageal dysfunction can result from a primary esophageal disorder or can be caused by a systemic disease that involves the esophagus. These are referred to, respectively, as primary and secondary esophageal motility disorders.

UPPER ESOPHAGUS

A significant challenge in understanding disorders of the pharyngoesophageal complex, including the UES, is that of obtaining useful physiologic information. Cine radiographic studies are very helpful in evaluating and elucidating the oropharyngeal phase of swallowing. It is more difficult to analyze the function of the UES. Radiographic studies are usually not very helpful except when a Zenker's diverticulum is identified. Both the vertical movement of the UES during swallowing and its asymmetry limit the accuracy and reproducibility of manometric analysis. Accordingly, discussion of pathophysiology and diagnosis of UES dysfunction is somewhat speculative and based on inferences from available information.

The act of swallowing is divided into three stages: (1) the voluntary preparatory/oral phase, (2) the involuntary pharyngeal stage, and (3) the esophageal stage. The oral phase involves chewing and mixing of food with saliva and positioning the bolus on the tongue. During the pharyngeal phase, food is transferred from the pharynx, through the UES, and into the esophagus. This process entails sequential contraction of the pharyngeal constrictor muscles and simultaneous relaxation of the cricopharyngeus muscle, which is the anatomic structure that constitutes the UES. This complex process is initiated by voluntary activity but becomes involuntary when the food bolus activates sensory receptors in the oropharynx. To consider dysfunction of the upper esophagus, the important points are that UES function cannot be arbitrarily separated from oropharyngeal function, and disorders of both the UES and the pharynx cause oropharyngeal dysphagia. This discussion focuses on the UES with a limited analysis of the full spectrum of the causes of oropharyngeal dysphagia, which are listed in Table 16–1.

Nervous System Causes of Oropharyngeal Dysphagia

Dysphagia frequently accompanies cerebrovascular accidents (CVA) as a result of interference with triggering of the swallowing reflex, pharyngeal peristalsis, or coordination of UES relaxation. This can occur acutely and resolve with time or may become a chronic problem. In one report, nearly 50% of patients had early dysphagia after a CVA, but the dysphagia resolved within 2 weeks in 86% of the patients.[32] Aspiration also can occur after a CVA and was documented in approximately 30% of patients in the same report.[32] With abnormalities of both pharyngeal and UES function, these unfortunate patients are not candidates for surgical correction. Performance of any surgical procedure on the upper sphincter simply interferes further with pharyngeal function and may actually increase the possibility of aspiration.

Other central and peripheral nervous system causes of oropharyngeal dysphagia are listed for completeness in Table 16–1. Clearly, these diseases and their sequelae are not amenable to surgical treatment. If significant oropharyngeal dysfunction is identified in a patient with normal esophageal function and one of these processes is suspected, then appropriate consultation with a neurologist should be sought.

Table 16–1. Causes of Oropharyngeal Dysphagia

Causes
Nervous System
Central nervous system disease
Cerebrovascular accident
Parkinson's disease
Multiple sclerosis
Amyotrophic lateral sclerosis
Brain tumors
Wilson's disease
Peripheral nervous system disease
Myasthenia gravis
Poliomyelitis
Neuropathies
Muscular
Primary myositis
Muscular dystrophy
Systemic lupus erythematosus
Metabolic myopathy
UES
Hypertensive UES
Hypotensive UES
Premature closure
Delayed relaxation
Incomplete relaxation

UES = upper esophageal sphincter.

Muscular Causes of Oropharyngeal Dysphagia

Muscular diseases tend to interfere predominantly with the effectiveness of pharyngeal muscular contraction. In patients with poliomyelitis or dermatomyositis, dysphagia is the predominant symptom, and weakness of pharyngomuscular contraction secondary to inflammation of the striated muscle is the cause. Myotonic dystrophy and oculopharyngeal muscular dystrophy can cause oropharyngeal dysphagia. The latter disease is seen frequently in the French Canadian population and it is an autosomal dominant inherited disease, characterized by abnormalities in amplitude, duration, and frequency of pharyngeal contraction with relatively normal UES function. Even though the primary pathology is in the muscles of the oropharynx, cricopharyngeal myotomy enhances pharyngeal clearance by reducing UES resistance. This allows the weakened pharynx to propel a bolus into the cervical esophagus, and this translates into symptomatic improvement.[69] Involvement of pharyngeal muscle may also occur in patients with thyrotoxicosis or collagen vascular diseases such as systemic lupus erythematosus.

UES Causes of Oropharyngeal Dysphagia

The UES causes of oropharyngeal dysphagia listed in Table 16–1 are difficult to demonstrate in any particular patient. When oropharyngeal function is normal, dysfunction of the UES must be inferred. Manometric studies are limited and radiographic findings are usually not diagnostic. The finding on barium swallow of a cricopharyngeal bar, illustrated in Figure 16–1, a posterior indentation at the introitus of the cervical esophagus caused by cricopharyngeal contraction, is nonspecific, because only the minority of individuals with this finding actually have symptoms. A mild controversy exists regarding patients who complain of oropharyngeal dysphagia but in whom no definite UES abnormality can be identified. Cricopharyngeal myotomy is a reasonable therapeutic option for selected patients. Careful clinical and cine radiographic assessment is essential to identify and exclude from operative consideration patients with oropharyngeal dysfunction caused by nervous system or primary muscle disease. When patients are carefully selected, cricopharyngeal myotomy safely and effectively improves swallowing.[19,56]

Pharyngoesophageal ("Zenker's") Diverticulum

Dysfunction of the UES is thought to be responsible for the entity of Zenker's diverticulum and the symptoms associated with it. It is really the sphincteric dysfunction that is of pathogenetic significance rather than one of its manifestations, which is the diverticulum.

This diverticulum is a "false" diverticulum and is a mucosal and submucosal outpouching that arises at the junction of the pharynx and esophagus in the posterior midline between the inferior constrictor of the pharynx and the cricopharyngeus. The anatomy is depicted in Figure 16–2, and the radiographic appearance is shown

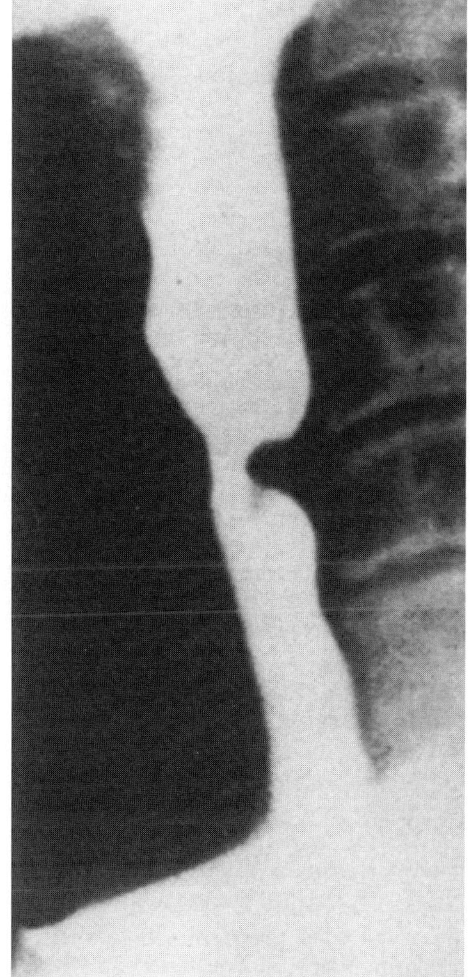

Figure 16–1. This barium swallow depicts the so-called cricopharyngeal bar or impression. This posterior indentation is presumably caused by contraction of the cricopharyngeus muscle, which constitutes the physiologic upper esophageal sphincter. Most patients with this finding are free of symptoms and it therefore does not constitute a significant pathologic condition.

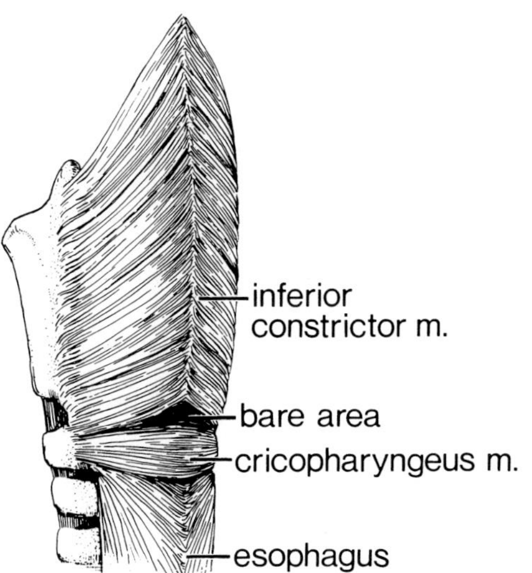

Figure 16–2. This drawing depicts the posterior anatomy of the pharynx and esophagus. A Zenker's or pharyngoesophageal diverticulum arises in the posterior midline in the "bare area" between the lowest of the pharyngeal constrictor muscles and the cricopharyngeus muscle. The diverticulum arises as a result of discoordination between these muscles. This motor dysfunction is the primary process responsible for both the patient's symptoms and the diverticulum.

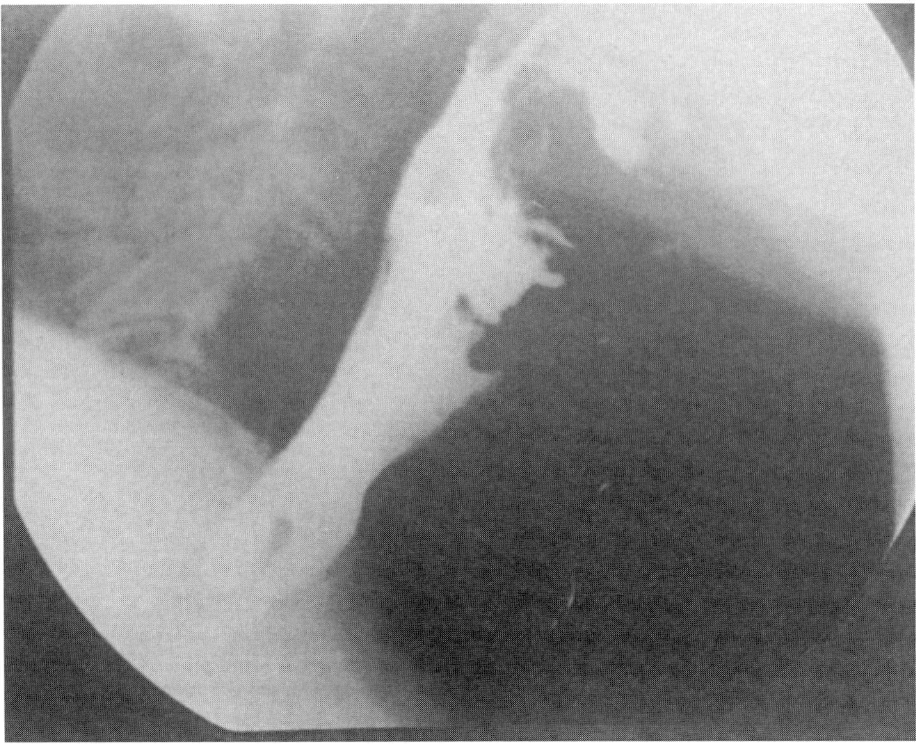

Figure 16–3. This radiograph shows a typical appearance of a moderate-size Zenker's or pharyngoesophageal diverticulum.

in Figure 16-3. Although the diverticulum is thought to be due to dysfunction of the upper sphincter, UES dysfunction cannot be demonstrated conclusively manometrically in every instance because of the limitations of the technique in this location. In approximately 50% of patients, either a hypertensive sphincter or, more commonly, absence of proper coordination between pharyngeal contraction and UES relaxation can be found.[67] As illustrated in Figure 16-4, the most frequently identified abnormality is premature cricopharyngeal relaxation. As the patient swallows, the UES relaxes prior to pharyngeal contraction. This discoordination results in an increase in pressure in the hypopharynx as rising pressure in the pharynx is opposed by a closing UES. It is presumably

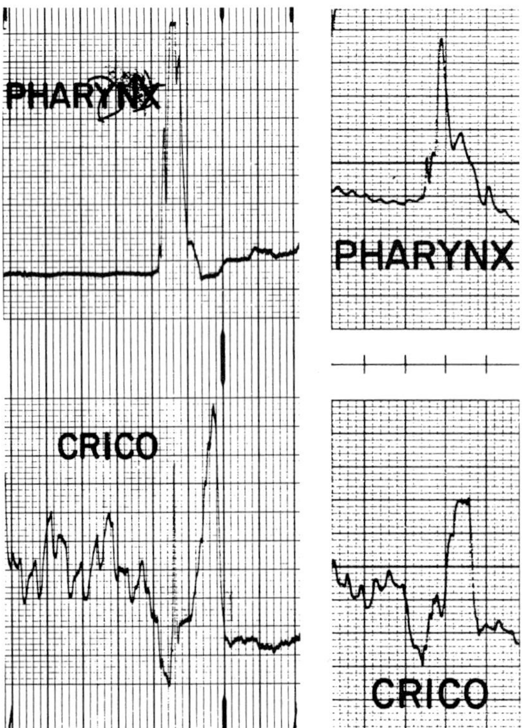

Figure 16–4. These manometric tracings show the most frequently identified motility abnormality in patients with Zenker's diverticulum. On the left is a normal manometric sequence. Simultaneous recordings show that the cricopharyngeus (crico) relaxes at the same time as the pharyngeal contraction occurs. In contrast, the simultaneous pressure recordings on the right are from a patient with a Zenker's diverticulum. The abnormality is that the cricopharyngeal or upper esophageal sphincter relaxation is premature, so that this sphincter is beginning to contract just as the pharynx begins its own contraction. This results in functional resistance to pharyngeal clearance, which causes the sensation of dysphagia and results in increased hypopharyngeal pressure that results in the formation of this "pulsion" diverticulum.

this increase in hypopharyngeal pressure that begins to distend the posterior mucosa and finally produces this pulsion diverticulum. Once formation of the pouch has begun, Laplace's law determines that the diverticular sac will continue to enlarge.

Patients with a Zenker's diverticulum invariably have dysphagia that is typically described as hesitancy and difficulty with clearing food from the oropharynx. It is this symptom that the patient is most aware of, but a careful history will identify the presence of cough and/or hoarseness, both of which are highly suggestive of aspiration as well. The dysphagia is clearly caused by the obstructive dysfunction of the sphincter. Aspiration may be caused by either diversion of a swallowed bolus into the larynx or regurgitation and subsequent inhalation of retained contents from the diverticulum.

It has been speculated that this disorder may be secondary to gastroesophageal reflux.[6] It is hypothesized that a reflexive spasm of the UES would protect against regurgitation and aspiration of the refluxed material. In fact, symptomatic, radiologic, or esophageal pH monitoring evidence for pathologic reflux can be found in approximately 40% of patients with Zenker's diverticulum.[6,23,67] Obviously, not all Zenker's diverticula are related to reflux, but this does suggest that reflux may be a causal or exacerbating factor in a substantial minority of patients.

Treatment of this disorder is surgical and is indicated to relieve dysphagia and prevent the sequelae of chronic aspiration. The latter benefit is of particular importance to the elderly who have a decreased cough reflex and diminished physiologic reserve and are, therefore, both prone to and devastated by episodes of aspiration pneumonia. Figure 16-5 illustrates the traditional surgical approach to the treatment of Zenker's diverticulum. Exposure of the cervical esophagus requires a neck incision and dissection to the deep neck compartment. Cricopharyngeal myotomy, division of the muscular fibers of the cricopharyngeus muscle, is an absolutely essential feature of operative management. Diverticulectomy alone fails because symptoms persist owing to the untreated cricopharyngeal dysfunction, and, in fact, the diverticulum itself will ultimately recur. Treatment of the diverticulum after cricopharyngeal myotomy is optional and should be based on the surgeon's experience. Diverticulopexy functionally removes the diverticular sac from the food stream, whereas diverticulectomy constitutes anatomic removal.[46]

My own group's experience with 30 patients undergoing myotomy and diverticulopexy resulted in no perioperative deaths, demonstrating that this operation can be performed safely even in elderly patients.[67] Significant morbidity is uncommon. Three of our patients had temporary vocal cord palsy related to recurrent laryngeal nerve injury, but all eventually had return of normal function. Wound infections occurred in two patients and both resolved with local wound care and antibiotic administration. Long-term follow-up demonstrated that 24 (80%) of these patients remained completely asymptomatic. Six patients had residual, mild dysphagia but no further clinical evidence of regurgitation or aspiration. These are typical results replicated by several centers and justify surgical treatment for most patients, both to restore the ability to swallow and to prevent aspiration and its associated risk of pneumonia.[5,18,24]

Despite these very good results with the open techniques, my opinion is that an even better approach now is becoming established. This is the transoral endoscopic stapling technique illustrated in Figure 16-6. This approach requires the use of a specialized diverticuloscope. With the patient intubated and under general anesthesia, the scope is positioned through the mouth with the larger blade in the esophagus and the smaller blade in the diverticulum. Although it takes a few moments to locate the anatomy, this is actually a straightforward and controlled undertaking and does not appear to risk perforation of the esophagus. I place a small, rigid viewing telescope within the diverticuloscope as it is being advanced, and this provides a video display both for the operating surgeon and for participating personnel. When the diverticuloscope is in its appropriate final location, it is balanced on a Mayo stand or the patient's chest, which frees the operator's hands. The contents of the diverticulum are aspirated until it is clean. Under video observation, an endoscopic GIA stapler is introduced through the diverticuloscope. The short limb is placed in the diverticulum and the longer limb into the esophagus. The firing of the stapler divides the common wall between the diverticulum and the esophagus. By definition, the cricopharyngeus muscle is divided at the same time. Subsequent stapler firings may be required to reach the bottom of the diverticulum. At the completion of the procedure, the diverticulum and the upper esophagus have become a common channel and the obstructive cricopharyngeus muscle has been dealt with.

Peracchia and his group[62] have among the largest reported experiences with this procedure to date in 95 patients with a median follow-up of 23 months. Although there was no postoperative morbidity or mortality, a conversion to an open operation was required in three patients (3.1%). Patients began oral feeding the day after their operation, and the median hospital stay was 3 days. Short- to medium-term results arc at least equivalent to those obtained with the open procedure. With a median follow-up of 23 months, dysphagia had either completely resolved or become mild in all patients. Similarly, regurgitation also either ceased or was classified as mild in all patients. My limited experience with six patients treated in this way confirms this larger experience. The procedure is straightforward, is simple to perform, and achieves complete resolution of the patient's symptoms without the need for an external incision. Although the transoral approach cannot be unequivocally declared the operation of choice without additional clinical reports to document both safety and efficacy, it certainly has theoretical appeal, and results to date are extremely promising.

ESOPHAGEAL BODY AND LOWER ESOPHAGEAL SPHINCTER

Achalasia

Achalasia is an idiopathic condition that is the most frequently encountered primary motor disorder of the

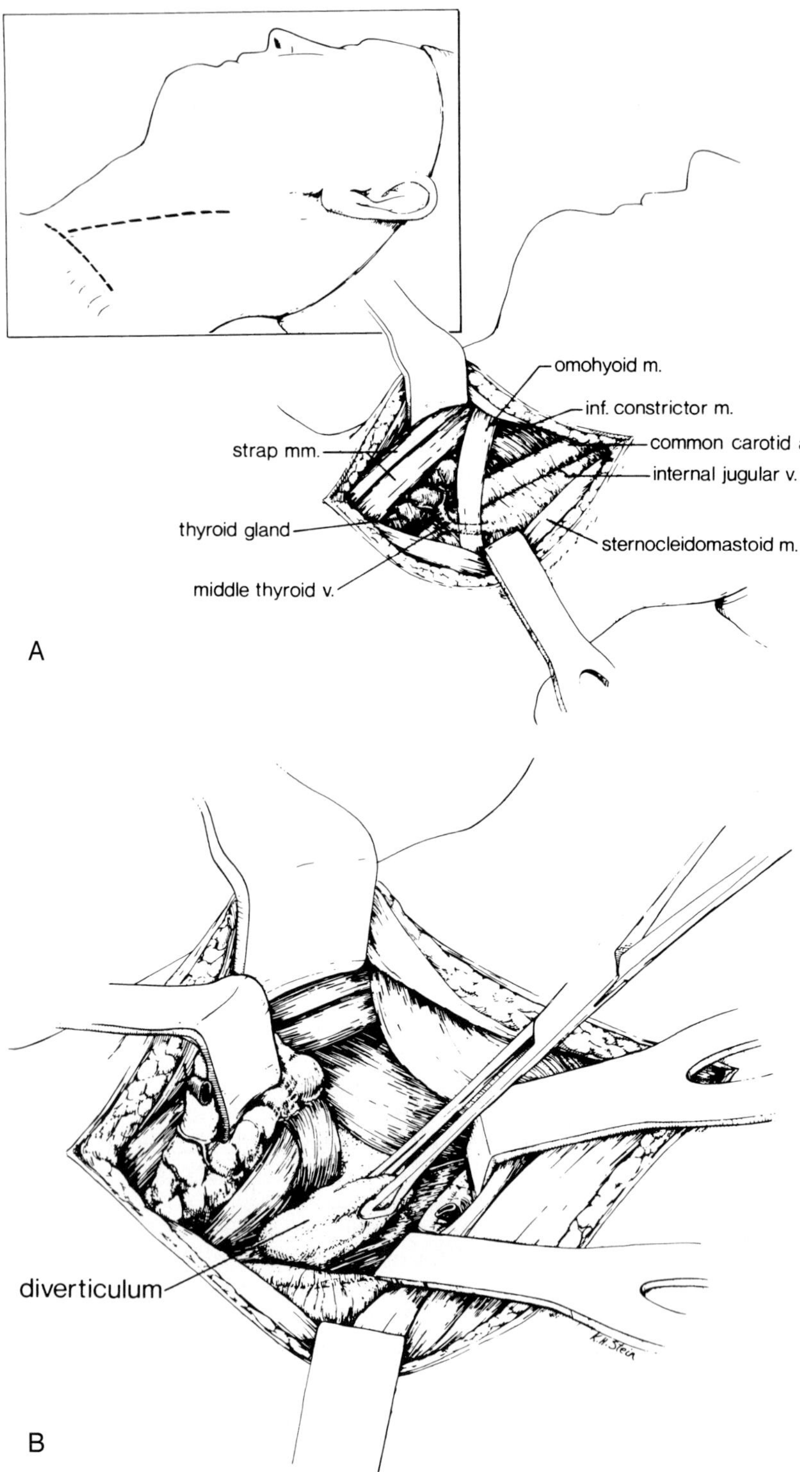

Figure 16–5. This sequence of illustrations represents the operative approach to Zenker's diverticulum. *A,* The inset shows that operative access to the cervical esophagus can be gained through either a vertical or a transverse incision that is subsequently deepened. The dissection is between the midline compartment and the carotid sheath laterally. Division of the omohyoid muscle is optional but improves exposure without any functional sequelae. Both the middle thyroid vein and the inferior thyroid artery may require division for complete access to the esophagus. *B,* The diverticulum is found posterior to the esophagus. If small, it may be quite adherent to the esophagus. The diverticular sac must be dissected and completely freed up to its neck.

Illustration continued on opposite page

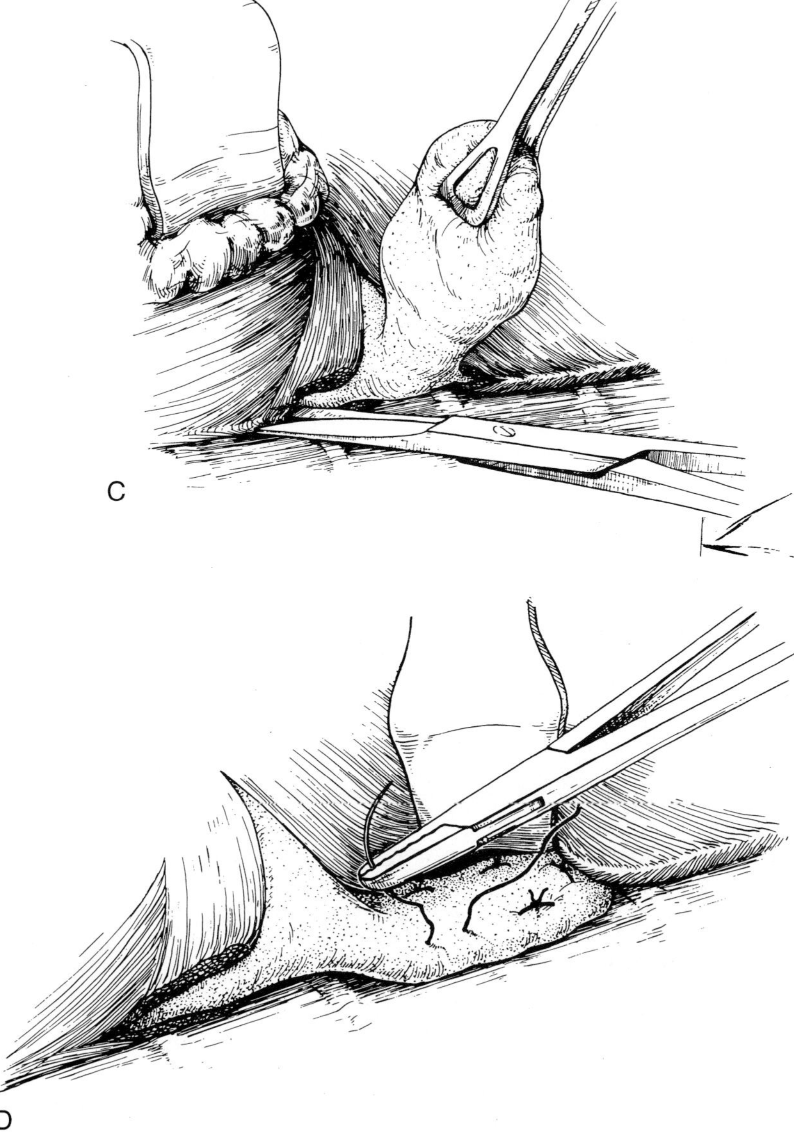

Figure 16–5 *Continued. C,* Cricopharyngeal myotomy is an essential operative maneuver. The myotomy either can be started on the esophageal body and extended cephalad, which is the author's preference, or can begin at the base of the diverticulum and extended caudally. The length of the myotomy is 3 to 4 cm. *D,* Following the myotomy, there are three options for handling the diverticulum. This illustration depicts the technique of diverticulopexy in which through-and-through sutures are placed to suspend the diverticulum from the prevertebral fascia behind the pharynx. A small (<3 cm) diverticulum may require no specific handling if it becomes just a mucosal bulge after the myotomy. The final alternative is to staple the neck and excise the diverticular sac.

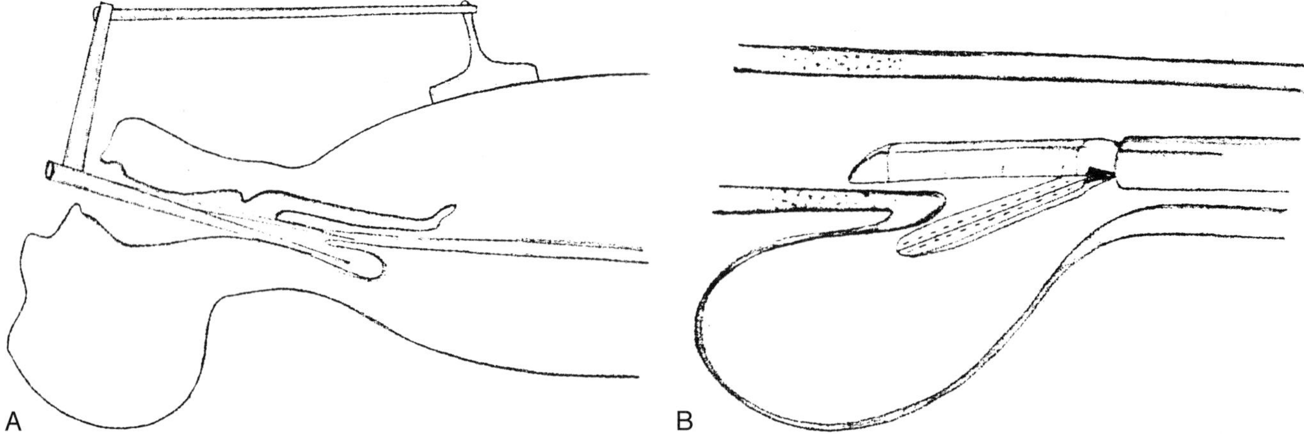

Figure 16–6. *A,* This illustration depicts the appearance when the diverticuloscope is properly positioned through the mouth. The upper blade has just entered the esophagus, and the lower blade is within the diverticulum. The scope is held by a mechanical arm that is on the patient's chest, which allows the operator's hands to be free. *B,* This illustration shows how the endoscopic GIA stapler is placed through the diverticuloscope so that one anvil is within the esophagus and the other is within the diverticulum. When the stapler is fired, the common wall is divided and the cricopharyngeus muscle is part of the divided tissue. This creates a common cavity between the diverticulum and the esophagus and removes the functional obstruction caused by the cricopharyngeus muscle.

esophagus. Both the esophageal body and the LES are involved. Histopathologically, this condition is one in which there is a diminution in or even an absence of the myenteric neural plexi. Also found is hypertrophy of esophageal nerves and associated hypertrophy of esophageal muscle.[9] The esophagus functions as though it has become denervated. This can be demonstrated by a hypersensitivity-type exaggerated response to cholinergic stimulation. Chagas' disease is a pathophysiologically similar condition seen in South America and known to be caused by the parasite *Trypanosoma cruzi.* In this condition, the parasite invades the nervous system, and this results in achalasia-like esophageal function. Based on this model, it is speculated that achalasia may be secondary to a viral or autoimmune process that affects the esophageal nerves somewhere along the neural visceromotor axis. Although this theory is supported by the observation that creation of neurologic deficits in animals produces the same esophageal dysfunction that is seen in achalasia, this etiology has not been proved in humans.[7,33,40]

Clinical Features

Achalasia occurs equally in both sexes and has a typical onset in the third or fourth decades, although it can occur both earlier and later in life. All patients have dysphagia, but the development of this symptom tends to be gradual and insidious. By the time the patient presents to a physician, he or she may have learned to accommodate to difficulty in swallowing, but will be aware that food, particularly solid foods such as meat and bread, tends to pass slowly. Over time, the esophagus is dilated by food retention and slowly enlarges. As this occurs, the sensation of dysphagia may subside and even disappear as the esophagus becomes another reservoir organ. In this situation, regurgitation of esophageal contents is quite common. Nighttime regurgitation leads to aspiration, which may be manifested by a nocturnal cough or even aspiration pneumonia.[10,28]

A diagnosis of achalasia is suggested by a clinical presentation featuring the symptoms of dysphagia and regurgitation and is supported by radiographic appearances such as those shown in Figure 16–7. Typically, the esophagus is dilated and tapers down smoothly at the gastroesophageal junction, producing a characteristic "bird's beak" appearance rather than the "apple core" configuration caused by stenosis from esophageal cancer. The esophagus may be mildly dilated or it may be extremely enlarged with a sigmoid configuration, the so-called megaesophagus, depending on the severity and duration of the disease.

Ultimately, the diagnosis of achalasia rests on manometric findings. Even when the clinical picture seems unequivocal, an esophageal motility examination should be performed prior to therapy to avoid diagnostic error. The two pathognomonic abnormalities are a nonrelaxing or incompletely relaxing LES and the complete absence of peristalsis in the smooth muscle portion of the esophagus where contractions are simultaneous and nonpropulsive rather than sequential/peristaltic and propulsive. These manometric features are illustrated in Figure 16–8. The poorly relaxing sphincter produces a functional obstruction of the distal esophagus, and this condition is exacerbated by the absence of effective esophageal contractions. For the esophagus to empty, the patient must accumulate a food column that exerts enough hydrostatic pressure at its bottom to force food through the sphincter.

During endoscopy, which should routinely be performed, the esophageal mucosa is usually normal. Food retention is common, and pre-endoscopic cleansing aids the examination. Distal esophagitis may be encountered, but this is more likely to be due to retention of food and oral bacteria than to gastroesophageal reflux. The LES usually remains closed, but the endoscope can be passed through it easily, because this is not a fixed obstruction caused by stricture. During the endoscopic procedure, it is important to look for a tumor of the distal esophagus

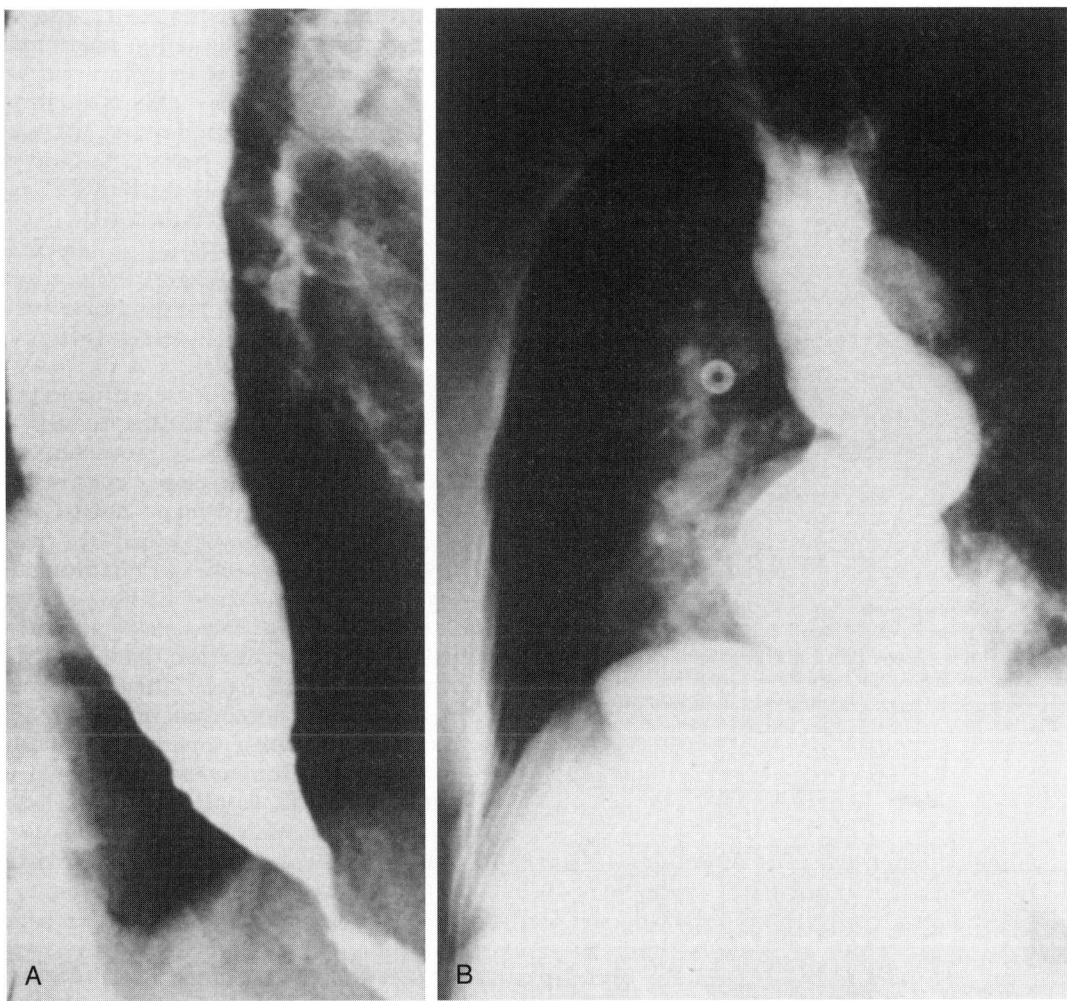

Figure 16–7. *A,* This radiograph shows the typical appearance of relatively early achalasia. The esophageal body is moderately dilated and it tapers at the gastroesophageal junction, producing the typical "bird's beak" appearance. *B,* This radiograph shows advanced achalasia with an extremely enlarged esophagus that has assumed a sigmoid configuration owing to the pressure created by the retained contents.

or gastroesophageal junction, which can cause a clinical and manometric picture identical to that of primary achalasia and is called pseudoachalasia.[39] The mechanism by which these tumors, which may be primary or metastatic from another site, reproduce both the clinical and manometric features of achalasia is unclear but seems to involve neural invasion by a tumor that is primarily extraluminal. In addition, endoscopic examination is necessary, because achalasia is a premalignant condition and is associated with a higher than expected incidence of squamous cell carcinoma.[8] Because the enlarged lumen allows a longer growth period before a cancer produces obstructive symptoms and also makes radiologic diagnosis more difficult, careful endoscopic analysis is important.

Vigorous Achalasia

A distinct subset of achalasia is formed by patients with what is termed vigorous achalasia.[53] In contrast to the routine achalasia patients, those with vigorous achalasia regularly experience a squeezing type of chest pain as an important symptom along with dysphagia. The manometric findings include the typical dysfunction of the LES with incomplete relaxation. The unique feature is that the simultaneous esophageal contractions are of a normal, or even elevated, pressure. This is clearly different from the routine achalasia patient in whom esophageal contractions are so weak that the adjective feeble is apt. Whether vigorous achalasia represents early achalasia or a variant of "normal" achalasia is not established. In fact, vigorous achalasia even bears some similarity to diffuse esophageal spasm but does differ by having no normal peristalsis and an abnormal sphincter.

Treatment

The treatment of achalasia is directed at the LES, which, in addition to having incomplete or no relaxation, is frequently hypertensive. Medical management aimed at decreasing this sphincteric resistance includes the use of smooth muscle relaxants such as nitrates and calcium-channel blocking agents.[54,71] The calcium slow channel blockers, such as nifedipine, have been shown to reduce LES pressure. Unfortunately, a modest reduction in sphincter pressure usually does not result in a significant improvement in the patient's clinical status.

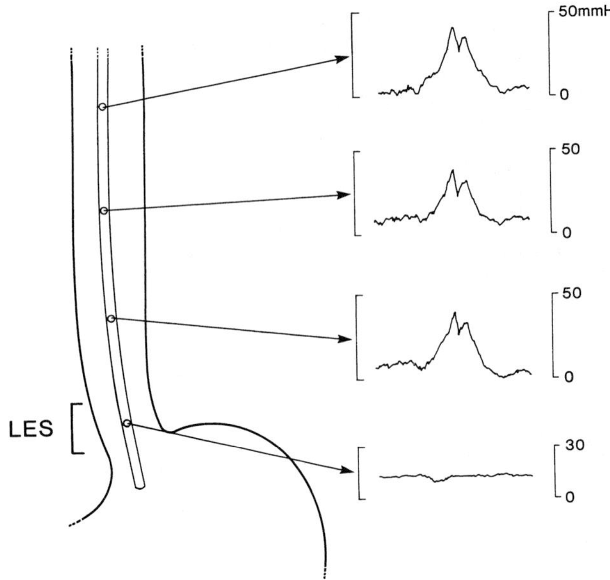

Figure 16–8. This representation of a motility tracing shows the classic manometric features of achalasia. The lower esophageal sphincter fails to relax with a swallow, creating a functional distal esophageal obstruction. Swallows also initiate simultaneous rather than peristaltic contractions, thus depriving the esophagus of its normal stripping, propulsive action.

The most effective treatment choices are directed at relieving the functional obstruction at the LES and consist of pneumatic dilation, open surgical myotomy, or a minimally invasive type of approach with either thoracoscopic or laparoscopic esophageal myotomy.

Pneumatic dilation is a reasonable initial therapy of choice for most patients. This technique involves placement of a balloon catheter across the region of the lower sphincter under fluoroscopic control. The balloon is inflated to a designated pressure and to a diameter of 3 or 4 cm. When inflation occurs, the patient usually experiences chest or epigastric pain, and when the balloon is removed, it usually is blood tinged. This suggests that balloon dilation results in forceful rupture of the lower esophageal musculature. Despite this mechanism of action, perforation occurs in only 3 to 5% of patients.[25,37,73,75]

Table 16-2 provides results from representative reports on the use of pneumatic dilation in the treatment of achalasia. The range of symptomatic improvement is 48 to 78%, and the risk of procedure-related mortality is quite low. The development of late postoperative reflux is an important issue but does not vitiate the good early results. Accordingly, because this procedure can be performed in the outpatient setting and without the need for general anesthesia or an operation, it is the choice for most patients. Patients who are not good candidates for dilation include those with an extremely dilated esophagus in whom it is difficult to pass the balloon through the LES, patients with so-called vigorous achalasia and relatively high-pressure contractions who seem to be at a somewhat higher risk for perforation, and younger patients in whom a more definitive approach can be defended. Two pneumatic dilation sessions constitute a reasonable trial of this therapeutic approach. For the third and subsequent dilations, results worsen and the risk of perforation increases. Therefore, when symptoms persist after two sessions, it is time to move to surgical treatment.

Table 16–2. Treatment of Achalasia: Pneumatic Dilation

Reference	Year	Improved (%)	Mortality (%)	Postoperative GERD (%)
Vantrappen and Hellemans[72]	1980	77	0.2	—
Fellows et al.[27]	1983	58	0	27
Robertson et al.[65]	1988	48	0	26
Barnett et al.[4]	1990	78	0	7
Wehrmann et al.[75]	1995	88	0	5

GERD = gastroesophageal reflux disease.

Surgical treatment is an esophagomyotomy through the musculature that creates the lower sphincter. This operation can be performed through either an open or minimally invasive approach. Heller described the first myotomy, and his original technique of a transabdominal double myotomy has been modified to the current one in which a single myotomy is carried out through a left thoracotomy.[60] The necessary proximal extent of the myotomy is undefined. It appears not to be important except in patients with vigorous achalasia and in those with fairly small esophagi that have not yet developed significant dilation. Ambulatory manometry performed while patients are eating has documented an almost fibrillatory motility pattern with frequent esophageal body repetitive contractions that are thought to be responsible for food holdup in the mid esophagus.[45] An example of this type of manometry finding is shown in Figure 16-9. This suggests a benefit to extending the myotomy to the aortic arch in this subgroup of patients. The real key to this operation, however, is clearly extending the myotomy distally. It must completely traverse the musculature of the lower sphincter and go onto the stomach. Some surgeons who regularly perform this operation believe that a carefully performed myotomy alone can be accomplished and is sufficient. Results in selected series are provided in Table 16-3. In the experienced hands of these reporting groups, dysphagia is relieved in more than 80% of patients. Development of iatrogenic gastroesophageal reflux appears to be uncommon in the reports; however, this conclusion is based primarily on clinical assessment alone rather than on objective testing

Table 16–3. Treatment of Achalasia: Esophagomyotomy

Reference	Year	Improved (%)	Mortality (%)	Postoperative GERD (%)
Ellis et al.[23]	1980	92	0	3
Goulbourne and Walbaum[34]	1985	80	0	5
Ellis et al.[20]	1988	92	0	6
Ellis et al.[24]	1992	88	0	8

GERD = gastroesophageal reflux disease.

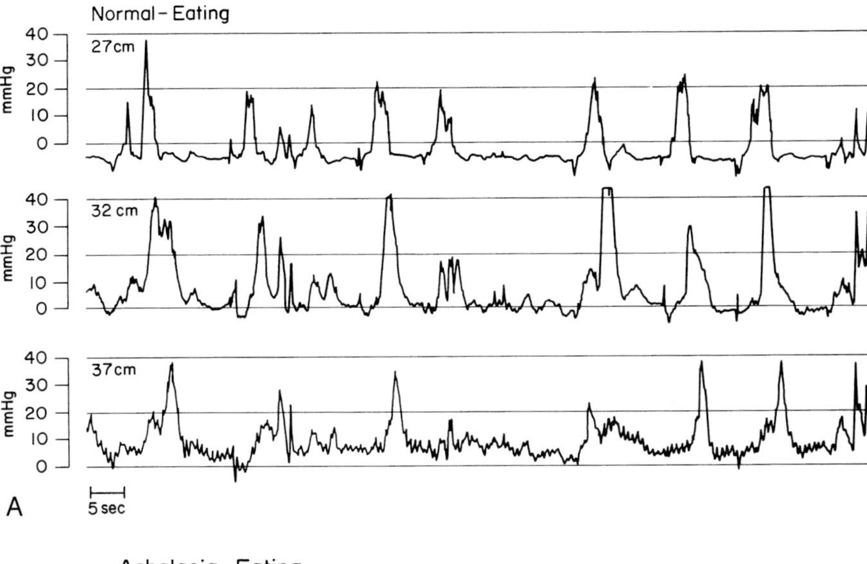

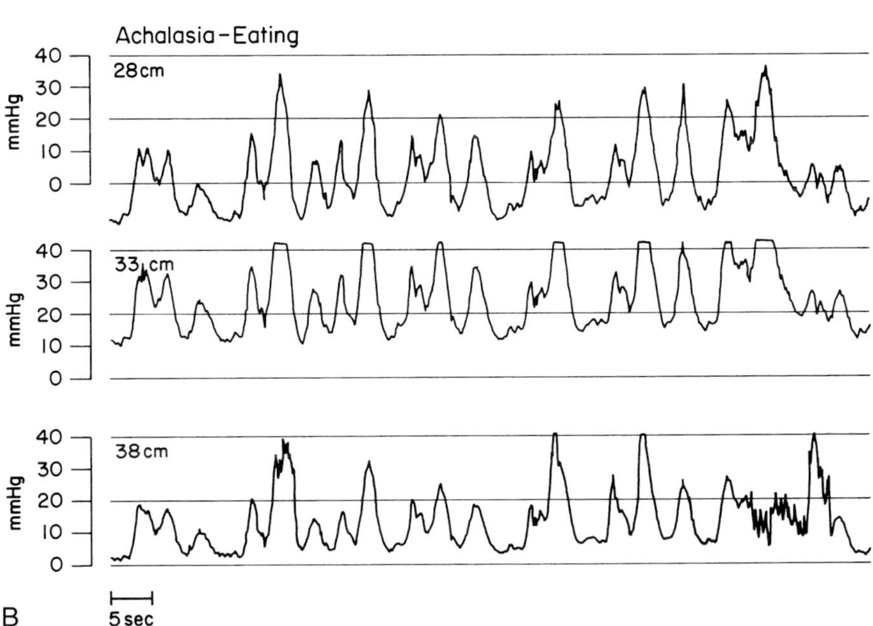

Figure 16-9. *A,* This manometry tracing was obtained from a normal volunteer while eating a meal. All contractions are sequential and peristaltic, and there are no more than three or four contraction waves a minute. *B,* This manometry tracing was obtained from a patient with achalasia while the patient was eating a meal. This nearly fibrillatory pattern of muscular contractions is in striking contrast to the normal tracing.

with pH monitoring. The reported range of patients who develop clinically significant reflux is higher according to other reports and ranges from 5 to 25% of patients.[21,22,52,70,77]

The open approach that the author favors is depicted in Figure 16-10 and is based on the belief that a complete myotomy is more ensured with complete dissection of the stomach and gastroesophageal junction from the hiatus and excision of the gastroesophageal fat pad.[1] When these maneuvers are accomplished, the myotomy can be performed with ideal exposure of the gastroesophageal junction, which helps to ensure a complete and, therefore, adequate myotomy. When this approach is chosen, it is necessary to reconstruct both the hiatus and the gastroesophageal junction to avoid development of iatrogenic reflux. This is accomplished by closing the hiatus posteriorly and performing a modified Belsey Mark IV fundoplication. The thickened esophageal muscle in patients with achalasia greatly aids the surgeon in performing the fundoplication by providing a secure purchase for the esophageal sutures.[47] The Belsey reconstruction, described as modified because four instead of the usual six sutures are used, is preferred to the Nissen procedure, because it does not produce as great a distal esophageal high-pressure zone and, therefore, does not cause dysphagia. The myotomy and Belsey approach has also been shown to relieve dysphagia in more than 80% of patients and incorporates operative features to prevent development of reflux. The author favors this technique because it both ensures a complete myotomy, which is the primary goal of the operation, and the unique hypertrophy of the muscle maximizes the conditions for construction of an effective Belsey-type reconstruction. When esophagomyotomy alone fails, the failure is due either to an inadequate myotomy, so that the patient has persistent dysphagia, or to iatrogenic gastroesophageal reflux due to excessive weakening of the sphincteric antireflux mechanism. The combined approach is a more involved operation but addresses both types of potential operative failure and is, therefore, my preference. Table

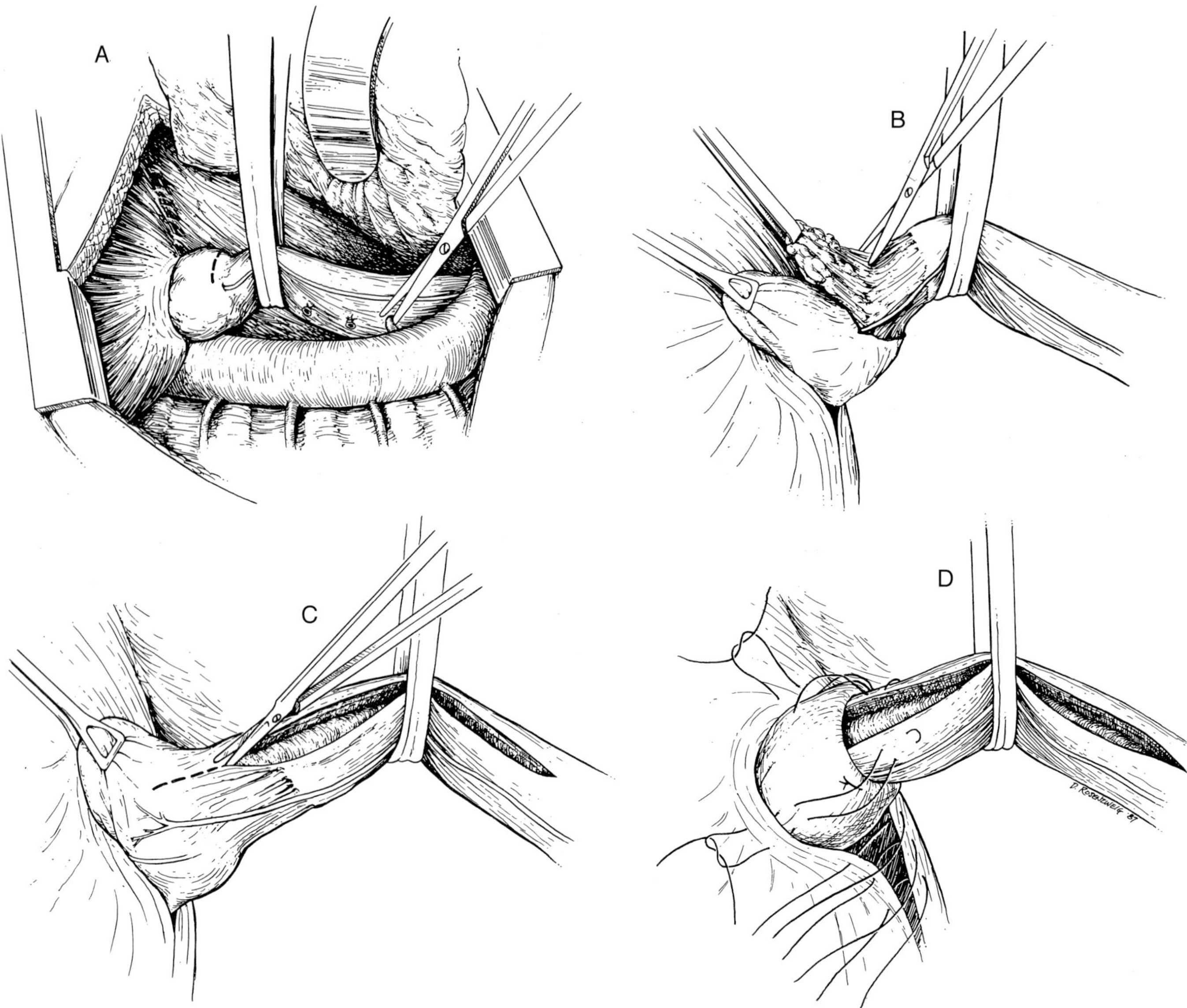

Figure 16–10. This series of drawings depicts the left thoracotomy operative approach for esophageal achalasia. *A,* The left lung is collapsed using a single-lung ventilation technique for the right lung. The inferior pulmonary ligament is released and the esophagus dissected from its mediastinal bed. Ligation and division of the lower esophageal arteries is usually required. The dotted line in the drawing locates the point of entry into the peritoneal cavity. A true hiatal hernia is not usually present, but dissection inside the muscular edges of the hiatus exposes the phrenoesophageal membrane and a "cap" of peritoneum through which abdominal access is gained. *B,* The esophageal hiatus is dissected to completely free up the gastroesophageal junction. The anterior fat pad at the gastroesophageal junction is removed. These two maneuvers result in uncompromised exposure of the anatomy. *C,* The esophagomyotomy is begun at a convenient location on the esophageal body. The correct submucosal plane is identified by cutting the muscle between forceps that grasp and suspend the muscle. Scissors with relatively blunt tips, such as Mayo scissors, are ideal for this maneuver. The myotomy is then extended through the gastroesophageal junction/LES region and onto the stomach. This complete myotomy ensures successful reduction of the LES pressure. *D,* Following the myotomy, the muscular edges of the hiatus are closed. A competent but nonobstructive antireflux mechanism is established by performing a modified (i.e., four-stitch) Belsey fundoplication. The thickened muscle of achalasia provides a secure purchase for the esophageal sutures.

Table 16–4. Treatment of Achalasia: Esophagomyotomy and Fundoplication

Reference	Year	Improved (%)	Mortality (%)	Postoperative GERD (%)
Nelems et al.[51]	1980	90	0	12
Little et al.[47]	1988	88	0	0
Csendes et al.[14]	1989	95	0	28
Stipa et al.[68]	1990	85	0	15
Malthaner et al.[48]	1994	95 (1 yr) 77 (5 yr) 69 (10 yr)	0	18

GERD = gastroesophageal reflux disease.

16-4 provides an overview of results obtained using this combined operation. A report by Malthaner and the Toronto group is particularly revealing.[48] They document the extent to which results deteriorate over time, a paradigm that is undoubtedly equally true for the other treatment options. In addition, they found that even with a fundoplication as part of the myotomy, the late development of reflux complications occurred in some patients. This was responsible for the deterioration of results over time and necessitated reoperation in the four patients with reflux at 7, 19, 23, and 23 years after the original procedure.

Although the open transthoracic and transabdominal approaches are more traditional, the last few years have seen a strong movement toward the use of minimally invasive surgical techniques in the treatment of achalasia.[2,5,35,41,59,61,62,74] Particularly encouraging has been the experience with a laparoscopic procedure, which has come to be my preferred approach for these patients. Five ports are placed in the abdomen with the orientation that is routine for a laparoscopic antireflux procedure. Only the anterior surface of the esophagus is dissected free from the hiatus, and the fat pad of the gastroesophageal junction is excised. Using scissors connected to the electrocautery, the lower esophageal muscle is divided until the submucosal plane is found. Then, using either scissors or an electrocautery hook, the muscle is divided both superiorly and inferiorly. Inferiorly, it is important to be sure that the myotomy has been carried onto the stomach, ensuring the complete division of the lower esophageal sphincter. With this approach, the majority of the gastroesophageal junction remains attached to the hiatus and presumably retains its intrinsic antireflux capability. However, the performance of a Dor procedure, in which the anterior fundus is sutured over the abdominal esophagus, adds further reflux protection by creating a flap valve mechanism at the gastroesophageal junction and is a further deterrent to reflux development.

There is not enough follow-up to document the long-term results of this operation. Several reports document that the laparoscopic procedure is associated with minimal morbidity and less than 1% mortality in patient series reported to date. Early relief of dysphagia is good, and up to 5 years the relief obtained by patients is equal to that obtained with the open procedure.[5,35,41,59,62,74]

Diffuse Esophageal Spasm

Diffuse esophageal spasm (DES) is a rare primary motor disease of the esophagus of unknown etiology that causes chest pain or dysphagia or both. Historically, the term DES has been applied to many types of abnormal esophageal motility disorders, especially those characterized by high-pressure contractions. The diagnostic focus has tightened over the past decade, and DES is now defined by the manometric feature of simultaneous contractions; the minimum frequency is more than 10 to 20% of all esophageal contractions following wet swallows.[12,63] Accordingly, older references must be read carefully to be sure they address the motor disorder as defined here. There must also be the presence of at least some normal peristalsis, distinguishing this condition from achalasia where all contractions are simultaneous and there is no normal peristalsis. As shown in Figure 16–11, these contractions are usually normotensive, but occasionally high-pressure contractions occur. It is the pattern of contractions that is abnormal, not their amplitude. Both the UES and LES are usually normal.

The clinical picture always includes chest pain. The pain is frequently described as squeezing or even crushing and, therefore, a cardiac etiology must be considered and appropriately evaluated. Esophageal dysphagia also occurs but is usually a minor symptom compared with the pain. The diagnosis of DES is based on manometric criteria; however, the radiographic picture can be dramatic. As shown in Figure 16–12, the simultaneous contractions cause a segmentation phenomenon that results in an appearance that has been said to resemble a corkscrew or rosary beads. This radiographic appearance is not specific, because asymptomatic, particularly elderly

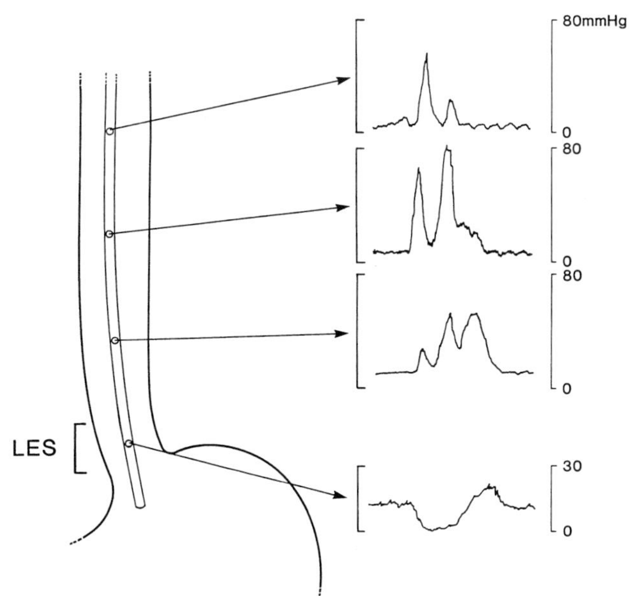

Figure 16–11. This manometric tracing was obtained from a patient with diffuse esophageal spasm. The hallmark feature is the finding of simultaneous contractions that are similar to those seen in achalasia. Frequently, as here, the contractions are also repetitive. There are always some normal peristaltic contractions, and the lower esophageal sphincter function is usually normal.

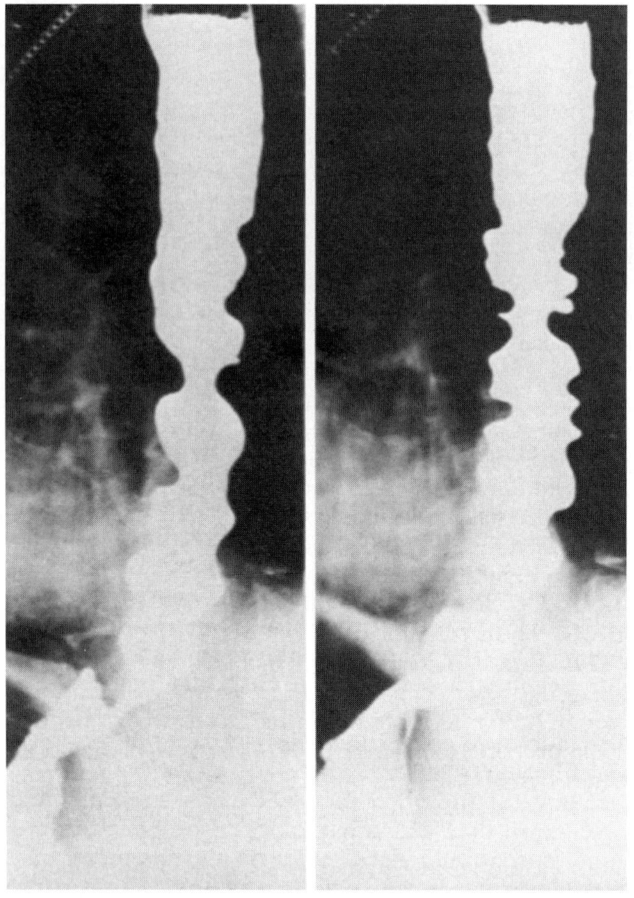

Figure 16–12. This is a typical radiograph from a patient with diffuse esophageal spasm. The multiple simultaneous contractions are causing segmentation of the barium column, resulting in a picture that has been said to resemble a corkscrew or even rosary beads. This radiographic appearance is not pathognomonic, as it can be found in asymptomatic, presumably normal, individuals.

people can have similar-appearing barium swallow radiographs, and only about one third of DES patients demonstrate this radiographic finding.[31,44]

Some patients with this motility abnormality that defines DES have gastroesophageal reflux disease. Patients generally fall into either a predominantly gastroesophageal reflux disease (GERD) pattern (in which heartburn is the dominant symptom, reflux is proven by pH monitoring, and frequent simultaneous contractions are attributed to reflux-induced spasm) or the DES category (in which crushing chest pain is prominent, reflux is not demonstrated, and simultaneous contractions are present).[43] The reflux is the primary disease in the first patient group, and it is the first priority for treatment. Control of reflux results in relief of symptoms.

Patients with the primary DES motor disorder are uncommon, constituting only 4% of all patients seen in one busy esophageal function laboratory, but they represent a clinical challenge.[15] They have symptoms and the presence of an abnormal motility pattern can be demonstrated, but the connection between the two is obscure. Delayed esophageal clearance with intraesophageal shuttling of fluid boluses has been demonstrated and presumably is responsible for dysphagia. However, for most patients, chest pain is the predominant symptom and dysphagia is absent or mild.[30] Not only is it unclear how simultaneous contractions cause pain, but also the chest pain frequently occurs between meals rather than with eating.

This uncertain pathophysiology makes treatment choices difficult. Initial therapy should be supportive, and reassurance and explanation are said to be the most important elements in the management of patients with DES.[65] This approach is derived from the observed relationship between DES and chronic emotional states.[66] In addition, smooth muscle relaxants including nitrates and calcium-channel blocking agents, such as nifedipine, are effective and constitute the second line of medical therapy. Long myotomy of the esophageal body, both with and without an associated antireflux procedure, has been reported to give good results.[26,38,42] However, surgical results are more predictable for relief of dysphagia than for relief of the most troublesome complaint, which is chest pain. Consequently, a selective and conservative approach to operative therapy is recommended.

High-Amplitude Peristaltic Contractions

This motility disturbance is characterized by high-pressure or -amplitude esophageal contractions (HAPC), which usually are peristaltic, although occasional simultaneous contractions are seen.[29] In this disorder, in contrast to DES, the pattern of contractions is usually normal, but their amplitude is abnormal. An example of HAPC motility findings is shown in Figure 16–13.

A difficulty with this disorder is that there is a wide range of normal esophageal contraction pressures, and pressures as high as those seen in symptomatic patients can be found in asymptomatic, presumably normal volun-

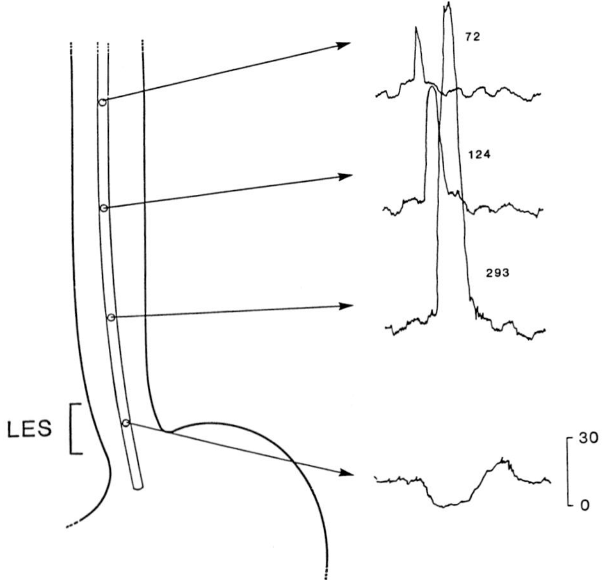

Figure 16–13. This is the manometric tracing of a patient with high-amplitude peristaltic contractions. These contractions are sequential and therefore peristaltic, but the pressure or amplitude is elevated, approaching 300 mmHg in the distal esophagus. The LES is normal.

teers.[21] Is a manometric abnormality that is associated with no symptoms a disease? Obviously not; therefore, an individual with this motility pattern but without symptoms does not have a motor disorder and represents a normal variant.

Like DES, the clinical picture of HAPC is predominated by angina-like chest pain, although dysphagia can be present. Because of the high pressure of the esophageal contractions, this disorder is also referred to as the nutcracker esophagus. However, the relationship between this disordered motility and the symptoms is unclear. There is no temporal relationship between the abnormal contractions and the chest pain.[55] The origin of the symptoms is undoubtedly related to the finding that patients with motor disorders and chest pain have a high prevalence of psychiatric disturbances that affect their pain perception.[11]

Treatment for patients with HAPC is generally problematic. One group reported that patients treated with the smooth muscle relaxant nifedipine experienced symptomatic improvement.[64] However, this was felt to be due more to the supportive patient-doctor relationship than to the effectiveness of the drug. Pain relief did not correlate with changes in contraction pressure. Not surprisingly, it is believed that only a small number of patients are candidates for surgical therapy. A long myotomy does reduce the pressure/amplitude of esophageal contractions and produces at least a reduction in the chest pain, but it should be reserved for patients whose symptoms resist maximum medical and supportive care.[29]

MISCELLANEOUS FUNCTIONAL DISORDERS

Collagen Vascular Diseases

The esophagus can be involved in any of these systemic diseases, but scleroderma is the one that most frequently affects the function of the esophagus by its involvement of the smooth muscle of the lower esophagus and LES. Depending on the severity of the disease and the degree of esophageal involvement, the result is impaired function of the esophageal body and a weak or completely patulous LES. The ineffective LES allows free reflux of gastric contents, and mucosal injury is potentiated by the inability of the esophagus to respond with secondary peristalsis to clear the noxious material.[57,78] Consequently, these patients suffer with severe heartburn and are prone to development of esophagitis and fibrous stricture.

If surgical antireflux therapy is considered, its timing is of more than the usual importance. Specifically, intervention should occur before development of advanced, erosive esophagitis or stricture. These complications necessitate more extensive surgical procedures, and even resection of an undilatable stricture may be required.[49] Performance of these procedures may be a challenge for which a scleroderma patient is unfit. In contrast, performing antireflux surgery at an earlier stage is both safer and more efficacious.

Vagotomy Sequelae (Postvagotomy Dysphagia)

The vagus nerve is an essential participant in the visceromotor neural control of esophageal function.[12] Both afferent and efferent vagal neurons connect to the central swallowing center in the medulla and pons, and the vagal fibers innervate the UES, the esophageal body, and the LES. Although the neurohumoral control of esophageal function is complex and incompletely defined, it is clear that both sensory and motor functions are provided by the vagus. In this context, it is more surprising that vagotomy usually does not produce symptoms than that dysphagia occasionally appears after performance of a truncal vagotomy. The reported incidence of this complication was only 0.7% in a report of a population of 1,298 patients undergoing vagotomy.[3] Because esophageal manometry is essentially normal in these patients, and since the dysphagia usually resolves spontaneously, it is more likely that dysphagia is owing to periesophageal edema or hematoma than to disruption of esophageal motor function.[36] Occasionally, esophageal dilation is required to relieve the dysphagia that follows injury of the vagus nerves.

Congenital Tracheoesophageal Fistula

Swallowing is frequently abnormal following and in spite of successful surgical correction of all types of tracheoesophageal fistula (TEF). This appears to be due to a congenital motor disorder rather than being a sequela of the TEF repair.[76] The few reports of motility studies in these patients suggest that distal esophageal function is abnormal and is characterized by weak or even absent contractions of the esophageal body and a hypotensive LES.[58] These findings are speculated to be related to a developmental failure of innervation of this segment of the esophagus rather than to surgical denervation during the TEF repair, because dysfunction has been shown to antedate surgical intervention. Not surprisingly, many of these patients develop reflux as they age. With both an ineffective reflux barrier and an impaired ability to clear the esophagus, it is not surprising that surgical antireflux procedures are frequently required.[58]

References

1. Altorki, N. K., and Little, A. G.: Achalasia and diffuse spasm of the esophagus. *In* Nyhus, L. M., and Baker, R. J. (eds.): Mastery of Surgery, 2nd ed. Boston, Little, Brown, 1992, p. 494.
2. Ancona, E., Peracchia, A., Zaninotto, G., et al.: Heller laparoscopic cardiomyotomy with antireflux anterior fundoplication (DOR) in the treatment of esophageal achalasia. Surg. Endosc. *7P:*459, 1993.
3. Anderson, H. A., Schlegel, J. F., and Olsen, A. M.: Postvagotomy dysphagia. Gastrointest. Endosc., *12:*13, 1966.
4. Barnett, J. L., Eisenman, R., Nostrant, T. T., and Elta, G. H.: Witzel pneumatic dilation for achalasia: Safety and long-term efficacy. Gastrointest. Endosc., *36:*482, 1990.
5. Beckingham, I. J., Callanan, M., Louw, J. A., and Bornman, P. C.: Laparoscopic cardiomyotomy for achalasia after a failed balloon dilation. Surg. Endosc., *13:*493, 1999.
6. Belsey, R.: Functional disease of the esophagus. J. Thorac. Cardiovasc. Surg., *52:*164, 1968.

7. Burgess, J. N., Schlegel, J. F., and Ellis, F. H.: The effect of denervation on feline esophageal function and morphology. J. Surg. Res., *12:*24, 1972.
8. Carter, R., and Brewer, L. A., III: Achalasia and esophageal carcinoma. Am. J. Surg., *130:*114, 1975.
9. Cassella, R. R., Brown, A. L., Sayre, G. P., and Ellis, F. H.: Achalasia of the esophagus: Pathologic and etiologic considerations. Ann. Surg., *160:*474, 1964.
10. Chakkaphak, S., Chakkaphak, K., Ferguson, M. K., and Little, A. G.: Disorders of esophageal motility. Surg. Gynecol. Obstet., *172:*325, 1991.
11. Clouse, R. E., and Lustman, P. J.: Psychiatric illness and contraction abnormalities of the esophagus. N. Engl. J. Med., *309:*1337, 1983.
12. Cohen, S.: Classification of the esophageal motility disorders. Gastroenterology, *84:*1050, 1983.
13. Collard, J. M., Otte, J. B., and Kestens, P. J.: Endoscopic stapling techniques of esophagodiverticulostomy for Zenker's diverticulum. Ann. Thorac. Surg., *56:*573, 1993.
14. Csendes, A., Braghetto, I., Henriquez, A., and Cortes, C.: Late results of a prospective randomized study comparing forceful dilation and esophagomyotomy in patients with achalasia. Gut, *30:*299, 1989.
15. Dalton, C. B., Castel, D. O., Hewson, E. G., et al.: Diffuse esophageal spasm. Dig. Dis. Sci., *36:*1025, 1991.
16. Donahue, P. E., Schlesinger, P. K., and Samelson, S.: Achalasia of the esophagus. Ann. Surg., *203:*505, 1986.
17. Duranceau, A., LaFontaine, E. R., and Vallieres, B.: Effects of total fundoplication on function of the esophagus after myotomy for achalasia. Am. J. Surg., *143:*22, 1981.
18. Duranceau, A., Rheault, M. J., and Jamieson, G. G.: Physiologic response to cricopharyngeal myotomy and diverticulum suspension. Surgery, *94:*655, 1983.
19. Ellis, F. H., and Crozier, R. E.: Cervical esophageal dysphagia: Indications for and results of cricopharyngeal myotomy. Ann. Surg., *194:*279, 1981.
20. Ellis, F. H., Crozier, R. E., and Watkins, E.: Esophagomyotomy for achalasia. Dis. Esophagus, *1:*81, 1988.
21. Ellis, F. H., Crozier, R. E., and Watkins, E.: Operation for esophageal achalasia. J. Thorac. Cardiovasc. Surg., *88:*344, 1984.
22. Ellis, F. H., Gibb, S. P., and Crozier, R. E.: Esophagomyotomy for achalasia of the esophagus. Ann. Surg., *192:*157, 1980.
23. Ellis, F. H., Schlegel, J. F., Lynch, V. P., and Payne, W. S.: Cricopharyngeal myotomy for pharyngoesophageal diverticulum. Ann. Surg., *170:*340, 1969.
24. Ellis, F. H., Watkins, E., Gibb, S. P., and Heatley, G. J.: Ten to 20-year clinical results after short esophagomyotomy without an antireflux procedure for esophageal achalasia. Eur. J. Cardiothorac. Surg., *6:*86, 1992.
25. Elta, G. H., Nostrant, T. T., and Wilson, J. A. P.: Treatment of achalasia with the Witzel pneumatic dilator. Gastrointest. Endosc., *2:*101, 1987.
26. Eypasch, E. P., DeMeester, T. R., Klingman, R. R., and Stein, H. J.: Physiologic assessment and surgical management of diffuse esophageal spasm. J. Thorac. Cardiovasc. Surg., *104:*859, 1991.
27. Fellows, I. W., Ogilvie, A. L., and Atkinson, M.: Pneumatic dilation in achalasia. Gut, *24:*1020, 1983.
28. Ferguson, M. K.: Achalasia: Current evaluation and therapy. Ann. Thorac. Surg., *52:*336, 1991.
29. Ferguson, M. K., and Little, A. G.: Angina-like chest pain associated with high-amplitude peristaltic contractions of the esophagus. Surgery, *104:*713, 1988.
30. Gillies, M., Nicks, R., and Skyring, A.: Clinical, manometric, and pathological studies in diffuse oesophageal spasm. BMJ, *2:*527, 1967.
31. Gonzalez, G.: Diffuse esophageal spasm. Am. J. Roentgenol., *117:*251, 1973.
32. Gordon, C., Hewer, B. L., and Wade, D. T.: Dysphagia in acute stroke. BMJ, *295:*411, 1987.
33. Goto, S., and Grosfeld, J. L.: The effect of a neurotoxin (benzalkonium chloride) on the lower esophagus. J. Surg. Res., *47:*117, 1989.
34. Goulbourne, I. A., and Walbaum, P. R.: Long-term results of Heller's operation for achalasia. J. R. Coll. Surg. Edinb., *30:*101, 1985.
35. Graham, A. J., Finky, R. J., Worsley, D. F., et al.: Laparoscopic esophageal myotomy and anterior partial fundoplication for the treatment of achalasia. Ann. Thorac. Surg., *64:*785, 1997.
36. Guelrud, M., Zambrano-Rincones, V., Simon, C., et al.: Dysphagia and lower esophageal sphincter abnormalities after proximal gastric vagotomy. Am. J. Surg., *149:*232, 1985.
37. Heimlich, H. J., O'Conner, T. W., and Flores, D. C.: Case for pneumatic dilatation in achalasia. Ann. Otol., *87:*519, 1978.
38. Henderson, R. D., Ryder, C., and Marryatt, G.: Extended esophageal myotomy and short total fundoplication hernia repair in diffuse esophageal spasm: Five-year review in 34 patients. Ann. Thorac. Surg., *43:*25, 1987.
39. Herrera, A. F., Colon, J., Valdes-Dapena, A., and Roth, J. L. A.: Achalasia or carcinoma? The significance of the mecholyl test. Dig. Dis., *15:*1073, 1970.
40. Higgs, B., Kerr, F. W. L., and Ellis, F. H.: The experimental production of esophageal achalasia by electrolytic lesions in the medulla. J. Thorac. Cardiovasc. Surg., *50:*613, 1968.
41. Hunter, J. G., Trus, T. L., Branum, G. D., and Waring, J. P.: Laparoscopic Heller myotomy and fundoplication for achalasia. Ann. Surg., *225:*655, 1997.
42. Little, A. G.: Motor disturbances of the esophagus. *In* Skinner, D. B., and Moody, F. (eds.): Surgical Treatment of Digestive Disease. Chicago, Year Book Medical Publishers, 1989, p. 122.
43. Little, A. G.: What is the incidence of associated hiatal hernia or gastroesophageal reflux in patients with diffuse esophageal spasm? *In* Giuli, R. (ed.): Primary Esophageal Motility Disorders. Berlin, Springer-Verlag, 1991, p. 643.
44. Little, A. G., and Bandt, P. D.: Are there specific radiographic features of diffuse esophageal spasm? *In* Giuli, R. (ed.): Primary Esophageal Motility Disorders. Berlin, Springer-Verlag, 1991, p. 643.
45. Little, A. G., Chen, W., Ferguson, M. K., et al.: Physiologic evaluation of esophageal function in patients with achalasia and diffuse esophageal spasm. Ann. Surg., *203:*500, 1986.
46. Little, A. G., and Skinner, D. B.: The management of Zenker's diverticulum: Cricopharyngeal myotomy and diverticulopexy. *In* Kittle, C. F. (ed.): Current Controversies in Thoracic Surgery. Philadelphia, W. B. Saunders, *3:*15, 1986.
47. Little, A. G., Soriano, A., Ferguson, M. K., et al.: Surgical treatment of achalasia: Results with esophagomyotomy and Belsey repair. Ann. Thorac. Surg., *45:*489, 1988.
48. Malthaner, R. A., Todd, T. R., Miller, L., and Pearson, F. G.: Long-term results in surgically managed esophageal achalasia. Ann. Thorac. Surg., *54:*1343, 1994.
49. McLaughlin, J. S., Roig, R., and Woodruff, M. F. A.: Surgical treatment of strictures of the esophagus in patients with scleroderma. J. Thorac. Cardiovasc. Surg., *61:*641, 1971.
50. Nair, L. A., Reynolds, J. C., Parkman, H. P., et al.: Complications during pneumatic dilation for achalasia or diffuse esophageal spasm. Dig. Dis. Sci., *10:*1893, 1993.
51. Nelems, J. M. B., Cooper, J. D., and Pearson, F. G.: Treatment of achalasia: Esophagomyotomy with antireflux procedure. Can. J. Surg., *23:*588, 1980.
52. Okike, N., Payne, W. S., Neufeld, D. M., et al.: Esophagomyotomy versus forceful dilation for achalasia of the esophagus: Results in 899 patients. Ann. Thorac. Surg., *28:*119, 1979.
53. Olsen, A. M., Ellis, F. H., and Creamer, B.: Cardiospasm (achalasia of the cardia). Am. J. Surg., *93:*299, 1957.
54. Orlando, R. C., and Bozymski, E. M.: Clinical and manometric effects of nitroglycerin in diffuse esophageal spasm. N. Engl. J. Med., *289:*23, 1973.
55. Orr, W. C., and Robinson, M. G.: Hypertensive peristalsis in the pathogenesis of chest pain: Further exploration of the "nutcracker" esophagus. Am. J. Gastroenterol., *77:*607, 1982.
56. Orringer, M. B.: Extended cervical esophagomyotomy for cricopharyngeal dysfunction. J. Thorac. Cardiovasc. Surg., *80:*669, 1980.
57. Orringer, M. B., Dabich, L., Zarafonetis, C. J. D., and Sloan, H.: Gastroesophageal reflux in esophageal scleroderma: Diagnosis and implications. Ann. Thorac. Surg., *22:*120, 1976.
58. Orringer, M. B., Kirsh, M. M., and Sloan, H.: Long-term esophageal function following repair of esophageal atresia. Ann. Surg., *186:*431, 1977.
59. Patti, M. G., Arcerito, M., De Pinto, M., et al.: Comparison of thoracoscopic and laparoscopic Heller myotomy for achalasia. J. Gastrointest. Surg., *2:*561, 1998.
60. Payne, W. S.: Heller's contribution to the surgical treatment of achalasia of the esophagus. Ann. Thorac. Surg., *48:*876, 1989.
61. Pellegrini, C., Wetter, L. A., Patti, M., et al.: Thoracoscopic esophagomyotomy. Initial experience with a new approach for the treatment of achalasia. Ann. Surg., *216:*291, 1992.

62. Peracchia, A., Bonavina, L., Narne, S., et al.: Minimally invasive surgery for Zenker diverticulum. Arch. Surg., *133:*695, 1998.
63. Richter, J. E., and Castell, D. O.: Diffuse esophageal spasm: A reappraisal. Ann. Intern. Med., *100:*242, 1984.
64. Richter, J. E., Dalton, C. B., Bradley, L. A., and Castell, B. O.: Oral nifedipine in the treatment of noncardiac chest pain in patients with the nutcracker esophagus. Gastroenterology, *93:*21, 1987.
65. Robertson, C. S., Fellows, I. W., Mayberry, J. F., and Atkinson, M.: Choice of therapy for achalasia in relation to age. Digestion, *40:*244, 1988.
66. Schuster, M. M.: Esophageal spasm and psychiatric disorder (Editorial). N. Engl. J. Med. *309:*1382, 1983.
67. Skinner, D. B., Altorki, N., Ferguson, M., and Little, A. G.: Zenker's diverticulum: Clinical features and surgical management. Dis. Esophagus. *1:*19, 1988.
68. Stipa, S., Gegiz, G., Iascone, C., et al.: Heller-Belsey and Heller-Nissen operations for achalasia of the esophagus. Surg. Gynecol. Obstet., *170:*212, 1990.
69. Taillefer, R., and Duranceau, A. C.: Manometric and radionuclide assessment of pharyngeal emptying before and after cricopharyngeal myotomy in patients with oculopharyngeal muscular dystrophy. J. Thorac. Cardiovasc. Surg., *95:*868, 1988.
70. Thomson, D., Shoenut, J. P., Trenholm, B. G., and Teskey, J. M.: Reflux patterns following limited myotomy without fundoplication for achalasia. Ann. Thorac. Surg., *43:*550, 1987.
71. Traube, M., Hongo, M., Magyar, L., and McCallum, R. W.: Effects of nifedipine in achalasia and in patients with high-amplitude peristaltic esophageal contractions. JAMA, *252:*1733, 1984.
72. Vantrappen, G., and Hellemans, J.: Treatment of achalasia and related motor disorders. Gastroenterology, *79:*144, 1980.
73. Vantrappen, G., Hellemans, J., Deloof, W., et al.: Treatment of achalasia with pneumatic dilations. Gut, *12:*268, 1971.
74. Vogt, D., Curet, M., Pitcher, D., et al.: Successful treatment of esophageal achalasia with laparoscopic Heller myotomy and Toupet fundoplication. Am. J. Surg., *174:*709, 1997.
75. Wehrmann, T., Jacobi, V., Jung, M., et al.: Pneumatic dilation in achalasia with a low-compliance balloon: Results of a 5-year prospective evaluation. Gastrointest. Endosc., *42:*31, 1995.
76. Werlin, S. L., Dodds, W. J., Hogan, W. J., et al.: Esophageal function in esophageal atresia. Dig. Dis. Sci., *26:*796, 1981.
77. Yon, J., and Christensen, J.: An uncontrolled comparison of treatments for achalasia. Ann. Surg., *182:*672, 1975.
78. Zamost, B. J., Hirschberg, J., Ippoliti, A. F., et al.: Esophagitis in scleroderma. Gastroenterology, *92:*421, 1987.

CHAPTER

17 Surgical Management of Esophageal Diverticula

CLAUDE DESCHAMPS • PETER C. PAIROLERO • VICTOR F. TRASTEK

PHARYNGOESOPHAGEAL (ZENKER'S) DIVERTICULUM

Nature and Pathophysiology

Pharyngoesophageal diverticulum was first described in 1769 by Ludlow[67] of Bristol, England, who noted a "preternatural bag formed in the pharynx" of a patient with symptoms who was followed through death and autopsy. By 1878, Zenker[111] had collected 27 additional autopsy cases and had added seven new cases. His precise and perceptive clinicopathologic correlations have stood the test of time and account for his name becoming associated eponymically with the condition. In 1908, Killian[57] defined the anatomic site of potential mucosal diverticular protrusion as a point in the posterior midline of the lower pharynx between the oblique fibers of the inferior constrictor of the pharynx just above the transverse fibers of the cricopharyngeus muscle. This presumed congenitally weak point for diverticular protrusion has become known as *Killian's triangle*. Thus, in all the early descriptions, this diverticulum was in fact realized to be lower hypopharyngeal in location, acquired, progressive in size, and a consequence of intraluminal pressures that caused a herniation of mucosa through the usually supporting muscular fibers.

Subsequently, the obstructive role of the cricopharyngeus muscle became increasingly apparent to endoscopists and radiologists, but the nature or mechanism of this obstruction remained elusive.[23,51,74,93] These observations of a prominent, partially obstructing posterior indentation below the neck of the sac led to the loose application of the term *achalasia of the cricopharyngeus*. Manometric studies of patients with Zenker's diverticulum, however, have often shown normal relaxation of the sphincter, a finding that belies the concept of achalasia. Hunt and colleagues[49] and Smiley and associates[92] found that the mean resting pressure in the upper sphincter of patients with pharyngoesophageal diverticula was more than double that in healthy subjects; they implicated a reflex spasm of the cricopharyngeus muscle that was the consequence of esophageal distention due to presumed gastroesophageal reflux. Furthermore, most of their patients without diverticula but with hiatal hernia and reflux had a similar hypertonicity. No one has been able to confirm these findings. In particular, Winans and Harris,[108] unable to define hypertonicity of the upper esophageal sphincter, pointed out the special technical problems that exist in studying the upper esophageal sphincter manometrically.

Ellis and co-workers[29] subsequently defined a significant incoordination in pharyngeal and cricopharyngeal activity and found that 14 to 90% of swallows in these patients showed temporal premature contractions of the upper esophageal sphincter. Incoordination was found in patients with all sizes of sacs. In retrospect, Kodicek and Creamer's[59] published manometric recording demonstrated this incoordination. Duranceau and colleagues[26] defined such incoordination in only 4 of 10 patients studied, whereas Lichter[65] substantiated incoordination in all 6 of his patients. Henderson and Marryatt[41] also defined incoordination but believed that it was a response to hiatal hernia and gastroesophageal reflux.

A more recent evaluation of the characteristics of the muscles making up the upper esophageal sphincter area by Lerut and colleagues[62] suggests that myogenic degeneration and neurogenic disease are not limited to the cricopharyngeal muscle but affect the striated muscles as well. Therefore, incoordination of the cricopharyngeal muscle could be considered only one aspect of a more complex functional problem, rather than a disease on its own, and a pharyngoesophageal diverticulum could be just one expression of this process. More recently, Cook and colleagues[14] studied and compared patients with Zenker's diverticula with controls using simultaneous videoradiography and manometry. They were able to document significantly reduced sphincter opening and greater intrabolus pressure in patients with Zenker's diverticulum. They concluded that the primary abnormality in patients with Zenker's diverticula is one of incomplete upper esophageal sphincter opening rather than abnormal coordination between pharyngeal contraction and upper esophageal sphincter relaxation or opening.

Thus, the act of swallowing in the presence of cricopharyngeal dysfunction, combined with the usual pressure phenomena during deglutition, is believed to generate sufficient transmural pressure to allow mucosal herniation through an anatomically weak point in the posterior pharynx above the cricopharyngeus muscle. Because of the recurrent nature of pressures involved and the constant distention of the sac with ingested material, the established diverticulum enlarges progressively and descends dependently. The neck of the diverticulum hangs over the cricopharyngeus, and the sac becomes interposed between the esophagus and the vertebrae.

Indeed, the advanced diverticulum may come to lie in the same vertical axis as the pharynx, permitting selective filling of the sac, which may compress and angulate the adjacent esophagus anteriorly. These anatomic changes obstruct swallowing. Moreover, because the mouth of the diverticulum is above the cricopharyngeus, spontaneous emptying of the diverticulum is unimpeded and often associated with laryngotracheal aspiration as well as regurgitation into the mouth.

Several investigators have commented on the high incidence of anatomic sliding esophageal hiatal hernia in association with Zenker's diverticulum[84]; however, contrary to the findings of Henderson and Marryatt,[41] few except Belsey,[4] Hunt and associates,[49] and Smiley and coworkers[92] noted clinically significant symptoms or complications of gastroesophageal reflux in patients with a diverticulum. Unfortunately, a diverticulum has posed technical difficulties in the accomplishment of detailed preoperative manometric and pH studies, and the available information in this regard is limited.

Furthermore, various cricopharyngeal and oropharyngeal functional abnormalities have been identified secondary to a host of neurologic conditions.[28,76] These abnormalities have not been associated with pharyngoesophageal diverticulum. Indeed, patients with a Zenker's diverticulum rarely have any definable neurologic deficit or disease. Other than the fact that a neurologic deficit can produce abnormalities in the pharyngeal phase of swallowing that can be managed by cricopharyngeal myotomy, the inclusion of such cases in a discussion of patients with a diverticulum may be a seriously misleading non sequitur.

In summary, a Zenker's diverticulum is currently defined as an acquired pulsion diverticulum of the hypopharynx that develops near the midline just cephalad to the transverse fibers of the cricopharyngeus muscle. Transient obstructive abnormalities probably contribute to the generation of increased intraluminal forces that lead to herniation of pharyngeal mucosa through muscle fibers that are usually supportive.

Symptoms and Diagnosis

Although the diverticulum may be asymptomatic, most patients develop symptoms early in the course of the disease. When the condition is established, it progresses in size (Figs. 17-1 and 17-2), frequency, and severity of symptoms and complications. Characteristically, the symptoms consist of high cervical esophageal dysphagia, foul breath, noisy deglutition, and spontaneous regurgitation with or without coughing or choking episodes. The regurgitated food is characteristically fresh and undigested and is not bitter, sour, or contaminated by gastroduodenal secretions. If the condition is neglected, weight loss, hoarseness, asthma, respiratory insufficiency, and pulmonary sepsis leading to abscess are all potential complications. A palpable cervical mass is rarely noted. The chief complications of pharyngoesophageal diverticulum are nutritional and respiratory. Carcinoma arising in a pharyngoesophageal diverticulum is extremely uncommon.[55, 69, 109] Diverticular perforation may occur with any

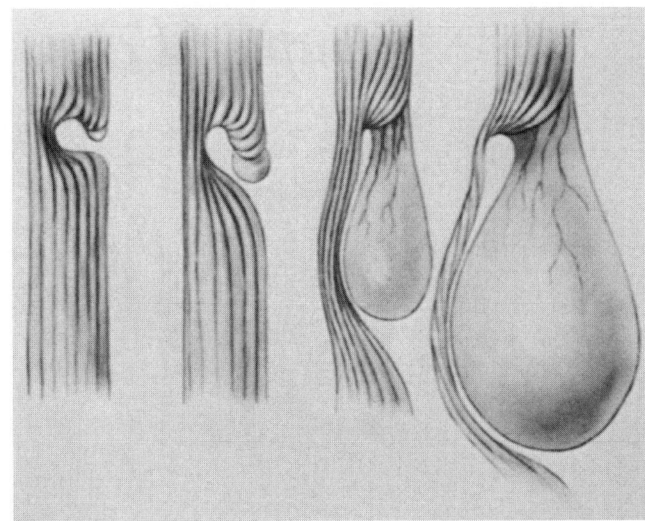

Figure 17–1. Evolution of pharyngoesophageal diverticulum from small to large. Note the prominence of the cricopharyngeus muscle within the spur between the esophagus and the diverticulum.

esophageal intubation or instrumentation or with the accidental ingestion of a foreign body.

Diagnosis is confirmed by radiographic barium swallow, which demonstrates the sac (see Fig. 17-2). Manometry and endoscopy are of little clinical value in this setting. If an endoscopy is indicated for other reasons, the endoscopist should be warned of the possibility of a pharyngoesophageal diverticulum because of the risk for instrumental perforation.

Treatment

The treatment of a pharyngoesophageal diverticulum is surgical. There is no medical therapy for this condition, and all patients with such diverticula should be considered candidates for surgical treatment, irrespective of the size of the diverticulum. Nutritional and chronic respiratory complications are not contraindications to the surgery. To the contrary, operation in such patients should be performed promptly because recurrent hypoxic episodes of aspiration are poorly tolerated in this elderly population.[79] Nor is advanced age a contraindication to surgical treatment. A recent review from the Mayo Clinic of patients 75 years or older who underwent surgical treatment of a Zenker's diverticulum demonstrated an improvement rate of 94% with no operative death.[15] Treatment is best done on an elective basis while the pouch is small or of moderate size and before complications have occurred. When nutritional or respiratory complications are present or when neoplasia is suspected, surgical intervention becomes urgent. Diverticular perforation is a surgical emergency.

Evolution of Current Management

In its early history, the surgical removal of Zenker's diverticulum universally resulted in failure.[7,31,37] Wheeler[106] re-

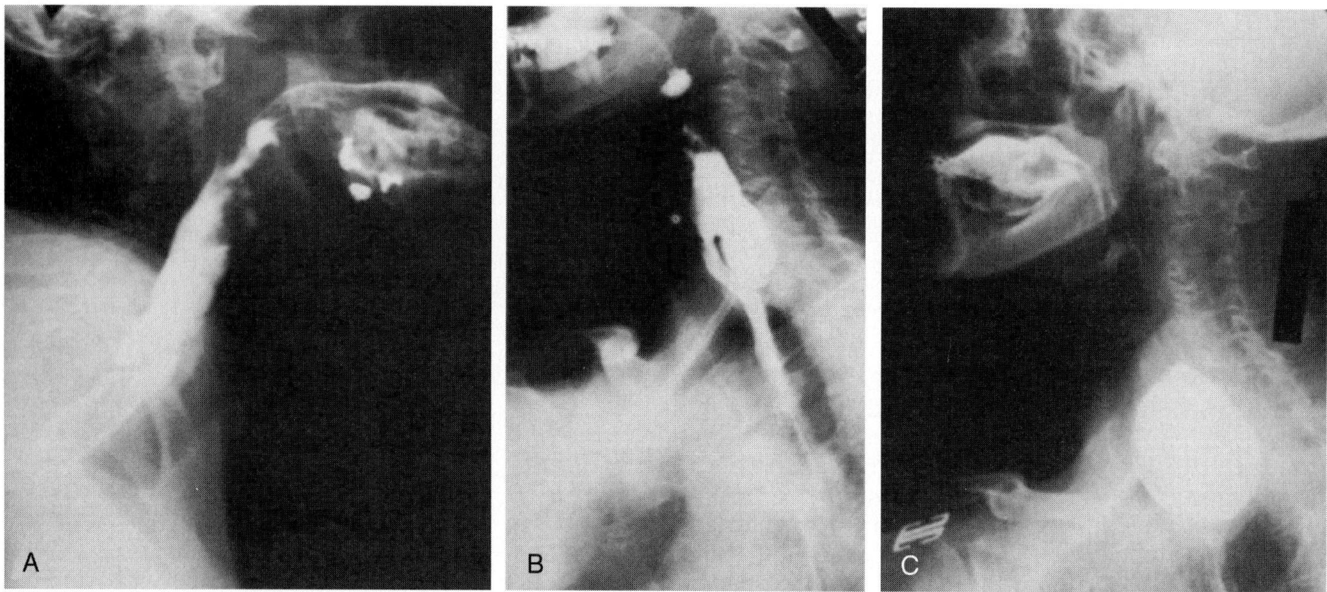

Figure 17–2. Radiographic appearance of various sizes of pharyngoesophageal diverticula. *A*, Small. *B*, Moderate. *C*, Large. (*A* and *C* from Payne, W.S.: Diverticula of the esophagus. *In* Payne, W.S., and Olsen, A.M. [eds.]: The Esophagus. Philadelphia, Lea & Febiger, 1974, with permission; *B* from Payne, W.S., and Clagett, O.T.: Pharyngeal and esophageal diverticula. Curr. Probl. Surg., 1-31, Apr., 1965, with permission of Year Book Medical Publishers.)

ported the first diverticulectomy in 1886, although von Bergmann[104] is generally credited with the first planned extirpation as a one-stage procedure. Subsequently, Kocher[58] reported two additional cases. By 1910, Mayo[70] had reported the successful one-stage removal of diverticula in six patients. About the same time, Goldmann[33] introduced a two-stage operation designed to minimize the danger of operative leak. Murphy[73] further improved the two-stage procedure. The first stage entailed mobilization of the sac, which was brought to the skin surface of the neck wound. As a result of this initial operation, fascial planes in the neck became sealed, and 2 weeks later the diverticulum could be safely extirpated without fear of spreading fatal cervical mediastinitis should a leak occur. Lahey and Warren[60] described an elaborate modification of the two-stage procedure, which Lahey championed until his death.[61]

Surgical treatment has evolved from the two-stage diverticulectomy to the highly successful one-stage diverticulectomy.[9,11,39,40,52,77,89,94] Because of our experience, reported by Ellis and associates,[29] and that of others[25-26,76,90] with cricopharyngeal myotomy, we recommend this procedure alone for small diverticula and reserve the one-stage diverticulectomy combined with cricopharyngeal myotomy for larger sacs.

Other approaches have also been used successfully.[44,53,72,87,88,91,97,107] Dohlman and Mattsson[22,23] performed a perioral endoscopic diathermic division of the septum or common wall between the diverticulum and the esophagus. This technique was popularized in the United States by Holinger and Schild[45,46] and in the Netherlands by van Overbeek and colleagues.[98-101] Collard in 1993[13] reported the use of an endoluminal stapling device to effect the cricopharyngeal myotomy endoscopically. Sutherland[93] used cricopharyngeal myotomy alone; Cross and associates[16] used it as an adjunct to extirpation, and Belsey,[4,5] Duranceau,[26] and Lerut and associates[63,64] used it as an adjunct to diverticulopexy.

Most patients undergoing surgical treatment require little or no preoperative preparation. Rarely are nutritional deficiencies severe enough to require preoperative parenteral hyperalimentation or gastrostomy. Prompt repair of the diverticulum provides the best means of correcting most deficiencies. Suppurative lung diseases, too, often require definitive resolution of the diverticular problem before they can be managed effectively. Occasionally, esophageal bougienage improves esophageal obstructive symptoms and may temporarily palliate nutritional and respiratory complications, but the patient is usually best served by prompt surgical treatment of the diverticulum.

Of the many methods described, only one-stage procedures are widely used, and of these, the following remain competitive: diverticulectomy alone or with myotomy, and myotomy alone or with diverticulopexy. Our experience is limited to diverticulectomy with or without myotomy for large diverticula and myotomy alone[80] for small diverticula. Our bias remains strong for these methods.

Surgical Technique

Either regional cervical blocks[42] or general anesthesia can be used satisfactorily, but almost all patients receive general anesthesia with a cuffed endotracheal tube. This technique controls not only the inspired gas concentrations and ventilation but also the airway, and it prevents intraoperative respiratory aspiration. Various incisions can be used to obtain surgical exposure, whether myotomy or diverticulectomy is planned. Right-handed surgeons find the left cervical approach easiest for exposing most diverticula, unless an uncommon right-sided origin of the diverticulum is noted before operation. Usually, an oblique incision is used along the anterior border of the sternocleidomastoid, extending from the level of the hyoid bone to a point 1 cm above the clavicle. After the incision has been deepened, surgical exposure of the retropharyngeal space and the diverticulum is obtained by retracting the sternocleidomastoid muscle and carotid sheath laterally and the thyroid gland and larynx medially. The diverticulum can be recognized promptly as arising from the posterior wall of the pharynx at a point just above the level where the omohyoid muscle crosses the incision (Fig. 17-3).

After the diverticulum is identified, it is mobilized and elevated with a Babcock or an Allis clamp. At this point, a No. 36 French Maloney bougie may be introduced in the esophagus to facilitate the dissection. The area of the neck is freed from surrounding fibrofatty tissue. Dissection of the neck of the diverticulum must be performed carefully so as not to injure the mucosa. The surgeon must thoroughly dissect out the diverticulum, identifying the margins of the pharyngeal muscular defect through which the mucosal sac protrudes. The myotomy is performed with a No. 15 blade with the dilator in place. Most sacs smaller than 2 cm simply disappear after the myotomy (Fig. 17-4). For diverticula between 2 and 4 cm, the myotomy is initiated at the neck of the diverticulum and is extended inferiorly for about 4 cm (Fig. 17-5*A*). Simultaneously, the surgeon uses a small peanut dissector to retract the divided muscle layer laterally. The myotomy is placed so that it is oriented roughly 135 degrees laterally from the anterior aspect of the esophagus. The diverticulum may be transected by the cut-and-sew technique and the mucosal defect closed with interrupted 4-0 silk sutures. Larger diverticula should be removed using a TA stapling device, which improves the speed and accuracy of closure[43] (see Fig. 17-5*B* and *C*). To avoid stricture, the bougie is left in place while the stapler device is applied and fired. The bougie is removed, the mucosal closure is left uncovered, and a small suction drain (Jackson-Pratt) is placed in the retropharyngeal space. The neck incision is closed, and the patient is sent to the regular ward after the recovery room.

Radiographic examination of the esophagus using contrast study is done the following day and, if satisfactory, diet is resumed. The drain is removed 2 days after the operation and the patient discharged home on the third postoperative day. If evidence of a mucosal leak is found on radiographic study, or if signs of excessive wound drainage develop, the drains are left in place, and the patient is fed nothing by mouth for 7 to 10 days. If repeat radiographs still show persistent leakage, a parenteral alimentation line is inserted and parenteral nutrition instituted to restore a positive nitrogen balance. Within 10 to 14 days, it is usually possible, with either sealing or a well-established drainage tract, to begin oral feedings. The drains can be removed eventually with the expectation that the fistula will close spontaneously.

Results

As Clagett and Payne[11] reported, the results of the one-stage pharyngoesophageal diverticulectomy have been most gratifying. From 1944 through 1971, 809 patients were treated at the Mayo Clinic by this means, and the operative mortality rate was 1.4%. The chief complications were recurrent nerve palsy (2.8%) and esophagocutaneous fistula (2.5%). Generally, both of these complications are only temporary problems that clear spontaneously in a matter of days or weeks. In a 5- to 14-year follow-up of 164 surgical patients, Welsh and Payne[105] found that 93% either were asymptomatic or had such rare and mild symptoms that they could be classified as having an excellent (82%) or a good (11%) result. Only 11 (7%) of the 164 had poor results, with or without anatomic recurrence, and required additional treatment. During the past 25 years, cricopharyngeal myotomy has been incorporated with equally satisfactory results. Payne and Reynolds'[78] late follow-up results show little change in the incidence of late diverticular recurrence, which has been minimal in either event. Any radiographic recurrence is less likely to be symptomatic if the initial diverticulectomy was accompanied by myotomy. Lerut and associates[63] reported similar results with no postoperative mortality, minimal morbidity, and very good to excellent results in 96% of patients.

Crescenzo and associates[15] recently reported the Mayo Clinic experience in patients 75 years and older. The

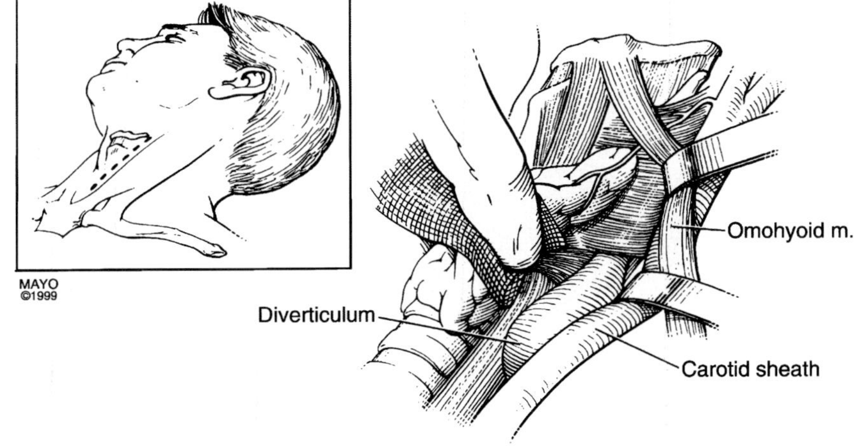

Figure 17-3. Surgical exposure of the retropharyngeal space is gained through an oblique left cervical incision oriented along the anterior border of the sternomastoid muscle *(inset)*. Retraction of the sternomastoid and carotid sheath laterally and the thyroid, pharynx, and larynx medially provides necessary exposure of the diverticulum, which is located at a cervical level where the omohyoid crosses the surgical field. (Note that the omohyoid has been retracted cephalad to show the diverticulum.)

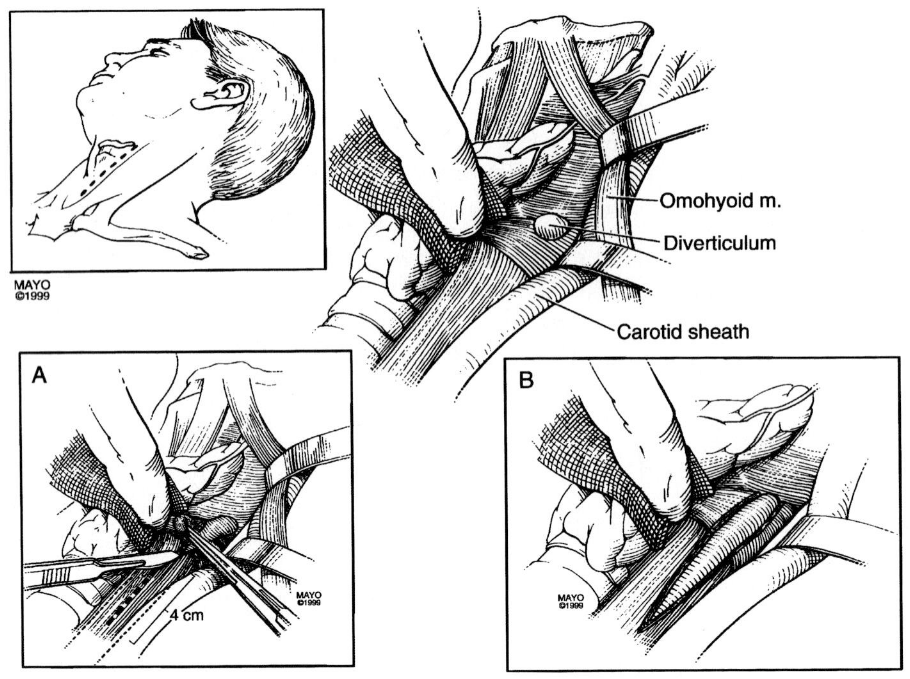

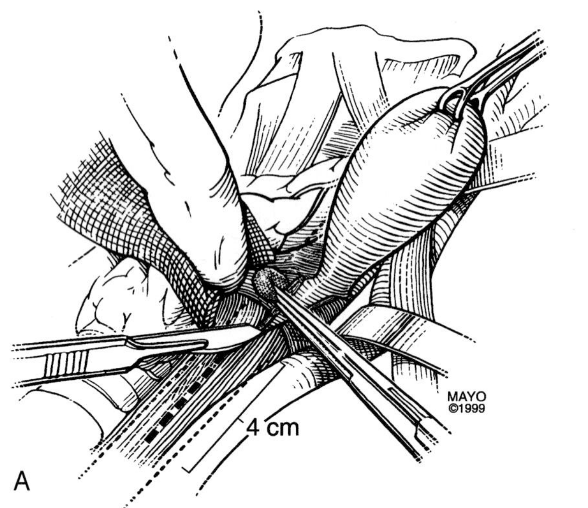

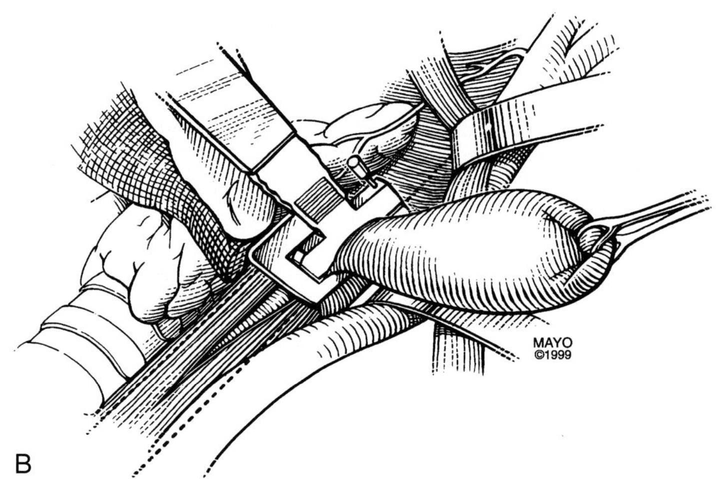

Figure 17–4. After connective tissue is dissected from the mucosal sac to identify the defect in the posterior pharyngeal wall, a posterior midline extramucosal myotomy is effected with a scalpel from the neck of the small sac inferiorly for a distance of 4 cm *(A)*. After retraction of the edges of the cut muscle with a peanut dissector, an almond-shaped diffuse bulge of mucosa through the myotomy is seen *(B)*. A small Jackson-Pratt drain is brought from the region of the myotomy and retropharyngeal space through a counterincision to the outside, and the platysma and skin are closed in layers.

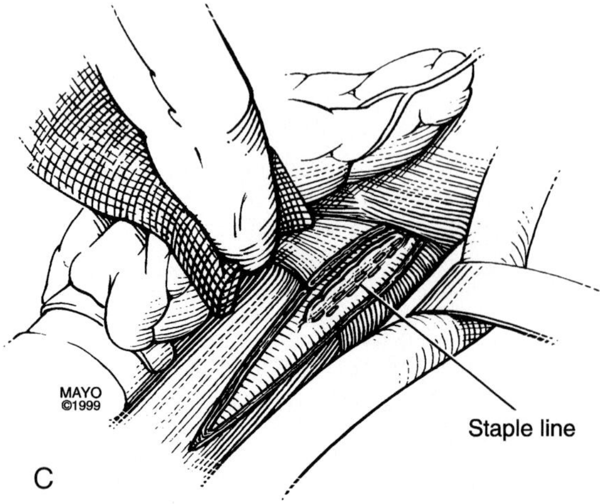

Figure 17–5. One-stage pharyngoesophageal diverticulectomy with myotomy. This procedure is used in the management of medium and large diverticula. Medium diverticulum exposed through a left cervical incision, as for myotomy alone *(A)*. Note that the omohyoid has been retracted cephalad and that a finger is used to retract the thyroid, rather than a metal instrument, to avoid injury to the recurrent nerve. The diverticulum has been dissected out to its neck, and its apex is held cephalad; with a No. 36 French catheter in the esophagus, an extramucosal myotomy with the scalpel is completed for a distance of 4 cm *(B)*. Depending on the size of the diverticulum, a TA-15, TA-30, or TA-55 stapling device has been selected. Most require TA-30 with 4.8-mm staples. Note that the staple line is oriented along the long axis of the esophagus and that an indwelling No. 36 French esophageal catheter is used to prevent stenosis and minimize the length of any luminal narrowing *(C)*. The mucosal closure is left uncovered. Drainage and closure are effected, as with myotomy alone.

median age was 79 years (range, 75 to 91 years). Preoperative symptoms included dysphagia in 69 patients (92%), regurgitation in 61 (81%), pneumonia in 9 (12%), halitosis in 3 (4%), and weight loss in 1 (1%). Gastroesophageal reflux symptoms were noted in 27 patients (36%). Diagnosis was made by barium swallow in 63 patients, esophagoscopy in 5, and a combination of both in 7. Surgical procedures included both diverticulectomy and myotomy in 57 patients (76%), myotomy alone in 9 (12%), diverticulopexy and myotomy in 5 (7%), and diverticulectomy alone in 4 (5%). There was no in-hospital mortality. Complications occurred in 8 patients (11%) and included esophagocutaneous fistula in 4, pneumonia and urinary tract infection in 1, and wound infection, myocardial infarction, and persistent diverticulum in 1 each. Follow-up was available in 72 patients (96%) and ranged from 8 days to 17 years (median, 3.3 years). At follow-up, 64 patients (88%) were symptom free, and 4 (6%) were improved with minimal symptoms. The remaining 4 patients (6%) have had varying degrees of dysphagia, and all have been treated with periodic esophageal dilatations. The authors concluded that surgery for symptomatic Zenker's diverticulum in the elderly is safe and effective and will result in resolution of symptoms and improved quality of life in most patients.

A word of caution on reoperation for recurrent pharyngoesophageal diverticulum: a review of Huang and associates[47] and more recently of Rocco and associates[83] of this aspect of diverticular surgery clearly indicated an increased risk for early postoperative morbidity. Patients who underwent previous operation for Zenker's diverticulum should be considered for reoperation only if they have progressively disabling or life-threatening symptoms. Reoperation on the upper esophageal sphincter can be a technical challenge. Previous surgery often results in obliterated tissue planes and friable esophageal mucosa. The use of an indwelling bougie is particularly helpful both as a landmark for the esophagus and as a mandrel over which esophageal repair can be accomplished without fear of luminal compromise.[79] We believe that diverticulectomy and cricopharyngeal myotomy is the treatment of choice for symptomatic patients with recurrent Zenker's diverticulum. Resolution of symptoms occurs in most patients.

Cancer arising in Zenker's diverticulum is rare; it appears to occur in chronically neglected or retained diverticula. Huang and associates[48] reported that in two patients with cancer totally confined to the sac, simple diverticulectomy provided long-term survival. More aggressive management would seem indicated if the malignancy extends beyond the sac.

EPIPHRENIC DIVERTICULUM

Epiphrenic diverticula arise within the distal 10 cm of the thoracic esophagus and are rare. However, the exact prevalence of this condition is unknown because asymptomatic cases are usually not discovered. Most of these diverticula are found in middle-aged or elderly patients, and male patients have a slight predominance. The relative incidence of epiphrenic to pharyngoesophageal diverticula at the Mayo Clinic since the 1950s has been 1 to 5.[95]

Pathophysiology

Mondiere, as early as 1833,[71] postulated that pulsion diverticula were mucosal herniations occurring through the muscularis wall associated with some form of obstruction to swallowing. Although it is not surprising that symptoms were attributed solely to the saccular abnormality of the distal esophagus in the past, the role of esophageal motility disorders in the genesis of this condition was not implicated until the 1930s.[103] With the advent of manometric studies, it has become evident that functional obstruction of the distal esophagus may be not only the cause of the diverticulum[34-36] but also a major cause of symptoms. Achalasia, diffuse esophageal spasm, hypertensive lower esophageal sphincter, and nonspecific motor abnormalities have all been seen in conjunction with epiphrenic diverticula.[6] However, motility disorders are not found in every patient, and, when present, both the type of manometric disturbances and the severity of symptoms vary.[8,18,21,56] Our most recent experience is consistent with these past observations, namely, that the cause of symptoms is multifactorial.[6]

Symptoms and Diagnosis

Symptoms in patients with epiphrenic diverticula are variable. Many patients do not have symptoms, and others have only mild dysphagia that is readily managed with simple methods such as thorough mastication and adequate fluids at mealtime. Most patients are in this category,[6] and the diverticulum is often an incidental finding on barium swallow done for unrelated reasons. Still other patients, however, have worsening and frequently incapacitating symptoms, most often severe dysphagia, chest pain, food retention, regurgitation, and subsequent aspiration. These latter symptoms may become life-threatening because repeated episodes of pneumonia may result in progressive destruction of lung parenchyma. In our experience, the ratio of patients with absent or only minimal symptoms to those with incapacitating symptoms was 1.7 to 1.

All patients with suspected epiphrenic diverticulum should undergo barium upper gastrointestinal radiographic examination. Barium swallow provides proof of diagnosis (Fig. 17-6), serves as a baseline if the patient does not have symptoms, provides clues to any associated motility disorder, and may detect other lesions, such as cancer, stricture, or hiatal hernia, that are causing symptoms. Patients with incapacitating symptoms should have further evaluation with both esophagoscopy and esophageal manometry. Esophagoscopy allows careful evaluation of the esophageal mucosa for esophagitis and the rare presence of cancer. However, endoscopy is not 100% sensitive. Esophagoscopy may also be of value in removing retained debris from the sac before operation in patients with severe retention and regurgitation. Manom-

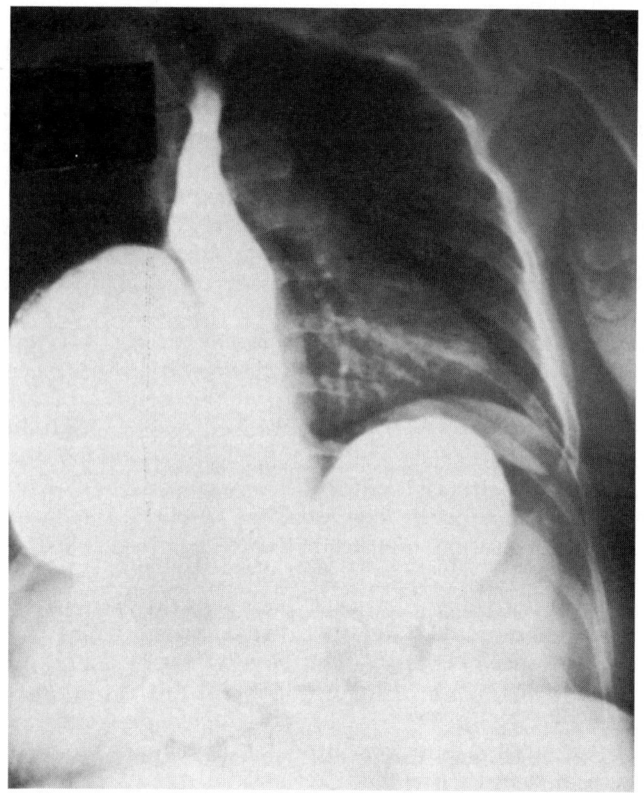

Figure 17–6. Esophagus with huge epiphrenic diverticulum occupying about half of the right thorax. Note the associated sliding esophageal hiatal hernia. (From Payne, W.S.: Esophageal diverticula. *In* Shields, T.W. [ed.]: General Thoracic Surgery, 3rd ed. Philadelphia, Lea & Febiger, 1983, p. 859, with permission.)

etry is mandatory to define associated motility disorders. These manometric findings may help determine the length of esophagomyotomy required to relieve functional obstruction. However, manometry may underestimate the extent of abnormal motility because of the difficulty in passing the probe into the stomach. If gastroesophageal reflux is suspected, a 24-hour pH study can also be performed to confirm reflux before proceeding with an antireflux procedure on clinical findings alone.[30,102] If not confirmed, the symptoms thought to be related to reflux may be caused by other conditions, such as abnormal motility or regurgitation of diverticular contents. Primary carcinoma has been noted with epiphrenic diverticula, as in the report of Allen and Clagett,[1] as have rare benign neoplasms, particularly leiomyoma and lipoma.

Treatment

The decision to proceed with surgical repair can be difficult. The surgeon must balance the risk of the procedure against the potential benefit when selecting surgical candidates. Simple medical measures often provide good temporary control in mildly symptomatic patients. In their publication describing 112 patients, Benacci and associates[6] had 47 patients who did not have symptoms and were thus not treated surgically. Twenty of these patients were followed for a median of 4 years (range, 1 to 17 years), and all remained symptom free without surgical intervention. Fifteen additional patients had mild symptoms without surgical intervention, and none of these patients developed incapacitating symptoms during follow-up (median, 11 years; range, 1 to 25 years). Although only half of patients with asymptomatic or mildly symptomatic disease had long-term follow-up available for review, progressive symptoms did not develop in any of them. Thus, we believe that patients with minimal symptoms should be managed conservatively and followed at regular intervals. If symptoms are incapacitating, an operation should be advised, if the patient is otherwise in good health. Diverticulectomy should also be considered when an operation is planned for the management of associated esophageal conditions, even when symptoms cannot be definitely attributed to the diverticulum. Neither size nor dependent location of the diverticulum correlated with symptoms in Benacci's report.[6] In contrast, based on their experience, Altorki and associates[2] have recommended operative treatment in all patients with epiphrenic diverticula.

Surgical Technique

Clairmont[12] performed the first extirpation of an epiphrenic diverticulum in 1927, using an extrapleural approach. A transpleural approach was first reported by Barrett in 1933.[3] The technique currently used at the Mayo Clinic is a transthoracic diverticulectomy, usually with a long extramucosal esophagomyotomy (Fig. 17–7). The sac is mobilized and the diverticulectomy performed longitudinally over a No. 50 French dilator. We prefer to use a stapling device and to close the muscular wall over the diverticular stump. An esophagomyotomy must be performed not only to prevent suture line leak and diverticular recurrence but also to relieve the symptoms from the associated condition. The esophagomyotomy is performed opposite the site of the diverticulectomy and should be carried onto the stomach for a few millimeters and extended cephalad through all regions of the esophagus documented to have abnormal motility. If motility is normal, the esophagomyotomy should be carried to a level above the diverticulum, which is usually between the inferior pulmonary vein and the arch of the aorta. Some surgeons have suggested that all patients undergoing an esophagomyotomy should have a concomitant antireflux procedure.[4,30,66] We do not routinely add an antireflux procedure in the absence of preoperative gastroesophageal reflux or hiatal hernia. If either is present, a less obstructive antireflux procedure, such as a modified Belsey Mark IV fundoplication, should be performed.[66]

Results

Benacci and associates[6] reviewed the Mayo Clinic experience with surgical treatment of epiphrenic diverticulum from 1975 to 1991. Among the 33 patients undergoing surgical resection during these years, 3 operative deaths occurred. Two patients had a clinically significant leak.

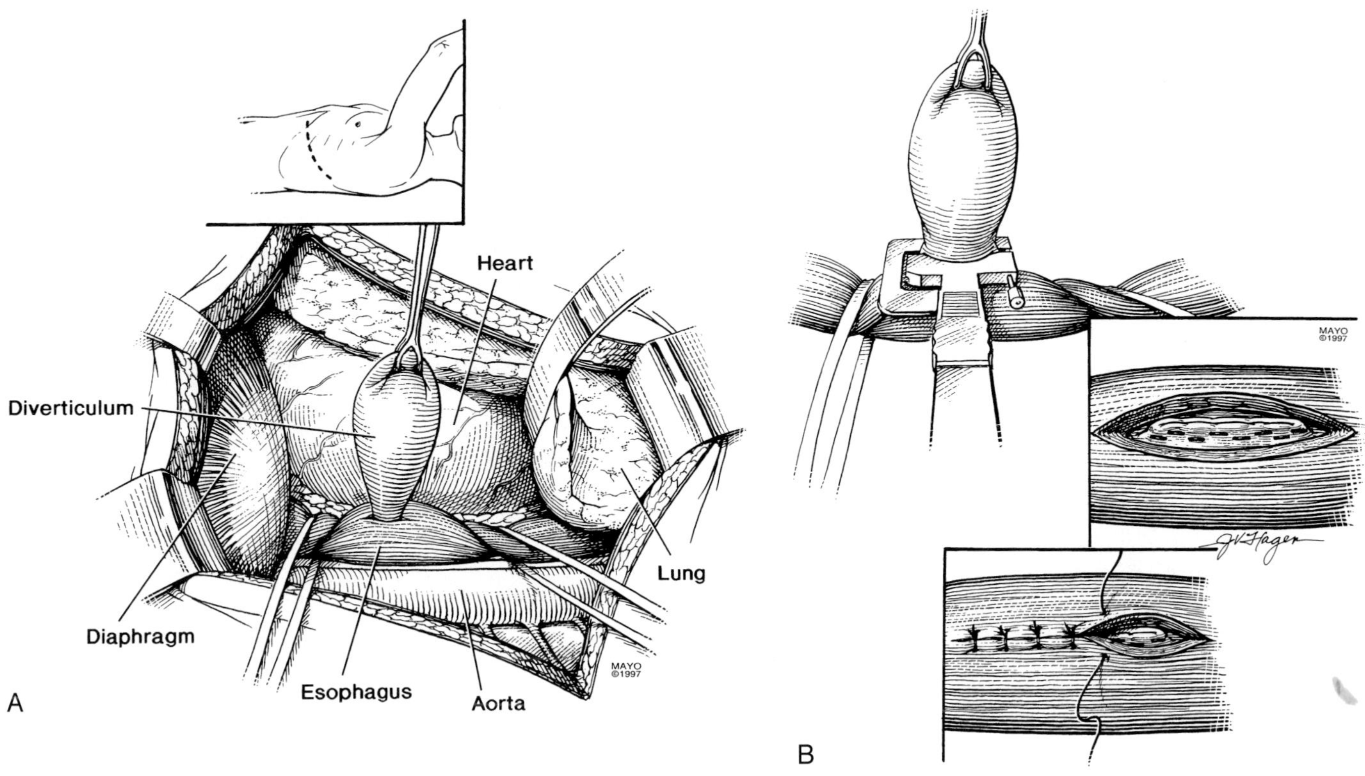

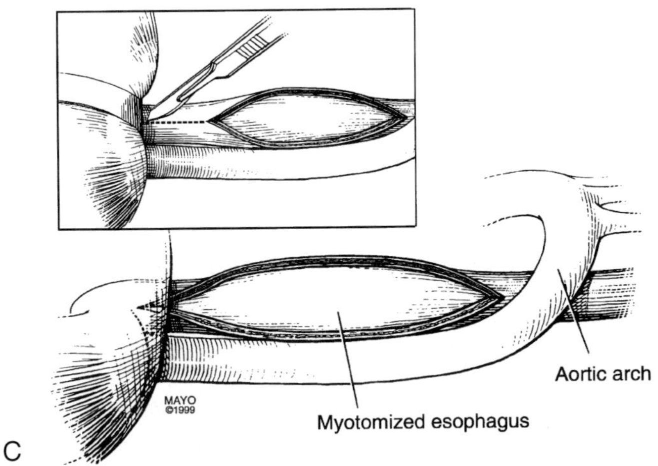

Figure 17–7. Surgical management of pulsion diverticulum of the lower portion of the esophagus. Placement of left posterolateral thoracotomy incision *(inset)*. Exposure of diverticulum is obtained when the chest is entered through the bed of the unresected left eighth rib. Note that the esophagus has been delivered from its mediastinal bed, tapes have been passed around the esophagus, and the esophagus has been rotated to bring the diverticulum into view. The neck of the mucosal diverticulum has been dissected, identifying the defect in the esophageal muscular wall *(A)*. A TA stapling device is used to transect and close the diverticulum followed by closure of esophageal musculature over mucosal suture line *(B)*. The site of the diverticular incision has been rotated back to the right and is not visible. A long esophagomyotomy, extending from the esophagogastric junction to the aortic arch, has been performed. The musculature of the esophagus has been freed from about 50% of the circumference of the esophageal mucosal tube to allow mucosa to bulge through the muscular incision *(C)*.

The third death was attributed to respiratory failure from aspiration during a Gastrografin swallow. Six esophageal leaks occurred, of which four were benign and asymptomatic. The need for meticulous surgical technique in these patients has been stressed by Orringer[75] and cannot be re-emphasized enough. Careful reapproximation of tissue and relief of distal obstruction are paramount in achieving a good result.

Although the failure to use esophagomyotomy in conjunction with diverticulectomy may be associated with recurrence or suture line complication and postoperative death, these sequelae are not inevitable results of its omission. One may infer from the data, however, only that every effort should be made to correct associated esophageal conditions to minimize postoperative complications and symptoms. Early radiographic examination of the esophagus using absorbable contrast medium (Gastrografin) before starting an oral diet is particularly valuable in the postoperative management of these patients. This examination permits an assessment of the suture line at the diverticulectomy site and evaluation of the esophagogastric lumen. When leak or obstruction is encountered, parenteral hyperalimentation is continued for 3 weeks before restudy and resumption of oral diet. Patients generally are symptom free postoperatively if associated esophageal conditions have been adequately dealt with during the operation. Follow-up in the 33 patients reported by Benacci and associates[6] ranged from 4 months to 15 years, with a median of 6.9 years. All patients did well immediately after repair. Recurrent diverticulum has not developed in this group to date. Overall results were good or excellent in 22 patients (76%), fair in 5 (17%), and poor in 2 (7%).

Surgical treatment of epiphrenic diverticulum results

in resolution of symptoms in most patients. Operative risks, however, are significant and portend to the difficulties in performing multiple concomitant procedures on the esophagus. Nonetheless, long-term results are acceptable and durable. Further understanding of the pathophysiology of epiphrenic diverticula may allow better selection of patients, reduced morbidity, and improved long-term results.

TRACTION MIDESOPHAGEAL DIVERTICULA

As noted in the previous sections of this chapter, acquired diverticula in the cervical and epiphrenic regions are thought to be pulsion or "false" diverticula because these sacs are thought to result from the generation of abnormal intraluminal esophageal pressures that cause a protrusion or herniation of mucosa and submucosa through defects in the normal supporting musculature of the esophageal wall. The term "false" was coined because not all layers of the normal esophageal wall are present in the wall of the sac, just mucosa and submucosa. Traction diverticula, on the other hand, are thought to result from localized external pulling or contracting inflammatory forces that draw all layers of the esophagus into a diverticular configuration. Because all layers are affected, these diverticula are considered to be "true." This line of reasoning becomes more cumbersome when various forms of foregut malformations (e.g., enterogenous cysts, foregut duplication) are found to communicate with the esophagus with or without duplication of muscular and epithelial elements.

Although most traction diverticula are associated with specific granulomatous disease of the subcarinal lymph nodes (Figs. 17-8 and 17-9), they can, in fact, occur at any point along the entire course of the esophagus wherever pulmonary, bronchial, or paraesophageal nodes are affected by granulomatous disease. The specific granulomatous process need not be old and burned out or inactive.[20,24,68,85] Furthermore, the whole process involved in creating a traction diverticulum cannot be fully divorced from broncholithiasis[81,96] or acquired nonmalignant esophagotracheobronchial fistula.[110] Indeed, increasing circumstantial evidence suggests that traction alone may not necessarily be the only mechanism causing these diverticula. Some cases, at least, appear to be epithelialized, spontaneously draining sinus tracts arising from more active granulomas.

The incidence of mediastinal granulomatous disease and the parallel incidence of traction diverticula appear to be related to the incidence of specific granulomatous disease, especially tuberculosis and histoplasmosis. The esophageal manifestations may be extrinsic compression, stricture, diverticulum, fistula, or a draining blind sinus tract leading from the esophagus.[24,68]

Regardless of the potential manifestations of traction diverticula, most are totally asymptomatic and likely to remain so and are of only passing notice during esophageal radiography or endoscopy. It is thought that because of their chronicity, configuration, and often dependent drainage, they remain stable in size and rarely cause symptoms.

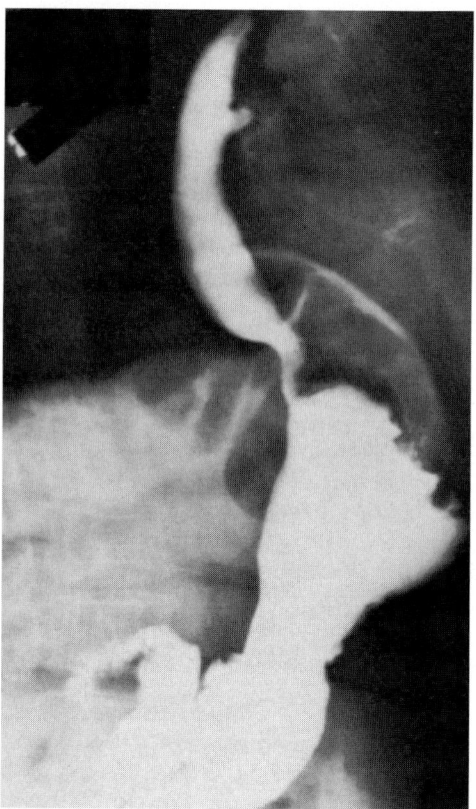

Figure 17–8. Esophagus with traction diverticulum in the middle third of the thoracic portion in relation to subcarinal lymph nodes. Patient was asymptomatic. (From Payne, W.S.: Diverticula of the esophagus. *In* Payne, W.S., and Olsen, A.M. [eds.]: The Esophagus. Philadelphia, Lea & Febiger, 1974, p. 207, with permission.)

Nevertheless, traction diverticula can produce striking manifestations. Because of their rarity, precise diagnosis is often delayed or entirely missed. Demonstration of such a complication as an acquired tracheobronchial esophageal fistula may be delayed when the manifestation is recurrent pneumonia without the classic "swallow-cough" sequence. Esophageal radiography sometimes fails to define such a fistula unless the patient is in the prone position during examination. Other techniques are simultaneous instillation of methylene blue or air in the esophagus during bronchoscopy and probing or catheterization of the sinus tract for either sinography or direct observation during either bronchoscopy or esophagoscopy.

Erosion of neighboring major blood vessels can produce massive upper gastrointestinal bleeding. Most bleeding, however, is more likely to be caused by friable granulation tissue or erosion of small bronchial or esophageal vessels by calcific debris.[10,82] Local excision of the diverticulum and adjacent inflammatory mass and closure in layers of the esophagus over an indwelling No. 40 to 50 French catheter are usually all that is required to care for a symptomatic, uncomplicated traction diverticulum. Fistulas to the respiratory tract or blood vessels require similar excisions and closure of the airway or vessel as well (Fig. 17-10). Recurrence of a fistula is minimized by the interposition of viable pleural pedicle, connective tissue, or muscle. As with any esophageal suture line,

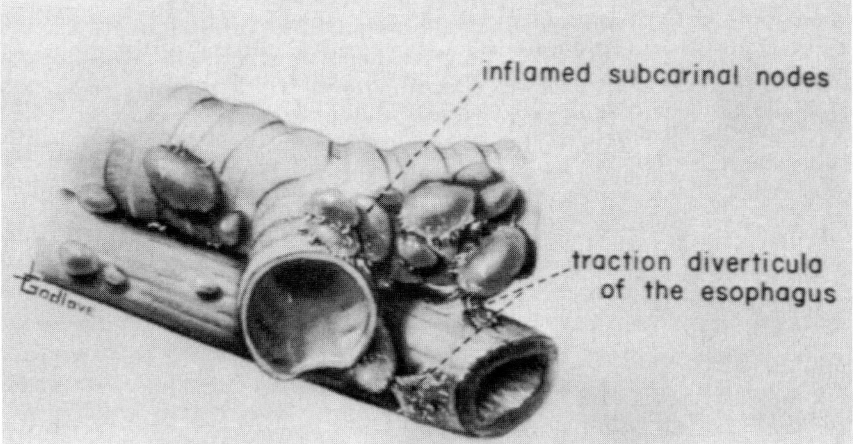

Figure 17–9. Traction diverticula of the esophagus occur most commonly in the middle third of the thoracic portion of the esophagus in relation to granulomatous subcarinal lymph nodes. Note how the esophageal wall is tented by inflammatory lymph nodes. (From Payne, W.S., and Clagett, O.T.: Pharyngeal and esophageal diverticula. Curr. Probl. Surg., 1–31, Apr., 1965, with permission of Year Book Medical Publishers.)

care should be taken to eliminate any distal esophageal obstruction.

Among the causes of acquired, nonmalignant esophagorespiratory fistulas seen at the Mayo Clinic, Wychulis and colleagues[110] found that late sequelae of infection due to tuberculosis or fungi were second only to trauma in frequency. Others, including Davis and colleagues[17] and Hutchin and Lindskog,[50] have commented on the occurrence of this occult and common cause of acquired benign tracheoesophageal fistula. The chance that such a fistula will develop in a patient with a traction diverticulum of the esophagus is probably remote, yet such a possibility should be considered in a patient with chronic recurrent suppurative lung disease or symptoms of cough after swallowing. In the evaluation of such patients, the esophagus should be examined radiographically. Cinefluoroscopy (or videofluoroscopy) during ingestion of contrast medium usually defines the site and size of a communication and aids in screening many other patients thought to have a fistula. Many patients suspected of having a fistula are actually aspirating ingested material through the larynx as a consequence of some mechanism other than a fistula. Specific study directed at the swallowing mechanism will assist in providing a more precise diagnosis in such cases. Endoscopic examination of both the esophagus and the tracheobronchial tree is indicated, and the orifices of the fistula can usually be identified. The introduction of methylene blue or other dye into the esophagus during bronchoscopy may facilitate this identification. Biopsy material should be obtained for histopathologic and microbiologic study, although viable organisms are rarely identified. If symptoms suggest chronic pulmonary suppuration, computed tomography for identification of bronchiolitis and bronchography for delineation of the extent of bronchiectasis may be indicated unless parenchymal resection is planned anyway.

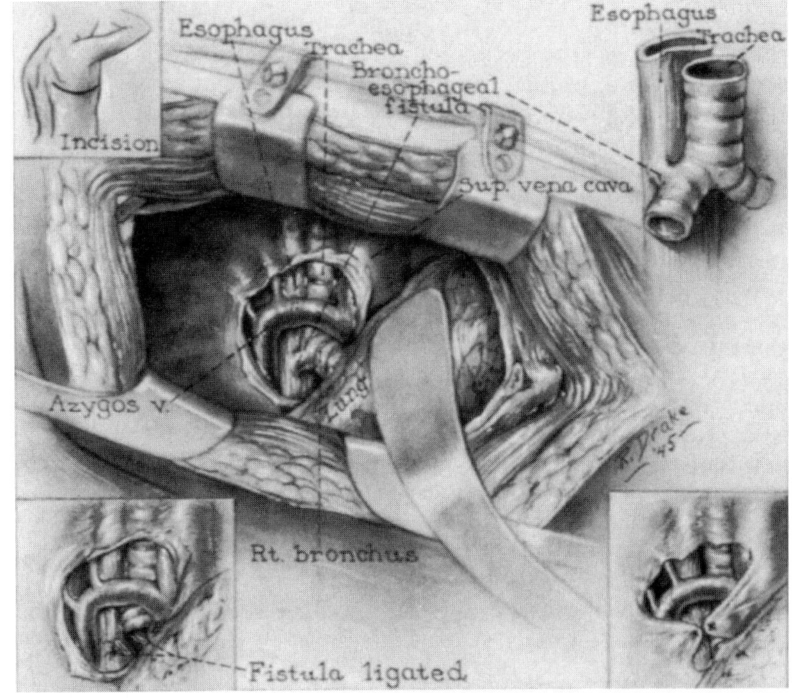

Figure 17–10. Technique for closing acquired esophagobronchial fistula as a complication of a traction diverticulum of the esophagus. Right posterolateral thoracotomy incision *(upper left inset)*. Surgical exposure. Lung has been retracted anteriorly. Note the relationship of the esophagus, right main bronchus, and fistula to neighboring sutures *(center)*. Fistula before division and after division and ligation *(upper right and lower left insets)*. Method of interposing pedicles of mediastinal pleura between esophageal and bronchial closures *(lower right inset)*. (From Payne, W.S., and Clagett. O.T.: Pharyngeal and esophageal diverticula. Curr. Probl. Surg., 1–31, Apr., 1965, with permission of Year Book Medical Publishers.)

In addition to division of the fistula and repair of the esophagus and airway, attention must be paid to correction of the distal esophageal obstruction, whether it is organic or one of the specific esophageal motility disturbances. A particularly useful maneuver under such circumstances is the passage of a No. 40 to 50 French esophageal dilator over a previously swallowed thread as a guide. Easy passage of the dilator to the stomach ensures the absence of an organically obstructed esophagus. Although traction diverticula are rarely complicated by specific esophageal motility disturbances, esophageal manometry is the most reliable method of defining these conditions.

Esophagovascular fistulas, as reported by Schick and Yesner,[86] Powell,[82] and Jonasson and Gunn,[54] are extremely rare complications of traction diverticula. Impressive hemorrhage may occur without communication with a major vessel, and in such cases, additional time may be available for orderly study and treatment. All too often, initial bleeding is sudden, massive, and fatal when major vessels are involved. In addition to standard endoscopic and radiographic studies, selective arteriography during active bleeding can be helpful in defining the site of hemorrhage.

References

1. Allen, T.H., and Clagett, O.T.: Changing concepts in the surgical treatment of pulsion diverticula of the lower esophagus. J. Thorac. Cardiovasc. Surg., *50:*455, 1965.
2. Altorki, N.K., Sunagawa M., and Skinner, D.B.: Thoracic esophageal diverticula: Why is operation necessary? J. Thorac. Cardiovasc. Surg., *105:*260, 1993.
3. Barrett, N.R.: Diverticula of the thoracic oesophagus: Report of a case in which the diverticulum was successfully resected. Lancet, *1:*1009, 1933.
4. Belsey, R.: Functional disease of the esophagus. J. Thorac. Cardiovasc. Surg., *52:*164, 1966.
5. Belsey, R.: Recent progress in oesophageal surgery. Acta Chir. Belg., *71:*230, 1972.
6. Benacci, J.C., Deschamps, C., Trastek, V.F., et al.: Epiphrenic diverticulum: Results of surgical treatment. Ann. Thorac. Surg., *55:*1109, 1993.
7. Bevan, A.D.: Diverticula of the esophagus. J.A.M.A., *76:*285, 1921.
8. Bontempo, L., Corazziari, E., Mineo, T.C., et al.: Esophageal motor activity in patients with esophageal diverticula. *In* DeMeester, T.R., and Skinner, D.B., (eds.): Esophageal Disorders, Pathophysiology and Therapy. New York, Raven Press, 1985, pp. 427–429.
9. Boyd, D.P., and Adams, H.D.: Esophageal diverticulum. N. Engl. J. Med., *264:*641, 1961.
10. Cheitlin, M.D., Kamin, E.J., and Wilkes, D.J.: Midesophageal diverticulum: Report of a case with fistulous connection with the superior vena cava. Arch. Intern. Med., *107:*252, 1961.
11. Clagett, O.X., and Payne, W.S.: Surgical treatment of pulsion diverticula of the hypopharynx: One-stage resection in 478 cases. Dis. Chest, *37:*257, 1960.
12. Clairmont, cited by Moynihan, B.: Diverticula of the alimentary canal. Lancet, *1:*1061, 1927.
13. Collard, J.M., Otte, J.B., Kestens, P.J.: Endoscopic stapling technique of esophagodiverticulostomy for Zenker's diverticulum. Ann. Thorac. Surg., *56:*573, 1993.
14. Cook, J.J., Gabb, M., Panagopoulos, V., et al.: Pharyngeal (Zenker's) diverticulum is a disorder of upper esophageal sphincter opening. Gastroenterology, *103:*1229, 1992.
15. Crescenzo, D.G., Trastek, V.F., Allen M.S., et al.: Zenker's diverticulum in the elderly: Is operation justified? Ann. Thorac. Surg., *66:*347, 1998.
16. Cross, F.S., Johnson, G.F., and Gerein, A.X.: Esophageal diverticula: Associated neuromuscular changes in the esophagus. Arch. Surg., *83:*525, 1961.
17. Davis, E.W., Katz, S., and Peabody, J.W., Jr.: Broncholithiasis, a neglected cause of bronchoesophageal fistula. J.A.M.A., *160:*555, 1956.
18. Debas, H.T., Payne, W.S., Cameron, A.J., et al.: Physiopathology of lower esophageal diverticulum and its implications for treatment. Surg. Gynecol. Obstet., *151:*593, 1980.
19. Deguise, F.: Dissertation sur l'anévrismé, suivie de propositions médicales sur divers objets, et des aphorismes d'Hippocrate sur le spasme. Thesis, Paris, 1804.
20. Dines, D.E., Payne, W.S., Bernatz, P.E., et al.: Mediastinal granuloma and fibrosing mediastinitis. Chest, *75:*320, 1979.
21. Dodds, W.J., Stef, J.J., Hogan, W.J., et al.: Distribution of esophageal peristaltic pressure in normal subjects and patients with esophageal diverticulum. Gastroenterology, *69:*584, 1975.
22. Dohlman, G., and Mattsson, O.: The endoscopic operation for hypopharyngeal diverticula: A roentgencinematographic study. Arch. Otolaryngol., *71:*744, 1960.
23. Dohlman, G., and Mattsson, O.: The role of the cricopharyngeal muscle in cases of hypopharyngeal diverticula: A cineroentgenographic study. Am. J. Roentgenol., *81:*561, 1959.
24. Dukes, R.J., Strimlan, C.N., Dines, D.E., et al.: Esophageal involvement with mediastinal granuloma. J.A.M.A., *236:*2313, 1976.
25. Duranceau, A., Gregoire, J.: Surgical management of Zenker's diverticulum. Hepatogastroenterology, *39:*132, 1991.
26. Duranceau, A., Rheault, M.J., and Jamieson, G.G.: Physiologic response to cricopharyngeal myotomy and diverticulum suspension. Surgery, *94:*655, 1983.
27. Effler, D.B., Barr, D., and Groves, L.X.: Epiphrenic diverticulum of the esophagus: Surgical treatment. Arch. Surg., *79:*459, 1959.
28. Ellis, F.H., Jr., and Crozier, R.E.: Cervical esophageal dysphagia: Indications for and results of cricopharyngeal myotomy. Ann. Surg., *194:*279, 1981.
29. Ellis, F.H., Jr., Schlegel, J.F., Lynch, V.P., et al.: Cricopharyngeal myotomy for pharyngo-esophageal diverticulum. Ann. Surg., *170:*340, 1969.
30. Evander, A., Little, A.G., Ferguson, M.K., et al.: Diverticula of the mid- and lower esophagus: Pathogenesis and surgical management. World I. Surg., *10:*820, 1986.
31. Girard, C.: Du traitement des diverticules de l'oesophage. Procès Verbaux, Mem. Discuss. Assoc. Franc. Chirurg., *103:*92, 1896.
32. Giuli, R., Estenne, B., Richard, C. A., et al.: Les diverticules de l'oesophage: A propos de 221 cas. Ann. Chir., *28:*435, 1974.
33. Goldmann, E.E.: Die zweideutige Operation von Pulsionsdivertikeln der Speiserhre; nebst Bemerkungen dber den Oesophagusmund. Beit. Klin. Chir., *61:*741, 1980–1989.
34. Goodman, H.I., and Parnes, I.H.: Epiphrenic diverticula of the esophagus. J. Thorac. Cardiovasc. Surg., *23:*145, 1952.
35. Habein, H.C., Jr., Kirklin, J.W., Clagett, O.T., et al.: Surgical treatment of lower esophageal pulsion diverticula. Arch. Surg., *72:*1018, 1956.
36. Habein, H.C., Jr., Moersch, H.J., and Kirklin, J.W.: Diverticula of the lower part of the esophagus: A clinical study of 149 nonsurgical cases. Arch. Intern. Med., *97:*768, 1956.
37. Halstead, A.E.: Diverticula of the oesophagus: With the report of a case. Ann. Surg., *39:*171, 1904.
39. Harrington, S.W.: Pulsion diverticula of the hypopharynx: A review of 41 cases in which operation was performed and a report of two cases. Surg. Gynecol. Obstet., *69:*364, 1939.
40. Harrington, S.W.: Pulsion diverticulum of the hypopharynx at the pharyngoesophageal junction: Surgical treatment in 140 cases. Surgery, *18:*66, 1945.
41. Henderson, R.D., and Marryatt, G.: Cricopharyngeal myotomy as a method of treating cricopharyngeal dysphagia secondary to gastroesophageal reflux. J. Thorac. Cardiovasc. Surg., *74:*721, 1977.
42. Hiebert, C.A.: Surgery for cricopharyngeal dysfunction under local anesthesia. Am. J. Surg., *131:*423, 1976.
43. Hoehn, J.G., and Payne, W.S.: Resection of pharyngoesophageal diverticulum using stapling device. Mayo Clin. Proc., *44:*738, 1969.
44. Hoffmann, E., and Gerhardt, C.: Behandlung der Oesophagusdivertikel. Zentralbl. Chin., *98:*1501, 1973.
45. Holinger P.H., and Schild, J.A.: The Zenker's (hypopharyngeal) diverticulum. Ann. Otol. Rhinol. Laryngol., *78:*679, 1969.

46. Holinger, P.H., and Johnston, F-C.: Endoscopic surgery of Zenker's diverticula: Experience with the Dohlman technique. Ann. Otol. Rhinol. Laryngol., *70:*1117, 1961.
47. Huang, B., Payne, W.S., and Cameron, A.J.: Surgical management for recurrent pharyngoesophageal (Zenker's) diverticulum. Ann. Thorac. Surg., *37:*189, 1984.
48. Huang, B., Unni, K.K., and Payne, W.S.: Long-term survival following diverticulectomy for cancer in pharyngoesophageal (Zenker's) diverticulum. Ann. Thorac. Surg., *38:*207, 1984.
49. Hunt, P.S., Connell, A.M., and Smiley, T.B.: The cricopharyngeal sphincter in gastric reflux. Gut, *11:*303, 1970.
50. Hutchin, P., and Lindskog, G.E.: Acquired esophagobronchial fistula of infectious origin. J. Thorac. Cardiovasc. Surg., *48:*1, 1964.
51. Jackson, C., and Shallow, T.A.: Diverticula of the oesophagus, pulsion, traction, malignant and congenital. Ann. Surg., *83:*1, 1926.
52. Jackson, C.L., and Norris, C.M.: Pharyngoesophageal diverticulum and the technique of its surgical treatment. Laryngoscope, *65:*546, 1955.
53. Jesberg, N.: Bilobed pulsion diverticulum of the hypopharynx: A historical summary and a case report. Ann. Otol. Rhinol. Laryngol., *63:*39, 1954.
54. Jonasson, O.M., and Gunn, L.C.: Midesophageal diverticulum with hemorrhage: Report of a case. Arch. Surg., *90:*713, 1965.
55. Juby, H.B.: The treatment of pharyngeal pouch. J. Laryngol. Otol., *92:*1101, 1978.
56. Kaye, M.D.: Oesophageal motor dysfunction in patients with diverticula of the mid-thoracic oesophagus. Thorax, *29:*666, 1974.
57. Killian, G.: Ueber den Mund der Speiserhre. Ztschr. Ohrenh., *55:*1, 1908.
58. Kocher, T.: Das Oesophagusdivertikel und Dessenbehandlung. Cor-Bl Schweiz, Aertz (Basel), *22:*233, 1892.
59. Kodicek, J., and Creamer, B.: A study of pharyngeal pouches. J. Laryngol. Otol., *75:*406, 1961.
60. Lahey, F.H., and Warren, K.W.: Esophageal diverticula. Surg. Gynecol. Obstet., *98:*1, 1954.
61. Lahey, F.H.: Oesophageal diverticula. Boston Med. Surg. J., *188:* 355, 1923.
62. Lerut, T.: Does the musculus cricopharyngeus play a role in the genesis of Zenker's diverticulum? Enzyme histochemical and contractility properties. *In* Siewert, J.R., and Holscher, A.M., (eds.): Diseases of the Esophagus. New York, Springer, 1988.
63. Lerut, T., van Raemdonck, D., Guelincky, P., et al.: Pharyngo-oesophageal diverticulum (Zenker's): Clinical, therapeutic, and morphological aspects. Acta Gastroenterol. Belg., *53:*330, 1990.
64. Lerut, T., van Raemdonck, D., Guelincky, P., et al.: Zenker's diverticulum: Is a myotomy of the cricopharyngeus useful? How long should it be? Hepatogastroenterology, *39:*127, 1992.
65. Lichter, I.: Motor disorder in pharyngoesophageal pouch. J. Thorac. Cardiovasc. Surg., *76:*272, 1978.
66. Little, A.G., Soriano, A., Ferguson, M.K., et al.: Surgical treatment of achalasia: Results with esophagomyotomy and Belsey repair. Ann. Thorac. Surg., *45:*489, 1988.
67. Ludlow, A.: A case of obstructed deglutition, from a preternatural dilatation of, and bag formed in the pharynx. Med. Observ. Inq., *3:*85, 1769.
68. MacCarty, R.L., Dukes, R.J., Strimlan, C.V., et al.: Radiographic findings in patients with esophageal involvement by mediastinal granuloma. Gastrointest. Radiol., *4:*11, 1979.
69. Mackay, I.S.: The treatment of pharyngeal pouch. J. Laryngol. Otol., *90:*183, 1976.
70. Mayo, C.H.: Diagnosis and surgical treatment of esophageal diverticula: Report of eight cases. Trans. Am. Surg. Assoc., *28:*197, 1910.
71. Mondiere, J.T.: Notes sur quelques maladies de l'oesophage. Arch. Gen. Med. Paris, *3:*28, 1833.
72. Mosher, H.P.: Webs and pouches of the oesophagus, their diagnosis and treatment. Surg. Gynecol. Obstet., *25:*175, 1917.
73. Murphy, J.B.: Diverticulum of the esophagus: Conservative treatment. Surg. Clin. (Chicago), 391, 1916.
74. Negus, V.E.: Pharyngeal diverticula: Observations on their evolution and treatment. Br. J. Surg., *38:*129, 1950.
75. Orringer, M.B.: Epiphrenic diverticula: Fact and fable (Editorial). Ann. Thorac. Surg., *55:*1067, 1993.
76. Orringer, M.B.: Extended cervical esophagomyotomy for cricopharyngeal dysfunction. J. Thorac. Cardiovasc. Surg., *80:*669, 1980.
77. Payne, W.S., and Clagett, O.T.: Pharyngeal and esophageal diverticula. Curr. Probl. Surg., 1-31, Apr., 1965.
78. Payne, W.S., and Reynolds, R.R.: Surgical treatment of pharyngoesophageal diverticulum (Zenker's diverticulum). Surg. Rounds, *5:*18, 1982.
79. Payne, W.S.: The treatment of pharyngoesophageal diverticulum: The simple and complex. Hepatogastroenterology, *39:*109, 1992.
80. Payne, W.S.: Diverticula of the esophagus. *In* Payne, W.S., and Olsen, A.M. (eds.): The Esophagus. Philadelphia, Lea & Febiger, 1974, p. 207.
81. Potaris, K., Miller, D.L., Trastek, V.F., et al.: Role of surgical resection in broncholithiasis. Ann. Thorac. Surg., *70:*248, 2000.
82. Powell, M.E.A.: A case of aortic-oesophageal fistula. Br. J. Surg., *45:*55, 1957.
83. Rocco, G., Deschamps, C., Martel, E., et al.: Results of reoperation on the upper esophageal sphincter. J. Thorac. Cardiovasc. Surg., *117:*28, 1999.
84. Rosenberg, S.J., and Harris, L.D.: A single physiologic mechanism for changing strength of both esophageal sphincters (Abstract). Gastroenterology, *60:*798, 1971.
85. Sakulsky, S.B., Harrison, E.G., Jr., Dines, D.E., et al.: Mediastinal granuloma. J. Thorac. Surg., *54:*279, 1967.
86. Schick, A., and Yesner, R.: Traction diverticulum of esophagus with exsanguination: Report of a case. Ann. Intern. Med., *39:*345, 1953.
87. Schmid, H.H.: Vorschlag eines einfachen Operationsverfahrens zur Behandlung des Oesphagusdivertikels. Wien. Klin. Wochenschr., *25:*87, 1912.
88. Seiffert, A.: Zur Befiandlung beginnender Hypopharynxdivertikel. Ztschr. Laryngol. Rhinol. Otol., *23:*256, 1932.
89. Shallow, T.A., and Clerf, L.H.: One stage pharyngeal diverticulectomy: Improved technique and analysis of 186 cases. Surg. Gynecol. Obstet., *86:*317, 1948.
90. Shaw, D.W., Cook, I.J., Jamieson, G.G., et al.: Influence of surgery on deglutitive upper oesophageal sphincter mechanics in Zenker's diverticulum. Gut, *38:*806, 1996.
91. Skinner, E.F., and Page, G.: Esophago-diverticulostomy for stenosis of upper esophagus associated with Zenker's diverticulum. Am. Surg., *24:*806, 1958.
92. Smiley, T.B., Caves, R.I.C., and Porter, D.C.: Relationship between posterior pharyngeal pouch and hiatus hernia. Thorax, *25:*725, 1970.
93. Sutherland, H. D.: Cricopharyngeal achalasia. J. Thorac. Cardiovasc. Surg., *43:*114, 1962.
94. Sweet, R.H.: Pulsion diverticulum of the pharyngoesophageal junction: Technic of the one-stage operation; a preliminary report. Ann. Surg., *125:*41, 1947.
95. Trastek, V.F., and Payne, W.S.: Esophageal diverticula. *In* Shields, T.W. (ed.): General Thoracic Surgery. Philadelphia, Lea & Febiger, 1989, pp. 989–1001.
96. Trastek, V.F., Pairolero, P.C., Ceithaml, E.L., et al.: Surgical management of broncholithiasis. J. Thorac. Cardiovasc. Surg., *90:*842, 1985.
97. Trible, W.M.: The surgical treatment of Zenker's diverticulum: Endoscopic vs external operation. South. Med. J., *68:*1260, 1975.
98. van Overbeek, J.J.M.: Meditation on the pathogenesis of hypopharyngeal (Zenker's) diverticulum and a report of endoscopic treatment in 545 patients. Ann. Otol. Rhinol. Laryngol., *103:*178, 1994.
99. van Overbeek, J.J.M., and Hoeksema, P.E.: Endoscopic treatment of the hypopharyngeal diverticulum: 211 cases. Laryngoscope, *92:*88, 1982.
100. van Overbeek, J.J.M., Hoeksema, P.E., and Edens, E.T.: Microendoscopic surgery of the hypopharyngeal diverticulum using electrocoagulation or carbon dioxide laser. Ann. Otol. Rhinol. Laryngol., *93:*34, 1984.
101. van Overbeek, J.J.M.: The hypopharyngeal diverticulum. Amsterdam, Van Gorcum, 1977, p. 136.
102. Viard, H., Sala, J.J., Favre, J.P., et al.: Le traitement chirurgical des diverticules de pulsion de l'oesophage. J. Chir. (Paris), *124:*658, 1987.
103. Vinson, P.P.: Diverticula of the thoracic portion of the esophagus: Report of 42 cases. Arch. Otolaryngol., *19:*508, 1934.
104. von Bergmann, E.: Ueber den Oesophagusdivertikel und seine Behandlung. Arch. Klin. Chir. (Berlin), *43:*1, 1892.
105. Welsh, G.R., and Payne, W.S.: The present status of one-stage

pharyngoesophageal diverticulectomy. Surg. Clin. North Am., *53:*953, 1973.
106. Wheeler, W.I.: Pharyngocele and dilatation of pharynx, with existing diverticulum at lower portion of pharynx lying posterior to the oesophagus, cured by pharyngotomy, being the first case of the kind recorded. J. Med. Sci. (3rd series, Dublin), *82:*349, 1886.
107. White, I.L.: Endoscopic treatment of hypopharyngeal diverticula. Cal. Med., *109:*374, 1968.
108. Winans, C.S., and Harris, L.D.: Quantitation of lower esophageal sphincter competence. Gastroenterology, *52:*773, 1967.
109. Wychulis, A.R., Gunnlaugsson, G.H., Clagett, O.T.: Carcinoma occurring in pharyngo-esophageal diverticulum: Report of three cases. Surgery, *66:*976, 1969.
110. Wychulis, A.R., Ellis, F.H., Jr., and Andersen, H.A.: Acquired nonmalignant esophagotracheobronchial fistula: Report of 36 cases. J.A.M.A., *196:*117, 1966.
111. Zenker, F.A.: Diseases of the esophagus. *In* von Ziemssen, H. (ed.): Cyclopaedia of the Practice of Medicine, Vol. 8. New York, William Wood & Company, 1878, p. 46.
112. Zuckerbraun, L., and Bahna, M.S.: Cricopharyngeus myotomy as the only treatment for Zenker diverticulum. Ann. Otol., *88:*798, 1979.

CHAPTER

18 Laparoscopic Esophageal Surgery

THOMAS R. EUBANKS • CARLOS A. PELLEGRINI

Laparoscopy has dramatically changed the operative approach to the distal esophagus. A once difficult exposure has been improved with the use of videoendoscopy to view the esophageal hiatus and gastroesophageal (GE) junction. In addition to better exposure, the minimally invasive approach has made elective operations more palatable to patients and referring physicians. This change is based on the shorter hospital stay, smaller incisions, and decreased postoperative pain.

Gastroesophageal reflux disease (GERD) is routinely treated through a laparoscopic approach. Paraesophageal hernias and esophageal dysmotility syndromes, especially achalasia, may be approached videoendoscopically but are less common clinical entities. Epiphrenic diverticula and benign soft tissue tumors are even less common, but experience with the laparoscopic approach is being reported. Esophagectomy for benign or malignant conditions can be accomplished with laparoscopic assistance but is practiced at very few centers. All of these procedures require advanced laparoscopic skills, including suturing, control of bleeding, and two-handed operative techniques.

Because these disease processes are discussed in other chapters, only details relevant to the laparoscopic approach or findings that have resulted from increased operative volume due to minimally invasive procedures are discussed in detail here. The operative technique for antireflux procedures is described precisely; the approach to other pathologic entities is described only as it deviates from the standard antireflux operation.

GASTROESOPHAGEAL REFLUX DISEASE

Indications

The indications for the laparoscopic treatment of GERD are the same as those for the open approach; severe esophagitis, Barrett's esophagus, and incomplete resolution of symptoms or relapses while on medical therapy are the most common. The diagnosis of laryngeal or pharyngeal reflux has become a more frequent indication for surgery. Extraesophageal symptoms include wheezing, coughing, hoarseness, and aspiration. The relationship between GE reflux and extraesophageal symptoms is not easy to establish, but an improvement in symptoms while on proton pump inhibitors helps predict success of the operation.[1]

In the past, unsuccessful medical treatment was commonly listed as a reason to proceed with operative therapy. In the era of proton pump inhibitors, which are much more effective than H_2-blockers,[2] this may no longer be a clear indication to proceed with operative intervention. The lack of response to high-dose proton pump inhibitor therapy may call into question the diagnosis of GERD. Some authors have recommended using proton pump inhibitors as a diagnostic test for GERD and a screening method for surgical referral.[3] If symptoms are unchanged with medical treatment, objective documentation of GERD should be obtained before proceeding with operative therapy.

Evaluation

The preoperative evaluation of patients with GERD should include manometry, 24-hour pH monitoring, upper endoscopy, and esophagography. Each of these tests provides distinctly different information about the disease process. Manometry and pH testing are functional studies that characterize the motility of the esophagus and the amount of acid exposure in a 24-hour observation period, respectively. Of particular interest in the manometry is the efficacy of peristalsis. If progressive peristalsis occurs less frequently than 60% of the time or if the pressure generated by the distal esophagus is less than 30 mmHg, then the type of antireflux operation may have to be altered. In these circumstances, a partial fundoplication is indicated to avoid an insurmountable barrier to bolus transport, which may be induced by a total fundoplication. The 24-hour pH study is the gold standard for the diagnosis of GERD. In normal patients, the distal probe (located 5 cm above the GE junction) should detect pH less than 4.0 less than 4% of the time during the study. The proximal probe (10 cm above the lower probe) should detect less than 1% acid exposure. Patients with abnormal proximal acid exposure are more likely to have extraesophageal symptoms. The placement of one of the probes above the upper esophageal sphincter has been used to help predict the outcome of operative intervention for the treatment of extraesophageal symptoms.[1]

The upper endoscopy and esophagogram provide anatomic details that are necessary to direct therapy. Endoscopy will document the extent of esophageal injury, detect Barrett's esophagus (which will require surveillance after operative treatment), and exclude cancer. An esophagogram is helpful in defining the anatomic relationship of the GE junction to the hiatus, because many of these patients have a sliding hiatal hernia (Fig. 18–1). In patients with longstanding GERD, the esophagus may be

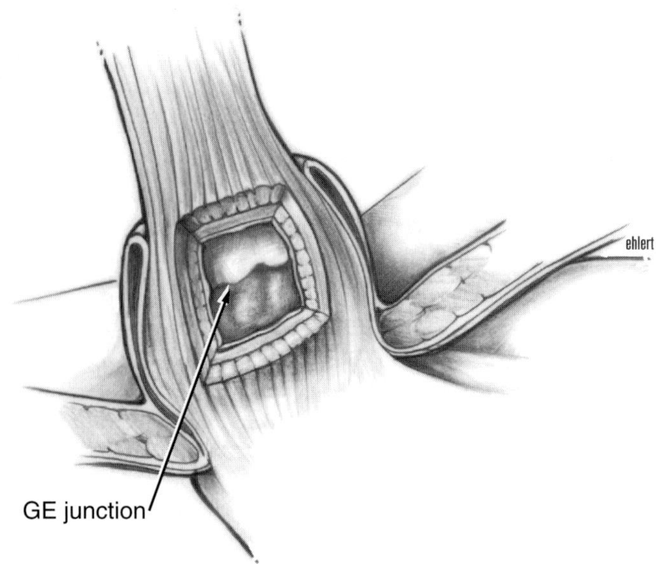

Figure 18–1. Schematic drawing of a sliding hiatal hernia, also referred to as a type I hernia. In this case the GE junction may move back and forth between the peritoneal cavity and the posterior mediastinum. (From Eubanks, T.R. and Pellegrini, C.A.: Hiatal hernia and gastrointestinal reflux disease. *In* Townsend, C.M., Jr. (ed.): Sabiston Textbook of Surgery, 16th ed. Philadelphia, W.B. Saunders, 2000, p. 755.)

shortened due to injury from acid exposure. These patients present an operative dilemma, because the fundoplication is likely to herniate through the hiatus if it is exposed to excessive tension from a shortened esophagus. In these situations, a lengthening procedure (Collis gastroplasty) may have to be performed, which changes the operative approach.[4]

Technique

The technique described here is the left crus approach to a total fundoplication. Fundus mobilization, crural closure, and gastropexy at the hiatus are essential to this technique. Although variations in technique may be encountered, the fundamentals of operative exposure and dissection are applicable to any approach.

The operation is facilitated long before access to the peritoneal cavity is established by proper patient positioning. The low lithotomy position provides access for the surgeon, who stands between the patient's legs, and the assistant, who stands to the patient's left. The angle between the left femur and the abdominal wall should be 180 degrees to allow the assistant full range of motion of the right hand instrument. The patient is fixed in position by the use of a bean bag or a special seat, so the operating table may be placed in the full reverse Trendelenburg position.

The video cart is placed at the head of the table so the surgeon, the assistant, and the scrub nurse can view the same monitor. Port placement is critical for its relative, if not its absolute, positioning. Two equilateral triangles are formed by the five ports (Fig. 18-2). The videoendoscope is placed 10 cm below the left costal margin, 3 cm to the left of the umbilicus. The assistant's right hand

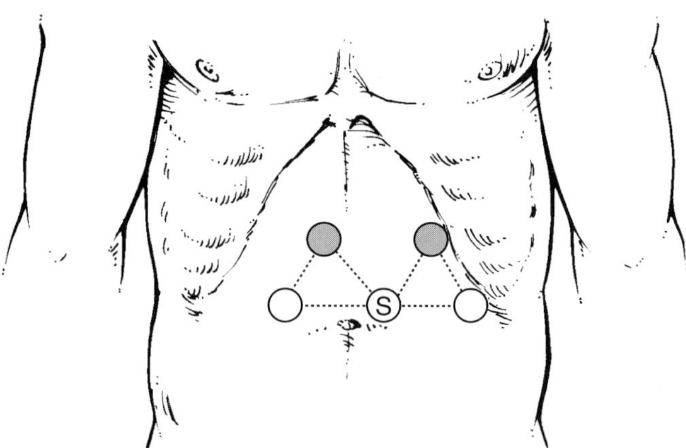

Figure 18–2. Schematic representation of port placement for the laparoscopic approach to the distal esophagus. (From Eubanks, T.R. and Pellegrini, C.A.: Hiatal hernia and gastrointestinal reflux disease. *In* Townsend, C.M., Jr. (ed.): Sabiston Textbook of Surgery, 16th ed. Philadelphia, W.B. Saunders, 2000, p. 755.)

port and the liver retractor complete the base of the two triangles. The apices of the triangles indicate the location of the surgeon's right and left hands (Fig. 18-2).

Once the ports are placed, the patient is placed in full reverse Trendelenburg position, and the liver retractor is positioned to expose the esophageal hiatus. The liver is held in position with a mechanical retractor, and the assistant operates the videoendoscope with the left hand and retracts with the right. The surgeon retracts with the left hand and performs the dissection with the right.

Initial dissection of the subhiatal fat pad is performed to identify the phrenoesophageal membrane along the left crus (Fig. 18-3). The lesser sac is then entered, and the short gastric vessels are transected with an ultrasonic dissector (Fig. 18-4). After the fundus is mobilized to the previously identified phrenoesophageal membrane, the peritoneal reflection and the membrane are incised anterior to the left crus. Once the mediastinal fat is identified,

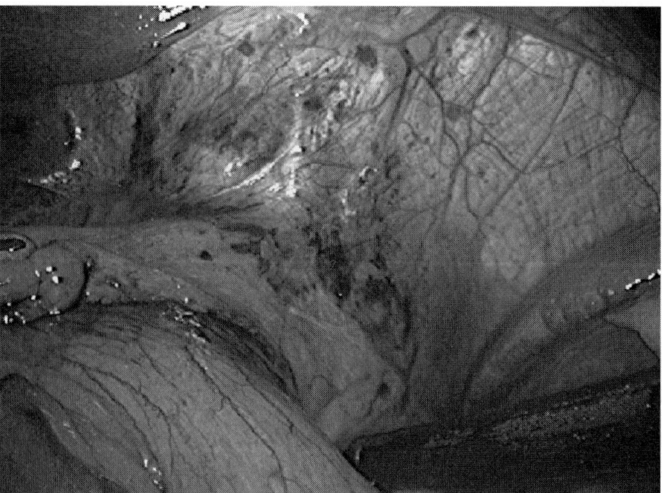

Figure 18–3. Subhiatal fat pad dissection reveals the phrenoesophageal membrane along the left crus *(bottom center)*. This initial dissection allows the short gastric vessel transection to be completed more easily.

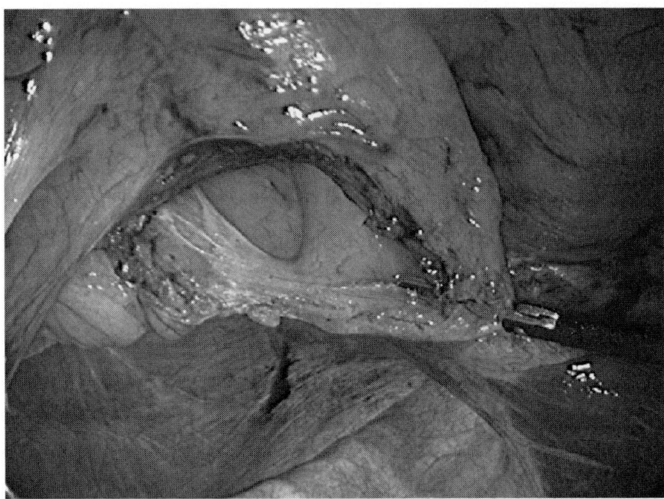

Figure 18–4. Transection of the short gastric vessels exposes the lesser sac and frees the fundus for creation of the antireflux procedure. The posterior aspect of the stomach is seen clearly in this photograph. This dissection is carried out towards the previously identified phrenoesophageal membrane at the left crus.

the phrenoesophageal membrane is incised circumferentially around the hiatus. The vagi will be preserved and visceral injury avoided if the dissection is carried out along the crural muscle fibers. A Penrose drain is passed around the esophagus to facilitate retraction.

Mediastinal mobilization of the esophagus is performed to allow at least 3 cm of intra-abdominal esophagus (Fig. 18–5). Crural closure is performed posteriorly (Fig. 18–6) and should allow easy passage of a No. 52 French bougie. This provides an excellent gauge of the degree of closure; the surgeon is unable to assess the closure through manual palpation.

When the fundoplication is fashioned, the bougie should be withdrawn from the GE junction. The posterior aspect of the fundus is passed posteriorly from left to right. The anterior aspect of the fundus is then passed from left to right anterior to the esophagus. The two are approximated with one suture. After the Penrose drain is removed and the bougie is advanced into the stomach, the fundoplication is completed with three or four interrupted silk sutures over a length of 2.5 to 3 cm. The bougie is removed, and the wrap is anchored to the hiatus and the esophageal wall at the left and right crura. The gastropexy helps prevent slipping and herniation (Fig. 18–7).

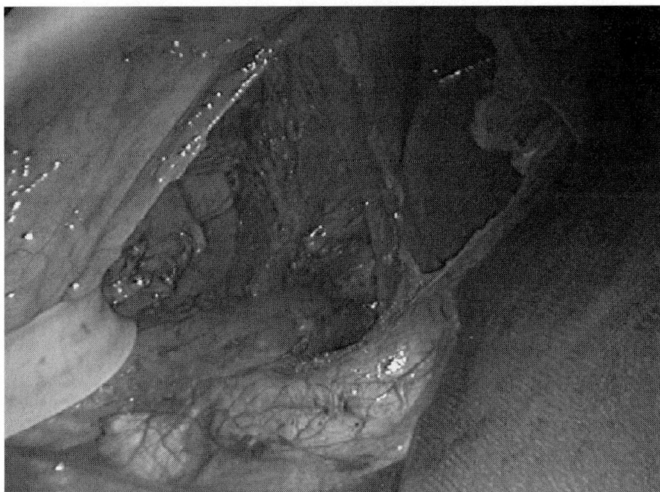

Figure 18–5. The mediastinal esophagus is mobilized to allow an adequate intra-abdominal length, prior to performing the fundoplication.

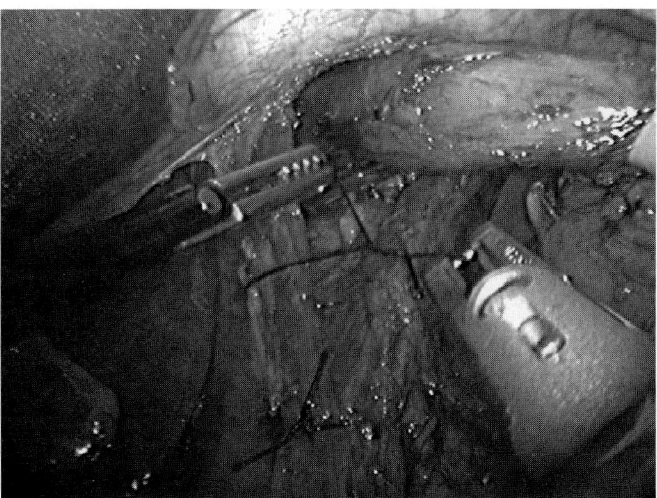

Figure 18–6. Posterior crural closure is completed in this case with a suturing device.

Results

Laparoscopic treatment of GERD is effective and well tolerated by patients. Control of typical symptoms of reflux ranges between 90 and 93%.[5-7] Atypical symptoms, such as aspiration, cough, and exacerbation of asthma, resolve in 75% of patients.[8] The median hospital stay is 2 days. The operation is less expensive than both long-term medical therapy (>10 years of single-strength proton pump inhibitor)[9] and the open technique.[10] Patient satisfaction is excellent, and quality-of-life measurements improve to a greater extent after operative intervention than they do after medical intervention.[11] Complications are uncommon, and when they do occur, they are usually minor (e.g., urinary retention, ileus, pneumothorax). Mortality rates from the operation are less than 1%.

During the past 7 years, 540 patients at the University of Washington underwent primary laparoscopic operations for GERD. Complete preoperative and postoperative evaluation (repeat manometry and pH studies) were available in 200 patients (37%). The primary symptoms, including heartburn, regurgitation, and abdominal pain, resolved in 186 patients (93%). Of the 14 patients who had persistent symptoms, about half had abnormal acid exposure on postoperative pH testing. Complications related to the laparoscopic approach include pneumothorax (4%), significant CO_2-induced subcutaneous emphysema (3%), and trocar site infection (0.5%). Two patients in our series died after the operation (0.4%). Both had primary pulmonary disease exacerbated by reflux-induced aspiration.

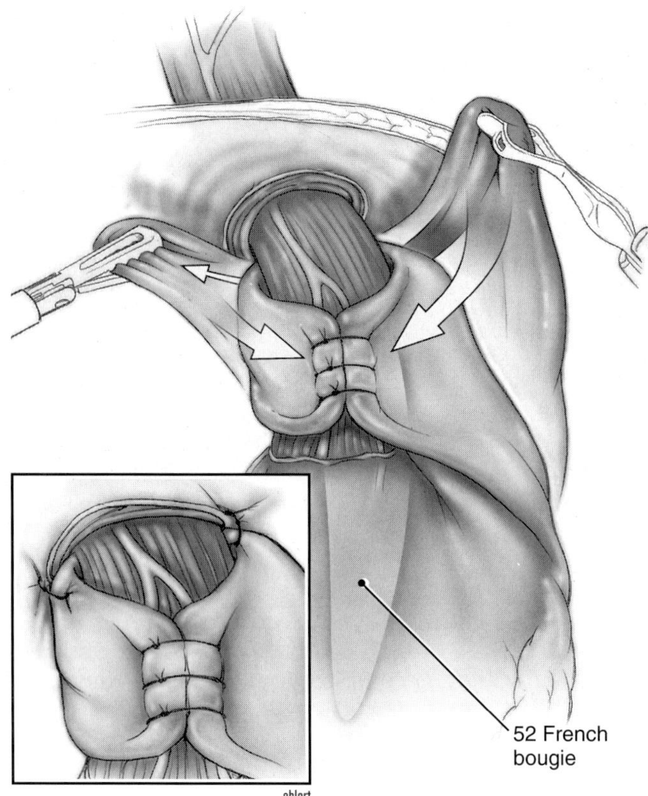

Figure 18–7. Total fundoplication completed. The fundus is anchored to the hiatus and esophagus at the left and right crura *(inset)*. (From Eubanks, T.R. and Pellegrini, C.A.: Hiatal hernia and gastrointestinal reflux disease. *In* Townsend, C.M., Jr. (ed.): Sabiston Textbook of Surgery, 16th ed. Philadelphia, W.B. Saunders, 2000, p. 755.)

Redo Antireflux Operations

Patients who present with persistent symptoms and physiologic evidence of abnormal acid exposure after an antireflux procedure may be candidates for a reoperation. The incidence of such a finding is about 5%, and the majority of patients can be treated with medical therapy. Before consideration of a second operation, an esophagogram is necessary to establish the integrity of the previous operation. The presence of an anatomic abnormality of the wrap, particularly a sizable herniation, is almost always best treated with surgery. Twenty-nine repeat antireflux procedures were completed laparoscopically at the University of Washington. Control of symptoms is less successful after the second procedure (80%), and the complication rates are higher (35%).

PARAESOPHAGEAL HERNIA

Paraesophageal hernias occur when the hiatal defect allows some structure other than the esophagus or cardia of the stomach to enter the mediastinum. Most commonly, the fundus of the stomach is in the hernia sac (Fig. 18-8). In extreme cases, the entire stomach may be located above the esophageal hiatus (Fig. 18-9). Although the indications for operative repair are different, the approach to paraesophageal hernias is similar to that of GERD. Several unique features of the operation distinguish it from a routine antireflux operation.

Indications

Paraesophageal hernias cause symptoms of abdominal pain, dysphagia, and heartburn. Paraesophageal hernias may induce chronic blood loss from the mucosa of the herniated fundus. The most impressive presentation of a paraesophageal hernia is gastric volvulus with vascular compromise; this requires emergent operative intervention. In the past, the mere presence of a paraesophageal hernia was an indication for operative repair due to the fear of such an episode.

The true incidence of gastric incarceration and ischemia is unknown. Of the 42 patients operated on at the University of Washington, only one required an emergency repair. All other patients had their hernias repaired because they were symptomatic. Interestingly, 11 patients were found to have gastric volvulus at the time of the operation. Thus, 25% of patients had the potential to develop vascular compromise and only one patient (2%) did.

Many patients are found to have paraesophageal hernias during a work-up for another medical problem. Patients who do not have symptoms in the proximal gastrointestinal tract but are found to have a paraesophageal

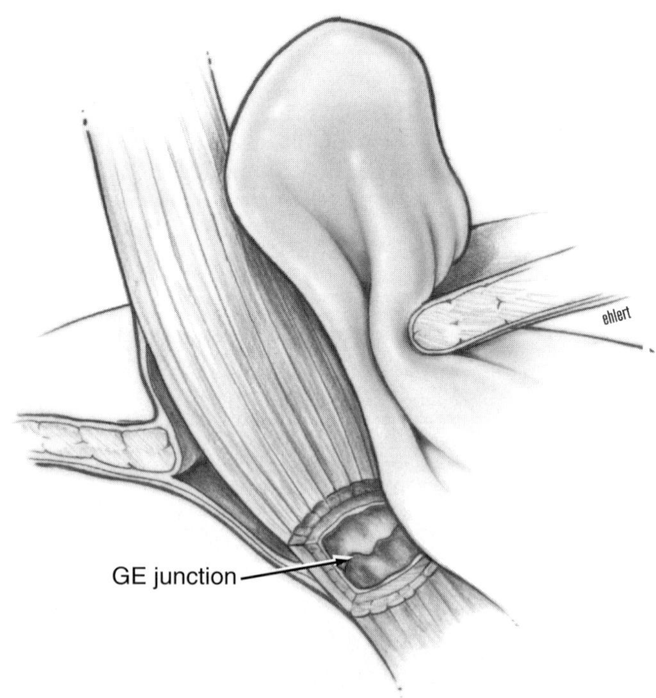

Figure 18–8. In this schematic representation of a hiatal hernia, the GE junction is fixed in the peritoneal cavity indicating a pure type II or rolling hiatal hernia. Paraesophageal hernias can present with a sliding component, where the GE junction is not fixed (type III or combined hiatal hernias). (From Eubanks, T.R. and Pellegrini, C.A.: Hiatal hernia and gastrointestinal reflux disease. *In* Townsend, C.M., Jr. (ed.): Sabiston Textbook of Surgery, 16th ed. Philadelphia, W.B. Saunders, 2000, p. 755.)

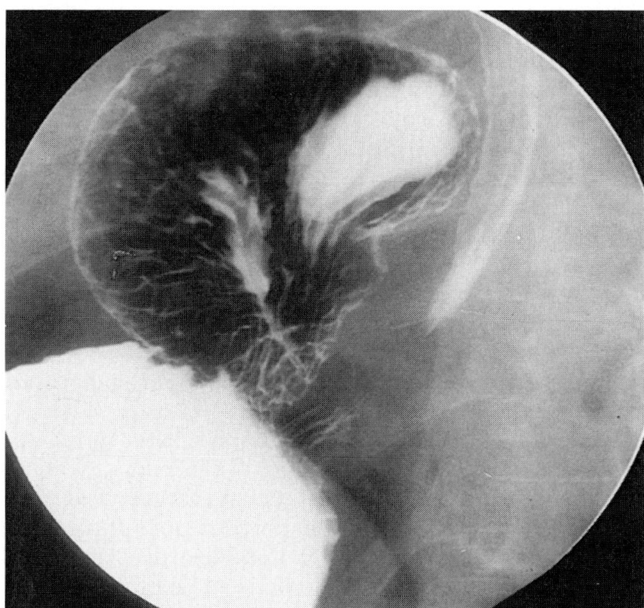

Figure 18–9. Contrast study revealing organoaxial volvulus of the stomach which is in the mediastinum, anterior to the esophagus.

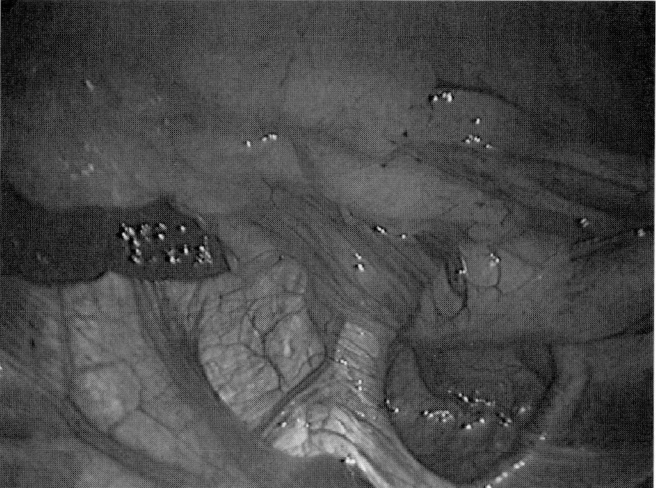

Figure 18–10. Elongation of the spleno-gastric ligament and short gastric vessels is demonstrated here. The urge to start the dissection along the left crus should be avoided as bleeding from the short gastric vessels will follow. If the short gastric vessels are transected first, starting at an accessible location of the fundus, bleeding will be avoided.

hernia may be observed without operative intervention. Patients who have symptoms that can be attributed to a paraesophageal hernia should have operative correction.

Evaluation

The preoperative evaluation is the same for these patients as it is for patients with GERD. Manometry, particularly the lower esophageal sphincter (LES) measurements, may be difficult to perform due to the angling of the GE junction; however, the distal esophageal amplitude and the degree of peristalsis should be obtainable. Twenty-four-hour pH monitoring is helpful if it influences the type of operation (i.e., whether an antireflux procedure is added to the operation); however, we advocate the routine use of an antireflux procedure as the hiatus is widely dissected during the repair. Endoscopy should be performed to assess esophageal and gastric mucosa and to determine the source of blood loss for patients with anemia. Upper gastrointestinal contrast studies provide the most valuable information because they show the size on the hernia, the amount of stomach involved, and whether the stomach is incarcerated in the mediastinum.

Technique

Patient positioning and port placement are the same as those described for GERD treatment. The initial dissection should be started at the greater curve in this operation. Dissection of the subhiatal fat pad along the left crus as described for GERD is difficult because the splenogastric ligament and the short gastric vessels are usually elongated and extend into the mediastinum (Fig. 18–10). These vessels are more safely taken if the lesser sac is entered early.

When the last short gastric vessel is divided at the hiatus, the only structures overlying the left crus are the sac and the phrenoesophageal membrane. A redundant sac often takes on the appearance of other structures, such as the vagi and the pleura. To avoid confusion, the left crural fibers should be exposed. This dissection plane is then continued anteriorly along the left crus toward the right. The stomach will be reduced into the peritoneal cavity and the hernia sac will be freed from the mediastinum in this manner. After the hernia sac has been transected along the crura, only the posterior sac dissection remains. Unfortunately, this is the most difficult part of the operation.

At this point, the hernia sac is intimately associated with the anterior wall of the esophagus and the anterior vagus (Fig. 18–11). Often, the location of the esophagus

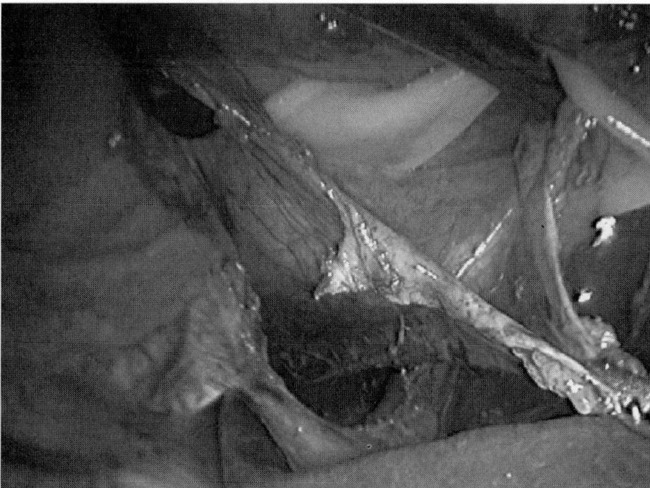

Figure 18–11. View from the left crus after initial dissection of the hernia sac in a paraesophageal hernia. The posterior aspect of the sac is intimately associated with the anterior esophagus and the anterior vagus, both of which are seen in the background.

is difficult to establish due to a redundant sac. A lighted bougie may be very helpful in these circumstances, because it facilitates identification of the esophagus. Once the plane between the esophagus and the sac is developed, the dissection proceeds into the mediastinum.

As much of the hernia sac as can safely be freed from the mediastinum should be removed. In most cases, the entire sac can be excised laparoscopically (Fig. 18–12). In very large paraesophageal hernias, the sac may extend to the inferior pulmonary veins. It is better to leave a small amount of sac in these cases than to risk injuring such mediastinal structures.

Once the sac is removed, the repair is the same as that for GERD. Occasionally, the hiatal defect will be too large to close by primary repair. In these cases, a relaxing incision may be made away from the hiatus on the right hemidiaphragm. This will allow apposition of the right and left crura. The relaxing incision is repaired with synthetic mesh to prevent iatrogenic diaphragmatic hernias. The mesh should be kept well away from the esophagus.

Results

Although the laparoscopic approach to paraesophageal hernias is more challenging than that of sliding hiatal hernias and GERD, a greater experience is being reported in the literature with this modality. Symptom resolution and patient satisfaction with the minimally invasive approach are similar to those of the operative repair of GERD. Symptoms of abdominal pain, dysphagia, and heartburn resolve in 90% of patients.[12,13] Acute blood loss and chronic anemia also respond to operative repair. The length of the hospital stay is 2 to 3 days. The complication rates for the paraesophageal hernia repairs are higher due to the more extensive mediastinal dissection. The incidences of pneumothorax, vagal injury, and extensive subcutaneous emphysema are higher. The incidence of recurrence of the hernia is about 8%.

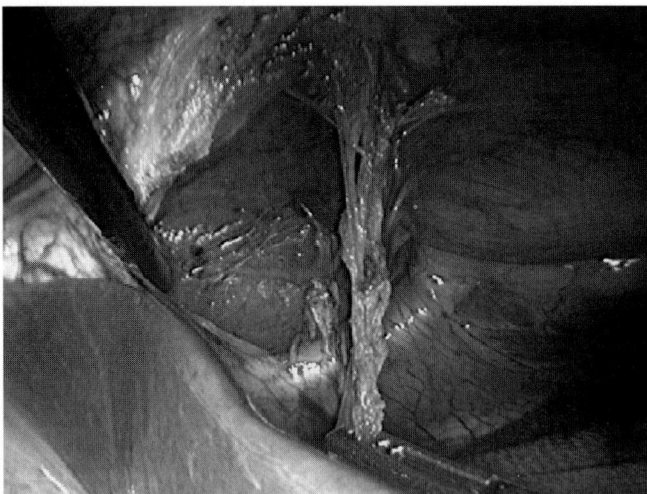

Figure 18–12. Operative view showing the complete reduction of a paraesophageal hernia sac. The esophageal hiatus may be seen in the background. The cut edges of the sac correspond to the circular dissection around the crura.

Of the patients operated on at the University of Washington, a total fundoplication was performed in 36 patients (86%); a partial fundoplication was used in 6 patients due to abnormal preoperative manometry. The operation was completed laparoscopically in 93% of cases. Three patients required conversion to an open procedure secondary to difficult dissection. All primary symptoms improved after the operation. Five patients had postoperative 24-hour pH studies performed. Four were normal with a mean acid exposure time of 0.8%. One patient had abnormal acid exposure (total percent time 16.6%) but had no symptoms. Anemia resolved in all patients. One patient had a recurrent hernia but is currently asymptomatic.

Pneumothorax was more common (7%). During the postoperative course, 20 patients (48%) had subcutaneous emphysema in the cervical region that resolved spontaneously. One patient died of portal venous thrombosis 7 days after the operation. He had been discharged but returned with an acute abdomen. At surgery, he was found to have extensive intestinal necrosis. Because this patient had a large hiatal hernia with a complete organoaxial volvulus, the dissection took a great deal of time. The total time of the operation was more than 8 hours. We suspect that the long duration of pneumoperitoneum contributed to the portal venous thrombosis.

ACHALASIA AND SPASTIC DYSMOTILITY

The operative approach to dysmotility of the esophagus consists of muscle transection to allow easier propelling of the food bolus toward the stomach. Accordingly, the operation palliates the symptoms but does not treat the underlying disease. The most common symptoms of achalasia include dysphagia, regurgitation of undigested food, and chest pain. Patients undergoing any treatment of dysmotility should obtain a high level of symptomatic relief with a low risk of adverse sequelae.

Indications

The most common motility abnormality for which surgery is performed is achalasia. The presence of the disease is an indication for operative treatment as long as the patient is a candidate to receive a general anesthetic agent. Although the nonoperative treatments for achalasia—dilation and botulinum toxin injection—can be effective, the results of operative therapy are superior. In a review article that analyzed weighted response rates of all published uncontrolled trials with more than 10 patients, initial therapy with laparoscopic treatment was superior to therapy with pneumatic dilation and botulinum toxin injection.[14] Furthermore, the only prospective, controlled trial that compared dilation with operative treatment favored surgical therapy.[15]

More nebulous indications for operative therapy are diffuse esophageal spasm and nutcracker esophagus. Because these diseases are relatively uncommon and few patients are referred to surgeons, it is difficult to acquire substantial knowledge about the results of operative intervention. Certainly, very few patients with spastic dysmotility will need operative treatment. Only those with unremitting dysphagia or persistent weight loss should be considered. Patients with symptoms of pain alone should not be treated surgically.

Evaluation

Manometry is essential to confirm the diagnosis of achalasia and spastic dysmotility. Although 24-hour pH monitoring results are normal in classic achalasia, we routinely obtain this study in dysmotility patients to document abnormal reflux and to differentiate it from the phenomenon of fermentation.[16] An esophagogram will help define the extent of the disease. It will demonstrate narrowing of the distal esophagus, and in advanced cases, a tortuous esophageal body may be found. These findings are important to the surgeon because they may guide operative decisions related to the length of the myotomy. Endoscopy is an essential preoperative procedure because it will help exclude other pathologic entities in the esophagus and the proximal gastrointestinal tract.

Technique

The following procedure incorporates a 7- to 10-cm esophagomyotomy with a partial posterior fundoplication. Because several of the barriers to GE reflux (e.g., phrenoesophageal membrane, crural apposition, and the intrinsic muscle fibers of the lower esophageal high-pressure zone) are disrupted during the operation, we believe it is necessary to perform an antireflux procedure during this operation.

Patients should be instructed to maintain a liquid diet for 2 days before the operation, because this will reduce the amount of particulate debris in the esophagus. Patient positioning and port placement are similar to those of an antireflux procedure with one exception; the camera port should be placed more laterally (to the left) for a myotomy than it is for treatment of GERD. This allows the operative view to be directed along the axis of the esophagus, which has a subtle right-to-left course as it passes from the mediastinum into the peritoneal cavity. Because the myotomy is carried out proximally, this view is essential.

Mobilization of the crura and fundus proceeds in a similar manner as that described previously. Once the phrenoesophageal membrane is freed from the esophagus, the anterior aspect of the esophagus is prepared for the myotomy. A No. 52 French bougie is placed into the lumen of the esophagus and stomach. The assistant maintains traction posteriorly on the stomach; this splays the anterior wall of the stomach over the bougie. The surgeon then mobilizes the subhiatal fat from the serosa of the stomach, avoiding injury to the anterior vagus (Fig. 18–13). As the dissection proceeds in a cephalad manner, the GE junction is encountered. The fat is then freed from the longitudinal muscle fibers of the esophagus. The anterior vagus will be elevated from the esophageal wall with this maneuver (Fig. 18–14). The vagus should be freed as proximally as the exposure allows (6 to 9 cm). Often, the anterior aspect of the hiatus is divided 1 to 2 cm to improve access to the mediastinum.

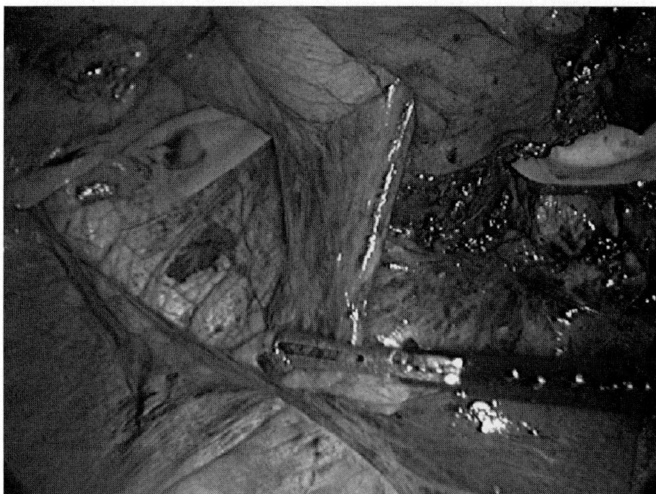

Figure 18–13. The subhiatal fat pad at the gastroesophageal junction is elevated from the anterior aspect of the stomach. This step allows exposure for the myotomy to be extended onto the stomach.

The myotomy is initiated at an area of the anterior esophagus, which does not appear to be affected by previous treatment (botulinum toxin injection or dilation). We use a cautery device with a right-angled tip to perform the myotomy. The heel of the device is used to divide the longitudinal fibers with electric current (Fig. 18–15). As the circular fibers are exposed, the tip of the device is used to create a space between the fibers and the submucosal plane. With the tip in the proper plane, the cautery device is used to elevate the fibers from the mucosa before they are transected (Fig. 18–16). The myotomy is carried out as proximally as is necessary based on preoperative manometry or to the limits of the

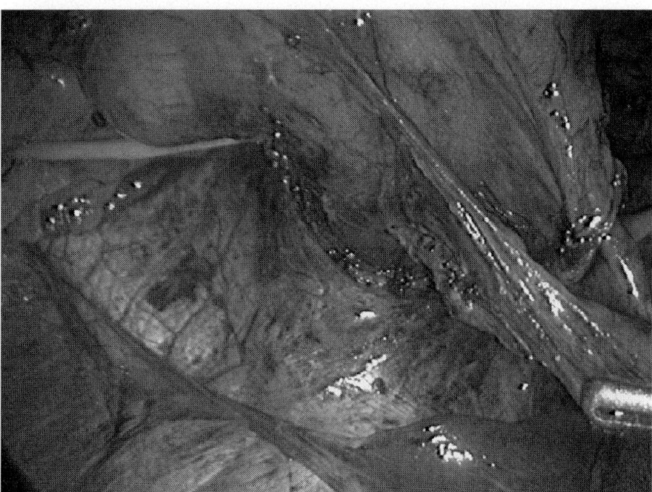

Figure 18–14. The subhiatal fat has been elevated in continuity with the anterior vagus, which may be seen entering the fat just left of center in the photograph. The anterior aspect of the esophagus, GE junction, and stomach are seen clearly.

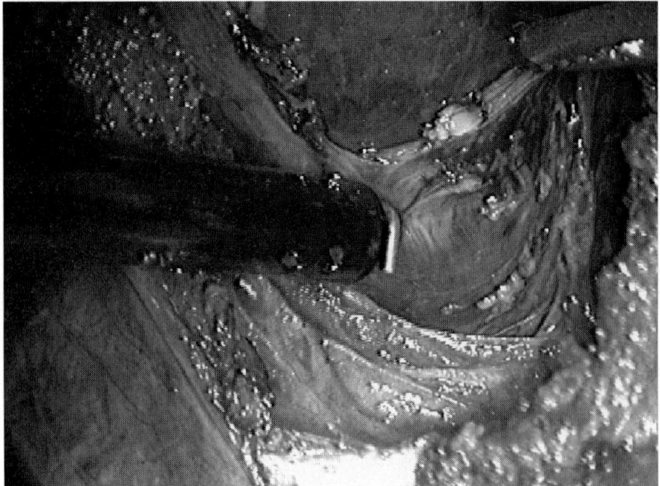

Figure 18–15. Division of longitudinal muscle fibers using the heel of the right-angle electrocautery device.

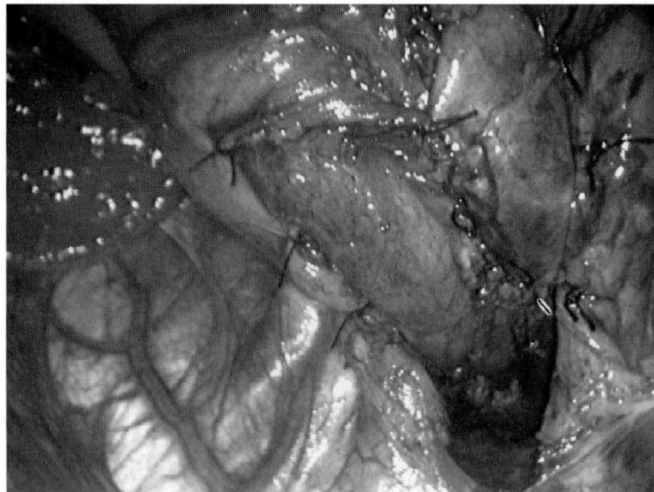

Figure 18–17. Posterior fundoplication completed after esophagomyotomy. The fundus is sutured to the cut edges of the myotomy. The anterior vagus can be seen traversing the esophageal mucosa from left to right in the upper left hand corner of the photograph.

operative exposure. The distal extent of the myotomy extends onto the stomach 1.5 cm. The transition between the circular fibers of the esophagus and the sling fibers of the stomach is readily apparent.

The posterior fundoplication is fashioned similarly to the total fundoplication. Instead of suturing the fundus to itself, the posterior aspect of the fundus (which has been passed from left to right behind the esophagus) is sutured to the right cut edge of the myotomy. The anterior fundus is similarly sutured to the left cut edge of the myotomy (Fig. 18–17). This not only creates a barrier to reflux but also directs lateral tension to the myotomy, which prevents apposition of the cut edges and rehealing. The crura are not reapproximated during this procedure.

An alternative to the posterior partial fundoplication is an anterior fundoplication (Dor). The advantage to this approach is that the fundus is used to cover the myotomy site, thus helping to prevent postoperative leaks and preventing the mucosa from adhering to the left lobe of the liver. We have performed more anterior partial fundoplications but have changed to a posterior fundoplication in an attempt to further reduce postoperative acid reflux.

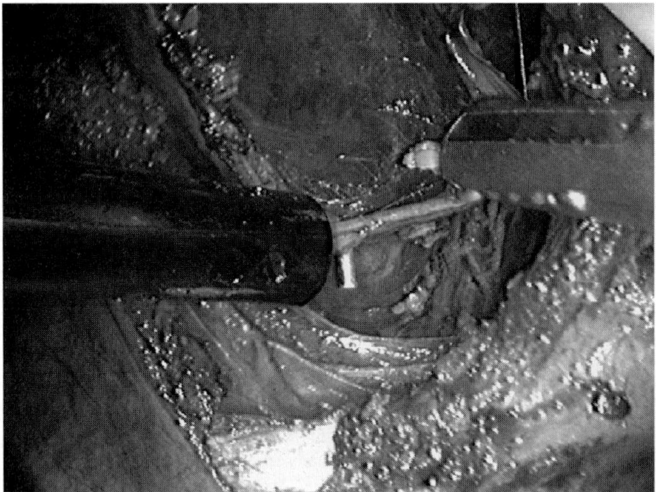

Figure 18–16. Transection of circular muscle fibers during myotomy for achalasia. The grasper is elevating the previously transected muscle, while the right-angle electrocautery device is used to separate the circular muscle from the submucosa. The anterior vagus is displaced to the right.

Results

The laparoscopic approach has been recognized as an excellent modality for the treatment of achalasia. Several small series have demonstrated the efficacy and the patient satisfaction. Although the thoracoscopic approach to the myotomy has been used, the laparoscopic approach allows for a more effective antireflux procedure.[17,18] Symptoms of dysphagia and regurgitation resolve completely in 80 to 90% of patients.[19-22] Long-term results regarding the resolution of symptoms are not yet available. The average length of the hospital stay is 2 days, and complications are uncommon.[23]

In our first report with minimally invasive techniques for achalasia, we used a thoracic approach and showed that 90% of patients had excellent or good results. Postoperative pH studies revealed that up to 50% of patients had abnormal, though asymptomatic, acid exposure.[24] Thus, we switched to a laparoscopic approach so we could add an antireflux procedure to the operation. Since then, 57 patients have had a laparoscopic myotomy performed at the University of Washington. The primary symptoms of dysphagia and regurgitation improved significantly in 93% of patients. When chest pain was present, 63% of patients responded to operative therapy. Postoperative pH testing reveals that abnormal acid exposure occurs in as many as 30% of patients, the majority of whom are asymptomatic. The laparoscopic approach not only provides better access for performing an antireflux procedure but also decreases the morbidity rate for the procedure (routine chest tube placement is not required) and allows the surgeon to work parallel to the plane of dissection instead of perpendicular to it, as in the thoracoscopic approach.

The unique complication of this procedure compared with the procedure for reflux disease is the risk of mucosal laceration, which occurred in 3 patients (5%). All perforations were repaired laparoscopically, and to date no adverse sequelae have occurred. Two of the patients had undergone botulinum toxin injection before surgery, which makes the dissection more difficult.[21] Recurrent symptoms have been found in 5 patients (9%) at a maximum follow-up of 6 years. Three patients had progressive dysmotility of the esophagus. Two other patients had functional obstructions of the distal esophagus secondary to the fundoplication. Both required operative correction, which was accomplished laparoscopically.

EPIPHRENIC DIVERTICULA

The majority of diverticula below the upper esophageal sphincter occur in the epiphrenic region. A diverticulum at this level should be operated on if the patient is experiencing significant symptoms and the risk of general anesthesia is not prohibitive. The most common symptoms include dysphagia and regurgitation of undigested food. Most diverticula within 10 cm of the GE junction can be approached laparoscopically.

Evaluation

Before surgery, manometry of the esophagus is necessary to detect abnormal motility of the esophagus. The most common motility disturbance that is detected is achalasia.[25] Other findings on manometry include diffuse esophageal spasm, hypertensive LES, nonspecific motility disorders, and normal motility. Other important information to be obtained from the manometry is the extent of the esophageal body that is involved with the motor abnormality. If a motility disorder is found, the operative procedure should include a myotomy in addition to the diverticulectomy. In addition to manometry, an esophagogram is essential in the preoperative evaluation. It will provide the surgeon with the size and location of the diverticulum relative to the GE junction.

Technique

As with dysmotility operations, the patient is instructed to maintain a liquid diet 2 days before surgery. Positioning, port placement, and initial dissection are the same as those described for achalasia. As the subhiatal fat is dissected free of the stomach serosa and the longitudinal fibers of the esophagus, the plane between the esophageal muscle fibers and the diverticulum will be revealed. Once the diverticulum is identified, it is dissected free from adjacent structures. Using the left hand to hold the diverticulum, the surgeon pushes away most of the surrounding structures and divides small vessels coming directly to the wall of the diverticulum. If the diverticulum is more cephalad, the hiatus may be opened as described previously to facilitate exposure of the mediastinum. Once the surface of the diverticulum has been freed, the neck is dissected down to the defect in the muscle of the esophagus. The neck should be freed of all surrounding tissue, which may be facilitated by downward traction of the diverticulum. When the diverticulum is fully mobilized, an automatic stapling and cutting device may be used to transect the neck of the sac flush along a No. 52 French bougie (Fig. 18-18). We approximate the muscle fibers at the diverticulectomy site as long as the caliber of the esophageal lumen will not be compromised.

A myotomy is then performed in a position along the anterior esophagus but well away from the diverticulectomy site in a similar manner as that described for achalasia. A posterior partial fundoplication is also added.

Results

The laparoscopic treatment of epiphrenic diverticula is uncommon. Three reports describe the treatment of a total of eight patients.[26-28] All of the patients had relief of primary symptoms, including regurgitation and dysphagia. No recurrences have been reported, although follow-up was not available for three patients. One patient required conversion to an open procedure.[26] Two complications, pneumothorax and atrial fibrillation, occurred.

At the University of Washington, we have evaluated six patients with symptomatic epiphrenic diverticula during the past 4 years. Four have undergone surgery to date. The symptoms of dysphagia, heartburn, and regurgitation were relieved by diverticulectomy and myotomy in three patients and by diverticulectomy and takedown of a vertical banded gastroplasty in the fourth. One patient had nutcracker esophagus with distal esophageal amplitudes of 240 mmHg and a mean resting LES pressure of 43 mmHg with complete relaxation. The second patient had

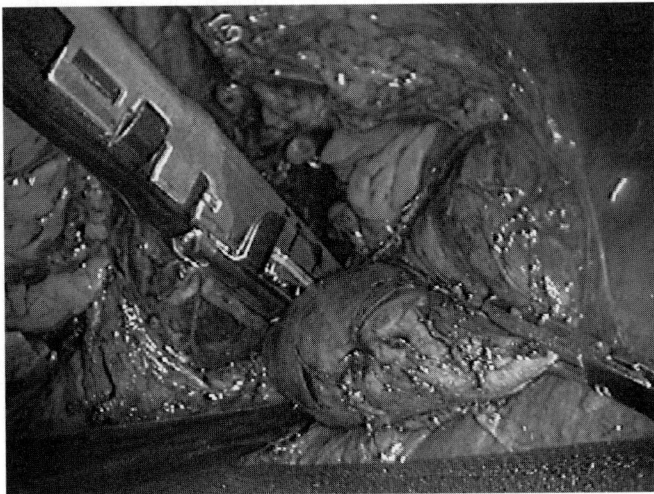

Figure 18–18. Transection of an epiphrenic diverticulum using an automatic stapling and cutting device. The diverticulum is being retracted to the right of the esophagus and a bougie is used to prevent compromise of the esophageal lumen.

severe dysphagia and normal esophageal motility, but the LES could not be negotiated with the manometry catheter. The third patient did not have a preoperative motility study. Due to the uncertainty of the function of the LES, a myotomy was performed in addition to the diverticulectomy. The fourth patient had normal motility and a normal LES pressure but had a pressure of 35 mmHg at a mesh band placed for a weight reduction operation. In three cases, a posterior partial fundoplication was performed; in the patient with a vertical banded gastroplasty, no antireflux procedure was added to the operation. Postoperative evaluation revealed normal manometry and the absence of acid reflux in the one patient who has completed follow-up; no recurrence was seen in the two patients with postoperative esophagograms.

Although few patients have been treated with a laparoscopic approach, the outcomes appear to be similar to those of the open repair.[29] No leaks have been reported, and at short-term follow-up, there has been no recurrence in the patients evaluated with postoperative studies.

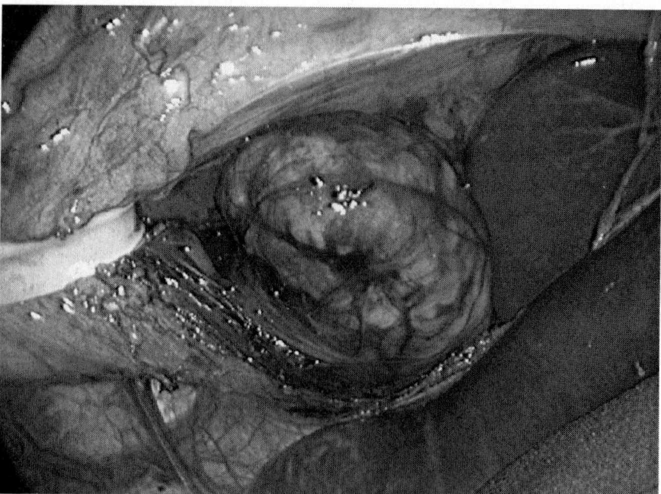

Figure 18-19. Large leiomyoma on the right anterior aspect of the distal esophagus. The Penrose drain is placing tension on the cardia. Note that a portion of the adventitial tissue is left on the tumor to facilitate traction.

BENIGN SOFT TISSUE TUMORS

Submucosal tumors of the distal esophagus may be treated with the laparoscopic approach. The presence of a tumor is an indication for operative resection to exclude malignancy. If benign tumors of the esophagus are uncommon, those that are within 10 cm of the GE junction, and therefore accessible by laparoscopy, are even less common. Due to the magnification of the laparoscope and camera, the improved view of the hiatus, and the less morbid access, these tumors are well suited for the laparoscopic approach.

Evaluation

The preoperative evaluation of a soft tissue tumor of the esophagus should include an esophagogram, upper endoscopy, and a computed tomography scan of the chest and upper abdomen. The esophagogram gives some idea of the size of the mass and its location relative to the hiatus, both of which aid in determining whether the lesion should be approached through the chest or abdomen. Upper endoscopy is necessary to exclude carcinoma arising from the mucosa. If the tumor is clearly submucosal, no attempt at biopsy should be made, because this will complicate an extramucosal excision. A computed tomography scan is helpful in determining the relation of the mass to surrounding structures and the presence of suspicious lesions in the lungs and liver.

Technique

Port placement and positioning are similar to those of the esophagomyotomy for achalasia. Access to intraoperative esophagoscopy to confirm the precise location of the tumor is also necessary.

The fundus and phrenoesophageal membrane are mobilized to access the distal esophagus. If the tumor is not clearly seen, intraoperative endoscopy will aid in directing the initial transection of the muscle fibers of the esophagus. When the mass is identified, the longitudinal and circular muscle fibers are incised as they are during an esophagomyotomy. It is helpful to maintain some areolar tissue attachments to the tumor to facilitate retraction (Fig. 18-19). As the dissection continues along the surface to the tumor, the submucosal plane will be encountered. Large vessels from the submucosal plexus may be peeled away from the tumor through careful dissection, allowing the tumor to be enucleated (Fig. 18-20). A bougie may be used to splay the mucosa; however, this often creates too much tension at the excision site and prevents manipulation of the mass.

When the tumor is freed, the myotomy may be closed

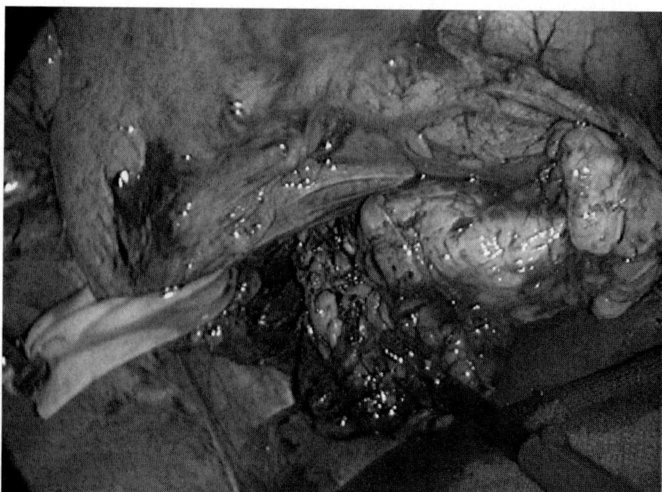

Figure 18-20. Completed enucleation of the tumor in Figure 18-19. This tumor was horseshoe shaped and circumscribed the distal esophagus.

primarily if doing so will not compromise the lumen. A total fundoplication is added to prevent GE reflux. If a large portion of the muscle has been disrupted, then closure of the myotomy is not possible and a partial fundoplication is used to prevent reflux and to buttress the excision site. If the mucosa is violated, a primary repair with fine permanent suture should be performed, and the area should be covered with a partial fundoplication.

Results

The thoracoscopic approach to resection of esophageal leiomyoma has been described by several authors.[30-32] Excision has been completed with a minimally invasive approach in all cases, no recurrences have been reported, and complications are uncommon. Although laparoscopic resection of gastric leiomyoma has been reported,[33,34] the leiomyoma of the distal esophagus and the GE junction are seldom approached laparoscopically due to the possibility of not having access to the proximal margin.

At the University of Washington, five patients have undergone laparoscopic excision of soft tissue tumors of the distal esophagus. The most common symptoms are heartburn, dysphagia, and abdominal pain. The diagnosis was suspected and the location of the tumor was confirmed with endoscopy. The most common manometry finding was a decreased LES pressure and normal motility. Four patients had resection with total fundoplication, and one patient had a partial fundoplication. The tumors were completely excised; all were benign, and none have recurred.

ESOPHAGEAL RESECTION

The role of minimally invasive surgery in the removal of the esophagus has not been completely defined. Although small series that describe the technical aspects of total esophagectomy have been reported, the experience is not broad enough to recommend its routine use.[35,36] No studies have compared the technique with the standard open procedure, so the benefits of the operation have not been demonstrated. In one series of nine patients, the average length of time for the operation was 6.5 hours and the blood loss was minimal at 290 ml. Two of nine patients required intensive care unit admission; the average length of stay was 6.4 days.[37] Although these results are quite remarkable, the advantage over the open procedure is not as apparent as it is for other esophageal procedures. For now, laparoscopic esophagectomy should only be performed in centers with a dedicated interest and access to a larger volume of patients.

SUMMARY

Minimal access surgery has changed the operative treatment of esophageal diseases. Through the use of videoendoscopic techniques, an equivalent operation can be performed with much less tissue destruction needed for access. Common diseases that can be treated include GERD, paraesophageal hernias, and esophageal dysmotility. Less common pathologic entities that may be approached laparoscopically include esophageal diverticula and leiomyomas. In the future, videoendoscopic techniques may be routinely used in esophagectomy for benign and malignant diseases.

References

1. So, J.B., Zeitels, S.M., and Rattner, D.W.: Outcomes of atypical symptoms attributed to gastroesophageal reflux treated by laparoscopic fundoplication. Surgery, *124*:28, 1998.
2. Hallerback, B., et al.: Omeprazole or ranitidine in long-term treatment of reflux esophagitis: Scandinavian Clinics for United Research. Gastroenterology, *107*:1305, 1994.
3. Lundell, L.R.: The knife or the pill in the long-term treatment of gastroesophageal reflux disease? Yale J. Biol. Med., *67*:233, 1994.
4. Jobe, B.A., Horvath, K.D., and Swanstrom, L.L.: Postoperative function following laparoscopic Collis gastroplasty for shortened esophagus. Arch. Surg., *133*:867, 1998.
5. Zaninotto, G., et al.: Laparoscopic treatment of gastro-esophageal reflux disease: Indications and results. Int. Surg., *80*:380, 1995.
6. Peters, J.H., and DeMeester, T.R.: Indications, benefits and outcome of laparoscopic Nissen fundoplication. Dig. Dis., *14*:169, 1996.
7. Horgan, S., and Pellegrini, C.A.: Surgical treatment of gastroesophageal reflux disease. Surg. Clin. North Am., *77*:1063, 1997.
8. Johnson, W.E., et al.: Outcome of respiratory symptoms after antireflux surgery on patients with gastroesophageal reflux disease. Arch. Surg., *131*:489, 1996.
9. Heudebert, G.R., et al.: Choice of long-term strategy for the management of patients with severe esophagitis: A cost-utility analysis. Gastroenterology, *112*:1078, 1997.
10. Blomqvist, A.M., et al.: Laparoscopic or open fundoplication? A complete cost analysis. Surg. Endosc., *12*:1209, 1998.
11. Velanovich, V., et al.: Quality of life scale for gastroesophageal reflux disease. J. Am. Coll. Surg., *183*:217, 1996.
12. Perdikis, G., et al.: Laparoscopic paraesophageal hernia repair. Arch. Surg., *132*:586; discussion 590, 1997.
13. Horgan, S., et al.: Repair of paraesophageal hernias. Am. J. Surg., *177*:354, 1999.
14. Spiess, A.E., and Kahrilas, P.J.: Treating achalasia: From whalebone to laparoscope. JAMA, *280*:638, 1998.
15. Csendes, A., et al.: Late results of a prospective randomised study comparing forceful dilatation and oesophagomyotomy in patients with achalasia. Gut, *30*:299, 1989.
16. Crookes, P.F., Corkill, S., and DeMeester, T.R.: Gastroesophageal reflux in achalasia: When is reflux really reflux? Dig. Dis. Sci., *42*:1354, 1997.
17. Raiser, F., et al.: Heller myotomy via minimal-access surgery: An evaluation of antireflux procedures. Arch. Surg., *131*:593; discussion 597, 1996.
18. Patti, M.G., Arcerito, M., and Pellegrini, C.A.: Thoracoscopic and laparoscopic Heller's myotomy in the treatment of esophageal achalasia. Ann. Chir. Gynaecol., *84*:159, 1995.
19. Collard, J.M., et al.: Heller-Dor procedure for achalasia: From conventional to video-endoscopic surgery. Acta Chir. Belg., *96*:62, 1996.
20. Corcione, F., et al.: Surgical laparoscopy with intraoperative manometry in the treatment of esophageal achalasia. Surg. Laparosc. Endosc., *7*:232, 1997.
21. Horgan, S., et al.: Does botox injection make esophagomyotomy a more difficult operation? Surg. Endosc., *13*:576, 1999.
22. Wang, P.C., et al.: The outcome of laparoscopic Heller myotomy without antireflux procedure in patients with achalasia. Am. Surg., *64*:515; discussion 521, 1998.
23. Holzman, M.D., et al.: Laparoscopic surgical treatment of achalasia. Am. J. Surg., *173*:308, 1997.
24. Pellegrini, C.A., et al.: Thoracoscopic esophageal myotomy in the treatment of achalasia. Ann. Thorac. Surg., *56*:680, 1993.

25. Streitz, J.M., Jr., Glick, M.E., and Ellis, F.H. Jr.: Selective use of myotomy for treatment of epiphrenic diverticula: Manometric and clinical analysis. Arch. Surg., *127:*585; discussion 587, 1992.
26. Myers, B.S., and Dempsey, D.T.: Laparoscopic resection of esophageal epiphrenic diverticulum. J. Laparoendosc. Adv. Surg. Tech. A., *8:*201, 1998.
27. Rosati, R., et al.: Diverticulectomy, myotomy, and fundoplication through laparoscopy: A new option to treat epiphrenic esophageal diverticula? Ann. Surg., *227:*174, 1998.
28. Chami, Z., et al.: Abdominal laparoscopic approach for thoracic epiphrenic diverticulum. Surg. Endosc., *13:*164, 1999.
29. Jordan, P.H., and Kinner, B.M.: New look at epiphrenic diverticulum. World J. Surg., *23:*147, 1999.
30. Bonavina, L., et al.: Surgical therapy of esophageal leiomyoma. J. Am. Coll. Surg., *181:*257, 1995.
31. Tamura, K., et al.: Thoracoscopic resection of a giant leiomyoma of the esophagus with a mediastinal outgrowth. Ann. Thorac. Cardiovasc. Surg., *4:*351, 1998.
32. Taniguchi, E., et al.: Thoracoscopic enucleation of a large leiomyoma located on the left side of the esophageal wall. Surg. Endosc., *11:*280, 1997.
33. Gurbuz, A.T., and Peetz, M.E.: Resection of a gastric leiomyoma using combined laparoscopic and gastroscopic approach. Surg. Endosc., *11:*285, 1997.
34. Taniguchi, E., et al.: Laparoscopic intragastric surgery for gastric leiomyoma. Surg. Endosc., *11:*287, 1997.
35. Yahata, H., et al.: Laparoscopic transhiatal esophagectomy for advanced thoracic esophageal cancer. Surg. Laparosc. Endosc., *7:*13, 1997.
36. Sammartino, P., et al.: Videoassisted transhiatal esophagectomy for cancer. Int. Surg., *82:*406, 1997.
37. Swanstrom, L.L., and Hansen, P.: Laparoscopic total esophagectomy. Arch. Surg., *132:*943; discussion 947, 1997.

VOLUME

I

Neoplasms and Cysts

CHAPTER

19 Carcinoma of the Esophagus and Cardia

MARK K. FERGUSON

Tumors of the esophagus and cardia are among the most challenging problems confronting the oncologic surgeon. Esophageal tumors are highly likely to result in early mortality owing to the likelihood of advanced disease at the time of diagnosis and the challenging nature of their treatment. Survival rates have not improved appreciably in 25 years despite the availability of new treatment modalities. This chapter reviews the current approaches taken in the diagnosis and management of esophageal cancer. It emphasizes the need for early diagnosis and improved therapeutic regimens if there is to be any positive impact on the course of this disease in the future.

EPIDEMIOLOGY

Cancer of the esophagus represents 1.0% of all cancers diagnosed in the United States and accounts for 2.1% of all deaths due to cancer.[122] An estimated 12,300 new esophageal cancers were diagnosed in 1998 and 11,900 deaths from esophageal cancer were predicted for the same year. Esophageal cancer accounts for 5.4% of all carcinomas of the digestive tract and causes 9.1% of all deaths due to these cancers. Cancer of the esophagus or cardia in the United States occurs in about 6 of 100,000 men and in 1.5 of 100,000 women.

Numerous geographic variations occur in the incidence of esophageal cancer throughout the world. The highest rates are found among the Turkoman of the Caspian Littoral of Iran, in whom the incidence is as high as 160 to 180 per 100,000 population.[76] High rates are also found in northern China, where there is an incidence of 109 per 100,000[44]; mortality is particularly high in the mountain provinces of northern China, ranging from 169 per 100,000 in regions of Shansi Province to 132 per 100,000 in areas of Hunan Province.[235] Esophageal cancer is also common in the Cape Province of South Africa, especially among the Bantu; in Ceylon; and in certain regions of Europe, particularly Normandy and Brittany.

ETIOLOGY

Social factors play an important role in determining the incidence of esophageal cancer among various cultural and ethnic groups. In the Western Hemisphere, a significant degree of alcohol use corresponds to a high rate of esophageal cancer in the United States, Britain, and France. The risk of developing carcinoma of the esophagus is increased 25 times in chronic drinkers of beverages containing a high percentage of alcohol and 10 times in people who drink a lot of beer.[139,140] The use of tobacco, particularly cigarettes, is also strongly associated with the development of esophageal cancer. Although alcohol consumption is a more potent risk factor than tobacco use, it is believed that the two potentiate each other in the development of esophageal cancer.

In geographic regions in which esophageal cancer is endemic, dietary factors are frequently implicated as etiologic agents. In Hunan Province in northern China, nitrosamines and polycyclic aromatic hydrocarbons discovered in food samples have been shown to induce esophageal carcinomas experimentally in animals.[235] Cocarcinogens extracted from the shrub *Croton flaveus* are probably related to the development of esophageal cancer in Curaçao, where the leaves and roots are chewed or used to brew tea.[231] In the Caspian Littoral of Iran, the high risk of esophageal cancer may be related to the high temperature at which tea is consumed, in addition to the possible carcinogenic effects of tannins and phenols in the tea.[76] Nutritional deficiencies are also related to the development of esophageal cancer. These deficiencies include the lack of certain trace elements in endemic areas, particularly Linhsien County in Hunan Province, China, and in South Africa, where smaller quantities of trace elements, such as molybdenum, manganese, iron, silicon, barium, titanium, selenium, and magnesium, are found than in areas with a low incidence of such tumors.[99,132,136] Deficiencies of riboflavin and vitamins A and C may also be significant.

Although mortality from cancer of the esophagus is higher in blacks than in whites in the United States, it is believed that increased exposure to other risk factors in the black population accounts for most of the observed differences. No definite etiologic relationship between genetic factors and the development of esophageal cancer has been established. The single exception to this statement is patients with tylosis, a syndrome of hyperkeratosis of the palms and plantar surfaces of the feet that is associated with papillomas of the esophagus.[82,185] The disease is determined by an autosomal dominant gene and carries a risk of squamous cell carcinoma of the esophagus of approximately 70%.

Some benign esophageal diseases predispose patients to the development of squamous cell carcinomas of the esophagus. Patients who have achalasia have a 5 to 10% lifetime risk, with carcinomas typically developing in the mid esophagus.[2,153,175,194] Patients with strictures caused by lye are said to have a 5% risk of developing esophageal cancer, although the accuracy of this number is questionable[74,91]; other information puts the likely incidence at less than 1%, with a latency period of 30 to 45 years.[13,188] Chronic esophagitis, whether owing to gastroesophageal reflux or to other inflammatory conditions, is also associated with a high incidence of esophageal cancer.[120]

Other benign esophageal disorders are associated with the development of adenocarcinomas of the esophagus. Congenital rests of columnar epithelium within the esophagus are found in a large number of patients at autopsy. These heterotopic islands of gastric mucosa can undergo degeneration to adenocarcinoma of the esophagus, although this entity is rare. On the other hand, persons with Barrett's esophagus (endobrachyesophagus), an acquired condition related to gastroesophageal acid reflux, are at risk of developing carcinoma of the esophagus that is more than 50 times that of the general population.[54]

PATHOLOGY

Squamous cell carcinomas are the most common malignancies of the esophagus worldwide. Squamous cell cancers are frequently multicentric, and second synchronous tumors are found in more than 25% of patients with an invasive primary cancer. Synchronous cancers are often found in the relatively early stages of development but invade the submucosa and beyond in more than 20% of cases. Intraepithelial carcinomas are also found contiguous with primary invasive cancers in almost 70% of patients. These findings suggest that field carcinomatous transformation may be a cause of the multicentricity of such tumors.[116,117] Invasion beyond the intramucosal stage apparently occurs by a variety of methods in patients with squamous cell cancers, including intraepithelial spread, direct stromal invasion, and intraductal spread, all of which are possible routes to deep tissue involvement.[219]

Variants of squamous cell carcinoma include rare polypoid tumors containing a prominent spindle cell component that demonstrates both carcinomatous and sarcomatous elements (Table 19-1). These tumors are sometimes referred to as pseudosarcomas or carcinosarcomas. Immunohistochemical staining demonstrates the presence of epithelial elements in sarcomatous areas and supports the concept that the spindle cells are of epithelial origin.[72,150]

The most distal parts of the esophagus and cardia are most commonly affected by adenocarcinomas rather than by squamous cell cancers (Fig. 19-1). These tumors arise from submucosal glands within the squamous-lined esophagus, from the columnar epithelium in the distal esophagus, or from the columnar epithelial lining of Barrett's esophagus. Adenocarcinomas of the esophagus and

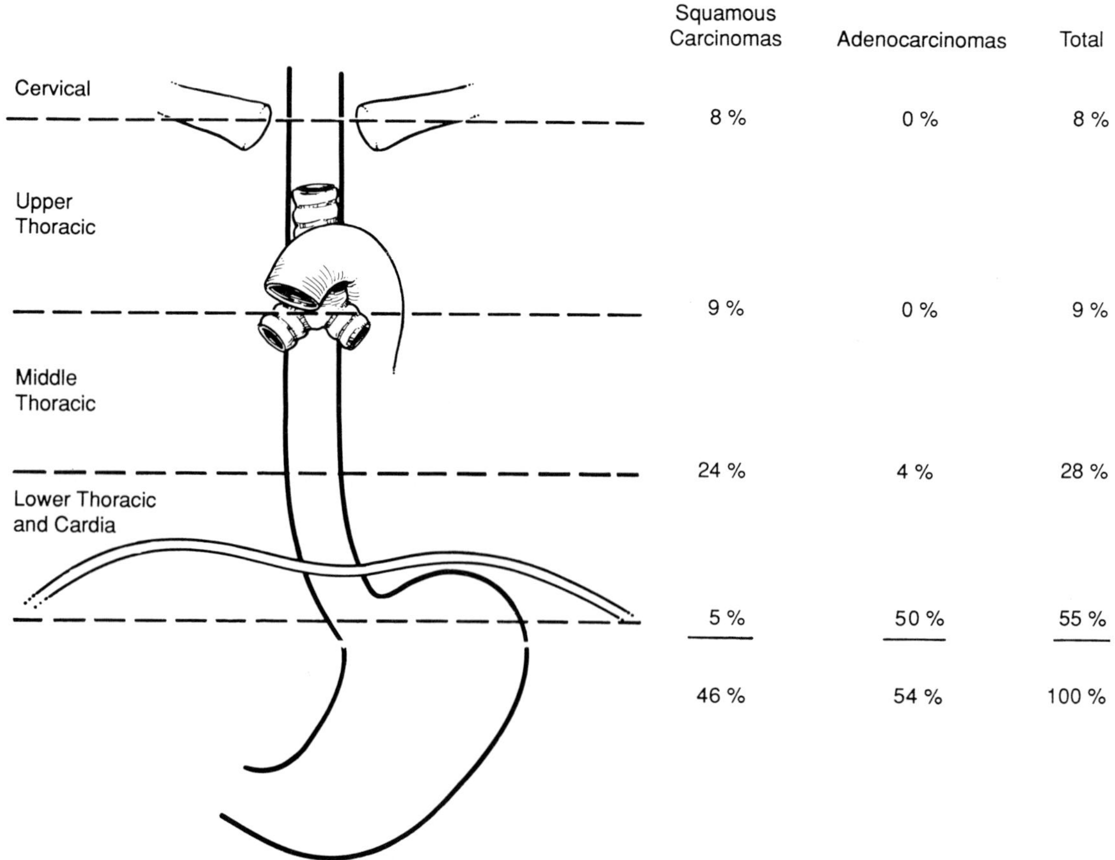

Figure 19–1. Distribution of squamous cell cancers and adenocarcinomas of the esophagus and cardia according to anatomic site.

Table 19–1. Malignant Tumors of the Esophagus

Epithelial
Squamous cell carcinoma
Spindle cell carcinoma
Carcinosarcoma
Pseudosarcoma
Adenocarcinoma
Adenoacanthoma
Adenosquamous carcinoma
Mucoepidermoid carcinoma
Adenoid cystic carcinoma
Carcinoid
Undifferentiated carcinoma
Small cell carcinoma
Nonepithelial
Leiomyosarcoma
Malignant melanoma
Rhabdomyosarcoma
Myoblastoma
Malignant lymphoma

cardia are relatively common, particularly in the Western Hemisphere. The reported incidence of these cancers is increasing in the United States at a rate surpassing that of any other cancer.[26,34,84,87,173] Adenocarcinomas are typically invasive at the time of discovery, although intraepithelial tumors are sometimes diagnosed in patients with Barrett's esophagus who are under surveillance screening.[32] In contrast to squamous cell cancers, adenocarcinomas are unlikely to be multicentric. However, proximal submucosal extension and distal subserosal extension are common.[146] Rare histologic variants exist, including mucoepidermoid tumors similar to those arising in the salivary glands and adenoid cystic carcinomas.

Numerous other unusual malignant tumors also may arise in the esophagus.[33] These tumors include malignant melanoma,[192] granular cell tumor,[77] lymphoma,[22] leiomyosarcoma,[50] undifferentiated tumors resembling oat cell carcinomas that are occasionally associated with paraneoplastic syndromes,[156,161] fibrosarcoma, rhabdomyosarcoma plasmacytoma, lymphosarcoma, and choriocarcinoma.[216,226]

PRESENTATION

Patients with esophageal cancer typically are in their sixth or seventh decade.[228] Most patients have a history of tobacco or alcohol use. The usual presenting complaint is dysphagia, which is found in 80 to 90% of patients (Table 19–2).[96,124] Cancers of the esophagus and cardia cause malignant strictures that result in progressive dysphagia. Such strictures initially cause problems in swallowing solids (meats and breads) and eventually result in difficulties with coarse vegetables and semisolids and, ultimately, liquids. These manifestations are typically present for several months before medical advice is sought.

The second most common presenting complaint is weight loss, which is experienced by more than half of patients diagnosed with esophageal cancer. The weight loss is often profound and is greater in patients with esophageal cancer than in those with most other malignancies, owing to the combined catabolic and obstructive effects of the tumor. Chest pain is frequently reported; it arises from esophageal spasms above a partially obstructing tumor, from irritation of the esophagus by malignant ulcerations, or from direct invasion of mediastinal structures including the spinal column or aorta. Other common symptoms or signs at presentation include regurgitation or vomiting, hoarseness due to recurrent laryngeal nerve involvement, cough secondary to tracheobronchial tree involvement, aspiration pneumonia associated with esophagorespiratory fistula, hematemesis, or melena.

DIAGNOSIS

When patients present with new complaints of dysphagia, a diagnosis of esophageal cancer should always be suspected. A systematic investigation in such patients begins with a careful history and physical examination. Valuable information can be gained from the presence of weight loss, abdominal pain or bone pain indicating possible metastatic spread, respiratory symptoms suggesting possible esophagorespiratory fistula formation, or hoarseness representing recurrent laryngeal nerve involvement. Supraclavicular or cervical lymphadenopathy and hepatic enlargement or nodularity may indicate metastatic spread.

Initial laboratory investigations include a red blood cell count to evaluate possible anemia and liver function tests and alkaline phosphatase level, the results of which may indicate metastatic spread to the liver or bone, respectively. No specific blood tests are available for the quantitation of tumor burden in squamous cell tumors, but measurement of carcinoembryonic antigen (CEA) may be valuable in patients with adenocarcinoma as a useful marker to evaluate treatment response and disease recurrence.

EVALUATION

Chest Radiography

Abnormalities of the esophagus are evident on plain chest radiograph in almost 50% of patients with esophageal

Table 19–2. Symptoms of Carcinoma of the Esophagus and Cardia*†

Symptom	Incidence (%)
Dysphagia	85.4
Weight loss	60.9
Pain	26.5
Regurgitation	22.8
Hoarseness	4.4
Cough	2.5

*Based on findings in 907 patients.

†Data from Galandiuk, S., Hermann, R. E., Cosgrove, D. M., et al.: Cancer of the esophagus. Ann. Surg., *203:*101, 1986; Launois, B., Paul, J. L., Lygidakis, N. J., et al.: Results of the surgical treatment of carcinoma of the esophagus. Surg. Gynecol. Obstet., *156:*753, 1983; Isolauri, J., Markkula, H., and Autio, V.: Colon interposition in the treatment of carcinoma of the esophagus and gastric cardia. Ann. Thorac. Surg., *43:*420, 1987.

cancer. These abnormalities include an air-fluid level in the prevertebral region, which signifies esophageal obstruction. Extensive local disease is indicated by the presence of a soft-tissue mass or by mediastinal lymphadenopathy with displacement or irregularity of the tracheal air shadow. More distant disease may be represented by a pleural effusion or pulmonary metastases.

Barium Esophagogram

The barium swallow film provides staging information about the location of the primary tumor and its probable overall length. Single-contrast studies are useful for identifying exophytic masses (Fig. 19-2). The double-contrast technique, which employs a high-density barium suspension with effervescent crystals, is more useful for delineating tumors of the infiltrating type (Fig. 19-3).[69] The identification of carcinoma in situ is difficult using either technique.

Barium studies allow an accurate estimate of the degree of obstruction caused by tumors of the esophagus. Such estimates are useful in selecting modes of palliative treatment to be used in patients ineligible for esophageal resection. The degree of obstruction is also a component of the stage of the primary tumor in some staging systems.

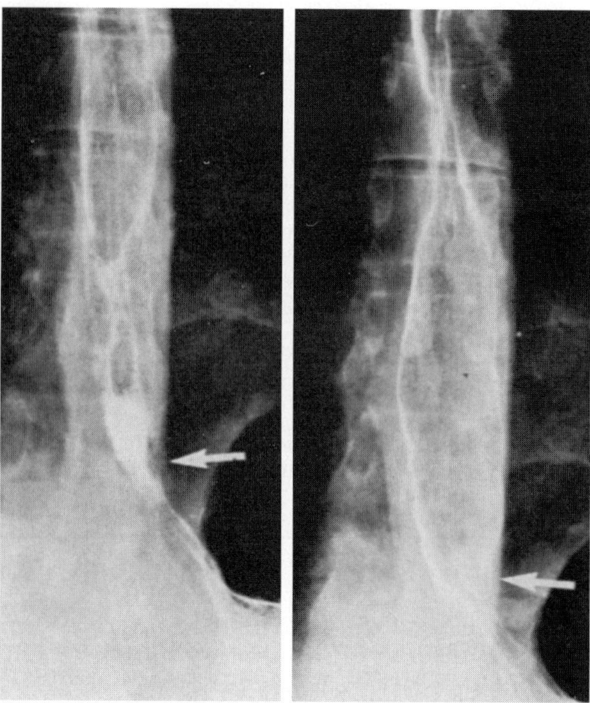

Figure 19–3. Superficial carcinomas may cause only small mucosal irregularities and are best demonstrated using double-contrast barium techniques. The only abnormality in this esophagogram was a persistent indentation 3 cm above the gastroesophageal junction *(arrows)*.

Esophagoscopy

Esophagoscopy is usually performed on every patient who is being evaluated for the presence of an esophageal carcinoma. The typical tumor is friable and exophytic, causing obstruction, or ulcerated with irregular raised borders. More subtle abnormalities include loss of esophageal wall motility caused by longitudinal submucosal infiltration. Close inspection for second synchronous primary tumors should be performed, particularly in patients with squamous cell cancers.

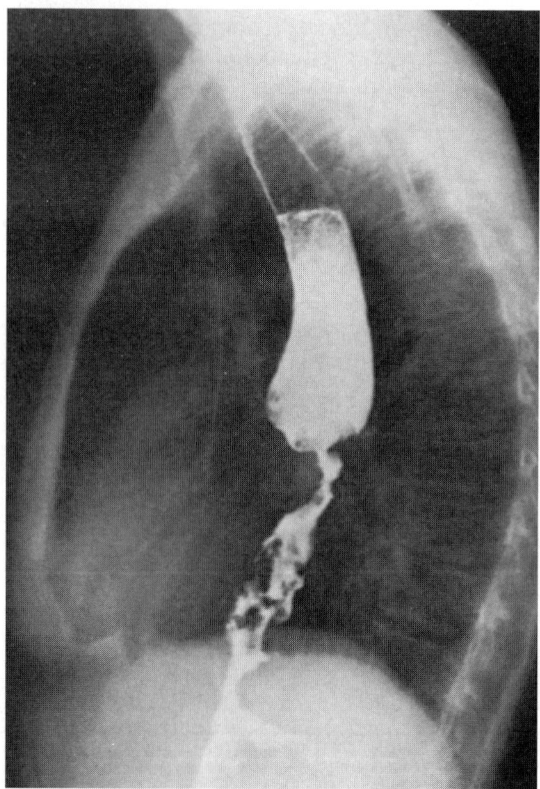

Figure 19–2. Barium swallow demonstrating gross destruction of mucosa in the distal esophagus with associated shouldering and proximal dilatation.

Measurement of the distance of the abnormalities from the incisors is valuable in planning therapy. Important reference landmarks include the cricopharyngeus, the aortic arch, the left mainstem bronchus, and the diaphragmatic hiatus. When the endoscope can be passed through the tumor, measurement of the overall length of involvement is also useful. A carefully performed retroflexion maneuver for a complete evaluation of the fundus and cardia is used to evaluate these structures for possible local involvement and to rule out additional pathology.

Histologic documentation of carcinoma of the esophagus or cardia is obtained routinely with cup forceps biopsies. Even when performed carefully, however, such biopsies are nondiagnostic in more than 7% of cases in which the flexible fiberoptic endoscope is used.[172] Rebiopsy using a rigid scope with a large angled cup forceps is indicated in such cases. On occasion, endoscopic dilation of malignant strictures is necessary to obtain a good biopsy specimen. The use of esophageal brush cytology can lead to a diagnosis of malignancy in some cases in which all biopsies are negative and serves as a valuable adjunct to the usual endoscopic techniques.

Endoscopic Ultrasound

The anatomy of the esophageal wall and the surrounding lymph nodes is assessed using endoscopic ultrasonography (EUS). Five distinct wall layers are identified in the normal esophagus, corresponding to the mucosa, lamina propria, muscularis mucosa, muscularis propria, and adventitia. Esophageal cancer appears as an irregularly delineated hypoechoic mass on EUS. The accuracy of EUS is greatest in patients with transmural tumors, particularly those invading adjacent structures. The overall accuracy of this technique for assessing depth of penetration is 70 to 85%.[37,66,157,176,187,214] Endoscopic ultrasonography is useful in evaluating mediastinal lymph nodes for metastatic involvement. Lymph nodes as small as 3 to 5 mm in diameter can be recognized; enlargement to 6 to 8 mm or greater in maximum diameter is often a sign of metastatic spread. However, qualitative criteria are more important in recognizing involved nodes, which are better circumscribed and have a more irregular hypoechoic internal pattern than that found in normal lymph nodes. The accuracy of detection of involved mediastinal lymph nodes using EUS is more than 75 to 90%.[40,66,157,176,187]

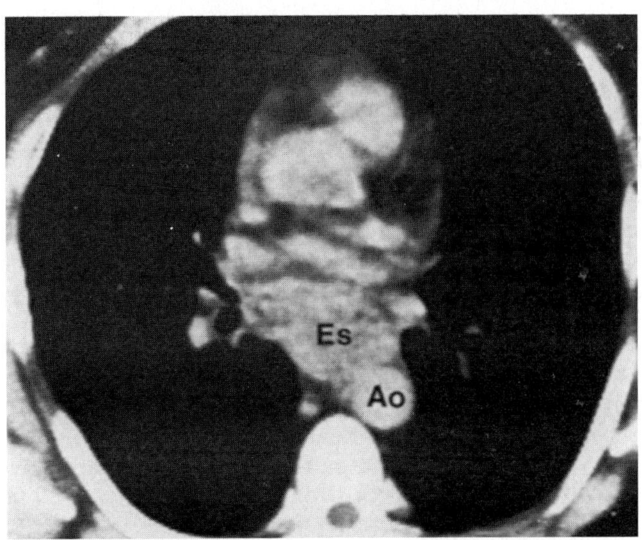

Figure 19–4. CT is useful in assessing technical resectability, such as in this patient with probable infiltration of the aorta *(Ao)* by an esophageal carcinoma *(Es)*.

Bronchoscopy

Bronchoscopic examination is mandatory in patients with esophageal carcinomas involving regions adjacent to the trachea or mainstem bronchi if esophagectomy is contemplated. The esophagus and tracheobronchial tree are in close proximity, and airway abnormalities are frequently detected, indicating possible transmural spread of tumor. Many patients with carcinomas located in the upper thoracic esophagus have airway abnormalities, including almost 10% with direct tracheobronchial invasion by the tumor.[184] A large tumor mass can cause anterior displacement of the membranous portion of the trachea, although this does not necessarily imply invasion of the tracheobronchial tree. Early findings that do indicate airway invasion include edema and elevation of the mucosa with contact bleeding.[42] Blunting of the carina is normally caused by metastatic involvement of subcarinal lymph nodes rather than by direct involvement of the carina by the primary tumor mass. Cytologic sampling of subcarinal lymph nodes is possible by means of transcarinal needle aspiration.

Computed Tomography of the Chest and Upper Abdomen

Computed tomography (CT) is currently the standard radiographic tool for evaluating esophageal carcinoma. Compared with the barium swallow, which is limited in its ability to detect extraesophageal spread of tumor, the cross-sectional imaging technique of CT makes it suitable for evaluating the esophageal wall and periesophageal structures. CT also provides useful information about lymph node enlargement and concomitantly evaluates the liver, lungs, and adrenal glands for metastatic spread.

Evaluation of the primary tumor by CT allows one to estimate esophageal wall thickness and tumor length. Maximum normal esophageal wall thickness is 5 mm, and asymmetric thickening is found in more than two thirds of patients with esophageal cancer.[182] CT also provides an estimate of the longitudinal extent of disease, although underestimations of length on the order of 2 to 3 cm often occur.[223]

Invasion of the primary esophageal tumor into the mediastinum is an important determinant of survival. Direct invasion with adjacent tissue destruction is an obvious finding on CT in some patients. More commonly, CT shows an esophageal mass that is inseparable from an adjacent structure such as the trachea, aorta, or heart (Fig. 19–4). One criterion of invasion is loss of the fat plane between the tumor and an adjacent structure. Cachexia, prior operation, or previous radiation therapy in patients with esophageal cancer may render interpretation of CT scans difficult owing to loss of fat planes or scarring. The cervical esophagus and gastroesophageal junction are particularly difficult to examine because of the absence of surrounding periesophageal fat planes.

The ability of CT to predict invasion of individual mediastinal structures is quite variable.[103,118,145,167,189,230] Tracheobronchial invasion is predicted with an overall accuracy of more than 85%, and aortic wall invasion is predicted with an overall accuracy of more than 80%. Unfortunately, the sensitivity of these two predictions is only 50 to 55%, rendering such predictions minimally useful for determining operability. Enhancement of scans with the use of continuous infusion or bolus injection of intravenous contrast material facilitates interpretation in some situations. The overall accuracy of CT in predicting mediastinal invasion by esophageal carcinoma is relatively good.

Regional adenopathy is detectable by CT scan only on the basis of lymph node enlargement (Fig. 19–5). Mediastinal lymph nodes are considered abnormally large when they are greater than 1 cm in maximum diameter, although the mediastinal location has some bearing on the normal nodal diameter.[73] Metastases from esophageal cancer to mediastinal lymph nodes are found frequently in normal-sized nodes. As a result, the accuracy of CT scanning in predicting regional node involvement by

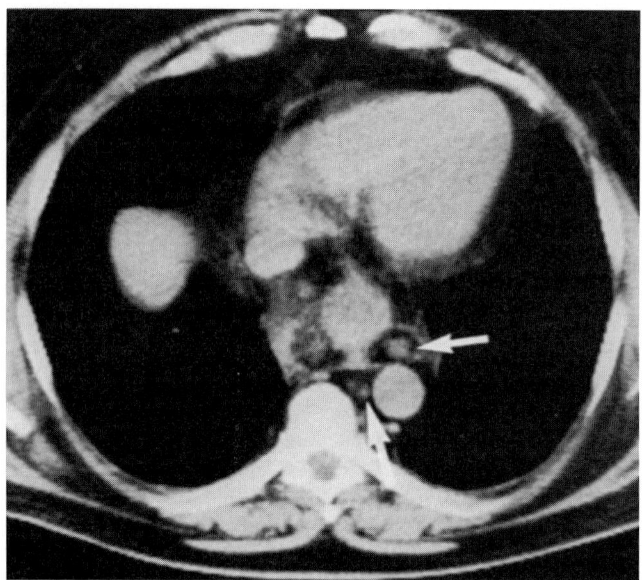

Figure 19–5. CT can illustrate the presence of enlarged regional nodes *(arrows).*

esophageal cancer is under 60%, and sensitivity is less than 30%.[103,118,145,189,230]

CT is particularly good for detecting liver, adrenal, pulmonary, and distant nodal metastases. Hepatic involvement appears as an irregular low-density lesion (Fig. 19–6), whereas adrenal metastases enlarge or obliterate the normal suprarenal "inverted Y" shape of the adrenal gland. Visceral metastases are detected with an overall accuracy of more than 95%, although sensitivity is poor (40%).[145,189] Metastases to distant lymph nodes, particularly the celiac axis nodes, are assessed with an overall accuracy of 82% and a sensitivity of more than 60%.

Magnetic Resonance Imaging

Magnetic resonance imaging (MRI) has considerable potential in the study of mediastinal structures, although few data are available about its applicability to the staging of esophageal neoplasms. MRI has many of the same problems as CT scanning in the evaluation of the esophagus and mediastinal structures. Measurement of esophageal wall thickness in the absence of intraluminal air or other contrast agents is difficult. Visualization of the middle third of the esophagus is complicated by artifacts resulting from respiratory and cardiac motion. MRI has no discernible advantage over CT in determining either extraesophageal spread of the primary tumor or regional nodal involvement.[128] Further technical advances in MRI are necessary before this technique can supplant CT for staging esophageal carcinoma.

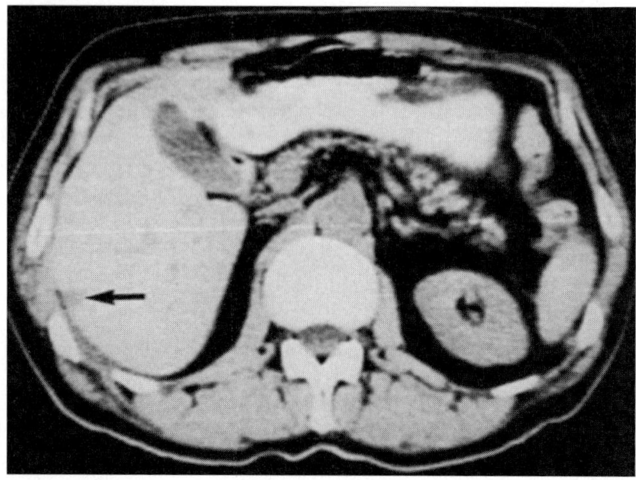

Figure 19–6. Liver metastases can often be discerned as being the initial site of distant spread in patients with esophageal cancer *(arrow).*

Positron Emission Tomography

Positron emission tomography (PET) is a promising investigative technique for staging patients with esophageal cancer. Patients are evaluated for areas of increased focal uptake after injection of ^{18}F-fluorodeoxyglucose. The accuracy of staging of regional disease is similar to that for computed tomography. However, PET facilitates selection of patients for operation by detecting distant disease that is not identified by conventional staging techniques. The overall accuracy for detecting distant metastases is in excess of 90%, and up to 20% of patients are found to have unsuspected distant metastases that are not detected with conventional staging.[25,143]

Scintigraphic Tests for Metastases

There is disagreement about the need for scintigraphic evaluation of metastases in patients with esophageal cancer. The organs most likely to harbor distant metastases are the lung, liver, adrenal glands, and bone. All these metastatic sites may be asymptomatic at the time the patient initially presents. Bone scans using ^{99m}Tc-labeled methylene diphosphonate commonly are used in staging patients with esophageal cancer and can be used to detect bone metastases in asymptomatic patients in the absence of elevated serum calcium or alkaline phosphatase levels.[95] Bone metastases are found at autopsy in, at most, 14% of patients[11,17] and are detected by bone scan as the only site of metastatic disease in fewer than 4% of patients. Benign bone abnormalities, which sometimes mimic metastases and require additional investigation to determine their cause, result in false-positive diagnoses in almost 30% of patients.[62]

Minimally Invasive Surgical Staging

Laparoscopy with or without laparoscopic ultrasonography has been used routinely in some centers since the early 1990s for the staging of carcinomas of the esophagus and esophagogastric junction. More recently, thoracoscopic staging has been added to the staging armamentarium. Laparoscopic staging permits detection of metastatic disease precluding resection in 10 to 20% of patients and is more accurate than EUS in abdominal staging.[21,142,167,208] Thoracoscopic staging is potentially valuable in permitting accurate stage assessment prior to neoadjuvant chemotherapy or chemoradiotherapy and provides the ability to assess direct tumor invasion into unresectable structures.[114,115] Laparoscopy, particularly as an initial step before formal resection, is likely to become a widely accepted technique for staging esophageal cancer. Whether thoracoscopic staging will enjoy a similar acceptance remains to be seen.

Other Studies

Mediastinoscopy is used by some as a staging procedure for carcinoma of the upper and middle thoracic esophagus to assess the status of the mediastinal lymph nodes. Mediastinoscopy may be used to predict the presence of unresectable tumor in some cases in which there are fixed perinodal metastases, but mediastinal spread of tumor is missed in as many as 50% of patients when this technique is used as a routine staging procedure.[158] Percutaneous needle biopsy of suspected extranodal metastases is highly accurate and may eliminate the need for an open biopsy procedure when this is indicated by other staging procedures, including the CT scan. In some cases, a "mini-laparotomy" is of value in documenting metastatic spread to subdiaphragmatic sites when suspicious findings are noted on CT scan.

Biological Staging

Some techniques for staging malignancies, including those of the esophagus and cardia, are nonanatomic. Measurements of oncogene expression and of cell DNA content and other histochemical analyses provide accurate determinants of prognosis in many studies. Preliminary results show that DNA content and degree of dispersion is related inversely to 5-year survival in patients with esophageal cancer.[209,237] Expression of *ras* oncogene p21 in esophageal squamous cell cancers correlates inversely with survival and is a better predictor than histologic grade or pathologic stage.[190]

Other oncogenes that have been reported to be indicators of long-term prognosis include cyclinD1 and MDM2 (murine double minute 2).[201] Mutations of the tumor suppressor genes p53 and possibly p73 may also be related to long-term prognosis.[51,201] The overexpression of c-erb and the *erb* B2 has been associated with improved survival in patients with esophageal cancer.[55]

STAGING SYSTEMS

In the TNM classification for staging esophageal cancer, the esophagus is divided into four sections.[10] The cervical esophagus commences at the lower border of the cricoid cartilage and ends at the thoracic inlet, approximately 18 cm from the upper incisor teeth. The upper thoracic esophagus extends from the thoracic inlet to the level of the carina, approximately 24 cm from the upper incisor teeth. The middle thoracic esophagus is made up of the proximal half of the esophagus between the carina and the esophagogastric junction. The lower thoracic esophagus begins approximately 32 cm from the upper incisor teeth and extends to the esophagogastric junction, approximately 40 cm from the upper incisor teeth. Although it is reasonable to include carcinomas of the cardia within this system, because they share many biologic similarities with adenocarcinomas of the lower esophagus, this staging system does not pertain to carcinomas of the cardia if it is strictly applied.

The primary tumor is classified according to its depth of invasion, designated by the letter T (Table 19-3). T_x represents a tumor demonstrated cytologically by the presence of cancer cells in brushings or washings but not evident endoscopically or radiographically. T_0 and T_{is} are other uncommonly used headings that indicate no evidence of primary tumor and carcinoma in situ, respectively.

T_1 designates a tumor that invades the submucosa but not beyond it. A tumor that extends into but not beyond the muscularis propria is labeled T_2. Tumors that invade the adventitia of the esophagus are labeled T_3, and tumors that invade contiguous structures such as the pericardium, tracheobronchial tree, aorta, or vertebral bodies are referred to as T_4.

The status of the regional lymph nodes is designated by the letter N with appropriate suffixes. Regional lymph nodes for tumors located primarily in the cervical esophagus include the cervical and supraclavicular nodes. Regional lymph nodes for tumors of the thoracic esophagus include the mediastinal and perigastric nodes, including

Table 19–3. Definitions of TNM Classification for Esophageal Cancer*

Code	Definition
Primary tumor (T)	
TX	Primary tumor cannot be assessed
T0	No evidence of primary tumor
Tis	Carcinoma *in situ*
T1	Tumor invades lamina propia or submucosa
T2	Tumor invades muscularis propia
T3	Tumor invades adventitia
T4	Tumor invades surrounding structures
Regional lymph nodes (N)	
NX	Regional lymph nodes cannot be assessed
N0	No regional lymph node metastasis
N1	Regional lymph node metastasis
Distant metastases (M)	
MX	Distant metastases cannot be assessed
M0	No distant metastases
M1	Distant metastases
	Tumors of the lower thoracic esophagus
M1a	Metastases in celiac lymph nodes
M1b	Other distant metastases
	Tumors of the midthoracic esophagus
M1a	Not applicable
M1b	Nonregional lymph nodes and/or other distant metastases
	Tumors of the upper thoracic esophagus
M1a	Metastases in cervical nodes
M1b	Other distant metastases

For tumors of midthoracic esophagus use only M1b, since these tumors with metastasis in nonregional lymph nodes have an equally poor prognosis as those with metastasis in other distant sites.

*From American Joint Committee on Cancer. Esophagus. Chpt. 9, AJCC Cancer Staging Manual, 5th ed. Philadelphia, Lippincott Williams & Wilkins, 1997, pp 65–69.

those along the lesser curve, the fundus, and the left gastric artery. N_0 represents an absence of demonstrable metastases to regional lymph nodes. N_1 represents metastases to regional lymph nodes, whereas N_x refers to situations in which the presence or absence of regional nodal involvement by tumor cannot be adequately assessed. The distribution of the regional nodes for tumors of the cervical and thoracic esophagus is shown in Figure 19–7, and the incidence of nodal involvement based on tumor location is presented in Table 19–4.

The presence or absence of distant metastases is designated by the letter M with modifying subscripts. M_x refers to situations in which the presence of distant metastases cannot be adequately assessed. M_0 indicates no known distant metastases. M_{1a} signifies the presence of metastases to proximate nonregional lymph nodes, such as celiac axis lymph nodes for tumors of the lower thoracic esophagus or cervical lymph nodes for tumors of the upper thoracic esophagus. M_{1b} is indicative of metastases to other nonregional lymph nodes or other distant metastases. Nonregional lymph nodes for cervical carcinomas include the mediastinal nodes, whereas nonregional nodes for carcinomas of the thoracic esophagus include the cervical or supraclavicular lymph nodes as well as omental, celiac, abdominal periaortic, common hepatic, and splenic nodes (see Table 19–4).[6,101] Autopsy studies show that metastases occur more often to lymph nodes, whether regional or distant, than to distant organs. Organ metastases occur most often in the liver, lung, peritoneum, and adrenal glands (Table 19–5). Combinations of the TNM categories have been grouped into stages (Table 19–6). Stage 0 includes carcinoma in situ with no evidence of invasion, regional node involvement, or metasta-

Table 19–4. Incidence of Lymph Node Involvement by Tumor*

	Cervical (%)	Upper Thoracic (%)	Middle Thoracic (%)	Lower Thoracic and Cardia (%)
Cervical	14	8	7	5
Superior mediastinal	11	29	11	11
Middle mediastinal	0	27	21	16
Lower mediastinal	0	29	18	28
Abdominal	3			
Superior gastric	—	32	33	55
Celiac artery	—	0	4	21
Common hepatic artery	—	0	2	10
Splenic artery	—	0	6	17

*Data from Sons, H. U., and Borchard, F.: Cancer of the distal esophagus and cardia: Incidence, tumorous infiltration and metastatic spread. Ann. Surg., *203*:188, 1986; Akiyama, H., Tsurumaru, M., Kawamura, T., et al.: Principles of surgical treatment for carcinoma of the esophagus. Ann. Surg., *194*:438, 1981; Kakegawa, T., Yamana, H., and Ando, N.: Analysis of surgical treatment for carcinoma situated in the cervical esophagus. Surgery, *97*:150, 1985.

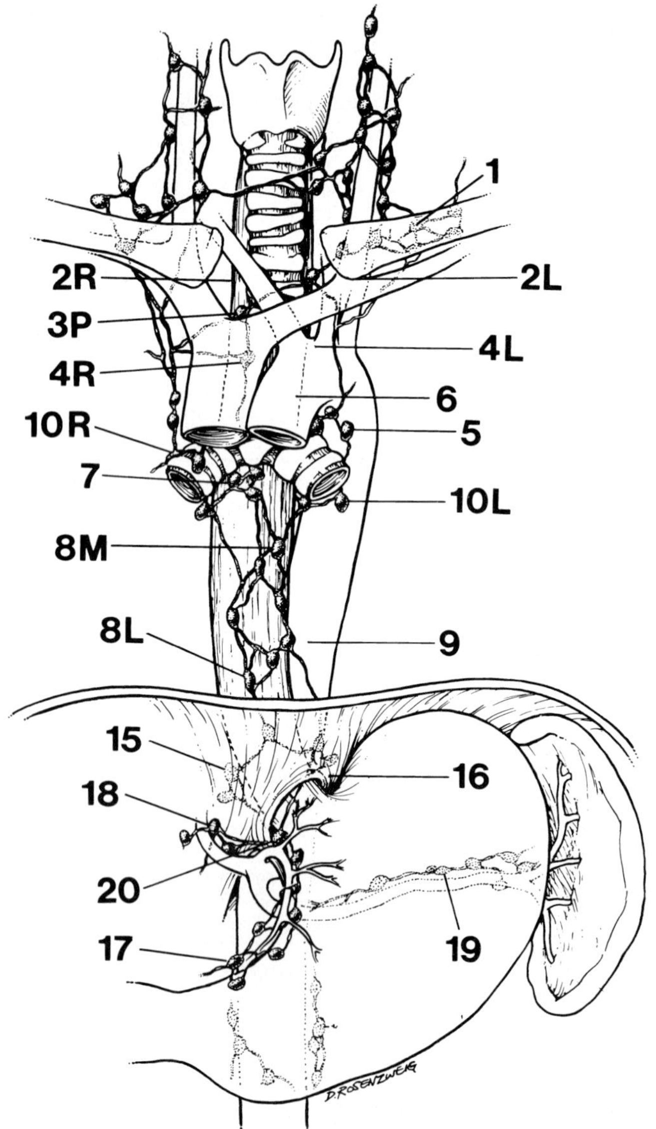

Figure 19–7. Sites of potential regional nodal involvement in esophageal cancer: 1, supraclavicular; 2R, right upper paratracheal; 2L, left upper paratracheal; 3P, posterior mediastinal; 4R, right lower paratracheal; 4L, left lower paratracheal; 5, aortopulmonary; 6, anterior mediastinal; 7, subcarinal; 8M, middle paraesophageal; 8L, lower paraesophageal; 9, pulmonary ligament; 10R, right tracheobronchial; 10L, left tracheobronchial; 15, diaphragmatic; 16, paracardial; 17, left gastric artery; 18, common hepatic artery; 19, splenic artery; 20, celiac axis.

Table 19–5. Sites of Metastatic Spread in Patients With Carcinoma of the Esophagus or Cardia*†

Site	Incidence (%)
Lymph nodes	72.3
Liver	31.8
Lung	25.5
Peritoneum	12.1
Adrenal glands	10.4
Bone	9.1
Kidney	8.8
Diaphragm	7.0
Pancreas	4.9
Thyroid	4.7
Spleen	4.7
Heart	3.8
Brain	1.5

*Based on results from 384 patients.

†Data from Sons, H. U., and Borchard, F.: Cancer of the distal esophagus and cardia: Incidence, tumorous infiltration and metastatic spread. Ann. Surg., *203*:188, 1986; Anderson, L. L., and Lad, T. E.: Autopsy findings in squamous-cell carcinoma of the esophagus. Cancer, *50*:1587, 1982; Attah, E. B., and Hajdu, S. I.: Benign and malignant tumors of the esophagus at autopsy. J. Thorac. Cardiovasc. Surg., *55*:396, 1968.

Table 19–6. TNM Staging Classification for Esophageal Cancer*

Stage 0	Tis	N0	M0
Stage I	T1	N0	M0
Stage IIA	T2	N0	M0
	T3	N0	M0
Stage IIB	T1	N1	M0
	T2	N1	M0
Stage III	T3	N1	M0
	T4	Any N	M0
Stage IV	Any T	Any N	M1
Stage IVA	Any T	Any N	M1a
Stage IVB	Any T	Any N	M1b

*From American Joint Committee on Cancer. Esophagus. Chpt. 9, AJCC Cancer Staging Manual, 5th ed. Philadelphia, Lippincott Williams & Wilkins, 1997, pp. 65–69.

sis. Stages I and II_a include invasive tumors without evidence of regional nodal metastases or distant metastases. Stage II_b consists of tumors with moderate invasion and involvement of regional nodes without distant metastases. Stage III tumors are those with a greater depth of invasion with or without regional nodal metastases, and stage IV disease includes any tumors with distant metastases. Using these stages, the Japanese Committee for Registration of Esophageal Carcinoma has analyzed survival in 3,211 patients who underwent surgical staging and resection. The stages as assigned provide an accurate differentiation among the five staging classifications and illustrate the prognostic value of pathologic staging (Fig. 19–8).[98]

EARLY DIAGNOSIS OF ESOPHAGEAL CARCINOMA

In geographic regions with a high incidence of esophageal tumors, particularly northern China, portions of Iran, South Africa, and Japan, early diagnosis of these tumors has been a subject of intense interest during the last 20 years. One of the primary causes for the overall poor prognosis in esophageal cancer is the fact that most tumors are diagnosed at a relatively advanced stage, often exhibiting metastatic spread. When early-stage carcinoma is diagnosed, the prognosis following definitive surgical treatment is excellent, and long-term cure rates sometimes exceed 90%.[59] This illustrates that the primary method by which significant improvements in survival from esophageal cancer will be made is the development of our ability to diagnose it at an early stage, before the tumor has penetrated the esophageal wall or spread to regional lymph nodes.

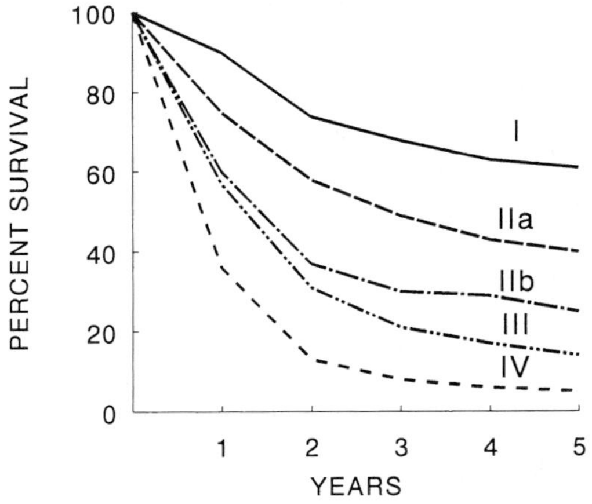

Figure 19–8. Actuarial survival by stage for cancer of the esophagus. (From Japanese Committee for Registration of Esophageal Carcinoma: A proposal for a new TNM classification of esophageal carcinoma. Jpn. J. Clin. Oncol., *14*:625, 1985.)

Screening examinations and other techniques of early diagnosis are not cost-effective on a large scale in the western world owing to the relatively low incidence of esophageal cancer in this population. However, such techniques are appropriate in selected populations, including men over 50 years of age who either smoke or drink in excess[52] and those with other diseases that carry an increased risk of esophageal cancer. Such diseases include head and neck cancer, bronchogenic carcinoma, gluten enteropathy, Plummer-Vinson syndrome, achalasia, chronic reflux esophagitis, lye stricture, and Barrett's epithelium. Blind cytologic screening is an accurate technique for selecting candidates for more definitive investigation and has been found to be cost-effective. The available techniques include panesophageal cytology using a brush,[16] an encapsulated sponge attached to a string, or an enmeshed inflatable balloon that is swallowed by the patient.[44] Another form of blind cytologic brushing is performed by inserting a standard cytology brush through an indwelling nasoesophageal tube, which yields specimens from the mid and distal thirds of the esophagus.[53]

The accuracy of these techniques depends on careful specimen preparation and on the availability of an experienced cytologist to analyze the samples. The techniques are safe and have good patient acceptance, and they are inexpensive in relation to other available diagnostic procedures. In groups of high-risk patients, the yield of marked dysplasia or frank carcinoma is as high as 3%, even in the absence of symptoms.[131] The overall accuracy rate for diagnosing cancers is 95%, with a false-positive rate of 2% in more than 2,000 cases.[202] As with all screening tests, the usefulness of this technique lies in its ability to detect esophageal cancer at an early stage. In most clinical series, less than 10% of patients with esophageal cancer are diagnosed at an early stage. Using the blind cytologic screening techniques just described in high-risk patients without symptoms, early-stage cancers are found in more than 75% of patients with documented malignancy.[23,44,80,202,235] Patients who have histologic changes that are known to be premalignant should undergo follow-up evaluation, including endoscopy.[35,46] Patients with dysplasia or frank carcinoma on blind cytologic examination should undergo directed endoscopic biopsy for staging and histologic diagnosis.

THERAPY

There is disagreement about what constitutes optimal therapy for patients with carcinoma of the esophagus and cardia. Despite efforts at early diagnosis, a large number of patients have either advanced regional disease or metastatic disease at the time of diagnosis. Complicating matters is our relatively poor ability to stage patients clinically, and many patients are found on surgical exploration to have more advanced disease than was originally thought. As a result, only a small percentage of patients truly have early-stage disease that is amenable to curative resection. Most patients have disease that is in an intermediate category, more advanced than an early stage but not metastatic. It is about these patients that the controversy over appropriate therapy is most heated.

Surgical Treatment

Surgical resection is the mainstay of curative therapy for carcinoma of the esophagus and cardia. Since resection was first demonstrated to be feasible on a routine basis, esophagectomy for carcinoma has remained a technical tour de force for the general and thoracic surgeon.

Patient Selection

Resection is the primary mode of therapy for most patients with carcinoma of the esophagus or cardia. Esophagectomy provides the best opportunity for cure in patients with limited disease and offers substantial palliation for patients with more advanced disease. A resection with curative intent is indicated in patients with stage I and stage II_a disease and is a controversial form of therapy for those with disease in stages II_b and III. When significant dysphagia or bleeding is present, palliative resection is often indicated, even in patients with advanced tumors in whom complete removal of gross disease is not possible. The percentages of patients with carcinoma of the esophagus and cardia who are surgically explored range from 50 to 80%, and there is also great variation in the rates of resectability among patients explored, ranging from 70 to over 95%.[89,141]

Although esophageal cancer occurs predominantly during the seventh and eighth decades of life, advanced age alone is not a specific contraindication to resection. Elderly patients, particularly those over 70 years of age, have a higher operative mortality than do younger patients.[63,127,177,225] This difference is accounted for somewhat by a high incidence of operative risk factors in the elderly population, including heart, liver, and kidney diseases. It is encouraging that the long-term prognosis in elderly patients, excluding operative mortality, is similar to that in younger patients.

Because esophageal cancer has strong etiologic ties to tobacco and alcohol use, it is not surprising that there is a high incidence of cardiovascular, pulmonary, and hepatic dysfunction in such patients. Forced expiratory volume at 1 second (FEV_1) is related to operative mortality, and a history of chronic bronchitis adversely affects the incidence of postoperative pulmonary complications.[39,79] At least 20 to 30% of patients have cardiovascular disease, including peripheral vascular obstructive disease and ischemic heart disease (with or without prior myocardial infarction).[58,113] With proper preoperative evaluation and perioperative management, most of these patients can undergo esophagogastrectomy without complication, making such cardiovascular problems only relative contraindications to operation. Cirrhosis in a patient with carcinoma of the esophagus is not an absolute contraindication to operation when a curative resection can be performed. The operative risk is acceptable in patients who are determined to be Child's class A and whose prothrombin time is no more than 150% of normal.[60]

Most patients with cancer of the esophagus or cardia, particularly those with advanced disease, have combined protein-calorie malnutrition. The degree of malnutrition correlates directly with the risk of operative complications, such as anastomotic leakage, wound dehiscence, or infections.[164] Preoperative nutritional repletion is possible in many cases by enteral or parenteral methods[31,163] and, when successful, reduces the incidence of postoperative complications and operative mortality.[47,193]

Perioperative Management

Appropriate perioperative management is vital to the success of surgical treatment of carcinoma of the esophagus and cardia. As a supplement to careful patient selection, optimization of cardiovascular status reduces problems of intraoperative management and improves the chances of operative survival. Esophageal cancer patients are often depleted of intravascular volume owing to dysphagia, lack of fluid intake necessitated by preoperative testing, and fluid losses sustained during preparation of the bowels for surgery. Volume repletion before surgery is thus an important safeguard.

Preparation of the colon before surgery is advisable, even when it is likely that the stomach will be used for reconstruction. Bowel preparation consists of a mechanical cleansing, using laxatives and enemas or a lavage technique, and antibiotic preparation with oral agents such as erythromycin base and neomycin sulfate. In patients in whom there is evidence of peripheral vascular obstructive disease, superior and inferior mesenteric angiography is sometimes useful to determine whether blood supply to the colon is sufficient to permit its use as an esophageal substitute.

Careful intraoperative management is essential to limit complications from esophageal resection. Radial artery catheterization is useful for monitoring blood pressure and obtaining arterial blood samples for blood gas measurement. For patients in whom a thoracotomy is performed, insertion of a double-lumen endotracheal tube allows deflation of the ipsilateral lung, facilitates dissection of the thoracic esophagus, and reduces the need for surgical assistants.

When major resections are undertaken, close observation in an intensive care unit is advisable for at least 24 hours postoperatively. Ventilatory support is sometimes necessary, particularly after prolonged procedures, although its routine use in patients in whom it is not required can lead to an increased incidence of respiratory complications postoperatively. Placement of an enteral feeding catheter intraoperatively, usually a needle catheter jejunostomy, facilitates early postoperative feeding, and the catheter can be used to provide supplemental nutrition as patients are adjusting to oral intake through a reconstructed esophagus.

Early mobilization is important to limit venous stasis and maximize recovery of the pulmonary system. Incentive spirometry and chest physical therapy performed by skilled nurses or designated physiotherapists aid in clearing secretions and expanding regions of atelectasis.

Broad-spectrum parenteral antibiotics are administered as a single preoperative dose followed by doses every 6 to 8 hours for 24 hours following the operation. For operations not involving the colon, a second-generation cephalosporin is sufficient. When esophageal reconstruction with the colon is performed, metronidazole, a third-generation cephalosporin, or a drug combination including an aminoglycoside is appropriate.

Selection of Operation

Appropriate selection of operation is important to maximize the benefits of surgical therapy for esophageal cancer and to minimize operative risks and complications. Selection depends in part on the location of the tumor and clinical staging but is also influenced by the philosophy of the surgeon performing the operation. Selection of the operation is determined in part by findings at the time of operation, and most procedures should begin with an exploration of the important anatomic regions for intraoperative staging before beginning resection.

STANDARD ESOPHAGECTOMY

Most esophageal cancers are resected through a combined thoracic and abdominal approach. For tumors involving the distal esophagus or cardia, a left lateral thoracotomy provides easy access to the esophagus as high as the aortic arch and permits access to the upper abdominal viscera through a peripheral incision in the diaphragm. For tumors of the mid and upper esophagus, access to the chest is gained through an anterolateral thoractomy while an abdominal approach is made simultaneously through an upper midline incision as popularized by Lewis[130] (Fig. 19–9).

For tumors of the lower thoracic esophagus and cardia, the patient is placed in the lateral position, and a left lateral thoracotomy is performed, entering the chest through the seventh or eighth intercostal space. An initial evaluation of the primary tumor is made, and particular attention is given to the possible involvement of contiguous structures (e.g., the pericardium, aorta, diaphragm). If the preliminary appraisal indicates that a resection can be performed, the diaphragm is divided peripherally from the sternum to the spleen, leaving a small margin of diaphragm attached to the chest wall for later reconstruction. The abdomen is then explored to assess the degree of stomach involvement and the presence or absence of metastases to the upper abdominal lymph nodes and the liver.

If conditions appear favorable for standard resection, the esophagus is mobilized from its bed beginning 5 cm proximal to the most cephalic extent of gross tumor. Squamous cell carcinomas of the esophagus are frequently multicentric and are best treated by a subtotal

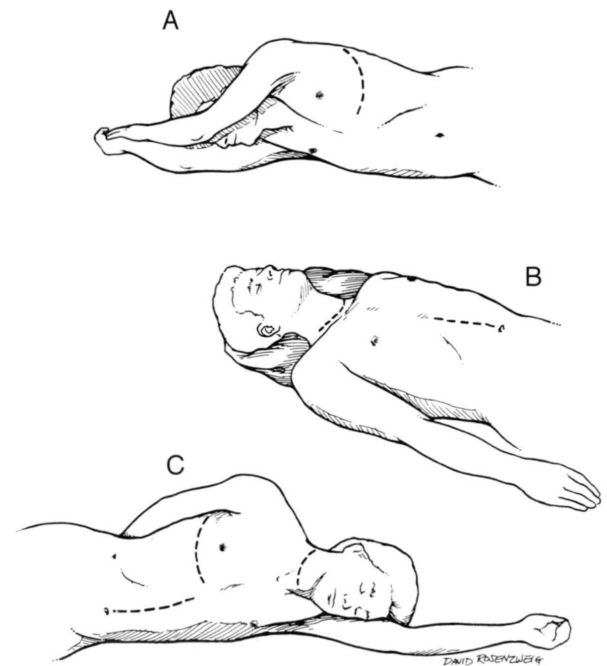

Figure 19–9. *A* through *C*, Incisions for resecting carcinomas of the esophagus or cardia.

esophagectomy.[116,117,211] The dissection includes soft tissues and lymph nodes abutting the esophagus, excluding pericardium and contralateral pleura; it requires division and ligation of two or three arterial branches extending from the aorta to the superficial esophageal vascular plexus as well as branches of the vagus nerve that descend from the level of the carina onto the esophagus. As the dissection is carried upward below the level of the arch, care must be taken to preserve the left recurrent laryngeal nerve, whereas damage to the right recurrent laryngeal nerve is unusual if one is careful to stay directly on the medial wall of the esophagus. The pleura is divided above the level of the arch, and a blunt dissection is extended up into the cervical prevertebral space. This aids in identifying the esophagus during the cervical portion of the operation.

For adenocarcinomas of the distal esophagus and cardia, tumor multicentricity is not a problem, and the proximal dissection can be limited to 5 cm above the gross level of the tumor.[57,85] The tumor mass itself is sharply dissected from the surrounding tissues including the aorta, prevertebral fascia, and pericardium. A 1- to 2-cm rim of diaphragm should be dissected free with the tumor using electrocautery if the tumor approaches within 5 cm of the hiatus. The diaphragm is reflected superiorly, and the dissection is continued within the abdomen.

If the stomach is to be used for reconstruction, all the short gastric vessels are divided, and the omentum is freed from the greater curvature, preserving the right gastric and gastroepiploic arteries on which the vascular supply to the stomach is based. After the stomach is reflected medially, the left gastric artery is divided at its origin, as is the coronary vein. If the stomach is not to be used for reconstruction, division of the omentum and short gastric vessels is not necessary. The gastrohepatic ligament is divided and the stomach transected with a stapling device, leaving a tumor-free margin 5 cm caudal to the most distal extent of tumor.

In patients in whom a distal esophagectomy and proximal gastrectomy are performed, reconstruction is accomplished with either a gastric pull-up, colon interposition (short segment), or small bowel interposition. Subtotal esophagectomy normally necessitates a cervical anastomosis using a gastric pull-up (if the fundus is intact) or a long-segment colon interposition.

Tumors of the mid and upper thoracic esophagus are approached by using a right lateral or anterolateral thoracotomy in combination with an upper abdominal incision for preparation of the organ selected for reconstruction. Tumors in these locations are usually squamous cell cancers and require a subtotal esophagectomy for adequate treatment. In these cases, the esophagus is encircled at least 5 cm distal to the most caudal extent of the tumor. The dissection of tumor is carried proximal from this point to separate the mass from the surrounding structures. The right recurrent nerve is usually easily identified as it separates from the vagus nerve and passes anterior to the innominate artery. The left recurrent nerve frequently originates inferior to this, and careful dissection of the vagus trunk is necessary to avoid injury to it. When a 5-cm margin of esophagus has been obtained proximal to the most cephalic extent of tumor, dissection can be carried out directly on the esophageal wall excluding the vagus nerves passing into the neck. The dissection is extended inferiorly on the esophageal wall through the esophageal hiatus, and the stomach is divided just distal to the cardia in order to include all squamous mucosa. Reconstruction is performed with either a gastric pull-up or a colon interposition, with the anastomosis made to the cervical esophagus through a separate neck incision or high in the right chest, above the level of the azygos vein.

Squamous cell carcinoma of the cervical esophagus is often difficult to treat owing to extension of the tumor into hypopharyngeal or laryngeal structures. To obtain adequate proximal margins, a total laryngectomy is sometimes necessary. In keeping with the concern about multicentric tumors, a total thoracic esophagectomy is also performed, but this can be done using a combined transhiatal and cervical approach. Reconstruction is performed using a long colon segment or gastric pull-up anastomosed to the posterior pharynx.

Routine postoperative care includes decompression of the reconstructed esophagus using an intermittent suction device connected to a tube passed transnasally to a point below the diaphragm. A barium swallow is performed 4 to 5 days postoperatively before beginning oral alimentation.

RADICAL EN BLOC ESOPHAGECTOMY

Some patients are candidates for an en bloc resection, which is performed to maximize the therapeutic benefit of surgical resection.[137] The objective of en bloc resection is complete removal of the digestive tract for 10 cm on either side of the tumor, accompanied by complete excision of the immediately adjacent tissues and the lymphatics draining the tumor. A left-sided thoracotomy is used to resect neoplasms whose proximal extent is 10 cm or more below the aortic arch. For en bloc resection of neoplasms of the middle and upper thoracic esophagus, a right lateral thoracotomy is performed through the fifth intercostal space. The radical dissection extends between 10 cm above and 10 cm below the palpable tumor. The object of an en bloc radical dissection is to remove all tissues that developmentally make up the "meso-esophagus." These include parietal pleura bilaterally, the azygos vein and thoracic duct, the posterior pericardium for tumors that lie immediately adjacent to it, and the right intercostal vessels adjacent to the tumor.[8,81]

Carcinomas of the cervical esophagus are treated with en bloc resection comprising total esophagectomy, bilateral modified radical neck dissection, and laryngectomy. These procedures are usually performed in conjunction with a head and neck surgeon. Tumor spread into the mediastinum is infrequent, although a right thoracotomy in the fourth intercostal space is sometimes necessary to perform an en bloc dissection of the esophagus to gain a satisfactory margin beyond the gross tumor. The remaining intrathoracic esophagus in most patients is removed by blunt dissection through the cervical incision using a transhiatal approach. The esophageal anastomosis is performed at the level of the mid pharynx or higher, depending on the level of transection necessary to gain a clear margin above the tumor.

THREE-FIELD NODAL DISSECTION

The appropriate extent of lymph node dissection accompanying radical esophagectomy is not agreed on. In 1981, Akiyama stressed the importance of a complete mediastinal and upper abdominal lymph node dissection in treating esophageal cancer.[6] Recent data indicate that upper mediastinal lymph nodes are involved by cancer in more than 10% of patients with lower esophageal tumors, and that 15 to 25% of patients with intrathoracic primary cancers have cervical nodal involvement. These data have prompted the use of three-field (abdominal, mediastinal, and cervical) nodal dissection in selected patients. Preliminary data suggest that long-term survival may be increased following a more extensive nodal dissection, but that the incidence of operative complications also may be increased.[105,174] No randomized, prospective studies have yet been performed that conclusively demonstrate the potential benefit of the approach.[7,9,18,29,71,129,151,162,204,218]

MINIMALLY INVASIVE ESOPHAGECTOMY

There is some preliminary experience with the use of laparoscopic gastric mobilization or thoracoscopic esophageal resection for management of esophageal cancer. Combinations of these techniques also have been used. Minimally invasive resectional procedures have been developed by some surgeons to enable a shortened hospital stay, a decreased incidence of postoperative complications and mortality, and a reduced cost of surgical management. The results to date are preliminary and do not demonstrate that minimally invasive techniques minimize complications or provide an adequate nodal and soft-tissue dissection. Additional data are necessary before these techniques will be widely adopted.[106,229]

Reconstruction

In most patients who undergo esophagectomy for malignancy, reconstruction is performed with a gastric pull-up. Other organs that can be used for reconstruction include the colon and small bowel. Although some surgeons prefer staged procedures, performing esophagectomy at one operation and reconstruction during a separate procedure, palliation is best achieved with immediate reconstruction. The advantages and disadvantages of each of the organs available for reconstruction are listed in Table 19–7.

The stomach is used most often for reconstruction, for a variety of reasons. It is partially mobilized during esophagectomy, particularly for neoplasms of the lower third of the esophagus and cardia, and further extensive dissection is usually unnecessary. When resection is performed with palliative intent, even distal tumors require only resection of the cardia and lesser curvature, preserving the fundus and thus the total length of the stomach. After dividing the short gastric vessels and left gastric artery, the stomach normally reaches to the distal pharynx after a carefully performed Kocher maneuver. The gastric blood supply is very dependable, and a single anastomosis is usually all that is required to restore continuity of the alimentary tract (Fig. 19–10). The disadvantages of using the stomach for reconstruction include its lack of peristaltic activity, the presence of a long suture line necessitated by resection of the lesser curvature, and some loss of gastric reservoir function. The stomach also retains its acid-secreting ability, which can result in severe acid reflux esophagitis and disabling aspiration. If an anastomotic leak occurs, the presence of acid-producing mucosa at the site of the leak may impair wound healing and promote fistula formation. Resection of more of the gastric body, forming a tube out of the greater curvature,

Table 19–7. Factors Affecting Choice of Organ Used for Esophageal Reconstruction

Organ	Advantages	Disadvantages
Stomach	Single anastomosis Reliable blood supply Convenient location Adequate length	Long suture lines Acid production Loss of reservoir function Aperistalsis Diameter mismatch
Left colon	No acid production Preservation of gastric reservoir Good diameter match Adequate length ? Peristalsis	Multiple anastomoses Less reliable blood supply
Jejunum	Best diameter match Peristalsis No acid production Preservation of gastric reservoir	Multiple anastomoses Least reliable blood supply Inadequate length

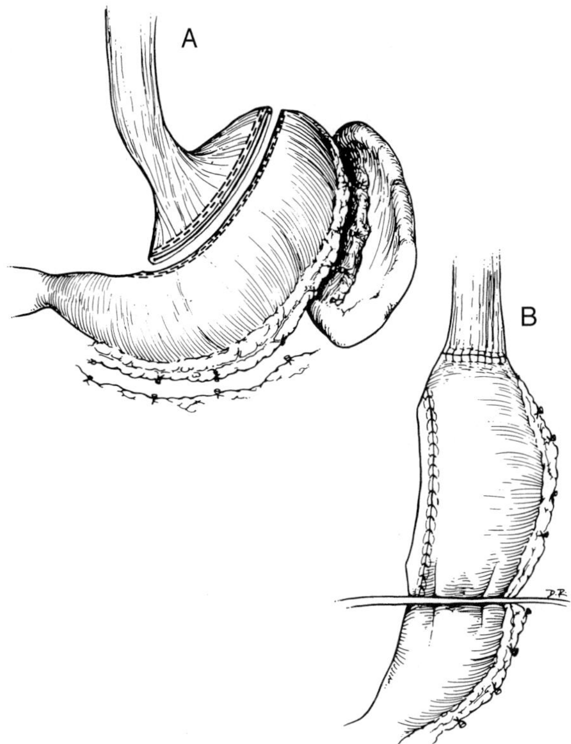

Figure 19–10. *A* and *B*, Reconstruction with a gastric pull-up following esophagectomy requires division of the short gastric vessels and left gastric artery with preservation of the right gastroepiploic arcade.

eliminates much of the acid-producing gastric mucosa and may reduce the incidence of esophagitis and aspiration but at the same time further reduces the reservoir capability of the stomach. A pyloroplasty is often performed, although emptying the intrathoracic stomach of either liquids or semisolids is often satisfactory without such a maneuver.[41,90]

Colon interposition is a useful alternative to gastric pull-up for reconstruction of the esophagus following esophagectomy, particularly after esophagogastrectomy. A variety of colon segments may be used, but an isoperistaltic segment of the left colon based on the ascending branch of the left colic artery provides the best functional results. The omentum is removed from the colon, and the marginal artery is divided distal to the ascending branch of the left colic artery. The length of colon segment necessary is measured, and the proximal portion of the marginal artery is divided at this point (Fig. 19–11). It is sometimes necessary to include a portion of the middle colic artery with the interposition segment to gain sufficient length to reach the cervical esophagus or pharynx because the vascular arcade from the marginal artery through the middle colic vessels must be preserved in this situation. A colon interposition provides advantages compared with gastric pull-up, including a better diameter match for the proximal esophageal anastomosis, preservation of the gastric reservoir function when gastrectomy is not necessary, and absence of acid production leading to improved healing of anastomotic leaks. The colon segment also displays peristalsis under some circumstances and provides excellent long-term relief of

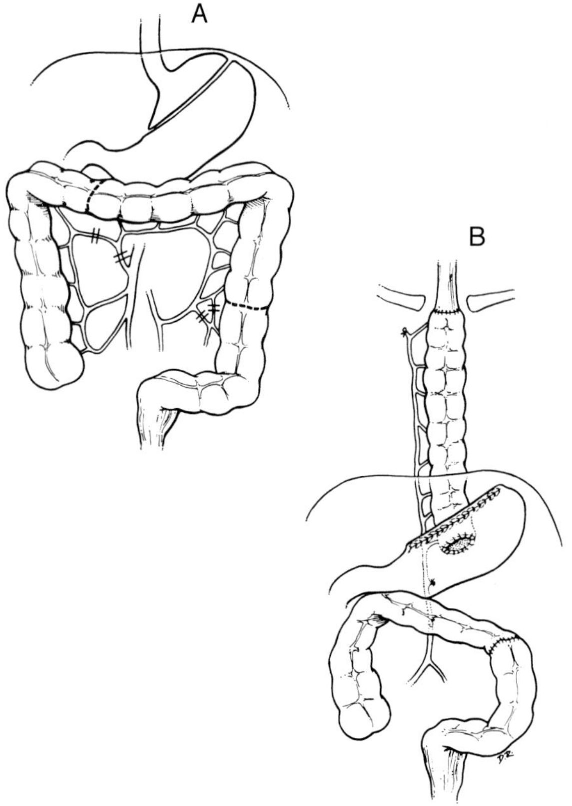

Figure 19–11. *A* and *B,* Reconstruction using a colon interposition is performed with the transverse and descending colon. The vascular supply is based on the ascending branch of the left colic artery and its confluence with the marginal artery.

dysphagia.[96,135] The isoperistaltic left colon segment provides more reliable function than right colon segments or the ileocolic segments proposed by others.[155] An antiperistaltic segment should not be used.

Jejunum is also sometimes used as an esophageal replacement. It offers advantages similar to those of the isoperistaltic left colon segment because it provides a good diameter match for the proximal esophageal anastomosis, displays peristaltic activity, does not secrete acid, and retains gastric reservoir function. However, the vascular architecture of the jejunum lacks a true marginal artery and is thus segmental. This factor severely limits the length of jejunum available for use in many cases. From a practical standpoint, jejunum is useful primarily for short segment interposition following resection of the distal esophagus and cardia (Fig. 19–12).

When esophageal resection entails leaving a segment of esophagus in the thorax, the organ used for esophageal replacement is brought through the bed of the esophagus in the posterior mediastinum. The anastomosis must be performed without tension, and this is done in a single layer using a monofilament suture, in multiple layers with an interrupted suture technique, or using stapling techniques.

When a cervical or pharyngeal anastomosis is necessary following total thoracic esophagectomy, either a posterior mediastinal or substernal route may be chosen as the passageway for the reconstructed organ. The posterior mediastinal route is shorter and should be used when there is concern about the length of organ available for reconstruction. When postoperative radiotherapy is planned, when there is gross residual tumor within the posterior mediastinum, or if there is gross contamination in the posterior mediastinum, a substernal route should be considered.

The choice between a cervical or an intrathoracic anastomosis for esophageal reconstruction is sometimes dictated by the site of disease and reconstructive options and is also influenced by the surgeon's preference. Anastomotic leaks complicating a cervical anastomosis are usually easily treated with simple drainage, whereas intrathoracic anastomoses complicated by leaks often result in severe mediastinitis or empyema that requires more aggressive intervention. The leak rates are higher for cervical anastomoses, possibly because of increased tension on the anastomosis. The likelihood of locoregional recurrence is not affected by the site of the anastomosis, assuming that surgical margins are negative. The site of the anastomosis does not appear to affect long-term survival.[121,183]

Complications

The incidence of morbidity and mortality following resection of neoplasms of the esophagus and cardia attests to

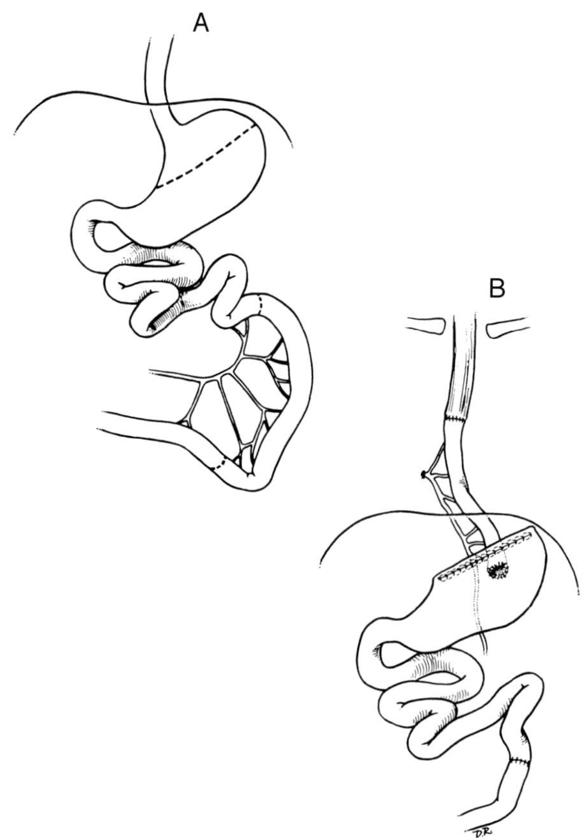

Figure 19–12. *A* and *B,* Jejunal segments, because of their regional blood supply, are useful primarily for short-segment esophageal reconstruction. As with colon interpositions, if a posterior mediastinal route is used, the jejunogastric anastomosis is best made on the posterior gastric wall.

Table 19–8. Postoperative Complications Following Esophagectomy*

Complication	Incidence (%)
Death†	5–14
Pulmonary	
Pneumonia	20
Respiratory insufficiency (ARDS‡)	14
Cardiovascular	
Myocardial infarction	2
Arrhythmia	30
Gastrointestinal	
Anastomotic leak	9
Gastric stasis or outlet obstruction	4
Infection	
Empyema	5
Subphrenic abscess	5
Other	
Vocal cord palsy	4
Chylothorax	2

*Based on data in references 63, 127, and 225.
†Hospital mortality.
‡Adult respiratory distress syndrome.

the magnitude of the operation, its technical difficulties, and the poor physiologic condition of many patients prior to operation (Table 19–8).[63,127,225] Operative mortality, defined as hospital deaths within 30 days of operation, ranges from zero to more than 20%. Because of the chronic nature of some operative complications and improvements in their management, estimates of operative mortality are more accurate 3 months postoperatively. Operative mortality is dependent on a number of factors, including tumor stage at the time of operation, the extent of resection, and the experience of the surgeon. Operative deaths are attributable to a variety of causes, but two stand out as the most common: pulmonary insufficiency due to pneumonia or the adult respiratory distress syndrome (ARDS), and anastomotic leaks.[63,127,225]

Pulmonary complications, including retained secretions, pneumonia (nosocomial or secondary to aspiration), or respiratory insufficiency due to ARDS, occur in more than 20% of patients following esophagectomy. Such complications can be minimized by keeping the patient in a semiupright position at all times to reduce the risk of aspiration. Vigorous pulmonary toilet exercises, including percussion and the use of incentive spirometers, lessen problems from retained secretions. Routine ventilatory support is not usually necessary and may contribute to the incidence of respiratory insufficiency and pneumonia.

Esophagovisceral anastomotic leaks are the bane of the thoracic surgeon. Overall mortality following an anastomotic leak ranges from less than 10 to 30% in most reports. Complications that occur following a leak from a cervical anastomosis are often managed by local drainage and do not carry an attendant high mortality. Intrathoracic anastomotic leaks, on the other hand, may result in a severe mediastinitis with or without an accompanying empyema. Negative intrathoracic pressures facilitate soilage following a mechanical anastomotic disruption, and further injury results if acid-producing mucosa is part of the anastomosis. Proper management in such cases requires adequate drainage of the affected spaces and may also necessitate removal of the reconstructive organ with proximal and distal diversion of the alimentary tract.

Results

Results of surgical therapy for carcinoma of the esophagus and cardia should be considered in terms of effective palliation of symptoms and of survival. All standard reconstructive techniques allow ingestion of a normal or slightly modified diet. The risk of occurrence of an anastomotic stricture that requires intermittent dilations is 5 to 10%. Palliation of swallowing until the time of death due to recurrent disease or 5 years from the time of resection is 80 to 90%.[96,220] More than half of patients who experience weight loss preoperatively regain the lost weight within 1 year following operation. Although less than 50% of patients are able to work at the time of diagnosis owing to poor performance status, more than 80% of survivors do sufficiently well to work between 2 and 5 years postoperatively.[212] Resection, whether palliative or potentially curative, also lessens the likelihood of chronic tumor pain, bleeding, local complications such as esophagobronchial or esophagotracheal fistula, and local recurrence.

Long-term survival depends less on tumor location than it does on disease stage. Patients with carcinomas of the cervical esophagus have a 5-year survival of 20% following resection,[38,101,148] whereas those with malignancies of the thoracic esophagus have a 5-year survival of 19%,[12,28,61,125,126,149,170,224] and those with adenocarcinomas of the distal esophagus and cardia have an overall 5-year survival following resection of 23%.[53,64,68,89,110,149,159,170,224,227]

Other Palliative Therapy

Malignant Bronchoesophageal Fistula

The development of a malignant fistula between the esophagus and the respiratory tract is a catastrophic complication of esophageal cancer. The incidence of this complication is about 5% of all patients with carcinoma of the esophagus.[30] Resection, even with palliative intent, is usually impossible because of the extent of local disease.[30] Significant palliation is possible, however, and provides relief from dysphagia and protection of the respiratory tract from continued soilage with saliva, food, and refluxed gastric material.

Most patients present with a history of coughing during eating, although some may have already developed a severe aspiration pneumonia at the time of diagnosis. The diagnosis is most easily made by barium swallow, and bronchoscopic examination often shows no conclusive evidence of a fistula even after it has been documented radiographically. The fistula involves the trachea in half of the patients, and in the majority of the remaining patients a mainstem bronchus is involved.[30,134] Most patients develop malignant respiratory fistulas during or after a course of mediastinal radiation therapy designed to treat the primary esophageal tumor. Such therapy is not a prerequisite for fistula formation because up to 40% of patients develop such fistulas without prior radiation treatment. A brief metastatic workup, including a CT scan and bone scan, reveals detectable metastases in fewer than 20% of patients with a malignant respiratory tract fistula who are in otherwise good condition.

Failure to provide palliative therapy or treatment by placement of a feeding tube results in a median survival of only 4 to 6 weeks. In patients with reasonable pulmonary reserve who have no evidence of distant metastases, aggressive management of this complication is warranted. Options include a surgical bypass procedure, esophageal exclusion, and intubation of the esophagus.

The bypass operation was described originally by Kirschner in 1920 and involved a gastric pull-up with an end-to-end cervical esophagogastrostomy in conjunction with a distal esophagojejunostomy to provide drainage for the isolated thoracic esophagus.[112] The latter anastomosis is unnecessary and is associated with many complications.[186] A preferable alternative is a red rubber catheter inserted percutaneously through the right side of the neck into the isolated thoracic esophagus for temporary decompression. As the fistula into the tracheobronchial tree enlarges, the esophagus decompresses its small volume of mucous secretions through the fistula into the airway, allowing the red rubber catheter to be removed. The bypass procedure may be performed using a gastric pull-up, as originally described, or a colon interposition.[134] Its use leads to a median survival of more than 20 weeks and good palliation of dysphagia and respiratory symptoms.

Esophageal exclusion is an alternative to the bypass operation and is particularly useful when no organ is readily available as an esophageal substitute. Isolation of the thoracic esophagus is performed similarly, using an end cervical esophagostomy and a decompressing tube. The gastroesophageal junction is divided, and a feeding tube is placed. This operation carries a moderate risk of morbidity and mortality and provides a median survival of 16 to 20 weeks without palliating dysphagia.

Esophageal intubation is also used in the management of malignant esophagorespiratory fistulas. Palliation of dysphagia is usually achieved, allowing ingestion of a semisolid diet. Most patients die of continued respiratory problems, often of reflux through the indwelling tube and pulmonary aspiration. Both pulsion and traction tubes have risks of other complications, such as erosion with bleeding or perforation.[168] Hospital mortality is 15 to 30%, similar to that for bypass operations. The use of coated, self-expanding wire mesh prostheses has become the treatment of choice for most patients with malignant esophagorespiratory fistulas. Placement is simple and is associated with a low hospital mortality rate (5–10%) and good palliation of symptoms with occlusion of the fistula noted in 80 to 90% of patients.[56,138]

Laser Therapy

Laser therapy has been used for the management of obstructing carcinomas of the esophagus and gastroesophageal junction since the early 1980s. The retrograde technique is superior to the prograde technique because the former requires one to two laser sessions to achieve palliation, whereas the latter often requires three or four sessions for the same results. The retrograde technique is performed by dilating the malignant stricture over a guidewire, followed by inserting the endoscope through the dilated tumor into normal esophagus or stomach. A flexible quartz fiber is passed through the working channel of the endoscope, and the scope is withdrawn until tumor comes within the view of the operator. The quartz fiber carries Nd:YAG laser energy at a wavelength of 1,064 nm and at energy levels of up to 120 watts; this laser energy is capable of causing tissue vaporization. Endoluminal tumor is coagulated during gradual withdrawal of the scope. Restoration of swallowing function is rapidly achieved, and frequently the procedure can be used on an outpatient basis.

Factors that increase the likelihood of successful palliation include a short length of tumor (<5 cm), location within the thoracic esophagus or cardia without significant angulation, good performance status, and a good appetite. Patients with tumors in the cervical esophagus, patients with poor performance status, or those with tumors longer than 8 cm are less likely to benefit from laser treatment.[3] When candidates are properly chosen, Nd:YAG laser therapy provides excellent palliation and may provide prolonged survival compared with other forms of palliative management of these tumors.[1,75,93,102,181,191,198,200] Nd:YAG laser palliation may be enhanced by combining laser therapy with other endoluminal modalities, such as stenting and external beam radiotherapy or brachytherapy.[45,97,208]

In addition to standard Nd:YAG laser therapy, photodynamic therapy (PDT) is available for the management of esophageal malignancies. A dihematoporphyrin derivative is injected intravenously and selectively retained in the tumor stroma. Between 48 and 72 hours after administration of the hematoporphyrin derivative, laser light at 630 nm is delivered through quartz fibers passed down the channel of a flexible esophagoscope. Energy at that wavelength activates the hematoporphyrin derivative to kill tumor cells by releasing singlet oxygen, resulting in local tissue destruction. Alternatively, aminolevulinic acid is administered systemically and is activated with a nonlaser light source with similar production of toxic oxygen metabolites.[104] Because this form of laser therapy produces tumoricidal effects by biochemical reaction rather than by heat coagulation or vaporization, it is potentially a more selective form of therapy. PDT provides excellent palliation and is associated with a low incidence of morbidity, primarily localized mediastinitis and dermal photosensitivity due to retention of the hematoporphyrin derivative in the skin.[83,133,147,152]

Intubation

Esophageal intubation for management of unresectable esophageal carcinoma was first used in the late nineteenth century and is currently a popular palliative technique. Pulsion (push-through) tubes employing a blind peroral insertion were first used successfully in the 1880s, and endoscopically guided insertion of these tubes became popular in the 1950s. Also during the fifties, traction (pull-through) tubes were first described, and came into widespread use in the 1960s. The introduction of Silastic and polyvinylchloride pulsion tubes reinforced with stainless steel wire coils enhanced the popularity of intubation during the 1970s and 1980s. The introduction of self-expanding metal stents in the 1990s revolutionized intubation for palliation of dysphagia. The stents are manufactured in a number of lengths and sizes and, in some cases, are coated with silicone or other similar material to prevent tumor ingrowth through the interstices of the stents. Use of these new stents has substantially reduced the complication rate associated with stent placement, and they are technically easier to place. Palliation of intrinsic and extrinsic obstructions is very good and is superior to that provided by laser therapy.[1,24,45,178,179,203]

Radiation Therapy

Radiation therapy has been a standard treatment modality for carcinoma of the esophagus and cardia for 50 years. Modern techniques, adopted during the 1970s, use anterior and posterior fields combined with oblique fields to limit radiation dosage to normal structures, including the heart, lungs, and spinal cord. The therapy is complex and demanding and normally requires a minimum of 6 weeks for completion. In patients whose expected median survival is only 25 to 30 weeks, this treatment represents a significant investment of time. Such treatment does offer the advantage of minimal acute mortality, but it carries the risk of long-term morbidity and failure of palliation in a significant number of patients.

Radiation therapy is used in some centers as the primary mode of therapy for esophageal cancer.[154] Prognostic factors that suggest a good response to radiation therapy include a tumor length of less than 5 cm, noncircumferential involvement of the esophageal wall, tumors in the upper thoracic esophagus, and female sex. Patients who are not operative candidates and are without metastatic disease have a relatively good prognosis and undergo curative therapy, consisting of 55 to 70 Gy delivered during 6 to 7 weeks in 200-cGy fractions. Contraindications to radiation treatment include the presence of a malignant bronchoesophageal fistula, mediastinitis owing to perforation of the tumor, and hemorrhage. Curative radiation therapy results in a median survival of 8 to 12 months, a 2-year survival in less than 20% of patients, and 5-year survival in less than 10%, except in patients with early-stage disease (Table 19-9).[14,19,49,86,88,100,205,206,215,217,232] Up to 75% of patients have at least temporary palliation of dysphagia, although only 50% of patients receiving radiation therapy alone experience long-term palliation of dysphagia.[169] More than 50% of patients develop strictures, half of which are due to local recurrence of tumor.[169] Other complications include pulmonary fibrosis, bronchoesophageal fistula, and bleeding. Palliative radiation therapy, using simple anterior and posterior treatment fields for a total of 40 to 50 Gy, is useful in most patients who are not candidates for operation or curative radiation therapy. Such patients include those with very poor performance status and those with widespread disease.

Intraluminal radiation therapy is an additional modality, particularly in patients who have already received the maximum dose of external beam radiation therapy with a poor response or local recurrence of tumor. Substances such as ^{192}Ir are afterloaded into an intraesophageal catheter periodically at weekly or biweekly intervals. This treatment delivers 90 to 100 Gy to a depth of 5 mm below the surface. A complete or partial response occurs in more than 50 to 90% of patients, and more than 90% experience significant relief of dysphagia. Nearly half develop benign or malignant strictures that require further therapy.[65,88] No reliable information is available on whether this modality prolongs survival.

Radiation therapy is used preoperatively in an effort to sterilize the tumor bed, improve resectability, decrease local recurrence, and improve survival. Five to 10% of patients undergoing preoperative radiation therapy never come to resection owing to the discovery of distant metastases during the interim period or to debilitation caused by the radiation therapy. Of patients receiving preoperative radiation therapy, 70 to 80% undergo resection, a percentage similar to that seen in patients treated by surgery alone. Surgical intervention is facilitated if it is performed between 10 and 20 days following completion of radiation therapy because the edema resulting from such therapy is reduced and radiation fibrosis has not yet occurred. Nevertheless, most surgeons agree that

Table 19–9. Results of Radiation Therapy Alone for Esophageal Cancer

Source	No. of Patients	Radiation Dose (Gy)	Median Survival (Mo)	2-Year Survival (%)	5-Year Survival (%)
John et al.[100]	35	56-61	8	13	—
Whittington et al.[232]	25	60-65	5	5	0
Araujo et al.[14]	31	50	16	22	6
Hishikawa et al.[88]	177	40-60	9	17	7
Herskovic et al.[86]	60	64	8.9	10	—
Sur et al.[215]	25	55	10	—	—
Sykes et al.[217]	101	45-52.5	15	30	21
Datta et al.[49]	108	35-50*	8	14	5
Smith et al.[206]	60	60	9	12	7
Slabber et al.[205]	36	40	5	3	3

*Some patients received intracavitary high-dose irradiation as part of their initial treatment.

Table 19–10. Results of Radiation Therapy Followed by Resection for Esophageal Cancer

Source	Radiation Dose (Gy)	Patients	Patients Operated On	Patients Undergoing Resection	Operative Mortality (%)	Median Survival (Mo)	2-Year Survival (%)	5-Year Survival (%)
Launois[123]	40	67	62	47	20	10	20	10
Sasaki[197]	40	43	43	43	—	—	45	27.3
Sasaki[196]	40	43	43	—	—	20	43	27.3
Huang[92]	40	168	168	151	3	17	—	35
Yadava[236]	30	68	68	68	15	32	—	17
Nygaard[166]	35	58	36	26	11	10	26	—

Table 19–11. Results of Surgical Resection Followed by Radiation Therapy for Esophageal Cancer

Source	Patients	Radiation Dose (Gy)	Median Survival (Mo)	2-Year Survival (%)	5-Year Survival (%)
Tanaka[221]	58	40–50	23	46	29
Iizuka[94]	103	50	21.3	52	—
Whittington[232]	19	54–63	14	34	—
FUASR[70]*	102	45–55	18	37	19
Fok[66]	30†	49	15	36	—

*French University Association for Surgical Research.
†Patients undergoing curative resection only.

Table 19–12. Response of Esophageal Cancer to Combination Chemotherapy

Source	Agents	Evaluable Patients	Complete Response* (%)	Clinical Response† (%)
Bedikian et al.[20]	5-FU, doxorubicin, VP-16, DDP	24	17	54
Iwatsuka and Yoshida[97]	DDP, methotrexate, bleomycin	14	0	50
Ajani et al.[4]	5-FU, VP-16, DDP	32	3	49
Kelsen et al.[111]	5-FU, vindesine, bleomycin	36	—	55
Schlag[199]	5-FU, DDP	27	7	38
Ajani et al.[4]	5-FU, VP-16, DDP, GM-CSF	23	0	50
Carey et al.[36]	5-FU, DDP	64	7	66
Kelsen et al.[110]	5-FU, DDP	213	3	17
Law et al.[125]	5-FU, DDP	60	7	58
Darnton et al.[48]	5-FU, DDP, mitomycin	18	0	56

*Response determined in surgical resection specimen.
†Response determined by computed tomography, barium swallow, and endoscopy.
5-FU = 5-fluorouracil, DDP = cisplatin, VP-16 = etoposide, GM-CSF = granulocyte macrophage colony-stimulating factor.

Table 19–13. Response of Esophageal Carcinoma to Combined Chemotherapy and Radiotherapy

Source	Agents	Radiation Dose (Gy)	Evaluable Patients	Complete Response* (%)
MacFarlane et al.[144]	5-FU, DDP, ± mitomycin C	30	22	36
Lackey et al.[119]	5-FU, DDP	30	28	29
Parker et al.[171]	5-FU, mitomycin C	30	41	27
Stewart et al.[210]	5-FU, DDP, mitomycin C	45	13	38
Gill et al.[78]	5-FU, DDP	36	46	24
Naunheim et al.[160]	5-FU, DDP	30–36	39	21
Forastiere et al.[68]	5-FU, DDP, vinblastine	45	41	24
Terz et al.[222]	5-FU, DDP	34	17	29
Wolfe et al.[234]	DDP and vincristine or 5-FU and DDP	45	165	21
Keller et al.[107]	5-FU, mitomycin	60	33	24
Raoul et al.[180]	5-FU, DDP	45	26	56
Walsh et al.[227]	5-FU, DDP	40	52	25
Naunheim et al.[159]	5-FU, DDP	30–36	24	17
Bosset et al.[28]	DDP	37	128	26

*Response determined in surgical resection specimen.
5-FU = 5-fluorouracil, DDP = cisplatin.

such operations are technically more difficult and time-consuming, and the differentiation between viable tumor and normal irradiated tissue is sometimes difficult to make. Although long-term local control is good, patients undergoing preoperative radiation therapy apparently have a higher incidence of nodal metastases outside the tumor bed and ultimately die of distant rather than local recurrences. Five-year survival is between 5 and 15% in most series and is not appreciably influenced by preoperative radiotherapy (Table 19-10).[15,92,123,166,196,197,213,233,236]

In patients in whom regional lymph nodes are involved with tumor or in whom there is transmural tumor invasion, local postoperative irradiation is used to decrease the likelihood of local recurrence. If resection was performed with curative intent, a total dose of 50 to 65 Gy is given over 5 to 6 weeks, whereas if resection was performed with palliative intent the total dose may be reduced to 45 to 55 Gy and given for a shorter time. Many patients are not able to complete such a course of postoperative therapy after withstanding the rigors of esophagectomy and reconstruction. The primary benefit of postoperative irradiation in resected patients is a reduction in the incidence of local recurrence. There is no survival benefit, and long-term survival remains poor (Table 19-11).[67,70,94,221,232]

Chemotherapy and Multimodality Therapy

Most patients with carcinoma of the esophagus have advanced disease, often with evidence of distant metastases, at the time of diagnosis. It is therefore reasonable to seek systemically active chemotherapeutic agents for the management of this disease. Unfortunately, results of such treatment have yielded conflicting results. Single-agent therapy using bleomycin, methotrexate, 5-fluorouracil (5-FU), doxorubicin, cisplatin, vindesin, mitomycin, and etoposide yields complete tumor response in only 5 to 15% of patients and partial response in an additional 10 to 25%, with a maximum overall response rate usually of under 40%.[108] Combination chemotherapy has been used as neoadjuvant, adjuvant, and single-modality therapy for treatment of esophageal cancer.[109] Few data exist regarding the utility of chemotherapy alone for management of potentially curable tumors. Chemotherapy as a neoadjuvant regimen results in a clinical response in 40 to 50% of patients and in a complete pathologic response in 5 to 15% of patients (Table 19-12).[4,5,20,36,48,97,110,111,125,199] In patients who experience a complete pathologic response, long-term survival is improved compared to that of patients who do not have a complete response. Preoperative chemotherapy does not appear to improve survival in resected patients compared to resection alone.[110] Similarly, postoperative adjuvant chemotherapy appears to provide no survival advantage in resected patients.[12]

Combination chemotherapy is also used preoperatively in conjunction with radiotherapy. About 25 to 30% of patients experience a complete pathologic response (Table 19-13).[28,68,78,107,119,144,159,160,171,180,210,222,227,234] It is not clear whether administration of chemoradiotherapy prior to resection improves survival compared to resection alone. Randomized studies fail to demonstrate a clear advantage to multimodality therapy.[28,227] Some authors suggest that adequate palliation can be achieved solely with combined radiotherapy and chemotherapy, particularly in patients whose disease is inoperable or unresectable or who refuse surgery. A combination of radiation therapy and chemotherapy results in palliation of dysphagia in 80% of patients, a radiographically determined complete response in 75 to 90%, and a 5-year actuarial survival of 15 to 30%.[14,43] Further investigation into multimodality therapy for esophageal cancer is ongoing.

References

1. Adam, A., Ellul, J., Watkinson, A. F., et al.: Palliation of inoperable esophageal carcinoma: A prospective randomized trial of laser therapy and stent placement. Radiology, *202:*344, 1997.
2. Aggestrup, S., Holm, J. C., and Sorensen, H. R.: Does achalasia predispose to cancer of the esophagus? Chest, *102:*1013, 1992.
3. Ahlquist, D. A., Gostout, C. J., Viggiano, T. R., et al.: Endoscopic laser palliation of malignant dysphagia: A prospective study. Mayo Clin. Proc., *62:*867, 1987.
4. Ajani, J. A., Roth, J. A., Ryan, B., et al.: Evaluation of pre- and post-operative chemotherapy for resectable adenocarcinoma of the esophagus or gastroesophageal junction. J. Clin. Oncol., *8:*1231, 1990.
5. Ajani, J. A., Roth, J. A., Ryan, M. B., et al.: Intensive preoperative chemotherapy with colony-stimulating factor for resectable adenocarcinoma of the esophagus or gastroesophageal junction. J. Clin. Oncol., *11:*22-28, 1993.
6. Akiyama, H., Tsurumaru, M., Kawamura, T., et al.: Principles of surgical treatment for carcinoma of the esophagus. Ann. Surg., *194:*438, 1981.
7. Akiyama, H., Tsurumaru, M., Udagawa, H., and Kajiyama, Y.: Radical lymph node dissection for cancer of the thoracic esophagus. Ann. Surg., *220:*364, 1994.
8. Altorki, N. K., Girardi, L., and Skinner, D. B.: En bloc esophagectomy improves survival for stage III esophageal cancer. J. Thorac. Cardiovasc. Surg., *114:*948, 1997.
9. Altorki, N. K., and Skinner, D. B.: Occult cervical nodal metastasis in esophageal cancer: Preliminary results of three-field lymphadenectomy. J. Thorac. Cardiovasc. Surg., *113:*540, 1997.
10. American Joint Committee on Cancer: Esophagus. AJCC Cancer Staging Manual, 5th ed. Philadelphia, Lippincott Williams & Wilkins, 1997, pp. 65-69.
11. Anderson, L. L., and Lad, T. E.: Autopsy findings in squamous-cell carcinoma of the esophagus. Cancer, *50:*1587, 1982.
12. Ando, N., Iizuka, T., Kakegawa, T., et al.: A randomized trial of surgery with and without chemotherapy for localized squamous carcinoma of the thoracic esophagus: The Japan Clinical Oncology Group Study. J. Thorac. Cardiovasc. Surg., *114:*205, 1997.
13. Appelquist, P., and Salmo, M.: Lye corrosion carcinoma of the esophagus. Cancer, *45:*2655, 1980.
14. Araujo, C. M. M., Souhami, L., Gil, R. A., et al.: A randomized trial comparing radiation therapy versus concomitant radiation therapy and chemotherapy in carcinoma of the thoracic esophagus. Cancer, *67:*2258, 1991.
15. Arnott, S. J., Duncan, W., Gignoux, M., et al.: Preoperative radiotherapy in esophageal carcinoma: A meta-analysis using individual patient data (Oesophageal Cancer Collaborative Group). Int. J. Radiat. Oncol. Biol. Phys., *41:*579, 1998.
16. Aste, H., Saccomanno, S., and Munizzi, F.: Blind pan-esophageal brush cytology. Endoscopy, *16:*165, 1984.
17. Attah, E. B., and Hajdu, S. I.: Benign and malignant tumors of the esophagus at autopsy. J. Thorac. Cardiovasc. Surg., *55:*396, 1968.
18. Baba, M., Aikou, T., Yoshinaka, H., et al.: Long-term results of subtotal esophagectomy with three-field lymphadenectomy for carcinoma of the thoracic esophagus. Ann. Surg., *219:*310, 1994.
19. Badwe, R. A., Sharma, V., Bhansali, M. S., et al.: The quality of swallowing for patients with operable esophageal carcinoma: A randomized trial comparing surgery with radiotherapy. Cancer, *85:*763, 1999.

20. Bedikian, A. Y., Deniord, R., and El-Akkad, S.: Value of preoperative chemotherapy in the management of locoregional esophageal carcinoma. *In* Siewert, J. R., and Hölscher, A. H. (eds.): Diseases of the Esophagus. Berlin, Springer-Verlag, 1988, p. 316.
21. Bemelman, W. A., van Delden, O. M., van Lanschot, J. J. B., et al.: Laparoscopy and laparoscopic ultrasonography in staging of carcinoma of the esophagus and gastric cardia. J. Am. Coll. Surg., *181*:421, 1995.
22. Berman, M. D., Falchuk, K. R., Trey, C., et al.: Primary histiocytic lymphoma of the esophagus. Dig. Dis. Sci., *24*:883, 1979.
23. Berry, A. V., Baskind, A. F., and Hamilton, D. G.: Cytologic screening for esophageal cancer. Acta Cytol., *25*:135, 1981.
24. Bethge, N., Sommer, A., Vakil, N.: Palliation of malignant esophageal obstruction due to intrinsic and extrinsic lesions with expandable metal stents. Am. J. Gastroenterol., *93*:1829, 1998.
25. Block, M. I., Patterson, G. A., Sundaresan, R. S., et al.: Improvement in staging of esophageal cancer with the addition of positron emission tomography. Ann. Thorac. Surg., *64*:770, 1997.
26. Blot, W. J., Devesa, S. S., Kneller, R. W., and Fraumeni, J. F., Jr.: Rising incidence of adenocarcinoma of the esophagus and gastric cardia. JAMA, *265*:1287, 1991.
27. Boring, C. C., Squires, T. S., Tong, T., and Montgomery, S.: Cancer statistics, 1994. CA Cancer J. Clin., *44*:7, 1994.
28. Bosset, J.-F., Gignoux, M., Triboulet, J.-P., et al.: Chemoradiotherapy followed by surgery compared with surgery alone in squamous-cell cancer of the esophagus. N. Engl. J. Med., *337*:161, 1997.
29. Bumm, R., and Wong, J.: More or less surgery for esophageal cancer: Extent of lymphadenectomy in esophagectomy for squamous cell esophageal carcinoma: How much is necessary? Dis. Esoph., *7*:151, 1994.
30. Burt, M., Diehl, W., Martini, N., et al.: Malignant esophagorespiratory fistula: Management options and survival. Ann. Thorac. Surg., *52*:1222, 1991.
31. Burt, M. E., Gorschboth, C. M., and Brennan, M. F. A controlled, prospective, randomized trial evaluating the metabolic effects of enteral and parenteral nutrition in the cancer patient. Cancer, *49*:1092, 1982.
32. Bytzer, P., Christensen, P. B., Damkier, P., et al.: Adenocarcinoma of the esophagus and Barrett's esophagus: A population-based study. Am. J. Gastroenterol., *94*:86, 1999.
33. Caldwell, C. B., Bains, M. S., and Burt, M.: Unusual malignant neoplasms of the esophagus. J. Thorac. Cardiovasc. Surg., *101*:100, 1991.
34. Cameron, A. J.: Epidemiology of columnar-lined esophagus and adenocarcinoma. Gastroenterol. Clin. N. Am., *26*:487, 1997.
35. Cameron, A. J., Ott, B. J., and Payne, W. S.: The incidence of adenocarcinoma in columnar-lined (Barrett's) esophagus. N. Engl. J. Med., *313*:857, 1985.
36. Carey, R. W., Hilgenberg, A. D., Wilkins, E. W., Jr., et al.: Long-term follow-up of neoadjuvant chemotherapy with 5-fluorouracil and cisplatin with surgical resection and possible postoperative radiotherapy and/or chemotherapy in squamous cell carcinoma of the esophagus. Cancer Invest., *11*:99, 1993.
37. Catalano, M. F., Van Dam, J., and Sivak, M. V. Jr.: Malignant esophageal strictures: Staging accuracy of endoscopic ultrasonography. Gastrointest. Endosc., *41*:535, 1995.
38. Chakkaphak, S., Krishnasamy, S., Walker, S. J., et al.: Treatment of carcinoma of the proximal esophagus. Surg. Gynecol. Obstet., *168*:307, 1989.
39. Chan, K.-H., and Wong, J.: Mortality after esophagectomy for carcinoma of esophagus: An analysis of risk factors. Dis. Esoph., *3*:49, 1990.
40. Chandawarkar, R. Y., Kakegawa, T., Fujita, H., et al.: Endosonography for preoperative staging of specific nodal groups associated with esophageal cancer. World J. Surg., *20*:700, 1996.
41. Cheung, H. C., Siu, K. F., and Wong, J.: Is pyloroplasty necessary in esophageal replacement by stomach? A prospective, randomized controlled trial. Surgery, *102*:19, 1987.
42. Choi, T. K., Siu, K. F., Lam, K. H., et al.: Bronchoscopy and carcinoma of the esophagus II. Am. J. Surg., *147*:760, 1984.
43. Coia, L. R., Paul, A. R., and Engstrom, P. F.: Combined radiation and chemotherapy as primary management of adenocarcinoma of the esophagus and gastroesophageal junction. Cancer, *61*:643, 1988.
44. Coordinating Group for Research on Esophageal Cancer: Early diagnosis and surgical treatment of esophageal cancer under rural conditions. Chin. Med. J., *2*:113, 1976.
45. Cottier, D. J., Carter, C. R., Smith, J. S., and Anderson, J. R.: The combination of laser recanalization and endoluminal intubation in the palliation of malignant dysphagia. J. R. Coll. Surg. Edinb., *42*:19, 1997.
46. Crespi, M., Grassi, A., Munoz, N., et al.: Endoscopic features of suspected precancerous lesions in high risk areas for esophageal cancer. Endoscopy, *16*:85, 1984.
47. Daly, J. M., Massar, E., Giacco, G., et al.: Parenteral nutrition in esophageal cancer patients. Ann. Surg., *196*:203, 1982.
48. Darnton, S. J., Ferry, D. R., Cullen, M. H., and Casson, A. G.: A phase II trial of preoperative mitomycin, cisplatin and 5-fluorouracil in adenocarcinoma of the oesophagus. Clin. Oncol., *10*:372, 1998.
49. Datta, N. R., Kumar, S., Nangia, S., et al.: A non-randomized comparison of two radiotherapy protocols in inoperable squamous cell carcinoma of the oesophagus. Clin. Oncol., *10*:306, 1998.
50. DeMeester, T. R., and Skinner, D. B.: Polypoid sarcomas of the esophagus. Ann. Thorac. Surg., *20*:405, 1975.
51. Dickman, S.: First p53 relative may be a new tumor suppressor. Science, *277*:1605, 1997.
52. Dowlatshahi, K., Lester, E., Bibbo, M., et al.: Brush cytology for the early detection of esophageal carcinoma among patients with upper aerodigestive malignancies. Laryngoscope *95*:971, 1985.
53. Dowlatshahi, K., Skinner, D. B., DeMeester, T. R., et al.: Evaluation of brush cytology as an independent technique for detection of esophageal carcinoma. J. Thorac. Cardiovasc. Surg., *89*:848, 1985.
54. Drewitz, D. J., Sampliner, R. E., and Garewal, H. S.: The incidence of adenocarcinoma in Barrett's esophagus: A prospective study of 170 patients followed 4.8 years. Am. J. Gastroenterol., *92*:212, 1997.
55. Duhaylongsod, F. G., Gottfried, M. R., Iglehart, J. D., et al.: The significance of c-*erb* B-2 and p53 immunoreactivity in patients with adenocarcinoma of the esophagus. Ann. Surg., *221*:677, 1995.
56. Dumonceau, J.-M., Cremer, M., Lalmand, B., and Deviere, J.: Esophageal fistula sealing: Choice of stent, practical management, and cost. Gastrointest. Endosc., *49*:70, 1999.
57. Ellis, F. H., Jr., Gibb, S. P., and Watkins, E., Jr.: Limited esophagogastrectomy for carcinoma of the cardia. Ann. Surg., *208*:354, 1988.
58. Elman, A., Guili, R., and Sancho-Garnier, H.: Risk factors of pulmonary complications following esophagectomy in carcinoma of the esophagus: Results of the prospective study conducted by the OESO group. *In* Siewert, J. R., and Hölscher, A. H. (eds.): Diseases of the Esophagus. Berlin, Springer-Verlag, 1988, p. 224.
59. Endo, M., Yoshino, K., Takeshita, K., and Kawano, T.: Analysis of 1,125 cases of early esophageal carcinoma in Japan. Dis. Esoph., *4*:71, 1991.
60. Fekete, F., Belghiti, J., Cherqui, D., et al.: Results of esophagogastrectomy for carcinoma in cirrhotic patients. Ann. Surg., *206*:74, 1987.
61. Fekete, F., Gayet, B., and Panis, Y.: Long-term results of transthoracic esophagectomy for squamous cell carcinoma. Dis. Esoph., *5*:105, 1992.
62. Ferguson, M. K., Little, A. G., Ryan, J. W., et al.: The value of scintigraphy in staging esophageal carcinoma. *In* Siewart, J. R., and Hölscher, A. H. (eds.): Diseases of the Esophagus. Berlin, Springer-Verlag, 1988, p. 143.
63. Ferguson, M. K., Martin, T. R., Reeder, L. B., and Olak, J.: Mortality after esophagectomy: Risk factor analysis. World J. Surg., *21*:599, 1997.
64. Ferguson, M. K., Reeder, L. B., Hoffman, P. C., et al.: Intensive multimodality therapy for carcinoma of the esophagus and gastroesophageal junction. Ann. Surg. Oncol., *2*:101, 1995.
65. Flores, A. D., Stoller, J. L., Nelems, B., et al.: Combined primary treatment of cancer of the esophagus and cardia by intracavitary and external irradiation. *In* Siewert, J. R., and Hölscher, A. H. (eds.): Diseases of the Esophagus. Berlin, Springer-Verlag, 1988, p. 745.
66. Fok, M., Cheng, S. W. K., and Wong, J.: Endosonography in patient selection for surgical treatment of esophageal carcinoma. World J. Surg., *16*:1098, 1992.
67. Fok, M., Sham, J. S. T., Choy, D., et al.: Postoperative radiotherapy

for carcinoma of the esophagus: A prospective, randomized controlled study. Surgery, *113:*138, 1993.
68. Forastiere, A. A., Orringer, M. B., Perez-Tamayo, C., et al.: Preoperative chemoradiation followed by transhiatal esophagectomy for carcinoma of the esophagus: Final report. J. Clin. Oncol., *11:*1118, 1993.
69. Freeny, P. C., and Marks, M. W.: Adenocarcinoma of the gastroesophageal junction: Barium and CT examination. AJR, *138:*1077, 1982.
70. French University Association for Surgical Research, Teniere, P., Hay, J.-M., et al.: Postoperative radiation therapy does not increase survival after curative resection for squamous cell carcinoma of the middle and lower esophagus as shown by a multicenter controlled trial. Surg. Gynecol. Obstet., *173:*123, 1991.
71. Fujita, H., Kakegawa, T., Yamana, H., et al.: Mortality and morbidity rates, postoperative course, quality of life, and prognosis after extended radical lymphadenectomy for esophageal cancer. Ann. Surg., *222:*654, 1995.
72. Gal, A., Martin, S. E., Kernen, J. A., et al.: Esophageal carcinoma with prominent spindle cells. Cancer, *60:*2244, 1987.
73. Genereux, G. P., and Howie, J. L.: Normal mediastinal lymph node size and number: CT and anatomic study. AJR, *142:*1095, 1984.
74. Gerami, S., Booth, A., and Pate, J. W.: Carcinoma of the esophagus engrafted on lye stricture. Chest, *59:*226, 1971.
75. Gevers, A. M., Macken, E., Hiele, M., and Rutgeerts, P.: A comparison of laser therapy, plastic stents, and expandable metal stents for palliation of malignant dysphagia in patients without a fistula. Gastrointest. Endosc., *48:*383, 1998.
76. Ghadirian, P.: Thermal irritation and esophageal cancer in northern Iran. Cancer, *60:*1909, 1987.
77. Giacobbe, A., Facciorusso, D., Conoscitore, P., et al.: Granular cell tumor of the esophagus. Am. J. Gastroenterol., *83:*1398, 1988.
78. Gill, P. G., Denham, J. W., Jamieson, G. G., et al.: Patterns of treatment failure and prognostic factors associated with the treatment of esophageal carcinoma with chemotherapy and radiotherapy either as sole treatment or followed by surgery. J. Clin. Oncol., *10:*1037, 1992.
79. Giuli, R., and Sancho-Garnier, H.: Diagnostic, therapeutic, and prognostic features of cancers of the esophagus: Results of the international prospective study conducted by the OESO group. Surgery, *99:*614, 1986.
80. Greenebaum, E., Schreiber, K., Shu, Y., et al.: Use of the esophageal balloon in the diagnosis of carcinomas of the head, neck and upper gastrointestinal tract. Acta Cytol., *28:*9, 1984.
81. Hagen, J. A., Peters, J. H., and DeMeester, T. R.: Superiority of extended en bloc esophagogastrectomy for carcinoma of the lower esophagus and cardia. J. Thorac. Cardiovasc. Surg., *106:*850, 1993.
82. Harper, P. S., Harper, R. M. J., and Howel-Evans, A. W.: Carcinoma of the esophagus with tylosis. Q. J. Med., *39:*317, 1970.
83. Heier, S. K., Rothman, K. A., Heier, L. M., and Rosenthal, W. S.: Photodynamic therapy for obstructing esophageal cancer: Light dosimetry and randomized comparison with Nd:YAG laser therapy. Gastroenterology, *109:*63, 1995.
84. Heitmiller, R. F., and Sharma, R. R.: Comparison of prevalence and resection rates in patients with esophageal squamous cell carcinoma and adenocarcinoma. J. Thorac. Cardiovasc. Surg., *112:*130, 1996.
85. Hennessy, T. P. J., and Keeling, P.: Adenocarcinoma of the esophagus and cardia. J. Thorac. Cardiovasc. Surg., *94:*64, 1987.
86. Herskovic, A., Martz, K., Al-Sarraf, M., et al.: Combined chemotherapy and radiotherapy compared with radiotherapy alone in patients with cancer of the esophagus. N. Engl. J. Med., *326:*1593, 1992.
87. Hesketh, P. J., Clapp, R. W., Doos, W. G., and Spechler, S. J.: The increasing frequency of adenocarcinoma of the esophagus. Cancer, *64:*526, 1989.
88. Hishikawa, Y., Kurisu, K., Taniguchi, M.: Radiotherapy for carcinoma of the esophagus in patients aged eighty or older. Int. J. Radiat. Oncol., *20:*685, 1991.
89. Holscher, A. H., Schuler, M., and Siewert, J. R.: Surgical treatment of adenocarcinomas of the gastroesophageal junction. Dis. Esoph., *1:*35, 1988.
90. Hölscher, A. H., Voit, H., Siewert, J. R., et al.: Function of the intrathoracic stomach. *In* Siewert, J. R., and Hölscher, A. H. (eds.): Diseases of the Esophagus. Berlin, Springer-Verlag, 1988, p. 660.
91. Hopkins, R. A., and Postlethwait, R. W.: Caustic burns and carcinoma of the esophagus. Ann. Surg., *194:*146, 1981.
92. Huang, G. J., Gu, X. Z., Wang, L. J., et al.: Combined preoperative irradiation and surgery versus surgery alone for squamous cell carcinoma of the midthoracic esophagus: A prospective randomized study in 360 patients. *In* Ferguson, M. K., Little, A. G., and Skinner, D. B. (eds.): Diseases of the Esophagus, Vol. I: Malignant Diseases. Mount Kisco, NY, Futura Publishing, 1990, p. 275.
93. Hurley, J. F., and Cade, R. J.: Laser photocoagulation in the treatment of malignant dysphagia. Aust. N. Z. J. Surg., *67:*800, 1997.
94. Iizuka, T., Ide, H., Kakegawa, T., et al.: Preoperative radioactive therapy for esophageal carcinoma. Chest *93:*1054, 1988.
95. Inculet, R. I., Keller, S. M., Dwyer, A., et al.: Evaluation of noninvasive tests for preoperative staging of carcinoma of the esophagus: A prospective study. Ann. Thorac. Surg., *40:*561, 1985.
96. Isolauri, J., Markkula, H., and Autio, V.: Colon interposition in the treatment of carcinoma of the esophagus and gastric cardia. Ann. Thorac. Surg., *43:*420, 1987.
97. Iwatsuka, M., and Yoshida, M.: A study of the clinicopathological effects of chemotherapy for human esophageal carcinoma. *In* Siewert, J. R., and Hölscher, A. H. (eds.): Diseases of the Esophagus. Berlin, Springer-Verlag, 1988, p. 319.
98. Japanese Committee for Registration of Esophageal Carcinoma: A proposal for a new TNM classification of esophageal carcinoma. Jpn. J. Clin. Oncol., *14:*625, 1985.
99. Jaskiewicz, K., Marasas, W. F. O., Rossouw, J. E., et al.: Selenium and other mineral elements in populations at risk for esophageal cancer. Cancer, *62:*2635, 1988.
100. John, M. J., Flam, M. S., Mowry, P. A., et al.: Radiotherapy alone and chemoradiation for nonmetastatic esophageal carcinoma. Cancer, *63:*2397, 1989.
101. Kakegawa, T., Yamana, H., and Ando, N.: Analysis of surgical treatment of carcinoma situated in the cervical esophagus. Surgery, *97:*150, 1985.
102. Karlin, D. A., Fisher, R. S., and Krevsky, B.: Prolonged survival and effective palliation in patients with squamous cell carcinoma of the esophagus following endoscopic laser therapy. Cancer, *59:*1969, 1987.
103. Kasbarian, M., Fuentes, P., Brichon, P. Y., et al.: Usefulness of computed tomography in assessing the extension of carcinoma of the esophagus and gastroesophageal junction. *In* Siewert, J. R., and Hölscher, A. H. (eds.): Diseases of the Esophagus. Berlin, Springer-Verlag, 1988, p. 185.
104. Kashtan, H., Konikoff, F., Haddad, R., and Skornick, Y.: Photodynamic therapy of cancer of the esophagus using systemic aminolevulinic acid and a nonlaser light source: A phase I/II study. Gastrointest. Endosc., *49:*760, 1999.
105. Kato, H., Watanabe, H., Tachimori, Y., and Iizuka, T.: Evaluation of neck lymph node dissection for thoracic esophageal carcinoma. Ann. Thorac. Surg., *51:*931, 1991.
106. Kawahara, K., Maekawa, T., Okabayashi, K., et al.: Video-assisted thoracoscopic esophagectomy for esophageal cancer. Surg. Endosc., *13:*218, 1999.
107. Keller, S. M., Ryan, L. M., Coia, L. R., et al.: High dose chemoradiotherapy followed by esophagectomy for adenocarcinoma of the esophagus and gastroesophageal junction: Results of a phase II study of the Eastern Cooperative Oncology Group. Cancer, *83:*1908, 1998.
108. Kelsen, D. P.: Chemotherapy of esophageal cancer. Semin. Oncol., *11:*159, 1984.
109. Kelsen, D., Hilaris, B., Coonley, C., et al.: Cisplatin, vindesine, and bleomycin chemotherapy of local regional and advanced esophageal carcinoma. Am. J. Med., *75:*645, 1983.
110. Kelsen, D. P., Ginsberg, R., Pajak, T. F., et al.: Chemotherapy followed by surgery compared with surgery alone for localized esophageal cancer. N. Engl. J. Med., *339:*1979, 1998.
111. Kelsen, D. P., Minsky, B., Smith, M., et al.: Preoperative therapy for esophageal cancer: A randomized comparison of chemotherapy versus radiation therapy. J. Clin. Oncol., *8:*1352, 1990.
112. Kirschner, M. B.: Ein neues Verfahren der Oesophagoplastik. Arch. Klin. Chir., *114:*604, 1920.
113. Konder, H., Poenitz-Pohl, E., Stahlknecht, C. D., et al.: Analysis of cardiopulmonary function in esophageal cancer patients prior to surgery. *In* Siewert, J. R., and Hölscher, A. H. (eds.): Diseases of the Esophagus. Berlin, Springer-Verlag, 1988, p. 249.

114. Krasna, M. J., Flowers, J. L., Attar, S., and McLaughlin, J.: Combined thoracoscopic/laparoscopic staging of esophageal cancer. J. Thorac. Cardiovasc. Surg., *111:*800, 1996.
115. Krasna, M. J., Reed, C. E., Jaklitsch, M. T., et al.: Thoracoscopic staging of esophageal cancer: A prospective, multiinstitutional trial. Ann. Thorac. Surg., *60:*1337, 1995.
116. Kuwano, H., Ohno, S., Matsuda, H., et al.: Serial histologic evaluation of multiple primary squamous cell carcinomas of the esophagus. Cancer, *61:*1635, 1988.
117. Kuwano, H., Matsuda, H., Matsuoka, H., et al.: Intra-epithelial carcinoma concomitant with esophageal squamous cell carcinoma. Cancer, *59:*783, 1987.
118. Laas, J., Scheller, E., Haverich, A., et al.: How accurate is the preoperative staging with computed tomography in esophageal cancer. *In* Siewert, J. R., and Hölscher, A. H. (eds.): Diseases of the Esophagus. Berlin, Springer-Verlag, 1988, p. 177.
119. Lackey, V. L., Reagan, M. T., Smith, R. A., and Anderson, W. J.: Neoadjuvant therapy of squamous cell carcinoma of the esophagus: Role of resection and benefit in partial responders. Ann. Thorac. Surg., *48:*218, 1989.
120. Lagergren, J., Bergstrom, R., Lindgren, A., and Nyren, O.: Symptomatic gastroesophageal reflux as a risk factor for esophageal adenocarcinoma. N. Engl. J. Med., *340:*825, 1999.
121. Lam, T. C. F., Fok, M., Cheng, S. W. K., and Wong, J.: Anastomotic complications after esophagectomy for cancer. J. Thorac. Cardiovasc. Surg., *104:*395, 1992.
122. Landis, S. H., Murray, T., Bolden, S., and Wingo, P. A.: Cancer Statistics, 1998. CA Cancer J. Clin., *48:*6, 1998.
123. Launois, B., Ben-Hassel, M., Delarue, D., et al.: Perioperative treatment of esophageal cancer. *In* Siewert, J. R., and Hölscher, A. H. (eds.): Diseases of the Esophagus. Berlin, Springer-Verlag, 1988, p. 308.
124. Launois, B., Paul, J. L., Lygidakis, N. J., et al.: Results of the surgical treatment of carcinoma of the esophagus. Surg. Gynecol. Obstet. *156:*753, 1983.
125. Law, S., Fok, M., Chow, S., et al.: Preoperative chemotherapy versus surgical therapy alone for squamous cell carcinoma of the esophagus: A prospective randomized trial. J. Thorac. Cardiovasc. Surg., *114:*210, 1997.
126. Law, S. Y. K., Fok, M., Cheng, S. W. K., and Wong, J.: A comparison of outcome after resection for squamous cell carcinomas and adenocarcinomas of the esophagus and cardia. Surg. Gynecol. Obstet., *175:*107, 1992.
127. Law, S. Y. K., Fok, M., and Wong, J.: Risk analysis in resection of squamous cell carcinoma of the esophagus. World J. Surg., *18:*339, 1994.
128. Lehr, L., Rupp, N., and Siewert, J. R.: Assessment of resectability of esophageal cancer by computed tomography and magnetic resonance imaging. Surgery, *103:*344, 1988.
129. Lerut, T., De Leyn, P., Coosemans, W., et al.: Surgical strategies in esophageal carcinoma with emphasis on radical lymphadenectomy. Ann. Surg., *216:*583, 1992.
130. Lewis, I.: The surgical treatment of carcinoma of the esophagus with special reference to a new operation for growths of the middle third. Br. J. Surg., *34:*18, 1946.
131. Li, F. P., and Shiang, E. L.: Screening for oesophageal cancer in 62,000 Chinese. Lancet, *2:*804, 1979.
132. Li, M. X., and Cheng, S. J.: Etiology of carcinoma of the esophagus. *In* Huang, G. J., and K'ai, W. Y. (eds.): Carcinoma of the Esophagus and Gastric Cardia. New York, Springer-Verlag, 1984, p. 25.
133. Lightdale, C. J., Heier, S. K., Marcon, N. E., et al.: Photodynamic therapy with porfimer sodium versus thermal ablation therapy with Nd:YAG laser for palliation of esophageal cancer: A multicenter randomized trial. Gastrointest. Endosc., *42:*507, 1995.
134. Little, A. G., Ferguson, M. K., DeMeeseter, T. R., et al.: Esophageal carcinoma with respiratory tract fistula. Cancer, *53:*1322, 1984.
135. Little, A. G., Scott, W. J., Ferguson, M. K., et al.: Functional evaluation of organ interposition for esophageal replacement. *In* Siewert, J. R., and Hölscher, A. H. (eds.): Diseases of the Esophagus. Berlin, Springer-Verlag, 1988, p. 664.
136. Liu, B. O., and Li, B.: Epidemiology of carcinoma of the esophagus in China. *In* Huang, G. J., and K'ai, W. Y. (eds.): Carcinoma of the Esophagus and Gastric Cardia. New York, Springer-Verlag, 1984, p. 1.
137. Logan, A.: The surgical treatment of carcinoma of the esophagus and cardia. J. Thorac. Cardiovasc. Surg., *46:*150, 1963.
138. Low, D. E., and Kozarek, R. A.: Comparison of conventional and wire mesh expandable prostheses and surgical bypass in patients with malignant esophagorespiratory fistulas. Ann. Thorac. Surg., *65:*919, 1998.
139. Lowe, W. C.: Survival with carcinoma of the esophagus. Ann. Intern. Med., *77:*915, 1972.
140. Lowenfels, A. B.: Alcohol and cancer. N. Y. State J. Med., *74:*56, 1974.
141. Lu, Y. K., Li, Y. M., and Gu, Y. Z.: Cancer of esophagus and esophagogastric junction: Analysis of results of 1,025 resections after 5 to 20 years. Ann. Thorac. Surg., *43:*176, 1987.
142. Luketich, J. D., Schauer, P., Landreneau, R., et al.: Minimally invasive surgical staging is superior to endoscopic ultrasound in detecting lymph node metastases in esophageal cancer. J. Thorac. Cardiovasc. Surg., *114:*817, 1997.
143. Luketich, J. D., Schauer, P. R., Meltzer, C. C., et al.: Role of positron emission tomography in staging esophageal cancer. Ann. Thorac. Surg., *64:*765, 1997.
144. MacFarlane, S. D., Hill, L. D., Jolly, P. C., et al.: Improved results of surgical treatment for esophageal and gastroesophageal junction carcinomas after preoperative combined chemotherapy and radiation. J. Thorac. Cardiovasc. Surg., *95:*415, 1988.
145. Maerz, L. L., Deveney, C. W., Lopez, R. R., and McConnell, D. B.: Role of computed tomographic scans in the staging of esophageal and proximal gastric malignancies. Am. J. Surg., *165:*558, 1993.
146. Mahoney, J. L., and Condon, R. E.: Adenocarcinoma of the esophagus. Ann. Surg., *205:*557, 1987.
147. Marcon, N. E.: Photodynamic therapy and cancer of the esophagus. Semin. Oncol., *21:*20, 1994.
148. Marmuse, J.-P., Koka, V. N., Guedon, C., and Benhamou, G.: Surgical treatment of carcinoma of the proximal esophagus. Am. J. Surg., *169:*386, 1995.
149. Mathisen, D. J., Grillo, H. C., Wilkins, E. W., Jr., et al.: Transthoracic esophagectomy: A safe approach to carcinoma of the esophagus. Ann. Thorac. Surg., *45:*137, 1988.
150. Matsusaka, T., Watanabe, H., and Enjoji, M.: Pseudosarcoma and carcinosarcoma of the esophagus. Cancer, *37:*1546, 1976.
151. Matsubara, T., Ueda, M., Yanagida, O., et al.: How extensive should lymph node dissection be for cancer of the thoracic esophagus? J. Thorac. Cardiovasc. Surg., *107:*1073, 1994.
152. McCaughan, J. S. Jr., Ellison, E. C., Guy, J. T., et al.: Photodynamic therapy for esophageal malignancy: A prospective twelve-year study. Ann. Thorac. Surg., *62:*1005, 1996.
153. Meijssen, M. A. C., Tilanus, H. W., van Blankenstein, M., et al.: Achalasia complicated by oesophageal squamous cell carcinoma: A prospective study in 195 patients. Gut, *33:*155, 1992.
154. Mendenhall, W. M., Parsons, J. T., Cassisi, N. J., et al.: Carcinoma of the cervical esophagus treated with radiation therapy. Laryngoscope, *98:*769, 1988.
155. Moreno Gonzalez, E., Calleja Kempin, I. J., Landa Garcia, J. I., et al.: Functional study of ileocolic interposition after esophagectomy and total esophagogastrectomy. *In* Siewert, J. R., and Hölscher, A. H. (eds.): Diseases of the Esophagus. Berlin, Springer-Verlag, 1988, p. 668.
156. Mori, M., Matsukuma, A., Adachi, Y., et al.: Small cell carcinoma of the esophagus. Cancer, *63:*564, 1989.
157. Murata, Y., Muroi, M., Yoshida, M., et al.: Endoscopic ultrasonography in the diagnosis of esophageal carcinoma. Surg. Endosc., *1:*11, 1987.
158. Murray, G. F., Wilcox, B. R., and Starek, P. J. K.: The assessment of operability of esophageal carcinoma. Ann. Thorac. Surg., *23:*393, 1977.
159. Naunheim, K. S., Petruska, P. J., Roy, T. S., et al.: Multimodality therapy for adenocarcinoma of the esophagus. Ann. Thorac. Surg., *59:*1085, 1995.
160. Naunheim, K. S., Petruska, P. J., Roy, T. S., et al.: Preoperative chemotherapy and radiotherapy for esophageal carcinoma. J. Thorac. Cardiovasc. Surg., *103:*887, 1992.
161. Nichols, G. L., and Kelsen, D. P.: Small cell carcinoma of the esophagus. Cancer, *64:*1531, 1989.
162. Nigro, J. J., Hagen, J. A., DeMeester, T. R., et al.: Prevalence and location of nodal metastases in distal esophageal adenocarcinoma confined to the wall: Implications for therapy. J. Thorac. Cardiovasc. Surg., *117:*16, 1999.
163. Nishi, M., Hiramatsu, Y., Hatano, T., et al.: Effect of nutritional

support as an adjunct to the treatment of esophageal cancer. *In* Siewert, J. R., and Hölscher, A. H. (eds.): Diseases of the Esophagus. Berlin, Springer-Verlag, 1988, p. 287.
164. Nishi, M., Hiramatsu, Y., Hioki, K., et al.: Risk factors in relation to postoperative complications in patients undergoing esophagectomy or gastrectomy for cancer. Ann. Surg., *207:*148, 1988.
165. Nishimaki, T., Suzuki, T., Suzuki, S., et al.: Outcomes of extended radical esophagectomy for thoracic esophageal cancer. J. Am. Coll. Surg., *186:*306, 1998.
166. Nygaard, K., Hagen, S., Hansen, H. S., et al.: Pre-operative radiotherapy prolongs survival in operable esophageal carcinoma: A randomized, multicenter study of pre-operative radiotherapy and chemotherapy. World J. Surg., *16:*1104, 1992.
167. O'Brien, M. G., Fitzgerald, E. F., Lee, G., et al.: A prospective comparison of laparoscopy and imaging in the staging of esophagogastric cancer before surgery. Am. J. Gastroenterol., *90:*2191, 1995.
168. Orel, J., Vidmar, S., and Hrabar, B.: Traction intubation of the esophagus for nonresectable carcinoma and malignant esophagobronchial fistula. Dis. Esoph., *3:*45, 1990.
169. O'Rourke, I. C., Tiver, K., Bull, C., et al.: Swallowing performance after radiation therapy for carcinoma of the esophagus. Cancer, *61:*2022, 1988.
170. Orringer, M. B., Marshall, B., and Stirling, M. C.: Transhiatal esophagectomy for benign and malignant disease. J. Thorac. Cardiovasc. Surg., *105:*265, 1993.
171. Parker, E. F., Reed, C. E., Marks, R. D., et al.: Chemotherapy, radiation therapy, and resection for carcinoma of the esophagus. J. Thorac. Cardiovasc. Surg., *98:*1037, 1989.
172. Patel, R., Bhogal, R., Kaymakcalan, H., et al.: Diagnosis of esophageal neoplasm by endoscopy and biopsy. Gastrointest. Endosc., *29:*159, 1983.
173. Pera, M., Cameron, A. J., Trastek, V. F., et al.: Increasing incidence of adenocarcinoma of the esophagus and esophagogastric junction. Gastroenterology, *104:*510, 1993.
174. Peracchia, A., Ruol, A., Bardini, R., et al.: Lymph node dissection for cancer of the thoracoesophagus: How extended should it be? Dis. Esoph., *5:*69, 1992.
175. Peracchia, A., Segalin, A., Bardini, R., et al.: Esophageal carcinoma and achalasia: Prevalence, incidence and results of treatment. Hepatogastroenterology, *38:*514, 1991.
176. Peters, J. H., Hoeft, S. F., Heimbucher, J., et al.: Selection of patients for curative or palliative resection of esophageal cancer based on preoperative endoscopic ultrasonography. Arch. Surg., *129:*534, 1994.
177. Poon, R. T. P., Law, S. Y. K., Chu, K. M., et al.: Esophagectomy for carcinoma of the esophagus in the elderly. Ann. Surg., *227:*357, 1998.
178. Raijman, I., Siddique, I., Ajani, J., and Lynch, P.: Palliation of malignant dysphagia and fistulae with coated expandable metal stents: Experience with 101 patients. Gastrointest. Endosc., *48:*172, 1998.
179. Ramirez, F. C., Dennert, B., Zierer, S. T., and Sanowski, R. A.: Esophageal self-expandable metallic stents—indications, practice, techniques, and complications: Results of a national survey. Gastrointest. Endosc., *45:*360, 1997.
180. Raoul, J. L., Le Prise, E., Meunier, B., et al.: Neoadjuvant chemotherapy and hyperfractionated radiotherapy with concurrent low-dose chemotherapy for squamous cell esophageal carcinoma. Int. J. Radiat. Oncol. Biol. Phys., *42:*29, 1998.
181. Reed, C. E., Marsh, W. H., Carlson, L. S., et al.: Prospective, randomized trial of palliative treatment for unresectable cancer of the esophagus. Ann. Thorac. Surg., *51:*552, 1991.
182. Reinig, J. W., Stanley, J. H., and Schabel, S. I.: CT evaluation of thickened esophageal walls. AJR, *140:*931, 1983.
183. Ribet, M., Debrueres, B., and Lecomte-Houcke, M.: Resection for advanced cancer of the thoracic esophagus: Cervical or thoracic anastomosis? J. Thorac. Cardiovasc. Surg., *103:*784, 1992.
184. Riedel, M., Hauck, R. W., Stein, H. J., et al.: Preoperative bronchoscopic assessment of airway invasion by esophageal cancer. Chest, *113:*687, 1998.
185. Ritter, S. B., and Petersen, G.: Esophageal cancer, hyperkeratosis, and oral leukoplakia: Follow-up family study. JAMA, *236:*1844, 1976.
186. Roeher, H. D., and Horeyseck, G.: The Kirschner bypass operation—a palliation for complicated esophageal carcinoma. World J. Surg., *5:*543, 1981.
187. Rosch, T., Lorenz, R., Zenker, K., et al.: Local staging and assessment of resectability in carcinoma of the esophagus, stomach, and duodenum by endoscopic ultrasonography. Gastrointest. Endosc., *38:*460, 1992.
188. Rosch, W., and Elster, K.: Gastrointestinal Prakanzerosen. New York, Witzstrock, 1977.
189. Ruol, A., Rossi, M., Ruffatto, A., et al.: Reevaluation of computed tomography in preoperative staging of esophageal and cardial cancers. *In* Siewert, J. R., and Hölscher, A. H. (eds.): Diseases of the Esophagus. Berlin, Springer-Verlag, 1988, p. 194.
190. Ruol, A., Stephens, J. K., Maiorana, A., et al.: Expression of ras oncogene p21 in esophageal squamous cell carcinoma. Surg. Forum *38:*445, 1987.
191. Rutgeerts, P., Vantrappen, G., Broeckaert, L., et al.: Palliative Nd:YAG laser therapy for cancer of the esophagus and gastroesophageal junction: Impact on the quality of remaining life. Gastrointest. Endosc., *34:*87, 1988.
192. Sabanathan, S., Eng., J., and Pradhan, G. N.: Primary malignant melanoma of the esophagus. Am. J. Gastroenterol., *84:*1475, 1989.
193. Saito, T., Zeze, K., Kuwahara, A., et al.: A prospective study on preoperative parenteral nutrition for patients with esophageal cancer. *In* Siewert, J. R., and Hölscher, A. H. (eds.): Diseases of the Esophagus. Berlin, Springer-Verlag, 1988, p. 268.
194. Sandler, R. S., Nyren, O., Ekbom, A., et al.: The risk of esophageal cancer in patients with achalasia. JAMA, *274:*1359, 1995.
195. Sargeant, I. R., Tobias, J. S., Blackman, G., et al.: Radiotherapy enhances laser palliation of malignant dysphagia: A randomised study. Gut, *40:*362, 1997.
196. Sasaki, T., Makuuchi, H., Sugihara, T., and Mitomi, T.: Evaluation of preoperative irradiation therapy for carcinoma of the esophagus. *In* Siewert, J. R., and Hölscher, A. H. (eds.): Diseases of the Esophagus. Berlin, Springer-Verlag, 1988, p. 313.
197. Sasaki, T., Makuuchi, H., Sugihara, T., et al.: Evaluation of preoperative irradiation therapy for carcinoma of the esophagus. *In* Siewert, J. R., and Hölscher, A. H. (eds.): Diseases of the Esophagus. Berlin, Springer-Verlag, 1988, p. 313.
198. Savage, A. P., Baigrie, R. J., Cobb, R. A., et al.: Palliation of malignant dysphagia by laser therapy. Dis. Esophagus, *10:*243, 1997.
199. Schlag, P. M.: Randomized trial of preoperative chemotherapy for squamous cell cancer of the esophagus. Arch. Surg., *127:*1446, 1992.
200. Segalin, A., Little, A. G., Ruol, A., et al.: Surgical and endoscopic palliation of esophageal carcinoma. Ann. Thorac. Surg., *48:*267, 1989.
201. Shimada, Y., Imamura, M., Shibagaki, I., et al.: Genetic alterations in patients with esophageal cancer with short- and long-term survival rates after curative esophagectomy. Ann. Surg., *226:*162, 1997.
202. Shu, Y.: Cytopathology of the esophagus. Acta Cytol., *27:*7, 1983.
203. Siersema, P. D., Hop, W. C. J., Dees, J., et al.: Coated self-expanding metal stents versus latex prostheses for esophagogastric cancer with special reference to prior radiation and chemotherapy: A controlled, prospective study. Gastrointest. Endosc., *47:*113, 1998.
204. Siewert, J. R., and Roder, J. D.: Lymphadenectomy in esophageal cancer surgery. Dis. Esoph., *5:*91, 1992.
205. Slabber, C. F., Nel, J. S., Schoeman, L., et al.: A randomized study of radiotherapy alone versus radiotherapy plus 5-fluorouracil and platinum in patients with inoperable, locally advanced squamous cancer of the esophagus. Am. J. Clin. Oncol., *21:*462, 1998.
206. Smith, T. J., Ryan, L. M., Douglass, H. O. Jr., et al.: Combined chemoradiotherapy vs. radiotherapy alone for early stage squamous cell carcinoma of the esophagus: A study of the Eastern Cooperative Oncology Group. Int. J. Radiat. Oncol. Biol. Phys., *42:*269, 1998.
207. Spencer, G. M., Thorpe, S. M., Sargeant, I. R., et al.: Laser and brachytherapy in the palliation of adenocarcinoma of the oesophagus and cardia. Gut, *39:*726, 1996.
208. Stein, H. J., Kraemer, S. J. M., Feussner, H., et al.: Clinical value of diagnostic laparoscopy with laparoscopic ultrasound in patients with cancer of the esophagus or cardia. J. Gastrointest. Surg., *1:*167, 1997.
209. Stephens, J. K., Bibbo, M., Dytch, H., et al.: Correlation between automated karyometric measurements of squamous cell carcinoma

of the esophagus and histopathologic and clinical features. Cancer, *64:*83, 1989.
210. Stewart, F. M., Harkins, B. J., Hahn, S. S., and Daniel, T. M.: Cisplatin, 5-fluorouracil, mitomycin C, and concurrent radiation therapy with and without esophagectomy for esophageal carcinoma. Cancer, *64:*622, 1989.
211. Sugimachi, K., Inokuchi, K., Ueo, H., et al.: Surgical treatment for carcinoma. Surg. Gynecol. Obstet., *160:*317, 1985.
212. Sugimachi, K., Maekawa, S., Koga, Y., et al.: The quality of life is sustained after operation for carcinoma of the esophagus. Surg. Gynecol. Obstet., *162:*544, 1986.
213. Sugimachi, K., Matsufuji, H., Kai, H., et al.: Preoperative irradiation for carcinoma of the esophagus. Surg. Gynecol. Obstet., *162:*174, 1986.
214. Sugimachi, K., Ohno, S., Fujishima, H., et al.: Endoscopic ultrasonographic detection of carcinomatous invasion and of lymph nodes in the thoracic esophagus. Surgery, *107:*366, 1990.
215. Sur, R. K., Singh, D. P., Sharma, S. C., et al.: Radiation therapy of esophageal cancer: Role of high dose rate brachytherapy. Int. J. Radiat. Oncol. Biol. Phys., *22:*1043, 1992.
216. Suzuki, H., and Nagayo, T.: Primary tumors of the esophagus other than squamous cell carcinoma—histologic classification and statistics in the surgical and autopsied materials in Japan. Int. Adv. Surg. Oncol., *3:*73, 1980.
217. Sykes, A. J., Burt, P. A., Slevin, N. J., et al.: Radical radiotherapy for carcinoma of the oesophagus: An effective alternative to surgery. Radiother. Oncol., *48:*15, 1998.
218. Tabira, Y., Okuma, T., Kondo, K., and Kitamura, N.: Indications for three-field dissection followed by esophagectomy for advanced carcinoma of the thoracic esophagus. J. Thorac. Cardiovasc. Surg., *117:*239, 1999.
219. Takubo, K., Takai, A., Takayama, S., et al.: Intra-ductal spread of esophageal squamous cell carcinoma. Cancer, *59:*1751, 1987.
220. Tam, P. C., Cheung, H. C., Ma, L., et al.: Local recurrences after subtotal esophagectomy for squamous cell carcinoma. Ann. Surg., *205:*189, 1987.
221. Tanaka, Y., Fujita, K., Miyama, T., et al.: An evaluation of postoperative prophylactic irradiation for esophageal cancer. *In* Siewert, J. R., and Hölscher, A. H. (eds.): Diseases of the Esophagus. Berlin, Springer-Verlag, 1988, p. 641.
222. Terz, J. J., Leong, L. A., Lipsett, J. A., and Wagman, L. D.: Preoperative chemotherapy and radiotherapy for cancer of the esophagus. Surgery, *114:*71, 1993.
223. Thompson, W. M., Halvorsen, R. A., Foster, W. L., Jr., et al.: Computed tomography for staging esophageal and gastroesophageal cancer. Re-evaluation. A. J. R., *141:*951, 1983.
224. Tilanus, H. W., Hop, W. C. J., Langenhorst, B. L. A. M., and van Lanschot, J. J. B.: Esophagectomy with or without thoracotomy. J. Thorac. Cardiovasc. Surg., *105:*898, 1993.
225. Tsutsui, S., Moriguchi, S., Morita, M., et al.: Multivariate analysis of postoperative complications after esophageal resection. Ann. Thorac. Surg., *53:*1052, 1992.
226. Turnbull, A. D., Rosen, P., Goodner, J. T., et al.: Primary malignant tumors of the esophagus other than typical epidermoid carcinoma. Ann. Thorac. Surg., *15:*463, 1973.
227. Walsh, T. N., Noonan, N., Hollywood, D., et al.: A comparison of multimodal therapy and surgery for esophageal adenocarcinoma. N. Engl. J. Med., *335:*462, 1996.
228. Wang, P. Y., and Chien, K. Y.: Surgical treatment of carcinoma of the esophagus and cardia among the Chinese. Ann. Thorac. Surg., *35:*143, 1983.
229. Watson, D. I., Davies, N., and Jamieson, G. G.: Totally endoscopic Ivor Lewis esophagectomy. Surg. Endosc., *13:*293, 1999.
230. Watt, I., Stewart, I., Anderson, D., et al.: Laparoscopy, ultrasound and computed tomography in cancer of the oesophagus and gastric cardia: A prospective comparison for detecting intra-abdominal metastases. Br. J. Surg., *76:*1036, 1989.
231. Weber, J., and Hecker, E.: Co-carcinogens of the diterpene ester type from *Croton flaveus L.* and esophageal cancer in Curacao. Experientia, *34:*679, 1978.
232. Whittington, R., Coia, L. R., Haller, D. G., et al.: Adenocarcinoma of the esophagus and esophago-gastric junction: The effects of single and combined modalities on the survival and patterns of failure following treatment. Int. J. Radiat. Oncol. Biol. Phys., *19:*593, 1990.
233. Wilson, S. E., Hiatt, J. R., Stabile, B. E., et al.: Cancer of the distal esophagus and cardia: Preoperative irradiation prolongs survival. Am. J. Surg., *150:*114, 1985.
234. Wolfe, W. G., Vaughn, A. L., Seigler, H. F., et al.: Survival of patients with carcinoma of the esophagus treated with combined-modality therapy. J. Thorac. Cardiovasc. Surg., *105:*849, 1993.
235. Wu, Y. K., Huang, G. J., Shao, L. F., et al.: Progress in the study and surgical treatment of cancer of the esophagus in China, 1940–1980. J. Thorac. Cardiovasc. Surg., *84:*325, 1982.
236. Yadava, O. P., Hodge, A. J., Matz, L. R., and Donlon, J. B.: Esophageal malignancies: Is preoperative radiotherapy the way to go? Ann. Thorac. Surg., *51:*189, 1991.
237. Yu, J.-M., Yang, L.-H., Guo-Qian, et al.: Flow cytometric analysis DNA content in esophageal carcinoma: Correlation with histologic and clinical features. Cancer, *64:*80, 1989.

CHAPTER

20 Radiation Therapy in Curative and Palliative Therapy of Esophageal Cancer

LAWRENCE R. KLEINBERG

This chapter explores the contribution of radiotherapy (RT) to the treatment of primary esophageal cancer. RT, with or without surgery and chemotherapy, is used in the curative and palliative treatment of esophageal cancer. Current knowledge about the appropriate role of RT is summarized in this chapter. An overview of the indications for RT is contained in Table 20-1.

Historically, primary RT served as the standard alternative to surgery in potentially curable esophageal cancer, but the results were quite disappointing. Consequently, RT as a single modality is now used only in limited circumstances. Randomized data show that the local control and survival outcome of RT administered concurrently with chemotherapy are superior to those of RT alone. Concurrent chemoradiotherapy is the standard nonoperative curative management.

Randomized trials that evaluated the role of neoadjuvant (preoperative) or adjuvant (postoperative) RT have also been conducted. Five randomized trials of preoperative RT have not demonstrated improved outcome. Similarly, randomized trials indicate that postoperative RT does not improve outcome. Postoperative therapy is, however, generally added when there are positive surgical margins or known residual disease. Although the trials of preoperative and postoperative RT have weaknesses, their results do provide convincing evidence that substantial improvements in survival are unlikely with these approaches. A growing body of evidence exists, including some randomized data, suggesting that preoperative concurrent chemoradiotherapy may improve the outcome of surgery. Trials to definitively evaluate the usefulness of this approach are under way. The role of postoperative chemoradiotherapy has not yet been rigorously evaluated.

Overall, current available data indicate that esophageal resection alone, preoperative chemoradiation, and concurrent definitive chemoradiotherapy are all appropriate curative therapies in properly selected patients. RT alone should be used only in patients who are not candidates for these treatment options. In addition, RT is important in the palliative therapy of esophageal cancer,

Table 20-1. Role of Radiation in Therapy of Esophageal Cancer

Indication	Recommendation	Evidence
Primary radiotherapy	Used only for patients who are not candidates for concurrent chemoradiation	Long-term survival rate of 0-10% for locally advanced disease and 15-25% for early disease; randomized trials have demonstrated a survival and local control benefit when chemotherapy is added
Primary chemoradiotherapy	Appropriate choice for nonoperative management	Randomized trials have demonstrated a 5-year survival rate of 9-27%
Preoperative radiotherapy	No known benefit	Five randomized trials
Postoperative radiotherapy	No known benefit; used for known residual disease	Two randomized trials
Preoperative chemoradiotherapy	Accepted alternative approach, although further data that demonstrate a benefit are needed	Benefit in two of three randomized trials and encouraging results in numerous phase II trials; a definitive large randomized U.S. Intergroup trial is under way
Brachytherapy	Useful for palliation and improved local control; no known survival benefit in curative therapy	Uncontrolled trials and single-institution experiences
Palliation	Radiotherapy is useful for palliation of swallowing difficulties and metastatic disease; the addition of chemotherapy should be strongly considered in patients with longer life expectancy; radiotherapy can be used for tracheoesophageal fistula	Uncontrolled trials and single-institution experiences
Postoperative chemoradiotherapy	Benefits not assessed; used for known residual disease	Very limited data

Table 20–2. Results From Treatment Arms From Selected Randomized Trials

	Survival Rate (%)				Median Survival Time (mo)	Local Failure Rate (%)
	1 yr	2 yr	3 yr	5 yr		
Surgery						
U.S. Intergroup[30]	60	37	26		14.9	
Bossett et al.[33]					18.6	
Walsh et al.[31]	42	26	6		11	
Urba et al.[32]			15		17.5	39
Radiotherapy						
RTOG[7,8,10]	34	10	0	0	9.3	68
ECOG[6] (surgery added in 24 of 56)	33	12	8	7	9.2	
Chemoradiotherapy						
RTOG[7,8,10]	52	36	30	26	14	46
RTOG[7,8,10] (nonrandomized confirmatory group)	62	35	26	14	16.7	58
ECOG[6] (surgery added in 21 of 58)	54	27	13	9	14.8	
Preoperative Chemoradiotherapy						
Walsh et al.[31]	52	37	32		16	
Bossett et al.[33]					18.6	
Urba et al.[32]			32		16.9	19

Randomized trials included in table are as follows (further details are given in the text): U.S. Intergroup: surgery with or without preoperative cisplatin/5-FU—no significant difference; RTOG: radiation with or without cisplatin/5-FU chemotherapy—significant benefit from chemotherapy; ECOG: radiation with or without mitomycin/5-FU chemotherapy—surgery also used at the discretion of the treating physicians—benefit from chemotherapy; Bossett et al.: surgery with or without preoperative cisplatin/radiotherapy—no benefit to neoadjuvant therapy; Walsh et al.: surgery with or without preoperative cisplatin/5-FU/radiotherapy—benefit to neoadjuvant therapy; Urba et al.: surgery with or without preoperative cisplatin/5-FU/vinblastine/radiotherapy—possible benefit to neoadjuvant therapy.

5-Fu = 5-fluorouracil; RTOG = Radiation Therapy Oncology Group; ECOG = Eastern Cooperative Oncology Group.

with the goal of maintaining or improving swallowing function.

The most significant data that outline the outcome of each of these treatment approaches are discussed in this chapter. Where available, the results of randomized trials are emphasized and critically discussed. The results achieved in selected recent important randomized trials are summarized in Table 20–2. Uncontrolled and retrospective studies are considered to the extent that important information that is unavailable from randomized trials is added. Additional topics that are covered include radiation technique and toxicities, brachytherapy, RT response assessment, RT in malignant tracheoesophageal fistula, and RT for palliation.

INTRODUCTION TO RADIOTHERAPY

RT involves the use of ionizing radiation in the treatment of malignant disease. Conventional external-beam treatments are administered with high-energy photon beams, typically with energy of 1.25 megaelectron volts (MV) to 15 MV or higher. These energies significantly exceed those of x-rays used in diagnostic radiology. The high energy of therapeutic radiation beams enables the treatment to penetrate the body and to be used to treat deep tissues. Depending on the actual energy, only several percent of the energy of the photon beam is absorbed per centimeter of tissue. Routine availability of high-energy radiation sources in the years after World War II dramatically increased the clinical usefulness of RT. Previously, only low-energy radiation sources, which emitted radiation that was absorbed to a significant extent by superficial tissues, were widely available. These low-energy beams required that an excessive (and often toxic) dose of radiation be delivered to the surface of the body so that a therapeutic dose could reach a deep tumor. For example, at a 10-cm depth in the patient, the radiation dose with a 6-MV beam might be more than 70% of the dose near the surface of the patient's body, but with only a 230-KV beam, the dose at 10 cm may only be approximately 30% of the surface dose.

Lower-energy radiation is still frequently used in brachytherapy. In brachytherapy, a radioactive material is placed in close proximity to the targeted area. Low-energy radiation is useful in brachytherapy because it does not penetrate tissues well, and therefore most of the dose is deposited in the targeted region around where the radioactive sources are placed. Brachytherapy thus allows high radiation doses to be administered to the tumor with exposure of only minimal volumes of surrounding tissues. In brachytherapy for esophageal cancer, a radioactive source can be placed into the esophageal lumen via a catheter to treat endobronchial tumors.

Weakly penetrating external radiation beams, such as electrons or low-energy photon beams as described, are still commonly used in appropriate situations. Weakly penetrating beams are indicated in the treatment of superficial tumors when it would be useful to spare deeper tissues, a situation that is rarely encountered in the treatment of primary esophageal cancer. Electron beam RT, which may penetrate up to several centimeters, is useful in the treatment of metastatic disease to supraclavicular nodes, skin, ribs, and other superficial sites but not in the therapy of primary esophageal cancer.

The success of radiation in the therapy of malignant disease is a consequence of several key properties. First, ionizing radiation has a higher tendency to kill malignant or rapidly dividing tissues than normal body tissues. Second, radiation beams have predictable characteristics that allow them to be aimed fairly precisely at the targeted tissue, so only nearby tissues or overlying normal tissues will be exposed to significant doses. Although the particular characteristics of the beam vary from machine to machine, important features such as heterogeneity over the cross section of the beam and penetrating characteristics can be measured precisely and used in precision treatment planning. Finally, it is well established that fractionation of the radiation into many small daily doses maximizes the capacity to administer a potentially curative dose. Fractionating RT reduces the risk of dose-limiting severe normal tissue toxicities while maintaining effectiveness in treating the tumor, providing the rationale for the lengthy RT courses used today.

PRIMARY RADIOTHERAPY

Primary Radiotherapy as a Single Modality

RT alone as definitive therapy for esophageal cancer provides palliation, temporary control of local disease, and a small chance of long-term control or cure. Historically, radiation served as the standard alternative to surgical therapy. Studies have demonstrated that the results of RT are not as good as those attained with concurrent chemoradiotherapy (see Table 20-2). Consequently, RT alone is used with decreasing frequency in both early and locally advanced disease.

Radiation as a single agent can be an effective, if not optimal, therapy for early lesions that are less than 5 cm in length, nonobstructing, and noncircumferential. The 5-year survival rate for such early lesions is reported to be 15 to 2%.[1-4] Specific local control data for those early stage lesions have not been reported. The outcome of RT for each stage of disease is difficult to compare with the results of surgery, because patients selected for RT generally have had poor prognostic features such as medically inoperable or surgical unresectable disease. Irradiated patients are not pathologically staged and may have unappreciated advanced or metastatic disease.

The importance of modern staging in the appropriate assessment of outcomes is demonstrated in a series from Christie Hospital,[4] Manchester, England, in which survival outcome was analyzed separately for 30 early-stage patients who had a pre-RT computed tomography (CT) scan and for 81 who were staged only with endoscopy, barium swallow, and liver ultrasound. Ninety-five percent of the tumors were less than 5 cm in length. The patients who had diagnostic CT had a 5-year survival rate of 42% versus a rate of 13% for those without CT scanning. In this study, it was impossible to determine how much of the benefit was the result of the exclusion of patients with advanced disease detected only on CT scan, how much was from better aim of RT, and how much was from other selection factors. However, the mean width of the irradiated area was larger in the patients who had a CT scan. The addition of endoscopic ultrasound to the routine evaluation of the patient with esophageal cancer, which further improves nonoperative staging and determination of tumor extent, will also enhance the ability to directly compare results of operative and nonoperative management and to develop better models for the selection of treatment options for individual patients.

Despite the limitations in the available data that compare the results of RT with other treatments for early-stage disease, it is clear that radiation alone is not an optimal therapy for patients with resectable disease. It may be appropriate to select RT alone for some patients with very small early-stage medically inoperable node-negative tumors, but even in this situation, strong consideration should be given to adding concurrent chemotherapy to improve survival outcome unless there are specific medical contraindications.

Most patients treated with definitive radiation do not have early disease as described here and present with larger lesions, swallowing dysfunction, and weight loss, all of which adversely affect outcome. As discussed later, the addition of chemotherapy to RT in this setting has been convincingly shown to increase survival[5-8] and is the recommended approach. However, even in locally advanced disease, definitive RT alone can be of palliative benefit and result in a cure rate of up to 10%.[1-3] Therefore, it is appropriate to use RT alone when there are medical contraindications to combined-modality therapy or if the patient refuses chemotherapy after informed discussion of the potential benefits. It is notable that even though previous trials have demonstrated long-term survival, two recent multi-institutional randomized trials conducted in the United States had no 3-year survivors in the RT control arm.[6-8] In contrast, these trials demonstrated that the 5-year survival rate with concurrent chemoradiotherapy is 9 to 27% with substantially improved local control.

When RT is used as a single modality in definitive treatment, a dosage of at least 60 to 64 Gy at 1.8 to 2.0 Gy/day should generally be used. The dose is limited by esophageal tolerance. Emani et al.[9] estimated that the radiation dose (with conventional fractionation) that would lead to a 5% rate of clinical stricture or perforation within 5 years would be 60 Gy when one third of the esophagus is treated, 58 Gy if two thirds are treated, and 55 Gy for all of the esophagus. Although escalation beyond the 60- to 64-Gy level might achieve a higher local control, the toxicity is likely to be excessive and survival is unlikely to be improved given the high rate of distant metastasis.

Combined Chemoradiotherapy as Primary Therapy: Improved Long-Term Survival

Chemotherapy administered concurrently with esophageal RT improves survival outcome and should be considered a potentially curative therapy. The rationale for adding chemotherapy to primary RT is two-fold. First, it may improve the cure rate by eradicating undetectable micrometastasis in some patients. In addition, systemic agents can have synergistic effects with RT, resulting in improved local control.

The Radiation Therapy Oncology Group (RTOG) trial 8501[7] definitively established concurrent therapy as a new standard of care in the nonoperative management of esophageal cancer. The outcome of 64-Gy RT alone was compared with 50-Gy administered concurrently with two cycles and followed by two cycles of 75 mg/m^2 cisplatin and 1000 mg/m^2/day 5-fluorouracil (5-FU) for 4 days. Only 54% of patients completed the planned post-RT chemotherapy. A lower RT dose was used in those receiving chemotherapy to minimize the risks of excessive toxicity. Eighty-seven percent of the patients had squamous cell carcinoma. Chest CT was not required, and 81% had tumors larger than 5 cm. The median survival rate was improved with the addition of chemotherapy from 9.3 to 14.1 months ($P < 0.001$). Most importantly, the 3- and 5-year survival rates improved to 30 and 27%, respectively, from 0% in this initial report. Despite the lower RT dose, local recurrence or persistent local disease as part of initial failure at a median follow-up of 18 months was reduced from 65 to 44% and distant failure was reduced from 26 to 12%. This study was closed before its accrual goals had been reached after a significant survival benefit was observed at a planned interim analysis, and an additional 69 nonrandomized patients were assigned to the concurrent chemotherapy arm to confirm the observed survival results. An update,[10] with a minimum follow-up of 5 years, reported that the 5-year survival rate in the randomized chemoradiotherapy group was 26% (95% confidence interval, 15 to 37%), and the rate was 14% (6 to 23%) in the confirmatory group. The 8-year survival rate was 22% in the randomized group, with no cancer-related deaths after 5 years. The incidence of local failure/persistent disease as part of initial failure was 53% and that of distant disease as part of initial failure was 22% in all patients treated in the combined-modality arms with mature follow-up. Although only 23 patients treated with combined-modality therapy had adenocarcinoma, it was reported that there was no statistically or clinically significant difference in outcome based on histology.

The Eastern Cooperative Oncology Group (ECOG) has also conducted a randomized trial to compare chemoradiation with radiation alone; the trial demonstrated a significant, albeit less dramatic, survival benefit.[6] Compared with the RTOG trial we described, a different chemotherapy regimen was used. All patients in this trial had squamous cell carcinoma, and surgery was permitted after 40 Gy at the discretion of the treating physicians. Patients received 60 Gy of RT in 30 fractions, although the option existed to assess the patient for surgery after 40 Gy. Those randomized to chemotherapy received 10 mg/m^2 mitomycin on days 2 and 29 of RT, and 96-hour infusions of 1000 mg/kg/day 5-FU were started on days 1 and 28. If surgery was performed, the second course of chemotherapy was not administered. Chemotherapy improved the median survival time from 9.2 to 14.8 months ($P =$ 0.03), and the 2-year survival rate was improved from 12 to 27%. Disappointingly, the 5-year survival rates were 7 and 9%, respectively. The results in this trial were confounded by the 45 patients (of 114) who were selected for surgery, because no patient in this trial treated with radiation alone survived 3 years without the addition of surgery. With chemoradiation, the median survival time for early lesions (< 5 cm, no extraesophageal spread, no involved lymph nodes) improved from 11.8 to 22.6 months, whereas for more advanced lesions, it was improved from 8.5 to 13.5 months. It should be noted that CT scan was not required for staging in this study.

These results are similar to those seen in a large pilot study from the Fox Chase Cancer Center in Philadelphia in which 60 Gy was administered concurrently with 5-FU (1 g/m^2/day) for 4 days on days 1 and 29 and mitomycin (10 mg/m^2) on day 2.[5] In this study, results were reported separately for tumors less than 5 cm in length (early) and those more than 5 cm. All patients had a CT scan as part of the staging evaluation. This study was limited to patients who had a tumor confined to the esophagus without suspicious nodes on the CT scan or radiologic/clinical evidence of extraesophageal extension to adjacent nerves or organs. For the tumors of 5 cm or less, the 3-year survival and local control rates were 73 and 100%, and for the group with tumors of more than 5 cm confined to the esophagus, the rates were 33 and 60%, respectively. A poor prognostic group with extraesophageal spread received the same chemotherapy with 50-Gy external radiation for palliation. The median survival time for those with extraesophageal spread in the absence of distant metastasis was 9 months, and the time for those treated palliatively with known distant metastasis was only 7 months.

There have been four other randomized trials that compared chemotherapy with chemoradiotherapy with negative results. A National Cancer Institute of Brazil trial[11] used only one cycle of chemotherapy and included only 59 patients; an EORTC[12] trial used subcutaneous methotrexate; in a Scandinavian trial,[13] low doses of cisplatin/bleomycin chemotherapy were used; and a South African trial[14] used an RT dose of only 40 Gy administered with a split-course regimen. However, each of those trials used suboptimal types or doses of chemotherapy or RT. Therefore, based on the RTOG and ECOG trials, concurrent chemoradiotherapy has become the standard of care for the nonoperative management of esophageal cancer.

The same factors that make it difficult to compare the results of surgical resection and the results of RT alone (i.e., selection bias, lack of pathologic staging, concurrent medical illness) also make comparison of surgery and chemoradiation unreliable, but the available data suggest that the outcome of chemoradiotherapy for these relatively advanced tumors may approach that achievable with esophageal resection. A recent U.S. Intergroup trial with a surgery-alone control arm demonstrated survival and local control rates similar to those seen in randomized studies with chemoradiation arms (see Table 20–2). In addition, some retrospective comparisons are similarly suggestive. A retrospective study of patients with locally advanced disease compared 82 patients treated at the Tom Baker Cancer Center in Calgary[15] with concurrent chemoradiotherapy on phase II protocols with 81 patients who had surgery during the same years. There was no difference in local failure, 3- or 5-year survival, or survival by stage or histology. In addition, a study conducted at Tenri, Hospital Japan[16] compared patients with early-stage tumors treated with chemoradiotherapy plus brachytherapy with a group treated with surgery with or without postoperative RT. The protocol patients received 60 mg/m^2 cisplatin on day 1, bolus of 400 mg/m^2 5-FU on days 1 to 4, and 44-Gy RT followed by high-dose-rate brachytherapy to a total RT dose of 70 Gy. Surgery was performed instead of brachytherapy in the 10% of patients who had no response to the initial part of treatment. The 1- and 3-year survival rates were similar in protocol patients and those treated initially with surgery.

Although comparisons of treatment results from different prospective and historical trials are only of limited use and must be interpreted extremely cautiously, these results do indicate that chemoradiotherapy may be an appropriate alternative to surgery under some circumstances. Clearly, studies that directly compare survival and quality-of-life outcome of surgery with chemoradiotherapy are needed to determine which patients are appropriate candidates for nonoperative management. However, at the present, chemoradiotherapy can be considered not only standard therapy for locally advanced unresectable disease but also an appropriate potentially curative alternative for resectable disease when operative risks are high, laryngectomy may be required, the patient refuses surgery, or the surgeon believes that there is a significant chance that negative margins may not be achieved.

When chemoradiotherapy is used, the standard RT dose is 50 Gy, which was demonstrated to be safe and beneficial in the landmark RTOG trial (8501).[7] Doses as high as 60 Gy can be considered safe based on the results of the ECOG trial[6] and the large pilot study carried out at Fox Chase Cancer Center.[5] Importantly, different chemotherapy regimens were used in these studies, which may potentiate the toxicities of radiation to differing extents. Caution should be used when deviating from these tested regimens, and new chemotherapy agents or substantial radiation dose escalation should occur only in the context of a clinical trial.

Current efforts to improve outcome with chemoradiotherapy center on improving both local control by increasing radiation dose and reducing distant spread by improving systemic therapy. For example, an ongoing RTOG randomized trial compared 64.8 Gy versus 50.4 Gy with concurrent chemotherapy to determine whether a higher local control and survival can be achieved without any benefit in preliminary analysis. Efforts to incorporate brachytherapy as means of dose escalation with chemoradiotherapy have not clearly improved outcome and have been associated with excessive toxicity.[17,18] A Southwest Oncology Group trial has shown that the use of continuous-infusion 5-FU throughout the entire RT course is not beneficial.[19] Neoadjuvant chemotherapy before concurrent chemoradiotherapy has been studied as a means to intensify the tolerated chemotherapy dose, because chemotherapy after concurrent chemotherapy was poorly tolerated in RTOG trial 8501. An ECOG trial[20] tested neoadjuvant 100 mg/m^2 cisplatin with 1,000 mg/m^2/day 5-FU for 5 days administered for three cycles followed by two cycles of 75 mg/m^2 cisplatin, the identical 5-FU dosing, and 64.8 Gy of esophageal RT at 1.8 Gy/day. However, with this regimen, 11% of patients had treatment-related death and there was no apparent survival benefit. Although other preliminary studies of neoadjuvant chemotherapy regimens have not resulted in such a high fatality rate, they have not clearly suggested a survival benefit.[21-23] Further improvement in outcome will likely depend on the development of improved systemic therapies. The high local failure rate seen after chemoradiotherapy alone also provides rationale for the use of trimodality therapy when esophagectomy is performed after neoadjuvant chemoradiotherapy to improve local control and survival.

NEOADJUVANT PREOPERATIVE RADIOTHERAPY

Preoperative Neoadjuvant Radiotherapy: No Benefit

In the past, preoperative RT has been advocated as a means for improving survival outcome. There are several possible benefits to preoperative RT: a reduction in tumor bulk, which might increase the chances of complete resection; sterilization of regional disease, which may not be effectively treated with surgery; improvement in nutritional state before esophagectomy through shrinkage of the obstructing tumor and devitalization of the tumor; and the reduced chances of viable tumor cell shedding during surgery.

Preoperative RT was been evaluated in five fully reported prospective randomized clinical trials,[24-28] with evidence of survival benefit in only one of these trials, in which half of the irradiated patients also received concurrent chemotherapy. These studies can be criticized because often the radiation dose was low, the interval between radiation and surgery did not allow sufficient time for tumor shrinkage (4 to 6 weeks is optimal), and the studies were too small to detect anything but a very large survival benefit. However, the consistency of the results of these trials provides substantial evidence that preoperative RT is not beneficial in improving survival. A meta-analysis[29] with individual patient data was undertaken to determine whether a small but significant benefit was overlooked. No significant survival benefit was identified in this meta-analysis, although there was a suggestion of a minimal survival benefit with a hazard ratio for death of 0.89 (95% confidence interval, 0.78 to 1.01), leading to an 11% reduction in the risk of death and an absolute survival benefit of 4% at 5 years of follow-up. To reliably detect an improvement in survival of this magnitude, a trial of approximately 2000 patients would be required. Such a trial is unlikely to be carried out given the small potential survival benefit and the promising results attained with preoperative combined chemoradiotherapy. At present, the available data do not support preoperative RT alone as a useful strategy.

Preoperative Neoadjuvant Chemoradiotherapy: Promising Results

Preoperative combined chemoradiotherapy is a promising approach that is under evaluation. Neither preoperative chemotherapy alone nor preoperative RT alone has proved to be of benefit by itself, but given that local recurrence (or unresectable disease at surgery) and distant failure are both significant problems, there is sound rationale to believe that a combined approach to address both problems has the potential to have a significant impact on outcome. A U.S. Intergroup randomized trial[30] that accrued patients from 1990 to 1995 had a control arm of 227 patients who were treated with surgery alone that provides benchmark data for survival and patterns of failure achieved nationally (see Table 20–2). Analysis of the results in this group demonstrated that of the patients thought to have surgically curable disease, only 59% were able to undergo total resection of the esophageal disease with negative margins and an additional 17% had local failure as a first site of failure, for an overall 58% rate of failure to control local disease. Curatively resected patients had a distant failure rate of 50%. Therefore, there clearly is a need to address both local and distant failure in surgically treated patients, providing rationale for the use of adjuvant chemotherapy and RT.

The concept of preoperative chemoradiotherapy has been tested in several recent randomized trials. One of these trials was clearly positive, one was positive on multivariate analysis and has been reported in abstract form only, and the third demonstrated no benefit to preoperative chemoradiotherapy. Therefore, the role of this approach remains controversial. An NCI-sponsored intergroup trial designed to definitely answer this question was terminated due to poor patient accrual. The randomized data are described here.

In a trial reported by Walsh et al.,[31] 113 patients with adenocarcinoma were randomized to surgery alone or surgery with preoperative chemotherapy and concurrent RT (40 Gy in 15 fractions). The chemotherapy, which began on the first day of RT, consisted of 15 mg/kg 5-FU for 5 days and 75 mg/m^2 cisplatin repeated again during week 6 after the completion of RT. The complete response rate to neoadjuvant therapy was 25%, and the incidence of positive nodes in the surgical specimen was reduced from 82 to 42% ($P < 0.001$). The median survival time was improved from 11 to 16 months ($P = 0.01$), with 1-, 2-, and 3-year survival rates improved from 44, 26, and 6% to 53%, 37%, and 32%, respectively. Despite the striking results, the trial has been criticized for the unexpectedly poor results with surgery alone and the relatively small size.

Urba et al.[32] has reported (in abstract form only) the results of a randomized trial at the University of Michigan that suggested a long-term survival benefit with preoperative therapy. One hundred patients were randomized to esophagectomy with or without preoperative chemoradiotherapy. The chemotherapy was 20 mg/m^2 cisplatin for 5 days and 1 mg/m^2 vinblastine for 4 days repeated for two cycles and 300 mg/m^2 5-FU for 21 days during RT. RT was 1.5 Gy administered twice a day to a total dose of 45 Gy. Seventy-five percent of patients had adenocarcinoma, and 25% had squamous cell carcinoma. Twenty-eight percent of those who received preoperative therapy had a complete response. Although median survival was similar in both arms, long-term survival was improved with preoperative therapy, with 3-year survival rates of 32% versus 15% (log-rank $P = 0.0734$; Cox regression value, 0.0402) reported at a median follow-up of 5.2 years for surviving patients. Site of first recurrence was locoregional for 39% of patients treated with surgery alone and 19% after this regimen of preoperative therapy. Tumors larger than 5 cm, age greater than 70 years, and squamous cell histology were associated with shorter survival times, after adjustment for other factors. Pathologic complete response (CR) was associated with improved survival ($P = 0.0060$). Although this trial is suggestive of a benefit of preoperative chemoradiotherapy, it is a relatively small trial in which the long-term survival benefit was significant only in multivariate analysis.

There also was a French multicenter randomized trial[33] that examined the role of preoperative chemoradiotherapy in 282 patients with squamous cell carcinoma. Although no survival benefit was demonstrated, there were prolonged disease-free survival and local recurrence-free survival times. The RT regimen was unconventional with 18.5 Gy administered in five fractions over 1 week and repeated after a 2-week break for a total dose of 37 Gy. Cisplatin 80 mg/m^2 was administered 0 to 2 days before each week of RT. Given the altered RT regimen and the use of single-agent chemotherapy that was not necessarily administered on the same day as RT, this trial did not test the therapeutic approach generally used in the United States.

In addition to these randomized trials, there have been multiple phase II studies that on the whole are suggestive of benefit for the approach of neoadjuvant chemoradiotherapy.[34–45] These trials have primarily differed in the chemotherapy regimen used but also occasionally in the RT details. These trials are discussed in Chapter 21. At Johns Hopkins University,[46–49] 92 patients (65 with adenocarcinoma and 27 with squamous cell carcinoma) were enrolled in two successive preoperative chemoradiotherapy protocols between 1989 and 1997. In both trials, the RT was 44 Gy in 22 fractions. In the initial trial, the chemotherapy consisted of 300 mg/m^2/day 5-FU for 30 days of continuous infusion with 26 mg/m^2/day cisplatin on days 1 to 5 and 20 to 30. In the second study, in an attempt to reduce hematologic toxicity, the daily 5-FU and cisplatin doses were reduced to 225 and 20 mg/m^2, respectively. In the second trial, patients also were administered postoperative paclitaxel and cisplatin chemotherapy. Of the initially enrolled patients, 93% were brought to resection, 87% had a complete resection, and 33% had a complete pathologic response. For those with pathologic CR, the 3-year survival rate was 77% versus 34% for those with residual disease. Patients with stage I disease at surgery had results similar to those with pathologic CR. The significant 3-year survival rate even in those without a complete response to neoadjuvant therapy suggests that surgery has an important role after combined chemotherapy. Isolated local failure as first failure occurred in only 6%, and concurrent distant/local first failure occurred in an additional 2%.

Although preoperative chemoradiotherapy should be

used with caution given the mixed results in randomized trials, the current evidence suggests that radiation dosages of 44 to 45 Gy at 1.8 to 2.0 Gy/day are optimum, followed by a 4- to 6-week interval before surgery. The isolated local failure rate is low (0 to 19%[32,45,50-53]), so there is no need to consider escalating the dose of RT or further intensifying the local therapy beyond 44 to 45 Gy at 1.8 to 2.0 Gy/day. Doses greater than 50 Gy are associated with increased surgical mortality rates,[51,54] and lower doses may be associated with increased local failure.[55] Improved outcome is likely to depend on the development of better systemic therapy.

ADJUVANT (POSTOPERATIVE) RADIOTHERAPY

Postoperative Radiotherapy: Limited Usefulness

Postoperative RT has several potential benefits in comparison with preoperative RT. Because the treatment is administered after recovery from surgery, operative complications will not be increased. The RT can be more effectively targeted as the full extent of disease is known. The decision on whether to administer radiation can be guided by pathologic findings. On the other hand, poorly vascularized tissues in the postoperative tumor bed may harbor hypoxic cells, which are resistant to RT.

Randomized data indicate that postoperative RT after complete resection is not beneficial. Although these trials suggested the possibility of some improvement in local control in some situations, the survival outcome was not improved in any subgroup of patients. In a trial reported by Teniere et al.,[56] 60 patients with curative resection were randomized to receive 49 Gy at 3.5 Gy/day or observation and 70 patients with palliative resection were randomized to receive 52.5 Gy at 3.5 Gy/day or observation. Patients had both adenocarcinoma and squamous cell carcinoma. Resections were considered curative when tumor had not invaded adjacent organs and all involved lymph nodes were discrete and less than 2 cm in size. In the palliative group, local failure was significantly improved by radiation from 46 to 20%, but no significant difference was seen in the curatively resected group (13 versus 10%). Radiated patients actually had a worse survival, in part due to a 37% complication rate in the gastric pull-up with 8% having fatal gastric bleeding, which may have resulted from the high daily dose of RT. In the other trial[57] performed by the French University Association for Cancer Research, patients were randomized after surgery to observation or to receive 45 Gy RT at 1.8 Gy/day. An additional 5 to 10 Gy was administered if mediastinal nodes were involved. There was no survival benefit overall or for any subgroup of patients. Local recurrence was significantly reduced only for node-negative patients (from 35 to 10%; $P < 0.002$), not for node-positive patients.

Therefore, the available evidence suggests that postoperative RT is not indicated, even in node-positive patients. On the other hand, when there is known gross residual disease or resection with positive margins, it is reasonable to administered postoperative RT with or without chemotherapy, because the risk of symptomatic local recurrence is assumed to be high. In the randomized trial of Fok et al.,[57] 2 of 29 (7%) patients with known residual disease in the mediastinum died of tracheobronchial obstruction after postoperative RT compared with 9 of 27 (33%) patients who did not receive RT. The dose should generally be limited to approximately 45 Gy at 1.8 to 2.0 Gy/day to limit the risk of toxicity to the gastric pull-up. When postoperative RT is administered, the dose should be limited to 45 Gy to avoid injury to the gastric pull-up or interposed bowel. We generally advocate chemotherapy along with RT when there is known residual disease based on the improved survival with this approach in patients who have had partial resection.

Postoperative Chemoradiotherapy: Little Data

The role of postoperative chemoradiotherapy has not yet been assessed in large trials. The advantages to this approach in contrast to preoperative therapy include the potential for using pathologic findings to guide therapy and possibly reduced surgical complications. On the other hand, if there is micrometastatic disease at the time of diagnosis, further growth can occur during the several months between diagnosis and the start of systemic therapy.

There are limited retrospective data that suggest this approach may be beneficial. A matched-pair analysis[58] of 67 patients with advanced-stage disease who were treated with postoperative RT and one cycle of cisplatin-based chemotherapy indicated that median survival improved from 18 to 33 months in comparison with patients treated with surgery alone. The data are limited, and this issue requires further study.[59] When postoperative RT is administered for positive margins or known residual tumor, it is reasonable to add chemotherapy given the superiority of this approach in newly diagnosed gross esophageal disease.

RADIOTHERAPY FOR PALLIATION

Radiotherapy for Palliation of Swallowing Difficulty

External radiation can improve swallowing function in a significant proportion of patients. Radiation alone improves dysphagia in approximately 46 to 89% of patients,[60-64] and chemoradiotherapy improves 59 to 88% of patients.[8,32,45,65-67] Relief is not immediate but is often relatively fast, with a median time to maximal improvement of 4 weeks (range, 2 to 21 weeks). High doses of RT (with chemotherapy when appropriate) are generally required for effective durable palliation[68] and should be used whenever life expectancy is greater than 3 months and Karnofsky performance status is 60 or greater. For

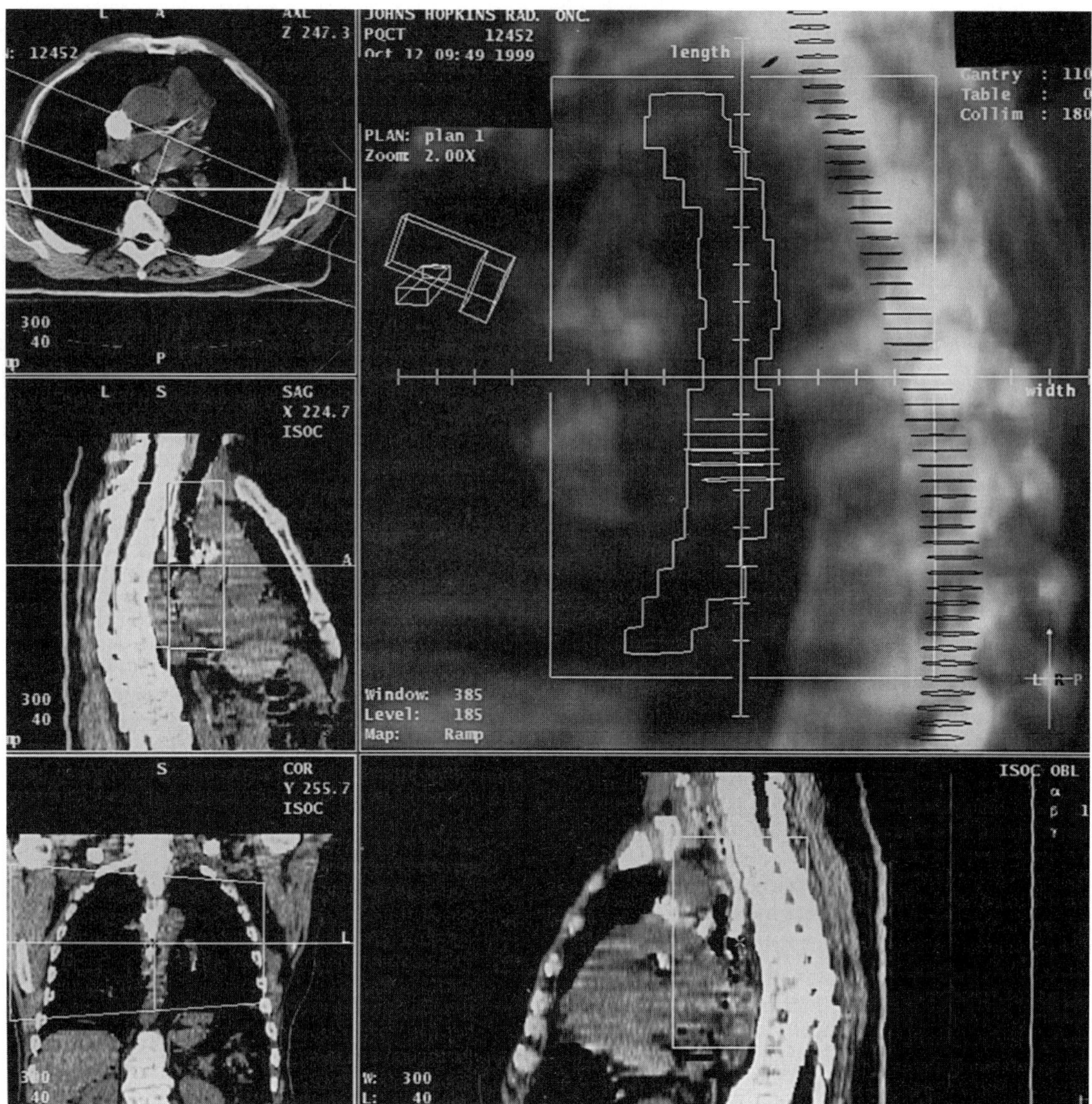

Figure 20–1. Demonstration of a beam's eye view treatment planning. The esophagus and spinal cord have been circled on the computed tomography scan and are superimposed onto the digitally reconstructed radiograph *(upper right)* created to show how the beam will "see" the body at an oblique angle. The computed tomography images on *left* and *bottom* also show how the beam will cross the body. The beam will be further shaped with alloy blocks to shield normal tissues, especially the spinal cord.

patients treated with such aggressive palliative regimens, relief of dysphagia for the remaining lifetime occurs in 51%[69] to 67%[66] of patients. However, the results of RTOG trial 8501[7] indicate a substantial incidence of persistent or recurrent local disease even in curatively treated patients that no doubt translates into a significant incidence of local symptoms even under optimal circumstances. When life expectancy is poor, less time-consuming regimens, such as 30 Gy × 10 fractions, may be more appropriate.

The relative roles of RT, laser therapy, electrocautery photodynamic therapy, and stenting in optimal palliative therapy are not well determined. It is possible that a combination of therapies might be used. Photodynamic therapy, electrocautery, or laser therapy can be used for quick palliation, with radiation added to delay regrowth of the tumor. This approach is often used in palliation of obstructive endobronchial lesions in lung cancer, but the safety and efficacy in esophageal cancer require further study.

Radiotherapy for Palliation of Tracheoesophageal Fistula

The use of definitive or palliative RT in the setting of tracheoesophageal fistula has been controversial. Tracheoesophageal fistula has historically been considered a contraindication to RT for fear that the fistula might worsen. However, there is evidence that RT can be beneficial and should not be withheld when it may be of palliative benefit. In a report from the Mayo Clinic,[70] lysis of tumor by RT could not be shown to be an important cause of TE fistula. In 22 patients who developed fistula after prior RT, recurrent tumor was the cause in all cases. For 10 irradiated patients with known TE fistula, the fistula did not worsen in any patient. Combined chemotherapy and RT has also been demonstrated to close the fistula in four of six patients in a series[71] of patients treated at the Washington, D.C., Veterans Affairs Medical Center. Patients were eligible for chemotherapy only if they were afebrile despite the fistula. Finally, in a series from the National Cancer Center Hospital, East Japan,[72] 17 of 24 fistulas closed after chemoradiotherapy.

RADIOTHERAPY TECHNIQUES AND PLANNING

In this section, the fundamentals of radiation treatment planning are discussed, including simulation, patient positioning, treatment planning, and treatment delivery.

The radiation planning process begins with a "simulation" or radiation planning session. The purpose of simulation is to define a reproducible patient position that can be used for daily treatment and to acquire anatomic imaging data that will allow the radiation beams to be correctly aimed at the tumor with the patient in that position. During the simulation, the patient will be appropriately positioned in a way that is likely to be highly reproducible from day to day. Frequently, custom molds are created to help immobilize the patient. Imaging data are then acquired with the patient in the treatment position. Reference marks are placed on the patient's skin that correspond to known points on the radiograph or CT scans that are taken during the simulation process. Standard simulation uses conventional radiography. Barium contrast is used for visualization of the esophagus, and CT data as well as information from endoscopy could be superimposed onto the radiograph to improve definition of the target area. Technology has become available that allows a CT scan to be obtained in the treatment position, followed by the creation of digitally reconstructed radiographs that contain not only the bony anatomy but also superimposed images of soft tissue anatomy. Typically, the radiation oncologist identifies normal anatomy and tumor on each slice of the treatment-planning CT scan, and a computer program superimposes these data onto a standard radiograph (Fig. 20–1). When this is demonstrated from an angle at which the beam will be aimed at the body, this is said to be a "beam's eye view." The ability to precisely visualize the relationship of the beam to soft tissue anatomy and tumor has been a critical step forward in radiation treatment planning that provides greater assurance that the tumor is being fully enclosed in the treated area while enhancing the ability to exclude critical normal tissues.

Definition of the extent of the tumor requires integration of data obtained from a variety of radiologic studies and procedures. The use of CT scans can depict the radial extension of the primary disease that cannot be visualized on barium studies. In addition, because barium studies can also underestimate the longitudinal extent of disease, all available data from endoscopy and ultrasound should be integrated into the planning process. The extent of nodal disease should be evaluated by CT and endoscopy with ultrasound. When appropriate, pathologic assessment of nodal disease can be obtained by ultrasound-guided needle biopsy, laparoscopy, or both. It is unknown whether there is a benefit to elective treatment of clinically uninvolved supraclavicular nodes for proximal lesions or celiac nodes for distal lesions.

Typical external-beam radiation treatments are produced by a linear accelerator or a cobalt radiation source contained in the treatment machine and delivered through the head of the machine. The beam is shaped to the targeted area by metal alloy blocks custom made for each patient's anatomy to appropriately shape the beam in the same way a light beam can be shaped by any opaque material placed in front of the bulb (Fig. 20–2). In simple situations, the beam may be aimed from the front and back of the patient. This approach limits the problem of excessive dose near the surface of the patient, which would occur when the beam is aimed from just

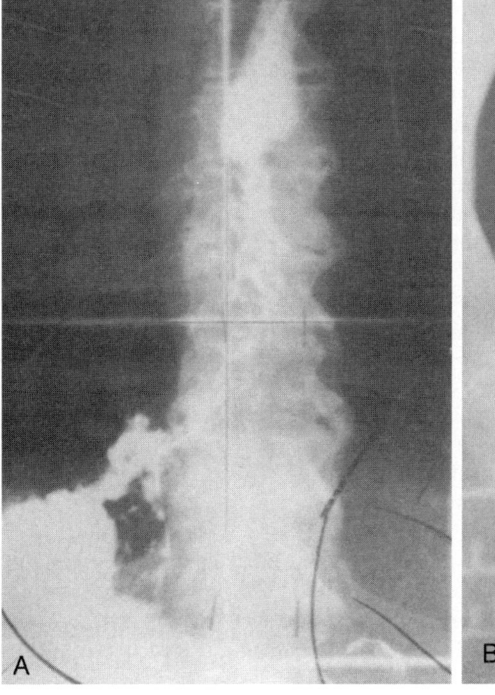

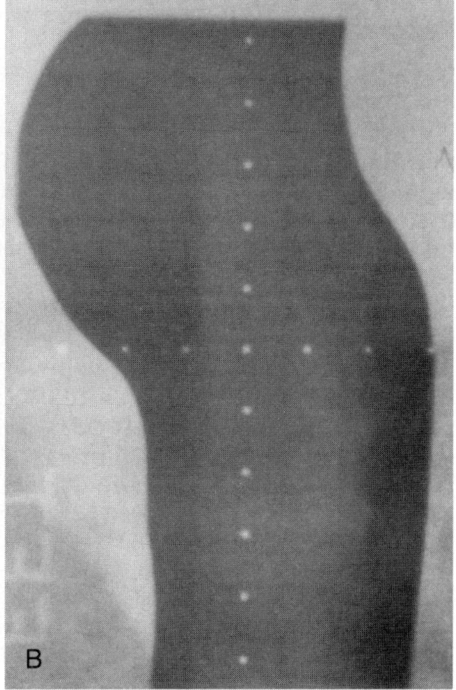

Figure 20–2. A conventional simulation radiograph showing an outline of the blocks that shield spinal cord and other normal tissue.

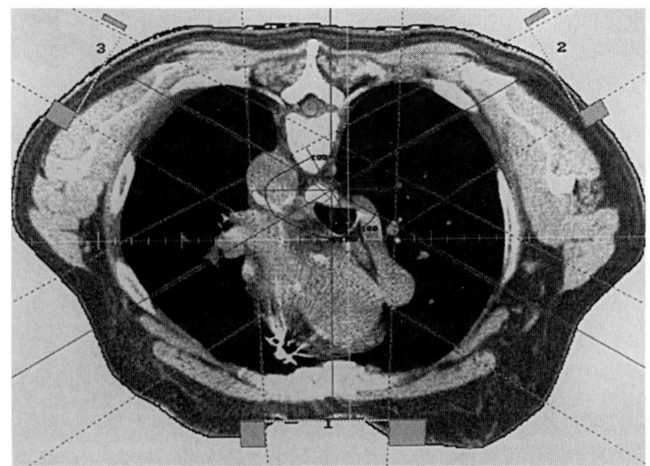

Figure 20–3. A treatment plan showing radiation beams aimed from three directions. *Circled area*, The region to which the prescribed dose of radiation will be prescribed. The irradiated regions of lung receive only 20 to 40% of the prescribed dose delivered to the esophagus.

one side (a high dose would have to be administered to that surface so the planned dose will penetrate to the tumor deep in the body). In more complex situations, the beam is aimed from multiple directions. Only at the point at which all of the beams overlap will the full radiation dose be deposited, and the normal tissues outside this area will receive only limited radiation doses (Fig. 20–3).

When possible, patients should be simulated and treated in the prone position, which has been documented to increase the distance between the esophagus and the spinal cord by a mean of 1.3 to 1.9 cm depending on the position along the thoracic esophagus. The difference tended to be greater for lesions distal to the carina.[73] Increasing the distance between the esophagus and spinal cord enhances the ability to deliver an adequate dose to the target while limiting the dose to the spinal cord. However, when the prone position is not tolerated, acceptable dose delivery is usually possible with the patient supine.

Computerized treatment planning systems depict the dose distribution within the patient. With standard "two-dimensional" treatment planning, the dose distribution is generally depicted on several representative selected planes or slices through the patient's anatomy. Information about the patient's surface shape, size, and internal anatomy; the position of the radiation field edges; and the characteristics of the beam of the treatment machine are used to determine how the dose will be distributed in the patient. If the dose distribution is not satisfactory, block positions, the proportion of dose contributed from each beam direction, and beam angles or number of beams can be altered to improve the treatment plan. Special devices (wedges and compensators) that attenuate radiation can be placed in the radiation beam to selectively alter the dose delivered to defined portions of the treatment area. Inaccuracies can be introduced because most treatment plans do not take account of the fact that different types of tissue (e.g., soft tissue, bone, lung) have different electron density and therefore attenuate the RT beam to differing extents. In addition, because the plan is only displayed for selected representative slices through the patient, the potential does exist for significantly underdosing of the tumor or overdosing of normal tissues in the areas that are not depicted.

The availability of inexpensive powerful computers allows the dosimetry problems described here to be solved through a depiction of dose distribution over the entire area of interest. With the availability of increased processing power on workstations or desktop computers, it is possible to make more extensive and sophisticated dose calculations. With traditional two-dimensional treatment planning. it is necessary to select several slices through the targeted area where the dose distribution would be calculated. The dose distribution is then extrapolated to the intervening areas by the physician. This technology also limits the possible radiation beam angles. because all fields must be treated in a single plane. With three-dimensional treatment planning, the dose is calculated at every pixel in the target volume, and therefore the dose to all portions of the tumor and normal tissues will be known more precisely. Pixel-by-pixel corrections for differing absorption of RT by different tissues can also be performed.

With inverse treatment planning, a newer technology that is under development, the physician can specify doses to a targeted area and dose limits for normal tissues, and then sophisticated computer algorithms are used to identify potential optimal solutions to blocking location, beam angle, number of beams, and dose from each beam direction. With intensity-modulated radiation therapy, another new technology under development, individual portions of the beam coming from a particular direction can be varied to allow more precise delivery of the expected dose.

Ultimately, improved targeting may improve outcome by ensuring that the target is effectively treated. It also may allow the ratio of dose to tumor surrounding normal tissue to be improved, allowing safe dose escalation, which may change the chances of tumor control. Finally, because the full three-dimensional anatomy of the patient is used in planning, it is possible to more accurately account for the differing attenuation of the RT beam by different body tissues. Clinical trials are ongoing for a variety of tumor types to determine whether the application of these technologies will actually improve outcome.

In any event, with all treatment plans and regardless of the technology is used, care must be taken to keep normal tissue doses and volumes within safe limits and to take account of varying thickness of the chest longitudinally. Wedges and compensators placed in the radiation beam should be used as needed to maintain homogeneity of the RT dose distribution by attenuating the radiation beam in areas where the body is thinner. The spinal cord should be limited to approximately 45 Gy, and the dose to large volumes of lung tissue should be minimized. Occasionally, it may be necessary to alter the beam arrangement to avoid excessive risk to the heart, but that is an unusual circumstance.

On each treatment day, the patient is precisely positioned with respect to the treatment machine using the reference marks placed on the skin at simulation. This ensures that the beam will be aimed properly. The head of the machine, as well as the treatment couch, can be rotated to allow the beam to be aimed from most directions. Generally, the beam will be turned on for only several minutes, and the patient will be in the treatment room for 15 to 30 minutes each day. Most of the time is spent in accurately positioning the patient and ensuring precise aim of the beam.

When definitive RT is used, treatment fields extend a minimum of 5 cm above and below the radiographically identifiable lesion to account for microscopic or submucosal tumor extension. If definitive RT is used to doses above 50 Gy with or without chemotherapy, a "cone-down" to a margin of 2 cm above and 2 cm below the tumor should be considered to limit toxicity while still focusing on the area of greatest tumor burden. A radial margin of 2.5 to 3.0 cm is generally used, but this may be limited posteriorly as needed to keep the spinal cord dose within tolerance. These margins are defined by the edges of the alloy blocks that shape the radiation field. It should be emphasized that the full dose of RT is not deposited at the block edge and the dose is actually about 50% at that point compared with the center of the field. The dose generally builds up to nearly 100% within 0.5 to 1 cm distant in from the block edge. In addition, it is generally possible to position the patient each day with an accuracy of only 0.25 to 0.5 cm. For these reasons, the radiation field as defined by the beam-shaping blocks must always be larger than the actual target.

A three- or four-field approach with an anterior and two posterior oblique off-cord fields with or without the addition of a fourth posterior field is a standard approach in the treatment of esophageal cancer and allows high doses to be delivered to the tumor while limiting the radiation dose delivered to the spinal cord and lung (see Fig. 20-3). When such arrangements with beams aimed from several directions are used, dose to normal tissues can be quite effectively limited: only where all of the beams cross will the full dose to be delivered. The dose delivered by the treatment fields should be weighted such that the maximal possible dose (that which delivers up to 45 Gy to the spinal cord) is delivered by the anterior and/or posterior fields, whereas only the remainder of the dose is delivered by the off-cord oblique fields to minimize dose to the lung tissue, which is sensitive to low doses of radiation. This beam arrangement can also be used for the treatment of upper esophageal tumors, because none of the beams enter laterally through the arms and shoulders. All fields can be treated from the first day of treatment, which has the advantage of delivering a lower fractional daily dose to uninvolved structures such as the lung. Alternatively, treatment can begin with anteroposterior/posteroanterior fields only, which may allow a quicker start to treatment while a more complex beam plan is developed, allow more margin for error in daily patient setup, and decrease daily treatment time. Under the latter circumstance, the multifield plan is generally implemented at a dose of no more than 30 to 36 Gy, well before tolerance of the spinal cord is approached.

When preoperative or postoperative RT is administered to the limited dose of 44 to 45 Gy, we generally use anteroposterior/posteroanterior fields to a total dose of 36 to 40 Gy, with the remainder of the dose given by opposed lateral off-cord fields. With this simple approach, the spinal cord dose is kept below tolerance levels. If all treatment is administered anteroposteriorly/posteroanteriorly, care must be taken that the spinal cord dose is kept to a safe limit. The spine can be relatively superficial and may receive a significantly higher dose than the "midplane" of the body, which received the planned 44 to 45 Gy.

Toxicities of Radiotherapy

In general, the actual administration of treatment is not associated with any discomfort at the time of RT administration, and the treatment of a given day is rarely associated with immediate worsening of any side effect. The acute toxicities of therapeutic radiation build gradually over weeks from a cumulative effect of the administered treatment on proliferating normal tissues. The late toxicities of RT do not seem to be related to whether the patient experienced significant acute effects, and they are thought to be the result of long-term radiation injury to microvasculature.

Each day, the patient is positioned on the treatment couch, which has a hard tabletop to enable precise positioning. The actual radiation treatment is not associated with any abnormal sensations, much like ordinary radiography. However, as the weeks of treatment proceed, short-term side effects develop.

Patients experience a marked esophagitis that increases during radiation treatment; this usually first occurs several weeks into therapy and clears within several weeks after the conclusion of therapy. In RTOG trial 8501,[7] toxicity data with both radiation alone and combined chemoradiotherapy were prospectively collected. Five percent of patients treated with 60 Gy RT alone developed grade III or greater acute esophagitis, whereas 20% of those treated with concurrent chemoradiotherapy developed these symptoms. Topical anesthetics, narcotics, and H_2-blockers are used to minimize discomfort during feeding. Oral nutritional supplements should be used to maintain nutritional state. Feeding tubes can be placed before therapy.

Other common mild short-term effects include redness, irritation, or darkening of the skin; fatigue; decreased blood counts; hair loss in the treated area; and chest discomfort. Nausea and vomiting is unlikely but possible if a significant portion of the stomach is treated. Pneumonitis is uncommon from radiation for esophageal cancer.

Esophageal stricture is the most common significant late toxicity of RT, potentially occurring months or years after treatment is completed. Benign stricture is reported to occur in 12 to 30% of curatively treated patients,[4,66,74,75] although experience shows that most long-term strictures are associated with recurrent tumor rather than with the radiation. Dilatation and/or stent placement can be used safely in the treatment of radiation stricture.[76] The median time to development of stricture is reported to be 6 months, although it can certainly occur much later.[74] In RTOG trial 8501,[7] late esophageal toxicity was observed in 10 of 53 patients treated only with radiation versus 11 of 51 patients treated with chemoradiation, but the nature of these events was not described.

Long-term esophageal toxicity includes not only strictures but also esophageal motility disorders, potentially leading to reflux, delayed emptying, or spasm. Motility disorders,[77-79] which can actually occur shortly after the completion of treatment, are common. These disorders rarely cause an atonic esophagus but are characterized by failure of the primary peristaltic wave in the area of RT with repetitive nonperistaltic waves occurring distal to the interruption. Failure of distal esophageal sphincter relaxation can occur. Prokinetic drugs such as metoclopramide can be used, potentially improving any resulting symptoms. If esophageal spasm occurs, nitrates, calcium channel antagonists, and anticholinergic drugs can be used. Other long-term radiation effects are uncommon but can include rupture of the esophagus, fistula formation, or lung fibrosis, causing shortness of breath. Radiation-induced malignancy is extremely rare.

It is important to note that patients treated with combined-modality therapies will also be at risk for other long- and short-term toxicities of chemotherapy, such as myelosuppression. In RTOG trial 8501,[7] severe and life-threatening acute complications occurred in 44 and 20% of patients who received chemoradiotherapy but only 25 and 3% of those who received RT alone, respectively. Most of those toxicities were acute esophagitis or hematologic toxicities. There was no observed increase in late severe complications.

Brachytherapy in Curative and Palliative Treatment

Brachytherapy involves the use of radioisotopes placed in the lumen of the esophagus to provide radiation to a small volume without any need to radiate overlying tissues. Typically, ^{192}Ir, with an average photon energy of 0.38 MeV, is used. Radiation emitted by iridium is 50% attenuated by 6.3 cm of tissue. More important, the dose of radiation falls inversely to the distance from a radioactive source, so the dose delivered 2 cm from a single radioactive iridium source will be less than 25% of the dose given at 1 cm. When there is a line of sources rather than a single point source, the dose falloff with distance is reduced but is still quite dramatic. In this way, large doses of RT can be administered without regard to other organs. However, dose escalation by brachytherapy is limited by the potential for injury resulting from the high dose of radiation administered to the esophagus itself. The techniques, potential benefits, and toxicities of brachytherapy are reviewed here.

First, a catheter of 0.6- to 1-cm width is inserted in the esophagus. The region to be treated is identified endoscopically or with barium. Radioactive sources are inserted into the catheter so as to treat the target with a 1- to 2-cm margin proximally and distally. The dose is prescribed at a distance of 1 cm from the radioactive sources, and dose falloff beyond this range is rapid with higher doses administered to closer areas. As discussed earlier, the dose rapidly falls with distance from the source by attenuation in tissue and, more importantly, by an inverse relationship with the square of the distance from the source. As a result, the dose delivered to any tissue abutting the radioactive source might be significantly higher than the dose prescribed at 1 cm from the source, whereas at farther distances, the dose might be subtherapeutic. This is in contrast to the situation with external-beam RT, where the dose throughout the target volume is fairly homogeneous (±5 to 10%). Therefore, only patients with tumor primarily confined to the esophageal wall and lumen itself can be effectively and durably treated or palliated with this approach.

Brachytherapy can be administered for esophageal cancer using high- or low-dose-rate techniques. High-dose-rate brachytherapy uses short intense applications (similar dose rate as external-beam RT) of several minutes, which are more convenient for the patient and do not require inpatient care. However, an expensive remote control device is required to automatically insert the radioactive source the appropriate distance down the endoluminal catheter. With the high doses of radiation emitted in just seconds from such an active source, manual loading is unsafe for medical personnel who would be at substantial risk from repeated exposures. In addition, because the consequences of misalignment of the source in the patient for even 1 minute or less can be significant, the remote device has many fail-safe features that cause immediate retraction if any abnormality is detected. Because high-dose-rate treatments may have a somewhat higher risk to normal tissues, treatment is frequently administered over several sessions or fractions, although the need for this precaution is controversial. With low-dose-rate brachytherapy, in which treatment is administered at 0.4 to 1.0 Gy/hr, treatment is administered with one to two insertions of the applicator but over a total treatment time of 24 to 48 hours. Although this approach does require overnight admission and prolonged esophageal intubation, fewer applications may be needed and the technology is more widely available. With low-dose-rate treatment, the radiation exposure from handling the low-activity sources for only a few minutes to insert it into the endoesophageal catheter is low. Therefore, manual insertion without the need for expensive automated equipment and special shielding is feasible.

Dose escalation, when RT is used as a single modality in curative therapy, has been safely carried out by the addition of brachytherapy, although there has been no clearly demonstrated benefit in survival and only a suggestion of improved local control[18,80-82] with the limited available data. Nevertheless, it is a reasonable option to add brachytherapy in patients treated with RT alone when the entirety of residual disease can be encompassed in the treated volume with the goal of improving local control. The American Brachytherapy Society Clinical Research Committee has published guidelines[83] suggesting that a good candidate for brachytherapy has tumor of 10 cm or less confined to the thoracic esophagus and without regional nodes. When brachytherapy is used, the external-beam dose is generally limited to 45 to 50 Gy in 1.8- to 2.0-Gy fractions, followed in 1 to 2 weeks by two or three weekly treatments of 5 Gy or by a single low-dose-rate brachytherapy application of 20 Gy over 24 to

48 hours. The dose is prescribed to 1 cm from the midpoint of the treatment catheter, as discussed earlier.

Brachytherapy can be most useful in selected cases for palliative treatment of esophageal cancer. For relief of obstructive symptoms, brachytherapy can be used in addition to, as an alternative to, or in patients previously treated with external-beam RT.[17] Several palliative regimens have been recommended as appropriate by the American Brachytherapy Society Consensus Guidelines panel.[17] In previously untreated patients, a limited dose of external-beam RT (i.e., 30 cGy) can be followed by high-dose-rate brachytherapy (10 to 14 Gy in one or two fractions) or low-dose-rate brachytherapy (20 to 25 Gy in a single application over 1 to 2 days). If life expectancy is judged to be 6 months or greater, conventional radiation doses of 45 to 50 Gy over 4 to 5 weeks can be used in hopes of increasing the durability of the response. Palliation occurs in 50 to 90% of cases with brachytherapy alone.[67,68,79] Dysphagia was palliated by external-beam RT followed by brachytherapy in 90% of patients in one series,[60] but the relative benefits of this approach compared with external-beam RT alone are unknown. On the other hand, brachytherapy alone can be used for palliation when life expectancy is short or when external-beam RT has been used in the past. Appropriate regimens for brachytherapy alone include high-dose-rate treatment of 15 to 20 Gy in two to four applications or low-dose-rate treatment of 25 to 40 Gy over 1 to 2 days. For patients with a poor prognosis, high-dose-rate brachytherapy of 15 Gy in one session, which also results in palliation in close to 70% of patients,[67,84] may also be an appropriate regimen. Therefore, another benefit to brachytherapy as an alternative to external-beam RT in palliative therapy is a reduced number of visits to the hospital.

The toxicities with brachytherapy have not been well quantified. One series of 148 patients treated with external-beam RT of 60 Gy over 6 weeks followed 1 week later by 12 Gy high-dose-rate brachytherapy in two fractions demonstrated 28% ulceration, 10% stricture, and 6% fistula. Except for fistula, which was generally fatal, the other complications were rarely severe.[85] In patients who are treated curatively with 60-Gy external-beam RT followed by high-dose-rate brachytherapy of 12 Gy in two fractions, one series with routine endoscopic follow-up found a 50% incidence of esophageal ulceration that usually healed with conservative management and rarely became severe.[86] Brachytherapy can be safely administered several weeks after laser therapy and may improve the dysphagia-free interval,[87-89] whereas its role with photodynamic therapy is uncertain.

In RTOG trial 9207,[17] the concept of adding brachytherapy of 5 Gy for three high-dose-rate treatments to chemoradiotherapy (as in RTOG trial 8501) was tested, but the incidence of fistula was 6 of 35, and this approach is not recommended. In that trial, chemotherapy was administered during the period when brachytherapy was also administered. There is limited information that brachytherapy, especially to a lower dose, after the completion of chemotherapy and RT may be safer[90] or that other less-intense regimens of concurrent chemotherapy, RT, and brachytherapy may be tolerable.[18,91]

CLINICAL AND RADIOLOGIC ASSESSMENT OF RESPONSE TO RADIOTHERAPY

Accurate post-RT staging could potentially be used in the selection of patients who might benefit from additional treatments with chemotherapy, surgery, or brachytherapy and in the identification of those who may not need further intervention. It is difficult to radiographically assess response to chemoradiation (or radiation) for esophageal cancer in the period immediately after treatment. The accuracy of postradiation imaging in the modern era has been examined for patients treated with preoperative chemoradiotherapy where pathologic correlation with imaging studies is available. Perhaps as a result of the gradual response to RT as well as inflammation and edema, neither CT nor ultrasound is accurate in the assessment of T stage or in the prediction of complete response.

In a prospective study of 50 patients,[92] CT after preoperative chemoradiotherapy proved inaccurate in determining T stage in the majority of patients—36% of patients were overstaged and 20% were understaged. Assessment of response using standard bidimensional tumor measurements was also highly inaccurate, with a sensitivity of 65%, a specificity of 33%, a positive predictive value of 58%, and a negative predictive value of 41%. Six of 12 patients who were thought to have stable disease on CT scan actually had pathologically complete response.

Endoscopy with ultrasound has also not proved to be helpful in assessment of the response, although it may be more helpful than CT or standard endoscopy with biopsy. In one series, 48% of patients with no evidence of tumor on standard endoscopy had positive pathologic specimens at surgery.[92a] This has lead to the search for ultrasound criteria that may be predictive. Investigators at the University of Verona[93] have reported a 48% accuracy rate in determining the extent of invasion and a 71% accuracy rate in assessing nodal stage after chemoradiotherapy. In a report from the Paoli-Calmettes Institute in Marseilles[94] that assessed response by ultrasound in T3 and T4 lesions, complete restitution of wall layers with or without an associated finding of echo-poor nodules located in the submucosa or muscularis propria was associated with a complete response in 78% of cases. Although more extensive disease on ultrasound could not be used to definitively assess actual T stage, residual tumor was histologically confirmed in 87% of the other cases. This same group found that in patients treated with chemoradiotherapy for squamous cell carcinoma, those with endoscopic complete response by this criterion had a mean survival of 49 months compared with 10 months for those with more advanced findings.[95] Another study has suggested that large decreases in measured cross-sectional area of tumor by ultrasound may be predictive of response.[96] These findings require independent corroboration in large series before they can be incorporated into clinical practice.

Therefore, radiographic or endoscopic response cannot be used at the present time to guide therapeutic decisions or provide prognostic information. Only surgical findings can be used to assess response with accuracy.

When patients are treated with definitive RT or chemoradiotherapy, we generally wait at least 3 months to perform endoscopy with or without ultrasound to allow inflammation to subside and completion of response to RT. Post-treatment scanning is performed at 4 to 6 weeks to obtain a new post-RT baseline, to determine whether bulky disease is shrinking, and to evaluate for progression of disease and development of distant metastasis. There have been no prospective studies to evaluate whether this is optimal timing.

References

1. Newaishy, G.A., Read, G.A., Duncan, W., Kerr, G.R.: Results of radical radiotherapy of squamous cell carcinoma of the oesophagus. Clin. Radiol., *33*:347, 1982.
2. De-Ren, S.: Ten-year follow-up of esophageal cancer treated by radical radiation therapy: Analysis of 869 patients. Int. J. Radiat. Oncol. Biol. Phys., *16*:329, 1989.
3. Okawa, T., Kita, M., Tanaka, M., and Ikeda, M.: Results of radiotherapy for inoperable locally advanced esophageal cancer. Int. J. Radiat. Oncol. Biol. Phys., *17*:49, 1989.
4. Sykes, A.J., Burt, P.A., Slevin, N.J., et al.: Radical radiotherapy for carcinoma of the oesophagus: An effective alternative to surgery. Radiother. Oncol., *48*:15, 1998.
5. Coia, L.R., Engstrom, P.F., Paul, A.R., et al.: Long-term results of infusional 5-FU, mitomycin-C, and radiation as primary management of esophageal carcinoma. Int. J. Radiat. Oncol. Biol. Phys., *20*:29, 1991.
6. Smith, T.J., Ryan, L.M., Douglass, H.Q., et al.: Combined chemotherapy vs. radiotherapy alone for early stage squamous cell carcinoma of the esophagus: A study of the Eastern Cooperative Oncology Group. Int. J. Radiat. Oncol. Biol. Phys., *42*:269, 1998.
7. Herskovic, A., Martz, K., Al-Sarraf, M., et al.: Combined chemotherapy and radiotherapy compared with radiotherapy alone in patients with cancer of the esophagus. N. Engl. J. Med., *326*:1593, 1992.
8. Al-Sarraf, M., Martz, K., Herskovic, L., et al.: Progress report of combined chemoradiotherapy versus radiotherapy alone in patients with esophageal cancer: An Intergroup study. J. Clin. Oncol., *15*:277, 1997.
9. Emami, B., Lyman, J., Brown, A., et al.: Tolerance of normal tissue of therapeutic irradiation. Int. J. Radiat. Oncol. Biol. Phys., *21*:109, 1991.
10. Cooper, J.S., Guo, M.D., Herskovic, A., et al.: Chemoradiotherapy of locally advanced esophageal cancer: long-term follow-up of a prospective randomized trial (RTOG 8501): Radiation Therapy Oncology Group. JAMA, *281*:1623, 1999.
11. Araujo, C.M.M., Souhami, L., Gil, R.A., et al.: A randomized trial comparing radiation therapy vs concomitant radiation therapy and chemotherapy in carcinoma of the thoracic esophagus. Cancer, *67*:2258, 1991.
12. Roussel, A., Jacob, J.H., Jung, G.M., et al.: Controlled clinical trial for the treatment of patients with inoperable esophageal carcinoma: A study of the EORTC gastrointestinal tract cancer cooperative group. *In* Schlag, P., Hohenberger, P., and Metzger, U. (eds.): Recent Results in Cancer Research, 1st ed. Berlin, Springer-Verlag, 1988, p. 21.
13. Nygaard, K., Hagen, S., Hansen, H.S., et al.: Pre-operative radiotherapy prolongs survival in operable esophageal carcinoma: A randomized, multicenter study of pre-operative radiotherapy and chemotherapy: The Second Scandinavian Trial in Esophageal Cancer. World J. Surg., *16*:1104, 1992.
14. Slabber, C.F., Nel, J.S., Schoeman, L., et al.: A randomized study of radiotherapy alone vs radiotherapy plus 5-fluorouracil and platinum in patients with inoperable, locally advanced squamous cell cancer of the esophagus. Am. J. Clin. Oncol. (CCT), *21*:462, 1998.
15. Chan, A., and Wong, A.: Is combined chemotherapy and radiation therapy equally effective as surgical resection in localized esophageal carcinoma? Int. J. Radiat. Oncol. Biol. Phys., *45*:265, 1999.
16. Murakami, M., Kuroda, Y., Nakajima, T., et al.: Comparison between chemoradiation protocol intended for organ preservation and conventional surgery for clinical T1–T2 esophageal carcinoma. Int. J. Radiat. Oncol. Biol. Phys., *45*:277,

16a. Minsky, B.D., Kelsen, D.P., Ginsberg, R., et al.: Preliminary results of Intergroup 0123 Randomized Trial of Combined Modality Therapy for esophageal cancer: standard vs. high dose radiation therapy. Proc. A.S.C.O. 927, 2000.

17. Gaspar, L.E., Qian, C., Kocha, W.I., et al.: A phase I/II study of external beam radiation, brachytherapy and concurrent chemotherapy in localized cancer of the esophagus (RTOG 92-07): Preliminary toxicity report. Int. J. Radiat. Oncol. Biol. Phys., *37*:593, 1997.
18. Yorozu, A., Takushi, D., and Oki, Y.: High-dose-rate brachytherapy boost following concurrent chemoradiotherapy for esophageal carcinoma. Int. J. Radiat. Oncol. Biol. Phys., *45*:271, 1999.
19. Poplin, E.A., Jacobson, J., Herskovic, A., et al.: Evaluation of multimodality treatment of locoregional esophageal carcinoma by Southwest Oncology Group 9060. Cancer, *78*:1851, 1996.
20. Minsky, B.D., Neuberg, D., Kelsen, D., et al.: Neoadjuvant chemotherapy plus concurrent chemotherapy and high-dose radiation for squamous cell carcinoma of the esophagus—A preliminary analysis of the phase II Intergroup trial 0122. J. Clin. Oncol., *14*:149, 1996.
21. Valerdi, J.J., Tejedor, M., Illarramendi, J.J., et al.: Neoadjuvant chemotherapy and radiotherapy in locally advanced esophagus carcinoma: Long-term results. Int. J. Radiat. Oncol. Biol. Phys., *27*:843, 1994.
22. Roca, E., Pennella, E., Sardi, M., et al.: Combined intensive chemoradiotherapy for organ preservation in patients with resectable and nonresectable oesophageal cancer. Eur. J. Cancer, *32A*:429, 1996.
23. Stuschke, M., Stahl, M., Wilke, H., et al.: Induction chemotherapy followed by concurrent chemotherapy and high-dose radiotherapy for locally advanced squamous cell carcinoma of the cervical oesophagus. Oncology, *57*:99, 1999.
24. Gignoux, M., Roussel, A., Paillot, B., et al.: The value of preoperative radiotherapy in esophageal cancer: Results of a study of the E.O.R.T.C. World J. Surg., *11*:426, 1987.
25. Arnott, S.J., Duncan, W., Kerr, G.R., et al.: Low dose preoperative radiotherapy for carcinoma of the oesophagus: Results of a randomized clinical trial. Radiother. Oncol., *24*:108, 1992.
26. Nygaard, K., Hagen, S., Hansen, H.S., et al.: Pre-operative radiotherapy prolongs survival in operable esophageal carcinoma: A randomized., multicenter study of pre-operative radiotherapy and chemotherapy: The second Scandinavian Trial in Esophageal Cancer. World J. Surg., *16*:1104, 1992.
27. Launois, B., Delarue, D., Campion, J.P., et al.: Preoperative radiotherapy for carcinoma of the esophagus. Surg. Gynecol. Obstet., *153*:690, 1981.
28. Huang, G.J., Gu, X.Z., Wang, L.J., et al.: Combined preoperative irradiation and surgery for esophageal carcinoma. *In* Delarue, N.C. (ed.): International Trends in General Thoracic Surgery, 1st ed. St. Louis, C.V. Mosby, 1988, p. 315.
29. Arnott, S.J., Duncan, W., Gignous, M., et al.: Preoperative radiotherapy in esophageal carcinoma: A meta-analysis using individual patient data (oesophageal cancer collaborative group). Int. J. Radiat. Oncol. Biol. Phys., *41*:579, 1998.
30. Kelsen, D.P., Ginsberg, R., Pajak, T.F., et al.: Chemotherapy followed by surgery compared with surgery alone for localized esophageal cancer. N. Engl. J. Med., *339*:1979, 1998.
31. Walsh, T.N., Noonan, N., Hollywood, D., et al.: A comparison of multimodal therapy and surgery for esophageal adenocarcinoma. N. Engl. J. Med., *335*:462, 1996.
32. Urba, S., Orringer, M., Turrisi, A., et al.: A randomized trial comparing surgery (S) to preoperative concomitant chemoradiation plus surgery in patients (pts) with resectable esophageal cancer (CA): Updated analysis. Proc. A.S.C.O., 983, 1997. Abstract.
33. Bossett, J.F., Gignoux, M., Triboulet, J.P., et al.: Chemoradiotherapy followed by surgery compared with surgery alone in squamous-cell cancer of the esophagus. N. Engl. J. Med., *337*:161, 1997.
34. Stahl, M., Wilke, H., Fink, U., et al.: Combined preoperative chemotherapy and radiotherapy in patients with locally advanced esophageal cancer: Interim analysis of a phase II trial. J. Clin. Oncol., *14*:829, 1995.
35. Orringer, M.B., Forastiere, A.A., Perez-Tamayo, C., et al.: Chemotherapy and radiation therapy before transhiatal esophagectomy for esophageal carcinoma. Ann. Thorac. Surg., *49*:348, 1990.
36. Ganem, G., Dubray, B., Raoul, Y., et al.: Concomitant chemoradiotherapy followed, where feasible, by surgery for cancer of the esophagus. J. Clin. Oncol., *15*:701, 1997.

37. Leichman, L., Steiger, Z., Seydel, H.G., et al.: Combined preoperative chemotherapy and radiation therapy for cancer of the esophagus: The Wayne State University Southwest Oncology Group and Radiation Therapy Oncology Group experience. Semin. Oncol., *11:*178, 1984.
38. Poplin, E., Fleming, T., Leichman, L., et al.: Combined therapies for squamous-cell carcinoma of the esophagus: A Southwest Oncology Group Study. J. Clin. Oncol., *5:*622, 1987.
39. Bates, B.A., Detterbeck, F.C., Bernard, S.A., et al.: Concurrent radiation therapy and chemotherapy followed by esophagectomy for localized esophageal carcinoma. J. Clin. Oncol., *14:*156, 1996.
40. Jones, D.R., Detterbeck, F.C., Egan, T.M., et al.: Induction chemoradiotherapy followed by esophagectomy in patients with carcinoma of the esophagus. Ann. Thorac. Surg., *64:*185, 1997.
41. Stewart, J.R., Hoff, S.J., Johnson, D.H., et al.: Improved survival with neoadjuvant therapy and resection for adenocarcinoma of the esophagus. Ann. Surg., *218:*571, 1993.
42. Malhaire, J.P., Labat, J.P., Lozac'h, P., et al.: Preoperative concomitant radiochemotherapy in squamous cell carcinoma of the esophagus: Results of a study of 56 patients. Int. J. Radiat. Oncol. Biol. Phys., *34:*429, 1996.
43. Algan, O., Coia, R.L., Keller, S.T., et al.: Management of adenocarcinoma of the esophagus with chemoradiation alone or chemoradiation followed by esophagectomy: Results of sequential nonrandomized phase II studies. Int. J. Radiat. Oncol. Biol. Phys., *32:*753, 1995.
44. Adelstein, D.J., Rice, T.W., Becker, M., et al.: Use of concurrent chemotherapy, accelerated fractionation radiation, and surgery for patients with esophageal carcinoma. Cancer, *80:*1011, 1997.
45. Gill, P.G., Denham, J.W., Jamieson, G.G., et al.: Patterns of treatment failure and prognostic factors associated with the treatment of esophageal carcinoma with chemotherapy and radiotherapy either as sole treatment or followed by surgery. J. Clin. Oncol., *10:*1037, 1992.
46. Forastiere, A.A., Heitmiller, R.F., Lee, D.J., et al.: Intensive chemoradiation followed by esophagectomy for squamous cell and adenocarcinoma of the esophagus. Cancer J. Sci. Am., *3:*155, 1997.
47. Heath, E.Z., Burtnesss, B.A., Heitmiller, R.F., et al.: Phase II evaluation of preoperative chemoradiation and post-operative adjuvant chemotherapy for squamous cell carcinoma and adenocarcinoma of the esophagus. J. Clin. Oncol., in press, 2000.
48. Kleinberg, L.R., Knisley, J.P.S., Heitmiller, R., et al.: Long term local control and survival with preoperative cisplatin, continuous infusion 5-FU, and 45 GY radiotherapy for esophageal cancer. Int. J. Radiat. Oncol. Biol. Phys., *45:*189, 1999.
49. Forastiere, A.A., Heitmiller, R., Kleinberg, L.R., et al.: Long follow-up of patients with esophageal cancer treated with preoperative cisplatin/5-FU and concurrent radiation. Proc. Am. Soc. Clin. Oncol., 1999.
50. Macfarlane, S.D., Hill, L.D., Jolly, P.C., et al.: Improved results of surgical treatment for esophageal and gastroesophageal junction carcinomas after preoperative combined chemotherapy and radiation. J. Thorac. Cardiovasc. Surg., *95:*415, 1988.
51. Kavanagh, B., Anscher, M., Leopold, K., et al.: Patterns of failure following combined modality therapy for esophageal cancer, 1984. Int. J. Radiat. Oncol. Biol. Phys., *24:*633, 1992.
52. Whittington, R., Coia, L.R., Haller, D.G., et al.: Adenocarcinoma of the esophagus and esophago-gastric junction: The effects of single and combined modalities on the survival and patterns of failure following treatment. Int. J. Radiat. Oncol. Biol. Phys., *19:*593, 1990.
53. Chidel, M.A., Rice, T.W., Adelstein, D.J., et al.: Resectable esophageal carcinoma: Local control with neoadjuvant chemotherapy and radiation therapy. Radiology, *213:*67, 1999.
54. Keller, S.M., Ryan, L., Coia, L.R., et al.: High-dose chemoradiotherapy followed by esophagectomy for adenocarcinoma of the esophagus and gastroesophageal junction: Results of a phase II study of the Eastern Cooperative Oncology Group. Cancer, *83:*1908, 1998.
55. Herskovic, A., Leichman, L., Lattin, P., et al.: Chemo/radiation with and without surgery in the thoracic esophagus: The Wayne State experience. Int. J. Radiat. Oncol. Biol. Phys., *15:*655, 1998.
56. Teniere, P., Hay, J.M., Fingerhut, A., et al.: Postoperative radiation therapy does not increase survival after curative resection for squamous cell carcinoma of the middle and lower esophagus as shown by a multicenter controlled trial. Surg. Gynecol. Obstet., *173:*123, 1991.
57. Fok, M., Sham, J.S.T., Choy, D., et al.: Postoperative radiotherapy for carcinoma of the esophagus: A prospective randomized controlled study. Surgery, *113:*138, 1993.
58. Nyambi, E., Kang, H.J., Millikan, K., et al.: Integration of surgery in multimodality therapy for esophageal cancer. Am. J. Clin. Oncol., *20:*11, 1997.
59. Yamamoto, M., Yamashita, T., Matsubara, T., et al.: Reevaluation of postoperative radiotherapy for thoracic esophageal carcinoma. Int. J. Radiat. Oncol. Biol. Phys., *37:*75, 1997.
60. Wara, W.M., Mauch, P.M., Thomas, A.N., and Phillips, T.L.: Palliation for carcinoma of the esophagus. Radiology, *121:*717, 1976.
61. O'Rourke, C., McNeil, R.J., Walker, P.J., and Bull, C.A.: Objective evaluation of the quality of palliation in patients with esophageal cancer comparing surgery, radiotherapy and intubation. Aust. N.Z. J. Surg., *62:*922, 1992.
62. Roussel, A., Jacob, J.H., Jung, G.M., et al.: Controlled clinical trial for the treatment of patients with inoperable esophageal carcinoma: A study of the EORTC Gastrointestinal Tract Cancer Cooperative Group. *In* Schlag, P., Hohenberger, P., and Metzger, U. (eds.): Recent Results in Cancer Research, lst ed. Berlin, Springer-Verlag, 1988, p. 21.
63. Petrovich, Z., Langholz, B., Formenti, S., et al.: Management of carcinoma of the esophagus: The role of radiotherapy. Am. J. Clin. Oncol. (CCT), *14:*80, 1991.
64. Badwe, R.A., Sharma, V., Bhansali, M.S., et al.: The quality of swallowing for patients with operable esophageal carcinoma: A randomized trial comparing surgery with radiotherapy. Cancer, *85:*763, 1999.
65. Urbe, S.G., and Turrisi, A.T.: Split-course accelerated radiation therapy combined with carboplatin and 5-fluorouracil for palliation of metastatic or unresectable carcinoma of the esophagus. Cancer, *75:*435, 1995.
66. Coia, L.R., Soffen, E.M., Schultheiss, T.E., et al.: Swallowing function in patients with esophageal cancer treated with concurrent radiation and chemotherapy. Cancer, *71:*281, 1993.
67. Jager, J., Langendijk, H., Pannebakker, M., et al.: A single session of intraluminal brachytherapy in palliation of esophageal cancer. Radiother. Oncol., *37:*237, 1995.
68. Flesichman, E.H., Kagan, A.R., Bellotti, J.E., et al.: Effective palliation for inoperable esophageal cancer using intensive intracavitary radiation. J. Surg. Oncol., *44:*234, 1990.
69. Caspers, R.J., Welvaart, K., Verkes, R.J., et al.: The effect of radiotherapy of dysphagia and survival in patients with esophageal cancer. Radiother. Oncol., *12:*15, 1988.
70. Gschossman, J.M., Bonner, J.A., Foote, R.L., et al.: Malignant tracheoesophageal fistula in patients with esophageal cancer. Cancer, *72:*1513, 1993.
71. Ahmed, H.F., Hussain, M.A., Grant, C.E., and Wadleigh, R.G.: Closure of tracheoesophageal fistulas with chemotherapy and radiotherapy. Am. J. Clin. Oncol., *21:*177, 1998.
72. Muto, M., Ohtsu, A., Miyamoto, S., Muro K. et al.: Concurrent chemoradiotherapy for esophageal carcinoma patients with malignant fistulae. Cancer, *86:*1406, 1999.
73. Corn, B.W., Coia, L.R., Chu, J.C.H., et al.: Significance of prone positioning in planning treatment for esophageal cancer. Int. J. Radiat. Oncol. Biol. Phys., *21:*1303, 1991.
74. O'Rourke, M.B., Tiver, K., Bull, C., et al.: Swallowing performance after radiation therapy for carcinoma of the esophagus. Cancer, *61:*2022, 1988.
75. Meng Ng, T., Spencer, G.M., Sargeant, I.R., et al.: Management of strictures after radiotherapy for esophageal cancer. Gastrointest. Endosc., *43:*584, 1996.
76. Ng, T.M., Spencer, G.M., Sargeant, I.R., et al.: Management of strictures after radiotherapy for esophageal cancer. Gastrointest. Endosc., *43:*584, 1996.
77. Goldstein, H.M., Rogers, L.F., Fletcher, G.H., et al.: Radiological manifestations of radiation-induced injury to the normal upper gastrointestinal tract. Radiology, *117:*135, 1975.
78. Coia, L.R., Myerson, R.J., and Tepper, J.E.: Late effects of radiation therapy on the gastrointestinal tract. Int. J. Radiat. Oncol. Biol. Phys., *31:*1213, 1995.
79. Lepkea, R.A., and Libshitz, H.I.: Radiation-induced injury of the esophagus. Radiology, *148:*375, 1983.
80. Caspers, R.J.L., Zwinderman, A.H., Griffioen, G., et al.: Combined external beam and low dose rate intraluminal radiotherapy in esophageal cancer. Radiother. Oncol., *27:*7, 1993.

81. Sur, R.K., Deepinder, P.S., Sharma, S.C., et al.: Radiation therapy of esophageal cancer: Role of high dose rate brachytherapy. Int. J. Radiat. Oncol. Biol. Phys., *22:*1043, 1992.
82. Hishikawa, Y., Kurisu, K., Taniguchi, M., et al.: High-dose-rate intraluminal brachytherapy for esophageal cancer: 10 years experience in Hyogo College of Medicine. Radiother. Oncol., *21:*107, 1991.
83. Gaspar, L.E., Subir, N., Herskovic, A., et al.: American Brachytherapy Society (ABS) consensus guidelines for brachytherapy for esophageal cancer. Int. J. Radiat. Oncol. Biol. Phys., *38:*127, 1997.
84. Rowland, C.G., and Pagliero, K.M.: Intracavitary irradiation in palliation of carcinoma of oesophagus and cardia. Lancet, *2:*981, 1985.
85. Hishikawa, Y., Kurisu, K., Taniguchi, N., et al.: High-dose-rate intraluminal brachytherapy for esophageal cancer: 10 years experience in Hyogo College of Medicine. Radiother. Oncol., *21:*107, 1991.
86. Hishikawa, Y., Izumi, M., Kurisu, K., et al.: Esophageal ulceration following high-dose-rate intraluminal brachytherapy for esophageal cancer. Radiother. Oncol., *28:*252, 1993.
87. Sander, R., Hagenmueller, F., Sander, C., et al.: Laser versus laser plus after loading with iridium-192 in the palliative treatment of malignant stenosis of the esophagus: A prospective, randomized, and controlled study. Gastrointest. Endosc., *37:*433, 1991.
88. Shmueli, E., Srivastava, E., Dawes, P.J.D.K., et al.: Combination of laser treatment and intraluminal radiotherapy for malignant dysphagia. Gut, *38:*803, 1996.
89. Spencer, G.M., Thorpe, S.M., and Sargeant, I.R.: Laser and brachytherapy in the palliation of adenocarcinoma of the oesophagus and cardia. Gut, *39:*726, 1996.
90. Montravadi, R.V.P., Gates, J.O., Bajpai, D., et al.: Combined chemotherapy and external radiation therapy plus intraluminal boost with high dose rate brachytherapy for carcinoma of the esophagus. Endocuriether./Hypertherm. Oncol., *11:*223, 1995.
91. Calais, G., Dorval, E., Louisot, P., et al.: Radiotherapy with high dose rate brachytherapy boost and concomitant chemotherapy for stages IIB and III esophageal carcinoma: Results of a pilot study. Int. J. Radiat. Oncol. Biol. Phys., *38:*769, 1997.
92. Jones, D.R., Parker, L.A., Detterbeck, F., et al.: Inadequacy of computed tomography in assessing patients with esophageal carcinoma after induction chemoradiotherapy. Cancer, *85:*1026, 1999.
92a. Bates, B.A., Detterbeck, F.C., Bernard, S.A., et al.: Concurrent radiation therapy and chemotherapy followed by esophagectomy for localized esophageal carcinoma. J. Clin. Oncol., *14:*156, 1996.
93. Laterza, E., de Manzoni, G., Guglielmi, A., et al.: Endoscopic ultrasonography in the staging of esophageal carcinoma after preoperative radiotherapy and chemotherapy. Ann Thorac Surg., *67:*1466, 1999.
94. Giovannini, M., Seitz, J.F., Thomas, P., et al.: Endoscopic ultrasonography for assessment of the response to combined radiation therapy and chemotherapy in patients with esophageal cancer. Endoscopy, *29:*4, 1997.
95. Giovannini, M., Bardou, V.J., Moutardier, V., et al.: Relation between endoscopic ultrasound evaluation and survival of patients with inoperable thoracic squamous cell carcinoma of the oesophagus treated by combined radio- and chemotherapy. Endoscopy, *31:*593, 1999.
96. Isenberg, G., Chak, A., Canto, M.I., et al.: Endoscopic ultrasound in restaging of esophageal cancer after neoadjuvant chemoradiation. Gastrointest. Endosc., *48:*158, 1998.

CHAPTER

21 Multimodality Therapy for Esophageal Carcinoma

ARLENE A. FORASTIERE

Medical recognition of the morbidity and mortality of esophageal cancer dates from the time of Galen in the second century. The intrathoracic location, lack of serosal membrane with a propensity for invasion of adjacent organs, extensive lymphatic drainage, and the fact that cancer of the esophagus is usually advanced when symptoms develop (predominantly dysphagia) account for the difficulties experienced today in curing this disease. Epidemiologic studies have documented a long latency period of 3 to 4 years from the development of carcinoma in situ until invasive cancer is diagnosed. By then, owing to the rich lymphatic network, clinically detectable or occult metastatic disease is usually present. In contrast to patients in high-risk areas of China where screening can detect early lesions, most patients in the Western world have advanced disease (stage II_b or III) at the time of presentation.

In 1998, 12,300 cases and 11,900 deaths from esophageal cancer were predicted in the United States.[22] Although squamous cell carcinoma accounted for nearly 90% of cases in the 1960s, more than 50% of referrals now include adenocarcinoma of the distal esophagus, gastroesophageal junction (GEJ), or cardia. From 1974 to 1994, the annual rates of adenocarcinoma per 100,000 population increased by more than 350%.[9] This change in epidemiology is being observed in Sweden and the United Kingdom as well.[15,30] Middle-class white males primarily account for this increase; associated risk factors include gastroesophageal reflux disease, smoking, obesity, and Barrett's dysplasia.

In the last 40 years, 5-year survival from esophageal carcinoma has remained at less than 10% owing to the fact that the disease is usually disseminated at the time the patient presents for medical attention. Even when successful control of local-regional disease is achieved with surgery or radiotherapy, patients often succumb to distant metastases. Efforts to improve survival have focused on improved local control—because this leads to much of the morbidity associated with this tumor—and more effective treatment of occult metastatic disease.

Combined-modality strategies include two types: surgical and nonsurgical approaches. Surgical approaches comprise preoperative radiotherapy, preoperative chemotherapy, and both chemotherapy and radiotherapy administered sequentially or concomitantly. Randomized trials of these preoperative therapies (termed induction or neoadjuvant) have been conducted over the past 2 decades to assess the favorable results observed in small nonrandomized series. Adjuvant chemotherapy and/or radiotherapy after esophagectomy has not been evaluated to the same extent as have the preoperative approaches. Nonsurgical treatment consists of sequential or concomitant chemotherapy and radiotherapy as definitive treatment for patients with localized disease. This approach has been evaluated in patients with clearly unresectable disease and in populations with mixed stages of disease, with differing results.

Only recently have trials included patients with adenocarcinoma of the distal esophagus, GEJ, and cardia. In studies to date, squamous cell carcinoma and adenocarcinoma histologic types do not appear to differ in median or overall survival rates but do have a somewhat different pattern of failure.[35] Local recurrence as a site of first failure is more frequent for squamous cell histology, whereas distant metastasis is a more frequent site of first failure for adenocarcinoma.

The rationale for chemotherapy used in the neoadjuvant setting includes the reduction of local and micrometastatic tumor burden, thus downstaging the tumor; exploitation of data pointing to 5-fluorouracil, cisplatin, and other cytotoxins as radiosensitizers; and the prevention of drug-resistant clones and enhanced delivery of chemotherapy to the local tumor owing to an intact vasculature. Preoperative treatment also allows for an in vivo assessment of tumor sensitivity to chemotherapy and aids in decision making regarding postoperative management. Preoperative radiotherapy similarly has the potential advantage of downstaging tumor, sterilizing tumor in areas that are not affected by surgery, and occasionally resulting in a pathologically negative resection specimen. Both modalities could potentially prevent the release of tumor cells intraoperatively to decrease, in theory, the rate of distant metastases.

MULTIMODALITY THERAPEUTIC STRATEGIES THAT INCLUDE SURGERY

Surgery and Adjuvant Radiotherapy

Following the rationale just outlined and with the knowledge that esophagectomy would remove residual disease, five randomized, controlled trials of preoperative radiotherapy were conducted between 1973 and 1988. Each prospectively compared radiotherapy followed by esophagectomy with surgery alone.[4,14,23,29,42] Only one of these trials showed a survival benefit from the addition of preoperative radiotherapy.[29] To study this further, a meta-analysis of updated individual patient data, including a total of 1,147 patients from these five trials, was performed by the Medical Research Council (MRC) Oesophageal Collaborative Group. The results of this meta-analysis showed that after a median follow-up of 9 years, preoperative radiotherapy afforded an absolute survival benefit of 4% at 2 years and 3% at 5 years, $P = 0.062$.[3] Thus, based on this updated survival analysis of these five randomized trials, no clear evidence exists to support the use of preoperative radiotherapy as a strategy to improve survival.

Postoperative adjuvant radiotherapy also has been evaluated in randomized trials with the rationale that improvement in local control may influence survival. Three randomized trials compared observation with adjuvant radiotherapy in patients who had undergone resection, and all reported no survival benefit.[10,39,43] In the largest of the three trials, reported by Teniere,[39] 221 patients who had a curative resection were randomized along with stratification based on the extent of lymph node involvement. After follow-up, ranging from 3 to 9 years, no differences in survival were observed in any of the treatment groups, although patients with N0 disease had a significantly better survival rate than that of N+ patients, regardless of treatment group. Radiotherapy did decrease local failure from 35% to 10% but only in the subset of patients with N0 disease.

A smaller trial from Hong Kong included 130 patients who had undergone either palliative or curative resection.[10] Local recurrence and death from tracheobronchial obstruction were significantly reduced in those who had a palliative resection. The entire group of patients treated with radiotherapy showed a significant increase in complication rate in the intrathoracic stomach and a significant shortening of the time to development of distant metastases. The investigators attributed these factors to a significantly shorter survival observed for the radiotherapy-treated group compared with the observation group. On the basis of this experience, postoperative radiotherapy was recommended only for patients undergoing a palliative resection with residual tumor in the mediastinum.

In a much smaller trial from Germany (68 patients), Zieren and colleagues[43] found no difference in overall or disease-free survival in curatively resected patients with squamous cell carcinoma. The incidence of fibrotic anastomotic strictures was significantly increased after radiotherapy and contributed to a delay in patients' recovery of their swallowing function and decreased their overall quality of life. In summary, the available data indicate no role for postoperative radiotherapy in patients who have undergone a complete resection.

Preoperative Chemotherapy

Cisplatin-based combination chemotherapy has been evaluated in numerous phase II trials as induction or neoadjuvant therapy prior to esophagectomy. Because of the frequency of distant metastatic disease, the addition of a systemic therapy is logical. Approximately 50% of patients demonstrate at least a 50% reduction in tumor mass after two or three courses of cisplatin and infusional 5-fluorouracil (5-FU), a well-established regimen in the treatment of this disease.[17] Occasional patients (<5%) have no evidence of tumor in the resection specimen.

Five randomized, controlled trials evaluating preoperative chemotherapy have been reported (Table 21–1).[21,25,29,33,36] Two of the trials also compared the sequential administration of chemotherapy and radiotherapy followed by surgery with immediate surgery.[25,29] These studies showed no significant difference in 3-year survival rates. Two other trials of note were conducted by Roth[33] in the United States and Schlag[36] in Germany. Roth compared cisplatin plus vindesine plus bleomycin followed by surgery with surgery alone, and Schlag employed the same design but used cisplatin plus 5-FU chemotherapy. Both combination regimens yielded similar response rates, similar median survival rates of 9 and 10 months, and no difference in overall survival compared with surgery only. However, Roth observed that the subset of patients who responded to preoperative chemotherapy had longer survival and no increase in operative mortality.

Because these trials enrolled only small numbers of patients and were limited to patients with squamous cell carcinoma, a large, definitive trial that included patients with adenocarcinoma was conducted by the U.S. G-I Intergroup. Trial 0113 enrolled 440 patients with potentially resectable esophageal cancer and randomized them to receive either (1) immediate surgery only or (2) three cycles of cisplatin plus 5-FU chemotherapy followed by esophagectomy, and then two cycles of adjuvant cisplatin plus 5-FU in those demonstrating response to the induction chemotherapy.[21] No differences were observed in curative resection rate (59% versus 62%), treatment mortality (6% versus 7%), median survival (16 months versus 15 months), or 3-year survival (26% versus 23%). The pattern of first failure was also similar between treatment groups for both local recurrence (31% versus 32%) and distant recurrence (50% versus 41%). The failure of this large multicenter trial to show benefit for either histology by the addition of chemotherapy to surgery has led investigators to conclude that, using our current best chemo-

Table 21–1. Randomized Trials of Induction Chemotherapy

Series	Treatment	No. Patients	Median (Mo)	3-Year Survival (%)
Nygaard[29]	Surgery	41		9
	DDP/Bleo → S	50		3
	DDP/Bleo → RT → S	47		17
Le Prise[25]	Surgery	45		14
	DDP/5-FU → RT → S	41		19
Roth[33]	Surgery	20	9	5
	DDP/VDS/Bleo → S	19	9	25
Schlag[36]	Surgery	41	10	
	DDP/5-FU → S	34	10	
Kelsen[21]	Surgery	227	16	26
	DDP/5-FU → S	213	15	23

DDP = cisplatin, Bleo = bleomycin, S = surgery, 5-FU = 5-fluorouracil, RT = radiotherapy, VDS = vindesine.

Table 21–2. Randomized Trials of Preoperative Chemoradiation

Series	Preoperative Treatment	Path CR	Survival	
			Median	*3 Years*
Forastiere[11]	DDP/5-FU/Vbl + RT 37.5-45 Gy	24% (10/41)	29 mo	47%
Naunheim[28]	DDP/5-FU + RT 30-36 Gy	21% (8/34)	23 mo	40%
Bates[5]	DDP/5-FU + RT 45 Gy	51% (18/35)	26 mo	41%
Forastiere[12]	DDP/5-FU + RT 44 Gy	40% (19/47)	35 mo	43%
Adelstein[1]	DDP/5-FU + RT 45 Gy (bid/split)	27% (18/67)		44%
Heath[16]	DDP/5-FU + RT 44 Gy	28% (11/39)	Not reached	62% (2 yr)

DDP = cisplatin, 5-FU = 5-fluorouracil, Vbl = vinblastine, RT = radiation therapy, Path CR = pathologic complete response.

therapy, this strategy of induction chemotherapy does not work as had been theorized.

Preoperative Concurrent Chemotherapy and Radiotherapy

The aim of treatment that includes all three modalities is improvement of survival through better local control and a decreased incidence of distant metastases. In studies in which chemoradiation alone was used, a significant proportion of patients failed locally.[18,20] Thus, the downstaging of disease with concurrent chemotherapy and radiotherapy followed by surgical removal of residual tumor has theoretical appeal. The results of single-institution phase II trials with the administration of preoperative cisplatin and 5-FU, with or without additional cytotoxic drugs, and concurrent with radiotherapy (40 to 50 Gy) have looked promising for improving survival compared with historic results of surgery alone. Details of selected studies are shown in Table 21–2.[1,5,11,12,16,28] These trials report pathologic complete response (path CR) in 21 to 51% of patients and 3-year survival rates in the 40% range. Furthermore, patients who achieve path CR have a significant survival advantage over those with residual tumor in the resected specimen. Approximately 60% of path CR patients and 25 to 30% of those with residual tumor in the resected esophageal specimen are alive at 5 years.[12] The long survival of the latter group supports the role of surgery in this trimodality approach.[5,11,12]

One recently published trial by Heath and colleagues[16] from Johns Hopkins carefully documented disease stage before treatment using CT scan, esophageal endoscopic ultrasound, and staging laparoscopy and then compared pretreatment staging with postoperative staging. Sixty-nine per cent of patients were downstaged, and their survival corresponded to their postoperative stage. Although 74% of patients had stages II_b, III, or IV ($M1_a$—celiac nodes positive) disease before treatment, after chemoradiotherapy and surgery 66% of patients had stage 0 (path CR), I, or II_a disease. Path CR was documented in patients with pretreatment stages II_a, II_b, and III disease. In this trial, the 2-year survival rate for all patients was 62% and that of path CRs was 91%. Thus, downstaging of patients with regional node involvement is possible and translates to long-term survival.

Three randomized, controlled trials that directly compared surgery alone with chemotherapy and concurrent radiotherapy followed by surgery are shown in Table 21–3.[6,40,41] All three trials reported similar pathologic CR rates of 28%, 25%, and 26% and similar 3-year survival rates of 32%, 32%, and 36% for patients treated with the multimodality approach. Three-year survival results after surgery alone, however, varied from 6 to 36%. Only one study reported a statistically significant difference in median and overall survival to demonstrate benefit from multimodality treatment.[41]

Walsh and colleagues[41] randomized 113 patients with adenocarcinoma of the esophagus to surgery alone or cisplatin plus 5-FU and concurrent RT (40 Gy) followed by surgery. There was a significant difference in median survival (11 months versus 16 months) and 3-year survival (6% versus 32%), favoring multimodality treatment. The study has been criticized for the poor survival outcome of the surgically treated group, which was 6%. Survival data from major centers in the United States and from

Table 21–3. Randomized Trials of Preoperative Chemoradiation

Series	Histology	Treatment	No. Patients	Path CR (%)	Survival	
					Median	*3 Years*
Urba[40]	Adeno + squamous	Surgery	50		1.48 yr	15%
		Pre-op chemo* + 45 Gy	50	28	1.36 yr	32%
Walsh[41]	Adeno	Surgery	55		11 mo	6%
		Pre-op chemo* + 40 Gy	58	25	16 mo†	32%
Bossett[6]	Squamous	Surgery	139		18.6 mo	36%
		Pre-op chemo‡ + 37 Gy	142	26	18.6 mo	36%

*Cisplatin/5-FU–based chemotherapy.
†Difference statistically significant.
‡Cisplatin.
Path CR = pathologic complete response.

the control arm of the recently completed Intergroup trial 0113 indicate that a 3-year survival proportion in the 20 to 30% range would generally be expected for patients considered to be candidates for curative resection.[21,31]

On the basis of encouraging results from a prior phase II trial,[12] Urba and colleagues[40] from the University of Michigan randomized 100 patients (75 with adenocarcinoma, 25 with squamous cell carcinoma) to surgery alone or to a 3-week course of protracted infusion 5-FU plus cisplatin plus vinblastine and concurrent twice-daily RT (45 Gy). The survival curves did not separate until after 2 years, so that no difference in median survival was observed (1.48 years versus 1.36 years). The 3-year survival rate was 15% for surgically treated patients versus 32% for those in the multimodality treatment group ($P = 0.07$), thus showing only a trend for benefit from preoperative chemoradiation. Within the multimodality treatment group, patients achieving path CR had significantly improved 3-year survival compared with those with residual tumor in the resected specimen (63% and 23%, respectively; $P = 0.006$). The pattern of first failure did not differ between the two treatment groups with respect to distant metastases, but local-regional failure was significantly decreased in the preoperative chemoradiation group with 19% recurrence versus 41% in the control group.

The third randomized trial reported by Bossett for the EORTC (European Organization for Research and Treatment of Cancer)[6] was limited to patients with stage I or II squamous cell carcinoma, which does not constitute the bulk of patients presenting with esophageal carcinoma in the United States. The patients enrolled in this trial likely had a better prognosis owing to their less advanced stage compared with that of the patients enrolled in the trials conducted by Walsh[41] and Urba.[40] This may explain the better survival rate achieved with surgery alone than was reported for the other two randomized trials. Two hundred and ninety-seven patients were randomized to receive surgery alone or single-agent cisplatin and concurrent radiotherapy (RT) (37 Gy). Despite the relative low intensity of the preoperative regimen, significant improvement in disease-free survival, curative resection rate, and local control as well as a lower rate of cancer-related deaths were observed in the multimodality group. A difference in overall survival, however, was not observed, perhaps because more postoperative deaths occurred in the group who received preoperative cisplatin and RT.

In summary, the randomized trials have shown the following:

1. 25 to 28% of patients achieve path CR in response to cisplatin-based chemotherapy and concurrent radiotherapy (RT);
2. 32 to 36% of all patients who received multimodality treatment are surviving at 3 years;
3. path CR patients have a significant survival advantage;
4. 25 to 30% of patients with residual tumor in the resected surgical specimen have long-term survival; and
5. local-regional control is improved.

The comparative survival results are conflicting, however, owing to a lack of uniformity in survival outcome of patients in the surgery-alone control arms. This disparity most likely reflects differing proportions of locally advanced stage patients enrolled in each of the trials. Nevertheless, at this time, the benefit of adding preoperative chemoradiotherapy to surgery is not clearly proven and this therapy remains investigational.

MULTIMODALITY THERAPY WITHOUT SURGERY

Concurrent Chemotherapy and Radiotherapy

Concern over the mortality and morbidity associated with esophagectomy led investigators in the late 1970s to evaluate combined chemoradiotherapy as definitive treatment. This approach is attractive for several reasons. The cytotoxins 5-FU, cisplatin, bleomycin, and mitomycin, which have established activity in esophageal cancer, also act to enhance radiation cell kill. Chemotherapy can provide a systemic effect for micrometastatic disease outside the radiation port, including distant micrometastases. The local failure rate may be reduced by chemotherapy effects on radioresistant cells.

Nonrandomized trials of concurrent chemotherapy and RT suggested that the approach was feasible, although acute toxicity was clearly increased over that expected from RT alone.[7,19,24,32] Survival and local and distant failure rates varied depending on the stage of the disease.[7] Five randomized, controlled trials that compared concurrent chemotherapy and RT with RT alone have been published (Table 21–4).[2,18,34,37,38] The patient populations, chemotherapy and RT dosage, and scheduling differed among the trials. The EORTC trial reported by Roussel[34] and the trial from Pretoria reported by Slabber[37] were limited to patients with locally advanced, unresectable squamous cell carcinoma. Median and overall survival rates showed no benefit from the addition of concomitant chemotherapy. Both of these trials, however, used suboptimal doses of RT. The trial from the National Cancer Institute of Brazil reported by Araujo[2] was limited to patients with stage II squamous cell carcinoma of the esophagus. No difference in survival was observed but the chemotherapy—one cycle of 5-FU, mitomycin-C, and bleomycin—was suboptimal. The two cooperative group trials from the United States, RTOG 85-01 and ECOG 1282, enrolled patients with no evidence of distant metastases without specifying resectability status.[18,38] Both trials utilized chemotherapy regimens that had been tested in phase II trials and an adequate (50 Gy) RT dose. The ECOG trial included an option for surgery after 40 Gy. Approximately half the patients in each arm underwent surgery; operative mortality was substantial at 17%. A significant difference in median survival was observed, favoring chemoradiotherapy (15 months versus 9 months), but 5-year survival rates were similar for both treatment groups (9% versus 7%). The only trial that adequately tested the concept of definitive chemoradiotherapy was the RTOG trial.

RTOG 85-01 compared RT alone (64 Gy) with combined chemoradiotherapy consisting of four courses of

Table 21–4. Randomized Trials of Radiotherapy Versus Radiotherapy Plus Chemotherapy

Trial		No. Patients	Local Failure	Median Survival (Mo)	Survival (%)
Herskovic*[18]	RT	62	68%	9	0 (5 yr)
(RTOG)	RT + CDDP/5-FU	61	47%†	14†	27†
Smith*[38]	RT	60		9	7 (5 yr)
(ECOG)	RT + 5-FU/mito 59			15†	9
Araujo‡[2]	RT	31	84%		6 (5 yr)
(NCI Brazil)	RT + CDDP/mito/5-FU	28	61%		16
Roussel§[34]	RT	111	66%	8	10 (4 yr)
(EORTC)	RT + CDDP	110	59%	10	8
Slabber§[37]	RT	36		5	
(Pretoria)	RT + CDDP/5-FU	34		6	

*Resectability not specified.
†Difference statistically significant.
‡Stage II only (1982 AJCC).
§Unresectable.

RT = Radiotherapy.
CDDP = Cisplatin.
5-FU = 5-Fluorouracil.
mito = Mitomycin.

cisplatin plus 5-FU (two concurrent with RT and two following RT) and 50 Gy of RT using single daily fractions of 2 Gy.[18] Randomization was terminated after the first interim analysis showed a significant difference in survival. An updated analysis with a minimum follow-up of 5 years has now been published.[8] The median survival rates for RT alone and for the combined treatment are 9 months and 14 months ($P < 0.001$), respectively, and 5-year survival rates are 0 and 26% ($P < 0.0001$), respectively. Local failure and distant metastases as sites of first failure were significantly lower in the chemotherapy-treated patients. However, local recurrence or persistence of disease at 12 months was still unacceptably high in the chemoradiotherapy arm at 47%. The positive results of this trial clearly demonstrate the superiority of chemoradiotherapy as the nonsurgical treatment of choice, and this has become the standard of care.

Attempts to improve on the results of RTOG 85-01, and on local control rates in particular, led to trials intensifying RT or intensifying chemotherapy. The Intergroup conducted trial 0122, in which cisplatin and 5-FU chemotherapy was intensified by administering three courses as induction chemotherapy and then two courses concurrent with RT (total dose 64.8 Gy). Thus, both chemotherapy and RT were intensified.[26] Toxicity was substantial and the survival results were not improved over those achieved in RTOG 85-01, and thus the regimen was not studied further.[26,27] Another strategy to improve local control is the addition of brachytherapy. The RTOG conducted a phase II trial of high dose rate brachytherapy added to the regimen tested in protocol 85-01 (four courses of cisplatin plus 5-FU and 50 Gy of RT). This approach resulted in a high rate of acute toxicity, including a treatment-related death rate of 8% and a cumulative incidence of fistula formation of 18% per year, and was therefore abandoned.[13]

On the basis of these experiences, the Intergroup decided to test an increased dose of external-beam RT alone as its follow-up randomized trial after 85-01. This trial (INT 0123) compared four courses of cisplatin plus 5-FU and concurrent RT (50.4 Gy) using single daily fractions of 1.8 Gy with the same exact regimen but including a higher total dose of RT, 64.8 Gy. The trial was opened in 1994 and closed in 1999 after the first interim analysis showed that the higher RT dose regimen was unlikely to prove superior with continued accrual. The high RT dose regimen was also associated with more toxicity.

In summary, the standard of care for nonsurgical therapy is concurrent chemoradiotherapy consisting of four courses of cisplatin plus 5-FU and 50.4 Gy of RT. Local failure (persistence plus recurrence) is high, and therefore this approach as definitive therapy must be considered investigational for patients who are candidates for resection. Increasing the intensity of current chemotherapy regimens or the intensity of RT (external beam or brachytherapy) has been shown to add toxicity without improving survival.

CONCLUSION

Over the last decade, surgical and nonsurgical multimodality approaches have evolved for treating cancer of the esophagus that has not overtly metastasized to distant sites. The demonstration that 27% of patients will be cured (i.e., disease-free at 5 years) after definitive chemoradiotherapy compared with 0 after RT alone is a major advance. Without doubt, this treatment option has influenced the selection of patients for surgical management, because it provides an alternative for restoring swallowing function in patients with local-regional disease for whom resection would likely be palliative. For patients with earlier stage disease, definitive chemoradiotherapy may also have an important role; however, trials prospectively comparing this approach to surgery with stratification for histology and stage have yet to be performed.

Multimodality treatment as part of surgical management remains investigational at this time. Preoperative or postoperative RT clearly does not add to the results of surgery, nor does preoperative chemotherapy either alone or administered in sequence with RT. The administration of chemotherapy concurrent with RT followed by surgery is most promising for improving survival. Our current cisplatin-based chemotherapy regimens result in path CR in 25 to 30% of patients, and it is clear that patients whose tumors are most sensitive to chemotherapy and RT have a survival advantage. Local control is improved, but the distant metastatic rate appears unaffected. The acute toxicities of these regimens are at the upper limit of tolerability.

Thus, new systemic therapeutics are needed that, when combined with RT, will substantially increase path CR rates. Cytotoxins that show activity in other gastrointestinal malignancies, such as the taxanes docetaxel and paclitaxel, irinotecan, gemcitabine, Navelbine, and capecitabine, are under investigation in esophageal cancer. Drugs with novel mechanisms, such as the signal transduction inhibitors, are also coming into clinical trials and many are associated with less toxicity than that of conventional cytotoxins. The specific class of matrix metalloproteinase inhibitors and angiogenesis inhibitors offers promise, in the adjuvant phase of treatment, to delay or prevent the development of distant metastases, which is now the primary cause of death from esophageal cancer. Last, it is essential to identify tumor markers that are predictive of response to multimodality therapies.

References

1. Adelstein, D.J., Rice, T.W., Becker, M., et al.: Use of concurrent chemotherapy, accelerated fractionation radiation, and surgery for patients with esophageal cancer. Cancer, *80:*1011, 1997.
2. Araujo, C.M.M., Souhami, L., Gil, R.A., et al.: A randomized trial comparing radiation therapy versus concomitant radiation therapy and chemotherapy in carcinoma of the thoracic esophagus. Cancer, *67:*2258, 1991.
3. Arnott, S.J., Duncan, W., Gignoux, M., et al.: Preoperative Radiotherapy for Esophageal Carcinoma. Cochrane Database Syst. Rev., *2:*CD001799, 2000.
4. Arnott, S.J., Duncan, W., Kerr, G.R., et al.: Low dose preoperative radiotherapy for carcinoma of the oesophagus: Results of a randomized clinical trial. Radiother. Oncol., *24:*108, 1992.
5. Bates, B.A., Detterbeck, F.C., Bernard, S.A., et al.: Concurrent radiation therapy and chemotherapy followed by esophagectomy for localized esophageal carcinoma. J. Clin. Oncol., *14:*156, 1996.
6. Bossett, J.F., Gignoux, M., Triboulet, J.P., et al.: Chemoradiotherapy followed by surgery compared with surgery alone in squamous cell cancer of the esophagus. N. Engl. J. Med., *337:*161, 1997.
7. Coia, L.R., Engstrom, P.F., Paul, A.R., et al.: Long-term results of infusional 5-FU, mitomycin-C and radiation as primary management of esophageal carcinoma. Int. J. Radiat. Oncol. Biol. Phys., *20:*29, 1991.
8. Cooper, J.S., Guo, M.D., Herskovic, A., et al.: Chemoradiotherapy of locally advanced esophageal cancer: Long-term follow-up of a prospective randomized trial (RTOG 85-01). J.A.M.A., *281:*1623, 1999.
9. Devesa, S.S., Blot, W.J., and Fraumeni, J.F., Jr.: Changing patterns in the incidence of esophageal and gastric carcinoma in the United States. Cancer, *83:*2049, 1998.
10. Fok, M., Sham, J.S., Choy, D., et al.: Postoperative radiotherapy for carcinoma of the esophagus: A prospective, randomized controlled study. Surgery, *113:*138, 1993.
11. Forastiere, A.A., Heitmiller, R.F., Lee, D.-J., et al.: Intensive chemoradiation followed by esophagectomy for squamous cell adenocarcinoma of the esophagus. Cancer J. Sci. Am., *3:*144, 1997.
12. Forastiere, A.A., Orringer, M.B., Perez-Tamayo, C., et al.: Preoperative chemoradiation followed by transhiatal esophagectomy for carcinoma of the esophagus: Final report. J. Clin. Oncol., *11:*1118, 1993.
13. Gaspar, L.E., Nag, S., Herskovic, A., et al.: A phase I/II study of external beam radiation, brachytherapy and concurrent chemotherapy in localized cancer of the esophagus (RTOG 92-07): Preliminary toxicity report. Int. J. Radiat. Oncol. Biol. Phys., *38:*127, 1997.
14. Gignoux, M., Roussel, A., Paillot, B., et al.: The value of preoperative radiotherapy in esophageal cancer: Results of a study by the EORTC. Recent Results Cancer Res., *110:*1, 1988.
15. Hansson, L.-E., Sparen, P., and Nyren, O.: Increasing incidence of both major histological types of esophageal carcinoma among men in Sweden. Int. J. Cancer, *54:*402, 1993.
16. Heath, E.I., Burtness, B.A., Heitmiller, R.F., et al.: Phase II evaluation of preoperative chemoradiation and postoperative adjuvant chemotherapy for squamous cell and adenocarcinoma of the esophagus. J. Clin. Oncol., *18:*868, 2000.
17. Heitmiller, R.F., Forastiere, A.A., and Kleinberg, L.: Esophageal Cancer. *In* Abeloff, M.D., Armitage, J.O., Lichter, A.S., and Niederhuber, J.E. (eds.): Clinical Oncology, 2nd ed. New York, Churchill-Livingstone, 2000, pp. 1517–1544.
18. Herskovic, A., Martz, K., Al-Sarrag, M., et al.: Combined chemotherapy and radiotherapy compared with radiotherapy alone in patients with cancer of the esophagus. N. Engl. J. Med., *326:*1593, 1992.
19. John, M.J., Flam, M.S., Mowry, P.A., et al.: Radiotherapy alone and chemoradiation for nonmetastatic esophageal carcinoma: A critical review of chemoradiation. Cancer, *63:*2397, 1989.
20. Kavanagh, B., Anscher, M., Leopold, K., et al.: Patterns of failure following combined modality therapy for esophageal cancer 1984–1990. Int. J. Radiat. Oncol. Biol. Phys., *24:*633, 1992.
21. Kelsen, D.P., Ginsberg, R., Pajak, T., et al.: Chemotherapy followed by surgery compared with surgery alone for localized esophageal cancer. N. Engl. J. Med., *339:*1979, 1998.
22. Landis, S.H., Murray, T., Bolden, S., et al.: Cancer statistics, 1998. CA Cancer J. Clin., *48:*6, 1998.
23. Launois, B., DeLa Rue, D., Campion, J., et al.: Preoperative radiotherapy for carcinoma of the esophagus. Surg. Gynecol. Obstet., *153:*690, 1981.
24. Leichman, L., Herskovic, A., Leichman, C.G., et al.: Non-operative therapy for squamous cell cancer of the esophagus. J. Clin. Oncol., *5:*365, 1987.
25. Le Prise, E., Etienne, P.L., Meunier, B., et al.: A randomized study of chemotherapy, radiation therapy, and surgery versus surgery for localized squamous cell carcinoma of the esophagus. Cancer, *73:*1779, 1994.
26. Minsky, B.D., Neuberg, D., Kelsen, D., et al.: Neoadjuvant chemotherapy plus concurrent chemotherapy and high dose radiation for squamous cell carcinoma of the esophagus—a preliminary analysis of the phase II intergroup trial 0122. J. Clin. Oncol., *14:*149, 1996.
27. Minsky, B.D., Neuberg, D., Kelsen, D.P., et al.: Final report of intergroup trial 0122(ECOG PE-289, RTOG 90-12): Phase II trial of neoadjuvant chemotherapy plus concurrent chemotherapy and high-dose radiation for squamous cell carcinoma of the esophagus. Int. J. Radiat. Oncol. Biol. Phys., *43:*517, 1999.
28. Naunheim, K.S., Petruska, P.J., Roy, T.S., et al.: Preoperative chemotherapy and radiotherapy for esophageal carcinoma. J. Thorac. Cardiovasc. Surg., *5:*887, 1992.
29. Nygaard, K., Hagen, S., Hansen, H.S., et al.: Pre-operative radiotherapy prolongs survival in operable esophageal carcinoma: A randomized, multicenter study of pre-operative radiotherapy and chemotherapy. The second Scandinavian trial in esophageal cancer. World J. Surg., *16:*1104, 1992.
30. Powell, J., and McConkey, C.C.: Increasing incidence of adenocarcinoma of the gastric cardia and adjacent sites. Br. J. Cancer, *62:*440, 1990.
31. Reed, C.E.: Surgical management of esophageal carcinoma. Oncologist, *4:*95, 1999.
32. Richmond, J., Seydel, H.G., Bae, Y., et al.: Comparison of three treatment strategies for esophageal cancer within a single institution. Int. J. Radiat. Oncol. Biol. Phys., *13:*1617, 1987.
33. Roth, J.A., Pass, H.I., Flanagan, M.M., et al.: Randomized clinical trial of preoperative and postoperative adjuvant chemotherapy with cisplatin, vindesine and bleomycin for carcinoma of the esophagus. J. Thorac. Cardiovasc. Surg., *96:*242, 1988.
34. Roussel, A., Haegele, P., Paillot, B., et al.: Results of the EORTC-GTCCG phase III trial of irradiation vs. irradiation and CDDP in inoperable esophageal cancer. Proc. Am. Soc. Clin. Oncol., *13:*199, 1994.
35. Salazar, J.D., Doty, J.R., Lin, J.W., et al.: Does cell type influence post-esophagectomy survival in patients with esophageal cancer? Dis. Esoph., *11:*168, 1998.
36. Schlag, P., for the CAO Study: Preoperative chemotherapy in localized squamous cell carcinoma of the esophagus: Results of a prospective randomized trial. Eur. J. Cancer, *37:*576, 1991.

37. Slabber, C.F., Nel, J.S., Schoeman, L., et al.: A randomized study of radiotherapy alone versus radiotherapy plus 5-fluorouracil and platinum in patients with inoperable, locally advanced squamous cell cancer of the esophagus. Am. J. Clin. Oncol., *21:*462, 1998.
38. Smith, T.J., Ryan, L.M., Douglass, H.O., et al.: Combined chemoradiotherapy vs. radiotherapy alone for early stage squamous cell carcinoma of the esophagus: A study of the Eastern Cooperative Oncology Group. Int. J. Radiat. Oncol. Biol. Phys., *42:*269, 1998.
39. Teniere, P., Hay, J.M., Fingerhut, A., et al.: Postoperative radiation therapy does not increase survival after curative resection for squamous cell carcinoma of the middle and lower esophagus as shown by a multicenter controlled trial. French University Association for Surgical Research. Surg. Gynecol. Obstet., *173:*123, 1991.
40. Urba, S., Orringer, M., Turrisi, A., et al.: A randomized trial comparing surgery to preoperative concomitant chemoradiation plus surgery in patients with resectable esophageal cancer. Proc. Am. Soc. Clin. Oncol., *16:*277, 1997.
41. Walsh, T.N., Noonan, N., Hollywood, D., et al.: A comparison of multimodal therapy and surgery for esophageal adenocarcinoma. N. Engl. J. Med., *335:*462, 1996.
42. Wang, M., Gu, X.Z., Yin, W.B., et al.: Randomized clinical trial on the combination of preoperative irradiation and surgery in the treatment of esophageal carcinoma: Report on 206 patients. Int. J. Radiat Oncol. Biol. Phys., *16:*325, 1989.
43. Zieren, H.U., Muller, J.M., Jacobi, C.A., et al.: Adjuvant postoperative radiation therapy after curative resection of squamous cell carcinoma of the thoracic esophagus: A prospective randomized study. World J. Surg., *19:*444, 1995.

CHAPTER

22 Esophageal Carcinoma: Palliation with Intubation and Laser

CAROLYN E. REED

A majority of patients (50 to 60%) with esophageal cancer have locally advanced and/or metastatic disease that is not amenable to curative therapy. For these patients, palliation of distressing symptoms such as dysphagia, regurgitation, and hypersalivation secondary to obstruction should be the predominant goal. An esophagorespiratory fistula may be present in up to 5% of patients with esophageal cancer, and symptoms of incessant coughing and ensuing pulmonary aspiration result in early death in 4 to 6 weeks.

The principal goal of palliation is to maintain a patent esophageal lumen, because dysphagia has been shown to be the most important factor affecting quality of life. The method of palliation should be quick, efficient, and cost-effective and have low morbidity and mortality. The mode of palliation may depend on tumor location, tumor characteristics, patient performance status, patient preferences, availability of treatment options, and physician experience. The three most common methods of palliation in the United States are radiation therapy, intubation, and laser treatment. This chapter focuses on esophageal intubation and laser therapy, including the use of photodynamic therapy (PDT).

Radiation therapy (RT) is still considered the gold standard of palliation by many. Dysphagia can be relieved in 50 to 70% of patients.[3,4,12,33,54] For good-performance patients with bulky local disease and multiple levels of lymph node involvement, radiation therapy is combined with chemotherapy in an attempt to relieve dysphagia and prolong survival. Although good palliation was achieved in a small series of patients reported by Coia et al.,[13,14] this chapter focuses on patients in whom prolongation of survival is not a primary goal.

Palliation with RT requires 4 to 6 weeks for effect, and higher doses of radiation (>45 Gy) have been associated with better results.[4,12,54] Recurrence of dysphagia owing to tumor regrowth or radiation fibrosis is reported in 30 to 50% of patients.[4,12,17] Brachytherapy has been added to increase local control, but with apparent increases in esophagitis, ulceration, and late stricture formation.[2,4,53]

PRELIMINARY CONSIDERATIONS

A moribund patient is not a candidate for laser treatment, PDT, or intubation. Comfort measures and dilatation with or without placement of a percutaneous endoscopic gastrostomy may allow the patient to live out his or her life at home. The necessity of interval endoscopies and laser retreatment for patients who must travel great distances may favor intubation.

Tumor characteristics and location may dictate the choice of palliation. Actual or impending esophagorespiratory fistulas should be treated with intubation. Tumors that are short, exophytic, and in the mid esophagus are amenable to various palliative modes. Tumors that are infiltrative or extrinsic are treated with a technique other than the laser. Gastroesophageal junction (GEJ) lesions are more difficult to palliate because angulation is more frequent, reflux is a common side effect, and extension of a stent into the stomach increases the potential for migration. Tumors near the cricopharyngeus are particularly challenging. Stents may cause respiratory embarrassment and/or result in a foreign-body sensation, and laser treatment can be technically difficult. PDT may be the best option for these patients and is also useful when tumor completely obstructs the lumen. Cost is an important issue as well. Factors that affect the choice of palliative technique are summarized in Table 22-1.

Initial dilatation is often necessary before definitive palliation. It can be the cause of major early complications. Every esophageal surgeon must be familiar with the various types of dilators, the appropriateness of the dilator based on stricture characteristics, and the methods to decrease complications associated with malignant stricture dilatation.

Mercury-filled bougies (e.g., Maloney, Hurst) are the easiest and safest dilators to use. They are most useful for symmetrical, short strictures larger than 12 to 14 mm. Unfortunately, their applicability is usually limited by more complex tumor characteristics.

Wire-guided bougies or through-the-scope (TTS) balloons are usually needed for long, tight, or tortuous malignant strictures. Most surgeons are unfamiliar with TTS balloon dilators, which are expensive and fragile and require endoscopy. The purported safety advantage of balloon dilators (i.e., radially directed distension rather than a shearing force) has not been proved. Dilatation is most commonly performed with wire-guided bougies, either the Savary-Gilliard system (Wilson-Cook, Winston-Salem, NC) or the American (C.R. Bard, Billerica, MA). If possible, the marked guidewire is placed in the antrum of the stomach under direct vision using a pediatric endoscope. As the endoscope is withdrawn in 5-cm increments, the guidewire is simultaneously advanced. After

Table 22–1. Factors That Affect Choice of Palliative Method

		Intubation		
Characteristic	**Laser**	***Plastic Stent***	***Covered SEMS***	**PDT**
Tumor Location				
Cervical	±	−	−	+
Mid	+	+	+	+
Distal	+	+	+	+
GEJ	±	±	±	+
Tumor Type				
Exophytic	+	+	+	+
Infiltrating	−	±	±	+
Extrinsic	−	+	+	−
Tumor Length				
<5 cm	+	±	+	+
>5 cm	±	+	+	+
Obstruction				
Circumferential	±	+	+	+
Noncircumferential	+	+	+	+
TEF	−	+	+	−
Cost	$$	$	$$$	$$$

SEMS = self-expanding metal stents, PDT = photodynamic therapy, GEJ = gastroesophageal junction, TEF = tracheoesophageal fistula, + = suitable, − = unsuitable, ± = variable suitability, $ = low cost, $$ = moderate cost, $$$ = high cost.

the endoscope has exited the mouth, the wire position is checked and maintained constantly in reference to the markings (distal tip >60 cm from the incisors). If the stricture cannot be traversed by a small endoscope, the guidewire is placed with the use of fluoroscopy. Dilatation under fluoroscopy is generally favored for long strictures, for angulated strictures, and when the GEJ is involved. The guidewire must not be bent or kinked, because the bent part can perforate the esophageal wall and kinking prevents smooth passage of the bougie and increases pressure against the stricture.

The single greatest pitfall in dilatation is to dilate too much too quickly. The first dilator that meets resistance determines the stricture size. No more than three successively larger dilators, in increments of 3 French or 1 mm, should be used (i.e., the rule of threes).

LASER THERAPY

The neodymium:yttrium-aluminum-garnet (Nd:YAG) laser has been used since the early 1980s for the endoscopic palliation of esophageal cancer. Tumor ablation is performed by passing a laser fiber through the biopsy channel of a flexible endoscope. The laser is usually applied in a noncontact mode at high power settings (70 to 150 watts) and at a distance of 0.5 to 1 cm from the tumor. Initial dilatation and a retrograde technique are preferred to allow the entire tumor to be treated in one or two sessions (Fig. 22–1). For a totally obstructing tumor, an antegrade approach can be used, in which the clinician treats 1 to 2 cm at a time and then clears necrotic debris before continuing with the subsequent segment. Laser therapy is usually performed in an outpatient setting, but effective palliation has been described in one session through the use of a retrograde approach with the patient under general anesthesia.[44] The contact mode allows the use of lower power settings with decreased laser plume and tactile feedback, but a comparative study showed no advantage over the noncontact method in regard to the number of treatment sessions, relief of dysphagia, or complication rate.[59] The contact mode may be useful for anastomotic recurrences and tumor overgrowth of a stent.

Tumors that are relatively short (<6 cm), nonangulated, exophytic, and noncircumferential and are in the mid or distal esophagus are most amenable to laser treatment. Tumors that are predominantly submucosal or cause extrinsic compression are not suitable for safe laser therapy. Gastroesophageal junction tumors may be angulated, which results in difficulty with parallel firing. Circumferential tumors are more vulnerable to postlaser strictures.

The technical success of laser therapy ranges from 90 to 100%, but the functional success averages 75 to 80%.[60] About one third to one half of treated patients develop recurrent dysphagia; therefore, repeat endoscopies at 4 to 6 weeks are advised. Up to 25% of patients may eventually require intubation.[68] Predictors of successful laser therapy have been studied.[8,10,38,48,49] Successful palliation of cervical lesions is low (30 to 50%). Naveau et al.[49] evaluated 11 variables as prognostic signs of symptomatic improvement. At 3 months, a good response to initial laser treatment and a tumor length of less than 6 cm correlated with a better prognosis. At 6 months, four variables indicated a more favorable prognosis: the initial symptomatic response, a tumor length of less than 6 cm, adenocarcinoma, and a tumor location of more than 27 cm from the incisors. The majority of series do not reveal a relationship between histology and response.[48] Poor performance status (often secondary to anorexia), general debility, and pain portend a poorer functional result.[6]

An advantage of laser therapy is its low complication rate. In a review of series totaling 431 patients, the perforation rate was 3%, formation of a fistula within 2 weeks of therapy occurred in 2.3% of patients, and significant hemorrhage occurred in 1.4%.[61] Perforation frequently was the result of prelaser dilatation. Combined treatment with chemotherapy and radiation or radiotherapy alone has been reported to increase the risk of fistula formation.[20,52] Ell and Demling[20] conducted a survey of 1,359 patients in 59 laser centers. The rates of major complications were perforation, 4.1%; fistula, 2.1%; bleeding, 0.7%; and sepsis, 0.6%. Treatment mortality was 1.0%.

Both brachytherapy and external-beam radiation therapy (EBRT) have been added to laser treatment in an attempt to improve palliation. In a prospective study that compared laser versus laser plus brachytherapy, the initial dysphagia-free interval was twice as long in patients with squamous cell carcinoma who received adjuvant brachytherapy.[63] The addition of brachytherapy (10 Gy high dose rate iridium-192) after laser recanalization of obstructing adenocarcinoma in 19 patients resulted in a longer dysphagia-free interval when compared with historical controls treated with laser alone.[71] In another study, 67 patients with unresectable esophageal or gastric cardia cancer were randomized to observation versus

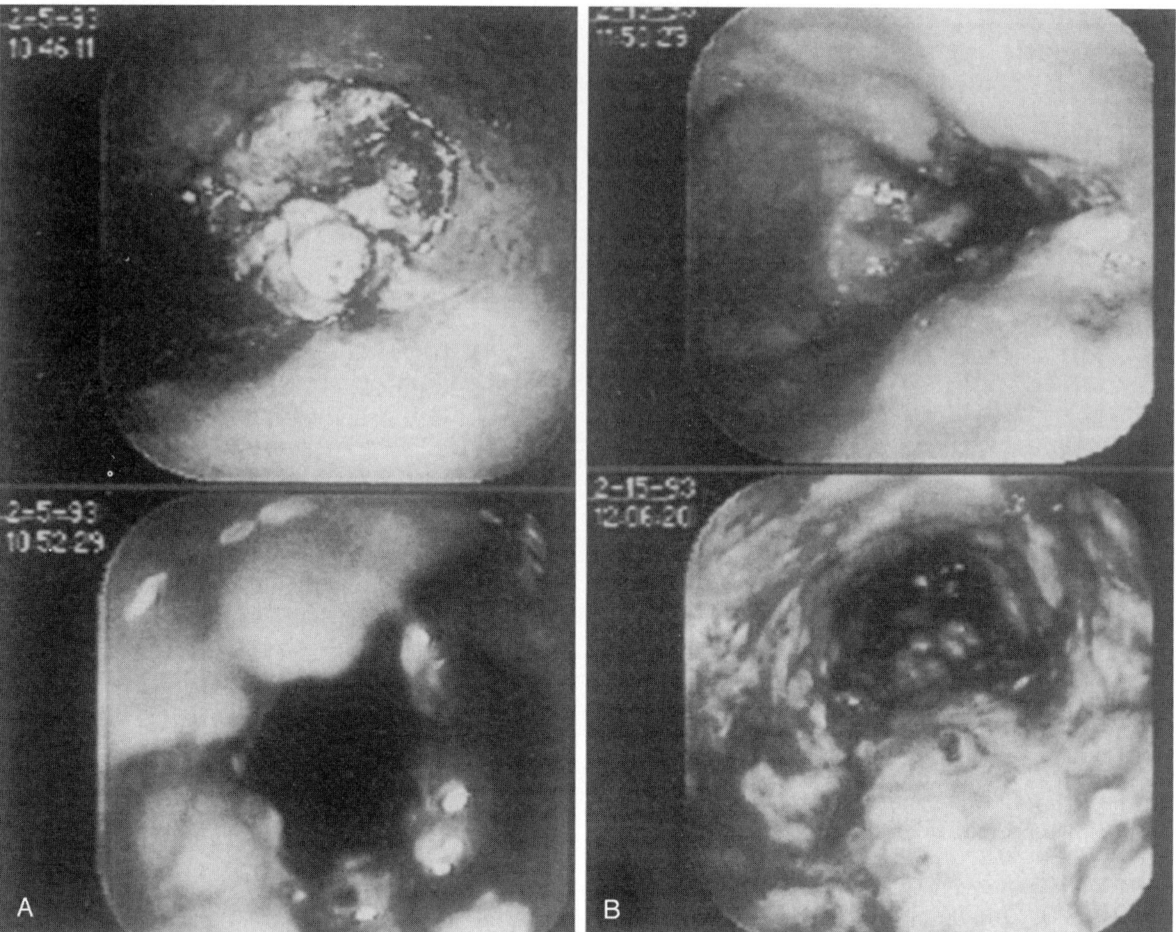

Figure 22–1. Endoscopic appearance of a distal adenocarcinoma before (*A*) and 3 days after (*B*) a single laser session. The views are proximal to (*top*) and within (*bottom*) the tumor stenosis.

EBRT (30 Gy in 10 fractions) after successful laser recanalization. The initial dysphagia-controlled interval and the duration between repeat laser therapy (treatment interval) increased significantly from 5 to 9 weeks.[64]

PHOTODYNAMIC THERAPY

Photodynamic therapy (PDT) is a nonthermal technique that can selectively necrose malignant tissue. A light-sensitive drug (photosensitizer) is intravenously injected and selectively concentrated in the malignant tumor. When activated by light of the proper wavelength, the drug produces cytotoxic singlet oxygen and other reactive radicals that lead to tissue destruction. At present, PDT for malignant esophageal strictures is performed using the Food and Drug Administration–approved photosensitizer Photofrin. The most common dose of Photofrin is 2 mg/kg, and light is usually administered 48 to 72 hours after drug administration with a laser delivering 690 nanometers of light. The laser beam is coupled to a flexible quartz fiber with a cylindrical diffuser tip in various lengths for uniform illumination of the target tissue. Normal tissue is not significantly affected, and there is no cumulative and little systemic toxicity.[62]

PDT may be particularly useful for long tumors, narrow and angulated lesions, totally obstructing tumors, and cervical strictures as well as for flat infiltrating tumors.[69] The most common complication of PDT is skin photosensitivity. With present photosensitizers, patients are told to avoid sunlight and strong indoor lighting for 30 days. Other side effects include transient fever, chest pain, and pleural effusions. Major complications including perforation, fistulas, and strictures have been reported in 10 to 20% of patients.[69]

PDT therapy is costly and the technology needs to be refined. Newer photosensitizers will require decreased time between drug administration and laser delivery, will be activated by longer wavelengths that penetrate deeper, and will have little cutaneous photosensitivity. Light delivery systems need to be improved to enhance the effectiveness of PDT. The benefit of adding therapy, such as local and systemic chemotherapy and radiation, to PDT requires further investigation.

Two randomized trials have compared PDT to the Nd:YAG laser. First, Heier et al.[26] randomized 22 patients to PDT and 20 patients to laser therapy. At 1 month, PDT was associated with a significantly greater improvement in dietary performance, Karnofsky status, and esophageal grade, regardless of tumor location, histology, or history of prior treatment. Second, in a large multicenter trial,

218 patients were randomized to either Nd:YAG laser therapy or PDT.[34] Palliation of dysphagia was equivalent for both therapies. Of note is that 25% of patients showed no improvement. At 1 month, the response was statistically higher for patients who had PDT than for those who underwent laser therapy (3.2% versus 20%, P = 0.05). Analysis revealed a better response to PDT in subgroups of patients with tumors of the cervical and distal esophagus, with tumors longer than 10 cm, and with a history of prior treatment.

INTUBATION—PLASTIC PROSTHESES

Peroral intubation with a plastic prosthesis is probably the most common method used worldwide for palliation of esophageal cancer. The tubes (Fig. 22-2) usually have an internal diameter of 10 to 12 mm, an external diameter of 14 to 17 mm, a proximal funnel design to anchor on the tumor and prevent caudal migration, and a distal flange or collar to prevent cephalad movement. The use of a plastic prosthesis is simple, quick, and inexpensive and leads to immediate relief of dysphagia. These tubes are especially useful for long asymmetric or tortuous tumors, tumors with extrinsic compression, and esophagorespiratory fistulas. Intubation is often performed when other methods of palliation fail. A general contraindication to intubation has been the presence of a tumor within 2 to 3 cm of the cricopharyngeus. However, the placement of a tube with or without modification has been tolerated by patients with cervical tumors.[24,35] Airway compression necessitates immediate removal of the tube.

A major drawback of palliation with a plastic prosthesis has been the initial need to dilate the tumor to a diameter greater than 45 French. Based on many series, the early perforation rate averages 6%.[43,60,73] Other early complications include hemorrhage (3.5%), aspiration pneumonia (0 to 2%), and tube migration (15%). Late complications include tube obstruction (9.5%), tube dislocation (8%), pressure necrosis (3%), and gastroesophageal reflux (which occurs almost universally when the tube crosses the GEJ).[43,61,73] Occlusion can result from food impaction, tumor overgrowth of either end, or angulation of the tube with impingement of the distal end on the gastric or esophageal wall. Both early and late tube migration occurs when the tube is not anchored properly or when subsequent therapy (i.e., RT) shrinks the tumor.

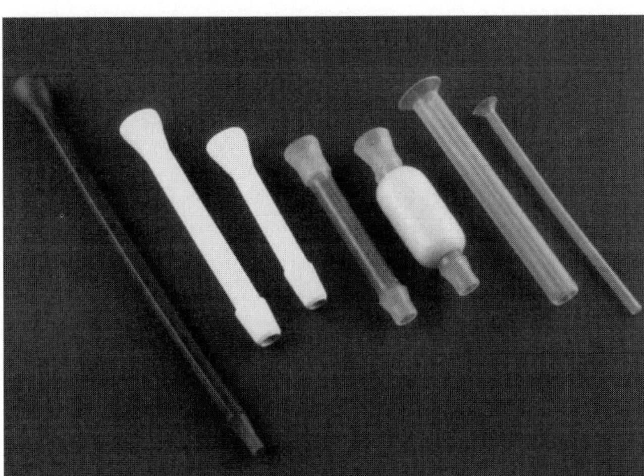

Figure 22-2. Plastic prostheses. From left to right: Celestin tube (Medoc Ltd. Tetbury, UK); Atkinson tubes (Key Med Inc.; Spring Valley, NY); uncuffed and cuffed Wilson-Cook silicone tubes (Wilson-Cook; Winston-Salem, NC); Montgomery salivary tubes (E. Benson Hood Laboratories; Pembroke, MA).

Success rates of greater than 90% are usually reported. In a review of several series, hospital mortality averaged 8%.[60] About one third of patients can eat solids after intubation, but the majority are restricted to semisolids. Patients must be instructed to chew food thoroughly, remain upright while eating, and drink large amounts of liquids with their meals.

In more recent series,[42,51] morbidity and mortality have been lower. A prospective study of 265 patients in India reported immediate complications in 4.3% of patients, late problems in 12.7%, and a procedure-related mortality of 3.9%.[42] These improved results were attributed to slow and gradual tumor dilatation, use of a small-diameter pusher tube for prosthesis insertion, and use of a modified soft prosthesis. Cost was estimated at U.S.$15! Trials comparing plastic and self-expanding metal stents are discussed later.

INTUBATION—SELF-EXPANDING METAL STENTS

Self-expanding metal stents (SEMS) for the palliation of esophageal cancer have gained popularity because of the technical ease of placement and the reported low early complication rate. Initial enthusiasm must now be tempered with the knowledge that late reintervention rates are significant.

The most commonly used stents in various series have been (1) the Gianturco Z-stent (Wilson-Cook), (2) the Wallstent (Boston Scientific, Natick, MA), (3) the Ultraflex (Boston Scientific), and (4) the EsophaCoil (Instent, Eden Prairie, MN) (Fig. 22-3). (The previous manufacturer of the Wallstent, The Schneider Division, was purchased by Boston Scientific in 1998.) The characteristics of these four stents are summarized in Table 22-2. The early stents were uncovered, but their rates of tumor ingrowth were unacceptable and led to development of stents coated with polyurethane. Each of the designs is unique: stainless steel mesh (Wallstent); knitted coat-of-mail (Ultraflex), connected segments of stainless steel with zigzag configuration (Gianturco Z-stent), and a coiled design (EsophaCoil). The radial forces of SEMS vary according to the metal used and the design. SEMS increase in radial force as follows: EsophaCoil, Wallstent, Gianturco Z, and Ultraflex.

The advantage of SEMS is the ability to compress and restrain the stent onto a delivery catheter to reduce the size of the delivery device. Tumor dilatation is frequently unnecessary. Stents are positioned and released within the malignant stricture under endoscopic, fluoroscopic, or combined endoscopic-fluoroscopic control. There ap-

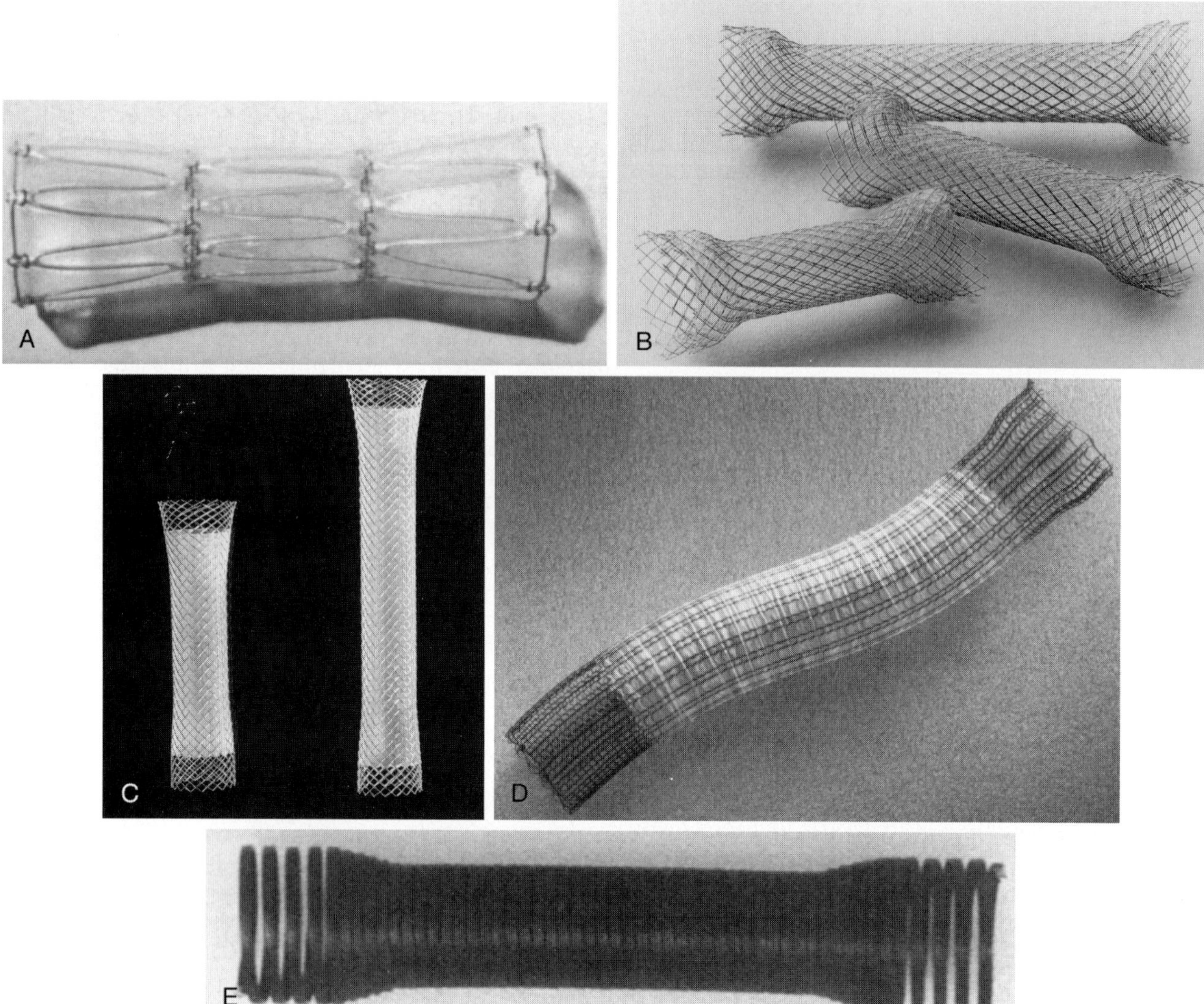

Figure 22–3. Self-expanding metal stents: *A,* Gianturco Z-stent (Wilson-Cook, Winston-Salem, NC); *B,* Wallstent I (Boston Scientific); *C,* Wallstent II (Boston Scientific); *D,* Ultraflex (Boston Scientific); *E,* EsophaCoil (Instent).

Table 22–2. Self-Expanding Metal Stents

	Covered Schneider Wallstent				
Characteristic	***I***	***II***	**Covered Ultraflex Stent**	**EsophaCoil**	**Gianturco Z-stent**
Stent material	Elgiloy	Elgiloy	Nitinol	Nitinol	Stainless steel
Structure	Mesh	Mesh	Knitted coat-of-mail	Spiral	Segmental, zig-zag configuration
Diameter of deployment system (Fr)	38	38	24 24	32	28
Internal diameter expanded (mm)	18	19	18 18	14, 16, 18, 20	18
Proximal flare outer diameter (mm)	28	28	23 28	18, 21, 24, 25.5	25
Total stent length (mm)	80, 100, 130	100, 150	100, 120, 150	75, 100, 150	60, 80, 100, 120, 140
Covered stent length (mm)	60, 80, 110	80, 130	70, 90, 120	Uncovered	60, 80, 100, 120, 140
Stent shortening (>20%) with deployment	Yes	Yes	Yes	Yes	No

pears to be little difference in the success and complication rates between the two methods.[46] With the covered Ultraflex and Wallstent SEMS, the length of the diseased segment determines the stent length that is used. To accommodate shortening after expansion, a stent that is at least 4 to 6 cm longer than the stricture should be chosen. The proximal and distal ends of the tumor are marked by mucosal contrast injections, by endoclipping, or by placing radiopaque markers on the patient's skin. After deployment, the stent gradually expands atraumatically (Fig. 22-4). The Z-stent is completely covered and does not shorten. With the Schneider stent, proximal position adjustment must be made before half the stent is released. The Ultraflex stent may be adjusted proximally by pulling with biopsy forceps after expansion. Although SEMS are not impossible to remove, the procedure is very difficult. If the tumor is not adequately covered, a second stent can be inserted into the first (Fig. 22-5).

The design of SEMS has undergone frequent changes, and therefore, the data comparing stent types is difficult to interpret. The Ultraflex stent is deployed by pulling a string that causes the stent to be unbraided. Both proximal and distal release systems are available. The stent progressively expands to its maximum diameter, usually over 2 to 4 days. A recent review of the Ultraflex stent summarizes its characteristics and performance.[46] Earlier versions of the Ultraflex had weaker radial force, and many endoscopists routinely used a balloon to dilate the stent after its release. A newer version of the Ultraflex has greater radial force and expansion is more complete. The Wallstent also has undergone modification, with a decrease in the size of its delivery system, and a change has been made in the shape of the uncovered ends of the Wallstent II. Expansion problems have not been reported with Gianturco Z-stents or Wallstents. Although covering SEMS decreased the rate of tumor ingrowth, the probability of migration has increased. To combat this problem, an uncovered proximal flare exists in both the Ultraflex and Wallstent. Depending on the overall length of the completely covered Gianturco Z-stent, one or two rows of small wire hooks are attached to the exterior of the stent's midsection to aid in preventing migration.

There are many problems when reviewing the results of palliation with the use of SEMS. Stent designs have continually changed, and many series include stents of varying designs or include both uncovered and covered stents. There is no commonly accepted definition of early and late complications, and the types and rates of reintervention are not always discussed. Comparisons that take into account tumor characteristics, location, the presence of esophagorespiratory fistulas, and so forth are lacking.

Despite limitations in the SEMS literature, studies have consistently reported high rates of technically successful deployment (>90 to 95%). As documented in a review of many early series from 1992 to 1997, early complications have been low.[21] The majority of reported series have dealt with uncovered stents. Relief of dysphagia is excellent, which is attributable to the large lumen size achieved with SEMS. An early complication that is not always reported is chest pain, which is usually mild and transient. A high incidence of incomplete expansion has been reported in a series of Ultraflex stents[32,40]; this is the result of the weaker radial force of these products as well as the type of tumor being stented. Late complications of SEMS include tumor ingrowth or overgrowth, stent migration, food impaction, bleeding, and fistula formation. Unfortunately, late complications and the need for reintervention are significant, averaging 36% in a review of many series.[21] More recent studies of all types of SEMS have confirmed that late complications and reintervention (i.e., stent reinsertion, percutaneous endoscopic gastrostomy [PEG] placement, endoscopic control of bleeding) rates are high.[15,30,56,57,76]

Location and characteristics of the tumor may dictate the best type of SEMS to use.[50] Placement of a stent within 2 cm of the cricopharyngeus is problematic, but cervical esophageal strictures have been successfully treated with Ultraflex stents.[55,66] Stent migration can be a problem when palliating cardial stenoses, and there may be a role for uncovered stents.[74] In very tortuous and irregular tumors, the flexible Ultraflex may conform better to the axis of the tumor. SEMS that provide a higher expansile force may be more effective for bulky and extrinsic tumors.

Placement of SEMS after chemotherapy, RT, or combined treatment has been reported to increase late complications.[7,28,70] However, other studies have shown no increased risk.[31,58] To lessen the potential for pressure necrosis of the esophageal wall, it has been recommended that more than 4 weeks elapse between tumoricidal intraluminal treatment and stent placement.[37]

Comparative studies of different types of SEMS have suffered from poor design, small numbers of patients, heterogeneous tumor characteristics, and changing stent modifications.[46] Obviously, comparison of uncovered and covered stents reveals increased tumor ingrowth in the former, and the overall reintervention rate depends on the rate of stent migration that occurs.[1,27] Comparison of the uncovered Wallstent and Ultraflex in one study revealed a higher reintervention rate with Ultraflex stents.[18] In another comparative study of these two uncovered stents, procedure-related mortality and early complication rate were higher with the Wallstent, but stent dysfunction and reintervention rates were significantly higher in the Ultraflex group.[65]

PLASTIC PROSTHESIS VERSUS SEMS

With the introduction of SEMS in 1990, enthusiasm for plastic prostheses waned in the United States. The need for only mild preliminary dilatation, which avoided the risk of perforation, and reduced procedure-related morbidity and mortality were factors that made SEMS attractive in the management of malignant strictures. However, the cost of SEMS is high, and the long-term morbidity is not negligible.[67]

Several prospective studies have compared SEMS to traditional prostheses. Knyrim et al.[29] randomly assigned 42 patients to a covered Wallstent or a Wilson-Cook silicone tube (Wilson-Cook). Complications related to device placement and function were significantly less in the SEMS group. Long-term morbidity was the same, and

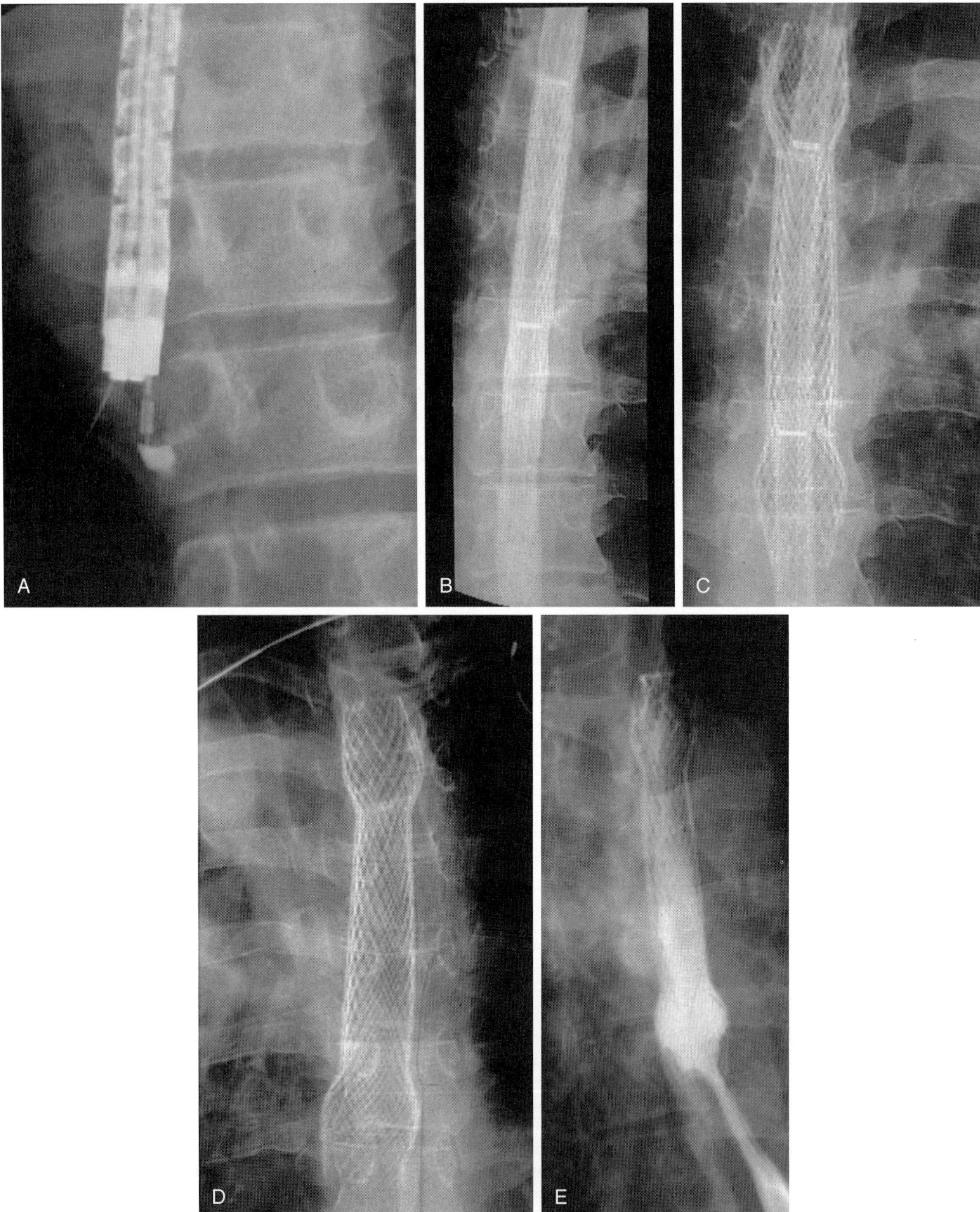

Figure 22–4. Deployment of SEMS: *A,* Distal margin of tumor being marked with radiopaque dye; *B,* Compressed stent delivery system advanced under fluoroscopic guidance into the tumor; *C,* Stent released; *D,* Delivery device removed and stent fully expanded, *E,* Esophagram 1 day after stent fully deployed.

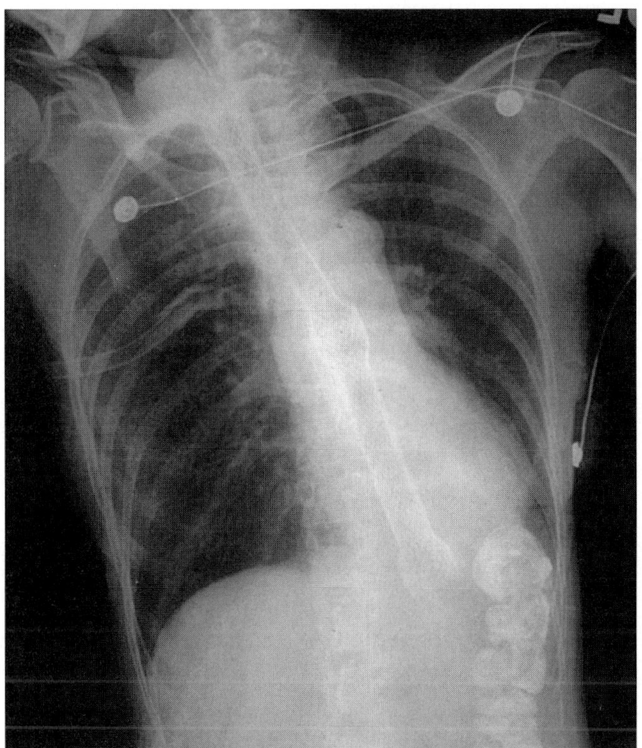

Figure 22–5. Two overlapping stents spanning a very long malignant tumor.

dysphagia relief was similar. DePalma and associates[16] compared the Wilson-Cook prosthesis with the Ultraflex stent and found early and late complications to be significantly higher with traditional tubes. Siersema et al.[70] randomized patients to the Gianturco Z-stent or the Celestin tube (Medoc, Tetbury, UK). Technical success and improvement in dysphagia were similar, but major complications occurred significantly more frequently with the latex Celestin procedure.

INTUBATION VERSUS LASER THERAPY

Laser therapy has been compared with conventional plastic stents in several trials.[5,11,22,25,36] In terms of swallowing ability, better palliation was experienced in the laser group in three studies,[5,11,36] and functional success was equivalent in another study.[22] There was a higher complication rate in the stent group reported in some series,[9,25] but this was not uniform. The laser group required more procedures.

When laser treatment was compared with both coated and uncoated SEMS in one study,[1] improvement in the dysphagia score was higher with SEMS. However, migration occurred in 26% of the coated SEMS group, and tumor ingrowth occurred in 26% of the uncoated SEMS. Better dysphagia relief with SEMS was confirmed in another report.[39] A study that compared laser with SEMS and plastic stents revealed significantly more minor and major complications in both the SEMS and the plastic stent groups compared with the laser group.[23]

PALLIATION OF ESOPHAGORESPIRATORY FISTULAS

A malignant esophagorespiratory fistula (ERF) results in early death as a consequence of constant pulmonary

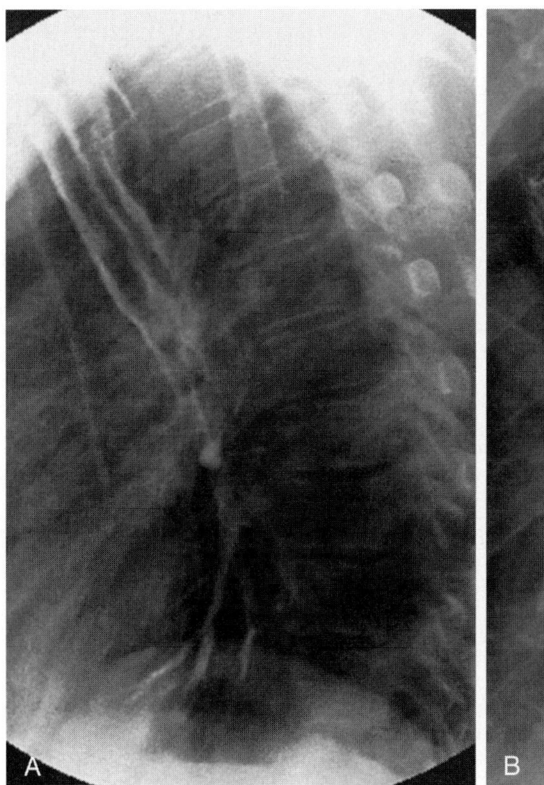

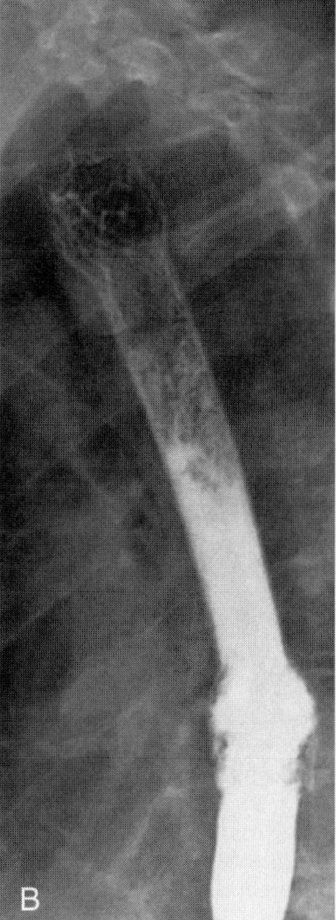

Figure 22–6. *A,* Esophagorespiratory fistula, *B,* Sealing of fistula with a self-expanding metal stent.

soilage. Options for palliation include esophageal exclusion and bypass, intubation, and radiation therapy. Supportive care may sometimes be most appropriate. Esophageal intubation with plastic prostheses has been the preferred approach in most circumstances.[72] The use of SEMS for closure of a fistula appears promising[75] (Fig. 22-6). Reports about the use of covered SEMS for closure of ERFs document a closure rate ranging from 70 to 100%.[41,45,47,56] Rates of reported closure may vary based on a clinical versus a radiologic definition of success.[56] Complete sealing with the Ultraflex stent has been attributed to its high degree of flexibility, which allows it to adhere to the esophageal wall.[19]

References

1. Adam, A., Ellul, J., Wakinson, A.F., et al.: Palliation of inoperable esophageal carcinoma: A prospective randomized trial of laser therapy and stent placement. Radiology, *202*:344, 1997.
2. Agrawal, R.K., Dawes, P.J.D.K., Clague, M.D.: Combined external beam and intracavitary radiotherapy in oesophageal carcinoma. Clin. Oncol. (R. Coll. Radiol.), *4*:222, 1992.
3. Ahmad, N., Goosenberg, E.B., Frucht, H., et al.: Palliative treatment of esophageal cancer. Semin. Radiat. Oncol., *4*:202, 1994.
4. Albertsson, M., Ewers, S.-B., Widmark, H., et al.: Evaluation of the palliative effect of radiotherapy for esophageal carcinoma. Acta Oncol., *28*:267, 1989.
5. Alderson, D., Wright, P.D.: Laser recanalization versus endoscopic intubation in the palliation of malignant dysphagia. Br. J. Surg., *77*:1151, 1990.
6. Alexander, G.L., Wang, K.K., Ahlquist, D.A., et al.: Does performance status influence the outcome of Nd:YAG laser therapy of proximal esophageal tumors? Gastrointest. Endosc., *40*:451, 1994.
7. Bethge, N., Summer, A., von Kleist, D., et al.: A prospective trial of self-expanding metal stents in the palliation of malignant esophageal obstruction after failure of primary curative therapy. Gastrointest. Endosc., *44*:283, 1996.
8. Brunetaud, J.M., Maunouy, V., Cochelard, D., et al.: Parameters affecting laser palliation in patients with digestive cancers. Laser Surg. Med., *9*:169, 1989.
9. Buset, M., des Marez, B., Baize, M., et al.: Palliative endoscopic management of obstructive esophagogastric cancer: Laser or prosthesis? Gastrointest. Endosc., *33*:357, 1987.
10. Carter, R., Smith, J.S., and Anderson, J.R.: Palliation of malignant dysphagia using the Nd:YAG laser. World J. Surg., *17*:608, 1993.
11. Carter, R., Smith, J.S., and Anderson, J.R.: Laser recanalization versus endoscopic intubation in the palliation of malignant dysphagia: A randomized prospective study. Br. J. Surg., *79*:1167, 1992.
12. Caspers, R.J., Welvaart, K., Verkes, R.J., et al.: The effect of radiotherapy on dysphagia and survival in patients with esophageal cancer. Radiother. Oncol., *12*:15, 1988.
13. Coia, L.R., Engstrom, P.F., Paul, A.R., et al.: Long-term results of infusional 5-FU, mitomycin-C, and radiation as primary management of esophageal carcinoma. Int. J. Radiat. Oncol. Biol. Phys., *20*:29, 1991.
14. Coia, L., Soffen, E.M., Schultheiss, T.E., et al.: Swallowing function in patients with esophageal cancer treated with concurrent radiation and chemotherapy. Cancer, *71*:281, 1993.
15. Cwikiel, W., Tranberg, K.-G., Cwikiel, M., et al.: Malignant dysphagia: Palliation with esophageal stents—long-term results in 100 patients. Radiology, *207*:513, 1998.
16. DePalma, G.D., di Matteo, E., Romano, G., et al.: Plastic prosthesis versus expandable metal stents for palliation of inoperable esophageal thoracic carcinoma: A controlled prospective study. Gastrointest. Endosc., *43*:478, 1996.
17. Desa, L., Raghunath, A.S., Chawla, S.L., et al.: Treatment policy for management of carcinoma of the esophagus. Br. J. Surg., *75*:275, 1988.
18. Dorta, G., Binek, J., Blum, A.L., et al.: Comparison between esophageal Wallstent and Ultraflex stents in the treatment of malignant stenoses of the esophagus and cardia. Endoscopy, *29*:149, 1997.
19. Dumonceau, J.M., Cremer, M., Laimand, B., et al.: Esophageal fistula sealing: Choice of stents, practical management, and cost. Gastrointest. Endosc., *49*:70, 1999.
20. Ell, C., and Demling, L.: Laser therapy of tumor stenoses in the upper gastrointestinal tract: An international inquiry. Lasers Surg. Med., *7*:491, 1987.
21. Ell, C., and May, A.: Self-expanding metal stents for palliation of stenosing tumors of the esophagus and cardia: A critical review. Endoscopy, *29*:392, 1997.
22. Fuchs, K.H., Freys, S.M., Schaube, H., et al.: Randomized comparison of endoscopic palliation of malignant esophageal stenoses. Surg. Endosc., *5*:63, 1991.
23. Gevers, A.M., Macken, E., Hiele, M., et al.: A comparison of laser therapy, plastic stents, and expandable metal stents for palliation of malignant dysphagia in patients without fistula. Gastrointest. Endosc., *48*:383, 1998.
24. Goldschmid, S., Boyce, H.W., Nord, H.J., et al.: Treatment of pharyngoesophageal stenosis by polyvinyl prosthesis. Am. J. Gastroenterol., *83*:513, 1988.
25. Hahl, J., Salo, J., Ovaska, R., et al.: Comparison of Nd:YAG laser therapy and oesophageal tube in palliation of oesophagogastric malignancy. Scand. J. Gastroenterol., *26*:103, 1991.
26. Heier, S.K., Rothman, K.A., Heier, L.M, et al.: Photodynamic therapy for obstructing esophageal cancer: Light dosimetry and randomized comparison with Nd:YAG laser therapy. Gastroenterology, *109*:63, 1995.
27. Hills, K.S., Chopra, K.B., Pal, A., et al.: Self-expanding metal oesophageal endoprostheses, covered and uncovered: A review of 30 cases. Eur. J. Gastroenterol. Hepatol., *10*:371, 1998.
28. Kinsman, K.J., DeGregorio, B.T., Katon, R.M., et al.: Prior radiation and chemotherapy increase the risk of life-threatening complications after insertion of metallic stents for esophagogastric malignancy. Gastrointest. Endosc., *43*:196, 1996.
29. Knyrim, K., Wagner, H.J., Bethge, N., et al.: A controlled trial of an expansile metal stent for palliation of esophageal obstruction due to inoperable cancer. N. Engl. J. Med., *329*:1302, 1993.
30. Kozarek, R.A., Raltz, S., Marcon, N., et al.: Use of the 25 mm flanged esophageal Z stent for malignant dysphagia: A prospective multicenter trial. Gastrointest. Endosc., *46*:156, 1997.
31. Kozarek, R.A., Ball, T.J., Brandabur, J.J., et al.: Expandable versus conventional esophageal prostheses: Easier insertion may not preclude subsequent stent-related problems. Gastrointest. Endosc., *43*:204, 1996.
32. Lagattolla, N.R.F., Rowe, P.H., Anderson, H., et al.: Restenting malignant oesophageal strictures. Br. J. Surg., *85*:261, 1998.
33. Langer, M., Choi, N.C., Orlow, E, et al.: Radiation therapy alone or in combination with surgery in the treatment of carcinoma of the esophagus. Cancer, *58*:1208, 1986.
34. Lightdale, C.J., Heier, S.K., Marcon, N.E., et al.: Photodynamic therapy with porfimer sodium versus thermal ablation therapy with Nd:YAG laser for palliation of esophageal cancer: A multicenter randomized trial. Gastrointest. Endosc., *42*:505, 1995.
35. Loizou, L.A., Rampton, D., Bown, S.G.: Treatment of malignant strictures of the cervical esophagus by endoscopic intubation using modified endoprosthesis. Gastrointest. Endosc., *38*:158, 1992.
36. Loizou, L.A., Grigg, D., Atkinson, M., et al.: A prospective comparison of laser therapy and intubation in endoscopic palliation for malignant dysphagia. Gastroenterology, *100*:1303, 1991.
37. Maier, A., Pinter, H., Freihs, G.B., et al.: Self-expandable coated stent after intraluminal treatment of esophageal cancer: A risky procedure? Ann. Thorac. Surg., *67*:781, 1999.
38. Mason, R.C., Bright, N., McColl, I.: Palliation of malignant dysphagia with laser therapy: Predictability of results. Br. J. Surg., *78*:1346, 1991.
39. Mason, R.: Palliation of malignant dysphagia: An alternative to surgery. Ann. R. Coll. Surg. Engl., *78*:457, 1996.
40. May, A., Selmaier, M., Hochberger, J., et al.: Memory metal stents for palliation of malignant obstruction of the oesophagus and cardia. Gut, *37*:309, 1995.
41. May, A., and Ell, C.: Palliative treatment of malignant esophagorespiratory fistulas with Gianturco-Z stents. Am. J. Gastroenterol., *93*:532, 1998.
42. Maydeo, A.P., Bapaye, A., Desai, P.N., et al.: Endoscopic placement of indigenous plastic esophageal endoprostheses—does it have a role in the era of expandable metallic stents? A prospective Indian study in 265 consecutive patients. Endoscopy, *30*:532, 1998.

43. Mehran, R.J., and Duranceau, A.: The use of endoprosthesis in the palliation of esophageal carcinoma. Chest Surg. Clin. North Am., *4:*331, 1994.
44. Mitty, R.D., Cave, D.R., and Birkett, D.H.: One-stage retrograde approach to Nd:YAG laser palliation of esophageal carcinoma. Endoscopy, *28:*350, 1996.
45. Mohammed, S., and Moss, J.: Palliation of malignant tracheo-esophageal fistula using covered metal stents. Clin. Radiol., *51:*42, 1996.
46. Mokhashi, M.S., and Hawes, R.H.: The Ultraflex stent for malignant esophageal obstruction. Gastrointest. Endosc. Clin. N. Am., *9:*413, 1999.
47. Morgan, R.A., Ellul, J.P.M., Denton, E.R.E., et al.: Malignant esophageal fistulas and perforations: Management with plastic-covered metallic endoprostheses. Radiology, *204:*527, 1997.
48. Narayan, S., and Sivak, M.V.: Palliation of esophageal carcinoma. Chest Surg. Clin. North Am., *4:*347, 1994.
49. Naveau, S., Chiesa, A., Poynard, T., et al.: Endoscopic Nd:YAG laser therapy as palliative treatment for esophageal and cardial cancer. Dig. Dis. Sci., *35:*295, 1990.
50. Neuhaus, H.: The use of stents in the management of malignant esophageal strictures. Gastrointest. Endosc. Clin. North Am., *8:*503, 1998.
51. O'Hanlon, D.M., Callanan, K., Karat, D., et al.: Outcome, survival, and costs in patients undergoing intubation for carcinoma of the esophagus. Am. J. Surg., *174:*316, 1997.
52. Overholt, B.F.: Laser and photodynamic therapy of esophageal cancer. Semin. Surg. Oncol., *8:*191, 1992.
53. Pakisch, B., Kohek, P., Poier, E., et al.: Iridium-192 high dose rate brachytherapy combined with external beam irradiation in nonresectable oesophageal cancer. Clin. Oncol. (R. Coll. Radiol.), *27:*7, 1993.
54. Petrovich, Z., Langholz, B., Forment, S., et al.: Management of carcinoma of the esophagus: The role of radiotherapy. Am. J. Clin. Oncol., *14:*80, 1991.
55. Pocek, M., Maspes, F., Masala, S., et al.: Palliative treatment of neoplastic strictures by self-expanding nitinol Strecker stent. Eur. Radiol., *6:*230, 1996.
56. Portwood, G.L., and Reed, C.E.: The use of lasers and stents in malignant esophageal disease. *In* Franco, K.L., and Putnam, J.B. (eds.): Advanced Therapy in Thoracic Surgery. Hamilton, Ontario, BC Decker, 1998, p.441.
57. Raijman, I., Siddique, I., Ajani, J., et al.: Palliation of malignant dysphagia and fistulae with coated expandable metal stents: Experience with 101 patients. Gastrointest. Endosc., *48:*172, 1998.
58. Raijman, I., Siddique, I., and Lynch, P.: Does chemoradiation therapy increase the incidence of complications with self-expanding coated stents in the management of malignant esophageal strictures? Am. J. Gastroenterol., *92:*2192, 1997.
59. Redford, C.M., Ahlquist, D.A., and Gostout, C.G.: Prospective comparison of contact with noncontact Nd:YAG laser therapy for palliation of esophageal carcinoma. Gastrointest. Endosc., *35:*394, 1989.
60. Reed, C.E.: Comparison of different treatments for unresectable esophageal cancer. World J. Surg., *19:*828, 1995.
61. Reed, C.E.: Endoscopic palliation of esophageal carcinoma. Chest Surg. Clin. North Am., *4:*155, 1994.
62. Saidi, R.F., and Marcon, N.E.: Nonthermal ablation of malignant esophageal strictures. Gastrointest. Endosc. Clin. North Am., *8:*465, 1998.
63. Sander, R., Hagenmueller, F., Sander, C., et al.: Laser versus laser plus afterloading with iridium-192 in the palliative treatment of malignant stenosis of the esophagus: A prospective randomized and controlled study. Gastrointest. Endosc., *37:*433, 1991.
64. Sargeant, I.R., Tobias, J.S., Blackman, G., et al.: Radiotherapy enhances laser palliation of malignant dysphagia: A randomized study. Gut, *40:*362, 1997.
65. Schmassmann, A., Meyerberger, C., Knuchel, J., et al.: Self-expanding metal stents in malignant esophageal obstruction: A comparison between two stent types. Am. J. Gastroenterol., *92:*400, 1997.
66. Segalin, A., Granelli, P., Bonavina, L., et al.: Self-expanding esophageal prosthesis: Effective palliation for inoperable carcinoma of the cervical esophagus. Surg. Endosc., *8:*1343, 1994.
67. Segalin, A., Bonavina, A., Carazzone, A., et al.: Improving results of esophageal stenting: A study on 160 consecutive unselected patients. Endoscopy, *29:*701, 1997.
68. Shmueli, E., Myszor, M.F., Burke, D., et al.: Limitations of laser treatment for malignant dysphagia. Br. J. Surg., *79:*778, 1992.
69. Siersma, P.D., Dees, J., and Van Blankenstein, M.: Palliation of malignant dysphagia from oesophageal cancer. Scand. J. Gastroenterol., *35(Suppl. 225):*75, 1998.
70. Siersma, P.D., Hop, W.C.J., Dees, J., et al.: Coated self-expanding metal stents versus latex prostheses for esophagogastric cancer with special reference to prior radiation and chemotherapy: A controlled, prospective study. Gastrointest. Endosc., *47:*113, 1998.
71. Spencer, G.M., Thorpe, S.M., Sargeant, I.R., et al.: Laser and brachytherapy in the palliation of adenocarcinoma of the esophagus and cardia. Gut, *39:*726, 1996.
72. Spivak, H., Katariya, K., Lo, A.Y., et al.: Malignant tracheo-esophageal fistula: Use of esophageal endoprosthesis. J. Surg. Oncol., *63:*65, 1996.
73. Tygat, G.N.J.: Endoscopic therapy of esophageal cancer: Possibilities and limitations. Endoscopy, *22:*263, 1990.
74. Vakil, N., Morris, A., Segalin, A., et al.: Prospective, controlled, randomized, multicenter comparison of covered and uncovered expandable metal stents in malignant GE junction obstruction (Abstract). Gastrointest. Endosc., *47:*AB77, 1998.
75. Wallace, M.B., and Van Dam, J.: Endoscopic management for malignant tracheoesophageal fistulas. J. Crit. Illness, *13:*759, 1998.
76. Wengrower, D., Fiorini, A., Valero, J., et al.: EsophaCoil: Long-term results in 81 patients. Gastrointest. Endosc., *48:*376, 1998.

CHAPTER

23 Benign Tumors and Cysts of the Esophagus

RICHARD F. HEITMILLER

OVERVIEW

Benign tumors and cysts of the esophagus are rare. Patterson[1] identified only 62 reported cases of benign esophageal tumors over the 215-year period of 1717 to 1932. In separate autopsy series, Moersch and Harrington[2] and Plachta[3] reported a prevalence of benign esophageal tumors or cysts of 0.59% (44/7,459) and 0.45% (90/19,982), respectively. The autopsy review by Plachta best summarizes the overall characteristics of benign esophageal tumors and cysts. In that review, of the total 504 esophageal tumors identified at autopsy, 82% were malignant and 18% benign. Benign tumors were more common in males than in females. The mean age of patients was 45 and 68 years for symptomatic and asymptomatic patients, respectively, although the age range was broad (22 to 92 years). Of the 90 benign esophageal tumors, the most common were 49 (54%) leiomyomas, 23 (27%) polyps, 3 (3%) cysts, 3 (3%) hemangiomata, and 2 (2%) papillomata. There was a slightly increased prevalence of benign tumors involving the lower third of the esophagus.

Although these lesions may attain significant size, most reports note that they infrequently cause symptoms. Vinson et al.[4] evaluated 4,000 patients presenting to the Mayo Clinic for dysphagia and identified only 3 patients with benign esophageal tumors. The most common symptoms associated with benign esophageal tumors and cysts are dysphagia, regurgitation, odynophagia, cough, and wheezing.

Ten per cent (9 of 90) of patients with benign tumors required surgical treatment in Plachta's series.[3] More recent reports suggest that benign esophageal tumors and cysts are an infrequent indication for esophagectomy. Davis and Heitmiller[5] performed 45 esophagectomies for benign disease in which benign tumor was the indication in only 2 (5%) patients. The pathology for those two cases was leiomyoma and melanotic schwannoma. Benign tumor was not an indication for transhiatal esophagectomy in any of the 166 cases reviewed by Orringer and Stirling.[6] In an operative series of 20 patients by Mansour et al.,[7] there were 13 leiomyomas, 4 cysts, 2 polyps, and 1 patient with granular cell myoblastoma. The infrequent occurrence of benign esophageal tumors and cysts requires that esophageal surgeons be particularly vigilant in searching for them.

HISTORY

Sussius[8] is credited with the first description of a benign esophageal tumor, a leiomyoma, in 1559. Since that time, there has been a slowly accumulating experience with benign esophageal tumors and cysts, reflecting the infrequent occurrence of this pathology. The first pathologic description of a leiomyoma is attributed by Seremetis[9] to Virchow in 1863. One of the earliest studies evaluating the low prevalence of benign esophageal tumors was by Vinson et al.[4] from the Mayo Clinic in 1926. Of 4,000 patients who presented to the clinic with dysphagia, only 3 were found to have benign esophageal tumors as the cause for their symptoms. The infrequent occurrence was further established by Patterson[1] in 1932, who identified only 61 reported cases of benign esophageal tumors and cysts over the preceding 215 years. This fact is now a well-known characteristic of these tumors.

Although the majority of patients with benign esophageal tumors are asymptomatic, many of the early reports involved symptomatic patients. Arrowsmith (1877)[10] described a patient with a benign polypoid esophageal growth resulting in such severe dysphagia that the patient died of malnutrition. Moersch and Harrington (1944)[2] noted that only 1 of 15 patients was asymptomatic. This undoubtedly reflects that these reports antedated modern endoscopic and radiographic methods, which have since increased the probability of diagnosis of asymptomatic lesions.

One of the first reports of treatment was by Vater (cited in reference 11), in 1750, who described a patient whose esophageal polyp spontaneously separated and was regurgitated. In 1818, Dubois (quoted in reference 12) successfully ligated a polypoid intraluminal esophageal neoplasm, which later separated while the patient was sleeping and led to regurgitation, aspiration, and asphixiation. Mackenzie[11] described 2 patients whose tumors were removed with a probang, which is a long, flexible rod with a sponge at one end. The first open surgical removal of a benign tumor is generally attributed to Oshawa[13] in 1933; however, Storey and Adams[14] identified a report from one year earlier by Sauerbruch[15] of a transpleural resection of a leiomyoma. The first successful surgery in the United States is attributed to Churchill[16] in 1937.

CLASSIFICATION

Three classification schemes have been proposed. They are summarized in Table 23–1. The first classification system, advocated by both Sweet et al.[17] and Moersch and Harrington,[2] is based on both clinical and gross pathologic findings. They organized tumors according to the esophageal layer, mucosa, submucosa, and muscularis, from which they originated. The second, an anatomic classification attributed to Nemir et al.,[18] organizes esophageal tumors by cell of origin into epithelial, non-epithelial, and heterotopic tumors. The third approach classifies benign tumors and cysts by location and clinical (radiographic and endoscopic) appearance. One example of this third approach, cited by Reed[19] and attributed to Herrera,[20] classifies tumors as intraluminal, intramural, and extramural. Another example, advocated by Avezzano et al.,[21] classifies tumors into two groups, intramural-extramucosal, and mucosal-intraluminal. These two similar schemes are combined into the third classification based on clinical findings. The following description of the specific benign tumors and cysts of the esophagus are organized by this last classification scheme.

INTRAMURAL-EXTRAMUCOSAL

Leiomyoma

Leiomyoma of the esophagus is the most common benign esophageal tumor. The frequency of diagnosis of esophageal leiomyoma is increasing as a consequence of improved diagnostic methods and not because of an increase in overall prevalence. Currently, most single cases of leiomyoma go unreported. The characteristic clinical features of patients with these tumors, described in earlier reviews by Storey and Adams,[14] Seremetis et al.,[9] Sweet et al.,[17] and Postlethwaite and Lowe,[8] remain remarkably consistent and valid today. New developments include the application of cytogenetic markers for classification and staging, the use of endoscopic ultrasound for diagnosis, and the introduction of minimally invasive techniques for surgical management of these tumors.

Table 23–1. Proposed Classification Schemes for Benign Esophageal Tumors

I. Classification by esophageal layer or origin[2,17]
   a. Mucosal
   b. Submucosal
   c. Muscularis
II. Classification by anatomic site of origin[18]
   a. Epithelial
   b. Non-epithelial
   c. Heterotopic
III. Classification by location and clinical appearance[19,20,55]
   a. Intramural-extramucosal
   b. Intraluminal-mucosal
   c. Cysts and duplications

Esophageal leiomyomas are uncommon. Many are undoubtedly small and remain undetected. The frequency of these tumors as estimated by autopsy series varies considerably from 1:63.6 to 1:18,847 patients. Some of the variation in reported frequency is undoubtedly related to the pathologist's zeal in searching for leiomyomas. As an example, Postlethwait and Musser[22] identified 51 leiomyomas in 1,000 unselected autopsy specimens (1:19.6 patients) using a compulsive histologic evaluation of each esophagus. Most of the tumors they found were small, 1 to 4 mm in diameter, and might have been missed by gross inspection alone. Lortat-Jacob[23] estimated that leiomyomas represents 0.4% of all esophageal tumors. Leiomyomas make up approximately two thirds of all benign esophageal tumors, and only 6% of all gastrointestinal leiomyomas arise in the esophagus. Esophageal cancer is 50 times more common than leiomyoma.

Patient characteristics are similar from reported series. In a review of 838 patients with leiomyomas, Seremetis et al.[9] found the mean age to be 44 (12 to 80) years. Male patients outnumbered female patients 1.9:1. Storey and Adams,[14] in an earlier review, demonstrated that the incidence of leiomyoma was similar (21 to 24.7%) for each of the four decades between the ages of 20 and 60 years. In their series, the percentage of male and female patients was 64.6 and 35.4%, respectively. In a smaller series, Sweet et al.[17] demonstrated the mean age to be 41.2 (range 19 to 67) years and the distribution of male and female patients to be similar to the figure reported by Storey and Adams.

Postlethwait and Lowe[8] have proposed a leiomyoma classification system based on gross findings. Tumors are classified as 1, round or oval (solitary or multiple); 2, solitary with extension; and 3, confluent (limited or leiomyomatosis). Grossly, esophageal leiomyomas are firm, well-circumscribed masses that have a whorled appearance on the cut surface, which may be smooth or exhibit nodularity. There is no specific fibrous encapsulation. These tumors are usually intramural, and the esophageal mucosa overlying the tumor is generally intact. However, some leiomyomas arise entirely outside the esophageal wall (2%) and are connected by a connective tissue stalk. A small subset (1%) present as an intraluminal polypoid tumor. Although larger tumors may become adherent to adjacent structures, they are not invasive. Tumors exhibit calcification in 1.8 to 3.9% of cases. Microscopically, leiomyomas reveal uniform spindle cells arranged in fascicles or whorls as illustrated in Figure 23–1. Fibrous tissue may be absent but its presence tends to increase in prevalence with tumor size. Fibrous encapsulation is absent.

Usually, leiomyomas are 2 to 5 cm in diameter, although tumors have been reported in sizes of several millimeters to 22 cm in length. Tumors exceeding 1,000 g are generally termed giant. Tumors can assume many shapes—some uniform, others bizarre. Round, oval, spiral, and horseshoe shapes have all been described. The vast majority of leiomyomas (97%) are solitary; the re-

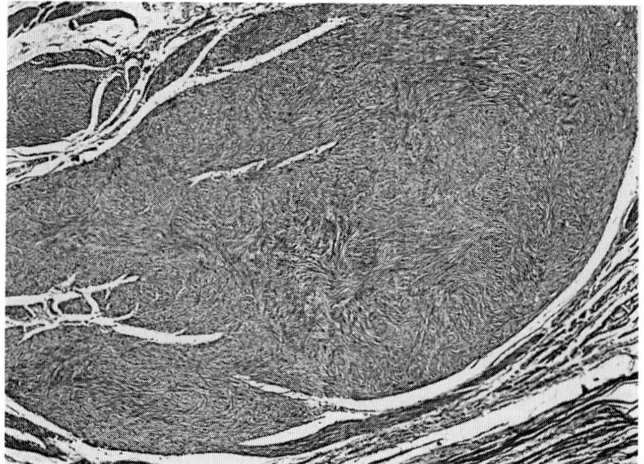

Figure 23–1. Photomicrograph of an intramural circumscribed leiomyoma demonstrating uniform spindle cells arranged in fascicles or whorls.

mainder are multiple. In some cases, the entire smooth muscle portion of the esophagus is filled by confluent small tumors; this condition is termed leiomyomatosis. According to Seremetis et al.,[9] the distribution of leiomyomas in the lower, middle, and upper esophagus is 56%, 33%, and 11%, respectively.

Originally, it was speculated that leiomyomas arose from smooth muscle cells of the muscularis mucosa, muscularis propria, blood vessel wall, or embryonic rest cells within the esophageal wall. Current cytogenetic studies, however, suggest that leiomyomas arise from the interstitial cells of Cajal (ICC), which regulate gut peristalsis. These cells have the potential to develop into smooth muscle cells, creating leiomyomas; into neural cells, creating schwannomas; or into undifferentiated mesenchymal tumors with stromal cell features, creating gastrointestinal stromal cell tumors (GIST). Specific cytogenetic markers have been identified that both differentiate these three tumors and demonstrate a common site of origin. These cytogenetic findings help explain the histologic similarity often seen among these three tumors and why these tumors have been reported to occur together in a single patient.[24, 25]

The symptoms related to leiomyomas, comprehensively reviewed by Seremetis et al.[9] continue to be valid today and are listed in Table 23–2. Approximately half of patients with leiomyomas are asymptomatic. When symptoms are present, dysphagia and pain predominate. The pain is usually retrosternal or epigastric and is often described as a feeling of pressure. Unlike the case of leiomyomas originating in the stomach, bleeding from esophageal leiomyomas is rare. Patients' symptoms are of long duration. Sixty per cent of patients reported the presence of symptoms over 2 years or more. The remaining 40% of patients had symptoms for an average of 11 months. Storey and Adams[14] emphasized that, in a symptomatic patient, multiple symptoms were the rule. They also noted that respiratory symptoms, including cough, dyspnea, or both, occurred in 10% of patients. Sweet et al.[17] identified tumor size as the single most important factor in determining the likelihood and severity of symptoms. The case of a 13-year-old girl with hypertrophic osteoarthropathy and an esophageal leiomyoma has been reported.[28] The osteoarthropathy rapidly regressed after removal of the leiomyoma.

Table 23–2. Esophageal Leiomyoma: Major Symptoms

Symptom	Prevalance
Dysphagia	47.5%
Pain	45%
Pyrosis	40%
Weight Loss	24%
Duration of Symptoms	30% > 5 yrs
	30% > 2 yrs
	40% 11 mos*

*Average length of symptoms.
From Seremetis M.G., Lyons, W.S., DeGuzman, V.C., and Peabody, J.W.: Leiomyomata of the esophagus: An analysis of 828 cases. Cancer, *38*:2166, 1976.

Conditions that historically have been associated with esophageal leiomyoma include hiatal hernia, diverticula, and achalasia. Amer et al.[27] documented esophageal motility disorders, distinct from achalasia, in four patients whose motility patterns normalized after leiomyoma removal. The association of leiomyoma with esophageal motility disorders might be expected given that these tumors originate from ICC cells, which are responsible for gastrointestinal motility. Other disorders that should be considered in the differential diagnosis of leiomyoma include esophageal cancer, other benign esophageal tumors or cysts, vascular anomalies, and lung and mediastinal tumors.

No symptoms specifically indicate that a patient has a leiomyoma. Fifty per cent of patients are asymptomatic. Symptomatic patients have indolent and often vague symptoms. Similarly, there are no physical findings that are characteristic for esophageal leiomyoma. If a tumor is larger sized—especially if it extends outside the esophageal wall—it may be visualized on plain chest film. The barium swallow features characteristic of leiomyoma have been well described.[8, 28–30] Contrast esophagogram demonstrates a segmental lesion that focally impinges on the column of swallowed contrast medium (Fig. 23–2). The crescent-shaped mass generally shows half the mass to be in the esophageal wall and the rest extending into the lumen. The junction of the mass and the esophageal wall demonstrates sharp margins (approaching 90 degrees). There is little obstruction to the flow of the contrast medium. The mucosa overlying the mass is intact but smooth, as though it is stretched over the tumor. The mucosa on the opposite wall is intact. Proximal esophageal dilatation is unusual. Tumors near or involving the esophagogastric margin are often larger, angulate the esophagus, and flatten the lumen. These tumors may demonstrate proximal esophageal dilatation and may simulate achalasia. Computed tomography (CT) may be used to image leiomyomas, which are seen to be submucosal masses. Administration of oral contrast material helps in visualizing these tumors. CT scanning is most helpful in evaluating larger tumors, especially those that extend outside the esophageal wall, for the assessment of the interface between the tumor and the mediastinum. The endoscopic characteristics of leiomyomas have also been

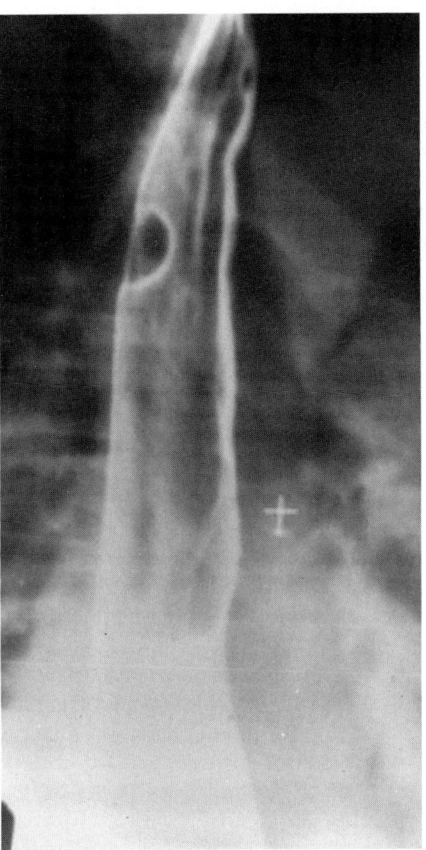

Figure 23–2. Contrast esophagogram demonstrating the characteristic findings of a leiomyoma.

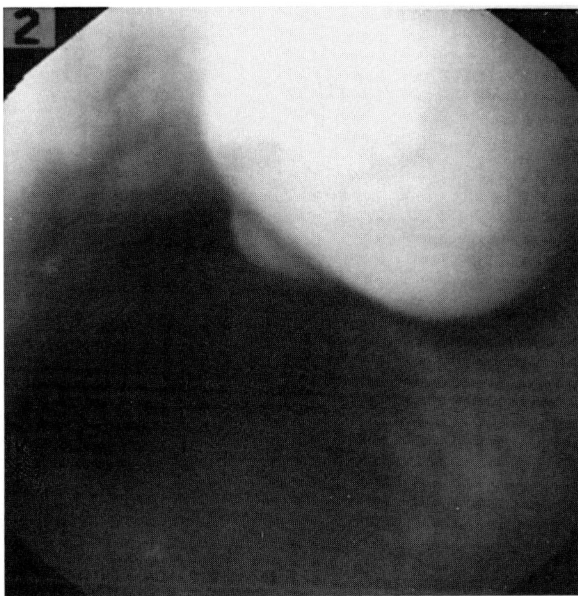

Figure 23–3. Endoscopic appearance of a leiomyoma illustrating the segmental tumor bulge, intact overlying mucosa, and luminal narrowing without obstruction.

well described[23, 33] and include (1) segmental tumor bulge into the lumen, (2) an intact overlying esophageal mucosa, (3) narrowing of the esophageal lumen without obstruction, and (4) a movable mass (Fig. 23–3). Finally, endoscopic ultrasound (EUS) has been shown to be useful in the diagnosis and staging of leiomyoma. EUS confirms the diagnosis by demonstrating that the mass arises from the submucosa (Fig. 23–4). It can also easily rule out a cystic mass that may be masquerading as a leiomyoma. Internal echo patterns of the tumor help to differentiate between benign and malignant tumors.[32, 33] In one study, Kawamoto et al.[34] showed that 98% of benign leiomyomas were anechoic, were of intermediate echogenicity, or were hypoechoic. EUS also defines the extent of tumor margins accurately.

The treatment of choice continues to be removal of the tumor by splitting the esophageal musculature and extracting the leiomyoma without injuring the underlying mucosa. If the mucosa is unexpectedly opened, it should be closed with a standard inverting suture technique. The divided musculature is then reapproximated over the defect. This procedure is termed enucleation[8, 17, 19] and is illustrated in Figure 23–5. Most cases of enucleation have been performed using thoracotomy. For tumors in the lower third of the esophagus, a left thoracotomy is employed, whereas a right thoracotomy is recommended for more proximal intrathoracic tumors. More recently, enucleation has been described using videothoracoscopic techniques.[35-37] Simultaneous intraoperative flexible esophagoscopy helps to localize the lesion, stabilize the esophagus, and protect the mucosa from inadvertent injury. Enucleation of lower-third leiomyomas has been reported using laparotomy and a transhiatal approach. In the series reported by Seremetis et al.,[9] esophageal resection was required in 10% of patients. The indications for resection were large tumors (>8 cm in diameter), annular tumors, dense adherence to the underlying mucosa, and extensive accidential damage to the esophageal wall during dissection. In rare cases, the tumor presents as an intraluminal polyp and may be resected endoscopically.

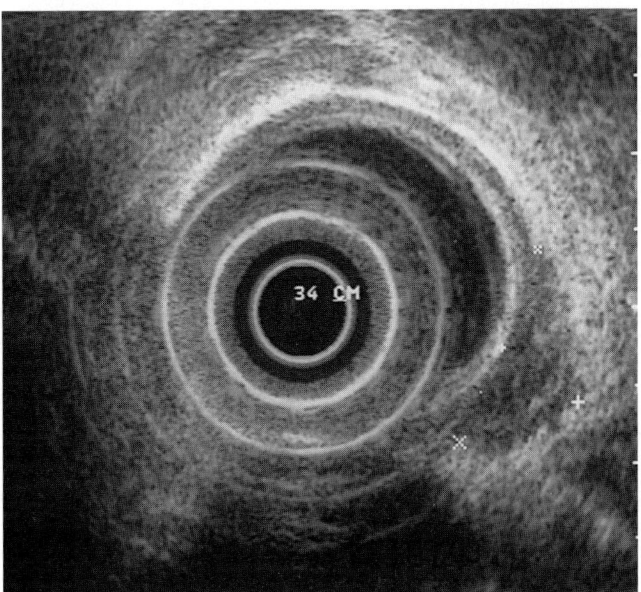

Figure 23–4. Endoscopic ultrasound of a leiomyoma demonstrating the size and location of the tumor. The tumor borders are marked by the three scan markers (*, x, +).

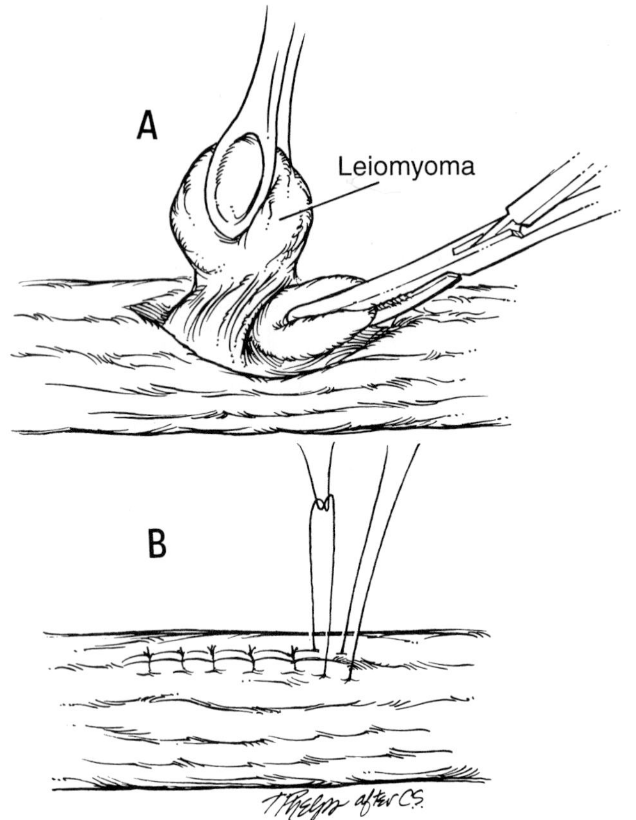

Figure 23–5. The technique of enucleation is illustrated. *A,* The esophageal muscular fibers are split and the leiomyoma is bluntly extracted from the esophageal wall. *B,* Once removed, the muscular defect is reapproximated.

Esophageal reconstruction following resection should be performed in accordance with the fact that the patient has benign disease.

Published results indicate that the surgical therapy for esophageal leiomyoma is safe.[8, 19] Rendina et al.[38] reported an operative mortality rate of 1.3% and 10.5% for enucleation and esophagectomy, respectively. In a more recent series by Bonavina et al.[39] of 66 patients, 95.5% of patients were managed by enucleation and 4.5% required esophagectomy. Enucleation was performed by thoracotomy in 50 (79%), laparotomy in 5 (8%), and videothoracoscopy in 8 (13%) patients. Indications for esophagectomy were either diffuse disease or large size. In their series, there were no deaths. The data suggest a continued decline in operative mortality in the management of these tumors in adults. Operative mortality for pediatric patients is higher (21%), undoubtedly reflecting the higher percentage of esophagectomies required for younger patients.[19, 40]

Leiomyoma rarely occurs in patients below the age of 10 to 12 years.[19, 40] In the pediatric age group, leiomyoma is more common in females and there is diffuse esophageal involvement in over 91% of all patients. Dysphagia is the most common presenting symptom. Patients are often thought to have achalasia. Because of the diffuse nature of the disease in children, treatment for the majority of them requires esophagectomy.

Granular Cell Tumor

Granular cell tumors (GCTs), also known as granular cell myoblastoma, are rare submucosal tumors that infrequently involve the esophagus. Esophageal GCTs and leiomyomas are both intramural submucosal tumors that share many clinical features, including presenting symptoms, diagnostic work-up, and treatment options. Abrikossof is credited with the first description of this tumor in 1926, and the first description of an esophageal GCT in 1931.[8] GCTs may occur in any organ system but are most commonly seen in the submucosa of the tongue, breast, respiratory system, and gastrointestinal tract. Most cases of GCT are benign. Malignant GCTs make up only 2 to 3% of overall cases. Reports have documented both a male[41] and a female[42] predominance with this tumor. More likely, GCT occurs equally in both sexes.[8] The average age at the time of diagnosis is 40 to 44 years. Although experience is accumulating with GCT, there is still controversy regarding its specific cell of origin, differentiation of benign and malignant tumors, and recommendations for optimal management.

The prevailing opinion is that GCT arises from neural cells within the esophageal wall. GCT cells have electron microscopic features similar to those of Schwann cells and stain for the neural proteins S-100 and neuron-specific enoslase (NSE).[8, 19] Only 1 to 2% of GCTs are found in the esophagus. Most GCTs, 50 to 63%, are located in the distal esophagus. Multiple esophageal GCTs are reported in 20% of patients. When the esophagus is involved, it is the sole organ site in the majority of cases; however, in 5 to 14% of patients GCTs are identified in multiple organ sites.[42] Grossly, the tumor arises in the submucosa and protrudes into the esophageal lumen. GCTs have a characteristic pale yellow color. The overlying esophageal mucosa is intact, but it is often so translucent that it seems absent. Microscopically, these tumor cells are pale staining with small nuclei and abundant cytoplasm, which is characteristically granular in appearance (Fig. 23-6). The overlying mucosa shows pseudoepitheliomatous hyperplasia. No characteristic histologic

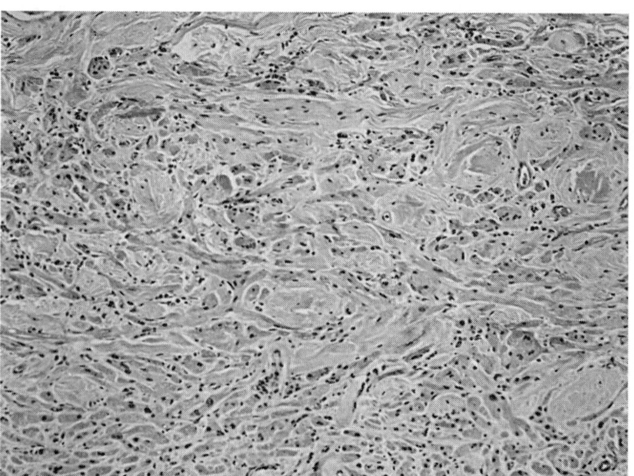

Figure 23–6. Photomicrograph of a granular cell tumor that shows relatively uniform plump spindle cells containing coarsely granular eosinophilic cytoplasm.

findings define malignant GCT. The diagnosis of benign versus malignant GCT is made on the basis of both clinical and histologic findings. Both local invasion and metastases have been reported with malignant GCT.

There are great similarities in the symptoms produced by esophageal GCT and leiomyoma. Symptoms include dysphagia, retrosternal pain or vague discomfort, and, less frequently, nausea and vomiting. Fifty per cent of GCT patients are asymptomatic. Coutinho et al.[41] have demonstrated nicely that the frequency of symptoms is directly related to tumor size as shown in Figure 23-7. In their series, the frequency of symptoms for patients with tumor sizes of 10 mm or less, 11 to 20 mm, 21 to 30 mm, and 31 to 40 mm was 25%, 52.2%, 77.7%, and 80%, respectively. The differential diagnosis for patients with suspected GCT includes other benign esophageal tumors and carcinoma.

As with patients with leiomyoma, the diagnosis is best made by contrast esophagogram and endoscopy. Barium esophagogram demonstrates a smooth-walled filling defect impinging on the esophageal lumen. Smaller tumors are difficult to identify radiographically, but larger tumors may result in high-grade esophageal obstruction. Endoscopically, the tumor is visible as a yellowish "molar-shaped" polypoid lesion protruding into the lumen.[43] Endoscopic biopsies of these tumors are often nondiagnostic. Endoscopic ultrasound is helpful to define the site of origin and the extent of these tumors. Tada et al.[43] describe the EUS findings of esophageal GCT as hyperechoic solid tumors surrounded by hypoechoic submucosa without continuity with the muscularis propria.

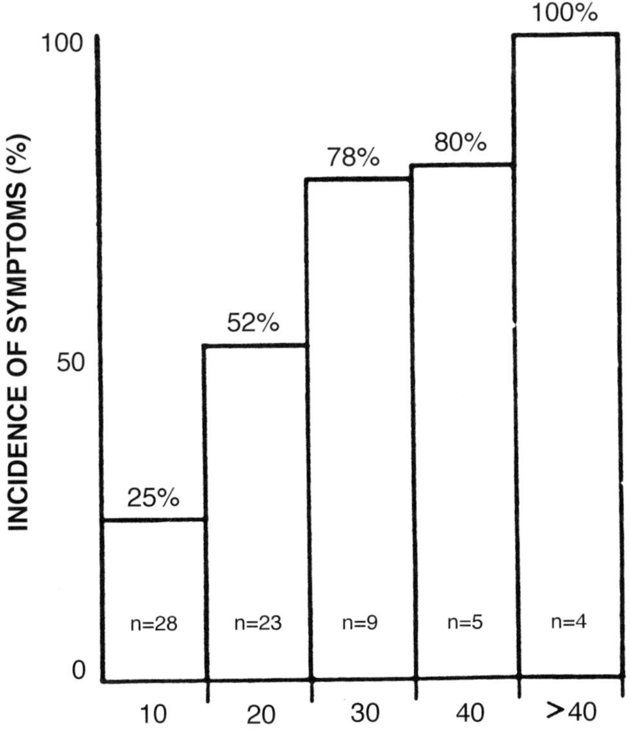

Figure 23-7. Incidence of symptoms as a function of granular cell tumor size. (From Coutinho, D.S. de S., Soga, J., Yoshikawa, T., et al.: Granular cell tumors of the esophagus: A report of two cases and review of the literature. Am. J. Gastroenterol., 80:758, 1985, with permission.)

The management of patients with GCT remains controversial. Postlethwait and Lowe[8] have argued that these tumors should be treated aggressively, with surgical removal on diagnosis, because of the inability to distinguish between benign and malignant tumors. Others have advocated conservative management with endoscopic follow-up for smaller, asymptomatic tumors. These authors cite the low frequency of malignancy and the availability of the tumor for endoscopic surveillance as justification for conservative management. This issue remains unresolved. There is agreement that symptomatic tumors and any tumor demonstrating rapid growth are indications for tumor removal. Transthoracic local resection of GCT is the gold standard of therapy. There are no reports of using videothoracoscopic methods. Operative mortality is approximately 2%. Endoscopic removal has been described but is reportedly associated with a possibility of local recurrence. One case of endoscopic alcohol injection of a GCT under EUS guidance has been reported.[45]

Hemangioma

Hemangiomas are benign vascular tumors that originate from the esophageal submucosa. They are rare, with fewer than 100 reported cases in the literature. In Plachta's series,[3] hemangioma accounted for 3% of all benign esophageal tumors. Gentry et al.[46] found that only 11 of 261 (4.2%) of gastrointestinal vascular tumors were located in the esophagus. The first description of an esophageal hemangioma, treated by radium application, is credited to Vinson et al.[47] in 1926. No data define the demographics of patients with esophageal hemangioma. Riemenschneider and Klassen[48] noted a slight male predominance and an age range from newborn infants to 72 years.

The gross appearance of hemangioma is a bluish-colored polypoid mass arising from the submucosa of the esophageal wall. Some hemangioma are small and form simple cystic masses. Others can become quite large with multinodularity. The tumor is noncircumferential and may involve the esophagus anywhere along its length. In a review of 58 patients, Govoni[49] noted that the majority of hemangiomas were located in the middle or distal esophagus. Microscopically, there is proliferation of benign vascular spaces of a cavernous nature. Multinodular masses demonstrate fibrous septation. The overlying mucosa is intact.

Symptoms include dysphagia, hemorrhage, and substernal pain or discomfort. In adults, symptoms may be of relatively short duration (2 months) or may be chronic (7 years).[48] Dysphagia tends to be mild even with larger tumors owing to the compressible, noncircumferential nature of these tumors. The hemorrhage produced by rupture may be massive and even fatal. Approximately one third to one half of patients with hemangiomas are asymptomatic.

Hemangiomas appear as well-defined submucosal tumors on barium esophagogram. A bluish, polypoid submucosal lesion is seen endoscopically. The mass is compressible endoscopically, and biopsies are not recommended.[50] EUS has been used to identify and "stage" these vascular tumors. In contrast to its use for leiomyomas or granular cell tumors, CT is particularly helpful in making the diagnosis of and planning the treatment for hemangiomas.[51] Magnetic resonance imaging also has been described in the diagnosis of hemangioma. This is especially true for larger tumors.

A wide variety of treatments have been proposed to manage esophageal leiomyoma, including endoscopic resection,[52] fulguration, sclerotherapy,[53] radiation therapy, and open or videothoracoscopic resection.[54] Removal usually can be performed either by local resection or enucleation, although esophagectomy is occasionally required. The surgical procedures are safe, with a mortality of approximately 2%.[8] There are no reports of recurrence following resection. The results of endoscopic resection are limited to case reports but seem reasonable over a limited follow-up.

Other Intramural Tumors

All benign esophageal tumors are uncommon. The most common intramural tumors, leiomyomas, granular cell tumors, and hemangioma, have been discussed separately. Other rare intramural esophageal tumors have been reported. These are covered briefly in this section.

Rhabdomyomas are tumors of the striated skeletal muscle of the upper third of the esophagus and are rare. Not enough patients have been identified to determine the clinical characteristics of these tumors. Lipomas and fibromas usually protrude into the esophageal lumen as polyps but may form submucosal masses. Schwannomas share many pathologic and clinical features with leiomyoma. Both tumors arise from the interstitial stem cells of Cajal. Schwannomas produce the same symptoms as leiomyomas and are diagnosed in the same manner. Recommended treatment is surgical enucleation. Congenital ectopic rests of pancreatic, thyroid, and parathyroid tissue have been reported in the esophageal wall.[8] In some cases, this tissue has been hormonally active. Treatment is local resection or enucleation.

INTRALUMINAL/MUCOSAL

Fibrovascular Polyp

Fibrovascular polyps are the second most common benign esophageal tumor and the most common intraluminal tumor. Fibrovascular polyp is a term that includes a broad range of specific intraluminal polyps, including fibromas, fibrolipomas, myomas, myxofibromas, pedunculated lipomas, and fibroepithelial polyps. The pathogenesis, clinical features, workup, and treatment options are similar regardless of the specific histologic type of polyp. Although not proved, it is hypothesized that these polyps begin as a region of submucosal thickening that elongates into the esophageal lumen as a result of esophageal peristaltic action to form a polyp. Polyps most commonly originate from the proximal esophagus just distal to the cricopharyngeus. They may achieve large size, resulting in esophageal dilatation, or be long enough to reach into the stomach. The most dramatic clinical feature of fibrovascular polyps is their potential for regurgitation out through the oropharynx, where they may be reswallowed, severed by biting and expectorated, or aspirated. Avezzano et al.[21] reported a male predominance (75%) and a peak prevalence in the sixth and seventh decades. Postlethwait and Lowe[8] commented that polyps were seen in older men (average age 54.7 years) and younger women (average age 43.4). In their series, 69% of patients were men (Table 23-3).

Grossly, these polyps are cylindrical-shaped masses attached by a stalk to the esophageal wall, usually of the proximal esophagus. Polyps range in length from less than 1 cm to greater than 20 cm. The average size is 5 cm.[57] Polyps may be long enough that they extend into the stomach, where acid results in focal ulceration. The diameter of a polyp may be wide enough that it results in esophageal dilatation. Multiple polyps have been reported. The site of origin within the esophagus is cervical, upper thoracic, middle, and lower esophageal in 80%, 2%, 8%, and 10% of patients, respectively.[8] Histologically, these polyps are composed of mature fibrous tissue with varying amounts of vascularity and adipose tissue. Which of these three components is most prominent determines the specific name for the polyp (e.g., fibrolipoma, myxofibroma). Polyps are covered by intact smooth mucosa. No malignant degeneration of these polyps has been reported, although at least one case of a coexisting squamous cell carcinoma has been identified.[55]

Aside from a regurgitated polyp, no physical findings are characteristic of these tumors. Potential symptoms include intermittent dysphagia, regurgitation of the polyp, and respiratory symptoms. Polyps that extend into the stomach may ulcerate and bleed, resulting in anemia and related symptoms. Levine et al.[56] reported that dysphagia (87%) and respiratory (25%) symptoms were most common. Regurgitation of the polyp into the mouth was noted in only 12% of patients. In Levine and colleagues' experience, the average duration of symptoms was 17 months; however, 44% of patients had symptoms for 6 months or less. Up to 30% of patients have been reported to be asymptomatic. Barium esophagogram demonstrates a polypoid filling defect that may be seen to move within

Table 23–3. Age and Sex of 55 Patients with Fibrovascular Polyps

Age (Yr)	Men	Women
20–29	3	5
30–39	3	3
40–49	6	1
50–59	11	4
60–69	8	4
70–79	5	0
80–89	2	0

From Postlethwait, R.W., and Lowe, J.E.: Benign tumors and cysts of the esophagus. *In* Zuidema, G.D. [ed.]: Shackelford's Surgery of the Alimentary Tract, Vol. I, 4th ed. Philadelphia, W.B. Saunders, 1996, pp. 369–386.

the esophageal lumen with a swallow. High-grade obstruction is uncommon. Larger polyps may cause esophageal dilatation that mimics achalasia. Polyps may be missed on endoscopy because most originate in the proximal esophagus and because they are covered by normal mucosa. EUS demonstrates an echo-dense intraluminal polyp.[55] Computed tomographic findings are of an intraluminal mass with heterogeneous density.[57] The differential diagnosis for a patient suspected of having a fibrovascular polyp includes polypoid schwannoma, leiomyoma, and hamartoma.

Treatment is resection of the polyp, including its point of origin and attachment. Failure to completely remove the polyp may result in recurrence. Historically, resection has been accomplished by open surgical techniques in which the esophageal wall is opened, preferably 180 degrees opposite the base of the polyp, and the polyp and stalk excised along with a small cuff of mucosa. The mucosal defect is reapproximated and the esophagotomy closed. The procedure is performed via cervical incision for proximal tumors and thoracotomy for more distal lesions. Endoscopic removal has been reported for polyps without excessive vascularity. Unless the polyp base is completely removed, however, local recurrence is possible. Treatment by either method is safe. No treatment-related deaths have been reported.[21]

Squamous Papilloma

Papilloma is a benign neoplastic disorder involving the esophageal mucosa. It is rare. Autopsy series show a frequency of 0.01 to 0.04% of the general population.[57] Adler et al.[58] are credited with the first histologic description in 1959. Papillomas occur in males more frequently than in females (2:1). The age on diagnosis ranges from 40 to 70 years. The etiology of papillomas is unknown. Gastrointestinal reflux or other chronic mucosal irritation has been proposed as a potential cause. More recently, Politoske[59] has reported on one case of esophageal papilloma associated with the human papillomavirus. The significance of this lesion is unclear. There is no documented premalignant transformation of papillomas; however, cases of progressive, fatal systemic dissemination have been reported.

Papillomas are usually solitary, sessile lesions involving the distal esophagus. Most lesions are small, measuring less than 1 cm in diameter. Microscopically, papillomas are composed of a central core of connective tissue covered with hyperplastic squamous cells (Fig. 23–8).

The majority of patients with papillomas are asymptomatic. Some patients may complain of mild dysphagia. There is an association of papillomas with gastroesophageal reflux and peptic ulcer disease.[58] Therefore, some patients may present indirectly with symptoms of these associated disorders. There are no characteristic findings on physical examination. Endoscopically fleshy pink-colored lesions, either sessile or pedunculated, are seen usually in the distal esophagus. Visually, the lesions may be mistaken for squamous carcinoma. The diagnosis is confirmed by biopsy. No further diagnostic or staging workup has been advocated.

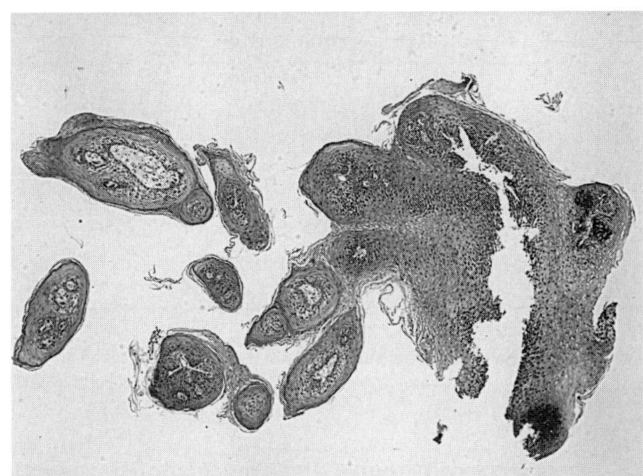

Figure 23–8. Photomicrograph of squamous papilloma showing no dysplastic squamous epithelium with a central core of connective tissue.

On the basis of published reports, it is not clear as to whether these lesions should be followed or aggressively resected. Certainly, the diagnosis must first be confirmed and cancer ruled out by biopsy. If a lesion is localized and pedunculated, most likely it should be resected endoscopically and the patient followed. Papillomas have been noted to recur and spread after treatment by laser fulguration, endoscopic resection, or surgical excision. Because of the risk of seeding, recurrence, or proliferation of disease, Politoske[59] concludes that papillomas should be removed with as little manipulation as possible.

CYSTS AND DUPLICATIONS

Cysts and duplications are included together because they share similar etiology, clinical and radiographic findings, and treatment options. Autopsy studies of the general population estimate the incidence of esophageal cysts to be 1:8,200 patients.[60] Ten to fifteen per cent of all gastrointestinal duplications are esophageal in origin. Cysts are more commonly diagnosed in males than in females and in children than in adults. Cysts and duplications account for approximately 0.5 to 3.3% of all benign esophageal tumors. In children, however, duplications have been shown to account for 12% of mediastinal masses. It is estimated that only 25 to 30% of patients with cysts occur in adults. Posthlethwaite and Lowe[8] demonstrated a biphasic age distribution for patients with cysts. Forty-one per cent of patients presented before age 9, and 38% presented between the ages of 20 and 49 years. The first description of a cyst is credited to Blassius in 1711, and the first resection of a cyst was reported by Sauerbruch and Fick in 1931.[15]

Arbona et al.[62] proposed a classification for esophageal cysts, which is most commonly cited and which is included in Table 23–4.

Cysts and duplications are congenital in origin. One theory states that the early foregut is lined with ciliated columnar epithelium that grows and obliterates the lumen. Vacuoles then are secreted that coalesce, line up,

Table 23–4. Classification of Esophageal Cysts

I. Congenital
  a. Duplication
  b. Bronchogenic
  c. Gastric
  d. Inclusion
II. Other
  a. Neuroenteric
III. Acquired
  a. Retention (single or multiple)

Data from Arbono, J.L., Fazzi, G.F., and Mayoral, J.: Congenital esophageal cysts: Case report and review of the literature. Am. J. Gastroenterol., *79*:177, 1984.

and form the bowel lumen. It is postulated that single vacuoles become separated and remain within the esophageal wall and develop into duplications or cysts.[19, 61, 62] Another theory has been advocated by Hutchison and Thomson.[63] Because the endodermal tube, which is destined to form the gut, is a part of the yolk sac or archenteron, they propose that all developmental gastrointestinal cysts should be labeled as archenteric cysts. According to their theory, at an early stage in development, a segment of endoderm becomes separated and fails to become incorporated into the developing gut. This segment retains its endodermal competence and therefore directs the mesoderm to form surrounding muscular wall. However, being displaced, its histologic differentiation is less precise, accounting for the diversity of mucosal linings noted in these developmental cysts.

Esophageal cysts are classified as duplications[19, 61, 62] if the cyst (1) is located within the esophageal wall, (2) is covered by two muscular layers, and (3) is lined by squamous epithelium or embryonic epithelium (columnar, pseudostratified, ciliated). Duplications are usually round but may be elongated tubular structures. The average diameter of spherical duplications is 4.5 cm. They are most frequently found in the lower esophagus. In the collective series by Arbona et al.,[62] the location was lower, middle, and upper esophagus in 60%, 17%, 23%, respectively. A case of an esophageal duplication cyst presenting as an abdominal mass has been reported. Esophageal duplications can be associated with duplications elsewhere in the gastrointestinal tract. Duplication cysts are not associated with vertebral abnormalities. Malignancies arising in duplications are rare.

Bronchogenic cysts arising from the esophagus are rare.[62] These cysts arise from an abnormality in lung bud separation from the primative foregut. Cells from this evolving lung bud become sequestered within the esophageal wall and develop into a bronchogenic cyst. Pathologically, these cysts are located within the esophageal wall and contain cartilage (Fig. 23-9). These cysts are found within the middle and lower thirds of the esophagus and are not associated with vertebral anomalies. No neoplastic changes have been reported.

Gastric cysts are postulated to arise from cells that are destined to become stomach but that fail to descend and remain within the esophageal wall. To be classified as a gastric cyst, a cyst must be located within the esophageal wall, contain a muscular wall, and be lined with gastric mucosa.[62] Mucosal hydrochloric acid and enzyme production with ulceration and hemorrhage has been described.

Inclusion cysts are intramural cysts that contain respiratory or squamous epithelium, are not covered by muscle, and do not contain cartilage. They can therefore be differentiated from bronchogenic and duplication cysts. Arbona et al.[62] reported inclusion cyst location to be in the lower, middle, or upper esophagus in 66%, 24%, and 10% of patients, respectively. Cyst size ranged from 0.5 cm to 20 cm. They are not associated with vertebral abnormalities.

Neuroenteric cysts, also known as posterior mediastinal duplication cysts, arise during notochord separation from the foregut endoderm. In this separation, an endodermal diverticulum may form that remains fused to the esophagus or attached to it by a stalk and develops into a cyst. Neuroenteric cysts are found in the posterior mediastinum, are covered by muscle, and are lined by a variety of gastrointestinal mucosa.[62] They are associated with vertebral abnormalities, which may not be at the same level as the cyst.

The normal esophagus contains mucosal and submucosal glands that may coalesce to form acquired cysts. They may be single or multiple. If multiple, the cysts are referred to as esophagitis cystica. These cysts range in size from a few millimeters to 3 cm in diameter and are located in the upper third of the esophagus.

No findings on physical examination are characteristic of cysts and duplications. Symptoms are related to size, location, and patient age. Respiratory symptoms, including cough and wheezing, are more common in children. Gastrointestinal symptoms, including dysphagia, epigastric and substernal pain, or anorexia and nausea, are more common in adults. The prevalence of gastroesophageal reflux seems to be increased in patients with cysts and duplications. According to Cioffi et al.,[64] 37% of patients are asymptomatic on presentation. Findings on contrast esophagography and esophagoscopy are similar to those seen in patients with leiomyoma in which a smooth-walled submucosal mass is identified. EUS is helpful to define the anatomy and establish the diagnosis. Com-

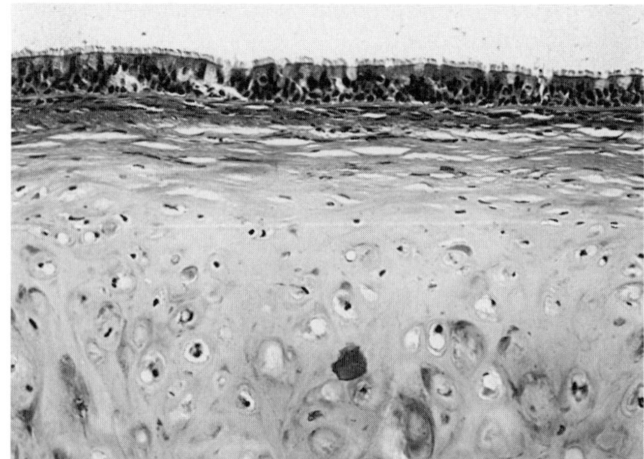

Figure 23–9. Photomicrograph of a bronchogenic cyst wall showing mature cartilage and respiratory-type pseudostratified ciliated columnar epithelium.

puted tomography is also helpful both for making the diagnosis and for planning surgical therapy.

Management options include observation, aspiration, and surgical resection. There are advocates for each option. Indications for resection include symptom control, increase in cyst size, and to rule out malignancy. Surgically, cysts may be enucleated in a manner similar to that used with leiomyomas. The procedure has been performed both through open thoracotomy as well as video-assisted thoracoscopic techniques.

References

1. Patterson, E.J.: Benign neoplasms of the esophagus: Report of a case of myxofibroma. Ann. Otol. Rhinol. Laryngol., *41:*942, 1932.
2. Moersch, H.J., and Harrington, S.W.: Benign tumor of the esophagus. Ann. Otol. Rhinol. Laryngol., *53:*800, 1944.
3. Plachta, A.: Benign tumors of the esophagus. Am. J. Gastroenterol., *38:*639, 1962.
4. Vinson, P.P., Moore, A.B., and Bowing, H.H.: Hemangioma of the esophagus. Am. J. Med. Sci., *172:*416, 1926.
5. Davis, E.A., and Heitmiller, R.F.: Esophagectomy for benign disease: Trends in surgical results and management. Ann. Thorac. Surg., *62:*369, 1996.
6. Orringer, M.B., and Stirling, M.C.: Transhiatal esophagectomy for benign and malignant disease. J. Thorac. Cardiovasc. Surg., *105:*265, 1993.
7. Mansour, K.A., Hatcher, C.R., and Haun, C.L.: Benign tumors of the esophagus: Experience with 20 cases. South Med. J., *70:*461, 1977.
8. Postlethwait, R.W., and Lowe, J.E.: Benign tumors and cysts of the esophagus. *In* Zuidema, G.D. (ed.), Shackelford's Surgery of the Alimentary Tract, 4th ed., Vol. I. Philadelphia, W.B. Saunders Company, 1996, pp. 369–386.
9. Seremetis, M.G., Lyons, W.S., De Guzman, V.C., and Peabody, J.W.: Leiomyomata of the esophagus: An analysis of 838 cases. Cancer, *38:*2166, 1976.
10. Arrowsmith, R.: Fatal case dysphagia produced by pylorus growth in the esophagus. Med. Chir. Trans., *30:*229, 1877.
11. MacKenzie, M.: Manual of Diseases of the Nose and Throat, Vol. 2. London, Churchill, 1884, p. 1.
12. Mahoney, J.J.: Polypoid tumors of the esophagus: Report of two cases. Laryngoscope, *50:*1086, 1940.
13. Oshawa, T.: Surgery of the esophagus. Arch. F. Jap. Chir., *10:*605, 1933.
14. Storey, C.F., and Adams, W.C.: Leiomyoma of the esophagus. Am. J. Surg., *91:*3, 1956.
15. Sauerbruch, F.: Presentations in the field of thoracic surgery. Arch. F. Klin. Chir., *173:*457, 1932.
16. Churchill, E.D.: Case records of the Massachusetts General Hospital, case no. 23491. N. Engl. J. Med., *217:*955, 1937.
17. Sweet, R.H., Soutter, L., and Valenzuela, C.T.: Muscle wall tumors of the esophagus. J. Thorac. Surg., *27:*13, 1954.
18. Nemir, P., Jr., Wallace, H.W., and Fallahnejad, M.: Diagnosis and surgical management of benign disease of the esophagus. Curr. Probl. Surg., *13:*1, 1976.
19. Reed, C.E.: Benign tumors of the esophagus. Chest Surg. Clin. North Am., *4:*769, 1994.
20. Herrera, J.L.: Benign and metastatic tumors of the esophagus. Gastroenterol. Clin. North Am., *20:*775, 1991.
21. Avezzano, E.A., Fleischer, D.E., Merida, M.A., and Anderson, D.L.: Giant fibrovascular polyps of the esophagus. Am. J. Gastroenterol., *85:*299, 1990.
22. Postlethwait, R.W., and Musser, A.W.: Changes in the esophagus in 1000 autopsy specimens. J. Thorac. Cardiovasc. Surg., *68:*953, 1974.
23. Lortat-Jacob, J.L.: Localized myomas and diffuse myomas of the esophagus (Myomatoses localisees et myomatoses diffuses de l'oesophage). Arch. Mal. Appl. Dig., *39:*519, 1950.
24. Sircar, K., Hewlett, B.R., Huizinga, J.D., et al.: Interstitial cells of Cajal as precursors of gastrointestinal stromal tumors. Am. J. Surg. Pathol., *23:*377, 1999.
25. Emory, T.S., Sobin, L.H., Lukes, L., et al.: Prognosis of gastrointestinal smooth-muscle (stromal) tumors. Am. J. Surg. Pathol., *23:*82, 1999.
26. Massicot, R., Aubert, D., Mboyo, A., et al.: Localized esophageal leiomyoma and hypertrophic osteoarthropathy. J. Pediatr. Surg., *32:*646, 1997.
27. Amer, K.M., Payne, H.R., and Jeyasingham, K.: The relevance of abnormal motility patterns in intra-mural oesophageal leiomyomata. Eur. J. Cardiothorac. Surg., *10:*634, 1996.
28. Harper, R.A.K., and Tiscenco, E.: Benign tumor of the oesophagus and its differential diagnosis. Br. J. Radiol., *18:*99, 1945.
29. Schatzki, R., and Hawes, L.E.: The roentgenological appearance of extramucosal tumors of the esophagus. Am. J. Roentgenol., *43:*1, 1942.
30. Glantz, I., and Grunebaum, M.: The radiological approach to leiomyoma of the esophagus with long-term follow-up. Clin. Radiol., *28:*197, 1977.
31. Lewis, B., and Maxfield, R.G.: Leiomyoma of the esophagus: Case report and review of the literature. Int. Abstr. Surg., *99:*105, 1954.
32. Takada, N., Higashino, M., Osugi, H., et al.: Utility of endoscopic ultrasonography in assessing the indications for endoscopic surgery of submucosal esophageal tumors. Surg. Endosc., *13:*228, 1999.
33. Massari, M., De Simone, M., Cioffi, U., et al.: Endoscopic ultrasonography in the evaluation of leiomyoma and extramucosal cysts of the esophagus. Hepatogastroenterology, *45:*938, 1998.
34. Kawamoto K., Yamada Y., Utsunomiya T, et al.: Gastrointestinal submucosal tumors: Evaluation with endoscopic US. Radiology, *205:*733, 1997.
35. Tamura, K., Takamori, S., Tayama, K., et al.: Thoracoscopic resection of a giant leiomyoma of the esophagus with a mediastinal outgrowth. Ann. Thorac. Cardiovasc. Surg., *4:*351, 1998.
36. Bardini, R., and Asolati, M.: Thoracoscopic resection of benign tumours of the esophagus. Int. Surg., *82:*5, 1997.
37. Roviaro, G.C., Maciocco, M., Varoli, F., et al.: Videothoracoscopic treatment of oesophageal leiomyoma. Thorax, *53:*190, 1998.
38. Rendina, E.A., Venuta, F., Pescarmona, E.D., et al.: Leiomyoma of the esophagus. Scand. J. Thorac. Cardiovasc. Surg., *24:*79–82, 1990.
39. Bonavina, L., Segalin, A., Rosati, R., Pavanello, M., Perrachia A: Surgical therapy of esophageal leiomyoma. J. Am. Coll. Surg., *181:*257–62, 1995.
40. Bourque, M.D., Spigland, N., Bensoussan A.L., et al.: Esophageal leiomyoma in children: Two case reports and review of the literature. J. Pediatr. Surg. *24:*1103–7, 1989.
41. Coutinho, D.S. de S., Soga, J., Yoshikawa, T., et al.: Granular cell tumors of the esophagus: A report of two cases and review of the literature. Am. J. Gastroenterol., *80:*758, 1985.
42. Giacobbe, A., Faciorusso, D., Conoscitore, P., et al.: Granular cell tumor of the esophagus. Am. J. Gastroenterol., *83:*1398, 1988.
43. Tada, M., Iida, M., Yao, T., et al.: Granular cell tumor of the esophagus: Endoscopic ultrasonographic demonstration and endoscopic removal. Am. J. Gastroenterol., *85:*1507, 1990.
44. Mineo, T.C., Biancari, F., Francioni, F., et al.: Conservative approach to granular cell tumor of the oesophagus. Scand. J. Thorac. Cardiovasc. Surg., *29:*141, 1995.
45. Moreira, L.S., and Dani, R.: Treatment of granular cell tumor of the esophagus by endoscopic injection of dehydrated alcohol. Am. J. Gastroenterol., *87:*659, 1992.
46. Gentry, R.W., Dockerty, M.B., and Clagett, O.T.: Vascular malformations and vascular tumors of the gastrointestinal tract. Int. Abst. Surg., *88:*281, 1949.
47. Vinson, P.P., Moore, A.B., and Bowing, H.H.: Hemangioma of the esophagus: Report of a case. Am. J. Med. Sci., *172:*416, 1927.
48. Riemenschneider, H.W., and Klassen, K.P.: Cavernous esophageal hemangioma. Ann. Thorac. Surg., *6:*552, 1968.
49. Govoni, A.F.: Hemangiomas of the esophagus. Gastrointest. Radiol., *7:*113, 1982.
50. Cantero, D., Yoshida, T., Ito, T., et al.: Esophageal hemangioma: Endoscopic diagnosis and treatment. Endoscopy, *26:*250, 1994.
51. Taylor, F.H., Fowler, F.C., Betsill, W.L., Jr., and Marroum, M.C.: Hemangioma of the esophagus. Ann. Thorac. Surg., *61:*726, 1996.
52. Yoshikane, H., Suzuki, T., Yoshioka, N., et al.: Hemangioma of the esophagus: Endosonographic imaging and endoscopic resection. Endoscopy, *27:*267, 1995.
53. Aoki, T., Okagawa, K., Uemura, Y., et al.: Successful treatment of an esophageal hemangioma by endoscopic injection sclerotherapy: Report of a case. Surg. Today, *27:*450, 1997.

54. Ramo, O.J., Salo, J.A., Baradini, R., et al.: Treatment of a submucosal hemangioma of the esophagus using simultaneous video-assisted thoracoscopy and esophagoscopy: Description of a new minimally invasive technique. Endoscopy, *29*:S27, 1997.
55. Ming, S.: Tumors of the esophagus and stomach. *In* Firminger H.I. (ed.): Atlas of Tumor Pathology, fascicle 7. Washington, D.C., Armed Forces Institute of Pathology, 1971, p. 68.
56. Levine, M.S., Buck, J.L., Pantongrag-Brown, L., et al.: Fibrovascular polyps of the esophagus: Clinical, radiographic, and pathologic findings in 16 patients. Am. J. Roentgenol., *166*:781, 1996.
57. Weitzner, S., and Hentel, W.: Squamous papilloma of esophagus. Am. J. Gastroenterol., *50*:391, 1968.
58. Adler, R.H., Carberry, D.M., and Ross, C.A.: Papilloma of the esophagus. J. Thorac. Cardiovasc. Surg., *37*:625, 1959.
59. Politoske, E.J.: Squamous papilloma of the esophagus associated with the human papillomavirus. Gastroenterology, *102*:668, 1992.
60. Whitaker, J., Deffenbaugh, L., and Cooke, A.: Esophageal duplication cyst. Am. J. Gastroenterol., *73*:329, 1980.
61. Kolomainen, D., Hurley, P.R., and Ebbs, S.R.: Esophageal duplication cyst: Case report and review of the literature. Dis. Esoph., *11*:62, 1998.
62. Arbona, J.L., Fazzi, G.F., and Mayoral, J.: Congenital esophageal cysts: Case report and review of the literature. Am. J. Gastroenterol., *79*:177, 1984.
63. Hutchison, J., and Thomson, J.D.: Congenital archenteric cysts. Br. J. Surg., *41*:15, 1953.
64. Cioffi, U., Bonavina, L., De Simone, M., et al.: Presentation and surgical management of bronchogenic and esophageal duplication cysts in adults. Chest, *113*:1492, 1998.

VOLUME

I

Resectional Therapy and Complications of Esophageal Surgery

CHAPTER

24 Techniques of Esophageal Reconstruction

DOUGLAS J. MATHISEN • EARLE W. WILKINS, JR.

Esophageal resection and reconstruction remain a major therapeutic challenge for surgeons involved in the care of patients with benign and malignant disease of the esophagus. Despite major advances in postoperative care, operative mortality rates worldwide remain unacceptably high. Much of the operative mortality is related to the complications of anastomotic leak. "Acceptable" leak rates of 8 to 10% are still reported today. These two factors continue to influence the choice of esophageal substitute and the method of reconstruction. Suffice it to say that whatever option is chosen, the operation requires careful planning and preparation of the patient, strict attention to the technical details of the operation, and dedicated postoperative care. Resection and reconstruction are inevitable for malignant disease, but every attempt should be made to preserve the native esophagus in benign disease because no esophageal substitute achieves "normal" swallowing comparable to that of the esophagus.

In the final analysis, the general thoracic surgical clinician must be thoroughly familiar not only with the technical knowledge of the utilization of various visceral esophageal substitutes but also with the appropriate judgmental selection of which replacement is best under specific circumstances. Accordingly, this chapter is intended to provide both details of surgical technique and the physiologic concepts that constitute the basis for selection of a particular organ for creation of a replacement "esophagus" (esophagoplasty).

HISTORICAL BACKGROUND

The first successful resection of the cervical esophagus was reported by Czerny in 1877.[5] Torek is credited with the first resection of the thoracic esophagus in 1913.[25] Successful resection and intrathoracic reconstruction of the esophagus was reported by Oshawa in 1939.[18] Sweet and Churchill in 1942 reported a three-layer technique of anastomosis giving reliable results superior to many contemporary reports today.[24] Sweet's series in 1954 of 141 patients with an operative mortality rate of 15% and a leak rate of 1.4% was remarkable for its time and is still acceptable by today's standards.[23] In 1946, Ivor Lewis popularized the laparotomy and right thoracotomy for tumors of the middle third of the esophagus—an approach that still bears his name.[10] Mahoney and Sherman in 1954 published their results with colon replacement following total esophagectomy.[11] Replacement of the distal esophagus with a short-segment colon interposition was reported in 1965 by Belsey[3] and with jejunum by Brain in 1965.[4] In 1980, in a review of the entire world's literature, Earlam and Cunha-Melo stated that "esophagectomy is associated with the highest operative mortality of any commonly performed operation."[6] Muller reported as recently as 1990 in another collective review that the overall operation mortality rates for curative resection and for palliative resection were 11% and 19%, respectively.[13] Mathisen and associates reported an operative mortality rate of 2.9% and no leaks at the Massachusetts General Hospital.[12] Others have reported similar excellent results from single institutions, but it is obvious that the challenge still remains.

OPTIONS IN REPLACING THE ESOPHAGUS

Surgeons involved in the care of patients with esophageal disease should be familiar with all of the available conduits for esophageal replacement. Individual circumstances may dictate the choice of substitute, or unexpected operative findings may dictate a change in plan. The surgeon should be flexible enough to tailor the choice of substitute to suit the patient and the underlying disease process. Many factors dictate which option is chosen: benign or malignant disease, availability of conduit, comorbid conditions such as chronic obstructive pulmonary disease, vascular occlusive disease, steroid-dependent conditions, prior irradiation, and ultimately the surgeon's preference. Some methods of reconstruction, such as antethoracic skin tubes or prosthetic replacements, are primarily of historical significance but should be remembered for that rare patient for whom no other option is available. Some methods, such as the reversed gastric tube, are suitable alternatives but have never gained in popularity.

The three standard visceral substitutes used for replacing the esophagus, in the order of both frequency and preference of usage, are stomach, colon, and jejunum.

Stomach. The liberal blood supply of the stomach makes it the most reliable organ for use in the intrathoracic replacement of the esophagus. Of its five feeding arterial sources, the left gastric artery, the left gastroepiploic artery, and the short gastric arteries may be divided, leaving the right gastric and right gastroepiploic arteries to supply the entire transpositioned stomach. Division of these arteries is possible because of the presence of extensive intrinsic collaterals within the gastric wall. A second reason for the reliability of the stomach in replacement of the esophagus is its size and contour, which, after total division of the greater and lesser omenta and lateral peritoneal liberation of the duodenal sweep (Kocher's maneuver), permit elongation of the stomach that allows it to be brought to the neck. When maximum length is required, the true fundus of the stomach should be used for anastomosis rather than the gastroesophageal junction. Skeletonizing the lesser curve also gives added length with little ischemic risk.

The stomach can be transposed by either the posterior mediastinal route in the bed of the native esophagus or by the substernal route. The posterior mediastinal route is the preferred route in most patients.

Colon. The left or right hemicolon may be used for long distances of esophageal replacement or bypass (i.e., when it is necessary to reach to the neck). When the left colon is elected and placed in an isoperistaltic direction, it derives its blood supply from the inferior mesenteric artery through the left colic artery. If the antiperistaltic direction is used, the midcolic artery becomes the feeding source. When shorter segments of colon are required, the transverse colon based on the middle colic artery and the splenic flexure supplied by the left colic artery are the primary options.

Jejunum. The jejunum is most frequently used as a short segment replacing the distal esophagus, more often in benign disease and particularly for reflux acid-peptic stricture. In these cases, proximal jejunum is used, with a segment beginning just distal to the first jejunal arterial branch from the superior mesenteric artery. In asthenic patients with a long jejunal mesentery, the jejunum may be brought to a level above the aortic arch, and in young children particularly, it may even reach all the way to the cervical level. More often, however, when such a length is mandated by the lack of other available options, *arterial augmentation* may be necessary, such as an internal mammary artery-to-jejunal artery anastomosis. This must be accompanied, of course, by appropriate venous anastomosis. For short-segment replacement of the cervical esophagus, a free *autograft* of small intestine may be used; arterial and venous anastomoses are accomplished by conventional microvascular techniques to, for example, the superior thyroid artery and the anterior facial vein.

Specific factors come into play in the ultimate selection of the viscus used to replace the esophagus. These include (1) availability, related to prior surgical resection; (2) anomalous anatomic variants, particularly in blood supply; (3) possible pathologic processes in the viscus under consideration; (4) technical reliability of the vascular supply necessary for appropriate anastomotic healing; and (5) always, the experience of the operating surgeon.

Throughout this discussion, emphasis is placed repeatedly on blood supply. *The first and foremost requisite for successful replacement of the esophagus is adequate circulation, both arterial input and venous drainage, in the substituting organ.* An anastomosis cannot heal by primary intention in the absence of reliable circulation in both ends to be joined.

TECHNICAL VARIABLES

In addition to selection of the viscus to be used for esophageal replacement, the surgeon has three other choices to consider in planning the ideal technical operation: (1) the surgical approach, (2) the route for replacement of the new "esophagus," and (3) the level of the anastomosis.

Placement of Incision. For distal partial esophagectomy and anastomosis below the aortic arch, there is almost general agreement on the use of the left transthoracic or thoracoabdominal incision. With upward paravertebral extension and Sweet's double-rib resection (or double intercostal incisions), the left-sided approach can be extended to any level of the intrathoracic esophagus if necessary, although dissection of large carcinomas at the level of the aortic arch may pose technical challenges (Fig. 24-1).

For mid-esophageal carcinomas, the conventional approach is use of the double incisions of Lewis: a midline laparotomy for gastric mobilization and a high right-sided posterolateral thoracotomy for esophageal dissection and execution of a high intrathoracic anastomosis at the apex of the chest. This plan may be extended to include a third, cervical incision to allow greater length of proximal esophageal resection and a higher level of anastomosis.

Yet another choice of surgical approach is the transhiatal esophagectomy of Orringer, in which a high midline laparotomy permitting enlargement of the hiatus and transhiatal dissection is combined with a cervical incision allowing proximal esophageal dissection and performance of the appropriate replacement anastomosis.[17] Extensive division of the hiatus allows greater visualization of the distal esophagus. Partial resection of the manubrium and the first and second ribs (Fig. 24-2) allows better visualization and dissection of the cervicothoracic esophagus in some patients. Utilization of both these techniques allows esophagectomy to be done under direct visualization in most patients.

In any of these approaches in which a cervical incision is made, either a right- or left-sided presternocleidomastoid oblique incision or a transverse, thyroidectomy-type incision that is extended more toward the side chosen for approaching the cervical esophagus may be used.

Route of Replacement. There are four options in choosing the route of replacement: (1) posterior mediastinal through the bed of the resected esophagus; (2) anterior mediastinal in the retrosternal position; (3) either lateral transpleural placement, usually behind the lung root; and (4) the antethoracic or presternal subcutaneous route. The fourth choice has never achieved universal popularity, primarily because of cosmetic considerations.

The orthotopic posterior mediastinal route for placement of the substituting viscus is the most widely used if the esophagus has been removed. It is the shortest and most direct route and does not require dissection and preparation of the second port of access.

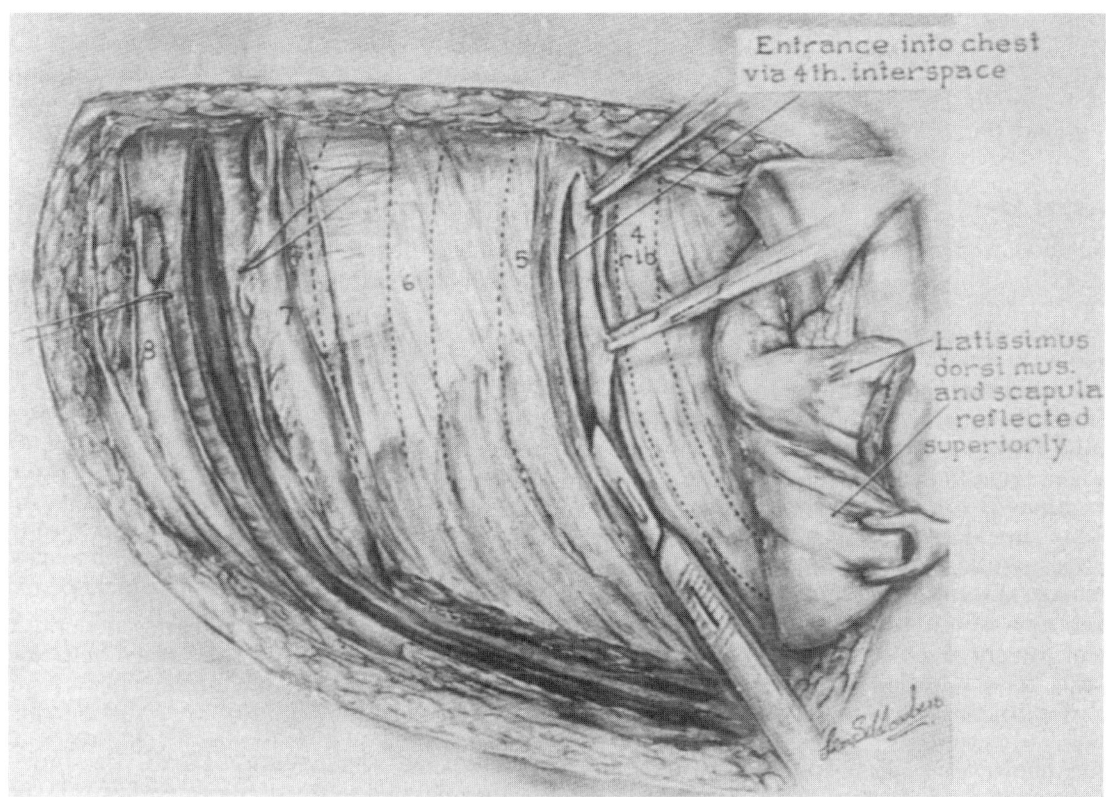

Figure 24–1. To perform a counterincision, the scapula is retracted off the chest wall and a higher interspace selected. A seventh and fourth interspace approach is illustrated. (From the Society of Thoracic Surgeons. Ann. Thorac. Surg., *46*:250, 1988, with permission.)

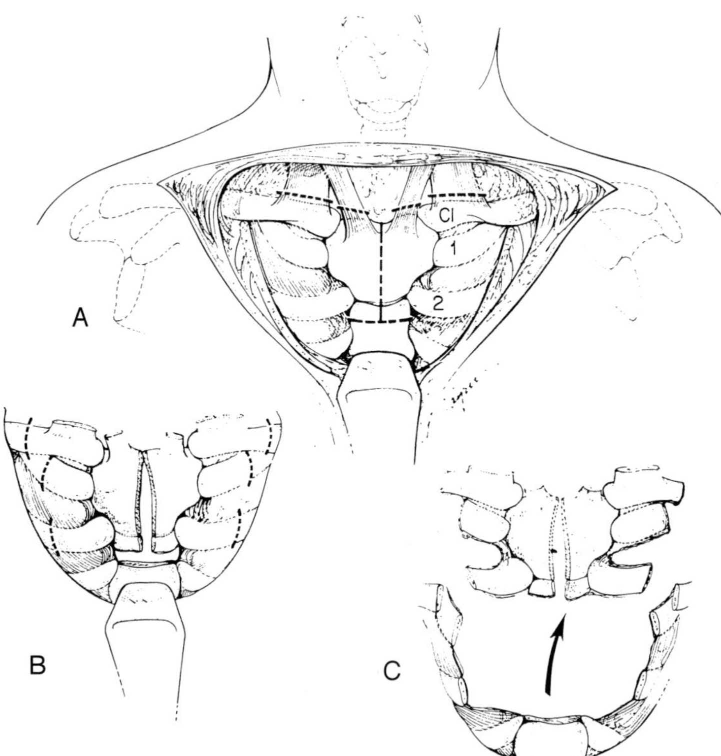

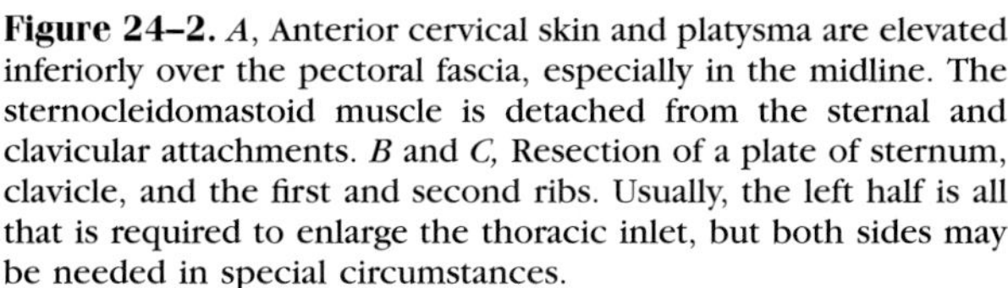

Figure 24–2. *A*, Anterior cervical skin and platysma are elevated inferiorly over the pectoral fascia, especially in the midline. The sternocleidomastoid muscle is detached from the sternal and clavicular attachments. *B* and *C*, Resection of a plate of sternum, clavicle, and the first and second ribs. Usually, the left half is all that is required to enlarge the thoracic inlet, but both sides may be needed in special circumstances.

The retrosternal route is used most commonly for bypass of the esophagus when it has been decided, because of tumor unresectability, condition of the patient, or staging, not to resect the esophagus. This choice may require enlarging the thoracic inlet by resecting the head of the clavicle and the anterior end of the first rib to ensure adequacy of room for the replacement and to be certain that there is no compression of the essential vascular supply (see Fig. 24–2).

The transpleural route is seldom used but may be necessary for a bypassing procedure if the usual anterior mediastinal route has been transgressed by a prior median sternotomy, particularly for an open cardiac surgical operation.

Level of Anastomosis. If the transhiatal approach to esophagectomy is used, there is no option; the anastomosis is always performed at the cervical level. Likewise, if the three-incision technique for near-total removal of the esophagus is planned, a cervical level is also chosen for the anastomosis. However, if a distal esophagectomy is planned, a decision about the level of the anastomosis is paramount. A level must be chosen that permits complete removal of the tumor and enough room for a resection margin that is free of even microscopic extension of carcinoma. This level must permit accomplishment of a safe anastomosis under ideal conditions of full visual exposure. Thus, in general, intrathoracic anastomoses at the middle to high level are better accomplished from the right-sided thoracic approach.

The most important aspect of a successful esophagectomy and replacement (at least in terms of postoperative recovery) is the performance of a safe, intact anastomosis. Next to blood supply, operative exposure and visibility for the surgeon are the most important requisites for success. *The technical goal of all esophageal surgeons is a zero anastomotic leakage rate.*

GUIDELINES IN MAKING THE CHOICE

For malignant disease in particular, the stomach is the most reliable replacement for the esophagus. Its intrinsic blood supply is the most extensive. Its pliability allows it to reach any necessary level. Its usage involves only one anastomotic suture line. It has stood the test of time and has now been in general use since the 1938 report of Adams and Phemister.[1] Its principal drawback is its association with the potential for development of reflux esophagitis resulting in possible stricture at or above the anastomosis. Although pyloric drainage procedures and anastomosis-wrapping techniques are used to minimize the possibility of damaging reflux, practice has shown that the higher the point in the esophagus at which the anastomosis is placed, the less likely the development of esophagitis. The fact that most of these patients do not survive a prolonged period of time should not be a factor in choosing the appropriate replacing viscus.

In patients with a nondilatable peptic stricture of the distal esophagus, interposition of a segment of intestine is the preferred method of replacement after esophageal resection. The choice between colon and jejunum is mainly one of the surgeon's preference and experience. Either organ can provide a satisfactory physiologic "barrier" against ongoing gastroesophageal reflux while maintaining the entire stomach in its normal abdominal anatomic location. An esophagogastric anastomosis, particularly at the distal esophageal level for reflux peptic disease, is fraught with a high incidence of postoperative esophagitis and the danger of possible life-threatening nocturnal tracheobronchial aspiration. On the other hand, in elderly or medically compromised patients, the esophagogastric distal anastomosis may be used because of the expedience of the procedure and the reliability of the circulation.

For long esophageal replacement in patients with benign disease (i.e., usually stricture, either peptic or corrosive), the colon is given first consideration. Its reliable marginal arterial circulation, especially between the left branch of the middle colic and the left colic arteries, permits isoperistaltic replacement of the left colon all the way through the posterior mediastinal esophageal bed to the level of the neck. An alternate route, even after resection, is placement through the retrosternal tunnel.

For esophageal bypass without resection, the colon is also the viscus of choice. It is placed behind the sternum unless obliteration of the anterior mediastinum by prior surgery, mediastinal irradiation, or malignant disease requires transpleural replacement. The side and position of placement (in front of or behind the root of the lung) are the surgeon's choice. Bypass rather than esophageal resection may be selected because of either the extent of an invasive carcinoma or the physiologic status of the patient, which militate against a successful transpleural resection. In addition, some general thoracic surgeons prefer to stage a procedure necessitated by corrosive destruction of the esophagus by using a looping esophageal bypass and later, esophageal resection.

STUDIES USEFUL IN THE DECISION-MAKING PROCESS

A viscus cannot be used to replace the esophagus unless it is intrinsically healthy (i.e., free of its own pathology) and provides an adequately nourishing arterial blood supply and an adequately draining venous return. There are three methods of assessing these characteristics: (1) endoscopy, (2) arteriography, and (3) barium contrast radiology.

Endoscopy. Endoscopy provides the greatest amount of information when it can be applied appropriately. For instance, if the fiberoptic esophagogastroscope can be negotiated through an esophageal carcinoma or stricture, it provides the necessary information about (1) the presence or absence of a second carcinoma, (2) the presence or absence of peptic ulceration or gastritis, and (3) the adequacy of the pyloric channel. In evaluating the colon for its use as a replacement of the esophagus, colonoscopy is essential. It provides the opportunity for total inspection and thus eliminates the possibility of the presence of a polyp, small carcinoma, or other unsuspected lesion in the substitute viscus, or for that matter in the residual colon that does not participate in the replacement. It may not provide information about diverticulitis unless it is extensive or actually obstructive.

Arteriography. There is room for a difference of opinion about the need for arteriography. The arterial supply of the stomach is abundant owing to its five primary sources, and its intrinsic network of interconnecting communications is so extensive that arteriography is not necessary. Anomalies in the source of arterial supply are neither too common nor sufficiently severe to arouse concern about adequacy of the arterial supply, even under the conditions of its necessary disconnection from the adjacent omentum, the spleen, the colon, and the celiac axis. For the colon, however, the situation is quite the opposite. The adequacy of segmental arterial supply and the incidence of anomalies are inconstant. First, atherosclerotic involvement of the colonic arteries is a major possibility, particularly in the older population that is so frequently affected by esophageal carcinoma; the origin of the inferior mesenteric artery is a particular site of atherosclerotic narrowing. Second, the variety and frequency of anomalies of colonic blood supply require a clear mapping of the several colonic arteries before a satisfactory decision can be made about (1) the utility of the colon as a replacement of the esophagus and (2) which portion thereof is to be used. Anomalous variants have been identified by careful anatomic dissections (Fig. 24-3), and major anomalies have been reported in more than 10% of patients studied by mesenteric arteriography by Sonneland and colleagues.[22] The principal point of

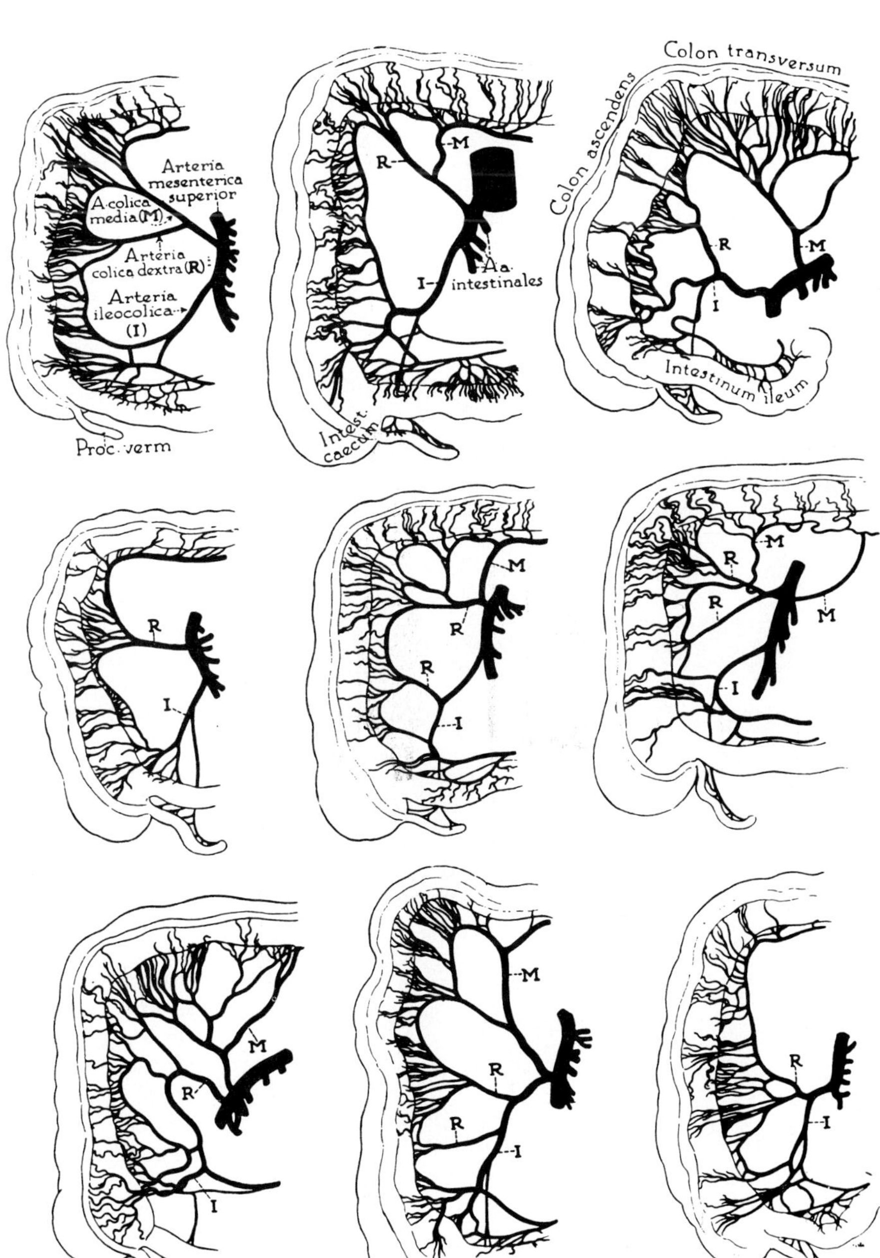

Figure 24–3. Anatomic variations in the distribution to the colon of branches of the superior mesenteric artery. The extreme variation and the inconstancy of a marginal artery connecting the right colic artery and the ileocolic artery branches make use of the right colon less reliable than use of the left colon. (From Sonneland, J., Anson, B.J., and Beaton, L.E.: Surgical anatomy of the arterial supply to the colon from the superior mesenteric artery based upon a study of 600 specimens. Surg. Gynecol. Obstet., *106*:385, 1958, with permission.)

strategic interest is the marginal communication between the left branch of the middle colic artery and the ascending portion of the left colic artery (Fig. 24–4). Successful use of the left colon depends on this critical marginal artery. The distribution of the right colic artery is in itself not consistent, and unreliable communications with the right branch of the middle colic artery or the ileocolic artery make selection of the right colon sometimes risky. The true benefit of colonic arteriography lies in the fact that it provides a clear anatomic "road map" *preoperatively* to eliminate any surprise or confusion at the operating table. The most common useful arteriographic findings are stenosis at the origin of the inferior mesenteric artery, inadequacy of the marginal artery, failure of communication of the right and left branches of the middle colic artery, and a short trunk of the middle colic artery precluding access and division. Knowledge of these findings before operation saves considerable time intraoperatively. The complete study includes transfemoral, retrograde catheter opacification of the inferior mesenteric artery, the superior mesenteric artery, *and* the celiac axis itself. Complications of such study in experienced radiographic hands are uncommon.

Barium Contrast Radiography. The contrast barium study, although the most frequently used, in some ways provides the least information to the surgeon making the decision. Its primary roles are (1) by means of the barium enema, demonstration of diverticulosis or diverticulitis and visual depiction of an estimate of colon length; and (2) by means of the barium swallow, a view of the stomach when passage of the esophagoscope through a tumor or stricture is not possible.

A concluding point in this section on diagnostic studies is that none of the three studies is actually applicable to the jejunum. The jejunum has a consistent blood supply and is always long enough, at least for short esophageal replacement. It is not accessible to endoscopy. The detail provided by a small bowel barium follow-through examination is marginal. For these reasons, indeed, many surgeons give it preference as the replacing viscus for the esophagus.

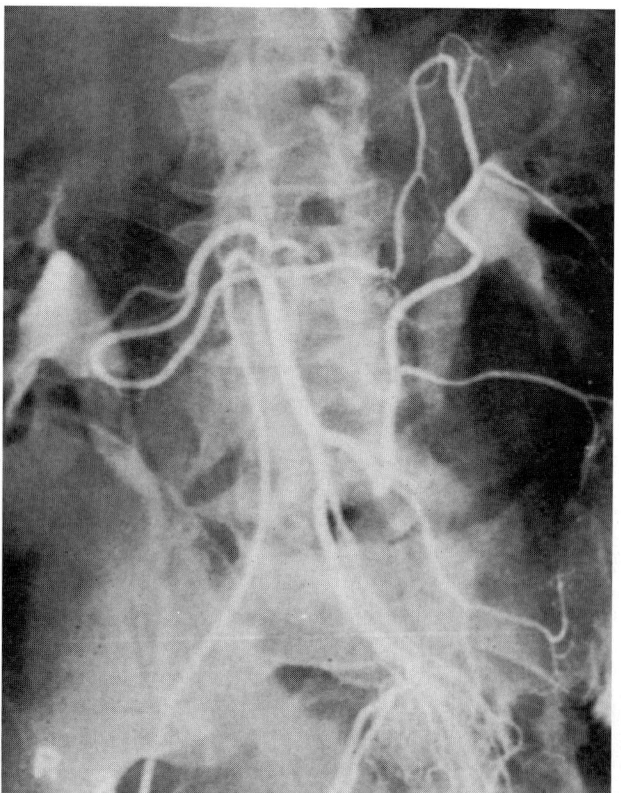

Figure 24–4. This inferior mesenteric arteriogram demonstrates filling of the left colic artery around the splenic flexure, through the anastomotic branch to the middle colic artery and even (overlying the right renal pelvis) to the right branch of the middle colic artery and the hepatic flexure. This anatomy ensures successful utilization of the left hemicolon for esophagocoloplasty.

ESOPHAGOGASTROSTOMY

The surgical technique for this esophageal replacement procedure is best considered by reducing it to its component steps: (1) mobilization of the stomach, (2) lengthening of the stomach, (3) drainage of the stomach, (4) transpositioning of the stomach, and (5) anastomosis. Each step is described here with a preferred method of performance and with the reason it is so performed. The actual esophageal dissection is described elsewhere.

Mobilization of the Stomach

Detaching the stomach from its complicated intra-abdominal anatomic relationships requires a full operative exposure. This is best achieved by performing a standard upper midline laparotomy (used for combined incisions, including the abdominal–right thoracic and the transhiatal–cervical) or by a left thoracoabdominal incision (used for distal esophageal resection). Although the stomach may be detached for distal esophagectomy using a strictly transthoracic, transdiaphragmatic approach, this method does not provide nearly the optimal exposure.

The initial step in detachment of the stomach is the division of the greater omentum outside the gastroepiploic arcade, which is formed by the right gastroepiploic artery from the gastroduodenal artery at the pyloric end of the stomach and the left gastroepiploic artery from the splenic artery toward the proximal stomach. This division is facilitated by grasping the transverse colon, lifting it out of the incision distally, and entering the lesser omental sac at a point where the omentum is thinnest and most transparent, usually at the midpoint of the stomach or slightly to its left. The dissection is carried all the way to the level of the pylorus, dividing the rather small omental branches of the epiploic arcade. These vessels may be coagulated, clipped, or tied. The use of fine ligatures is preferred to avoid any retrograde coagulum, which might compromise the integrity of the gastroepiploic arcade, and to avoid metal clips, which might compromise the clarity of detail of any subsequent computed tomography (CT) scan. The dissection is then directed toward the spleen, where the left gastroepiploic artery is ligated at the upper end of the arcade above the segmental artery to the stomach.

The short gastric (gastrolienal) arteries are divided carefully between hemostatic forceps and are ligated securely. The more proximal of these vessels may be quite short, requiring the application of suture ligatures. Ligatures on the stomach end must be tied securely; there have been times when these ties slipped off the stomach when it later became distended within the thorax. Finally, there is a posterior branch from the splenic artery to the back of the cardia of the stomach that is very constant; its division completes the liberation of the greater curvature.

The reflection of the peritoneum at the esophagogastric junction is divided, and blunt finger or right-angled forceps dissection permits the surgeon to encircle the abdominal esophagus. Circumferential passage of an empty Penrose rubber drain permits upward traction on this end of the stomach during dissection of the laser curvature. If the entire stomach is to be used to replace the esophagus, the vagus nerves are divided at this point. If the proximal stomach itself is to be resected, the branches of the vagus nerves are included when the stomach itself is transected. The rather avascular, thin gastrohepatic omentum is then entered low on the stomach, and a second Penrose drain is passed around the stomach at about the level of the incisura, permitting downward traction during dissection of the lesser curvature.

Attention is directed toward exposing the origin of the left gastric artery at the trifurcation of the celiac axis. This structure is approached most easily from behind the stomach, which is elevated to the right by the assistant applying traction on the two Penrose tapes. It is necessary to divide the filmy, avascular adhesions between the back of the stomach and the retroperitoneum, extending from the pylorus to the superior edge of the pancreas. At this point, the celiac axis and its three branches can be identified by palpation as the left thumb and forefinger encircle what is left of the lesser curvature attachments. The left gastric artery is exposed with this guidance using sharp dissection. It is doubly ligated at its origin from the celiac axis, using a heavy nonabsorbable suture material, such as No. 0 silk. The first ligature is placed and firmly tied before the artery is actually divided so that, should the ligature break during tying, a freely spurting major artery is avoided. Two hemostatic clamps are then applied distal to this first ligature, and the artery is divided between them. A second tie or transfixation stitch is placed on the left gastric artery 5 mm distal to the first tie. The artery on the gastric side is managed best with a secure stitch ligature. The left gastric vein is usually identifiable separately from the artery and is handled similarly. Alternatively, it may be included in the first arterial ligature; if so, the second ties should be secured separately on artery and vein. The tissue remaining now includes branches of the vagus nerves and sympathetic chains, extending upward to the Penrose tape previously placed to encircle the esophagogastric junction; this tissue is divided between clamps and suture-ligated because vessels frequently arise from the undersurface of the liver to this highest point on the lesser curvature.

The stomach is now free except for the duodenum with the right gastric and right gastroepiploic arteries and the esophagus with its two vagus nerves. Depending on the procedure contemplated, the stomach is now handled in one of two ways:

1. If the primary operation is a distal esophagogastrectomy, the nodes along the left gastric artery and celiac axis have been dissected carefully so that they remain in continuity with the stomach. The stomach is transected *from* a greater curvature point opposite the level of emergence of the left gastroepiploic artery *to* a point on the lesser curvature below the lowest branch of the left gastric artery using the GIA stapler (Fig. 24-5). The lesser curvature point of transection may actually be carried distally to a point below the incisura. The stapled gastric margin is turned in with interrupted Lembert No. 3-0 silk sutures.
2. If the operation planned is a more proximal esophagectomy of the Ivor Lewis type, nothing further need be done at this point. The transection of the stomach at the cardia, or with some of the left gastric tissue attached to the specimen, is carried out after the stomach is drawn through an enlarged hiatus into the right hemithorax following the right thoracic esophageal dissection. This method allows less opportunity for possible torsion of the stomach as it is drawn upward. The operator must be careful not to pull the stomach too tightly, which could result in compression by the hiatus or in redundancy of the stomach in the chest with resultant poor emptying.

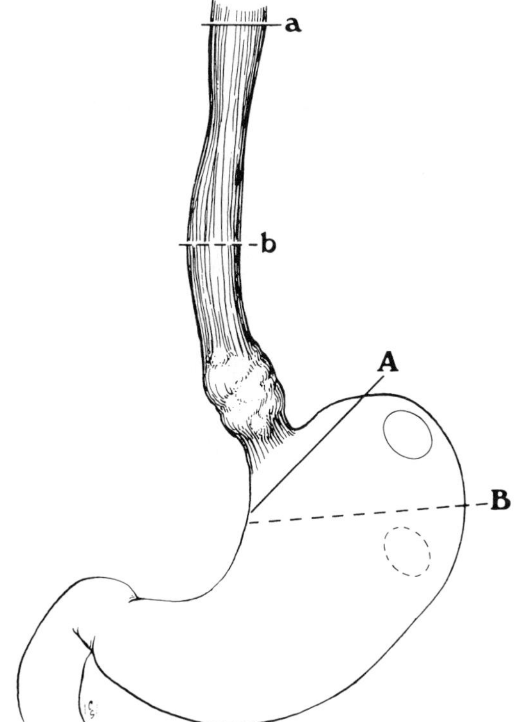

Figure 24–5. The gastric fundus should be preserved *(A)* to maximize gastric length, which will permit extension of the gastric tube to the neck (a) if needed. It is important not to assume adequate gastric length and to prematurely amputate the gastric fundus *(B)*. The proposed esophagogastric site is indicated by a circle.

Lengthening of the Stomach

Lengthening of the stomach is accomplished, following the dissection described, by right lateral peritoneal pancreaticoduodenal mobilization, so-called Kocher's maneuver (Fig. 24-6). This procedure is begun distal to the pylorus along the second portion of the duodenum, taking particular care to preserve the right gastric artery and to remain anterior to the common bile duct. It has not been necessary actually to expose or intubate the common bile duct during this maneuver. The peritoneum alone is divided, and the dissection is carried around the C curve of the duodenum along the inferior margin of its third portion. The duodenum can then be dissected free posteriorly by blunt dissection behind the pancreas just in front of the inferior vena cava. This entire maneuver permits the duodenum to assume almost a vertical axis as the stomach is drawn upward into the thorax. It thus permits the stomach to reach all the way to the cervical level; the pylorus then lies at the level of the diaphragmatic hiatus.

Akiyama has described resection of the lesser curvature of the stomach to gain additional length[2] (Fig. 24-7*A*). This maneuver may be needed to remove a lymphatic drainage siphon, but, aside from dividing both anterior and posterior branches of the left gastric artery individually as they ramify on the gastric wall, less curvature excision per se is not actually necessary to gain length. This procedure can be accomplished by the use of the linear stapler as well (see Fig. 24-7*B*).

Because of the peculiar shape of the stomach, maximal length is obtained by applying upward traction on a point high on the greater curvature of the stomach, actually the highest point of the fundus (see Fig. 24-7*A*). The actual location of this point is determined by moving the

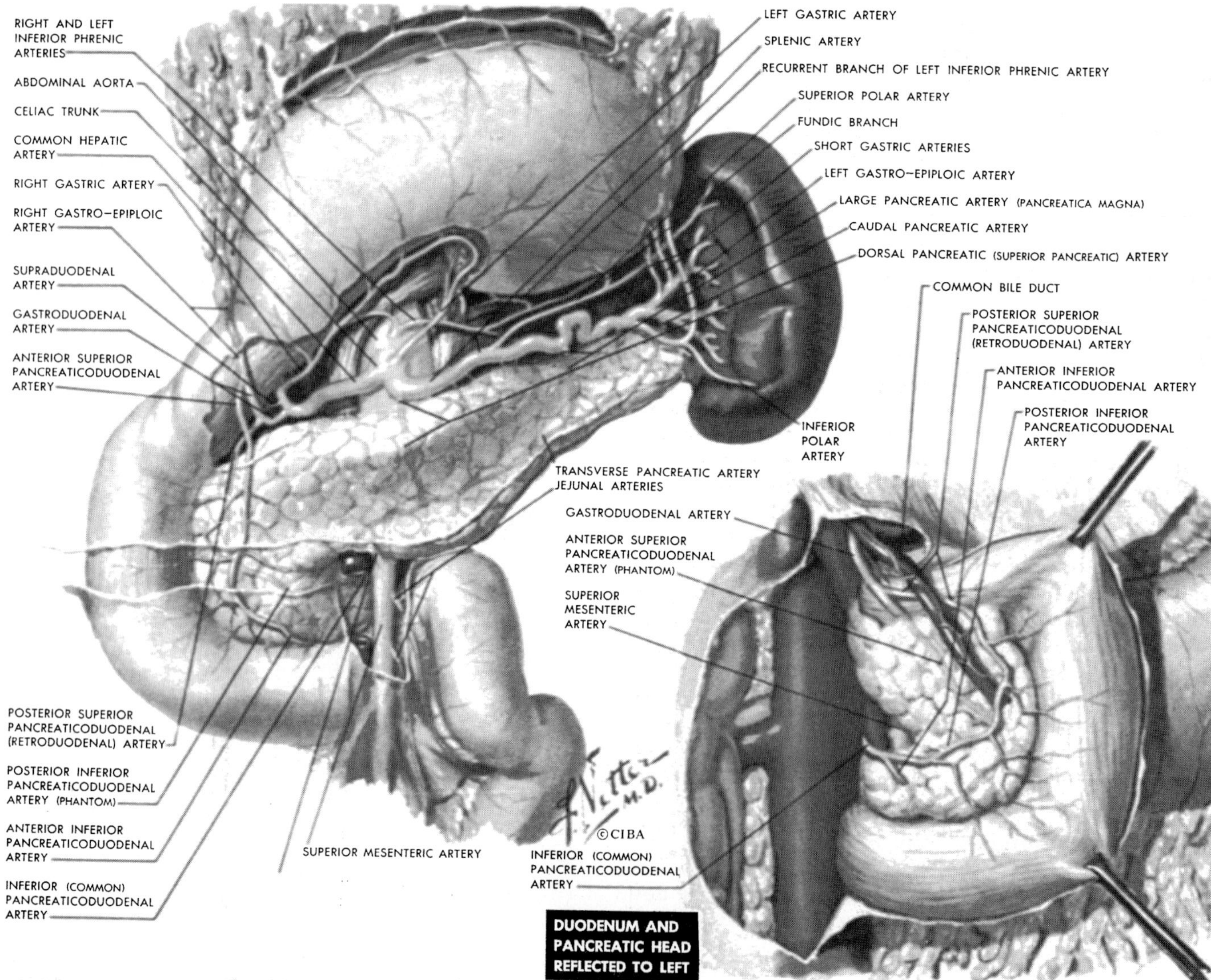

Figure 24-6. This illustration *(lower right)* illustrates peritoneal freeing of the outer aspect of the duodenal curve, permitting its retraction to the left and exposure of the retroduodenal structures. This permits maximal mobilization of the stomach upward in the thorax; thus, the pylorus actually lies at the level of the diaphragmatic hiatus. (From Netter, F.H.: The CIBA Collection of Medical Illustrations. Vol. 3: Digestive System. Part I: Upper Digestive System. New York, CIBA-GEIGY Corp., 1959, p. 58, with permission.)

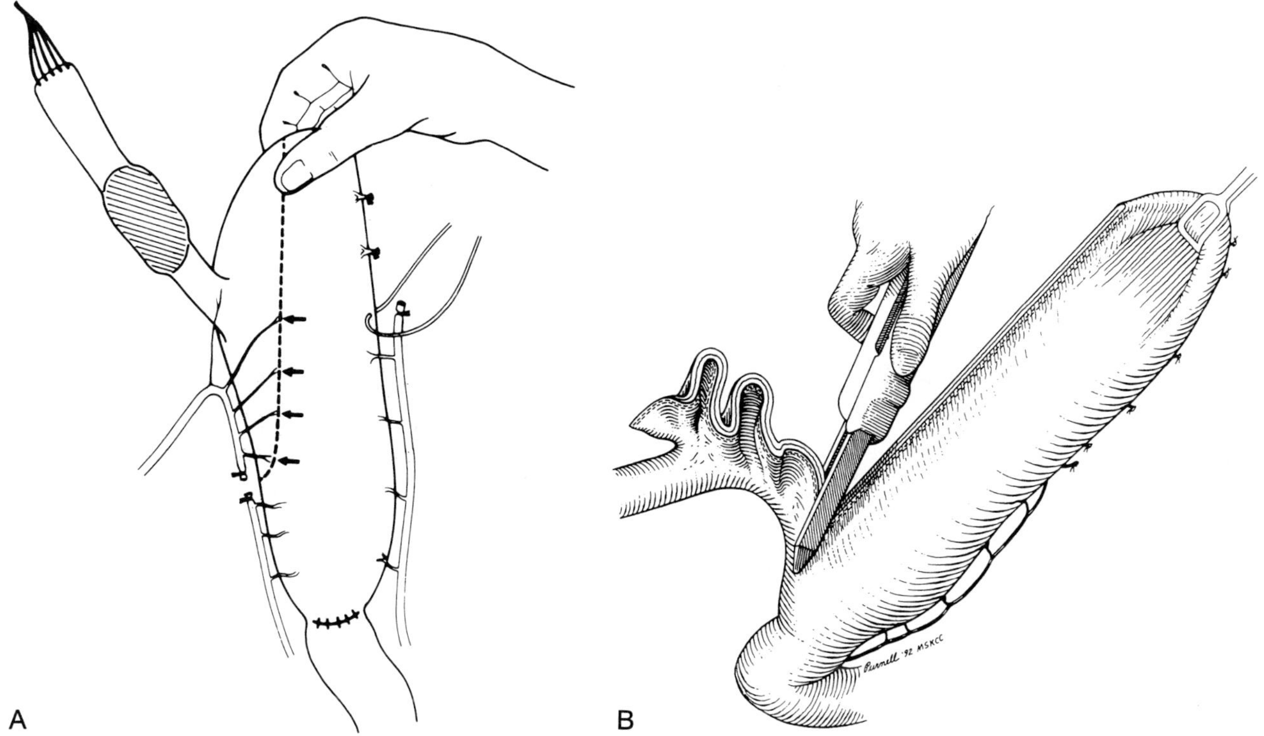

Figure 24–7. *A*, This illustration demonstrates both removal of the lesser curvature of the stomach and elongation of the stomach by traction on the greater curvature. The subsequent esophagogastric anastomosis will be made to a point toward the greater curvature from the surgeon's thumb. (From Akiyama, H.: Surgery for carcinoma of the esophagus. Curr. Probl. Surg., *17*:56, 1980, with permission.) *B*, Multiple applications of the GIA-60 stapler are used to "unfold" the lesser curvature and achieve maximal length of the gastric tube. (From Shriver, C.D., Spiro, R.H., and Burt, M.: A new technique of gastric pull-through. Surg. Gynecol. Obstet. *177*:519, 1993.)

grasping right thumb and forefinger up and down on this curvature, testing by applying upward traction to find the point providing maximal length.

Drainage of the Stomach

Opinion regarding the advisability of a drainage procedure after esophagectomy is varied. Actual practice is largely the result of personal experience. There are staunch supporters of a routine drainage procedure and those who favor it only when pyloric obstruction is encountered.

Huang and colleagues in a prospective study of pyloroplasty versus no pyloroplasty after esophagectomy showed no difference in gastric emptying time.[8] If gastric outlet obstruction at the level of the pylorus persists, surgical intervention is invariably required. This can be difficult in a patient after esophagogastrectomy, especially if an Ivor Lewis or transhiatal approach has been used, because the pylorus is usually located at or near the hiatus, making exposure difficult. Balloon dilation may be successful in patients who have had a pyloromyotomy and failed conservative measures for gastric outlet obstruction.

From a physiologic standpoint, a gastric drainage procedure makes eminently good sense. In the early years of clinical experience with vagotomy for peptic disease, it became clear very soon that obstructive symptoms were encountered frequently when vagotomy was carried out without a drainage procedure. After esophagectomy, gastric stasis may be observed when the anastomosis is examined radiologically at the initial postoperative study. Because gastroesophageal reflux is not uncommon after an intrathoracic anastomosis of the esophagus and stomach, and the threat of peptic stricture is therefore always a possibility, most experienced general thoracic surgeons now vote for a drainage procedure.

A pyloromyotomy is preferred by most. It does not detract from the length of the stomach when the stomach must be brought to the neck, and the pyloric muscle retains some of its barrier capacity against the reflux of bile and pancreatic juice into the stomach, which threatens alkaline gastritis (Fig. 24–8). Performance of a complete pyloromyotomy is not always an easy technical task. The best teachers of the proper technique are pediatric surgeons, who gain considerable experience from performance of the Ramstedt-Fredet operation for hypertrophic pyloric stenosis.

The myotomy is limited to 3 cm. Transfixion sutures of silk around the pyloric vein on either side of the myotomy site facilitate exposure by reducing bleeding and permitting lateral traction. With the left hand placed behind the gastroduodenal junction lifting the pyloric channel forward, the incision is begun directly over the easily palpable pyloric muscle using an unused No. 15 Bard-Parker blade. The surgeon's thumb retracts the muscle downward as it is divided while the assistant provides countertraction upward. When the submucosal plane is reached, the myotomy incision is carried onto the first

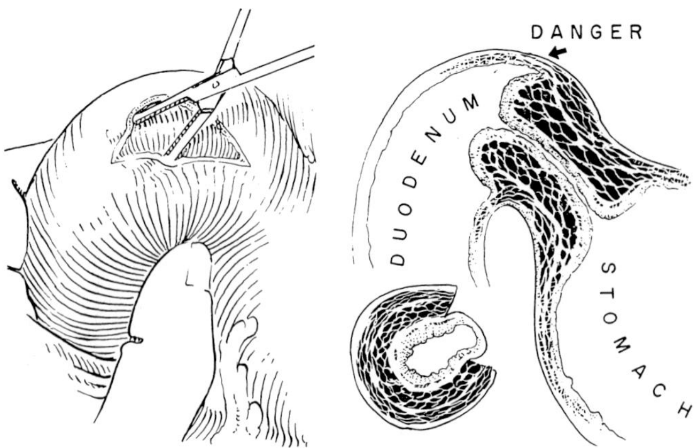

Figure 24–8. Pyloromyotomy. The 3-cm incision across the pylorus provides complete exposure of the sphincter muscle for division down to the mucosal layer. A fine hemostatic forceps is helpful in this dissection. The principal risk of entry into the duodenum is shown in the cross section at the right, where the duodenal mucosa covers the undersurface of the pyloric muscle at the duodenal aspect.

portion of the duodenum, which presents the only real danger of entry into the lumen. Duodenal mucosa tends to follow the inferior margin of the sphincter outward for 1 to 2 mm in an almost everting fashion. Thus, the last muscle fibers are often best separated, again with good exposure and light with loupe magnification, using fine, plastic, vertically cutting scissors.

If entry into the duodenum does ensue, the safest procedure is then to convert the maneuver to a pyloroplasty. The Heineke-Mikulicz method of vertical incisions and horizontal closure suffices, again limiting the length of vertical incisions to no more than 2 to 3 cm. Continuous fine inverting chromic catgut or polyglycolic acid sutures are used for an inner layer closure, and interrupted Lembert sutures of fine silk are used for the reinforcing outer layer. A single layer closure is also acceptable. Tacking a tab of adjacent residual omentum over the pyloromyotomy or pyloroplasty provides an additional safety device against possible subsequent leakage.

Transposition of the Stomach

If the esophagus has been removed, the stomach is placed in the posterior mediastinal or orthotopic position. If a bypassing conduit is planned, a retrosternal tunnel must be constructed to allow anterior mediastinal transpositioning of the stomach.[15]

In the orthotopic position, the shortest route is used. Ngan and Wong have measured the distances of the various routes used for gastric replacement.[14] The orthotopic route was an average of 2 cm less than the retrosternal route; the latter is an additional 2 cm less than the presternal subcutaneous route of passage. The Ivor Lewis right-sided thoracotomy approach to the esophageal dissection permits the now fully mobilized stomach to be drawn gently through the hiatus into the orthotopic position, and then, with certainty about the appropriate axis ensured, the cardia or more distal stomach is transected with the GIA stapler, and the staple line is inverted with interrupted fine silk for security. The use of a sterile plastic bag facilitates passage of the stomach in the orthotopic positions (Fig. 24–9).

If the bypassing route is used, the diaphragmatic attachments to the back of the sternum are sharply divided, and this avascular opening is gradually dilated from the width of two fingers to a size that permits upward passage of the entire hand (Fig. 24–10). The areolar tissue and pleural membrane are swept gently, palm upward, from the midline to the patient's left until the plane of dissection developed through a left oblique cervical incision is encountered. Blood pressure and pulse rate and rhythm must be monitored carefully during this procedure. If hypotension or dysrhythmia develops, the hand must immediately be withdrawn until normalcy is restored; then and only then is the blunt dissection continued. The left pleural membrane does not approach as close to the midline as the right, and therefore blunt dissection to the left is less likely to result in entering the pleura. If a pleural space is entered, a thoracostomy tube (No. 28 Argyle) is placed to allow underwater seal drainage. In any event, a portable chest radiograph is always taken before the patient is moved from the operating table; an unsuspected pneumothorax can then be managed promptly with chest tube evacuation.

Anastomosis

In patients undergoing esophageal resection, this anastomosis may be placed below the aortic arch (as in those

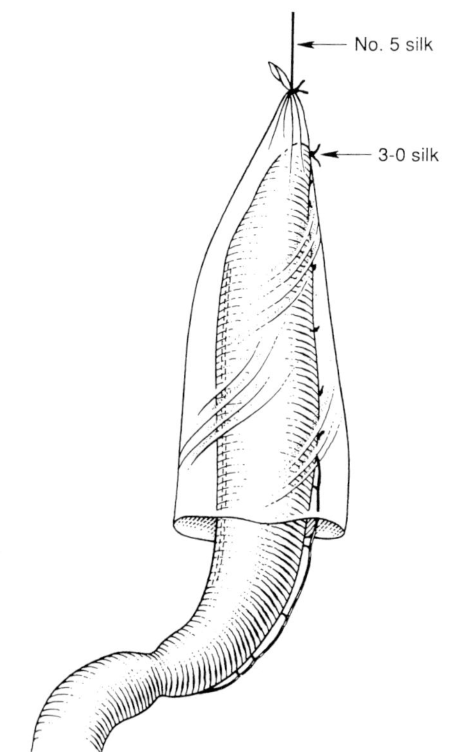

Figure 24–9. The gastric tube is secured to the plastic bag by a horizontal mattress suture, and the apex of the bag is tied to the No. 5 silk emerging from the posterior mediastinum through the hiatus. The tube is now ready for transposition to the neck. (From Shriver, C.D., Spiro, R.H., and Burt, M.: A new technique of gastric pull-through. Surg. Gynecol. Obstet. *177*:519, 1993.)

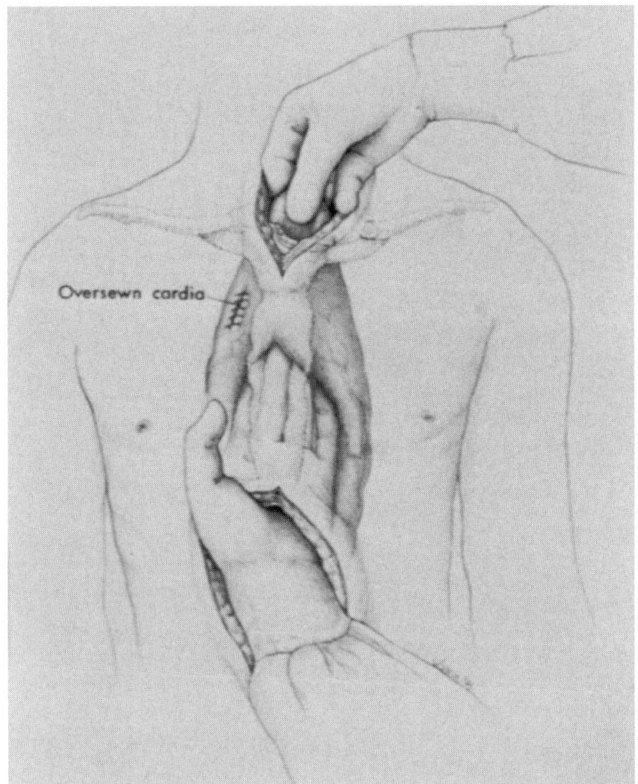

Figure 24–10. The retrosternal tunnel has been bluntly dissected with the finger so that the entire hand can be extended upward in the anterior mediastinum. This figure illustrates passage of the stomach through this tunnel to the thoracic inlet and the cervical incision. Note that the thoracic inlet has been enlarged by resection of the inner end of the clavicle and a portion of the manubrium. (From Orringer, M.B., and Sloan, H.: Substomal gastric bypass of the excluded thoracic esophagus for palliation of esophageal carcinoma. J. Thorac. Cardiovasc. Surg., *70*:836, 1975, with permission.)

needing a left-sided thoracotomy for a carcinoma of the cardia or very distal esophagus), at the apex of the right hemithorax (as in the conventional Ivor Lewis approach), or in the neck for subtotal esophagectomy. If an anterior mediastinal bypass is used, the anastomosis perforce must be in the neck. Wherever the anastomosis is located, exposure must be excellent. This procedure may actually be the most critical part of the operation. In our personal experience and that at the Massachusetts General Hospital, the esophagogastric anastomosis is sufficiently secure that placing it in the mediastinum is not a concern. Thus, placement of the anastomosis in the neck is dictated *solely* by the extent of pathology, not by fear of possible leakage at the anastomotic suture line.

For more than 50 years we have used a two-layer anastomosis of interrupted fine (4-0) silk. Meticulous attention to detail is required in this purely manual technique. No crushing clamps or clamps of any sort are permitted on the edges to be joined. The cutting cautery is not used to transect the esophagus; only a new sharp scalpel blade is used. There must be no tension on the respective edges of the esophagus and stomach. The edges are handled as little as possible with grasping forceps. Placement of a given stitch is guided by gentle traction on the preceding one. The interrupted technique prevents shirring or purse-stringing of the anastomosis and allows patent capillaries to extend to the precise edges of the anastomosed structures.

The details of the anastomosis have been previously described by Wilkins[27] and Mathisen and colleagues.[12] It is an end-to-side (esophagus-to-stomach) technique. A point on the stomach is selected on its anterior aspect at least 2 cm from the gastric closure line (made in freeing the stomach); this point lies in what was the fundus of the stomach and toward the greater curvature. A small circle (the size of a nickel) is scored with the scalpel in the gastric serosa. This maneuver exposes the intramural plexus of vessels that are then individually suture-ligated with fine silk, thus minimizing ooze and preserving an unobscured view for suture placement (Fig. 24–11). With esophageal resection, the specimen is still attached to the proximal esophagus at this point; the specimen is lifted proximally to expose the line of planned transection of the esophagus, and a long right-angled occluding clamp is placed just distal to the planned anastomosis line (i.e., toward the specimen). This assists in providing exact exposure of the anastomosis and at the same time prevents spillage of gastric contents or tumor cells from the specimen.

1. The first row of 4-0 silk sutures is an outer posterior row, placed in horizontal mattress fashion, between the muscularis of the esophagus and the musculoserosa of the stomach (see Fig. 24–11*A*). Four to six of these sutures are placed first and then tied carefully, always drawing the stomach upward to the esophagus by positioning the tying left forefinger above the point of actual approximation. The esophagus is a fixed structure that cannot be brought down distally; its serosaless muscular coats are also more fragile and do not hold sutures as well as the stomach. The outer posterior row of sutures covers only about one third of the circumference; this limitation permits more accessible exposure for the next layer. The corner ties are left long and marked with hemostats.

2. Only now is the esophagus opened, again with the scalpel, about 4 to 5 mm distal to the initial row of stitches, and the incision is extended around each corner. The mucosal layer of stomach is opened, and the scored button is excised. The pinkish gray esophageal mucosa is exposed carefully (it tends to retract) by spreading (not grasping) the opening in the esophagus. The inner posterior stitches, also of 4-0 silk, are placed and tied as one proceeds (see Fig. 24–11*B*). Each stitch is placed about 5 mm back from the cut edge. The gastric mucosa is then picked up for a similar bit of tissue. The needle must be pulled through each edge separately; trying to include both edges in one application of the needle causes tearing. The use of atraumatic grasping forceps is necessary to place this first stitch. Subsequent grasping of mucosa is usually unnecessary. Elevation of the prior stitch guides placement of the next. The full posterior mucosal row is completed, leaving the corner sutures uncut. Transection of the esophagus is now completed, and the specimen is removed (see Fig. 24–11*C*). The nasogastric tube is directed downward through the anastomosis to the level of the gastric antrum and is fixed by the anesthetist to the patient's nose.

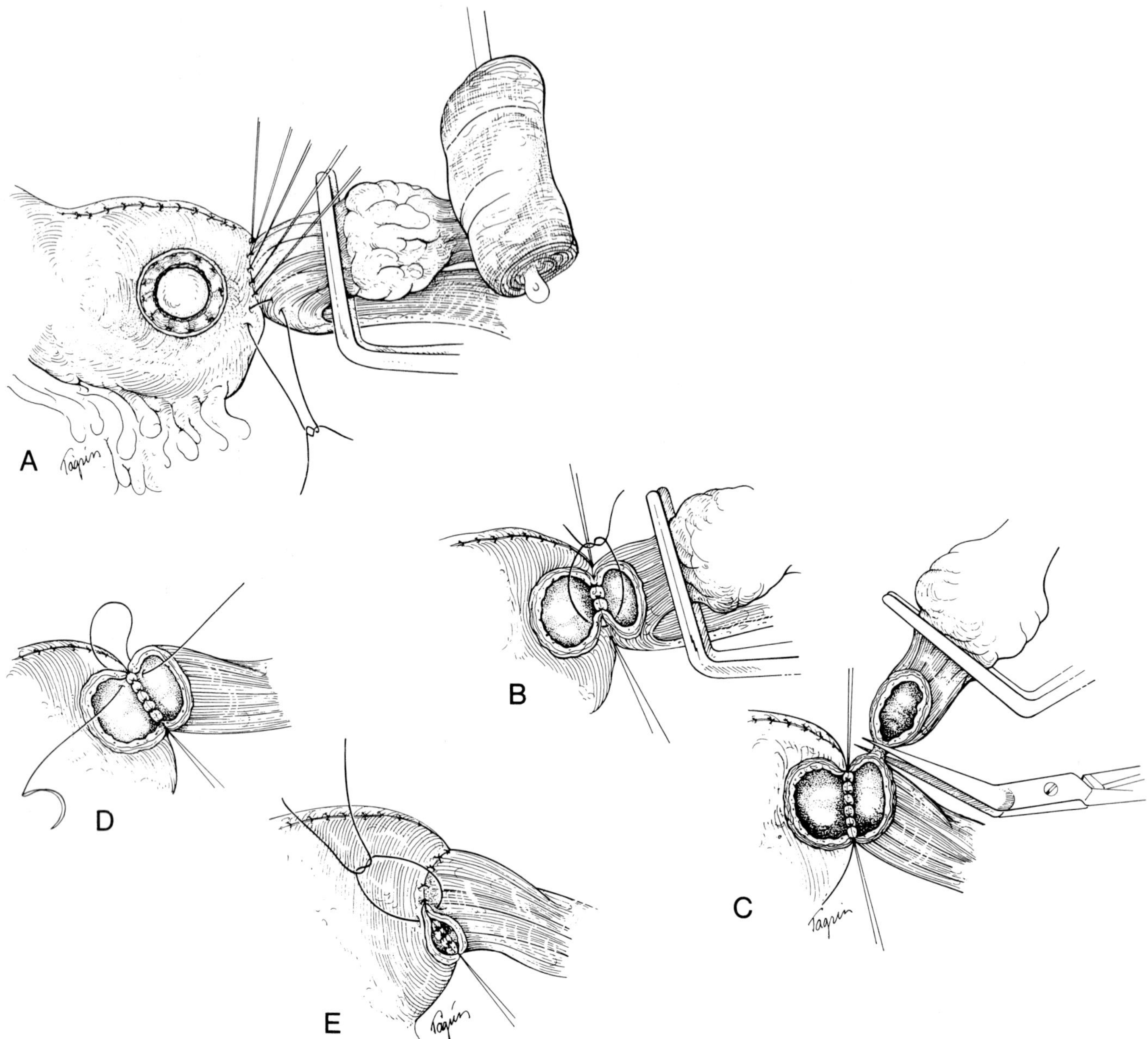

Figure 24–11. *A*, The first step in the Sweet anastomosis developed at the Massachusetts General Hospital. An end-to-side anastomosis is being initiated with excision of a button of gastric wall. This button must not be placed too close to the gastric turn-in. The button can actually be placed quite close to the greater curvature, often between the last two branches of the gastroepiploic arcade. The outer posterior row of the anastomosis is being performed with interrupted mattress sutures of fine silk placed across the longitudinal muscle fibers of the esophagus. My preference is to place all of these sutures before tying. *B*, The gastric button has been excised. With the specimen still attached and excluded with the right-angle clamp, the mucosae of the esophagus and stomach are approximated with interrupted fine silk sutures. *C*, Completion of the posterior inner row and excision of the specimen. *D*, The corner of the anastomosis is being turned to begin the anterior row of sutures. These are placed, again in interrupted fashion, with the knots tied on the inside. *E*, Completion of the anastomosis with mattress sutures of interrupted silk in the outer anterior row. Each suture approximates the muscle of esophagus to the musculoserosa of stomach. These sutures are placed in horizontal mattress fashion (not as actually shown) so that there is less risk of cutting through. (From Mathisen, D.J., Grillo, H.C., Wilkins, E.W. Jr., et al.: Transthoracic esophagectomy: A safe approach to carcinoma of the esophagus. Ann. Thorac. Surg., *45:*137, 1988, with permission.)

3. The anterior inner row is continued in interrupted fashion, placing the stitches so that the knots are always tied within the lumen (see Fig. 24–11*D*). The assistant holds the previous tie down and away as each subsequent stitch is secured. This method allows complete inversion of the mucosal layer. The prior suture is then cut after tying of each subsequent stitch. This row of sutures is tied from either end toward the middle so that a final horizontal mattress suture can be placed anteriorly to complete the anterior mucosal row.

4. The outer anterior row is placed in horizontal mattress fashion over what is left, which is about two thirds of the circumference (see Fig. 24–11*E*). The serosa of the stomach is brought as much as 1 cm above the inner mucosal layer. Because the anastomosis has been placed 2 cm or more down the apex of the stomach posteriorly

and the stomach has been folded upward anteriorly, a valve-like luminal orifice has been created that helps to minimize the possibility of gastroesophageal reflux. The stomach is suspended by a series of nonabsorbable sutures to the fascia overlying the thoracic spine. This minimizes the possibility of downward drag of a potentially full stomach on the fragile anastomosis.

Whether the esophagogastrectomy is performed as a replacement of the esophagus or as a bypass of it, it may be accompanied by placement of a feeding jejunostomy. The jejunostomy is used for feeding purposes if there is any difficulty with the anastomosis or with delay in postoperative gastric emptying. It also provides access for immediate postoperative substantive caloric feeding, obviates the need for total intravenous parenteral nutrition, and promotes healing at the anastomotic sites by providing a catabolic status for the patient.

One week after surgery, the esophagogastric anastomosis is checked by a barium swallow. If there is no difficulty with the anastomosis, the jejunostomy tube may be removed when the patient begins to tolerate oral feedings.

Functional Results

Despite the vast experience with stomach as an esophageal substitute, precious little information is available on long-term functional results. Orringer and associates have reported early and late functional results after transhiatal esophagectomy and cervical esophagogastric anastomosis in 138 patients for benign esophageal disease.[16] Sixty-eight per cent had excellent or good results, and 29% had fair results requiring dilation or antidiarrheal medications. True strictures requiring repeated dilations occurred in only 10%. Weight loss (mean, 11 pounds) occurred in 49%, whereas 41% weighed more (mean, 11 pounds), and 9% experienced no change in their weight. In 55 patients followed more than 5 years, 78% had no or only mild dysphagia, 20% had moderate dysphagia requiring occasional anastomotic dilation, and 2% had severe dysphagia requiring regular dilation. Dumping was experienced by 23%, with only 7% requiring treatment. Nocturnal regurgitation requiring sleeping on a wedge was experienced in 13% of patients followed beyond 5 years.

ESOPHAGOCOLOPLASTY

The term *esophagocoloplasty* is used arbitrarily in this section to denote either replacement or bypass of the esophagus by colon. As clearly described already, the stomach is the first choice for providing a substitute for the esophagus. However, when the stomach has previously been removed, even partially, the colon is the replacing viscus of choice. In addition, when bypass of an unresectable esophageal carcinoma is required, the colon offers the best possibility for providing successful palliation. The specific indications for esophagocoloplasty are given in Table 24-1.

Table 24–1. Indications for Esophagocoloplasty

Malignant tumors
1. Replacement of esophagus after gastrectomy
2. Bypass of unresectable carcinoma
3. Palliation of esophagotracheal or bronchial fistula
4. Staged complex esophageal resections

Benign conditions
1. Staged bypass of caustic esophageal stricture
2. Esophageal atresia (congenital) when primary anastomosis is not feasible
3. Bypass of long peptic esophageal stricture in physiologically impaired patient

Preoperative Preparation

Emphasis has already been placed on performing colon evaluation by colonoscopy, mesenteric arteriography, and barium enema, in that order. Of these, complete opacification of the colon arterial blood supply is the most important in providing a complete map of the several colic arteries for the abdominal surgeon. In older patients, the presence of atherosclerotic plaques, which might impair successful vascularity of the interposing colon, are identified by these studies. Any of the estimated 10% of major mesenteric arterial anomalies (see Fig. 24-3) may be identified. Although in most cases, the details of this anatomy can be worked out by intraoperative transillumination of the colon mesentery, arteriographic study saves both time and confusion in the actual conduct of the operation.

Mechanical cleansing of the colon to be placed in the chest is an important fundamental procedure. A clean colon is essential to primary healing of the esophagocolic anastomosis in the neck, where spillage of residual fecal contents must be avoided. The first step in providing a clean colon is the cleansing necessary for either the colonoscopy or the barium enema. If barium is used, its total evacuation must be verified by a preoperative plain abdominal radiograph. An elemental diet providing oral alimentation of essential amino acids is often satisfactory in patients with dysphagia. Mechanical cleansing of the colon (GoLYTELY) is the major element in assuming a clean colon. Enemas are rarely required and should not be administered within 12 to 18 hours before surgery. Oral intestinal antibiotics are favored by some, with 1 g of neomycin and 1 g of erythromycin every 4 hours times four doses the most common regimen. Broad-spectrum, so-called prophylactic, antibiotics are initiated parenterally on-call to the operating theater, and maintenance doses are continued in bolus intravenous fashion during the procedure and 48 hours after.

Operative Technique

The use of colon in a bypass procedure is described here. Its use as a replacement differs only in the orthotopic route of placement in the posterior mediastinum, the shortest distance to the neck. This avenue should not be chosen if gross residual carcinoma is left in the mediastinum. Many surgeons prefer to use the retrosternal position for the colon, whether as a replacement or as a bypass.

Colon esophageal bypass is ideally suited to the two-team approach. Because of the related amounts of dissection required, the cervical team can often delay its incision until the exploratory findings in the abdomen are clearly favorable: (1) an absence of major intra-abdominal metastatic disease, and (2) the presence of a suitable length of colon with a proper arterial blood supply and venous drainage.

Standard endotracheal anesthesia is used, and the patient is placed supine on the operating table with the head turned to the right. Hyperextension of the neck, as achieved with elevation of the shoulders by the so-called thyroid bag, is used. The operative field is prepared from the left mastoid process to the symphysis pubis. A Salem sump nasogastric tube is passed to the point of esophageal obstruction or into the stomach. Intraoperative monitoring is provided by a radial artery line, a central venous pressure line, and continuous electrocardiographic tracing.

Team One. A long midline or left paramedian laparotomy incision is used, extending from the xiphoid process to below the umbilicus. Careful exploration is needed to search for hepatic metastases, left gastric artery–celiac axis node metastases, peritoneal or omental implants of tumor, a possible second gastric carcinoma, or other unsuspected intra-abdominal process.

The colon is then mobilized, including its two flexures, from the ascending to the sigmoid colon level. Freeing the colon from the omentum and from the right and left peritoneal reflections is not difficult but must be accomplished carefully. The general surgical background of the thoracic surgeon is a helpful attribute. Points requiring particular care in this dissection are, in order of approach: (1) total detachment of the omentum, leaving it attached to the stomach but preserving the midcolic vessels as the posterior leaf of the omentum is peeled off the transverse mesocolon; (2) taking down the splenic flexure of the colon without injury to the spleen, a process that is more easily accomplished after the left peritoneal reflection has been incised, permitting downward traction on both transverse and descending colon; and (3) freeing the hepatic flexure off the duodenum and retroperitoneal structures in the right upper quadrant.

This subtotal freeing of the colon now permits it to be elevated for appropriate transillumination and visualization of all colic vessels. Because of a more satisfactory experience with its use and the greater reliability of its arterial supply, the left hemicolon is preferred to the right for use as the bypassing conduit. The marginal communication between the left branch of the midcolic artery and the ascending portion of the left colic artery is critical, and its presence and adequacy on the preoperative arteriogram must be verified (see Fig. 24–4). The ramification of the midcolic artery is no less critical. Because the length of the necessary colon bypass takes one to the hepatic fixture, a bifurcation of the midcolic artery well out from its superior mesenteric arterial source is required; a bifid separation origin of the right and left branches of the midcolic artery does not permit retrograde blood flow all the way from the left colic artery to the hepatic flexure. *An isoperistaltic placement of the colon segment is preferred* (Fig. 24–12).

To utilize the left colic artery as the source of blood supply, the midcolic vessels are now divided at their origin from the superior mesenteric vessels and doubly ligated (Fig. 24–13). For complete mobility of the hepatic flexure, the right colic vessels usually must also be divided. The distance from the point where the colon is tethered by the left colic artery is measured to the level of the midneck. The distance is then measured around the colon toward the hepatic flexure, and the point of appropriate transection is carefully identified. The colon is transected using the GIA stapler both at this point and at the juncture of the descending and sigmoid colons. The colon segment is attached only by its feeding left colic artery and draining vein at this point; the segment

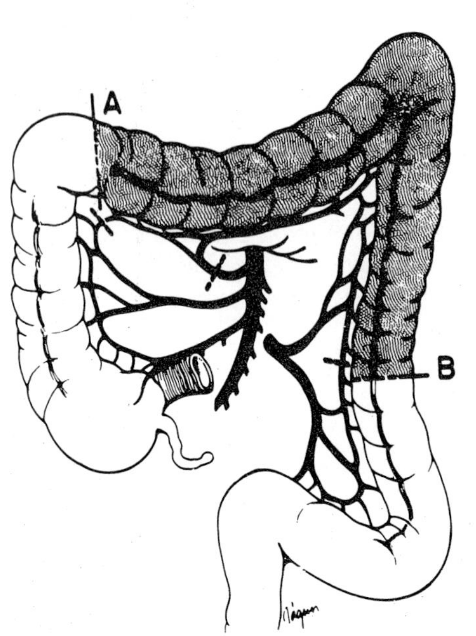

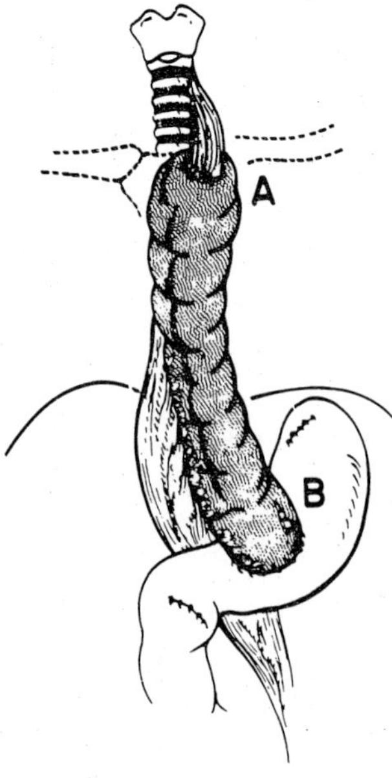

Figure 24–12. Schematic illustration showing use of the left colon to replace the esophagus. Points A and B are determined by the length of colon necessary to reach the neck. The left colic artery provides the blood supply. The middle colic artery is divided. The colon is placed, always, in isoperistaltic fashion so that the segment near the hepatic flexure is anastomosed to the esophagus in the neck and the end near the sigmoid colon is attached to the antrum of the stomach in the abdomen.

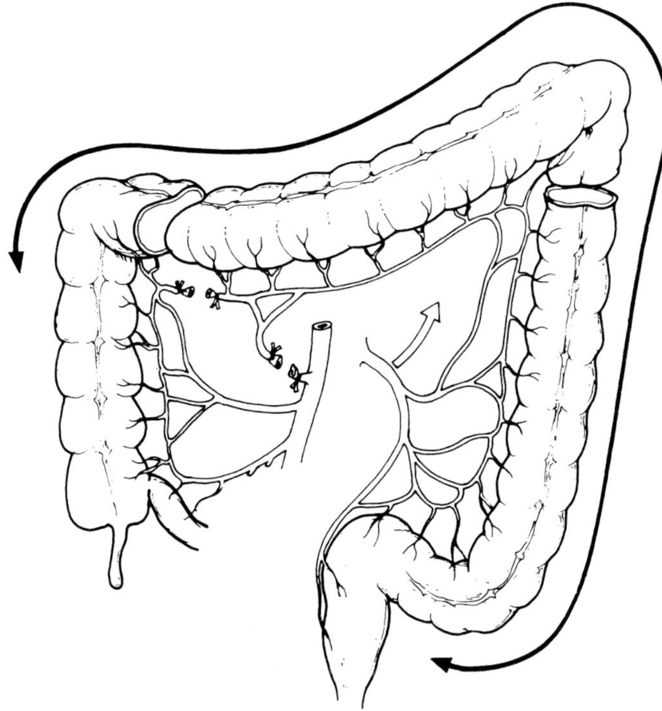

Figure 24–13. The long line with arrows at either end illustrates the extent of colon to be freed for left colon replacement of the esophagus. Blood supply is provided through the inferior mesenteric artery, the left colic artery, and the anastomotic branch connecting the middle colic artery. The middle colic artery has been divided near its origin from the superior mesenteric artery.

can then be passed behind the stomach through a wide aperture made in the avascular gastrohepatic omentum. This maneuver allows the left colic artery to extend the shortest distance in its new position, without angulation and without potential compression by a dependent full stomach (were the artery allowed to lie in front of the stomach).

The mobilized residual abdominal colon can now be reanastomosed. Our preference has been to use an end-to-end, two-layer, inverting anastomosis of interrupted fine silk. A most important detail is the closure of the colon mesentery to minimize the likelihood of internal herniation of small intestine. This closure usually lies slightly caudad from the ligament of Treitz and often requires closure by approximation of the mesentery to the posterior peritoneum.

Now that a viable colon bypassing segment has been demonstrated, the second team has begun the cervical incision. Meanwhile, the retrosternal tunnel is bluntly dissected by the first team, both from below and from the cervical incision as described subsequently. Particular attention is paid to the adequacy of the thoracic inlet portion of this tunnel; it should admit four fingers. The inlet can be enlarged if necessary as described earlier (see Fig. 24–2). The colon segment is then gently drawn upward by means of a guiding heavy silk thread, taking care to keep its mesentery on the right without any twist. The sterile plastic bag is helpful in passing the colon segment (see Fig. 24–9). Impediment of the venous return may threaten subsequent venous thrombosis and failure of the colon bypass. Viability of the upper end of the segment must be verified not only by visual inspection of its color but also by palpable observation of arterial pulsation, by application of a Doppler probe, or by incisional demonstration of actual arterial blood flow.

The cologastric anastomosis is carried out end-to-side to the anterior aspect of the midportion of the stomach, using an inner layer of running 4–0 atraumatic catgut and an outer layer of interrupted 4–0 silk sutures.

The pylorus is palpated to determine the need for a pyloric drainage procedure; an opportunity is available at the time of the cologastric anastomosis to palpate the pyloric channel from within. In general, pyloric drainage is required only if the esophagus is being removed and the vagus nerves are thus divided; simple bypass does not compromise gastric innervation, and stasis is not likely to be a problem.

Gastric decompression is provided by a Stamm gastrostomy placed proximal to the cologastric anastomosis. A 5-ml No. 18 Foley catheter works effectively and is brought out through a stab incision placed laterally in the left upper quadrant. The stomach is secured to the anterior peritoneum in four quadrants around the tube with 3–0 silk sutures.

Team Two. A left-sided oblique cervical incision is a useful approach to the cervical esophagus. It requires dividing the omohyoid muscle, retracting the sternocleidomastoid muscle laterally, dividing the inferior thyroid artery and often the middle thyroid vein, detaching the sternal insertions of the peritracheal muscles, and entering the avascular prevertebral plane. The esophagus is readily apparent by palpation of its inlaying nasogastric tube.

The esophagus is encircled, taking care not to damage the membranous portion of the trachea or the recurrent laryngeal nerves. Even a unilateral vocal cord palsy enhances the possibility of postoperative aspiration into the tracheobronchial tree. The mobilized esophagus is transected 2 to 3 cm distal to the cricopharyngeus sphincter, its proximal end marked with silk sutures at the corners and left open without clamping, and its distal end turned in with two layers, one stapled and the second with inverting 4–0 interrupted silk sutures.

The critical esophagocolic anastomosis is carried out in end-to-end fashion using two layers of inverting interrupted 4–0 silk. The actual suture material is not as important as the two-layer, interrupted technique. Use of the left colon bypass minimizes the possibility of any discrepancy in size between the two lumens being anastomosed. Proper interval spacing of the sutures or use of a short vertical incisional enlargement of the end of the esophagus permits a purely circumferential anastomosis without a T corner if the colon end seems too large and is partially closed before anastomosis. The nasogastric tube, withdrawn appropriately in transecting the esophagus, is replaced distally into the colon bypass before completing the anterior row of sutures: It provides evacuation of colonic air, monitors postoperative bleeding, and minimizes the possibility of tracheal aspiration. This tube must be left just overnight.

The neck is closed without drainage unless there is annoying ooze; if necessary, drainage should be provided by a closed system, such as a Jackson-Pratt device. (The abdominal incision has now been closed by team one.) A portable chest radiograph is obtained before the anesthesia tube is removed. Any pneumothorax is decompressed by means of a closed thoracostomy tube.

Postoperative Care

The most important detail of postoperative management is the need to be sure of viability of the colon bypass segment. The most reliable indication that something is amiss is a persistently high fever. Endoscopy is hazardous in assessing viability because of the fresh anastomosis. Furthermore, the appearance of the mucosa is not always a reliable indicator of viability. The best method in assessing viability is the so-called second-look operation. The neck incision can be opened easily under local anesthesia, and the upper end of the colon segment can be inspected directly. If the segment is nonviable, it must be removed totally from its retrosternal location promptly. A necrotic colon persisting in the anterior mediastinum is a source of possible death. In one case of failed colon bypass in our experience, the residual viable colon was brought up subcutaneously, and the resultant gap was ultimately bridged with a free jejunal autograft.

The nasogastric tube is removed on the day after surgery. Feedings are begun by gastrostomy on the second day, or when residual fluid as measured by daily drainage is minimal (i.e., less than 100 ml). The patient is fed in a semierect position to minimize possible gastrocolic reflux. A barium esophagram is carried out on about the seventh postoperative day. Oral feeding is then begun gradually if the anastomosis proves to be intact.

Results

Wain reported our results with long-segment colon substitution of the esophagus in 136 patients.[26] Indications for use were neoplasms in 88 and non-neoplastic disorders in 48 (Table 24-2). Left colon was used in 100 of 136 (74%) and right colon in 36 of 136 (26%). Major acute complications included graft ischemia (4 of 100 left colon, 8 of 36 right colon) and cervical anastomotic leak (Table 24-3). The 30-day operative mortality rates were 16% in the neoplastic group and 0% in the non-neoplastic group (Table 24-4). The differences in operative mortality between benign and malignant disease were corroborated by a review by Postlethwait[20] (Table 24-5). Late complications included proximal anastomotic stenosis (eight), graft redundancy (four), bile reflux (two), and esophageal mucocele (one). Among operative survivors, excellent function (no dysphagia, stable weight) was obtained in 88% (107 of 122), good function (mild dysphagia, stable weight) in 10% (12 of 122), and only three patients (2.5%) had poor results.

This operation requires precise attention to technical detail for successful outcome. The major complications and causes of operative mortality are related to technical failures. Strict adherence to these technical details should minimize these complications. When successful, the colon had proved to be an effective lasting viscus with which to replace the esophagus.

Table 24–2. Indications for Colon Esophageal Bypass*

Diagnosis	No. of Patients
Neoplastic	88
Esophageal cancer	78
Proximal gastric cancer	3
Laryngeal cancer	3
Thyroid cancer	3
Malignant carcinoid	1
Non-neoplastic	48
Stricture	35
Caustic	16
Peptic	14
Radiation	5
Congenital atresia	10
Motility disorder	3

*From Wain, J.C.: Long segment colon interposition. Semin. Thorac. Cardiovasc. Surg., *4*:336, 1992, with permission.

Table 24–3. Acute Complications of Colon Esophageal Bypass*

Diagnosis	No. of Patients
Technical	
Graft ischemia	12
Left colon	4
Right colon	8
Cervical anastomotic leak	8
Vocal cord paresis	3
Acute nonvascular perforation	1
Sternal necrosis	1
Other	
Pneumonia	15
Wound infection	9
Small bowel obstruction	4
Pulmonary embolism	2
Cholecystitis	1

*From Wain, J.C.: Long segment colon interposition. Semin. Thorac. Cardiovasc. Surg., *4*:336, 1992, with permission.

ESOPHAGOJEJUNOPLASTY

Jejunum represents the third alternative for esophageal replacement and is rarely used purely as a bypass. As a replacement, it can be used in one of three ways: (1)

Table 24–4. Cause of Operative Mortality in Long-Segment Colon Bypass for Neoplasm*

Cause	No. of Patients
Colon necrosis	7
Respiratory failure	5
Metastatic disease	1
Sudden cardiac death	1

*From Wain, J.C.: Long segment colon interposition. Semin. Thorac. Cardiovasc. Surg., *4*:336, 1992, with permission.

Table 24–5. Colon Interposition Operative Mortality*

	Benign		Malignant	
	No. of Patients	*Deaths (%)*	*No. of Patients*	*Deaths (%)*
Through 1961	54	11.1	78	21.8
Through 1971	655	7.5	245	24.5
Through 1981	474	4.9	367	16.6
TOTAL	1,183	6.8	690	20.0

*From Postlethwait, R.W.: Surgery of the Esophagus, 2nd ed. Norwalk, CT, Appleton-Century-Crofts, 1986, p. 505, with permission.

interposition, (2) Roux-en-Y limb, or (3) autograft. As an interposition, it retains its vascular supply and drainage with a jejunal branch from the superior mesenteric artery and, just as important, a jejunal venous tributary to the superior mesenteric vein. It is most frequently used as a short-segment interposition bridging the gap created by resecting a distal esophageal stricture, although it may also be used to restore continuity after distal esophagectomy for carcinoma when the stomach has previously been removed. The anatomy of its mesentery makes long-segment interposition difficult, although in children, a Roux-en-Y loop readily reaches the neck. As an autograft, it is used for resection of short cervical esophageal segments containing carcinoma, after extensive cervical trauma involving damage to the esophagus, or for augmentation of a failed colonic esophageal bypass.

Interposition. The short interposition for distal esophageal resection replacement is described here because it is the most common application of esophagojejunoplasty. A left-sided thoracoabdominal incision provides the necessary exposure for both the esophageal procedure and the preparation of the jejunum. The proximal jejunum is identified and lifted out of the abdomen for transillumination of its mesentery (Fig. 24–14). The first jejunal artery is identified and preserved to maintain the vascular integrity of the 10 to 12 cm of jejunum adjacent to the ligament of Treitz, which will be used for reanastomosis of the jejunum after isolation of the segment to be interposed.

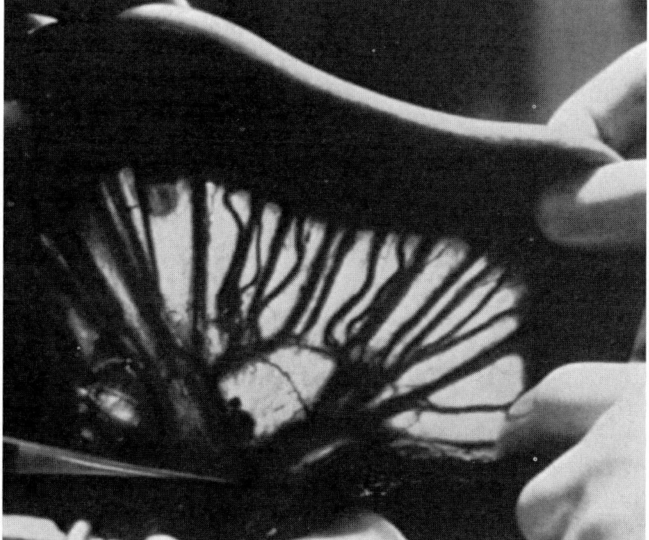

Figure 24–14. Transillumination of the jejunum demonstrates the jejunal branches of the superior mesenteric artery and permits selection of an appropriate one for reliable blood supply for the segment to be used in esophagojejunoplasty.

The appropriate length of the jejunum needed is determined, and the upper three or four jejunal arteries to this measured segment are exposed. With the help of the transilluminating light, these arteries are isolated and occluded sequentially with atraumatic bulldog clamps to test the reliability of one jejunal artery to provide circulation to this segment. The peritoneum is reflected carefully from either side of the mesentery outward to the primary anastomotic arcade, the tissue intervening between the jejunal arteries is incised, and the necessary jejunal arteries and veins are divided and securely ligated with 2-0 silk. For longer reaches of the jejunal segment, one or two points on the secondary anastomotic arcade may require division (Fig. 24–15).

The jejunal segment is now separated from its normal intestinal continuity with proximal and distal application of the GIA stapler. The pedicled segment to be interposed is then brought behind the colon, through the transverse mesocolon. Because the segment has a proclivity to retain its curved axis, the stapled proximal end of the segment is turned in with interrupted 3-0 silk Lembert sutures. The distal end of the jejunal segment is anastomosed first to the posterior aspect of the fundus of the stomach; here, the two-layer anastomosis is provided by an outer layer of interrupted 4-0 silk and an inner layer of continuous 4-0 chromic catgut or Dexon sutures. The esophagojejunal anastomosis is carried out end-to-side to a point some 2 cm away from the jejunal turn-in on its antimesenteric border (Fig. 24–16). This is done with the same inverting two layers of interrupted silk sutures described in the section on esophagogastrostomy. If the stomach has been removed, this distal anastomosis may be carried out to the duodenal stump. Jejunal continuity is restored by an end-to-end anastomosis done with an outer layer of silk and an inner running catgut layer.

Roux-En-Y Limb. When there is no stomach for jejunal interposition, the alternative technique of a Roux-en-Y jejunal limb may be used. This procedure actually entails just two anastomoses—esophagojejunal and end-to-side jejunojejunal—instead of the three needed for the technique using the interposed segment. The higher the jejunum must reach in the chest, or even in the neck, the more jejunal arteries must be divided to provide adequate length of the Roux-en-Y limb. Unfortunately,

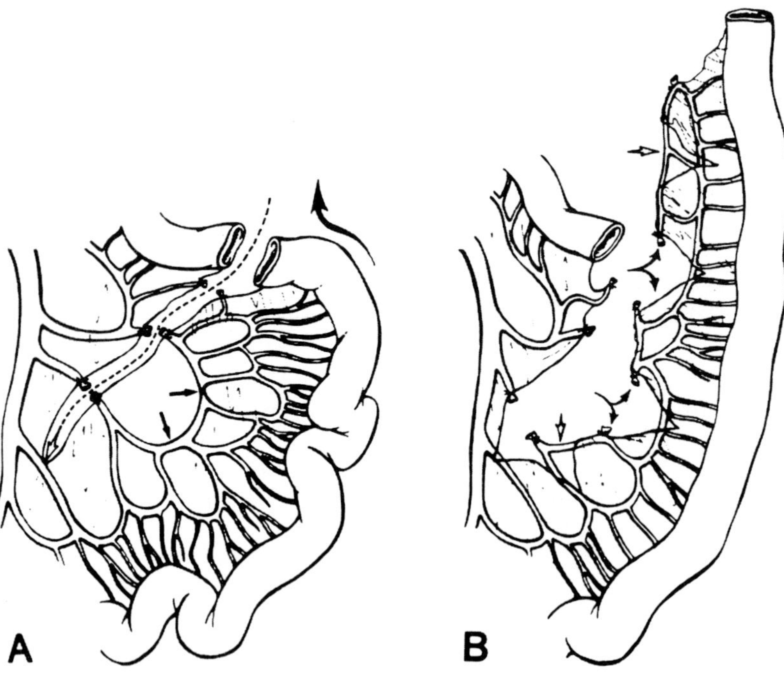

Figure 24–15. *A* and *B*, Diaphragmatic illustration of (1) preservation of the highest jejunal artery, (2) division of the next three jejunal arteries, and (3) two points of division of a secondary arcade in *B*. Particular care must be taken that an arcade exists from the feeding arterial source (in this case, the fourth jejunal artery) all the way to the transected margin. (From Ring, W.S., Varco, R.L., L'Heureux, P.R., et al.: Esophageal replacement with jejunum in children: An 18 to 33 year follow-up. J. Thorac. Cardiovasc. Surg., *83*:918, 1982, with permission.)

this requirement increases the possibility of vascular failure at the tip of the Roux jejunal segment. This particular unreliability explains why jejunum is generally considered only the third choice for esophageal replacement. Ring and associates[21] stated that jejunum is the first choice in children, but their illustrations (Fig. 24–17) show a process of staging the esophagojejunal anastomosis with an unanastomosed jejunal stoma in the neck in the first stage, planned presumably to be certain of its viability, with subsequent esophagojejunal anastomosis.

In cervical esophagojejunoplasty, there is always the possibility of vascular enhancement by microvascular anastomosis of the internal mammary artery or a branch of a carotid artery to the jejunal mesentery arterial arcade. A suitable draining vein must also be identified and anastomosed under these circumstances. Payne and Fisher have described a unique experience with "free jejunal transfer circulatory augmentation of pedicled intestinal interpositions using microvascular surgery," in which the details of a number of variants of esophagojejunoplasty are described to solve unusual problems of cervical esophageal replacement.[19] When the thoracic surgeon contemplates the use of jejunum for a long-segment replacement of the esophagus, such as to the cervical level, he or she would be well advised to consult a microvascular surgical practitioner to prepare for this possible need for circulatory augmentation.

Free Transfer. The free transfer procedure is accomplished most expeditiously by two teams. Attention in this discussion is focused on the abdominal procurement ("harvesting") team. Through a routine laparotomy, a suitable segment of jejunum is selected—more "downstream" than a segment used for interposition—some 40 cm distal to the ligament of Treitz (Fig. 24–18*B*). The principal determining point in the site of selection is an appropriate length of a jejunal artery and vein for later vascular anastomoses. The character of the bowel itself is an additional consideration; it must have adequate caliber and be free from intrinsic pathology. The length of needed jejunum is delineated, and the jejunum is transected proximally and distally with the GIA stapler.

A B C D

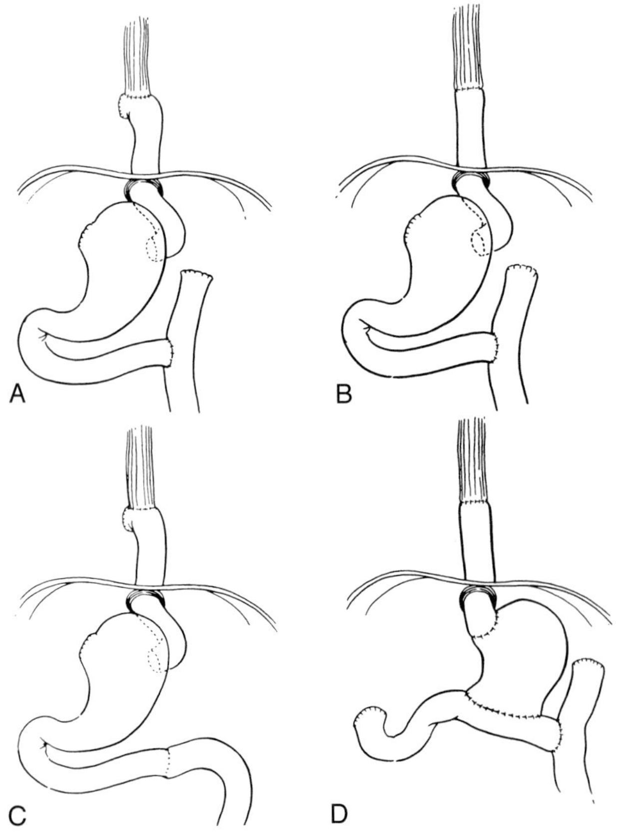

Figure 24–16. Methods of reconstruction using jejunum. (From Postlethwaite, R.W.: Surgery of the Esophagus, 2nd ed. Norwalk, CT, Appleton-Century-Crofts, 1986, p. 500, with permission.)

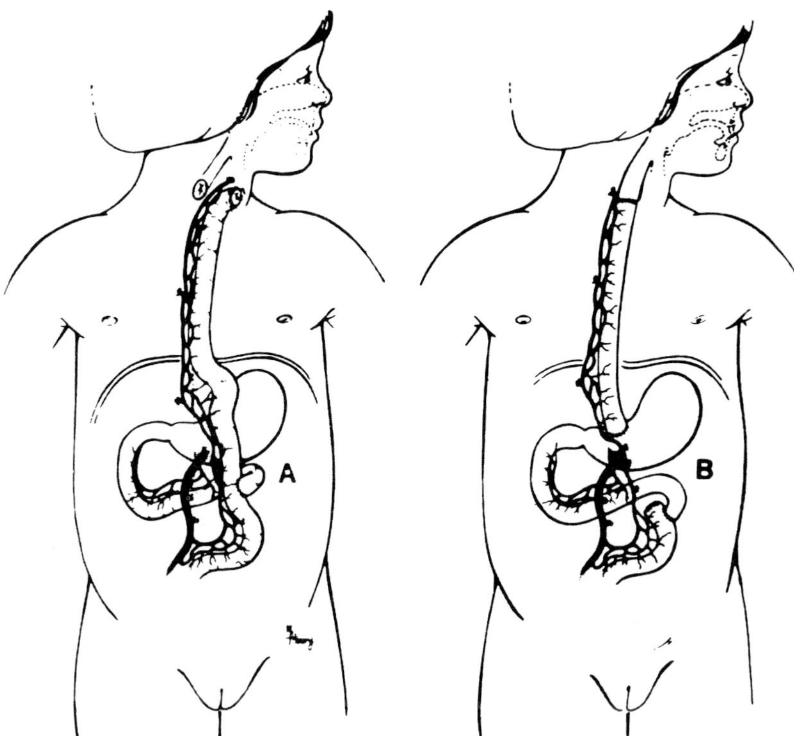

Figure 24–17. Use of the jejunum to replace the esophagus in a child. The jejunum readily reaches the neck. *A*, The proximal jejunum is brought out as a cervical stoma permitting secondary performance of the esophagojejunal anastomosis. *B*, The distal jejunum has been divided and anastomosed to the antrum of the stomach and the cervical anastomosis completed. (From Ring, W.S., Varco, R.L., L'Heureux, P.R., et al.: Esophageal replacement with jejunum in children: An 18 to 33 year follow-up. J. Thorac. Cardiovasc. Surg., *83*:918, 1982, with permission.)

The mesentery is divided in a V fashion to the origin of the perfusing vessels. The isolated segment is now allowed to perfuse until the cervical team is prepared to carry out the actual transfer (see Fig. 24–18*A*). Meanwhile, jejunal continuity is re-established by end-to-end anastomosis as described in the preceding section. Only the mesentery then requires closure, using a continuous 4-0 chromic catgut suture after the actual transfer has been carried out.

The jejunal autograft, with the artery and vein carefully occluded by noncrushing bulldog clamps, is moved to the cervical incision. The segment is placed, always in an isoperistaltic fashion, in the cervical esophageal bed, and the proximal jejunal anastomosis is performed first—cervical esophagus or hypopharynx is anastomosed to the jejunal segment with two layers of inverting interrupted 4-0 silk, just as for esophagogastrostomy (see Fig. 24–18*D*). This provides enough fixation and stability to allow performance of the two microvascular anastomoses without concern for tension or torsion. A suitable neck artery (the inferior thyroid, transverse cervical, or common carotid artery itself) is used for a standard vascular anastomosis with 10-0 nylon monofilament sutures, done under the operating microscope (see Fig. 24–18*E*). The microvascular bulldog clamps are then released, and the jejunal autograft is allowed to perfuse. The final step is the two-layer anastomosis of the distal jejunum to the esophagus, again using inverting, interrupted fine silk sutures (see Fig. 24–18*F*). Then, a venous anastomosis is accomplished using the facial vein, the middle thyroid vein, or one of the jugular veins.

The cervical incision is usually closed without drainage. A thermistor probe has been used as a method of monitoring the viability of the jejunal graft. Alternatively, a Silastic "window" can be used for direct observation of the jejunal segment for 24 to 48 hours and then primarily closed once viability is ascertained (see Fig. 24–18*G*). It is preferred not to allow a nasogastric tube to pass through the cervical jejunum; gastric drainage is accomplished more readily by a gastrostomy tube.

FREE JEJUNAL INTERPOSITION

Hundreds of jejunal transplants for cervical esophageal reconstruction have been performed. The graft survival rate is nearly 95%. Jurkiewicz and Paletta have reported their experience with 130 cases, with a similar graft survival and patient success rate of 92%.[9] The operative mortality rate was 5%. The main cause of graft failure is arterial or venous insufficiency. This part of the operation is technically demanding and requires careful attention in choosing suitable vessels for anastomosis, proper length, and careful positioning of the vascular pedicle. If graft failure occurs, a second attempt with another free jejunal graft should be made, with success rates of 50 to 75% expected. Pharyngocutaneous fistula is a common postoperative complication, reported in 33 of 101 patients in Jurkiewicz's series. Twenty-four of these cases closed spontaneously; the others were managed by a second graft or simple drainage.

SHORT-SEGMENT COLON INTERPOSITION

Short-segment colon interposition is an alternative to jejunal interposition of the distal esophagus. Preparation of

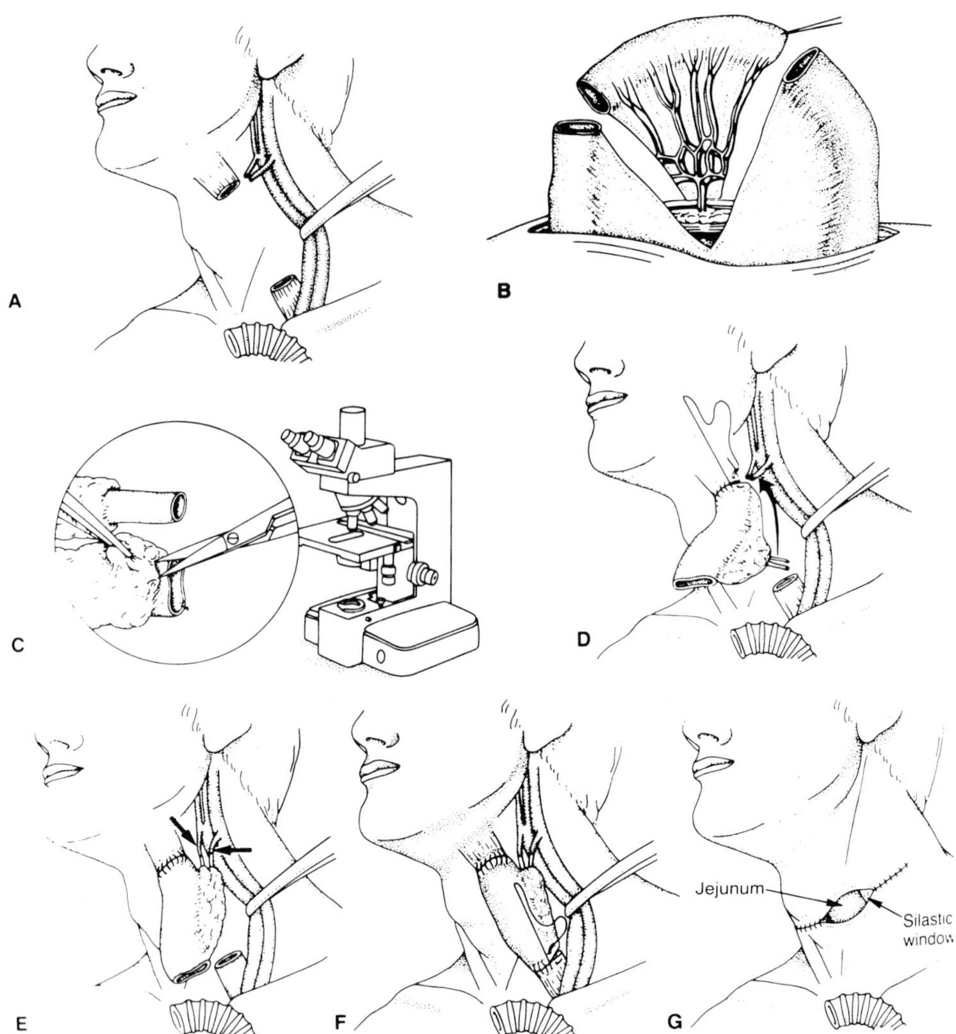

Figure 24–18. Reconstruction of cervical esophagus with free jejunal graft. Technique described by Hester et al. (1980). *A*, Tumor extirpation and neck dissection is completed. *B*, After abdominal exploration, a suitable segment of proximal jejunum is isolated on its pedicle, and the bowel is divided proximally and distally, ensuring that the only blood supply to the segment is through the pedicle. *C*, The artery and vein of the chosen segment are clean of adventitia using the operating microscope. *D*, The proximal bowel anastomosis is completed using interrupted 3–0 Vicryl sutures. *E*, The arterial and venous anastomoses to the chosen donor vessels are done. *F*, The distal bowel anastomosis is completed using interrupted 3–0 Vicryl sutures. *G*, A small window of dimethicone (Silastic) sheeting is left over the jejunum to allow close postoperative observation of the replant. (From Skinner, D.B., and Belsey, R.H.R.: Management of Esophageal Disease. Philadelphia, W.B. Saunders, 1988, with permission.)

the patient and colon is as described for long-segment colon interposition. Because extensive length is not required, more options exist, and arteriography is not as critical. The most popular segment of colon to use for distal esophageal replacement is an isoperistaltic segment of the distal transverse colon and descending left colon based on the ascending branch of the left colic artery.

The operation is usually performed through an extended left thoracoabdominal incision to allow mobilization of the colon segment, resection of the diseased distal esophagus, and anastomosis of the interposition to the distal esophagus and posterior wall of the stomach. The colon is carefully palpated for abnormalities. The choice of colon segment is determined. Left colon segments are based on the ascending branch of the left colic artery. Transverse colon segments are based on the middle colic artery. The colon segment should be isoperistaltic. In our experience, the left colon was used more commonly ($n = 19$) than the transverse colon ($n = 3$). The length of colon segment needed is then mobilized. The main vascular pedicle is identified but not skeletonized. Collateral blood supply along the artery of Drummond or the middle colic artery branch is isolated, carefully test-clamped with fine bulldog clamps, and ligated after the viability of the segment is ascertained. A 15-minute trial occlusion of collateral vessels is sufficient to determine viability. An appropriate length of colon is freed between noncrushing bowel clamps or with a linear stapling device. Colonic continuity is restored. The colon segment is placed in a posterior mediastinal position avoiding tension or torsion of the vascular pedicle. A two-layer anastomosis with interrupted 4–0 silk is preferred. The

Table 24–6. Indications for Short-Segment Intestinal Interposition of the Distal Esophagus*

Diagnosis	No. of Patients
Gastroesophageal reflux disease	34
Failed antireflux repair	21
Nondilatable stricture	9
Complication of treatment for achalasia	2
Complication of myotomy for motility disorder	1
Complication of intrathoracic esophagogastrostomy	1
Esophageal moniliasis with stricture	2
Barrett's esophagus with carcinoma in situ	2
Leak from esophagotomy	1
Carcinoma of the esophagus	1
Leiomyosarcoma of the esophagus	1

*From Gaissert, H.A., Mathisen, D.J., Grillo, H.C., et al.: Short segment intestinal interposition of the distal esophagus. J. Thorac. Cardiovasc. Surg., *106*:860, 1993, with permission.

proximal anastomosis is end to end. The distal anastomosis is end to side, most commonly to the posterior gastric wall. For short-segment interposition, anastomosis to the posterior gastric wall allows the colon to be positioned in a more direct, straight path than anastomosis to the anterior gastric wall. At least 12 cm of intra-abdominal length of colon is desirable to prevent reflux. A nasogastric tube through the colonic segment is used initially, and gastrostomy or jejunostomy is performed when indicated. The hiatus is carefully tacked to the colon to prevent herniation of abdominal contents. A drainage procedure is always done.

Table 24–7. Major Complications After Intestinal Interposition*

Complication	No. of Patients
Colon	
Pneumonia/ARDS	4†
Graft perforation	1
Colon perforation, subphrenic abscess	1
Chylothorax	1
Pulmonary edema	1
Pulmonary embolus	1
Deep vein thrombosis	1
Jejunum	
Pneumonia	3
Graft necrosis	1†
Gastric perforation	1
Paraparesis, aortoenteric erosion	1
Transient recurrent nerve injury	1
Myocardial infarction	1†

*From Gaissert, H.A., Mathisen, D.J., Grillo, H.C., et al.: Short segment intestinal interposition of the distal esophagus. J. Thorac. Cardiovasc. Surg., *106*:860, 1993, with permission.

†Cause of operative mortality.

ARDS, adult respiratory distress syndrome.

Results of Short-Segment Colon and Jejunal Interposition

Gaissert and associates published our results for jejunal (19 patients) and short-segment colon interposition (22 patients) of the distal esophagus.[7] Indications for intestinal interposition are listed in Table 24–6. Multiple prior operations were common in more than 75% of patients. Major complications occurred in 45% of patients (10 of 22) after colon interposition, and the hospital mortality rate was 4.5% (Table 24–7). Major complications following jejunal interposition occurred in 31% of patients, and the hospital mortality rate was 10.9%. Late functional results in 34 patients with a mean follow-up of 87 months were excellent in 26, fair in 5, and poor in 1.

Intestinal interposition is a technically demanding procedure and requires strict attention to the details of the operation to avoid catastrophic complications and ensure the greatest chance for success.

References

1. Adams, W.E., and Phemister, D.B.: Carcinoma of lower thoracic esophagus: Report of successful resection and esophagogastrostomy. J. Thorac. Surg., *7*:621, 1938.
2. Akiyama, H.: Surgery for carcinoma of the esophagus. Curr. Probl. Surg., *17*:56, 1980.
3. Belsey, R.: Reconstruction of the esophagus with left colon. J. Thorac. Cardiovasc. Surg., *49*:33, 1965.
4. Brain, R.H.F.: The place of jejunal transplantation in the treatment of simple strictures of the esophagus. Ann. R. Coll. Surg. Engl., *40*:100, 1967.
5. Czerny, V.: Neue Operationen. Zbl. Chir., *4*:443, 1877.
6. Earlam, R., and Cunha-Melo, J.R.: Oesophageal squamous cell carcinoma. I. A critical review of surgery. Br. J. Surg., *67*:381, 1980.
7. Gaissert, H.A., Mathisen, D.J., Grillo, H.C., et al.: Short segment intestinal interposition of the distal esophagus. J. Thorac. Cardiovasc. Surg., *106*:860, 1993.
8. Huang, G.J., Zhang, D.C., and Zhang, D.W.: A comparative study of resection of carcinoma of the esophagus with and without pyloroplasty. *In* DeMeester, T.R., and Skinner, D.B. (eds.): Esophageal Disorders: Pathophysiology and Therapy. New York, Raven Press, 1985, p. 383.
9. Jurkiewicz, M.J., and Paletta, C.E.L.: Free jejunal graft. *In* Current Therapy in Cardiothoracic Surgery. Philadelphia, B.C. Decker, 1989, p. 206.
10. Lewis, I.L.: The surgical treatment of carcinoma of the oesophagus. With special reference to a new operation for growths of the middle third. Br. J. Surg., *34*:18, 1946.
11. Mahoney, E.B., and Sherman, C.D., Jr.: Total esophagoplasty using intrathoracic right colon. Surgery, *35*:937, 1954.
12. Mathisen, D.J., Grillo, H.C., Wilkins, E.W., Jr., et al.: Transthoracic esophagectomy: A safe approach to carcinoma of the esophagus. Ann. Thorac. Surg., *45*:137, 1988.
13. Muller, J.M., Erasmi, H., Stelzner, M., et al.: Surgical therapy of oesophageal carcinoma. Br. J. Surg., *77*:845, 1990.
14. Ngan, S.Y.K., and Wong, J.: Lengths of different routes for oesophageal replacement. J. Thorac. Cardiovasc. Surg., *91*:790, 1986.
15. Ong, G.B.: The Kirschner operation—a forgotten procedure. Br. J. Surg., *60*:221, 1973.
16. Orringer, M.B., Marshall, B., and Stirling, M.C.: Transhiatal esophagectomy for benign and malignant disease. J. Thorac. Cardiovasc. Surg., *105*:265, 1993.
17. Orringer, M.B., and Orringer, J.S.: Esophagectomy without thoracotomy: A dangerous operation? J. Thorac. Cardiovasc. Surg., *85*:72, 1983.
18. Oshawa, T.: Surgery of the esophagus. Arch. Jap. Surg., *10*:605, 1933.

19. Payne, W.S., and Fisher, J.: Esophageal reconstruction: Free jejunal transfer or circulatory augmentation of pedicled interpositions using microvascular surgery. *In* Delarue, N.C., Wilkins, E.W., Jr., and Wong, J. (eds.): International Trends in General Thoracic Surgery, Vol. IV. Esophageal Cancer. St. Louis, C.V. Mosby, 1988.
20. Postlethwait, R.W.: Surgery of the Esophagus, 2nd ed. Norwalk, CT, Appleton-Century-Crofts, 1986, p. 505.
21. Ring, W.S., Varco, R.L., L'Heureux, P.R., et al.: Esophageal replacement with jejunum in children: An 18 to 33 year follow-up. J. Thorac. Cardiovasc. Surg., *83*:918, 1982.
22. Sonneland, J., Anson, B.J., and Beaton, L.E.: Surgical anatomy of the arterial supply to the colon from the superior mesenteric artery based upon a study of 600 specimens. Surg. Gynecol. Obstet., *106*:385, 1958.
23. Sweet, R.H.: Thoracic Surgery, 2nd ed. Philadelphia, W.B. Saunders, 1954, p. 309.
24. Sweet, R.H., and Churchill, E.D.: Transthoracic resection of tumors of the esophagus and stomach. Ann. Surg., *116*:566, 1942.
25. Torek, F.: The first successful case of resection of the thoracic portion of the esophagus for carcinoma. Surg. Gynecol. Obstet., *16*:614, 1913.
26. Wain, J.C.: Long segment colon interposition. Semin. Thorac. Cardiovasc. Surg. *4*:336, 1992.
27. Wilkins, E.W., Jr.: Esophageal anastomotic techniques: The esophagogastric anastomosis. *In* Wu, Y., and Peters, R. (eds.): International Practice in Cardiothoracic Surgery. Beijing, Science Press, 1985, p. 590.

CHAPTER

25 Transhiatal Esophagectomy Without Thoracotomy

MARK B. ORRINGER

Since the earliest reports of successful transthoracic esophagectomy and intrathoracic esophagogastric anastomosis for carcinoma,[1,9,64,70] this operation has become the most common surgical procedure for resectable malignancies of the esophagus. Dramatic improvements have been made in preoperative evaluation, nutritional support, anesthetic and operative techniques, and postoperative care, yet the physiologic insult of esophageal resection and reconstruction in patients with compromised nutritional and pulmonary status secondary to impaired swallowing remains great. Combined thoracoabdominal operations in debilitated patients result in postoperative respiratory embarrassment; a frequent need for prolonged mechanical ventilatory assistance; and a significant incidence of postoperative atelectasis, pneumonia, and respiratory insufficiency. Disruption of an intrathoracic esophagogastric anastomosis with resultant mediastinitis and sepsis remains among the most disastrous complications of esophageal surgery. Thus, respiratory insufficiency and mediastinitis due to anastomotic leak have been the leading causes of postoperative morbidity and mortality in most major reported series of esophageal resection and reconstruction and have been responsible for operative mortality figures that historically have ranged from 15 to 40%[27,38,92] and averaged 33%.[26] Although a few outstanding modern surgical series have reported operative mortality rates of less than 5%, in most contemporary reports published between 1980 and 1988,[4,28,66] the mean hospital mortality rate for esophageal resection for carcinoma is still 13%.[69] There is little question that esophageal resection and reconstruction remain among the most formidable of thoracic surgical procedures.

Against this backdrop of years of experience with transthoracic esophagectomy, transhiatal esophagectomy without thoracotomy has emerged as an alternative operative approach that, when appropriately applied, may be associated with substantially less risk and morbidity.[22,46,84,86,108,110,114] Not only does transhiatal esophagectomy avoid the morbidity of a thoracotomy in these patients, but also the routine cervical esophageal anastomosis that is performed almost eliminates mediastinitis resulting from anastomotic disruption as a cause of postoperative death. Further, the abdominal approach used for esophagectomy in these patients provides access to all portions of the gastrointestinal tract used for esophageal substitution, giving the surgeon the option of utilizing the stomach or any portion of the colon that might be needed for esophageal replacement.

HISTORY

Denk performed the first reported blunt transmediastinal esophagectomy without thoracotomy in 1913 in cadavers and experimental animals using a vein stripper to avulse the esophagus from the posterior mediastinum.[23] Turner, the British surgeon, carried out the first successful transhiatal blunt esophagectomy for carcinoma in 1933 and re-established continuity of the alimentary tract using an antethoracic skin tube at a second operation.[113] The advent of endotracheal anesthesia permitted transthoracic esophagectomy under direct vision, and transhiatal esophagectomy without thoracotomy became a seldom-used approach, finding occasional use as a concomitant procedure with laryngopharyngectomy for pharyngeal or cervical esophageal carcinomas when the stomach was used to restore continuity of the alimentary tract. Ong and Lee in 1960 and LeQuesne and Ranger in 1966 reported the first successful primary pharyngogastric anastomoses after laryngopharyngectomy and thoracic esophagectomy.[59,71] In these cases, and in the report by Akiyama and associates,[3] blunt resection of the *normal* thoracic esophagus was carried out. Kirk used this approach for palliation of incurable esophageal carcinoma in five patients.[54] Thomas and Dedo treated four patients with severe chronic pharyngoesophageal caustic strictures by blunt thoracic esophagectomy without thoracotomy, mobilization of the stomach through the posterior mediastinum, and pharyngogastric anastomosis.[109]

In 1975, Orringer and Sloan proposed the technique of substernal gastric bypass of the excluded thoracic esophagus as a method of palliation of incurable esophageal carcinomas, both those that were invading contiguous major structures, such as the trachea or aorta, and those that had metastasized to either cervical or abdominal lymph nodes.[85] This procedure was envisioned as a "simple" bypass to relieve dysphagia without the potential postoperative morbidity of a thoracotomy and intrathoracic esophageal anastomosis (Figs. 25-1 through 25-4). Unfortunately, further experience with this operation failed to substantiate its value as a worthwhile palliative procedure achievable with minimal morbidity.[72] The two major complications of this procedure were cervical anas-

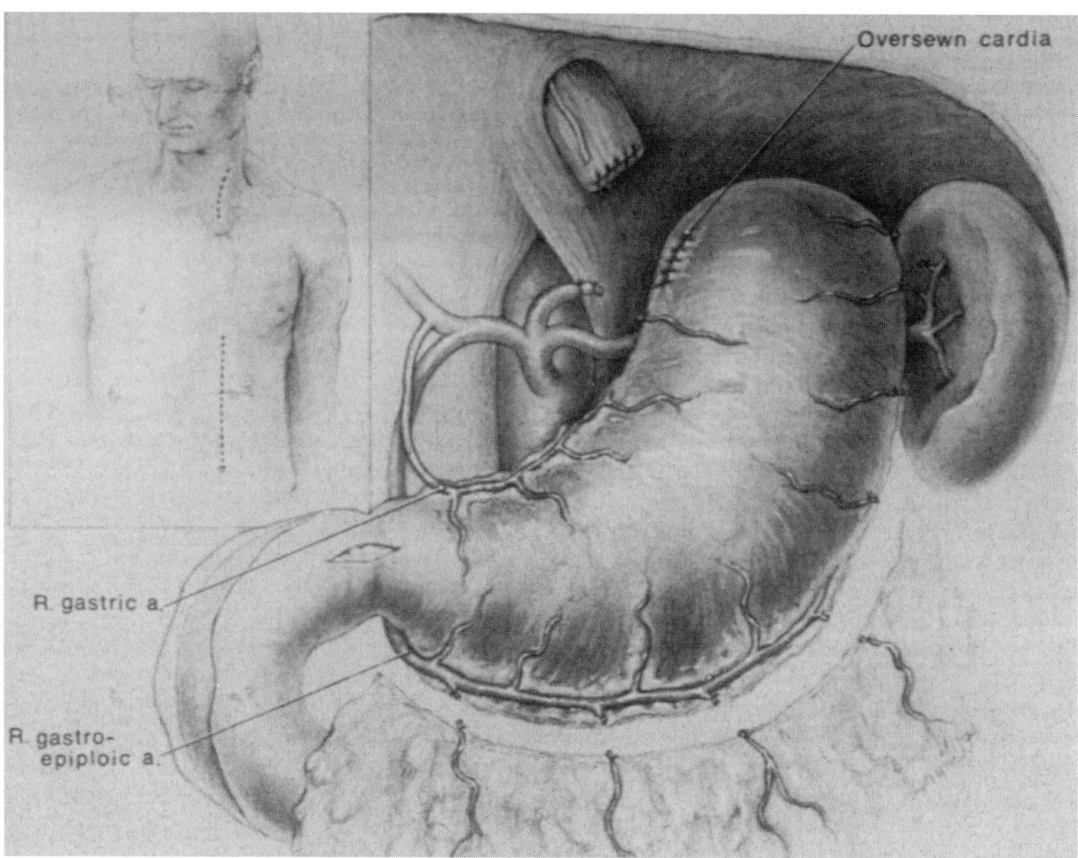

Figure 25–1. Routine mobilization of the stomach for esophageal replacement either in the substernal or posterior mediastinal position. The left gastric artery and left gastroepiploic vessels are divided, whereas the right gastric and right gastroepiploic arteries are preserved. A pyloromyotomy and generous Kocher maneuver are routine. The divided stapled cardia is always oversewn to reinforce the staple suture line. *Inset* shows the left cervical incision and the upper midline abdominal incision used both for substernal gastric interposition and for transhiatal esophagectomy and esophageal replacement with stomach in the posterior mediastinum. (From Orringer, M.B., and Sloan, H.: Substernal gastric bypass of the excluded thoracic esophagus for palliation of esophageal carcinoma. J. Thorac. Cardiovasc. Surg., *70*:836, 1975, with permission.)

tomotic leak and disruption of the excluded thoracic esophagus, particularly at the distal suture line. In 37 patients so treated, there were nine hospital deaths (24%), seven with anastomotic leak (19%) and six with disruption of the divided distal esophagus (17%). Major postoperative complications occurred in 59% of these patients. Only 15 (54%) of the 28 survivors left the hospital able to swallow within 3 weeks of operation, and 10 (36%) required hospitalization for 1 month or longer after operation. In those who survived the operation and left the hospital alive, the average length of survival was only 5.9 months. In only 7 patients (25% of the survivors) was good palliation achieved with the bypass operation. Generalized weakness and progressive cachexia in the remainder prevented adequate oral intake and necessitated tube feeding with diet supplements. It was concluded that substernal gastric bypass of the excluded thoracic esophagus is simply too drastic an operation for patients with unresectable esophageal cancer and a limited life expectancy of only several months. In the occasional vigorous patient with an unresectable esophageal carcinoma, substernal gastric bypass may be worthwhile, but the divided distal esophagus should be decompressed into a loop of jejunum as originally proposed by Kirschner[55] and more recently by others.[2,119]

Although the goal of substernal gastric bypass of the excluded thoracic esophagus was not realized, several important lessons were learned from this experience. First, with proper mobilization, the normal North American Caucasian stomach *always* reaches above the level of the clavicles for a cervical esophagogastric anastomosis. Second, the acute consequences of a cervical esophagogastric anastomotic leak, essentially a salivary fistula, are generally less severe than those associated with an intrathoracic anastomotic esophageal leak and mediastinitis. Third, owing to the anterior angulation at the thoracic inlet, subsequent esophagoscopy and dilation are much more hazardous and difficult after a substernal gastric interposition than is the case when the esophageal substitute is positioned in the posterior mediastinum in the original esophageal bed. On the basis of this experience, we adopted a routine policy of avoiding an intrathoracic esophagogastric anastomosis whenever possible. Regardless of the level of the esophageal pathologic lesions, the entire thoracic esophagus was resected, and a cervical esophageal anastomosis was performed. Although this necessitated three incisions (cervical, thoracic, and abdominal) in our patients with esophageal carcinoma, death from anastomotic disruption following esophagectomy almost disappeared.

In 1974, I performed an unplanned and my first transhiatal esophagectomy. In the process of mobilizing

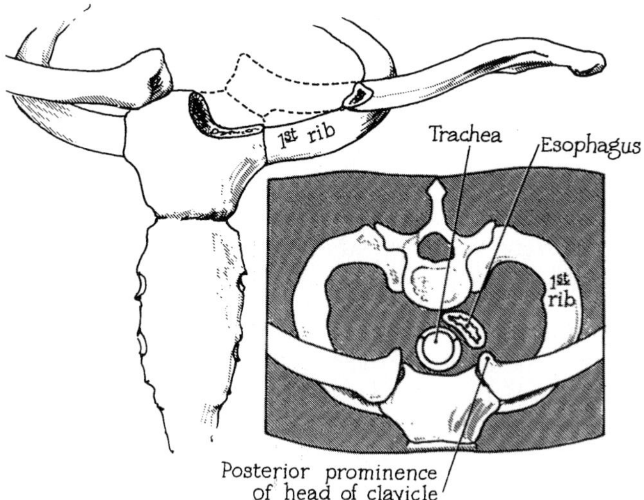

Figure 25–2. Enlarging the anterior opening into the superior mediastinum for esophageal bypass or replacement using the retrosternal route. *Inset* shows normal position of the cervical esophagus at the thoracic inlet, posterior and to the left of the trachea. When performing an anastomosis between the cervical esophagus and a retrosternal visceral esophageal substitute (either stomach or colon), compression of the graft by the posterior prominence of the head of the clavicle may occur. Thus, the medial clavicle and adjacent manubrium, and often the medial first rib as well, are routinely resected when using the *anterior* mediastinal route to allow more room for the transposed stomach (or colon) at the anterior thoracic inlet. (From Orringer, M.B., and Sloan, H.: Substernal gastric bypass of the excluded thoracic esophagus for palliation of esophageal carcinoma. J. Thorac. Cardiovasc. Surg., *70*:836, 1975, with permission.)

the stomach through the abdomen in an obese patient with a large sliding hiatal hernia and a small distal third esophageal adenocarcinoma in preparation for a standard transthoracic esophageal resection and esophageal reconstruction, I mobilized nearly 4 inches of esophagus out of the posterior mediastinum and into the abdomen through the diaphragmatic hiatus. I knew from experience with mediastinoscopy performed to evaluate patients with carcinoma of the lung that the index finger could reach through a cervical incision into the mediastinum to the level of the carina. Therefore, in this particular obese patient, who was regarded as a high risk for a thoracic procedure, I made a cervical incision and, with one hand in the abdomen inserted through the diaphragmatic hiatus into the posterior mediastinum and the other placed in the superior mediastinum through the cervical incision, carried out a "blunt" esophageal mobilization. After removing the esophagus, the mobilized stomach was positioned in the posterior mediastinum in the original esophageal bed, and a cervical esophagogastric anastomosis was performed. The surprisingly successful outcome in this patient was my initial experience with transhiatal esophagectomy without thoracotomy and was the basis for our subsequent 1978 report of the procedure in 28 patients, 4 of whom had benign disease of the intrathoracic esophagus and 22 of whom had carcinomas involving various levels of the esophagus.[86] Since then, our personal experience with more than 1200 patients undergoing transhiatal esophagectomy without thoracotomy[73,74,81,83] as well as reports by others,[9-11,21,22,35,47,100,104,105,107,108,112] have justified our current belief that few patients needing esophageal resection for either benign or malignant disease require a thoracotomy. This chapter describes the technical aspects of transhiatal esophagectomy, its indications and contraindications, and the results achieved to date.

Much has been learned about the cervical esophagogastric anastomosis (CEGA) since the 1980s. Our initial premise that the acute complications of a CEGA leak are less common than those of an intrathoracic anastomotic leak has been validated, for a CEGA is seldom associated with mediastinitis. Further, 98% of CEGA leaks are managed successfully with local wound care, which includes early institution of dilatation therapy,[80] and less than 2% are associated with disastrous complications such as gastric tip necrosis, cervical vertebral osteomyelitis, epidural abscess, tracheogastroesophageal anastomotic fistula, and so forth.[51] Unfortunately, the long-term sequelae of a CEGA leak have not been as minor as initially postulated because nearly half of CEGA leaks result in an anastomotic stricture as healing progresses. The need for lifelong esophageal dilatation therapy negates the merits of an operation intended to relieve dysphagia.

The most recent advance in the technical refinements of transhiatal esophagectomy and a CEGA has been the development of a side-to-side stapled anastomosis using

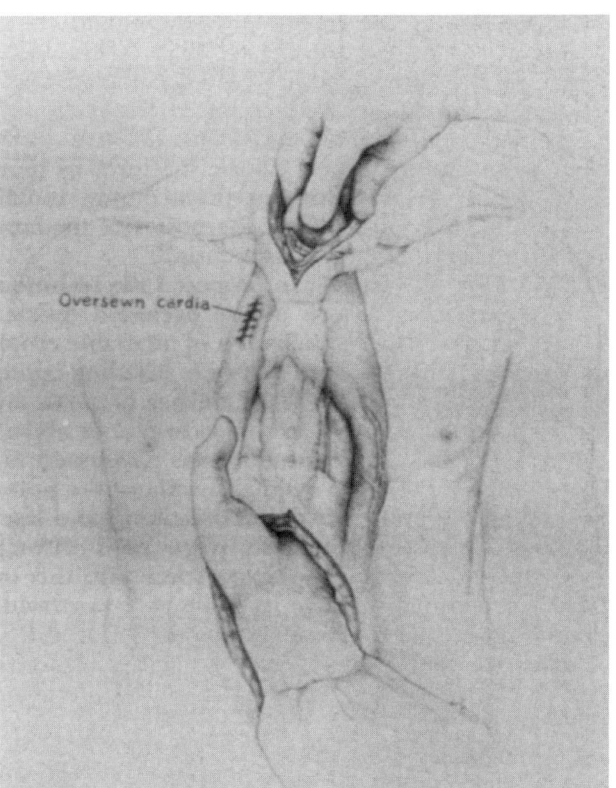

Figure 25–3. Positioning the mobilized stomach in the anterior mediastinum for substernal gastric bypass. The gastric fundus, not the divided cardia, reaches most superiorly, several centimeters above the level of the clavicles, for the esophagogastric anastomosis. The anterior opening into the superior mediastinum has been widened by resection of the clavicle and medial manubrium of the sternum. (From Orringer, M.B., and Sloan, H.: Substernal gastric bypass of the excluded thoracic esophagus for palliation of esophageal carcinoma. J. Thorac. Cardiovasc. Surg., *70*:836, 1975, with permission.)

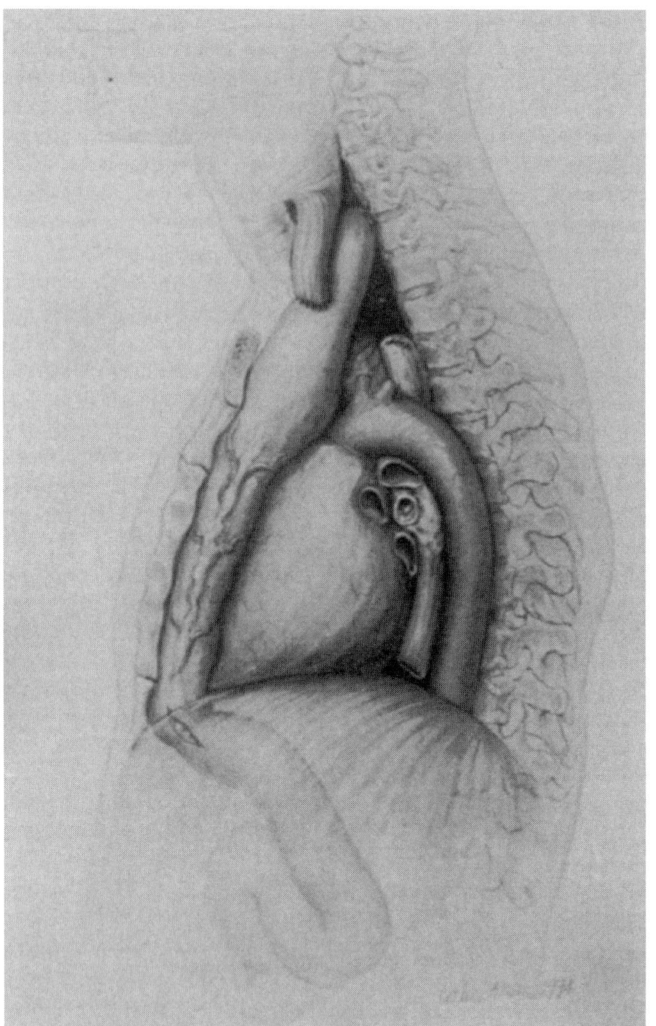

Figure 25–4. Lateral view showing final position of the retrosternal stomach and the excluded thoracic esophagus in the posterior mediastinum. The gastric fundus has been suspended from the prevertebral fascia; the anastomosis has been performed on the anterior wall of the stomach; and the esophagus, with its unresectable tumor, is excluded in the posterior mediastinum. (From Orringer, M.B., and Sloan, H.: Substernal gastric bypass of the excluded thoracic esophagus for palliation of esophageal carcinoma. J. Thorac. Cardiovasc. Surg., *70*:836, 1975, with permission.)

the Auto-Suture Endo-GIA 30-3.5 stapler applied directly through the cervical wound.[82] With this technique, the cervical esophagogastric anastomotic leak rate has decreased dramatically from the average of 10 to 15% to less than 3%, the need for postoperative anastomotic dilatations has decreased, and patient satisfaction with swallowing has improved.

INDICATIONS AND CONTRAINDICATIONS

Every patient requiring an esophagectomy for either benign or malignant disease is regarded as a potential candidate for transhiatal esophagectomy without thoracotomy. In patients with upper or middle thoracic esophageal carcinomas, bronchoscopic evidence of tracheobronchial *invasion* (not contiguity) is an absolute contraindication to transhiatal esophagectomy. In patients with cervicothoracic esophageal tumor involving the larynx or upper trachea, at least a 5-cm length of trachea above the carina is optimal for construction of an anterior mediastinal tracheostomy. (See later discussion of carcinomas involving the cervicothoracic esophagus.) Therefore, precise measurement of the distance between the distal margin of the tumor and the carina at esophagoscopy is important in assessing the resectability of these tumors.

Patients with thoracic esophageal carcinomas and *biopsy-proven* hepatic, supraclavicular lymph node, or distant metastatic disease have so short a life expectancy that we do not regard them as candidates for esophagectomy. We require a tissue diagnosis of distant metastatic disease before deeming an esophageal carcinoma unresectable. Although the computed tomographic (CT) scan provides unequaled radiographic assessment of the mediastinum, in our experience, this diagnostic modality is *not* a reliable indicator of *resectability* of esophageal carcinoma.[93] The CT scan may demonstrate *contiguity* of the esophageal tumor with the aorta or the prevertebral fascia, but this is *not* synonymous with invasion.

Although the CT scan is helpful in evaluating for metastatic disease, it has limited ability to accurately assess depth of tumor invasion or regional lymph node status. Esophageal endoscopic ultrasonography (EUS) has emerged as a more precise means for estimating the depth of tumor invasion and has proved more accurate than CT in identifying metastases to regional lymph nodes.[16,42,111,116,120] Reed and associates have demonstrated the efficacy of the combination of EUS and fine-needle aspiration biopsy in confirming celiac lymph node metastases in patients with esophageal carcinoma.[94]

Although general clinical assessment, including a barium swallow examination, endoscopy and a CT scan of the chest and upper abdomen, has allowed us to determine resectability of most esophageal cancers we have treated with a transhiatal esophagectomy since the 1980s, better documentation of distant metastatic disease that precludes resection may certainly be possible with the previously mentioned tests. Similarly, even though we have not used them on a routine basis, promising results with positron emission tomography (PET)[12,63] as well as minimally invasive thoracoscopic and laparoscopic staging of esophageal cancer have been reported.[56,62]

Transhiatal esophagectomy for benign disease of the esophagus has been possible even in patients who have undergone radiation therapy or who have periesophagitis associated with caustic injuries or prior operations, or megaesophagus of achalasia.[75,81,89] Obviously, a history of prior esophageal surgery, particularly a long esophagomyotomy or a resection of a midesophageal diverticulum, should alert the surgeon to the possibility of significant intrathoracic periesophageal adhesions. When undertaking a transhiatal esophagectomy for either benign or malignant disease, the surgeon *must* be prepared to open the thorax to resect the esophagus if local tumor invasion or periesophageal attachments prevent a safe transhiatal resection or if untoward intraoperative bleeding occurs. The most important contraindication to transhiatal esophagectomy is the surgeon's assessment on manual palpation of the esophagus through the diaphragmatic hiatus that mediastinal fixation of the esophagus due to either tumor or adhesions precludes a safe transhiatal resection.

PREOPERATIVE PREPARATION

Aggressive preoperative pulmonary physiotherapy is consistently rewarded by fewer postoperative pulmonary complications. Complete abstinence from cigarette smoking for at least 2 weeks before operation is insisted upon in all of our patients. Regular use of an incentive spirometer is begun and maintained on an outpatient basis at least 2 weeks before surgery. When possible, patients are encouraged to walk one to two miles a day to condition themselves for early postoperative ambulation. When weight loss is marked and the esophageal obstruction is high grade, a nasogastric feeding tube is inserted through the tumor and into the stomach to allow administration of 2,000 to 3,000 cal/day. Use of a percutaneous gastrostomy or jejunostomy feeding tube is avoided because these interfere with subsequent gastric mobilization. The patient and his or her family play an active role in preparation for surgery, and hospitalization is seldom required to maintain satisfactory caloric intake through the nasogastric feeding tube. Intravenous parental nutrition is seldom utilized in our patients. Because oral hygiene is often neglected in patients with esophageal carcinoma, and the presence of carious teeth and their associated pathogenic oral flora may adversely affect the outcome of an anastomotic leak, the patient's mouth is carefully examined preoperatively, and dental consultation for the repair or removal of carious teeth is obtained. In patients with a history of previous gastric disease or surgery resulting either in gastric scarring or size limitation that may preclude the use of the entire stomach as an esophageal substitute, a barium enema is performed to evaluate the suitability of the colon as an esophageal replacement. The colon is then prepared in the event that colonic interposition is required for esophageal replacement. A colonic bowel prep in transhiatal esophagectomy patients is not routine, however, because in patients with a normal stomach, the gastric fundus readily reaches above the level of the clavicles to allow a cervical anastomosis.

The patient with esophageal obstruction is invariably dehydrated. Before the need for concern with acquired immunodeficiency syndrome (AIDS), in order to minimize intraoperative vascular instability, we routinely transfused our patients with 1 pint of blood for every 10 lb of weight loss experienced preoperatively. This practice is of course no longer acceptable. In fact, more than 99% of our patients undergoing transhiatal esophagectomy are admitted to the hospital the day of scheduled surgery. However, because preoperative outpatient tube feedings as required or mandated increased oral intake of fluids have resulted in a better hydration status, intraoperative intravenous rehydration is far less of a problem. Perioperative blood transfusions are now the exception rather than the rule, and we are more tolerant of anemia in these patients postoperatively.

ANESTHETIC MANAGEMENT

Cardiac displacement by the surgeon's hand in the posterior mediastinum during transhiatal esophagectomy may produce hypotension. Therefore, intra-arterial blood pressure is monitored continuously intraoperatively with a radial artery catheter. This catheter is sutured in place and protected by padding because the patient's arms are kept at his or her sides during the operation to allow the surgeon and assistants access to the neck, chest, and abdomen without the inconvenience of negotiating arm boards. Two large-bore peripheral intravenous catheters are inserted to permit rapid volume replacement if required, although intraoperative blood loss generally averages less than 1,000 ml. We have not found it necessary to monitor central venous pressure routinely, but if it is required, it should be done through a right neck vein, away from the operative field on the left neck. Placement of a thoracic epidural catheter preoperatively has become routine. Epidural anesthesia not only minimizes the need for intraoperative inhalation anesthetic agents (thereby facilitating early removal of the endotracheal tube) but also greatly improves postoperative pulmonary hygiene by providing improved pain control.

An *unshortened* standard endotracheal tube is generally used so that if a membranous tracheal tear occurs during the transhiatal dissection, the endotracheal tube can be advanced into the distal trachea or left main-stem bronchus, placing the balloon beyond the tear and permitting direct repair. It should be recognized by both the anesthetist and the surgeon that patients who have tumors in the upper or middle third of the esophagus or who have a history of a long esophagomyotomy or resection of a mid esophageal diverticulum may require a thoracotomy to mobilize the esophagus. One option is to utilize a double-lumen endotracheal tube in these cases and, if necessary, carry out a right anterolateral thoracotomy, and deflate the right lung, allowing access to the posterior mediastinum for an esophagectomy under direct vision. However, the exposure of esophagus through an anterolateral thoracotomy is not optimal. Therefore, if the surgeon finds it necessary to convert to a transthoracic esophagectomy intraoperatively, I prefer to reposition and redrape the patient for a true right posterolateral thoracotomy, if need be, advancing the endotracheal tube into the left main-stem bronchus for institution of single-lung anesthesia. A double-lumen endotracheal tube is seldom needed in patients undergoing transhiatal esophagectomy. Inhalation anesthetic agents are discontinued, and inspired oxygen concentration is increased as the actual transhiatal dissection is performed to minimize the adverse effects of transient hypotension, which is not uncommon during the esophagectomy. The operation requires close cooperation between the anesthetist and the surgeon to minimize prolonged hypotension. Manual contact with the pericardium during the transhiatal dissection may induce artifactual electrocardiographic (ECG) changes that simulate ventricular arrhythmia but subside the moment the hand is removed from the posterior mediastinum. Cause for alarm here is more perceived than real. The endotracheal tube is typically removed at the end of the operation, epidural anesthesia having largely eliminated the need for mechanical ventilatory assistance after transhiatal esophagectomy.

OPERATIVE TECHNIQUE

The patient is placed in the supine position with a small folded sheet tucked beneath the scapulae to extend the neck. The head is turned toward the right and stabilized with a head ring beneath the occiput. The skin is prepared and draped from the mandibles to the pubis and anterior to both mid axillary lines. The arms are carefully padded, protecting the intravenous and arterial catheters, and are placed at the patient's side. When there is concern that a transthoracic esophagectomy may be required (e.g., in patients with upper- or middle-third esophageal tumors or those undergoing reoperation after a previous esophagomyotomy), the right side may be "bumped up" on a folded blanket, the right arm bent at the elbow, and the right hand placed in the small of the back. This position allows access for a right anterolateral thoracotomy should it be required. The operating table can then be rolled toward the right so that the abdomen is again parallel to the floor, and the abdomen can be approached through the usual upper midline incision. As indicated previously, however, I prefer the supine position for all patients undergoing transhiatal esophagectomy. Use of a table-mounted, self-retaining (upper hand) retractor greatly facilitates exposure. Transhiatal esophagectomy has three separate phases: abdominal, cervical, and mediastinal.

Abdominal Phase

The abdomen is entered through a midline supraumbilical incision (see Fig. 25-1, *inset*). After dividing the triangular ligament of the liver, the left hepatic lobe is retracted to the right. The stomach is examined carefully to be certain that there is no gastric scarring resulting from prior operations or disease that precludes its use as an esophageal substitute. The right gastroepiploic artery is identified early in the operation and is protected thereafter. This is particularly important in patients who have undergone prior abdominal surgery because the need to divide adhesions may jeopardize the gastric blood supply. Adhesions between the spleen and adjacent omentum are divided early to prevent splenic capsular tears.

Mobilization of the greater omentum from the stomach begins along the mid greater curvature, where the greater omentum is incised at an avascular point at which the right gastroepiploic artery terminates as it enters the stomach or anastomoses with small branches of the left gastroepiploic artery. The omentum is separated from the right gastroepiploic artery at least 1.5 to 2 cm inferior to the vessel to minimize the chance of injury to this artery. The left gastroepiploic and short gastric vessels are divided and ligated along the high greater curvature of the stomach, avoiding both injury to the spleen and gastric necrosis due to ligation of these vessels too near the gastric wall. Distally, the greater omentum is separated from the stomach to the level of the pylorus and the origin of the right gastroepiploic artery from the gastroduodenal.

After the greater curvature of the stomach has been mobilized, the peritoneum overlying the esophageal hiatus is incised and the esophagogastric junction encircled with a 1-inch rubber drain. Proceeding downward along the lesser curvature of the stomach, the gastrohepatic omentum along the high lesser curvature of the stomach is incised, and the left gastric artery is isolated, ligated, and divided. When the patient has carcinoma, celiac axis lymph nodes are resected and submitted to the pathologists for staging purposes. When possible, the left gastric artery is divided near its origin from the celiac axis. If there is a large celiac axis lymph node mass secondary to metastatic disease, cure is not possible, and unless resection of these lymph nodes is relatively easy, they should only be biopsied and not totally excised to lessen the risk for hemorrhage. The right gastric artery is protected as the remainder of the gastrohepatic omentum is divided inferiorly along the lesser curvature.

After the gastric mobilization has been completed, a generous Kocher maneuver is carried out until there is sufficient mobility of the duodenum to allow the pylorus to be displaced from its usual position in the right upper quadrant of the abdomen to the level of the xiphoid process in the midline. A pyloromyotomy is performed routinely because delayed gastric emptying is possible after the vagotomy that accompanies esophagectomy. The pyloromyotomy begins as a 1.5-cm incision through gastric muscle, which is then carried through the pylorus and then onto the duodenum for 0.5 to 1 cm (see Fig. 25-1). This procedure is carried out using the cutting current of a needle-tipped electrocautery and a fine-tipped vascular mosquito clamp to dissect the gastric and duodenal muscle away from the underlying submucosa. Silver clip markers are placed at the level of the pyloromyotomy to allow future radiographic assessment of gastric emptying.

As in the routine repair of a transabdominal hiatal hernia or a standard Ivor Lewis esophagogastrectomy, the distal 5 to 10 cm of esophagus is mobilized into the abdomen from the mediastinum by retracting the esophagogastric junction downward by its encircling rubber drain while dissecting upward into the mediastinum with the opposite hand (Fig. 25-5). The mobility of the esophagus within the posterior mediastinum is assessed at this time. In patients with esophageal tumors, the tumor is grasped and "rocked" from side to side to ascertain that the esophagus is not fixed to the prevertebral fascia, the aorta, or the adjacent mediastinal structures. Narrow Deaver retractors inserted into the diaphragmatic hiatus facilitate direct exposure and dissection of the lower half of the esophagus from the posterior mediastinum. Right-angle clamps, 13 inches long, are used to clamp and permit division and ligation of periesophageal tissues under direct vision virtually to the level of the carina. The mediastinal dissection is now temporarily discontinued. A No. 14 French rubber jejunostomy feeding tube is inserted 4 to 6 inches beyond the ligament of Treitz and secured in place using a Weitzel maneuver.[36] The jejunos-

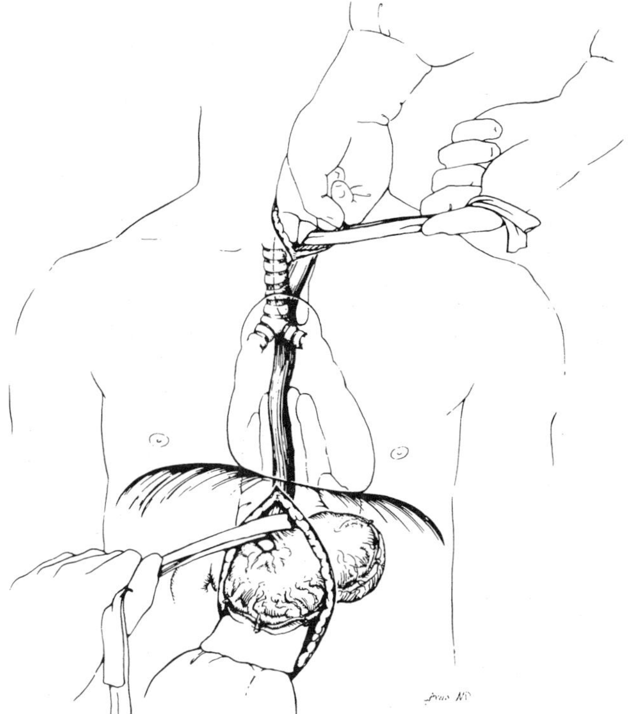

Figure 25–5. Transhiatal mobilization of the upper and lower esophagus from the posterior mediastinum is facilitated by traction on rubber drains placed around the esophagogastric junction and the cervical esophagus. The volar aspects of the fingers are kept against the esophagus to reduce the chance of injury to adjacent structures. (From Orringer, M.B.: Surgical options for esophageal resection and reconstruction with stomach. *In* Baue, A.E., Geha, A.S., Hammond, G.L., et al. [eds.]: Glenn's Thoracic and Cardiovascular Surgery, 6th ed. Stamford, CT, Appleton & Lange, 1996, p. 899, with permission.)

tomy is not brought out through the abdominal wall until the transmediastinal esophagectomy has been completed.

Cervical Phase

The cervical esophagus is mobilized through an oblique incision that parallels the anterior border of the left sternocleidomastoid muscle and extends from the suprasternal notch to the level of the cricoid cartilage (about 5 to 7 cm in length). The platysma and omohyoid fascial layer are incised, the sternocleidomastoid muscle and carotid sheath and its contents are retracted laterally, and the larynx and trachea are retracted medially. *No retractor* other than the surgeon's finger should be placed against the recurrent laryngeal nerve in the tracheoesophageal groove during the entire cervical portion of this operation. The middle thyroid vein is usually ligated and divided. The inferior thyroid artery may be ligated and divided as well.

The dissection is carried posteriorly directly to the prevertebral fascia, which is followed by blunt finger dissection into the superior mediastinum. The tracheoesophageal groove is developed by sharp dissection along the anterolateral surface of the esophagus, remaining posterior to the recurrent laryngeal nerve to prevent injury to it. The cervical esophagus is encircled with a 1-inch rubber drain, which is retracted superiorly as blunt dissection of the upper thoracic esophagus from the superior mediastinum is carried out (see Fig. 25–5). The volar aspects of the fingers are kept against the esophagus in the midline, and care is taken not to tear the posterior membranous trachea. Using this technique, the upper thoracic esophagus is mobilized almost to the level of the carina through the neck incision.

Mediastinal (Transhiatal) Dissection

Transhiatal esophagectomy is carried out in an orderly, sequential manner and is not simply a random wrenching of the esophagus from the posterior mediastinum. If on initial assessment of the esophagus through the diaphragmatic hiatus it is believed that the esophagus is mobile enough to be resected transhiatally, the surgeon inserts one hand through the diaphragmatic hiatus posterior to the esophagus as the other, inserted through the neck incision along the prevertebral fascia, proceeds downward. A half-sponge on a stick is inserted into the superior mediastinum through the cervical incision along the prevertebral fascia to facilitate this dissection (Fig. 25–6). The posterior esophageal dissection is thus carried out by sweeping the esophagus away from the prevertebral fascia from above until the sponge stick makes contact with the hand inserted through the diaphragmatic hiatus. Intra-arterial blood pressure is monitored continually throughout the intrathoracic esophageal dissection to avoid prolonged hypotension. Blood is evacuated from the posterior mediastinum by means of a No. 28 French Argyle Saratoga sump catheter inserted from the cervical incision downward into the mediastinum.

After the posterior mediastinal dissection has been completed, the anterior esophageal dissection is performed. The Penrose drain encircling the esophagogastric junction is retracted inferiorly as the surgeon's hand is inserted palm downward against the anterior esophagus and advanced into the mediastinum (Fig. 25–7). The esophagus is progressively mobilized away from the posterior aspect of the pericardium and the carina. Working simultaneously through the abdominal and cervical incisions along the anterior surface of the esophagus, the surgeon avulses the typically filmy attachments to the posterior trachea (Fig. 25–8). When the anterior and posterior esophageal dissections are complete, the remaining lateral esophageal attachments must be divided. The cervical esophagus is again retracted superiorly by its encircling Penrose drain, and the lateral esophageal attachments are gently dissected away from the esophagus as it is delivered into the neck wound. In this manner, about 5 to 8 cm of upper thoracic esophagus is mobilized circumferentially. One hand inserted through the diaphragmatic hiatus anterior to the esophagus is advanced into the superior mediastinum behind the trachea until the completely circumferentially mobilized upper esophagus and its intact lateral attachments are palpated (Fig. 25–9). The esophagus is thus "trapped" against the prevertebral fascia between the index and middle fingers, and a downward raking motion of the hand avulses the remaining periesophageal attachments (Fig. 25–10). At

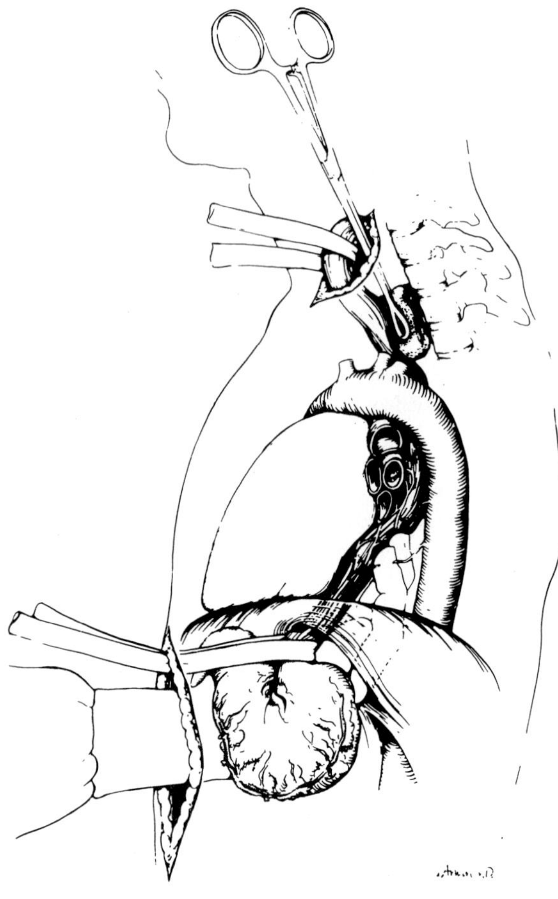

Figure 25–6. Transhiatal mobilization of the esophagus away from the prevertebral fascia is facilitated using a half-sponge on a stick inserted through the cervical incision and advanced until it makes contact with the hand inserted from below through the diaphragmatic hiatus. (From Orringer, M.B.: Surgical options for esophageal resection and reconstruction with stomach. *In* Baue, A.E., Geha, A.S., Hammond, G.L., et al. [eds.]: Glenn's Thoracic and Cardiovascular Surgery, 6th ed. Stamford, CT, Appleton & Lange, 1996, p. 899, with permission.)

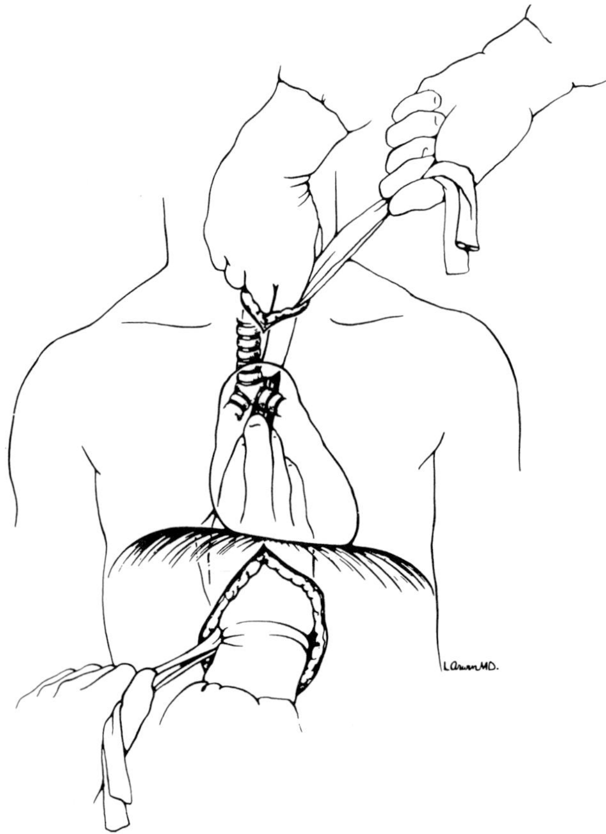

Figure 25–7. Anterior transhiatal esophageal mobilization carried out as a mirror-image of the posterior dissection, keeping the volar aspects of the fingers against the esophagus, particularly near the posterior membranous trachea and left mainstem bronchus. (From Orringer, M.B.: Surgical options for esophageal resection and reconstruction with stomach. *In* Baue, A.E., Geha, A.S., Hammond, G.L., et al. [eds.]: Glenn's Thoracic and Cardiovascular Surgery, 6th ed. Stamford, CT, Appleton & Lange, 1996, p. 899, with permission.)

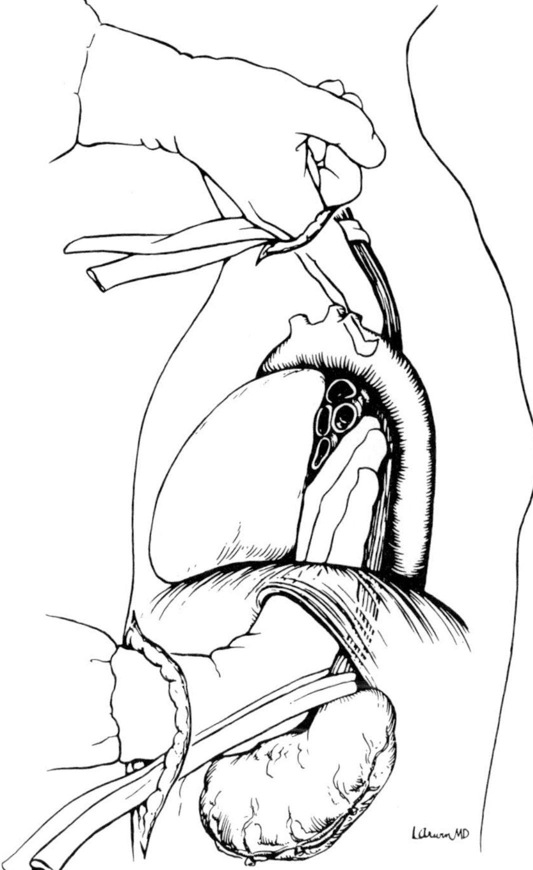

Figure 25–8. As the anterior esophageal dissection is performed, constant pressure should be exerted posteriorly against the esophagus to minimize the hemodynamic effects of cardiac displacement. (From Orringer, M.B.: Surgical options for esophageal resection and reconstruction with stomach. *In* Baue, A.E., Geha, A.S., Hammond, G.L., et al. [eds.]: Glenn's Thoracic and Cardiovascular Surgery, 6th ed. Stamford, CT, Appleton & Lange, 1996, p. 899, with permission.)

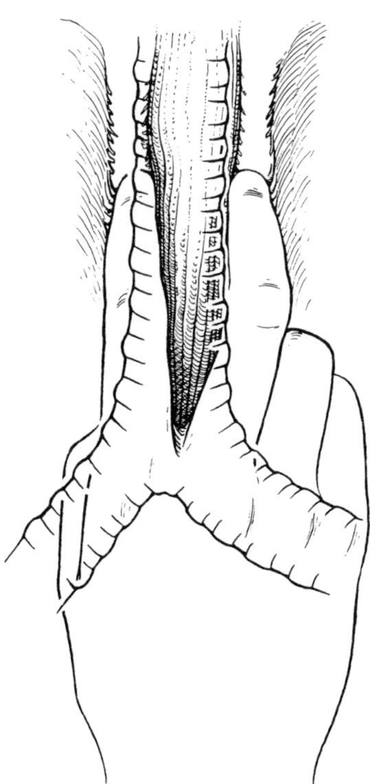

Figure 25–9. The right hand inserted through the diaphragmatic hiatus is advanced upward into the superior mediastinum until the undivided lateral esophageal attachments are felt. (From Orringer, M.B.: Transhiatal blunt esophagectomy without thoracotomy. *In* Cohn, L.H. [ed.]: Modern Technics in Surgery, Vol. 62. Cardiovascular Surgery. New York, Futura Publishing, 1983, p. 1, with permission.)

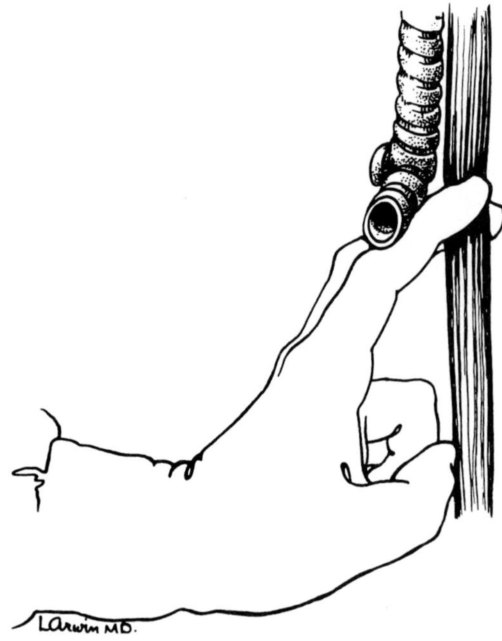

Figure 25–10. With the esophagus trapped between the index and middle fingers against the prevertebral fascia, a downward raking motion of the hand avulses the lateral periesophageal attachments. (From Orringer, M.B.: Transhiatal blunt esophagectomy without thoracotomy. *In* Cohn, L.H. [ed.]: Modern Technics in Surgery, Vol. 62. Cardiovascular Surgery. New York, Futura Publishing, 1983, p. 1, with permission.)

times, periesophageal adhesions or fibrosis impedes mobilization of the entire intrathoracic esophagus by restricting a 1- to 2-cm segment in the subcarinal or subaortic area. It may be necessary to compress this tissue firmly between the index finger and thumb, thus fracturing it. Alternatively, as originally described by Waddell and Scannell,[117] access to the upper thoracic esophagus to the level of the carina may be achieved by using a partial upper sternal split to allow the remaining periesophageal attachments to be divided under direct vision[73] (Fig. 25–11).

When mobilization of the entire intrathoracic esophagus is complete, several inches of esophagus are delivered into the cervical wound and the esophagus is then divided, the anterior tip being left slightly longer than the posterior corner (Fig. 24–12). In dividing the upper esophagus, some redundancy in length is intentionally left, because in later construction of the cervical esophagogastric anastomosis a variable length is amputated. In dealing with benign esophageal disease, particularly disease involving primarily the distal half of the esophagus, a generous length of cervical and upper thoracic esophagus should be left intact. If there is any difficulty getting the stomach to reach well into the neck wound, a partial upper sternal split can be performed, and the extra remaining length of upper esophagus will then easily reach to the gastric fundus. After dividing the esophagus in the neck, the stomach is retracted inferiorly through the abdominal incision, and the thoracic esophagus is thus drawn out of the posterior mediastinum through the diaphragmatic hiatus.

With the esophagus now removed from the posterior mediastinum, blood is evacuated from the posterior mediastinum using the Argyle Saratoga sump catheter inserted through the cervical incision. Narrow, deep Deaver retractors placed in the diaphragmatic hiatus allow direct inspection of the posterior mediastinum and the mediastinal pleura. If there is bleeding from a divided aortic esophageal artery, this is controlled with a long right-angle clamp and the vessel ligated. If entry into either chest cavity has occurred during the esophageal dissection, a No. 28 French chest tube is inserted into the appropriate chest in the mid axillary line and connected to underwater chest tube suction. One or two large abdominal packs are inserted into the posterior mediastinum through the diaphragmatic hiatus to tamponade any residual minor bleeding while the stomach is further prepared. The stomach and attached esophagus are placed on the anterior abdominal wall. The gastric fundus is retracted superiorly, and an area along the high lesser curvature of the stomach at the level of the second vascular arcade from the cardia is cleared of fat and blood vessels with clamps and ties. The upper stomach is then progressively divided with the GIA stapler applied initially to the lesser curvature (Fig. 25–13). When the partial proximal gastrectomy has been completed, the esophagus and attached upper stomach are removed from the field. The gastric staple suture line is oversewn with a running 4–0 polypropylene Lembert stitch. The posterior mediastinal abdominal packs placed earlier are now removed through the hiatus and a final inspection for bleeding is carried out.

Recently our focus has shifted from the actual technique of transhiatal esophagectomy to methods of avoiding a subsequent CEGA leak. To minimize trauma to the mobilized stomach, particularly to the gastric tip to which the cervical esophagus will be anastomosed, traction sutures in the tip of the stomach and suction devices to pull the stomach through the posterior mediastinum and into the neck wound are now avoided. The goal is to keep the tip of the stomach pink and healthy for the cervical anastomosis. The gastric submucosal collateral circulation is preserved by avoiding construction of a gastric "tube" as much as possible.

After identifying the most superior point along the greater curvature of the stomach (Fig. 25–14), this area

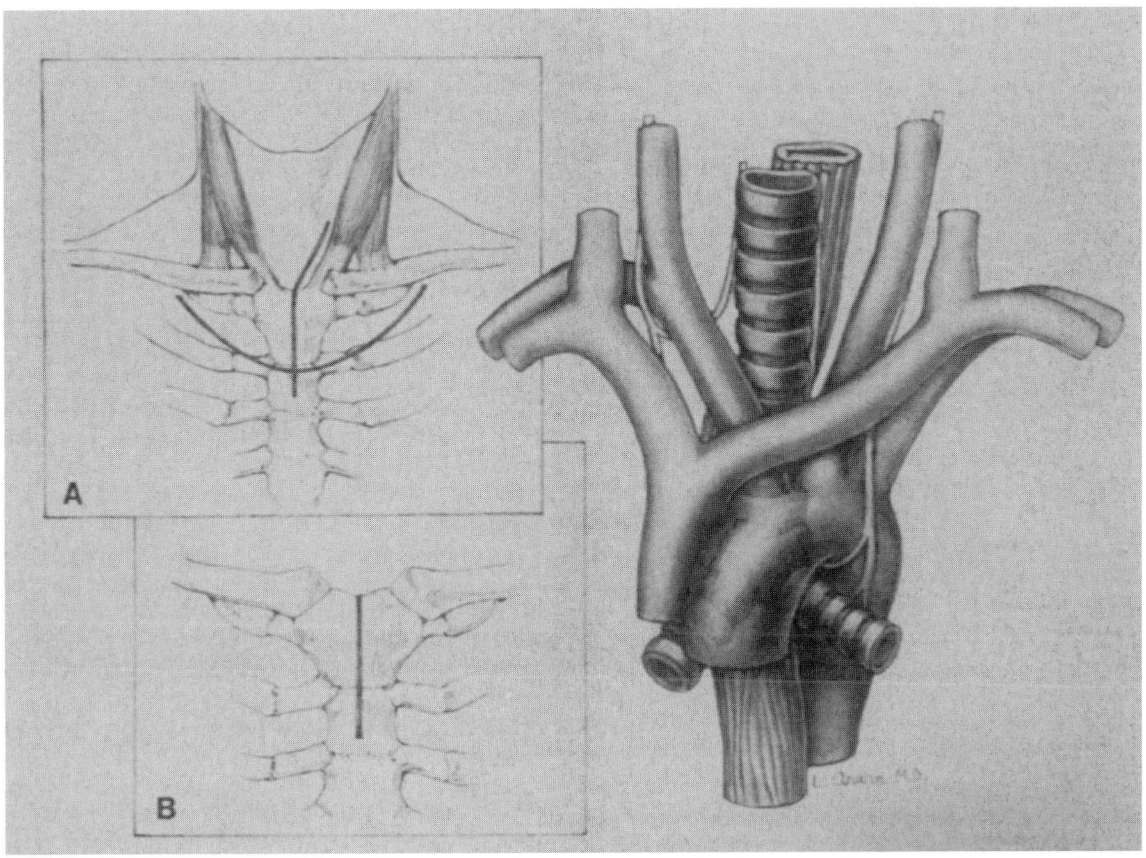

Figure 25–11. Exposure of the upper thoracic esophagus through a partial sternal split. Main illustration demonstrates the course of the left recurrent laryngeal nerve beneath the aortic arch and in the tracheoesophageal groove. *Inset A*, The left cervical incision is extended onto the anterior chest in the midline. Occasionally, a curved anterior thoracic incision may be used to avoid a scar on the low anterior neck. *Inset B*, The sternotomy incision extends from the suprasternal notch through the manubrium and across the angle of Louis. (From Orringer, M.B.: Partial median sternotomy: Anterior approach to the upper thoracic esophagus. J. Thorac. Cardiovasc. Surg., *87*:124, 1984, with permission.)

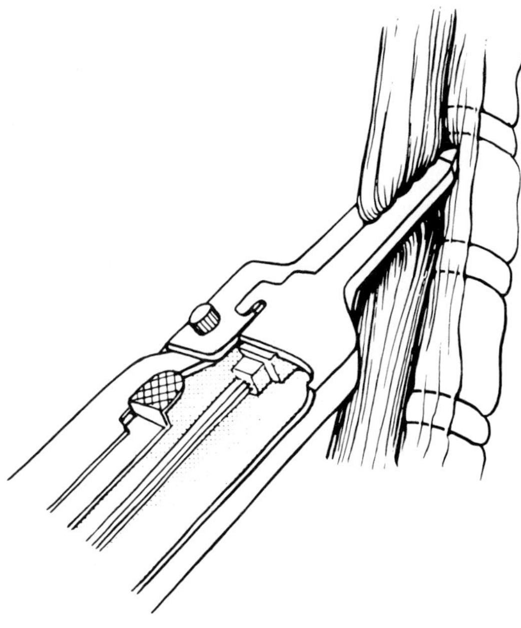

Figure 25–12. Oblique division of the upper esophagus in the cervical wound, the anterior tip being left slightly longer than the posterior corner. (From Orringer, M.B., and Sloan, H.: Esophageal replacement after blunt esophagectomy. *In* Nyhus, L.M., and Baker, R.J. [eds.]: Mastery of Surgery, 2nd ed. Boston, Little, Brown, 1992, p. 569, with permission.)

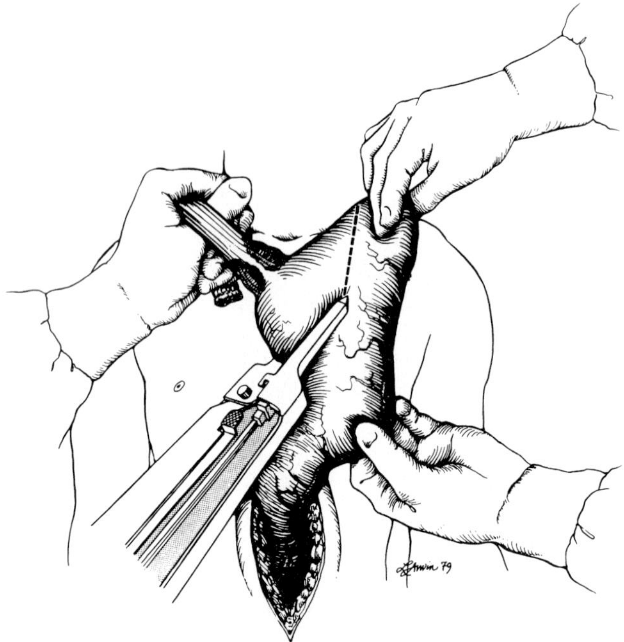

Figure 25–13. Partial proximal gastrectomy performed routinely in transhiatal esophagectomy and esophageal replacement with stomach. The mobilized stomach and attached distal esophagus are delivered from the abdominal incision and retracted superiorly as the surgical stapler is applied sequentially, beginning from the high lesser curvature and proceeding toward the high greater curvature (as indicated by the *dotted line*). This technique is also used for tumors of the cardia (as shown), where the stapler can be applied 4 to 6 cm distal to palpable tumor. (From Orringer, M.B., and Sloan, H.: Esophageal replacement after transhiatal esophagectomy without thoracotomy. *In* Nyhus, L.M., and Baker, R.J. [eds.]: Mastery of Surgery, 2nd ed. Boston, Little, Brown, 1992, p. 569, with permission.)

is grasped with one hand, and the mobilized stomach is gently manipulated upward through the diaphragmatic hiatus, under the aortic arch, and into the superior mediastinum until the gastric tip can be palpated by the other hand inserted into the cervical wound. A Babcock clamp inserted through the neck wound is then used to grasp the stomach gently and deliver the tip into the cervical field until it can be grasped by the fingertips and 4 to 5 cm drawn above the length of the clavicles (Fig. 25–15). "Suspension sutures" between the tip of the stomach and the cervical prevertebral fascia, as previously described, are now avoided to minimize gastric trauma and the potential for vertebral osteomyelitis, which may result from bacterial seeding of a cervical disc.

Care must be taken to avoid torsion of the stomach during its repositioning in the posterior mediastinum. When the stomach is in proper position, the gastric staple suture line can be seen along the right side of the gastric fundus in the neck wound. The anterior surface of the stomach is gently palpated from below through the hiatus and also from the neck incision to be certain that no twist in the stomach has occurred.

Before performing the cervical anastomosis, the abdominal phase of the operation is concluded to avoid contamination by oral bacteria that might occur after the cervical esophagus is opened. A saline moistened abdominal gauze pack is used to cover the cervical wound; the color of the stomach beneath it is assessed several times as the abdominal portion of the operation is completed. The diaphragmatic hiatus is narrowed with an average of one to three No. 0 silk sutures so that it easily admits three fingers alongside the stomach. The edge of the diaphragmatic hiatus is tacked to the anterior gastric wall with several 3-0 silk sutures, and as the retracted left hepatic lobe is returned to its normal location, the previously divided triangular ligament of the liver is sutured back over the hiatus with a single 3-0 silk suture to further prevent herniation of intraabdominal viscera into the chest through the hiatus, a complication that has been reported.[49,95] The pyloromyotomy is covered by adjacent omentum. The feeding jejunostomy tube is brought out through a separate left upper quadrant stab wound, and the jejunum is fixed to the anterior abdominal wall with several interrupted sutures. The abdominal incision is closed and excluded from the field by covering it with a sterile towel. The last major portion of the operation, the CEGA, is now performed.

Cervical Esophagogastric Anastomosis

When the stomach has been properly mobilized, a 4- to 5-cm length of gastric fundus rests in the neck wound above the level of the left clavicle (Fig. 25–16). The

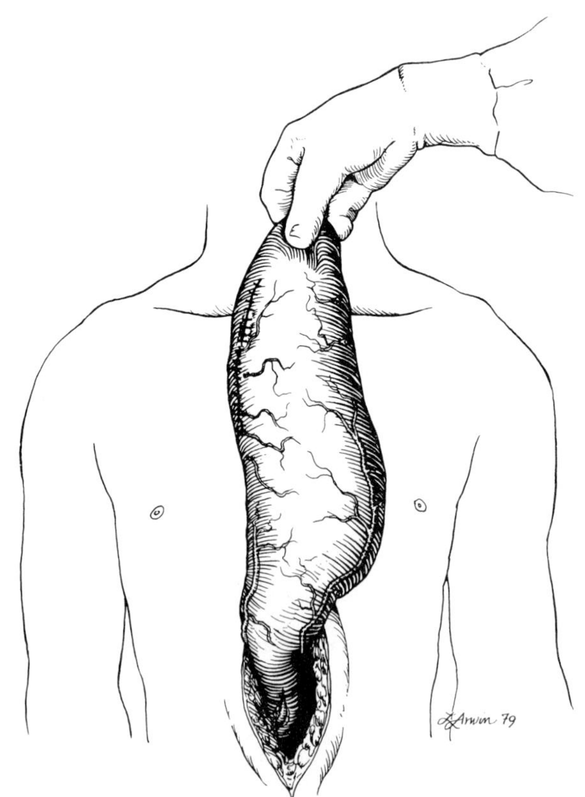

Figure 25–14. Identification of the site on the high greater curvature of the stomach that will reach most superiorly to the neck. The oversewn staple suture line where the cardia was divided is shown. (From Orringer, M.B., and Sloan, H.: Esophageal replacement after transhiatal esophagectomy without thoracotomy. *In* Nyhus, L.M., and Baker, R.J. [eds.]: Mastery of Surgery, 2nd ed. Boston, Little, Brown, 1992, p. 569, with permission.)

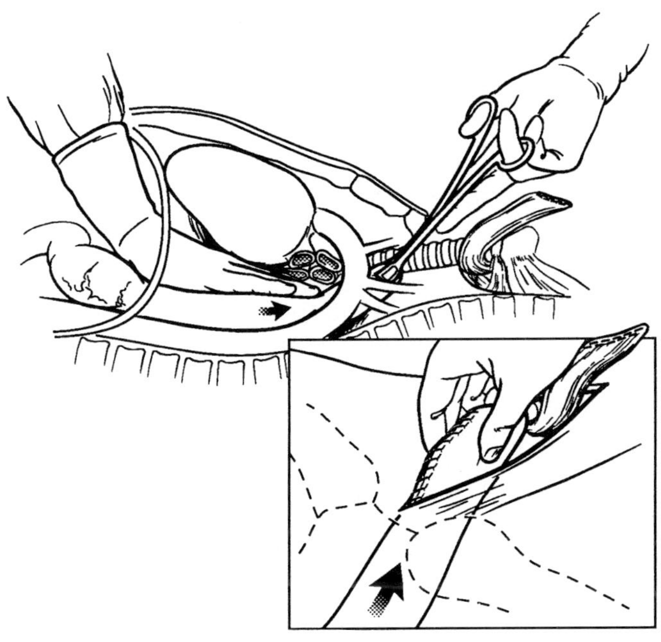

Figure 25–15. The mobilized stomach is gently manipulated through the diaphragmatic hiatus and into the posterior mediastinum in the original esophageal bed. Cardiac displacement is minimized by keeping the hand flat and as much against the spine as possible. After the stomach has reached the superior mediastinum beneath the aortic arch, the tip is grasped with a Babcock clamp inserted through the cervical incision and carefully drawn into the cervical field until it can be grasped by the finger tips *(inset)*. The clamp is not ratcheted closed completely to minimize gastric trauma. Four to five centimeters of stomach is delivered above the level of the clavicle primarily by pushing from below in the chest rather than applying traction in the neck. (From Orringer, M.B., Marshall, B., and Iannettoni, M.D.: Eliminating the cervical esophagogastric anastomotic leak with a side-to-side stapled anastomosis. J. Thorac. Cardiovasc. Surg., *119*:277, 2000.)

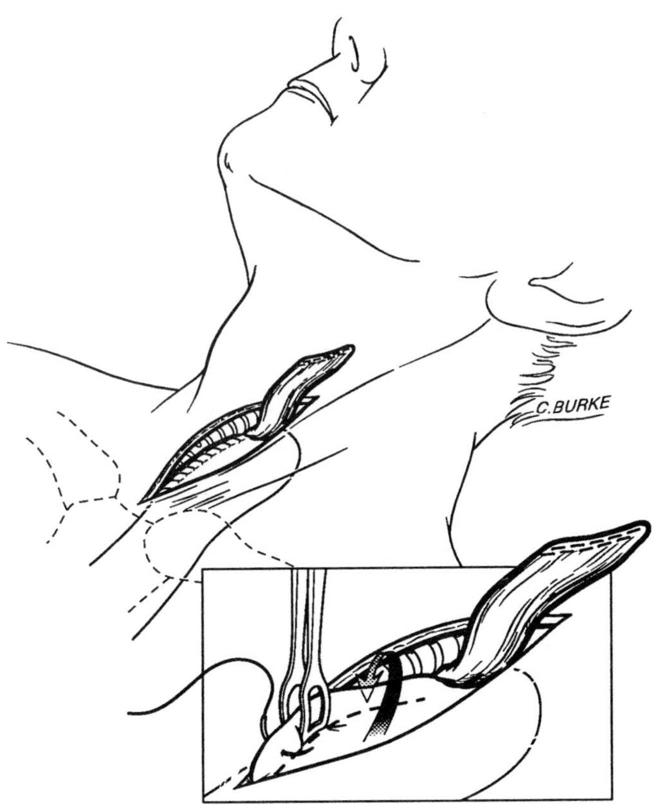

Figure 25–16. The tip of the mobilized stomach rests anterior to the prevertebral fascia in the neck, 4 to 5 cm above the level of the left clavicle and well behind the divided cervical esophagus. The end of the esophagus is retracted superiorly, the oversewn gastric staple suture line is rotated more medially toward the patient's right side, and a Babcock clamp is used to elevate the anterior gastric wall into the field. A 3-0 silk traction suture placed distal to the clamp is fixed to the drapes and elevates the stomach to the surface of the wound. (From Orringer, M.B., Marshall, B., and Iannettoni, M.D.: Eliminating the cervical esophagogastric anastomotic leak with a side-to-side stapled anastomosis. J. Thorac. Cardiovasc. Surg., *119*:277, 2000.)

divided end of the upper esophagus is retracted superiorly with an Allis clamp. As the oversewn gastric staple suture line is rotated even more medially with a Babcock clamp, a traction suture is placed in the anterior gastric wall behind the level of the clavicle and is used to elevate the stomach to the surface of the wound. A 1.5-cm vertical gastrotomy is made on the anterior gastric wall (Fig. 25-17). The gastrotomy must be sufficiently below the tip of the gastric fundus to allow the later full insertion of the 3-cm long staple cartridge. In estimating the optimal length of cervical esophagus that will be required, some redundancy should be planned because the stomach (and the anastomosis) will partially retract into the thoracic inlet after the traction suture is ultimately removed. The cervical esophageal staple suture line is amputated, again leaving the anterior tip of the esophagus longer than the posterior corner (Fig. 25-18). The amputated tip is submitted as the "proximal esophageal margin" for histologic evaluation.

Two anastomotic stay-sutures are placed to facilitate alignment of the esophagus and stomach for the anastomosis (Fig. 25-19). An Auto Suture Endo GIA II 30-3.5 staple cartridge loaded on a Versafine GIA stapler is inserted into the stomach and the esophagus (Fig. 25-20*A*). As the stapler is applied and the jaws approximated, proper alignment of the posterior wall of the esophagus and the anterior wall of the esophagus is crucial (see Fig. 25-20*B*). With the jaws of the stapler closed but before the cartridge is fired, two suspension sutures between the anterior gastric wall and the adjacent posterior esophageal wall are placed on either side (Fig. 25-21*A*). Firing the stapler creates a 3-cm long side-to-side anastomosis (see Fig. 25-21*B*). A No. 16 French nasogastric tube is inserted across the anastomosis and into the intrathoracic stomach by the anesthetist, and the anterior edges of the gastrostomy and open esophagus are approximated in two layers (Fig. 25-22). Hemostatic metallic clips are placed on either side of the anastomosis as markers to permit future radiographic assessment, and the wound is closed loosely with interrupted sutures over a small rubber drain. A portable chest radiograph is taken in the

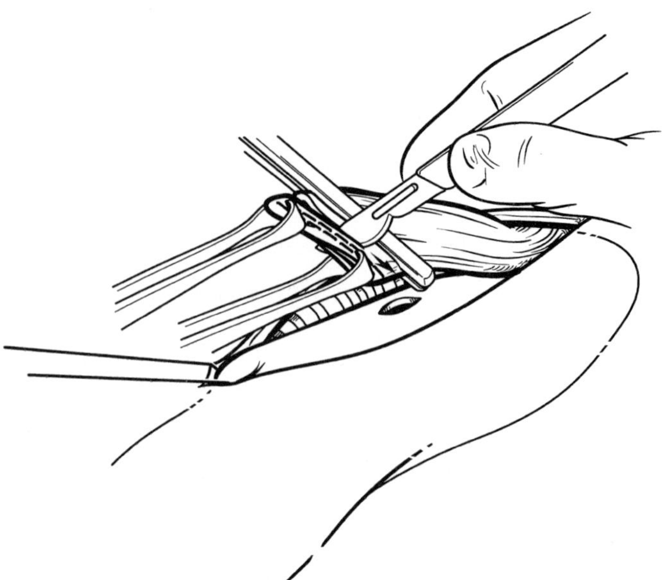

Figure 25-18. The esophageal staple suture line is amputated obliquely in an anterior to posterior orientation, again creating a longer anterior than posterior tip. An atraumatic vascular forceps is used as a guide for amputation of the staple suture line, which is submitted as the "proximal esophageal margin." (Modified from Orringer, M.B., Marshall, B., and Iannettoni, M.D.: Eliminating the cervical esophagogastric anastomotic leak with a side-to-side stapled anastomosis. J. Thorac. Cardiovasc. Surg., *119*:277, 2000.)

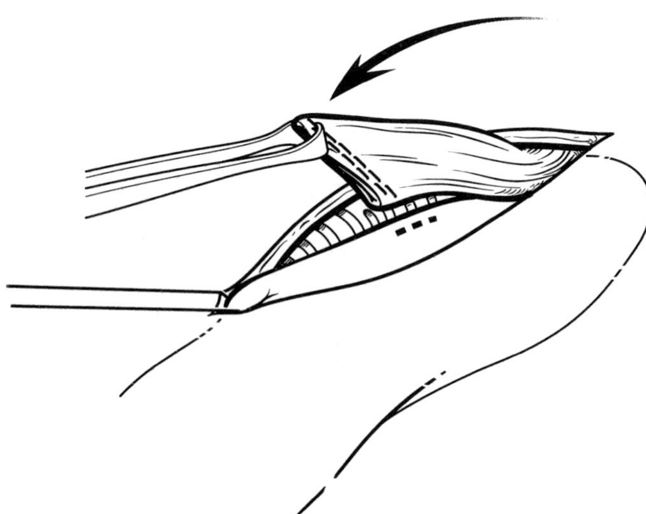

Figure 25-17. Using a needle-tip electrocautery, a 1.5-cm vertical gastrotomy is made on the anterior gastric wall, well away from the staple suture line and after carefully assessing where the end of the cervical esophagus will ultimately rest in a tension-free fashion when the traction suture is removed. (Modified from Orringer, M.B., Marshall, B., and Iannettoni, M.D.: Eliminating the cervical esophagogastric anastomotic leak with a side-to-side stapled anastomosis. J. Thorac. Cardiovasc. Surg., *119*:277, 2000.)

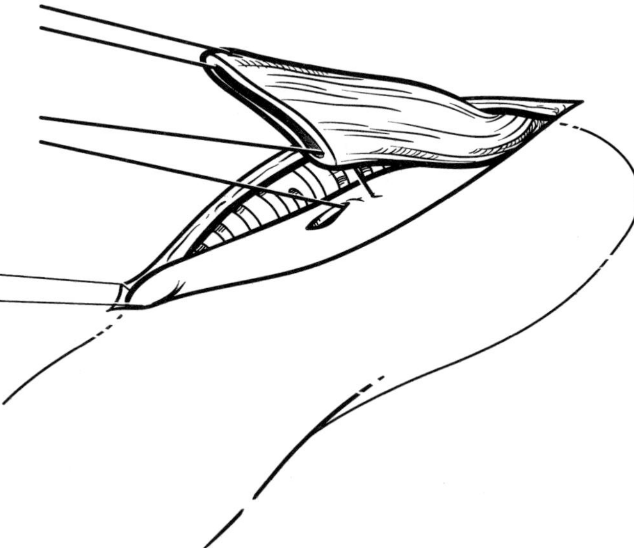

Figure 25-19. Two 4-0 polyglycolic acid stay sutures are placed, one at the tip of the anterior corner of the beveled esophagus and the other from the superior corner of the vertical gastrotomy and the posterior corner of the esophagus. (Modified from Orringer, M.B., Marshall, B., and Iannettoni, M.D.: Eliminating the cervical esophagogastric anastomotic leak with a side-to-side stapled anastomosis. J. Thorac. Cardiovasc. Surg., *119*:277, 2000.)

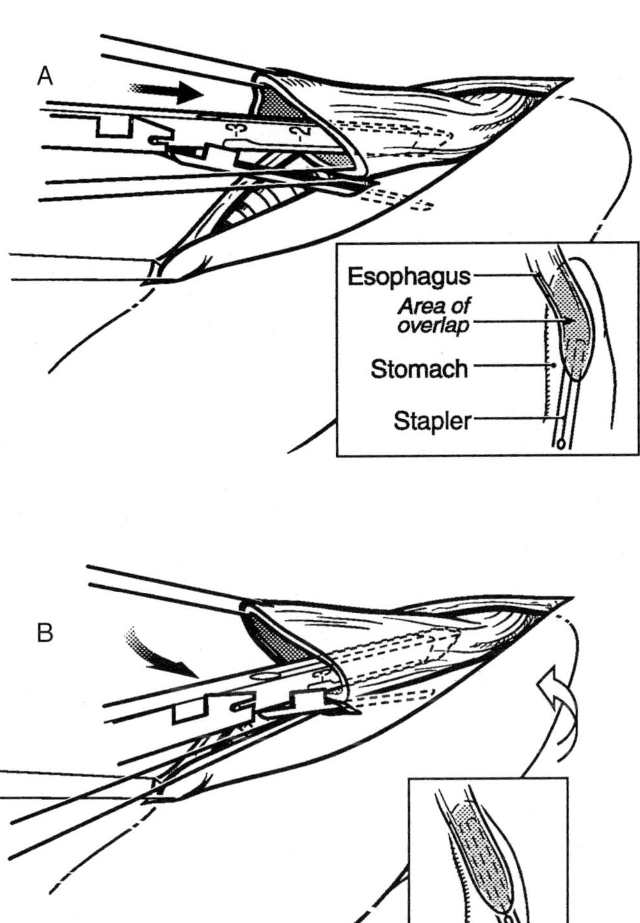

Figure 25–20. *A*, The two stay sutures are retracted inferiorly as the ENDO-GIA 30-3.5 staple cartridge is inserted, the thinner anvil portion into the stomach and the thicker staple-bearing portion into the esophagus. *B*, The staple cartridge is gradually rotated and pointed toward the patient's right ear as it is advanced into the esophagus and stomach *(inset)*. The posterior wall of the esophagus and the anterior wall of the stomach are carefully aligned in a parallel fashion, keeping the site of the anastomosis well away from the gastric staple suture line. (From Orringer, M.B., Marshall, B., and Iannettoni, M.D.: Eliminating the cervical esophagogastric anastomotic leak with a side-to-side stapled anastomosis. J. Thorac. Cardiovasc. Surg., *119:*277, 2000.)

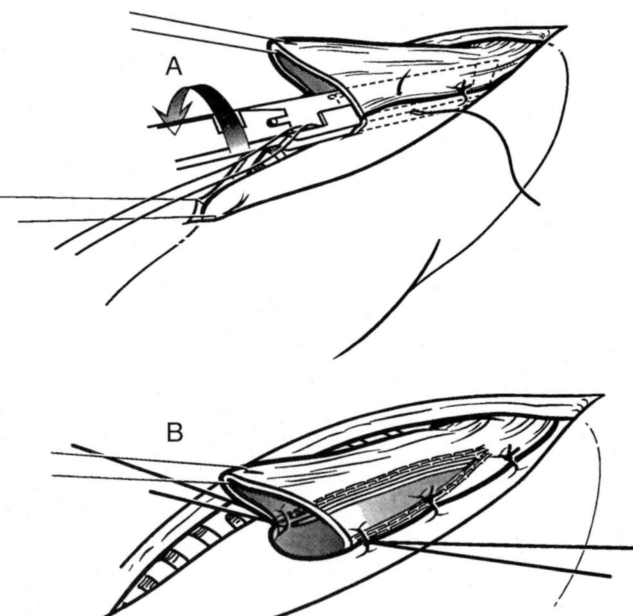

Figure 25–21. *A*, The jaws of the stapler are approximated by squeezing the handle, but before firing it, the stapler is rolled from one side to the other as two "suspension" sutures between the esophagus and adjacent stomach are placed on either side. *B*, A 3-cm long side-to-side anastomosis is created by firing the stapler and thereby advancing the knife assembly. The stapler is removed, the anastomosis inspected for bleeding, a nasogastric tube inserted, and "corner" sutures placed in preparation for completion of the anastomosis. (From Orringer, M.B., Marshall, B., and Iannettoni, M.D.: Eliminating the cervical esophagogastric anastomotic leak with a side-to-side stapled anastomosis. J. Thorac. Cardiovasc. Surg., *119:*277, 2000.)

operating room to be certain that no unrecognized hemothorax or pneumothorax is present and that the nasogastric and endotracheal tubes are in the proper position.

Transhiatal Esophagectomy for Carcinoma of the Esophagogastric Junction

The technique just described can be used in most patients with carcinoma of the cardia and proximal stomach (Fig. 25–23). The traditional proximal hemigastrectomy performed for such tumors "wastes" valuable stomach that can be used for esophageal replacement, contributes little to the patient's longevity, and commits the surgeon to an intrathoracic esophageal anastomosis. In most cases it is possible to divide the stomach 4 to 6 cm distal to gross tumor, thereby preserving the entire greater curva-

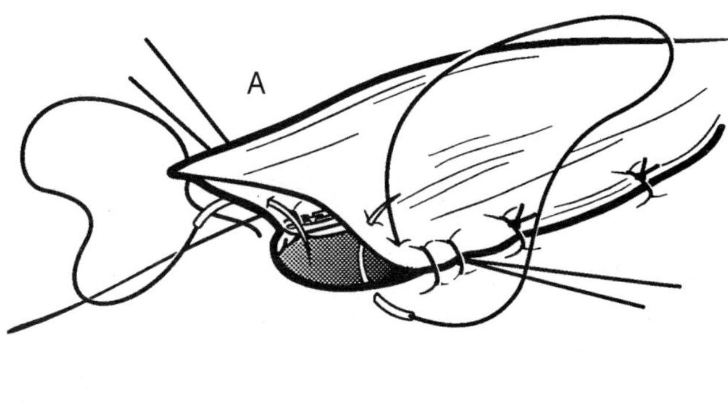

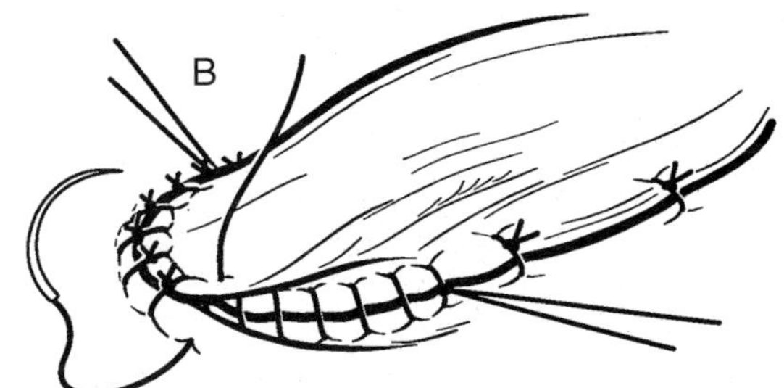

Figure 25–22. The gastrotomy and open esophagus are apposed in two layers: *(A)* a running inner layer of 4-0 monofilament absorbable suture, and *(B)* an outer interrupted layer. (From Orringer, M.B., Marshall, B., and Iannettoni, M.D.: Eliminating the cervical esophagogastric anastomotic leak with a side-to-side stapled anastomosis. J. Thorac. Cardiovasc. Surg., *119:*277, 2000.)

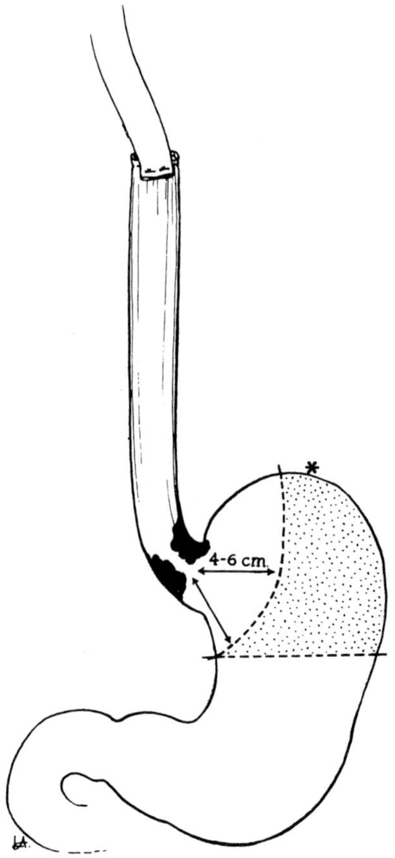

Figure 25–23. Transhiatal esophagectomy and proximal partial gastrectomy for lesions of the cardia and distal esophagus. A 4- to 6-cm gastric margin is obtained while preserving the entire greater curvature and that point *(asterisk)* that reaches most cephalad. The *stippled area* indicates the portion of stomach that is typically resected in a standard hemigastrectomy for distal esophageal carcinoma, thus eliminating the possibility of a cervical esophagogastric anastomosis. (From Orringer, M.B., and Sloan, H.: Esophagectomy without thoracotomy. J. Thorac. Cardiovasc. Surg., *76*:643, 1978, with permission.)

ture of the gastric fundus. The narrowed gastric "tube" that remains functions as a satisfactory esophageal substitute.

Particular care must be taken in assessing the feasibility of a transhiatal esophagectomy and proximal partial gastrectomy for tumors of the esophagogastric junction. The cervical esophagus should not be divided until the surgeon is convinced that adequate remaining stomach will remain to reach to the neck. If the cervical esophagus is divided and the thoracic esophagus is removed *before* the esophagogastric junction tumor is found to involve so much stomach that a proximal hemigastrectomy is required to remove it, there will not be sufficient gastric length to reach to the neck, and the patient will be left with a cervical esophagostomy and a feeding tube, the worst possible consequence of an esophageal operation intended to relieve dysphagia!

POSTOPERATIVE CARE

A postoperative portable chest radiograph in the operating room establishes proper position of the chest tube, excludes an unrecognized hemothorax or pneumothorax, and allows assessment of the mediastinum for inordinate widening suggesting mediastinal bleeding. Transhiatal esophagectomy without thoracotomy and a cervical esophagogastric anastomosis constitute a less severe physiologic insult to the patient than the traditional combined thoracoabdominal approaches for esophagectomy and esophageal reconstruction. The average operative time for transhiatal esophagectomy is 3 to 4 hours. Thoracic epidural anesthesia permits removal of the endotracheal tube immediately at the conclusion of the operation in most patients, provided that no significant contraindication is discovered on the postoperative chest radiograph in the operating room.

Preoperative teaching emphasizes to the patient the desirability and necessity for early postoperative ambulation and pulmonary hygiene. As soon as the endotracheal tube is removed, use of the incentive spirometer, which was begun preoperatively, is resumed. Ambulation is begun the evening of surgery. Postoperative ileus seldom lasts longer than 72 hours because transhiatal esophagectomy is essentially an upper abdominal operation. Nasogastric tube drainage generally amounts to less than 100 ml/8-hr nursing shift by the third postoperative day when the tube is removed. Feeding of 5% dextrose in water (D-5-W) through the jejunostomy tube at a rate of 30 ml/hr is begun on the third postoperative day. If this amount is tolerated for 12 hours, the volume is increased to 60 ml/hr. The following day, half-strength jejunostomy tube feedings are begun, followed by full-strength feedings the next day. Postoperative diarrhea may occur in response to either tube feedings or the vagotomy that accompanies transhiatal esophagectomy. This diarrhea is controlled with diphenoxylate (Lomotil) or paregoric.

Within 3 to 5 days of operation, intravenous lines, the arterial catheter, the cervical wound drain, the thoracic epidural anesthesia catheter, the Foley urethral catheter, and the nasogastric tube have been removed to facilitate unrestrained ambulation and vigorous respiratory physical therapy. When removal of the nasogastric tube has been well tolerated for 24 hours, oral liquid feedings are begun. As oral intake increases, the jejunostomy feedings are concomitantly decreased and then discontinued. On the seventh postoperative day, a barium swallow examination is performed to document that the anastomosis is intact and that gastric emptying through the pyloromyotomy is adequate (both areas having been marked with silver clips). There is little logic in not allowing the patient to take nourishment by mouth until after a postoperative barium swallow on the tenth postoperative day, when anastomotic healing is assured. The patient is swallowing saliva from the moment he or she awakes from the operation; the fact that the patient is not swallowing food does not mean that oral contents are not crossing the anastomosis. Further, there is usually a period of 1 week or so of "adjustment" during which the patient becomes accustomed to initial retrosternal fullness, early satiety, or the postvagotomy cramping and diarrhea ("dumping") that may occur with this procedure, and if oral feeding is delayed until after the barium swallow on the tenth postoperative day, another week of unnecessary hospitalization is usually required.

The patient is typically discharged on the seventh postoperative day after satisfactory results on the postoperative barium swallow have been observed (Figs. 25-24 to 25-26). The jejunostomy feeding tube is removed on an outpatient basis 2 weeks later, about 4 weeks after the operation. Occasionally, if the patient is anorectic immediately after surgery, he or she is encouraged to supplement his or her caloric intake with jejunostomy tube feedings at night for the first several weeks at home. Most patients, however, are able to eat satisfactorily when they leave the hospital without the need for supplemental jejunostomy tube feedings.

COMPLICATIONS OF TRANSHIATAL ESOPHAGECTOMY AND THEIR MANAGEMENT

The most common acute complications of transhiatal esophagectomy without thoracotomy can be classified into two broad categories: (1) those that occur intraoperatively (pneumothorax, tracheal tear, and hemorrhage), and (2) those that occur during the first "critical" 10 days after operation (hoarseness or impaired swallowing due to recurrent laryngeal nerve injury, anastomotic disruption, chylothorax, supraventricular tachyarrhythmias, and sympathetic pleural effusion). The late complications of transhiatal esophagectomy are relatively few: CEGA anastomotic stricture and herniation of abdominal viscera through the diaphragmatic hiatus. Less common early complications of transhiatal esophagectomy and a CEGA, occurring with an incidence of less than 1%, include gastric tip necrosis, vertebral body osteomyelitis, epidural abscess, pulmonary microabscesses from internal jugular vein abscess, and tracheogastric anastomotic fistula.[51] Delayed emptying of the intrathoracic stomach may result if an inadequate gastric drainage procedure has been performed, if the hiatus has been narrowed excessively, or if tumor recurs locally. Torsion of the intrathoracic stomach is avoidable as long as care is taken to ensure the proper orientation of the stomach within the posterior mediastinum.

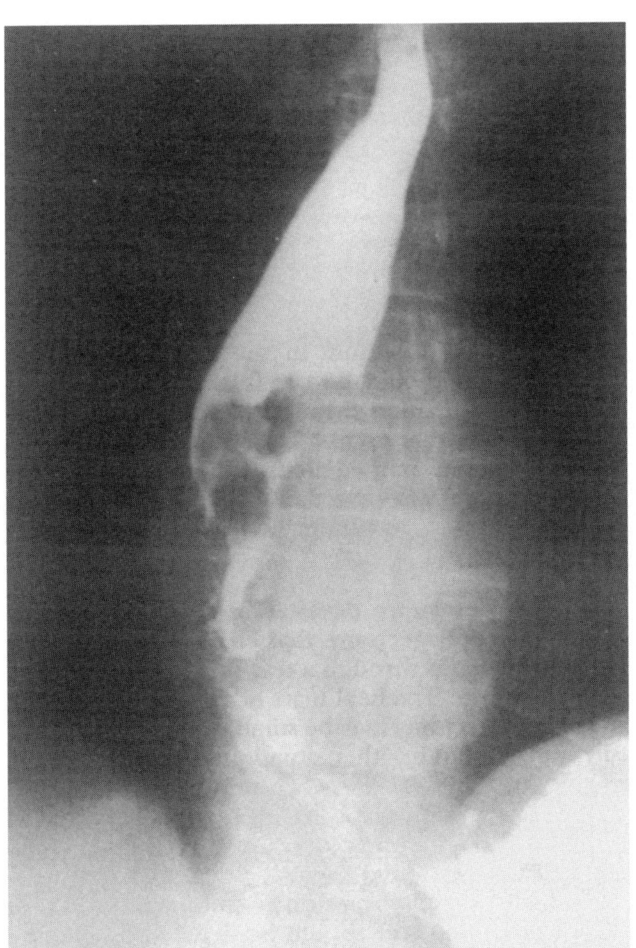

Figure 25-24. Preoperative barium swallow showing large tumor involving the middle and lower thirds of the esophagus.

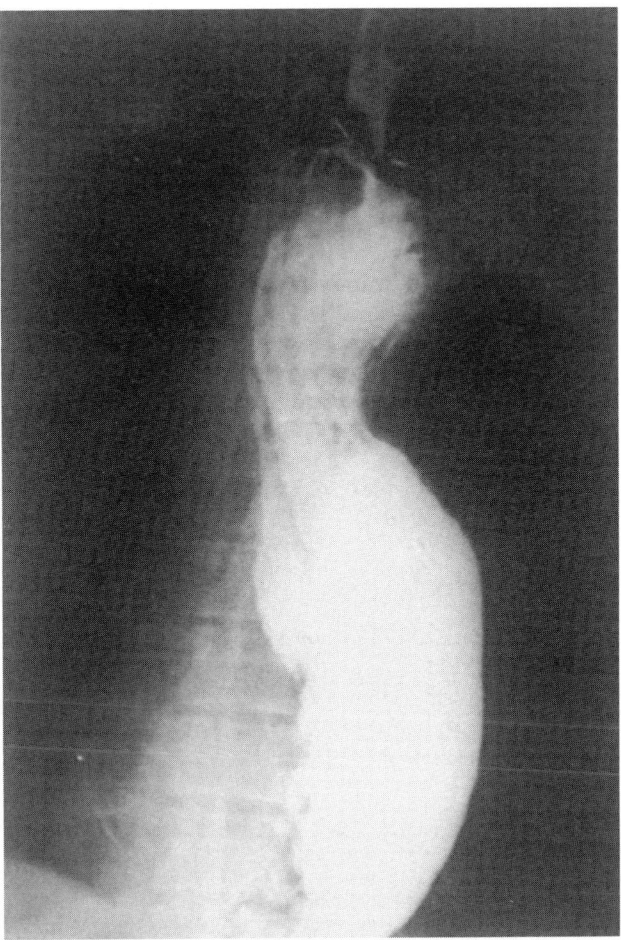

Figure 25-25. Postoperative barium swallow in patient shown in Figure 25-24 after transhiatal esophagectomy and cervical esophagogastric anastomosis. The two silver clips above the level of the clavicle mark the cervical esophagogastric anastomosis.

Pneumothorax

Entry into one or both pleural cavities during the mediastinal dissection occurs in nearly two thirds of patients undergoing transhiatal esophagectomy. After the esopha-

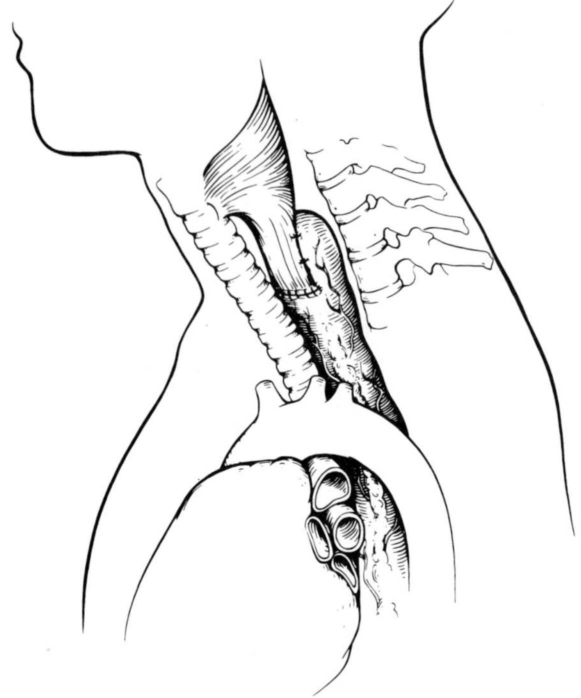

Figure 25–26. Final position of the mobilized stomach after transhiatal esophagectomy and cervical esophagogastric anastomosis. The stomach rests in the posterior mediastinum in the original esophageal bed. Two "suspension" sutures on either side of the anastomosis between the back of the cervical esophagus and the adjacent stomach limit tension on the anastomosis and are preferable to "tacking" sutures between the stomach and the prevertebral fascia. The pylorus (not shown) generally comes to rest several centimeters below the level of the diaphragmatic hiatus. (From Iannettoni, M.D., Whyte, R.I., and Orringer, M.B.: Catastrophic complications of the cervical esophagogastric anastomosis. J. Thorac. Cardiovasc. Surg., *110*:1493, 1995, with permission.)

gectomy has been completed and before positioning the stomach in the posterior mediastinum in the original esophageal bed, the pleura should be carefully inspected both visually and by palpation through the diaphragmatic hiatus to be certain that no tear has occurred. If the pleura has been violated, immediate insertion of a chest tube or tubes provides effective therapy.

Tracheal Tear

There are few more devastating experiences during transhiatal esophagectomy than feeling a rush of air from the ventilator through a tear in the posterior membranous trachea! Tracheal tears occurring during transhiatal esophagectomy may be small, linear, and relatively easily sutured, but in other situations, if the surgeon has wrongly attempted to resect a tumor that is densely adherent to or invading the trachea, and major tracheobronchial disruption occurs, the situation may be irreparable.

If a tracheal tear occurs during esophagectomy, the endotracheal tube cuff should be deflated by the anesthetist and the tube should be advanced, guided by the surgeon's hand in the posterior mediastinum, into the distal trachea or left main-stem bronchus so that the endotracheal tube cuff is distal to the tear. With control of the airway re-established, repair of the tear can be achieved in a more controlled manner. A partial upper sternal split (see Fig. 25–11) provides ample exposure of the upper trachea for direct repair. If possible, it is best to complete the transhiatal esophagectomy before attempting the tracheal repair because once the esophagus is removed, exposure of the posterior trachea is optimum. If the tracheal tear is extensive or involves the carina or main-stem bronchus, an anterior repair through a partial upper sternal split is not possible. In such a situation, one-lung anesthesia administered through the endotracheal tube inserted into the left main-stem bronchus should be continued and the abdomen closed quickly with several large full-thickness abdominal wall sutures. The cervical wound is also closed loosely, and both wounds are covered. The patient is then turned on the left side, and the right chest is prepared and draped. Through a fifth-interspace posterolateral thoracotomy, the tracheal tear should be identified and repaired and the esophagectomy completed, mobilizing the upper esophagus bluntly well up into the neck. After closing the chest, the patient is repositioned supine. The abdominal and cervical incisions are reopened, the mobilized stomach relocated into the posterior mediastinum, and the cervical esophagogastric anastomosis constructed as described previously.

Hemorrhage

The average intraoperative blood loss with transhiatal esophagectomy is less than 1,000 ml, and major intraoperative bleeding is the exception rather than the rule. The aortic esophageal arteries branch into very small vessels before they reach the wall of the esophagus, and when these smaller vessels are avulsed from the esophagus during transhiatal esophagectomy, natural hemostatic mechanisms of thrombosis and arterial contraction control bleeding.[61] As one gains experience with the technique of transhiatal esophagectomy, more and more of the dissection can be done under direct vision. For example, with narrow retractors placed on either side of the diaphragmatic hiatus, the lateral esophageal attachments can be divided using long right-angled clamps and ligated, often to the level of the carina. Major uncontrolled bleeding should simply not occur with this operation if the surgeon exercises judgment in selecting patients for the procedure. When palpation of the esophagus through the diaphragmatic hiatus indicates fixation of the esophagus to the aorta or periesophageal tissues, the transhiatal approach should probably be abandoned. If major intraoperative bleeding occurs during the transhiatal dissection, the No. 28 French Argyle Saratoga sump catheter should be inserted through the cervical incision to help evacuate the mediastinal bleeding from above, and with the aid of narrow deep retractors placed within the diaphragmatic hiatus, the mediastinum should be inspected in an effort to identify and control the point of bleeding. If hemostasis cannot be achieved under direct vision, there is little alternative but to tamponade the mediastinum with large abdominal packs inserted through the diaphragmatic hiatus. After waiting 5 to 10 minutes to allow natural hemostatic mechanisms to come into play and intravenous volume resuscitation if needed, the packs can be removed and the mediastinum inspected once again. If adequate control of bleeding is still not possible, the mediastinum should be tamponaded again with abdominal packs. A thoracotomy must then be performed to obtain hemostasis. If bleeding is encountered during dissection of the lower third of the esophagus, a left thoracotomy should be performed. Alternatively, if dissection of the mid or upper thoracic esophagus results in bleeding, a right thoracotomy is more appropriate for attempted control.

Recurrent Laryngeal Nerve Injury

Recurrent laryngeal nerve injury occurring during transhiatal esophagectomy and cervical esophagogastric anastomosis is a serious complication that may have more significance than simply a hoarse voice. Impaired cricopharyngeal motor dysfunction with resulting cervical dysphagia and aspiration may cause serious aspiration pneumonia. Transient recurrent laryngeal nerve injury occurred frequently in our early experience with this operation. The injury was attributed initially to unavoidable intraoperative stretching of the left recurrent laryngeal nerve beneath the aortic arch in the chest. However, it was subsequently realized that such an injury to the recurrent laryngeal nerve seldom actually occurs. Rather, recurrent laryngeal nerve paresis or paralysis almost inevitably results from injury to the nerve during the cervical portions of the operation. It is therefore a *preventable* complication that can be avoided by not placing *any* retractor against the tracheoesophageal groove. This complication now rarely occurs in our hands because we have adopted the policy of avoiding placement of metal retractors against the tracheoesophageal groove. Only the first assistant's index finger is used to retract the trachea and thyroid gland medially.

Anastomotic Leak

A cervical esophageal anastomotic leak seldom occurs after the tenth postoperative day, is typically associated with very little acute morbidity, and is rarely fatal. If the patient develops a temperature of 101°F or more 48 hours after transhiatal esophagectomy, an anastomotic leak is assumed until proved otherwise, and an immediate contrast study of the esophagus is performed. Water-soluble contrast material (Gastrografin) may result in serious chemical pneumonitis if aspirated and is therefore avoided. If a leak is suspected, dilute barium, which better defines the mucosal detail, is preferred. A cervical esophageal anastomotic leak is treated by opening the cervical wound in its entirety at the bedside and instituting regular packing of the wound. The patient may be asked to swallow water while a bedside suction catheter is used to evacuate the fluid issuing from the neck wound; swallowing helps to "flush" any associated debris. The neck wound is packed with moistened gauze at least three times a day, and nutrition is maintained with jejunostomy tube feedings. Leaks that occur 7 to 10 days after the operation are generally small. Each time the neck dressing is changed, the patient is asked to swallow water, and observation of the amount that exists through the wound provides an estimate of the size of the anastomotic leak. Once the fistula is small, the patient is permitted to swallow a soft diet while applying direct pressure to the cervical wound. Passage of a No. 46 French tapered Maloney dilator at the bedside is carried out at least once after opening the cervical wound and before the patient is discharged to be certain that there is no distal obstruction associated with the fistula and to minimize the chance of development of an anastomotic stricture. In our experience, passage of an esophageal dilator before the fistula has closed does not damage the anastomosis further and in fact is usually followed by total closure of the fistula in 2 to 5 days. The majority of cervical esophagogastric anastomotic leaks heal spontaneously within 2 to 3 weeks. However, at least 50% result in a subsequent anastomotic stricture for which chronic esophageal dilatation is necessary.[80]

Chylothorax

If excessive or prolonged chest tube drainage occurs after transhiatal esophagectomy, the diagnosis of chylothorax due to an injured thoracic duct must be considered. This diagnosis may not be readily apparent because the serous chest drainage does not become "milky" until oral intake of fats is resumed. However, if chest tube drainage exceeds 200 to 400 ml/8-hr shift more than 48 hours after transhiatal esophagectomy, the possibility of a thoracic duct injury must be considered. The diagnosis is established by administering 30 to 60 ml/hr of cream through the jejunostomy tube for 3 to 6 hours. If there is a concomitant change in the character of the chest tube drainage fluid from serous to milky, the diagnosis is established. Conservative management of chylothorax in the patient who has undergone an esophagectomy has little justification.[78] The loss of large amounts of fluid rich in protein and lymphocytes that occurs with a chylothorax is not tolerated by the already nutritionally compromised patient with esophageal obstruction. Unless there is a dramatic reduction in the chyle leak within 3 to 5 days after instituting elemental jejunostomy tube feedings, thoracotomy and ligation of the torn thoracic duct are the most effective methods of dealing with the problem and minimizing morbidity. The patient is given 60 to 90 ml/hr of cream in the jejunostomy tube for 6 hours, and when there is a sustained flow of milky chest tube drainage, a thoracotomy is performed on the side of the chest tube that is draining the chyle. A double-lumen endotracheal tube permits one-lung anesthesia and exposure of the mediastinum through a very limited thoracotomy. The thoracic duct injury is easily identified owing to the brisk flow of milky fluid from it, and direct suture ligation is a relatively simple undertaking. This approach entails a less severe physiologic insult to the patient than weeks of hospitalization and intravenous hyperalimentation given in the hope that the injury will heal spontaneously.

Sympathetic Pleural Effusion

When the pleural cavity is not violated during transhiatal esophagectomy, and no chest tube is therefore required, a sympathetic pleural effusion related to the mediastinal dissection may occur during the first postoperative week. So long as the effusion is asymptomatic and does not continue to enlarge, no treatment is necessary, and spontaneous resolution is usual. Alternatively, if significant dyspnea results from a large effusion, several thoracenteses may be beneficial. Recurrent pleural effusion must be differentiated from a chylothorax and treated accordingly.

RESULTS OF TRANSHIATAL ESOPHAGECTOMY FOR BENIGN AND MALIGNANT ESOPHAGEAL DISEASE

Since the 1980s, multiple published reports have described various surgeons' early experience with transhiatal esophagectomy and have debated the indications and relative morbidity and mortality of transhiatal esophagectomy versus transthoracic esophagectomy. In a comprehensive collective review of the complications of transhiatal esophagectomy in 1,353 patients (99% for esophageal cancer) reported in 23 papers published between 1981 and 1992, Katariya and colleagues indicated that only 1.3% had been converted to open thoracotomies for control of hemorrhage.[53] A rather amorphous list of "pulmonary complications," which occurred in half of patients, included pneumothorax, pleural effusions, pneumonia, emphysema, and respiratory failure. Additional complications included anastomotic leak (15.1%); recurrent laryngeal nerve injury (11.3%); cardiac arrhythmias, myocardial infarction, or tamponade (11.9%); incidental splenectomy (2.6%); chylothorax (0.7%); and tracheal injuries (0.67%). The reported 30-day mortality rate for the 1,353 patients was 7.1%. It is worth noting, however, that 16 of the 23 papers referenced in this review (69.5%) were surgical series of 50 or fewer patients and therefore were not a reflection of the type of results that more experienced teams can achieve.

A more recent collective review by Gandhi and Naunheim of the complications of transhiatal esophagectomy in 1,192 patients reported in eight papers published between 1992 and 1994[34] included four series of 100 patients or more (118, 131, 141, and 583), the latter from the University of Michigan.[83] The average mortality rate was 6.7%. Complications included mediastinal hemorrhage (3%), recurrent laryngeal nerve injury (9%), respiratory complications (12%), anastomotic leak (12%), and cardiac complication (16%).

In the largest reported transhiatal esophagectomy series, my associates and I have reported our 20-year experience with this procedure in 1,085 patients requiring an esophagectomy for disease of the intrathoracic esophagus.[81] Transhiatal esophagectomy without thoracotomy was performed in 1,085 patients with diseases of the intrathoracic esophagus, 285 (26%) of whom had benign tumors necessitating esophageal replacement; 800 (74%) patients had malignant disease[81] (Table 25-1). The patients with benign disease ranged in age from 14 to 89 years (mean, 52 years). In this group, esophagectomy was required for severe reflux strictures, multiple failed prior antireflux procedures, caustic injuries, various chronic strictures (secondary to radiation therapy, monilial esophagitis, postemetic injury, and so forth), epithelial dysplasia associated with a columnar-lined lower esophagus (Barrett's esophagus), scleroderma reflux esophagitis, alkaline esophagitis, and chronic esophagopleural cutaneous fistula. One third of the patients had neuromotor esophageal dysfunction (achalasia or spasm), and many of these patients had undergone earlier unsuccessful operations. Among the 800 patients with carcinoma, 651 (81%) were men, and 149 (19%) were women; these patients ranged in age from 29 to 92 years (mean, 64 years). Two hundred thirty-nine (22%) of this entire series of patients were 71 years of age or older. Included within this group of 800 esophageal carcinomas were 225 (28%) squamous cell carcinomas (28 of the upper esophagus, 121 involving the mid esophagus, and 76 affecting the lower third), and 555 (69%) adenocarcinomas (5 upper third, 53 in the middle third, and 497 in the lower third or cardia). There were 12 adenosquamous carcinomas, 11 signet ring cell, 2 anaplastic, 2 poorly differentiated, 2 small cell, and 1 undifferentiated carcinoma. Periesophageal fibrosis and mediastinal inflammation associated with prior esophageal surgery, perforations, or radiation therapy have not contraindicated transhiatal esophagectomy in most patients. One hundred and forty-six (52%) of the patients with benign disease had a history of one or more prior esophageal or periesophageal operations: antireflux repairs in 85; esophagomyotomy in 60; vagotomy in 15, and a variety of other operations in 23. Four patients with acute caustic esophageal injuries under-

Table 25-1. Indications for Transhiatal Esophagectomy (1085 Patients)*

Diagnosis	No. of Patients (%)
Benign Conditions	***285 (26)***
Neuromotor dysfunction	93 (33)
Achalasia	70
Spasm/dysmotility	22
Scleroderma	1
Stricture	75 (26)
Gastroesophageal reflux	42
Caustic ingestion	19
Radiation	4
Other	10
Barrett's mucosa with high-grade dysplasia	54 (19)
Recurrent gastroesophageal reflux	21 (7)
Recurrent hiatus hernia	14 (5)
Acute perforation	14 (5)
Acute caustic injury	6
Other	8
Carcinoma of Intrathoracic Esophagus	***800 (74)***
Upper third	36 (4.5)
Middle third	177 (28.0)
Lower third thoracic and/or cardia	587 (73.5)

*From Orringer, M.B., Marshall, B., and Iannettoni, M.D.: Transhiatal esophagectomy: Clinical experience and refinements. Ann. Surg., *230*:392–400, 1999, with permission.

Table 25–2. Esophageal Reconstruction After Transhiatal Esophagectomy (1085 Patients)*

Procedure	Benign (No. of Patients)	Carcinoma (No. of Patients)	Total (%)
Immediate			
Cervical esophagogastrostomy	258	782	1,040 (96)
Posterior mediastinal	256	777	
Retrosternal	2	5	
Cervical esophagocolostomy	22	17	39 (4)
Posterior mediastinal	16	10	
Retrosternal	6	7	
Delayed (2–8 wks)–retrosternal	4		4
None (esophagostomy, tube)	1	1	2
TOTAL	285	800	1,085

*From Orringer, M.B., Marshall, B., and Iannettoni, M.D.: Transhiatal esophagectomy: Clinical experience and refinements. Ann. Surg, *230*:392–400, 1999, with permission.

went emergency transhiatal esophagectomy, cervical esophagostomy, and feeding jejunostomy, followed by esophageal reconstruction 2 to 8 weeks later. One patient with a malfunctioning antiperistaltic retrosternal colonic bypass of a caustic stricture underwent removal of the restrosternal colon, transhiatal esophagectomy, and a CEGA. In the 22 years that I have been performing transhiatal esophagectomy, the operation has been possible in 98% of patients in whom it has been attempted, 15 requiring the addition of a thoracotomy for esophageal resection because of intrathoracic esophageal fixation or bleeding.

In all but 6 patients, esophageal resection and reconstruction were performed during the same operation (Table 25–2). Stomach was used as the visceral esophageal substitute in 1,040 (96%) of our patients undergoing immediate esophageal replacement. Among the 250 patients with acute or chronic caustic injuries, 6 required either partial or total gastric resections, and in these patients, colon was used to replace the esophagus. In 33 others, colon was used as the esophageal substitute when prior gastric resection for peptic ulcer disease precluded use of the stomach as an esophageal substitute. The stomach was positioned in the posterior mediastinum in the original esophageal bed in all but 20 patients in whom either residual posterior mediastinal tumor or fibrosis and narrowing prevented adequate positioning of the stomach for a tension-free cervical anastomosis. In these 20 patients, a retrosternal colonic interposition was performed. Generous mobilization of the duodenum from its retroperitoneal location (Kocher maneuver) is routine when the stomach is used for esophageal replacement. A pyloromyotomy is the usual gastric drainage procedure, and a feeding jejunostomy for postoperative nutritional support is used routinely in every patient undergoing esophageal reconstruction. At the time of esophagectomy, patients with carcinoma undergo routine resection of accessible subcarinal, paraesophageal, and celiac axis lymph nodes, but no attempt is made to perform an en bloc wide resection of the esophagus and its contiguous lymph node–bearing tissues. The generally dismal prognosis of esophageal carcinoma was confirmed in this series by the fact that postsurgical tumor-node-metastasis (TNM) staging of these carcinomas indicated that 46% were either transmurally invasive or metastatic beyond the regional lymph nodes (TNM stage III or IV) (Table 25–3). There was one intraoperative death in this series from mediastinal hemorrhage that could not be con-

Table 25–3. Postsurgical TNM Staging of 800 Intrathoracic Esophageal Carcinomas*

Stage	Tumor Site: *Upper*	*Middle*	*Lower*	Cardia	Total
0†	8	15	45	4	72 (9.0%)
I	2	25	57	10	94 (11.8%)
IIA	10	48	109	22	189 (23.6%)
IIB	2	19	46	12	79 (9.9%)
III	9	54	170	63	296 (37.0%)
IVA	—	2	15	11	28 (3.5%)
IVB	5	14	17	2	39 (4.9%)
Unstaged‡			2	1	3 (0.4%)
TOTAL	36 (4.5%)	177 (22.1%)	462 (57.8%)	125 (15.6%)	800 (100.0%)

*From Orringer M.B., Marshall B., Iannettoni M.D.: Transhiatal esophagectomy: Clinical experience and refinements. Ann. Surg, *230*:392–400, 1999, with permission. Staging data from Fleming, I.R., et al. (eds.): AJCC Cancer Staging Handbook. From AJCC Cancer Staging Manual, 5th ed., Philadelphia, Lippincott Williams & Wilkins, 1998, with permission.

†Includes 14 Tis + 59 T0 after prior chemotherapy and/or radiation.

‡Includes 1 intraoperative death, 1 stromal carcinoma, and 1 T0, Nx, M0 patient.

trolled. Measured intraoperative blood loss averaged 652 ml in patients with carcinoma and 795 ml in patients with benign disease (Table 25–4).

Intraoperative Complications

Entry into one or both pleural cavities occurred intraoperatively and was treated with a chest tube or tubes in 831 patients (77%). Intraoperative membranous tracheal lacerations occurred in four patients. Three involved the high membranous trachea and were repaired through a partial upper sternal split. One tear involved the membranous trachea and was managed by guiding the endotracheal tube into the left main-stem bronchus by palpation through the diaphragmatic hiatus, selectively ventilating one lung, and then performing a substernal gastric bypass. Then, through a right thoracotomy, the esophagectomy was completed, and the tracheal tear was successfully repaired. In 34 patients (3%), a splenectomy was required because of intraoperative injury. Entry into the duodenal or gastric mucosa during performance of the pyloromyotomy occurred in less than 2%. This was managed by suturing the hole and buttressing the repair with adjacent omentum.

Postoperative Complications

Five patients (two with a megaesophagus of achalasia and three with carcinoma) were reoperated on within 24 hours of transhiatal esophagectomy for control of mediastinal bleeding from the aortic esophageal arteries. Left recurrent laryngeal nerve injury occurred in 74 patients (7%); the hoarseness was transient in 50 of the patients and resolved spontaneously in 2 to 12 weeks. Of 24 patients (less than 1%) with true vocal cord paralysis, a vocal cord medialization procedure has been performed in 7. This complication was more common in our early experience with this operation and was initially believed to be an unavoidable result of blunt dissection in the subaortic area along the course of the left recurrent laryngeal nerve. However, after accumulating more experience with this procedure, it has become apparent that recurrent laryngeal nerve injury associated with transhiatal esophagectomy is an almost totally preventable iatrogenic complication. Since adopting a policy of avoiding placement of any retractor against the tracheoesophageal groove during the cervical portions of the operation, our incidence of recurrent laryngeal nerve injury after transhiatal esophagectomy has fallen to less than 3%. Injury to the thoracic duct resulting in postoperative chylothorax occurred in 18 patients (less than 1%), 12 of whom had carcinoma and 6 of whom had benign disease. Chylothorax occurring in a nutritionally depleted patient with esophageal obstruction must be treated aggressively. In all 18 of our patients, transthoracic ligation of the injured thoracic duct within 7 to 10 days of operation was carried out with a successful outcome in each case.[75]

The overall rate of anastomotic leak following cervical esophagogastric anastomosis has been 13% (146 patients); 36 (25%) occurred among the 258 patients with benign disease in whom the stomach was used to replace the esophagus; and 110 (75%) occurred among the 782 patients with CEGA for carcinoma. Among the 7 patients in whom the stomach was positioned *retrosternally*, there were 6 anastomotic leaks (86%). In contrast, among the 1,030 surviving patients in whom the stomach was positioned in the original esophageal bed in the posterior mediastinum, there were 137 leaks (13%). In all except 9 of the 146 anastomotic leaks in this series, opening the cervical wound at the bedside and local packing provided a successful outcome, and the fistulas healed spontaneously. As reported previously, initiation of esophageal bougienage within 7 to 10 days of opening the neck wound expedites healing and minimizes late severe stenosis.[80] In 9 patients, necrosis of the upper stomach at the thoracic inlet occurred, necessitating takedown of the stomach from the chest and a cervical esophagostomy.

Table 25–4. Measured Intraoperative Blood Loss With Transhiatal Esophagectomy*

Diagnosis	No. of Patients	Range (Average)
Benign disease	282†	100–4,000 ml (795 ml)
Carcinoma	794†	35–4,250 ml (652 ml)
Upper third	36	75–3,000 ml (820 ml)
Middle third	175†	50–4,250 ml (748 ml)
Lower third	586†	35–3,600 ml (613 ml)
Total	1,076	35–4,250 ml (689 ml)

*From Orringer, M.B., Marshall, B., and Iannettoni, M.D.: Transhiatal esophagectomy: Clinical experience and refinements. Ann. Surg, *230*:392–400, 1999, with permission.

†Excludes 3 intraoperative deaths due to hemorrhage, 2 with benign disease and 1 with carcinoma, and 6 surviving patients who experienced inordinate intraoperative blood loss ranging from 5,850 to 18,440 ml.

Mortality

The total hospital mortality rate among these 1,085 patients was 4% (44 deaths). Among the 250 patients with benign disease, there were 8 deaths (2.8%) resulting from sepsis (5), acute myocardial infarction (1), respiratory insufficiency (1), and portal vein thrombosis after splenectomy (1). There were 36 deaths (4.5%) among the 800 patients with carcinoma resulting from hepatic failure (6), respiratory insufficiency (5), myocardial infarction (4), intraoperative hemorrhage (3), pneumonia (3), sepsis (3), intestinal ischemia (3), sudden death/cardiac arrest (3), pulmonary embolus (2), and posterior mediastinal abscess, retroperitoneal abscess, unrecognized brain metastasis, and delayed pyloromyotomy leak (1 each).

FUNCTIONAL RESULTS OF VISCERAL ESOPHAGEAL SUBSTITUTION WITH STOMACH

Benign Disease

Follow-up information regarding functional results for up to 213 months (average 47 months) is available in 242 of the 251 hospital survivors of transhiatal esophagectomy and esophageal replacement with stomach. The functional results of esophageal substitution have been assessed by analyzing the presence and degree of (1) dysphagia, (2) regurgitation, and (3) postvagotomy diarrhea and cramping ("dumping"). Passage of a tapered Maloney esophageal dilator is utilized liberally for *any* degree of cervical dysphagia occurring after discharge from the hospital. With this liberal use of dilatation therapy, 186 of these patients (77%) have had at least one postoperative esophageal dilatation. At the time of their most recent follow-up 157 (65%) are eating a regular unrestricted diet; 38 (16%) have intermittent mild dysphagia that requires no treatment; 36 (15%) require an occasional esophageal dilatation but swallow well between treatments and are satisfied with their ability to eat; and 11 (4%) require regular dilatations (daily or weekly) for severe dysphagia.

Postoperative gastroesophageal reflux was completely denied by 146 (60%) of these patients, whereas on careful questioning, 77 (32%) acknowledged experiencing occasional regurgitation, primarily if they lay down shortly after eating. They sleep comfortably, horizontally, on only one or two pillows and do not feel that they have significant reflux. More regular and troublesome nocturnal regurgitation, however, has been experienced by 18 patients (7%) who must sleep with the head of their bed elevated at night. To date, only 1 (less than 1%) of our patients with a cervical esophagogastric anastomosis has experienced pulmonary complication secondary to aspiration. Postprandial abdominal cramping and diarrhea often occur after an esophagectomy with its accompanying vagotomy and CEGA. In most patients, these symptoms are transient and gradually subside over the course of the first year.

At the time of the last follow-up evaluation 147 (61%) of our patients with benign disease denied any diarrhea or cramping. "Mild" diarrhea (occasional, requiring no treatment) is experienced by 49 (20%); "moderate" diarrhea (periodically requiring medication for control) is experienced by 16 (7%); and "severe" diarrhea requiring regular medication, such as diphenoxylate, loperamide, or tincture of opium, is experienced by 10 (4%). Thirty-eight patients (16%) acknowledge experiencing mild intermittent postprandial cramping that requires no treatment, whereas 9 (4%) use an antispasmodic on a regular basis to control their moderate cramping. Some degree of "dumping syndrome" (postprandial nausea, cramping, diaphoresis, palpitations, diarrhea) has been experienced by 95 patients (40%) but fortunately subsides over time and is well controlled with diphenoxylate or tincture of opium.

The functional results of esophageal substitution with stomach have been scored as follows: excellent (completely asymptomatic); good (mild symptoms requiring no treatment); fair (symptoms requiring occasional treatment such as an esophageal dilatation or antidiarrheal medication); and poor (symptoms requiring regular treatment). At the time of the latest follow-up, 71 (29%) of the patients were rated as having an excellent result, 93 (39%) a good result, 68 (28%) a fair result, and 10 (4%) a poor result.

Carcinoma

Patients undergoing esophagectomy and esophageal replacement for carcinoma tend to have a shorter life expectancy than those with benign disease, and because they are often more debilitated preoperatively and have a slower recovery, they tend to register fewer complaints in follow-up than patients with benign disease. Of the 748 hospital survivors of transhiatal esophagectomy and esophageal replacement with stomach for carcinoma, 72 have follow-up information regarding functional results available for up to 194 months (average, 29 months) after surgery. As indicated previously, outpatient esophageal dilatations are performed liberally in patients with any complaint of cervical dysphagia in postoperative follow-up. In contrast to patients with benign disease, in whom only 23% have never undergone a postoperative esophageal dilatation, of the 721 patients with cancer who have had regular postoperative follow-up, 343 (48%) have never undergone an esophageal dilatation.

At the time of the last follow-up, 575 (80%) denied experiencing any dysphagia; 71 (10%) had mild dysphagia that required no treatment; 55 (8%) underwent an occasional dilatation for moderate dysphagia; and 20 patients (2%) had severe dysphagia that necessitated regular esophageal dilatations. Five hundred and seventy-one (79%) denied experiencing any regurgitation; 124 (17%) had mild regurgitation if they lay down shortly after eating, but they still sleep horizontally without difficulty; and 25 (3.5%) sleep with the head of the bed elevated to prevent nocturnal reflux. One patient (less than 1%) experienced pulmonary complications due to aspiration. Five hundred and thirty (74%) denied any postprandial cramping or diarrhea. One hundred ninety-one (26%) had dumping symptoms of varying degrees: 117 (16%) mild diarrhea requiring no treatment; 27 (14%), moderate diarrhea requiring occasional medication; and 6 (<1%), severe diarrhea necessitating regular medication. Eighty-three patients (11.5%) experienced postprandial cramping that was mild and required no treatment, whereas 13 (2%) used periodic antispasmodics to control their moderate cramping. The overall functional result at the time of latest follow-up in these patients with carcinoma was as follows: excellent (asymptomatic) in 389 (54%); good (mild symptoms requiring no treatment) in 204 (28%); fair (symptoms requiring occasional treatment) in 108 (15%); and poor (severe dysphagia requiring regular dilatation) in 20 (3%).

Survival of Patients With Carcinoma

There were 764 operative survivors among the 800 patients undergoing transhiatal esophagectomy for carcinoma. Thirty-one (4%) have been lost to follow-up. Patients were followed for up to 195 months (mean 27 months) after transhiatal esophagectomy. Figure 24–27 shows the Kaplan-Meier actuarial survival for the first 5 years after transhiatal esophagectomy for carcinoma of the intrathoracic esophagus and cardia and indicates an overall 2-year survival rate of 47% and a 5-year survival of 23%. The 5-year survival rate of patients with lower-third cancers was 26% compared with 13% in those with

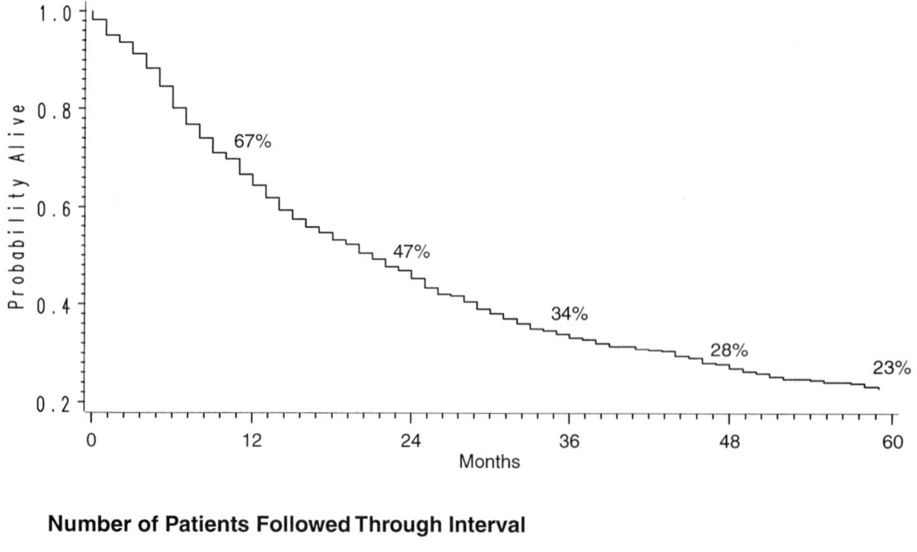

Figure 25–27. Kaplan-Meier actuarial survival curve of 800 patients undergoing transhiatal esophagectomy for carcinoma of the intrathoracic esophagus and cardia. (From Orringer, M.B., Marshall, B., and Iannettoni, M.D.: Transhiatal esophagectomy: Clinical experience and refinements. Ann. Surg., *230:* 392, 1999, with permission.)

middle-third carcinomas and 24% in those with upper-third tumors (Fig. 25–28). A total of 217 (27%) of our 800 patients undergoing a transhiatal esophagectomy for carcinoma have had preoperative chemotherapy and radiation therapy at either our Medical Center[31,79] or other facilities. Of these, 49 (23%) had T0 N0 tumors (complete responders) on assessment of the resected esophagus. For these 49 patients, the 2-year actuarial survival rate was 86%, and the 5-year actuarial survival rate, 48% (Fig. 25–29). Predictably, tumor stage has been an important determinant of survival after transhiatal esophagectomy, the survival rate with stage 0 and I tumors being considerably better than that associated with stage III and IV disease (Fig. 25–30; Table 25–5). Adenocarcinomas were associated with an overall statistically significant ($P <$ 0.01) survival advantage compared with squamous carcinomas, and this advantage approached statistical significance ($P = 0.06$) at 5 years (Fig. 25–31).

SUMMARY

In our experience, transhiatal esophagectomy has been applicable in almost every patient requiring esophagectomy for either benign or malignant disease. More difficult resections may be facilitated by placing narrow deep retractors within the diaphragmatic hiatus and dissecting the esophagus from the lower mediastinum under direct vision. Pinotti and associates of Brazil routinely incise the

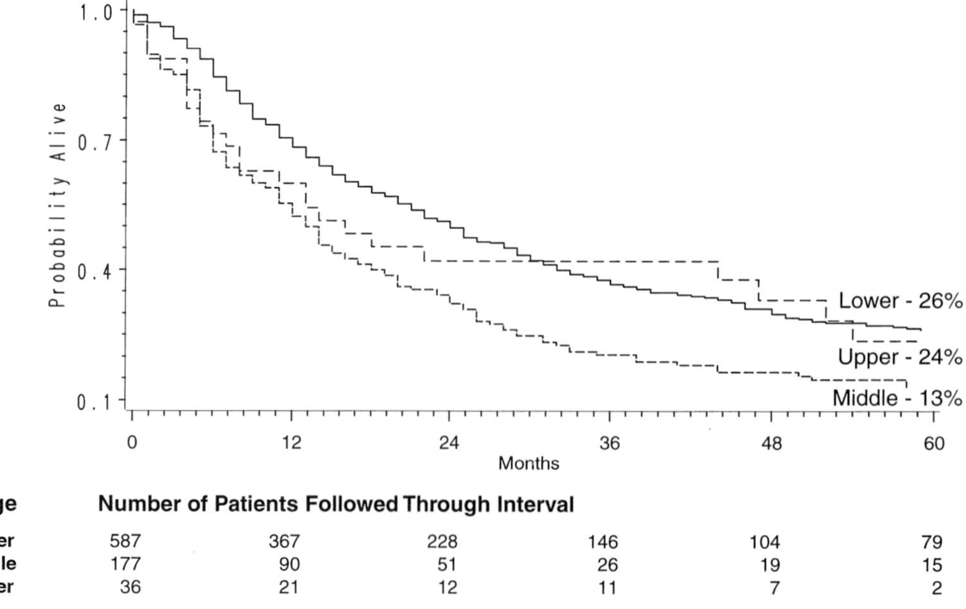

Stage	Number of Patients Followed Through Interval					
Lower	587	367	228	146	104	79
Middle	177	90	51	26	19	15
Upper	36	21	12	11	7	2

Figure 25–28. Site-dependent Kaplan-Meier survival curves in patients undergoing transhiatal esophagectomy for carcinoma of the intrathoracic esophagus and cardia. (From Orringer, M.B., Marshall, B., and Iannettoni, M.D.: Transhiatal esophagectomy: Clinical experience and refinements. Ann. Surg., *230:*392, 1999, with permission.)

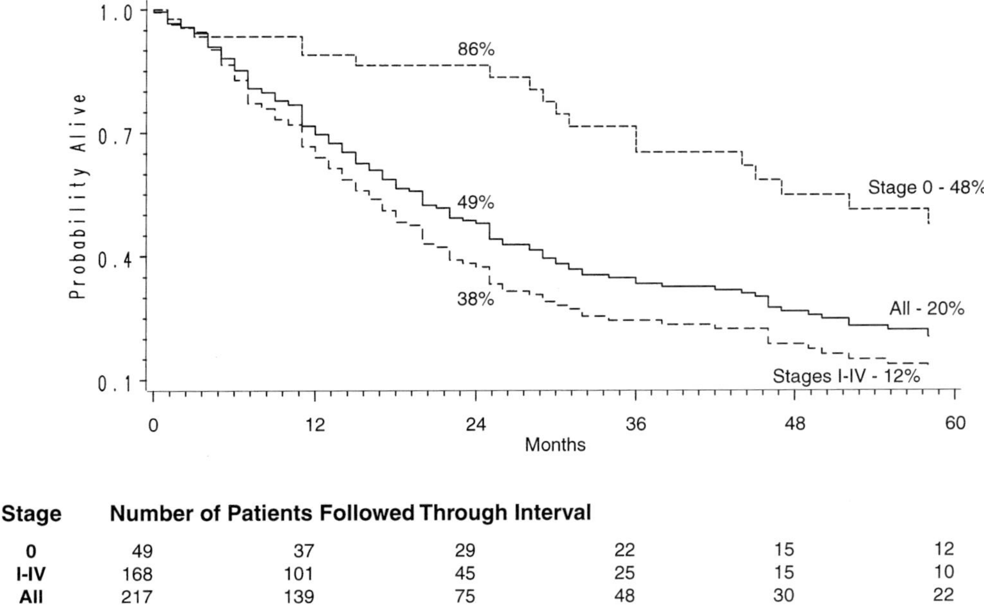

Stage	Number of Patients Followed Through Interval					
0	49	37	29	22	15	12
I-IV	168	101	45	25	15	10
All	217	139	75	48	30	22

Figure 25–29. Kaplan-Meier survival curve in patients receiving chemotherapy and radiation therapy before transhiatal esophagectomy. (From Orringer, M.B., Marshall, B., and Iannettoni, M.D.: Transhiatal esophagectomy: Clinical experience and refinements. Ann. Surg., *230*:392, 1999, with permission.)

diaphragm from the anterior hiatus toward the xiphoid to facilitate the esophagectomy in their patients with megaesophagus due to achalasia.[91] We have used this approach in only five of our patients. The surgeon undertaking a transhiatal esophagectomy without thoracotomy *must* be prepared to convert to a transthoracic esophageal resection if palpation of the esophagus through the diaphragmatic hiatus indicates marked fixation of the esophagus to adjacent structures. The single most important contraindication to this operation is the surgeon's judgment that this approach is unsafe. Nevertheless, among our last 1,100 consecutive patients with operable carcinoma of the intrathoracic esophagus, transhiatal esophagectomy has been possible in 1,085 (98.6%). The

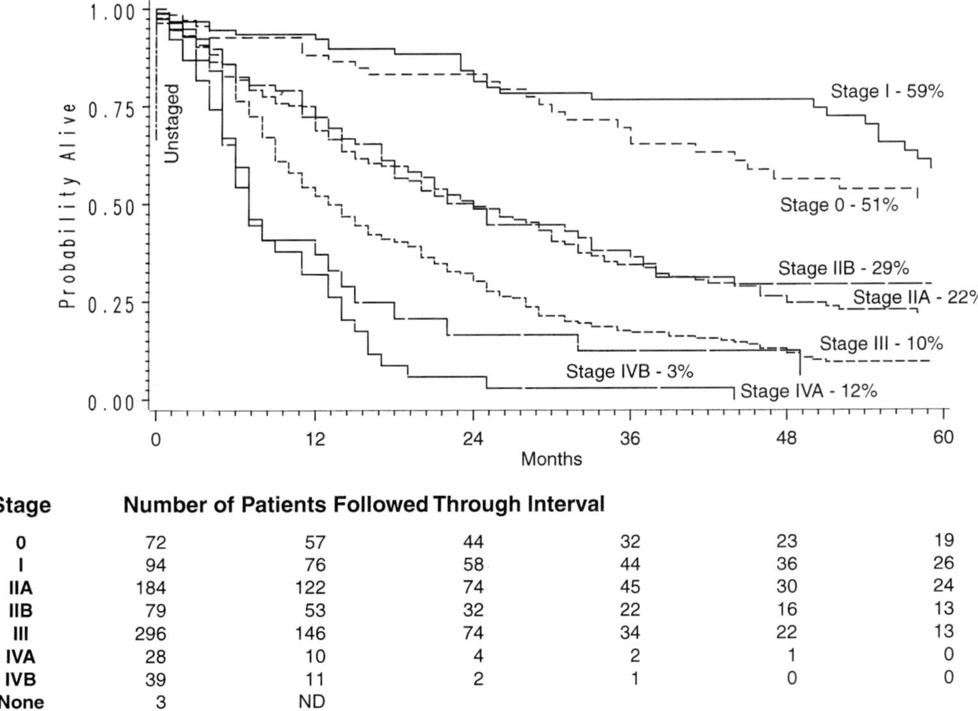

Stage	Number of Patients Followed Through Interval					
0	72	57	44	32	23	19
I	94	76	58	44	36	26
IIA	184	122	74	45	30	24
IIB	79	53	32	22	16	13
III	296	146	74	34	22	13
IVA	28	10	4	2	1	0
IVB	39	11	2	1	0	0
None	3	ND				

Figure 25–30. Stage-dependent Kaplan-Meier actuarial survival curves in patients undergoing transhiatal esophagectomy for carcinoma of the intrathoracic esophagus and cardia. (From Orringer, M.B., Marshall, B., and Iannettoni, M.D.: Transhiatal esophagectomy: Clinical experience and refinements. Ann. Surg., *230*:392, with permission.)

Table 25–5. Kaplan-Meier Survival After Transhiatal Esophagectomy by Tumor Stage*

TNM Stage	No. of Patients	Survival (%) 2 Years	Survival (%) 5 Years
0	72	83	51
I	94	84	59
IIA	189	50	22
IIB	79	51	29
III	296	32	10
IVA	28	17	7
IVB	39	6	0

*From Orringer, M.B., Marshall, B., and Iannettoni, M.D.: Transhiatal esophagectomy: Clinical experience and refinements. Ann. Surg., *230*:392–400, 1999, with permission.

addition of a partial upper sternal split is helpful in facilitating dissection of the upper and midthoracic esophagus in patients with tumors in both of these locations as well as in those with periesophageal fibrosis following prior surgery in this area.

I believe that the stomach is the preferred organ for esophageal replacement for both benign and malignant disease. Unlike thin-walled small or large intestine, the stomach is a resilient, thick-walled *upper* gastrointestinal organ that functions normally to transmit semisolid chewed food and is not prone to the redundancy that frequently occurs with intestinal esophageal substitutes. The extremely high incidence of significant gastroesophageal reflux and esophagitis that accompanies an *intrathoracic* esophagogastric anastomosis is seldom encountered with a properly performed *cervical* anastomosis. Based on my communications with several other esophageal surgeons, it appears that an anastomosis between the *end* of the cervical esophagus and the *end* of the amputated tip of the gastric fundus in the neck is associated with significant postoperative gastroesophageal reflux. In contrast, when the gastric fundus is mobilized as far superiorly as possible in the neck wound, and the end of the cervical esophagus is anastomosed to the anterior wall of the stomach several centimeters from the top, the resultant acute angle of entry from the esophagus into the stomach, as well as the retroesophageal gastric segment, tends to minimize subsequent gastroesophageal reflux. The stomach anastomosed to the cervical esophagus appears to be an excellent esophageal substitute. About 30% of these patients will experience occasional mild reflux, particularly if they lie down immediately after eating. Transient dumping syndrome (postprandial cramping, diarrhea, diaphoresis, palpitations, and so forth), seldom disabling, occurs in varying degrees in nearly 70%. Almost 70% of our patients have undergone at least one outpatient CEGA dilatation early after operation, but swallowing is ultimately regarded as good or excellent in about 80%. Patients who develop an anastomotic leak have at least a 50% incidence of subsequent anastomotic stricture. The dramatic reduction in anastomotic leak rate associated with our use of the side-to-side stapled cervical esophagogastric anastomosis has markedly reduced the need for postoperative anastomotic dilatation and resulted in improved swallowing for patients.[82]

Regardless of whether stomach or colon is used to replace the esophagus, the posterior mediastinum is preferred to the retrosternal route. First, the posterior mediastinum is the shortest distance between the neck and the abdomen. Second, because the cervical esophagus must form an angle anteriorly to meet the retrosternal stomach or colon, any subsequent endoscopic or dilatation procedures that are required are more difficult than when the instruments can be passed directly posteriorly into the esophageal substitute in the original esophageal bed. Finally, in the posterior neck in the esophageal bed,

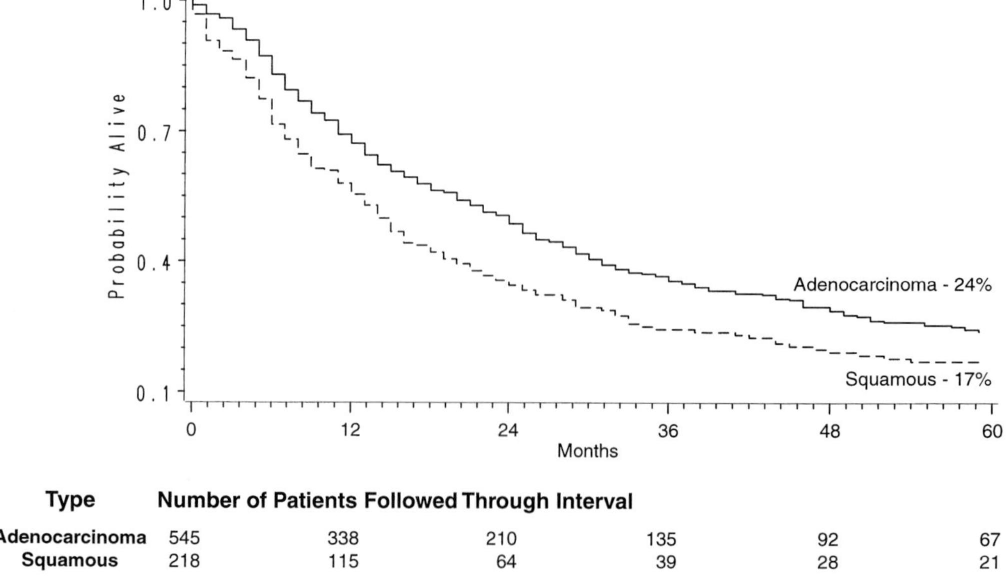

Figure 25–31. Histology-dependent Kaplan-Meier survival curves in patients undergoing transhiatal esophagectomy for carcinoma of the intrathoracic esophagus and cardia. (From Orringer, M.B., Marshall, B., and Iannettoni, M.D.: Transhiatal esophagectomy: Clinical experience and refinements. Ann. Surg., *230*:392, 1999, with permission.)

the cervical anastomosis is "buttressed" by the spine, the trachea, the carotid sheath, and the anterior cervical strap muscles. In contrast, in its relatively subcutaneous "unsupported" location, the anastomosis between the cervical esophagus and a retrosternal stomach or colon is more likely to leak in the early postoperative period. This fact is emphasized by our 13% rate of anastomotic leaks with the stomach positioned in the original esophageal bed, compared with the 86% leak rate with retrosternally positioned stomachs.

With the notable exception of some recent reported series of esophagectomies with operative mortality rates of less than 5%, in most contemporary Western series of esophageal resection and reconstruction between 1980 and 1988, the average reported mortality rate was 13%.[69] Transhiatal esophagectomy without thoracotomy is simply a less severe physiologic insult to the weakened patient with esophageal obstruction than the traditional combined thoracic and abdominal operation. Ninety-one per cent of our patients were discharged and able to eat within 3 weeks of operation. Recently, the average length of stay after an uncomplicated transhiatal esophagectomy has been reduced to 7 days. Postoperative pulmonary complications ("splinting," atelectasis, pneumonia, and respiratory insufficiency associated with incisional pain) and fatal mediastinitis due to anastomotic disruption are virtually eliminated when a thoracotomy and an intrathoracic esophageal anastomosis are avoided and pulmonary physiotherapy is given strict attention. Despite early expressed concerns about the potential for major intrathoracic hemorrhage, significant intraoperative blood loss does not occur with a properly performed transhiatal esophagectomy, and the average blood loss for this operation has been 689 ml. The need for a chest tube because of entry into one or both pleural cavities during the esophagectomy is easily managed. Recurrent laryngeal nerve injury should occur rarely. Thus, the most frequent complications of transhiatal esophagectomy can be avoided with proper surgical judgment and technique.

The greatest controversy about the use of transhiatal esophagectomy remains the appropriateness of this operation in patients with esophageal cancer. Proponents of traditionally held views of cancer surgery argue that transhiatal esophagectomy precludes an en bloc mediastinal lymphadenectomy and thus denies the patient with esophageal cancer both accurate tumor staging and the chance for potential cure. Unfortunately, only in countries where mass screening techniques provide a large population of patients with carcinoma limited to the mucosa and submucosa is this tumor frequently encountered in a localized, surgically curable form. In most esophageal cancer patients in Western countries, distant nodal metastases and transmural tumor invasion preclude cure. In our series, for example, 46% of the patients had either stage III or stage IV tumors on the basis of their postsurgical pathology, and cure of such "systemic" disease by any operation is unlikely. In addition, 217 of our patients have had preoperative radiation therapy and chemotherapy that likely "downstaged" their esophageal cancers.

Advocates of radical operations intended to "cure" cancer at other sites are becoming smaller in number as objective comparison of survival with less radical methods of treatment is made. For example, it is now generally agreed that the traditional Halsted radical mastectomy with en bloc dissection of regional lymph nodes in continuity with the breast primary for breast carcinoma offers no better survival than simple mastectomy followed by postoperative radiation therapy.[25,29,115] Similarly, a recently reported prospective randomized trial evaluating radical lymph node dissection for gastric cancer, with more than 300 patients in each arm of the study, found no survival benefit for the more radical procedure.[15] Radical esophagectomy with en bloc "complete" lymphadenectomy continues to be advocated by some.[5,6,45,60] However, our survival statistics after transhiatal esophagectomy for esophageal carcinoma are similar to those reported in most Western series of standard transthoracic esophagectomy[13,14,37,39,50,67] and to those reported after so-called radical en bloc esophagectomy with mediastinal lymphadenectomy.[101] It is the stage and biologic behavior of the tumor at the time of esophagectomy rather than the operative approach, the size of the specimen, or the number of lymph nodes dissected that determines survival in these patients. Altorki and Skinner have recently reported the presence of occult cervical lymph node metastases in 35% of patients undergoing a three-field lymph node dissection for carcinoma of the thoracic esophagus otherwise thought to be potentially "curable."[7] This finding simply reinforces our position that, in most of our patients, esophageal cancer is a *systemic* disease, and systemic therapy (e.g., chemotherapy or immunotherapy) is most likely required to cure it, if a cure is possible. Patients with stage I carcinomas confined to the esophageal mucosa are curable by any type of esophagectomy, and for this reason, in these patients, I prefer to avoid a thoracotomy and its attendant morbidity whenever possible.

A final word of caution is appropriate in this discussion of the merits of transhiatal esophagectomy, which, like many operations, is safe and well tolerated if it is performed carefully and with proper judgment. The esophagus is a *thoracic* organ, and most complications of esophageal resection and reconstruction are thoracic. The fact that a thoracotomy is not necessary in most patients requiring esophageal resection does not absolve the surgeon from the responsibility of having a sound knowledge of thoracic anatomy and the relevant surgical complications and their management. Control of thoracic aortic bleeding, the limits of pericardial resection, isolation and control of the thoracic duct, and use of selective one-lung ventilation are basic in the training of thoracic surgeons. Absence of the need for a thoracic incision in patients requiring esophageal resection does not relegate the performance of transhiatal esophagectomy to the general abdominal surgeon who has had no prior thoracic surgical experience.

RESECTION OF CARCINOMA INVOLVING THE CERVICOTHORACIC ESOPHAGUS—CERVICAL EXENTERATION

The cervicothoracic esophagus may be involved by malignancies of laryngotracheal, esophageal, or thyroid origin.

These tumors, which involve the esophagus and trachea at the thoracic inlet, compromise not only the ability to swallow but often the airway as well. Successful management of these tumors requires the application of techniques from a variety of surgical specialties, including thoracic surgery, otolaryngology, plastic surgery, and general surgery. Removal of the esophagus may be the least challenging part of the entire procedure. Laryngectomy and resection of the proximal trachea may be required, often with adjacent anterior cervical skin involved by local tumor recurrence (e.g., recurrence at a tracheal stoma after laryngectomy). Restoration of alimentary continuity, coverage of the great vessels of the neck and superior mediastinum, and establishment of a satisfactory airway pose a formidable challenge. Despite the magnitude of the operative undertaking required to treat these tumors successfully, gratifying palliation and sometimes cure can be achieved with a systematic and organized approach.

Since the 1980s, a variety of methods for reestablishing alimentary continuity after laryngopharyngectomy have been advocated, including myocutaneous flaps, free jejunal segments, stomach, and colon.[32,40,52,68,90,98,103,118] Many have advocated gastric transposition and a pharyngogastric anastomosis.[8,17,48,97,102] This procedure has been associated with mortality rates that have ranged from 5 to 31% and anastomotic leak rates ranging from 7 to 37%. In their experience with 157 pharyngogastric anastomoses after laryngopharyngoesophagectomy, Lam and associates reported a hospital mortality rate of 31% and an anastomotic leak rate of 23%.[58] Sullivan and associates have more recently reported an operative mortality rate of 12% and an anastomotic leak rate of 31% in a group of 32 patients undergoing pharyngogastric anastomoses.[106] Neither of these latter reports discussed the postoperative functional results of pharyngogastrostomy.

Growing experience and expertise in microvascular technique have resulted in free jejunal transfer becoming the most popular method of pharyngeal reconstruction when resecting proximal tumors of the hypopharynx, pharynx, larynx, and esophagus above the thoracic inlet.[18,20,30,52,90,96,98] Successful re-establishment of alimentary continuity has been achieved in nearly 95% of patients undergoing free jejunal transfer and with similar morbidity to that encountered after pharyngogastrostomy.

This has been corroborated by studies comparing free jejunal grafts and pharyngogastric anastomoses and demonstrating little difference in outcome.[24,99] A recent report by Fujita and associates found no significant difference in the incidence of local recurrence and a lower hospital mortality rate (13% versus 50%) in patients undergoing proximal esophagectomy with jejunal transfer and total esophagectomy with pharyngogastrostomy, respectively.[33] On the basis of such reports, it is now generally accepted that a free jejunal transfer is the procedure of choice in patients requiring short-segment reconstructions above the thoracic inlet. Alternatively, tumors that involve the esophagus at the level of the thoracic inlet or below are best treated with a total esophagectomy and either a gastric or colonic interposition.

If a tumor involves the esophagus at the thoracic inlet (Fig. 25-32), the high retrosternal trachea at the same level may also be involved. Therefore, if a concomitant laryngopharyngectomy is required, division of the cervical trachea for construction of a standard tracheostomy may not be possible because the remaining tracheal

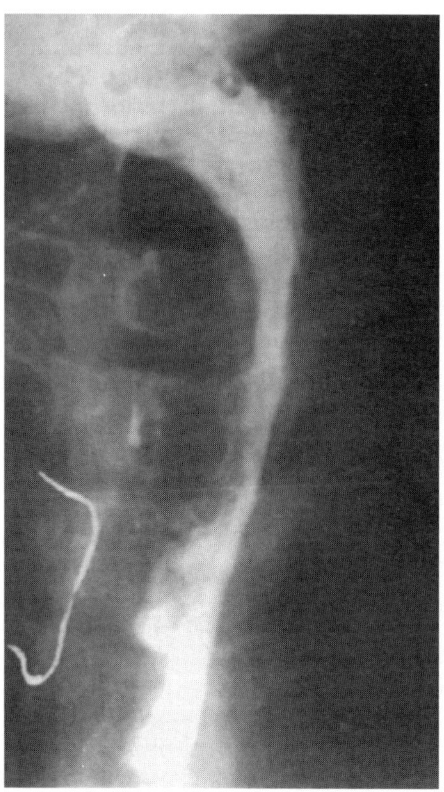

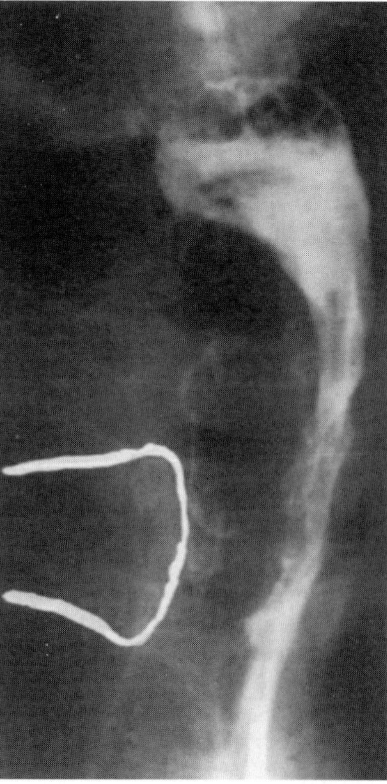

Figure 25-32. Cervical esophagogram in a patient with a large squamous cell carcinoma involving the cervicothoracic esophagus within the thoracic inlet. The head of the clavicle has been highlighted to emphasize how such tumors may straddle the thoracic inlet.

stump beyond the tumor will not reach to the level of the suprasternal notch. Resection of cervicothoracic esophageal malignancies is greatly facilitated by removing the anterior "breast plate," which includes the medial clavicles, upper manubrium of the sternum, and adjacent medial first (and occasional second) rib. With the anterior bony chest wall thus resected, wide exposure of the superior mediastinum and its contents is achieved (Figs. 25-33 and 25-34).[77,87] Using this approach, it is possible to divide the retrosternal trachea to construct an anterior mediastinal tracheostomy and carry out a laryngopharyngesophagectomy without thoracotomy. Alimentary continuity may be re-established using stomach (Figs. 24-35 and 24-36). It should be realized that in constructing a pharyngogastric anastomosis, the stomach is required to reach cephalad to its limit, and consequently every effort must be made to reduce tension on the anastomosis. This is facilitated by performing a generous Kocher maneuver and by creating a long gastric tube by sequential division with the stapler along the lesser curvature (see Fig. 25-13) to maximize the upward reach of the stomach. Despite these maneuvers, tension on the pharyngogastric anastomosis is not uncommon, and this is likely a major contributing factor to the about 30% incidence of anastomotic leaks that have been reported.

Most small, localized pharyngogastric anastomotic leaks are well controlled with continuous suction on subcutaneous drainage catheters placed at the time of surgery. Major disruption, on the other hand, may necessitate taking down the anastomosis, creating a pharyngostome, and later attempting to re-establish alimentary continuity. This is *not* the relatively innocuous course of a standard CEGA after transhiatal esophagectomy. A second serious concern with the pharyngogastric anastomosis is the long-term function result. Although clinically significant gastroesophageal reflux is the exception after a transhiatal esophagectomy and CEGA, resection of the upper esophageal (cricopharyngeal) sphincter, which occurs with a laryngopharyngoesophagectomy, results in nearly uniformly troublesome regurgitation of gastric contents with postural maneuvers such as bending and reclining and with Valsalva maneuvers such as coughing. Long-term survivors of a pharyngogastric anastomosis complain of this troublesome regurgitation. For this reason, I favor use of a colonic interposition to re-establish alimentary continuity after a laryngopharyngoesophagectomy, not because of insufficient gastric length to reach to the pharynx, but rather because a colonic interposition is associated with a lower anastomotic leak rate, less postoperative regurgitation, and therefore a better functional result.[77] Grillo and Mathisen also favor use of the colon to restore alimentary continuity after a cervical exenteration.[44]

Although we originally utilized the bipedicled upper thoracic "apron" flap described by Grillo and Mathisen[44] for resection of the breast plate and construction of the mediastinal tracheostomy, we have subsequently found that resection of the anterior chest wall can be achieved satisfactorily using an extended low collar incision (Figs. 25-37 and 25-38). Skin and subcutaneous tissue may have to be retracted vigorously during the chest wall resection, but the result is well-vascularized anterior thoracic skin rather than the bipedicled apron flap for construction of the tracheostomy. In patients with a tracheal

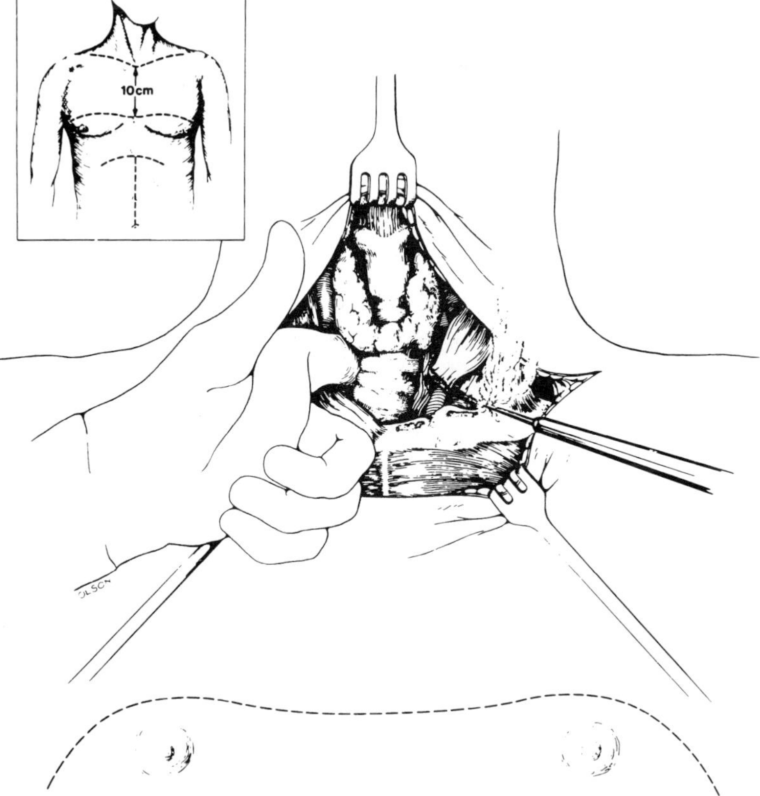

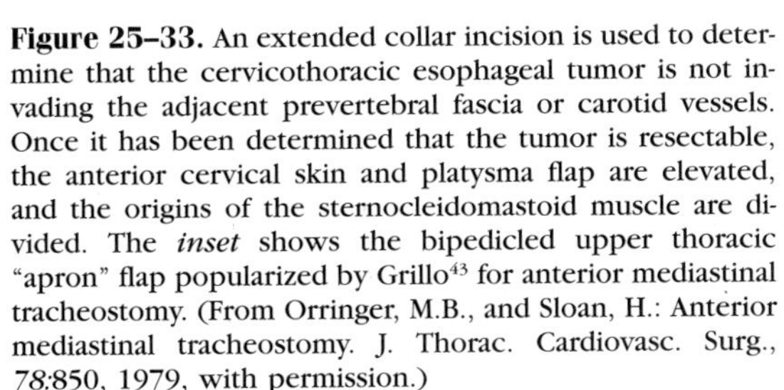

Figure 25-33. An extended collar incision is used to determine that the cervicothoracic esophageal tumor is not invading the adjacent prevertebral fascia or carotid vessels. Once it has been determined that the tumor is resectable, the anterior cervical skin and platysma flap are elevated, and the origins of the sternocleidomastoid muscle are divided. The *inset* shows the bipedicled upper thoracic "apron" flap popularized by Grillo[43] for anterior mediastinal tracheostomy. (From Orringer, M.B., and Sloan, H.: Anterior mediastinal tracheostomy. J. Thorac. Cardiovasc. Surg., *78*:850, 1979, with permission.)

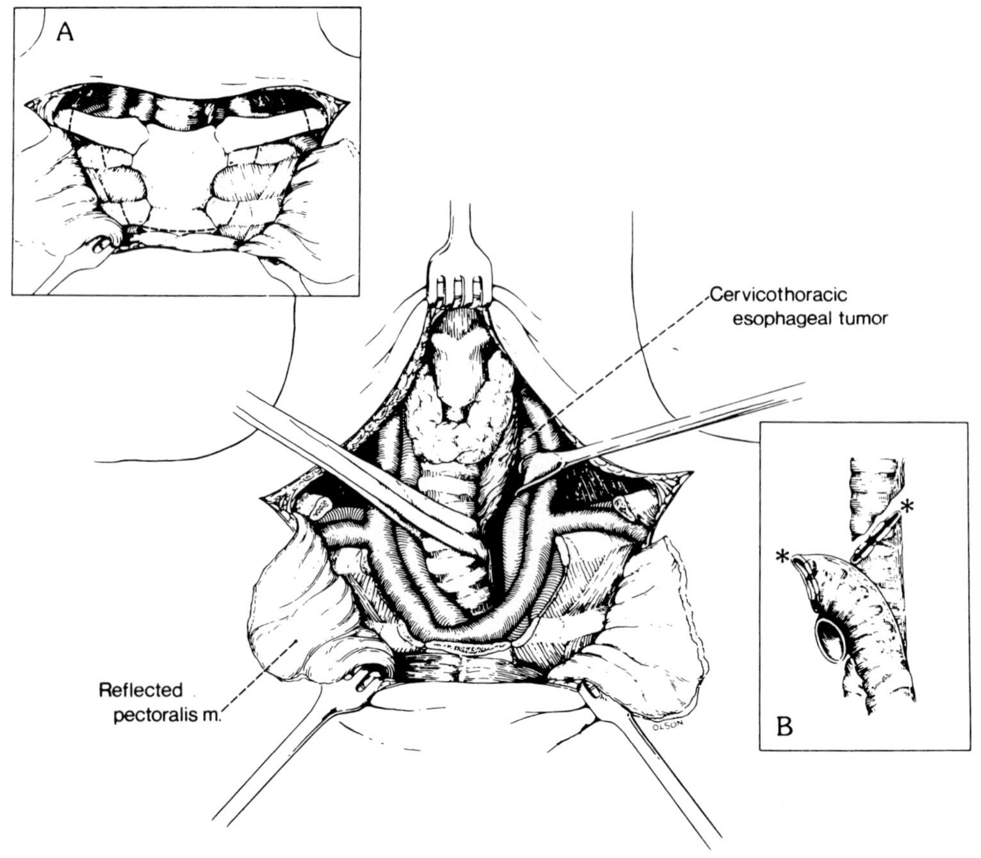

Figure 25–34. *Inset A*, Resection of the anterior thoracic "breast plate" (the medial thirds of the clavicles, short segments of the first and second costal cartilages, and the upper manubrium) permits exposure of the superior mediastinum and its contents, specifically, the trachea, cervicothoracic esophagus, and associated great vessels. *Inset B*, The oblique division of the trachea preserves as much of the posterior membranous portion *(asterisk)* as possible because this is the area that will have to reach most anteriorly when the trachea is brought forward over the innominate artery and sutured to skin. (From Orringer, M.B., and Sloan, H.: Anterior mediastinal tracheostomy. J. Thorac. Cardiovasc. Surg., *78*:850, 1979, with permission.)

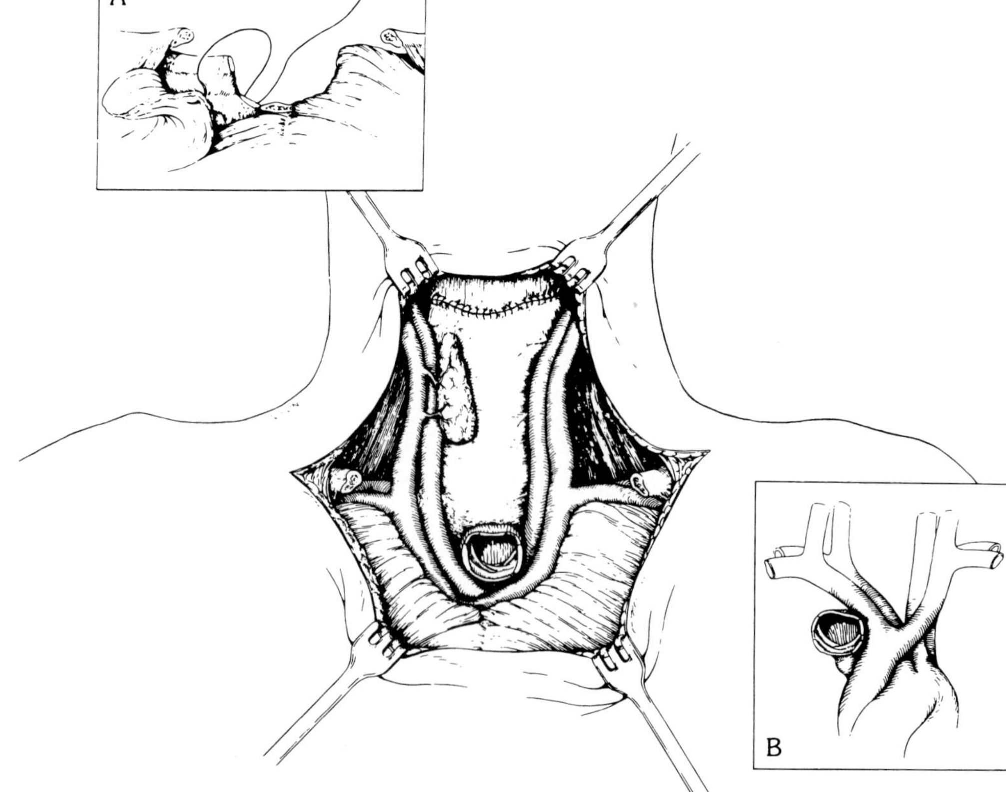

Figure 25–35. The completed pharyngogastric anastomosis. Thyroid and parathyroid function are preserved whenever possible. The divided trachea is positioned over the innominate artery for construction of the mediastinal tracheostomy. *Inset A*, Suturing of the pectoralis muscle over the edge of the divided bony chest wall is shown. *Inset B*, Transposition of the tracheal stump inferiorly and to the right of the innominate artery and vein minimizes tension when the trachea is sewn to the skin. This maneuver is utilized liberally to prevent postoperative innominate artery erosion. (From Orringer, M.B., and Sloan, H.: Anterior mediastinal tracheostomy. J. Thorac. Cardiovasc. Surg., *78*:850, 1979, with permission.)

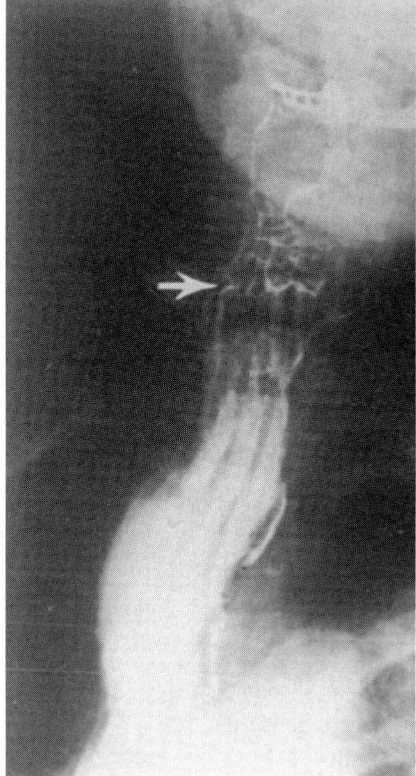

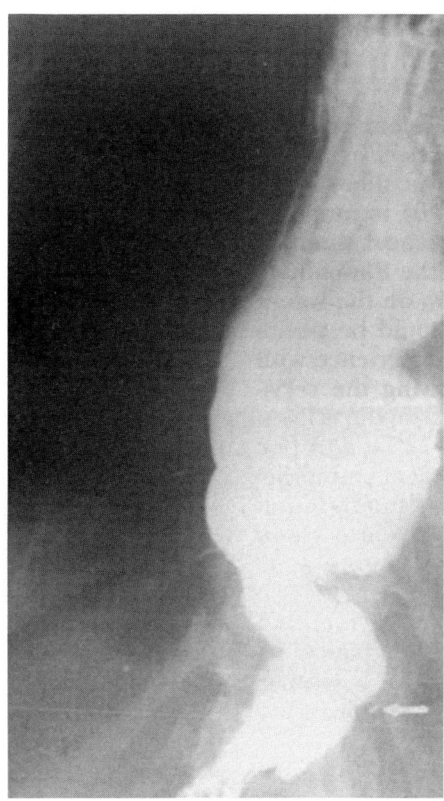

Figure 25–36. Postoperative esophagogram in patient shown in Figure 25–32 after laryngopharyngectomy, anterior mediastinal tracheostomy, and pharyngogastric anastomosis. *Left*, The pharyngogastric anastomosis is indicated by the *arrow*. *Right*, The level of the pyloromyotomy *(arrow)*.

Figure 25–37. The extended collar incision combined with vigorous downward retraction of the anterior upper thoracic skin in most cases permits resection of the anterior breast plate without the need for the additional transverse incisions and skin grafts on the upper chest and abdomen that are required with the Grillo bipedicled upper thoracic "apron" flap. (From Orringer, M.B.: Anterior mediastinal tracheostomy with and without cervical exenteration. Ann. Thorac. Surg., *54*:628, 1992, with permission.)

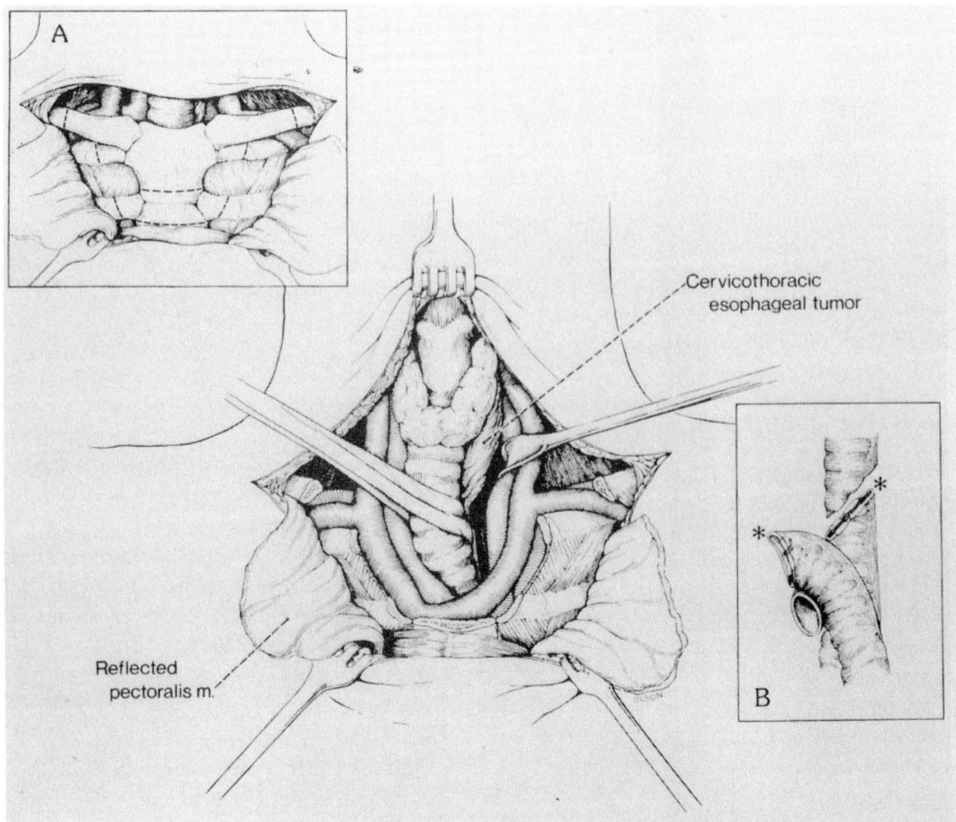

Figure 25–38. Resection of the anterior breast plate for anterior mediastinal tracheostomy. *Inset A* illustrates incision through the medial thirds of the clavicles, adjacent first costal cartilages, and sternum above the sternomanubrial junction *(upper dotted line)*. When a very low tracheal division is required, the second costal cartilages and sternum below the sternomanubrial junction (*lower dotted line* and *inset A* of Fig. 25–34) are resected. (From Orringer, M.B.: Anterior mediastinal tracheostomy with and without cervical exenteration. Ann. Thorac. Surg., *54*:628, 1992, with permission.)

stomal recurrence following a laryngectomy for carcinoma (Figs. 25–39 and 25–40) resection of a 3- to 5-cm margin of skin around the stoma and recurrence is required. In this situation, a thoracoacromial "nipple" flap is used to resurface the anterior neck and superior mediastinum after resecting the former tracheal stoma (Figs. 25–41*B* and *C* and 25–42). To construct an anterior mediastinal tracheostomy, a minimal residual length of 5 cm of distal trachea above the carina is ideal to reach to the skin. Precise preoperative bronchoscopic measurements are mandatory to establish the distance between the ca-

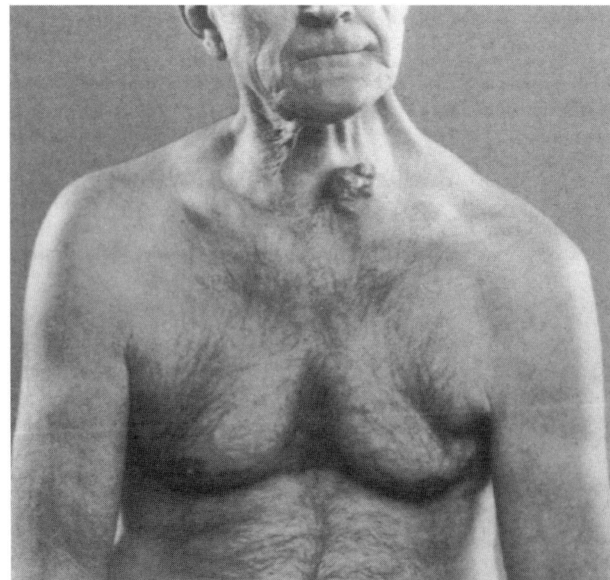

Figure 25–39. Recurrent squamous cell carcinoma of the tracheal stoma in a 60-year-old man who had undergone a laryngectomy for carcinoma 2 years earlier.

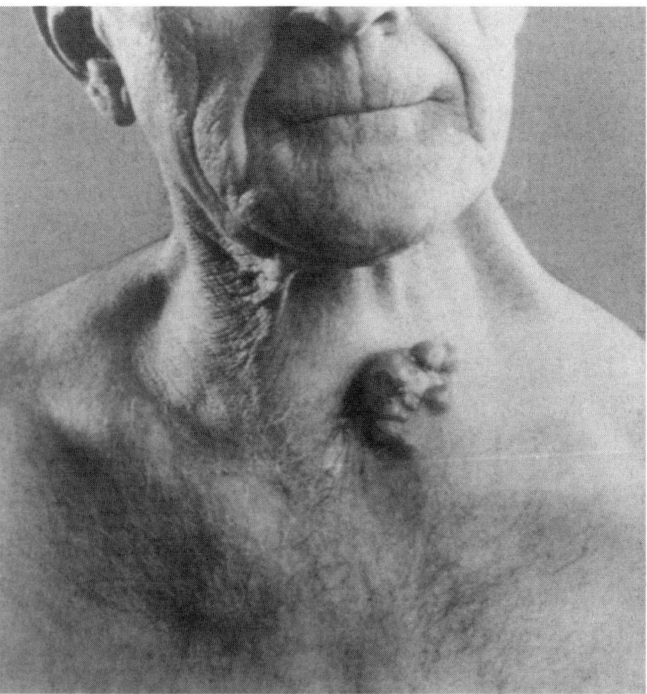

Figure 25–40. Recurrent squamous cell carcinoma; same patient as shown in Figure 25–39.

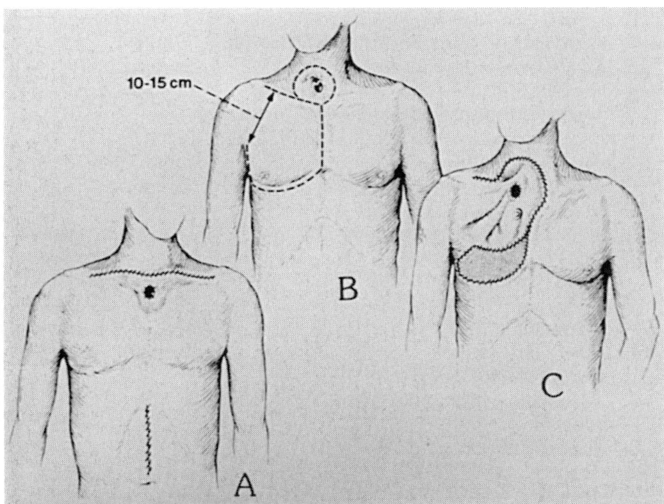

Figure 25–41. *A*, Extended collar incision, anterior mediastinal tracheostomy, and upper midline abdominal incision after cervical exenteration, transhiatal esophagectomy, and pharyngogastric anastomosis. *B*, Incisions for resection of tracheal stomal recurrences and skin involved by tumor and the thoracoacromial "nipple" flap used for reconstruction. *C*, Rotated thoracoacromial flap in position, mediastinal tracheostomy, and skin graft *(stippled area)* over anterior thorax. (From Orringer, M.B., and Sloan, H.: Anterior mediastinal tracheostomy with and without cervical exenteration. Ann. Thorac. Surg., *56*:628, 1992, with permission.)

rina and the tumor and assess operability. Early reports describing anterior mediastinal tracheostomy list subsequent innominate artery erosion as a major postoperative complication and cause of death.[43] This complication results because the divided trachea erodes into the innominate artery, where it has been pulled forward over the top of the artery and sutured to the skin. Grillo and Mathisen emphasized their concern about the possibility of innominate artery erosion after mediastinal tracheostomy by advocating prophylactic division of the innominate artery after preoperative aortic arch angiography and intraoperative electroencephalographic monitoring after clamping the vessel for 10 minutes before dividing it.[44] Mathisen and colleagues divided the artery in 7 of their 14 patients undergoing anterior mediastinal tracheostomy. In addition, they interposed the mobilized omentum between the mediastinal great vessels, the trachea, and the skin to eliminate erosion of the great vessels.[65]

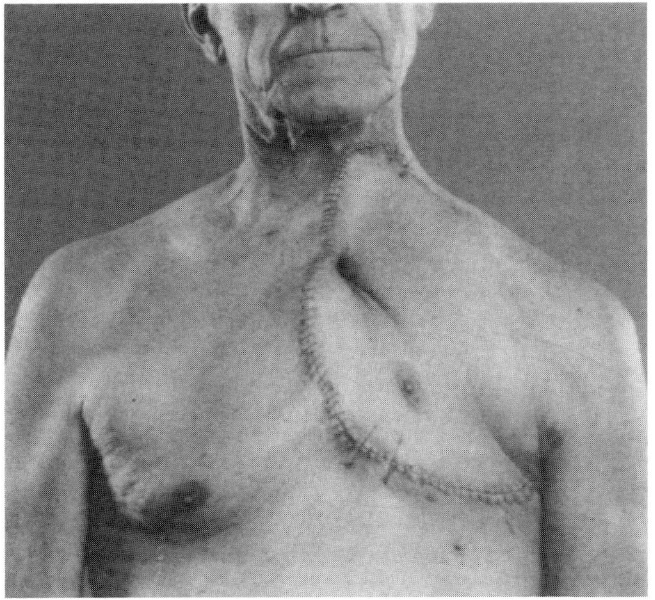

Figure 25–42. Completed left thoracoacromial "nipple" flap used to resurface the skin of the anterior neck following resection of the tracheal stomal recurrence shown in Figures 25-39 and 25-40.

I am convinced, however, that innominate artery erosion after mediastinal tracheostomy can be avoided without the need to divide the vessel or to mobilize omentum into the neck if, whenever there is the least concern about undue pressure on the innominate artery by the trachea, the remaining tracheal stump is transposed beneath and to the right of the innominate artery (see Fig. 25-35*B*). Without tension on the suture line between skin and trachea, there should be no innominate artery erosion. Thus, in our experience with 47 exenterations for malignancies involving the cervicothoracic esophagus, an anterior mediastinal tracheostomy has been required in 34 patients (72%), and one third have had transposition of the tracheal stump beneath the innominate artery. And with no interposition of either muscle or omentum between the artery and trachea, we have encountered only one postoperative innominate artery erosion in this group.[76]

The magnitude of the operative undertaking required to resect a cervicothoracic esophageal malignancy, re-establish alimentary continuity, and provide a satisfactory airway cannot be underestimated and requires considerable surgical expertise. The results of surgical therapy in these patients, many of whom represent failures of radiation therapy to control the primary tumor, are not nearly so good as those achieved when only an esophagectomy and visceral esophageal substitution are required.

Among our 47 patients requiring cervical exenterations for carcinoma involving the cervicothoracic esophagus, 39 (83%) had squamous carcinoma of either the hypopharynx, the postcricoid esophagus, or the cervicothoracic esophagus. In five (11%), the cervicothoracic esophagus was involved by laryngeal squamous carcinoma; in two (4%), by thyroid cancer; and in one (2%), by a high malignant tracheoesophageal fistula. An anterior mediastinal tracheostomy was required in 34 (72%) of these patients. A transhiatal esophagectomy without thoracotomy was performed in all. Alimentary continuity was re-established with a pharyngogastric anastomosis in 44 (94%) and with colon in 3 (6%), in whom a prior gastric resection for ulcer disease precluded use of the stomach as an esophageal substitute. Twenty-six (55%) of these patients had undergone preoperative head and neck radiation therapy. The resultant morbidity was high. Eight (17%) hospital-related deaths occurred. Thirteen patients (28%) sustained anastomotic leaks, most of which were well controlled with local drainage, but one of these resulted in major anastomotic dehiscence necessitating a free jejunal graft between the remaining pharynx and stomach, which had been mobilized into the neck. Whenever possible, the thyroid and parathyroid glands should be preserved, or the parathyroid glands should be dissected from the specimen and reimplanted into either adjacent pectoral muscle or the forearm. Unfortunately, given the degree of preoperative radiation therapy received by many of these patients, it was often impossible to identify the parathyroid glands within the fibrotic cervical tissues. Thus, 13 (28%) of these patients sustained iatrogenic hypoparathyroidism necessitating chronic calcium and vitamin D replacement. As might be expected from the substantial postoperative complication rate, these patients often had prolonged postoperative courses. Compared with the standard transhiatal esophagectomy patient undergoing a cervical esophagogastric anastomosis without the need for concomitant laryngectomy or pharyngogastric anastomosis whose typical postoperative hospitalization is 10 days, only 8 (21%) of the 39 hospital survivors undergoing cervical exenterations were discharged from the hospital within 7 to 14 days; 11 (28%) were discharged within 15 to 21 days. Twenty patients (51% of the operative survivors) required hospitalizations of between 22 and 50 days after surgery. It is also discouraging that 23 of the 39 survivors of the operation (59%) survived fewer than 12 months after surgery; 3 lived between 13 and 24 months. Thirteen of the 39 survivors (33%) have lived 24 months or more and have achieved gratifying palliation of dysphagia and airway obstruction.

It is clear that laryngopharyngectomy, combined with a transhiatal esophagectomy, anterior mediastinal tracheostomy, and restoration of alimentary continuity, constitutes an enormous undertaking in patients whose prognosis is poor. Nevertheless, as experience is gained, meaningful palliation can be achieved in a significant number of these patients with judicious patient selection, meticulous operative technique, and compulsive attention to postoperative care.[41,57,65,76,87,106,118]

References

1. Adams, W.E., and Phemister, D.B.: Carcinoma of the lower thoracic esophagus: Report of a successful resection and esophagogastrostomy. J. Thorac. Surg., *7:*621, 1988.
2. Akiyama, H., and Hiyama, M.: A simple esophageal bypass operation by the high gastric division. Surgery, *75:*674, 1974.
3. Akiyama, H., Sato, Y., and Takahashi, F.: Immediate pharyngogastrostomy following total esophagectomy by blunt dissection. Jpn. J. Surg., *1:*225, 1971.
4. Akiyama, H., Tsurumaru, M., Kawamura, T., et al.: Principles of surgical treatment for carcinoma of the esophagus: Analysis of lymph node involvement. Ann. Surg., *194:*438, 1981.
5. Akiyama, H., Tsurumaru, M., Udagawa, H., et al.: Radical lymph node dissection for cancer of the thoracic esophagus. Ann. Surg., *220:*364, 1994.
6. Altorki, N.K., Girardi, L., and Skinner, D.B.: En bloc esophagectomy improves survival for stage III esophageal cancer. J. Thorac. Cardiovasc. Surg., *114:*948, 1997.
7. Altorki, N.K., and Skinner, D.B.: Occult cervical nodal metastasis in esophageal cancer: Preliminary results of three-field lymphadenectomy. J. Thorac. Cardiovasc. Surg., *113:*540, 1997.
8. Azurin, D.J., Go, L.S., and Kirkland, M.L.: Palliative gastric transposition following pharyngolaryngoesophagectomy. Am. Surg., *63:*410, 1997.
9. Bains, M.S., and Spiro, R.H.: Pharyngolaryngectomy total extrathoracic esophagectomy and gastric transposition. Surg. Gynecol. Obstet., *149:*693, 1979.
10. Baker, J.W., and Schechter, G.L.: Management of panesophageal cancer by blunt resection without thoracotomy and reconstruction with stomach. Ann. Surg., *203:*491, 1986.
11. Barbier, P.A., Becker, C.D., and Wagner, H.E.: Esophageal carcinoma: Patient selection for transhiatal esophagectomy. A prospective analysis of 50 consecutive cases. World J. Surg., *12:*263, 1988.
12. Block, M.I., Patterson, G.A., Sundaresan, S., et al.: Improvement in staging of esophageal cancer with the addition of positron emission tomography. Ann. Thorac. Surg., *64:*770, 1997.
13. Bolton, J.S., Ochsner, J.L., and Abdoh, A.A.: Surgical management of esophageal cancer: A decade of change. Ann. Surg., *219:*475, 1994.
14. Bolton, J.S., Sardi, A., Bowen, J.C., et al.: Transhiatal and transthoracic esophagectomy: A comparative study. J. Surg. Oncol., *51:*249, 1992.
15. Bonenkamp, J.J., Hermans, J., Sasako, M., et al.: Extended lymph node dissection for gastric cancer. N. Engl. J. Med., *340:*908, 1999.
16. Botet, J.F., Lightdale, C.J., Zauber, A.G., et al.: Preoperative staging of esophageal cancer: Comparison of endoscopic US and dynamic CT. Radiology, *181:*419, 1991.
17. Cahow, C.E., and Sasaki, C.T.: Gastric pull-up reconstruction for pharyngolaryngoesophagectomy. Arch. Surg., *129:*425, 1994.
18. Carlson, G.W., Schusterman, M.A., and Guillamondegui, O.M.: Total reconstruction of the hypopharynx and cervical esophagus: A 20-year experience. Ann. Plast. Surg., *29:*408, 1992.
19. Churchill, E.D., and Sweet, R.H.: Transthoracic resection of tumors of the stomach and esophagus. Ann. Surg., *115:*897, 1942.
20. Coleman, J.J., Searles, J.M., Jr., Hester, T.R., et al.: Ten years experience with free jejunal autograph. Am. J. Surg., *154:*394, 1987.
21. Cordiano, C., Fracastoro, G., Mosciaro, O., et al.: Esophagectomy and esophageal replacement by gastric pull-through procedure. Int. Surg., *64:*17, 1979.
22. Daniel, T.M., Fleischer, K.J., Flanagan, T.I., et al.: Transhiatal esophagectomy: A safe alternative for selected patients. Ann. Thorac. Surg., *54:*686, 1992.
23. Denk, W.: Zur Radikaloperation des Osophaguskarfzentralbl. Chirurg, *40:*1065, 1913.
24. deVries, E.J., Stein, D.W., Johnson, J.T., et al.: Hypopharyngeal reconstruction: A comparison of two alternatives. Laryngoscope, *99:*614, 1989.
25. Donegan, W.L.: Surgical clinical trials. Cancer, *53:*691, 1981.
26. Earlam, R., and Cunha-Melo, J.R.: Oesophageal squamous cell carcinoma. I. A critical review of surgery. Br. J. Surg., *67:*381, 1980.
27. Ellis, F.H., Jr.: Carcinoma of the esophagus. Cancer, *33:*264, 1983.
28. Ellis, F.H., Jr., and Gibb, S.P.: Esophagogastrectomy for carcinoma: Current hospital mortality and morbidity rates. Ann. Surg., *190:*699, 1979.
29. Fisher, B., Redmond, C., and Fisher E.R., et al.: 10-Year results of a randomized clinical trial comparing radical mastectomy and total mastectomy with or without radiation. N. Engl. J. Med., *312:*674, 1985.
30. Flynn, M.B., Banis, J., and Acland, R.: Reconstruction with free bowel autografts after pharyngoesophageal or laryngopharyngeal resection. Am. J. Surg., *158:*333, 1989.
31. Forastiere, M., Orringer, M.B., Perez-Tamayo, C., et al.: Preoperative chemoradiation followed by transhiatal esophagectomy for carcinoma of the esophagus: Final report. J. Clin. Oncol., *11:*1118, 1993.
32. Frederickson, J.M., Wagenfeld, D.J.H., and Pearson, G.: Gastric pull-up vs. deltopectoral flap for reconstruction of the cervical esophagus. Arch. Otolaryngol., *107:*613, 1981.
33. Fujita, H., Kakegawa, T., Yamana, H., et al.: Total esophagectomy versus proximal esophagectomy for esophageal cancer at the cervicothoracic junction. World J. Surg., *23:*486, 1999.
34. Gandhi, S.K., and Naunheim, K.S.: Complications of transhiatal esophagectomy. Chest Surg. Clin. North Am., *7:*601, 1997.
35. Garvin, P.J., and Kaminski, D.L.: Extrathoracic esophagectomy in the treatment of esophageal cancer. Am. J. Surg., *104:*772, 1980.
36. Gerndt, S.J., and Orringer, M.B.: Tube jejunostomy as an adjunct to esophagectomy. Surgery, *115:*168, 1994.
37. Gertsch, P., Vauthey, J.N., Lustenberger, A.A., et al.: Long-term results of transhiatal esophagectomy for esophageal carcinoma: A multivariate analysis of prognostic factors. Cancer, *72:*2312, 1993.
38. Giuli, R., and Gignoux, M.: Treatment of carcinoma of the esophagus: Retrospective study of 2400 patients. Ann. Surg., *192:*44, 1980.
39. Gluch, L., Smith, R.C., Bambach, C.P., et al.: Comparison of outcomes following transhiatal or Ivor Lewis esophagectomy for esophageal carcinoma. World J. Surg., *23:*271, 1999.

40. Goldberg, M., Freeman, J., Gullane, P.J., et al.: Transhiatal esophagectomy with gastric transposition for pharyngolaryngeal malignant disease. J. Thorac. Cardiovasc. Surg., *97:*327, 1989.
41. Gomes, M.N., Krole, S., and Spear, S.L.: Mediastinal tracheostomy. Ann. Thorac. Surg., *43:*539, 1987.
42. Greenberg, J., Durkin, M., Van Drunen, M., et al.: Computerized tomography or endoscopic ultrasound in preoperative staging of gastric and esophageal tumors. Surgery, *11:*696, 1994.
43. Grillo, H.C.: Terminal or mural tracheostomy in the anterior mediastinum. J. Thorac. Cardiovasc. Surg., *51:*422, 1966.
44. Grillo, H.C., and Mathisen, D.J.: Cervical exenteration. Ann. Thorac. Surg., *49:*401, 1990.
45. Hagan, J.A., Peters, J.H., and DeMeester, T.R.: Superiority of extended en bloc esophagogastrectomy for carcinoma of the lower esophagus and cardia. J. Thorac. Cardiovasc. Surg., *106:*850, 1993.
46. Hankins, J.R., Atlar, S., Coughlin, T.R., et al.: Carcinoma of the esophagus: A comparison of the results of transhiatal versus transthoracic resection. Ann. Thorac. Surg., *47:*700, 1989.
47. Hankins, J.R., Miller, J.E., Attar, S., et al.: Transhiatal esophagectomy for carcinoma of the esophagus: Experience with 26 patients. Ann. Thorac. Surg., *44:*123, 1987.
48. Harrison, D.F., and Thompson, A.E.: Pharyngolaryngoesophagectomy with pharyngogastric anastomosis for cancer of the hypopharynx: Review of 101 operations. Head Neck Surg., *8:*418, 1986.
49. Heitmiller, R.F., Gillinov, A.M., Jones, B., et al.: Transhiatal herniation of colon after esophagectomy and gastric pull-up. Ann. Thorac. Surg., *63:*554, 1997.
50. Horstmann, O., Verreet, P.R., Becker, H., et al.: Transhiatal esophagectomy compared with transthoracic resection and systematic lymphadenectomy for the treatment of esophageal cancer. Eur. J. Surg., *161:*557, 1995.
51. Iannettoni, M.D., Whyte, R.I., and Orringer, M.B.: Catastrophic complications of the cervical esophagogastric anastomosis. J. Thorac. Cardiovasc. Surg., *110:*1493, 1995.
52. Jurkiewicz, M.J.: Reconstructive surgery of the cervical esophagus. J. Thorac. Cardiovasc. Surg., *88:*893, 1984.
53. Katariya, K., Harvey, J.C., Pina, E., et al.: Complications of transhiatal esophagectomy. J. Surg. Oncol., *57:*157, 1994.
54. Kirk, R.M.: Palliative resection of oesophageal carcinoma without formal thoracotomy. Br. J. Surg., *61:*689, 1974.
55. Kirschner, M.: Ein neues Verfahren der Oesophagoplastik. Arch. Klin. Chir., *114:*606, 1920.
56. Krasna, M.J., Flowers, J.L., Attar, S., et al.: Combined thoracoscopic/laparoscopic staging of esophageal cancer. J. Thorac. Cardiovasc. Surg., *111:*800, 1996.
57. Krespi, Y.P., Wurster, C.F., and Sisson, G.A.: Immediate reconstruction after total laryngopharyngectomy and mediastinal dissection. Laryngoscope, *95:*156, 1985.
58. Lam, K.H., Wong, J., Lim, S.T., et al.: Pharyngogastric anastomosis following pharyngolaryngoesophagectomy: Analysis of 137 cases. World J. Surg., *5:*509, 1981.
59. LeQuesne, L.P., and Ranger, D.: Pharyngogastrectomy with immediate pharyngogastric anastomosis. Br. J. Surg., *53:*105, 1966.
60. Lerut, T., DeLeyn, P., Coosemans, W., et al.: Surgical strategies in esophageal carcinoma with emphasis on radical lymphadenectomy. Ann. Surg., *26:*583, 1992.
61. Liebermann-Meffert, D.M.I., Luescher, U., Neff, U., et al.: Esophagectomy without thoracotomy: Is there a risk of intramediastinal bleeding. Ann. Surg., *206:*184, 1987.
62. Luketich, J.D., Schauer, P., Landreneau, R., et al.: Minimally invasive surgical staging is superior to endoscopic ultrasound in detecting lymph node metastases in esophageal cancer. J. Thorac. Cardiovasc. Surg., *114:*817, 1997.
63. Luketich, J.D., Schauer, P.R., Meltzer, C.C., et al.: The role of positron emission tomography in staging esophageal cancer. Ann. Thorac. Surg., *64:*765, 1997.
64. Marshall, S.F.: Carcinoma of the esophagus. Surg. Clin. North Am., *18:*643, 1938.
65. Mathisen, D.J., Grillo, H.C., Vlahakes, G.J., et al.: The omentum in the management of complicated cardiothoracic problems. J. Thorac. Cardiovasc. Surg., *95:*677, 1988.
66. Mathisen, D.J., Grillo, H.C., Wilkins, E.W., et al.: Transthoracic esophagectomy: A safe approach to carcinoma of the esophagus. Ann. Thorac. Surg., *45:*137, 1988.
67. Moon, M.R., Schulte, W.J., Haasler, G.B., et al.: Transhiatal and transthoracic esophagectomy for adenocarcinoma of the esophagus. Arch. Surg., *127:*951, 1992.
68. Moores, D.W.O., Ilves, R., Cooper, J.D., et al.: One-stage reconstruction for pharyngolaryngectomy: Esophagectomy and pharyngogastrostomy without thoracotomy. J. Thorac. Cardiovasc. Surg., *85:*330, 1983.
69. Muller, J.M., Erasmi, H., Stelzner, M., et al.: Surgical therapy of oesophageal carcinoma. Br. J. Surg., *77:*845, 1990.
70. Ohsawa, T.: The surgery of the esophagus. Arch. F. Jap. Chir., *10:*605, 1933.
71. Ong, G.B., and Lee, T.C.: Pharyngogastric anastomosis after oesophagopharyngectomy for carcinoma of the hypopharynx and cervical esophagus. Br. J. Surg., *48:*193, 1960.
72. Orringer, M.B.: Substernal gastric bypass of the excluded esophagus—results of an ill-advised operation. Surgery, *96:*467, 1984.
73. Orringer, M.B.: Partial median sternotomy: Anterior approach to the upper thoracic esophagus. J. Thorac. Cardiovasc. Surg., *87:*124, 1984.
74. Orringer, M.B.: Transhiatal esophagectomy without thoracotomy for carcinoma of the thoracic esophagus. Ann. Surg., *200:*282, 1984.
75. Orringer, M.B.: Transhiatal esophagectomy for benign disease. J. Thorac. Cardiovasc. Surg., *90:*649, 1985.
76. Orringer, M.B.: Anterior mediastinal tracheostomy with and without cervical exenteration. Ann. Thorac. Surg., *54:*628, 1992.
77. Orringer, M.B.: Anterior mediastinal tracheostomy with and without cervical exenteration—updated in 1998. Ann. Thorac. Surg., *67:*591, 1999.
78. Orringer, M.B., Bluett, M., and Deeb, G.M.: Aggressive treatment of chylothorax complicating transhiatal esophagectomy without thoracotomy. Surgery, *104:*720, 1988.
79. Orringer, M.B., Forastiere, A.A., Perez-Tamayo, C., et al.: Chemotherapy and radiation therapy before transhiatal esophagectomy for esophageal carcinoma. Ann. Thorac. Surg., *49:*348, 1990.
80. Orringer, M.B., and Lemmer, J.H.: Early dilatation in the treatment of esophageal disruption. Ann. Thorac. Surg., *42:*536, 1986.
81. Orringer, M.B., Marshall, B., and Iannettoni, M.D.: Transhiatal esophagectomy: Clinical experience and refinements. Ann. Surg., *230:*329, 1999.
82. Orringer, M.B., Marshall, B., and Iannettoni, M.D.: Eliminating the cervical esophagogastric anastomotic leak with a side-to-side stapled anastomosis. J. Thorac. Cardiovasc. Surg., *119:*277, 2000.
83. Orringer, M.B., Marshall, B., and Stirling, M.C.: Transhiatal esophagectomy for benign and malignant disease. J. Thorac. Cardiovasc. Surg., *105:*265, 1993.
84. Orringer, M.B., and Orringer, J.S.: Esophagectomy without thoracotomy—a dangerous operation? J. Thorac. Cardiovasc. Surg., *85:*72, 1983.
85. Orringer, M.B., and Sloan, H.: Substernal gastric bypass of the excluded thoracic esophagus for palliation of esophageal carcinoma. J. Thorac. Cardiovasc. Surg., *70:*836, 1975.
86. Orringer, M.B., and Sloan, H.: Esophagectomy without thoracotomy. J. Thorac. Cardiovasc. Surg., *76:*643, 1978.
87. Orringer, M.B., and Sloan, H.: Anterior mediastinal tracheostomy—indications, techniques, and clinical experience. J. Thorac. Cardiovasc. Surg., *78:*850, 1979.
88. Orringer, M.B., and Stirling, M.C.: Cervical esophagogastric anastomosis for benign disease—functional results. J. Thorac. Cardiovasc. Surg., *96:*887, 1988.
89. Orringer, M.B., and Stirling, M.C.: Esophageal resection for achalasia—indications and results. Ann. Thorac. Surg., *47:*340, 1989.
90. Paletta, C.E., and Jurkiewicz, M.J.: Esophageal replacement: Microvascular jejunal transplantation. *In* Baue, A.E., Geha, A.S., Hammond, G.L., et al. (eds.): Glenn's Thoracic and Cardiovascular Surgery, 5th ed. Norwalk, CT, Appleton & Lange, 1991, p. 819.
91. Pinotti, H.W., Zilberstein, B., Pollara, W., et al.: Esophagectomy without thoracotomy. Surg. Gynecol. Obstet., *154:*344, 1981.
92. Postlethwait, R.W.: Complications and deaths after operations for esophageal carcinoma. J. Thorac. Cardiovasc. Surg., *85:*827, 1983.
93. Quint, L.E., Glazer, G.M., Orringer, M.B., et al.: Esophageal carcinoma: CT findings. Radiology, *155:*171, 1985.
94. Reed, C.E., Mishra, G., Sahai, A.V., et al.: Esophageal cancer staging: Improved accuracy by endoscopic ultrasound of celiac lymph nodes. Ann. Thorac. Surg., *67:*319, 1999.

95. Reich, H., Lo, A.Y., and Harvey, J.C.: Diaphragmatic herniation following transhiatal esophagectomy. Scand. J. Thorac. Cardiovasc. Surg., *30:*101, 1996.
96. Salamoun, W., Swartz, W.M., Johnson, J.T., et al.: Free jejunal transfer for reconstruction of the laryngopharynx. Head Neck Surg., *96:*149, 1987.
97. Sasaki, C.T., Salzer, S.J., Cahow, C.E., et al.: Laryngopharyngoesophagectomy for advanced hypopharyngeal and esophageal squamous cell carcinoma: The Yale experience. Laryngoscope, *105:*160, 1995.
98. Sasaki, T.M., Baker, H.W., McConnell, D.B., et al.: Free jejunal graft reconstruction after extensive head and neck surgery. Am. J. Surg., *139:*650, 1980.
99. Schusterman, M.A., Shestak, K., deVries, E.J., et al.: Reconstruction of the cervical esophagus: Free jejunal transfer versus gastric pull-up. Plast. Reconstr. Surg., *85:*16, 1990.
100. Shahian, D.M., Neptune, W.B., Ellis, F.H., et al.: Transthoracic versus extrathoracic esophagectomy: Mortality, morbidity, and long-term survival. Ann. Thorac. Surg., *41:*237, 1986.
101. Skinner, D.B.: En bloc resection for neoplasms of the esophagus and cardia. J. Thorac. Cardiovasc. Surg., *85:*59, 1983.
102. Spiro, R.H., Bains, M.S., Shah, J.P., et al.: Gastric transposition for head and neck cancer: A critical update. Am. J. Surg., *162:*348, 1991.
103. Spiro, R.H., Shah, J.P., Strong, B.W., et al.: Gastric transposition in head and neck surgery: Indications, complications, and expectations. Am. J. Surg., *146:*483, 1983.
104. Steiger, Z., and Wilson, R.F.: Comparison of the results of esophagectomy with and without a thoracotomy. Surg. Gynecol. Obstet., *153:*653, 1981.
105. Stewart, J.R., Sarr, M.G., Sharp, K.W., et al.: Transhiatal (blunt) esophagectomy for malignant and benign esophageal disease: Clinical experience and technique. Ann. Thorac. Surg., *40:*343, 1985.
106. Sullivan, M.W., Talamonti, M.S., Sithanandam, K., et al.: Results of gastric transposition for reconstruction of the pharyngoesophagus. Surgery, *126:*666, 1999.
107. Szentpetery, S., Wolfgang, T., and Lower, R.R.: Pull-through esophagectomy without thoracotomy for esophageal carcinoma. Ann. Thorac. Surg., *27:*399, 1979.
108. Terz, J.J., Beatty, J.D., Kokal, W.A., et al.: Transhiatal esophagectomy. Am. J. Surg., *154:*42, 1987.
109. Thomas, A.N., and Dedo, H.H.: Pharyngogastrostomy for treatment of severe caustic stricture of the pharynx and esophagus. J. Thorac. Cardiovasc. Surg., *73:*817, 1977.
110. Tilanus, H.W., Hop, W.C.J., Langenhorst, B.L., et al.: Esophagectomy with or without thoracotomy: Is there any difference? J. Thorac. Cardiovasc. Surg., *105:*898, 1993.
111. Tio, T.I., Coene, P.P.L.O., Schouwink, M.H., et al.: Esophagogastric carcinoma: Preoperative TNM classification with endosonography. Radiology, *173:*411, 1989.
112. Tryzelaar, J.F., Neptune, W.B., Ellis, F.H., Jr.: Esophagectomy without thoracotomy for carcinoma of the esophagus. Am. J. Surg., *143:*486, 1982.
113. Turner, G.G.: Excision of thoracic esophagus for carcinoma with construction of extrathoracic gullet. Lancet, *2:*1315, 1933.
114. Ujiki, G.T., Pearl, G.J., Poticha, S., et al.: Mortality and morbidity of gastric "pull-up" for replacement of the pharyngoesophagus. Arch. Surg., *122:*644, 1987.
115. Veronesi, V., Saccozzi, R., Delvecchio, M., et al.: Comparing radical mastectomy with quadrantectomy, axillary dissection, and radiotherapy in patients with small cancers of the breast. N. Engl. J. Med., *305:*6, 1981.
116. Vilgrain, V., Mompoint, D., Palazzo, L., et al.: Staging of esophageal carcinoma: Comparison of results with endoscopic sonography and CT. Am. J. Roentgenol., *155:*277, 1990.
117. Waddell, W.R., and Scannell, J.G.: Anterior approach to carcinoma of the superior mediastinal and cervical segments of the esophagus. J. Thorac. Surg., *33:*663, 1957.
118. Withers, E.H., Davis, J.L., and Lynch, J.B.: Anterior mediastinal tracheostomy with a pectoralis major musculocutaneous flap. Plast. Reconstr. Surg., *67:*381, 1981.
119. Wong, J., Lam, K.W., Wei, W.I., et al.: Results of the Kirschner operation. World J. Surg., *5:*547, 1981.
120. Ziegler, K., Sanft, C., Zeitz, M., et al.: Evaluation of endosonography in TN staging of oesophageal cancer. Gut, *32:*16, 1991.

CHAPTER

26 Complications of Esophageal Surgery

MARK B. ORRINGER

ANATOMIC AND PHYSIOLOGIC CONSIDERATIONS

Many of the complications of esophageal surgery are related directly to the unique features of esophageal anatomy and physiology. A thorough understanding and appreciation of these characteristics allows the informed esophageal surgeon to think and act defensively, thus averting complications before they occur. In performing esophagoscopy, for example, one must bear in mind the three naturally occurring sites of esophageal narrowing: the upper esophageal introitus, or cricopharyngeal sphincter; the level of the aortic arch and left mainstem bronchus; and the esophagogastric junction (Fig. 26–1). The rigid esophagoscope must be manipulated appropriately through these points of narrowing to minimize the risk of injury during esophagoscopy. Another unique feature of esophageal anatomy is its unusually fatty submucosa, which allows relatively great mobility of the overlying squamous mucosa. In performing a manual esophageal anastomosis, particular care must be exercised to make sure that every suture transfixes the mucosal edge, which at times may retract more than 1 cm away from the cut esophageal margin (Fig. 26–2). Postoperative esophageal anastomotic leaks are most often related to technical errors, and there is simply no substitute for meticulous technique and attention to detail in esophageal surgery.

Suture line tumor recurrence after an esophagectomy for carcinoma is a terrible late complication of esophageal surgery that is related directly to anatomic considerations, in this case, the extensive submucosal lymphatic drainage of the esophagus. The well-known propensity of esophageal tumor cells to spread through the submucosal lymphatics 4 to 6 cm and more beyond gross neoplasm has justified the mandate that, whenever possible, a 6- to 10-cm margin be obtained beyond the tumor before constructing the anastomosis (Fig. 26–3). The esophagus is also unique in the gastrointestinal tract because it lacks a serosal layer. The rather soft and often tenuous esophageal muscle holds sutures poorly and cannot be relied on to maintain a fundoplication, for example, unless the associated submucosa is transfixed by the esophageal stitch.

The esophagus is nourished by four to six paired aortic esophageal arteries as well as collateral circulation from the inferior thyroid, intercostal and bronchial, inferior phrenic, and left gastric arteries. The segmental "poor" blood supply of the esophagus has frequently been incriminated as the cause of anastomotic disruption. This contention is simply unjustified. The submucosal collateral circulation of the esophagus is extensive, and even after the cardia has been divided and the intrathoracic esophagus mobilized completely out of the chest, the distal end of the esophagus maintains good arterial bleeding so long as the inferior thyroid arteries remain intact. Once again, poor technique, not poor blood supply, is the more likely explanation for the complication of esophageal anastomotic disruption. Finally, parasympa-

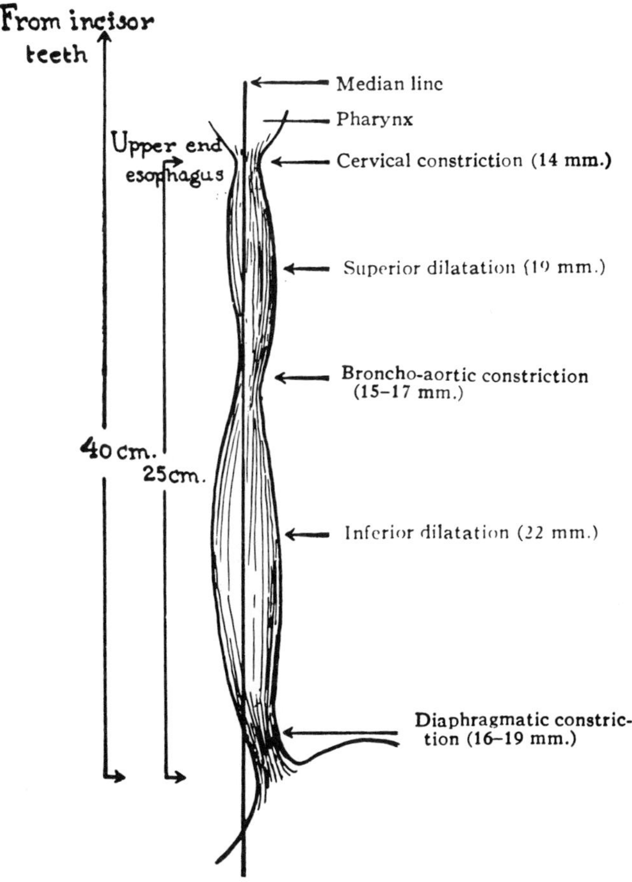

Figure 26–1. Normal esophageal constrictions, dilatations, and measurements. (From Shackelford, R.T. [ed.]: Surgery of the Alimentary Tract, Vol. 1, 2nd ed. Philadelphia, W.B. Saunders, 1978, p. 9, with permission.)

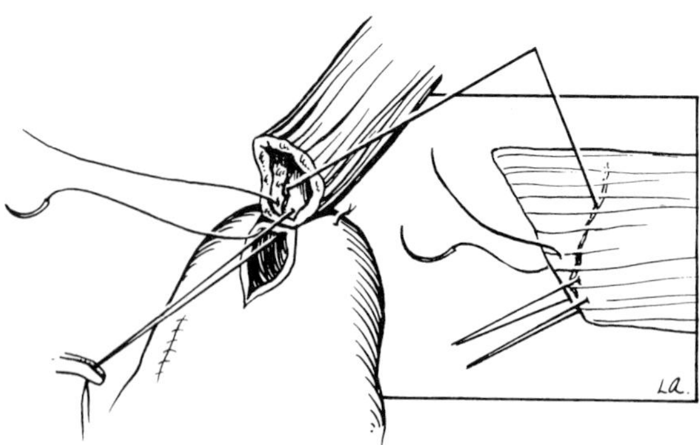

Figure 26–2. Failure of an esophageal anastomotic suture to transfix the mucosa is a function of the fatty submucosa, which permits mobility of the overlying mucosa and allows its retraction. The mucosa must be identified and deliberately transfixed with each suture placed to achieve mucosal apposition and avoid an anastomotic leak. (From Orringer, M.B.: Complications of esophageal surgery and trauma. *In* Greenfield, L.J. [ed.]: Complications in Surgery and Trauma. Philadelphia, J.B. Lippincott, 1984, p. 261, with permission.)

thetic innervation of the esophagus is supplied by the vagus nerves, and the recurrent laryngeal supplies the upper portion of the esophagus. Recurrent laryngeal nerve injury during esophageal surgery may result in one of the most devastating complications, cricopharyngeal muscle dysfunction with subsequent incapacitating cervical dysphagia and aspiration pneumonia.[30,48] Similarly, injury to the vagal nerve trunks in operations on the distal esophagus may produce neurogenic dysphagia or gastric atony and pylorospasm, which are very troublesome complications after esophageal surgery.

Physiologic considerations influence other complications of surgery on the esophagus. The pathophysiology of gastroesophageal reflux and secondary reflux esophagitis directly influences the results of antireflux surgery and hence the complication of recurrent reflux. For example, it has been demonstrated that the incidence of recurrent reflux in patients undergoing the standard Belsey Mark IV transthoracic hiatal hernia repair in the presence of esophagitis or a stricture is between 25 and 75%.[26,92,121] In the presence of the intramural inflammation and esophageal shortening that may accompany reflux esophagitis, the esophageal sutures of the Belsey repair may not be reliable, and tension on the repair to reduce the prerequisite 3 to 5 cm of distal esophagus below the diaphragm sets the stage for recurrence of the hernia (Fig. 26–4). These same considerations apply to the Nissen fundoplication and the Hill posterior gastropexy, which also aim to restore an intra-abdominal segment of distal esophagus and require esophageal or periesophageal sutures (Figs. 26–5 and 26–6). To avert the complication of disruption of the repair due to the need to suture inflamed esophagus and tension on the repair, the esophagus-lengthening Collis gastroplasty has been combined with a fundoplication (Figs. 26–7 through 26–9).[47,91,93-96,106,107,129] The gastroplasty tube functions as a new distal esophagus and provides healthy, resilient tissue—the gas-

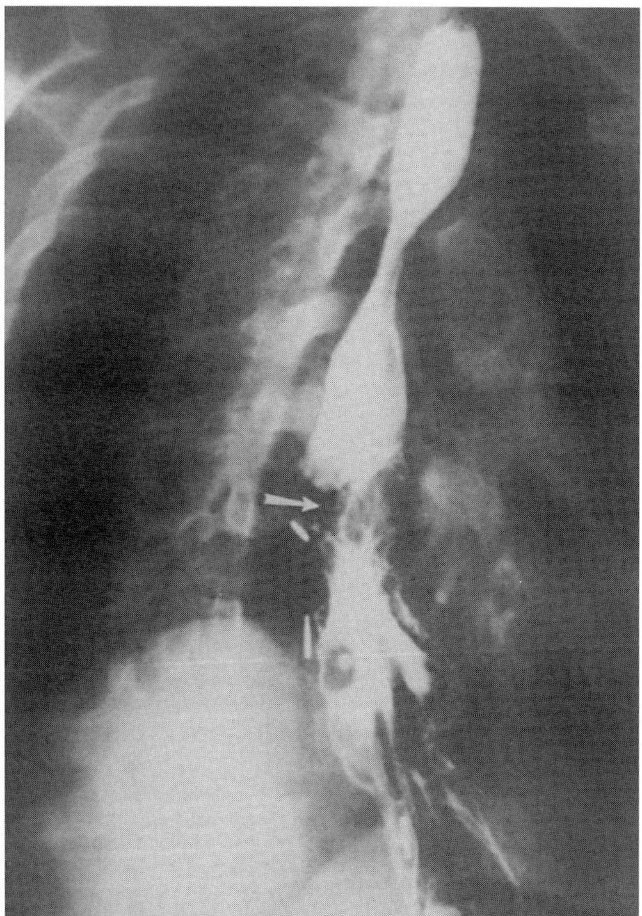

Figure 26–3. Intrathoracic esophagogastric anastomotic stricture *(arrow)* due to recurrent tumor at the suture line. This patient had undergone an esophagogastrectomy for a distal-third esophageal adenocarcinoma 7 months earlier. An insufficient 3-cm esophageal margin proximal to the tumor had been obtained, and palliation of dysphagia was short-lived.

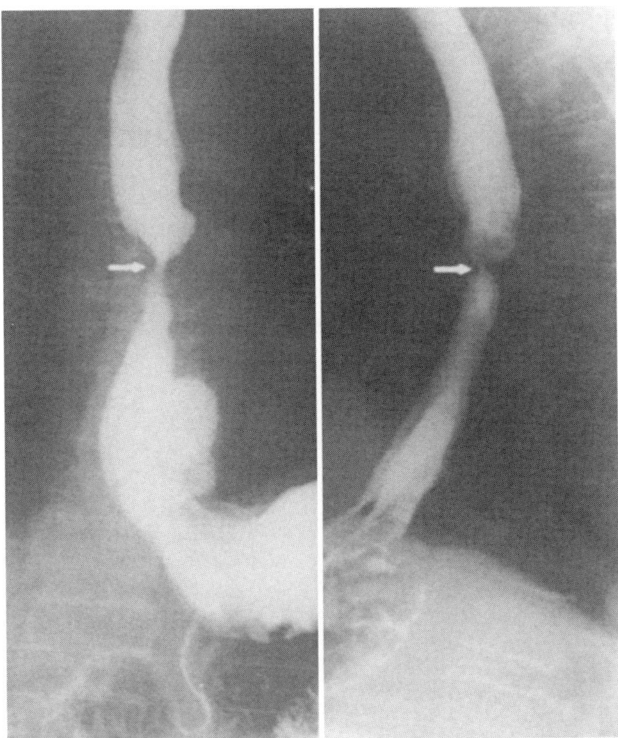

Figure 26–4. Posteroanterior *(left)* and lateral *(right)* views from a barium swallow examination showing a sliding hiatal hernia with a midesophageal stricture *(arrow)* at the squamocolumnar junction in a patient with Barrett's esophagus. Standard antireflux operations (Hill, Belsey, or Nissen) require reduction below the diaphragm of not only the esophagastric junction but also the distal 3 to 5 cm of esophagus. The esophageal shortening and periesophageal fibrosis due to reflux esophagitis in this patient prevented a tension-free standard repair.

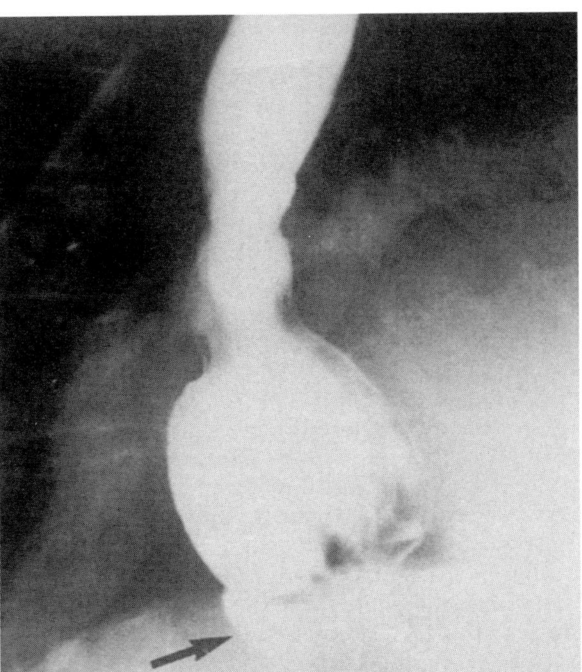

Figure 26–6. Slipped Nissen fundoplication in a patient who was operated on for reflux complicated by a short esophagus and stricture. Tension on the repair resulted in its subsequent disruption. The proximal stomach has herniated through the fundoplication *(arrow)* and is seen above the level of the diaphragm.

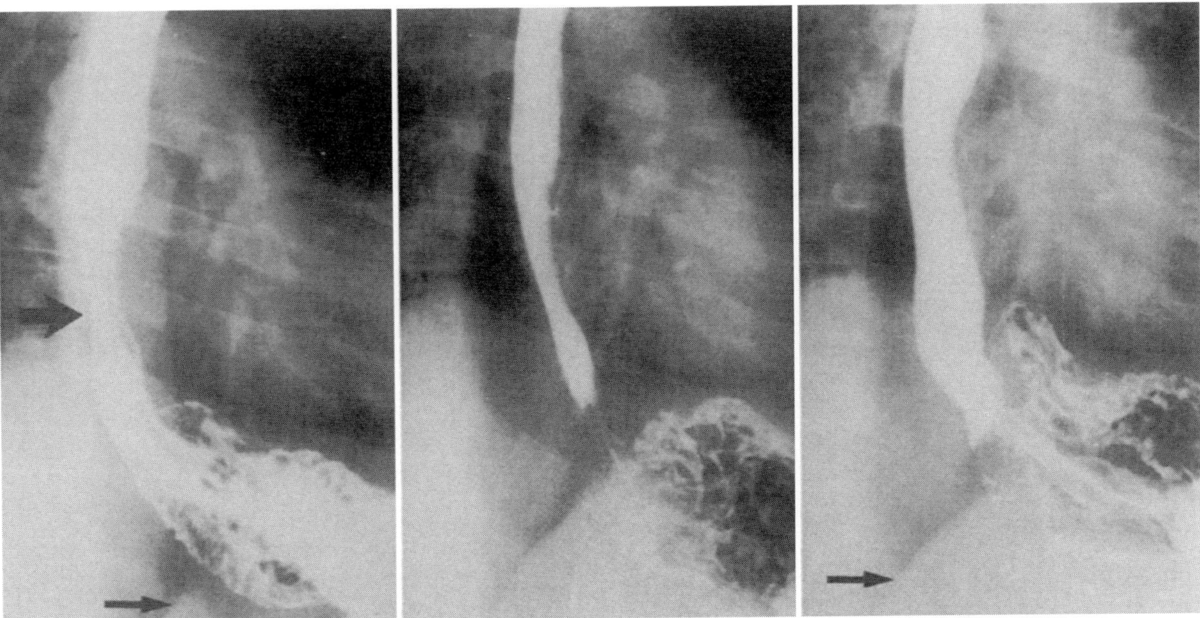

Figure 26–5. Development of a recurrent hiatal hernia after a Hill posterior gastropexy for reflux esophagitis with a stricture. *Left,* There is a sliding hiatal hernia above the diaphragm *(small arrow)* as well as a reflux stricture *(large arrow)*. This patient was obese and had distal esophagitis and associated esophageal shortening. *Center,* One week after a Hill repair, there already is little evidence of an intra-abdominal distal esophageal segment. *Right,* Within 1 year of performing this hiatal hernia repair under tension, disruption has occurred, and the stomach is seen above the diaphragm *(arrow)*. (From Orringer, M.B.: Complications of esophageal surgery and trauma. *In* Greenfield, L.J. [ed.]: Complications in Surgery and Trauma. Philadelphia, J.B. Lippincott, 1984, p. 262, with permission.)

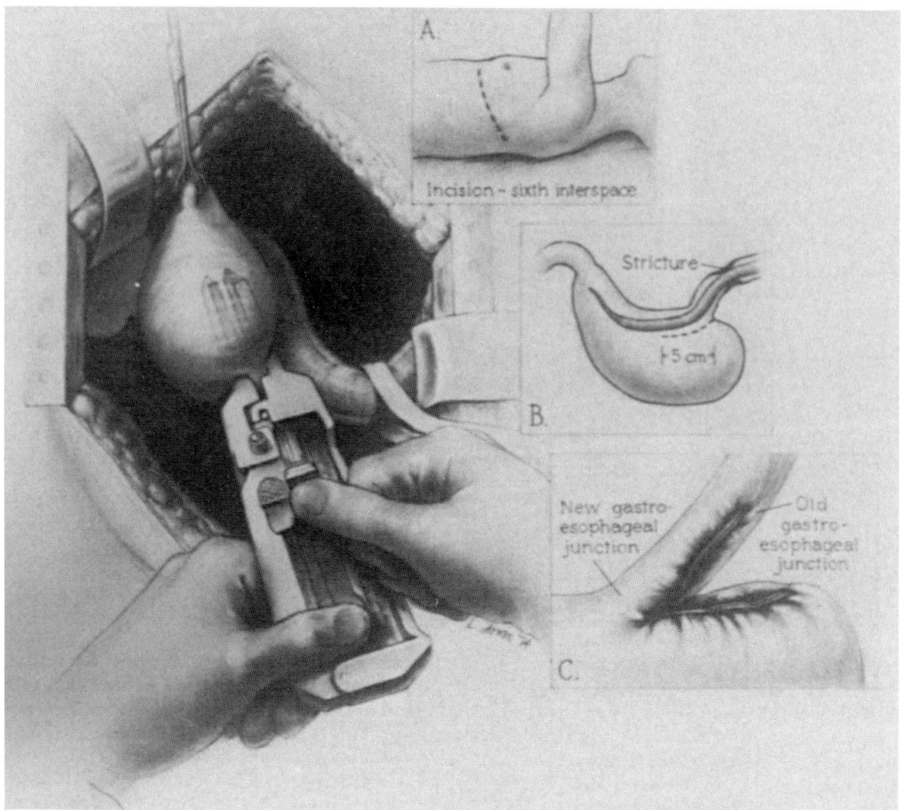

Figure 26–7. Construction of the Collis gastroplasty using the GIA surgical stapler. *A,* The sixth left interspace incision used. *B,* The esophageal dilator (No. 54 or 56 French) is displaced against the lesser curvature of the stomach; *dotted line* indicates where the stapler will be applied. *Main illustration,* Advancing the knife assembly for construction of the gastroplasty tube. *C,* The 5-cm gastric tube extension of the functional esophageal tube. (From Orringer, M.B., and Sloan, H.: An improved technique for the combined Collis-Belsey approach to dilatable esophageal strictures. J. Thorac. Cardiovasc. Surg., *68:*298, 1974, with permission.)

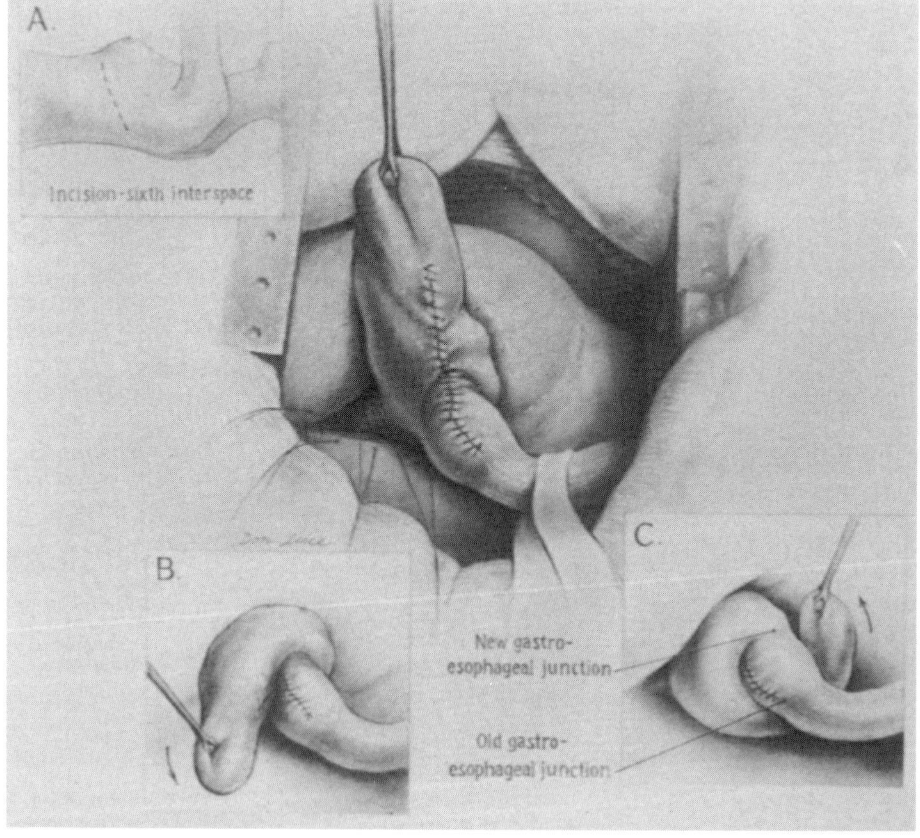

Figure 26–8. *A,* The elongated gastric fundus remaining after construction of the gastroplasty tube. The staple suture line has been oversewn. *B* and *C,* Positioning the gastric fundus posterior to the gastroplasty tube in preparation for the fundoplication. (From Orringer, M.B., and Sloan, H.: Combined Collis-Nissen reconstruction of the esophagogastric junction. Ann. Thorac. Surg., *25:*16, 1978, with permission.)

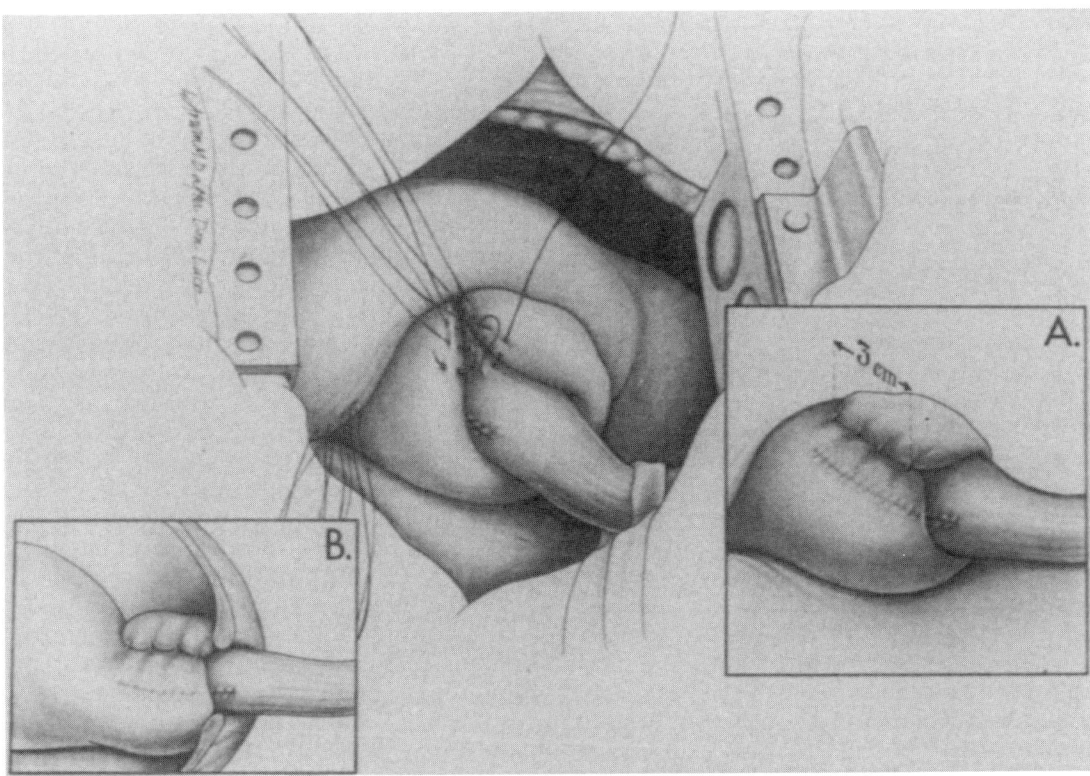

Figure 26–9. Construction of a 3-cm-long fundoplication to complete the Collis-Nissen operation. *A,* Four seromuscular 2–0 silk sutures placed 1 cm apart are used. *B,* The fundoplication is placed beneath the diaphragm, and the previously placed posterior crural sutures are tied. (From Stirling, M.C., and Orringer, M.B.: The combined Collis-Nissen operation for esophageal reflux strictures. Ann. Thorac. Surg., *45:*148, 1988, with permission.)

tric wall—around which to perform the fundoplication. Furthermore, the additional "esophageal length" provided by the gastroplasty tube reduces tension on the repair. The presence of reflux esophagitis and a peptic stricture also complicates an antireflux procedure if the stricture is perforated during attempted dilation.

An intrathoracic esophagogastric anastomotic leak, perhaps the most dreaded complication of esophageal surgery, in part owes its morbidity to associated gastroesophageal reflux. An intrathoracic esophagogastric anastomosis is associated almost invariably with the development of reflux esophagitis, compared with a cervical esophagogastric anastomosis, which is rarely associated with clinically significant reflux.[99] Although it has been argued that with appropriate attention to detail, an intrathoracic esophagogastric anastomosis can be performed reliably and with an exceedingly low morbidity rate,[35,77] the potential for an anastomotic leak and secondary mediastinitis cannot be eliminated totally, and this fact perhaps more than anything else has influenced our current "defensive posture" that the best esophagogastric anastomosis is a *cervical* anastomosis, with which the consequence of a leak is a salivary fistula and not life-threatening mediastinitis and sepsis.[97]

Gastroesophageal reflux after esophageal resection and an esophagogastric anastomosis may be responsible for life-threatening aspiration of gastric contents into the tracheobronchial tree in the early postoperative period. For this reason, initial decompression of the intrathoracic stomach with a nasogastric tube and placement of the patient in a 45-degree head-up position are important. Similarly, because of the potential for regurgitation and aspiration after eating, patients who have a fresh esophagogastric anastomosis should not be permitted to undergo postural drainage as part of their postoperative pulmonary physiotherapy within 1 to 2 hours of mealtime.

The potential pulmonary complications, primarily aspiration pneumonia, resulting from esophageal obstruction due to a variety of causes cannot be overestimated. Particularly in the patient with a megaesophagus of advanced achalasia, the risk of massive regurgitation and aspiration on induction of general anesthesia is enormous. Awareness of this possibility dictates the need for nasogastric tube esophageal decompression and emptying in these patients before a rapid sequence induction of general anesthesia and endotracheal intubation.

Esophageal Perforation

There are a variety of causes of esophageal perforation (Table 26–1), but regardless of the cause, the resultant mediastinitis poses a devastating threat. The urgent need for prompt recognition and treatment of disruption of esophageal continuity cannot be underestimated and requires virtually a race against the clock to institute appropriate drainage or repair. Repair of an acute esophageal tear in an otherwise normal esophagus within 6 to 8 hours of the injury carries a morbidity risk that is essen-

Table 26–1. Causes of Esophageal Perforation

Instrumental

- Endoscopy
  - Direct injury
  - Injury occurring during removal of a foreign body
- Dilatation
- Intubation (esophageal, endotracheal)

Noninstrumental

- Barogenic trauma
  - Postemetic
  - Blunt chest or abdominal trauma
  - Other (e.g., labor, convulsions, defecation)
- Penetrating neck, chest, or abdominal trauma
- Postsurgical
  - Anastomotic disruption
  - Devascularization after pulmonary resection, vagotomy, or repair of a hiatal hernia
- Corrosive injuries (acid or alkali ingestion)
- Erosion by adjacent infection with resultant fistula involving the tracheobronchial tree, pericardium, pleural cavity, or aorta

tially the same as that imposed by elective esophagotomy and primary esophageal closure. If surgery is delayed more than 6 to 8 hours from the time of injury, local inflammation greatly jeopardizes primary healing of the esophageal tear, and the mortality rate rises dramatically.[64,78,79,120,126]

DIAGNOSIS

There is no more important maxim in esophageal surgery than that stating that pain or fever after esophageal instrumentation or surgery represents an esophageal perforation until proved otherwise and dictates the need for an immediate esophagogram. Time is of the essence in establishing the diagnosis and instituting proper drainage or repair, and the esophageal contrast study cannot wait until a convenient morning hour or the routine scheduled radiologic studies for the day have been completed. If an esophageal perforation is suspected, a contrast study using a water-soluble agent (e.g., diatrizoate sodium [Gastrografin]) should be performed. Negative results of a diatrizoate sodium study, however, should be followed by a barium swallow, which provides better mucosal detail and may detect an injury that is missed by the diatrizoate sodium study (Fig. 26–10).

If the chest roentgenogram demonstrates air in the soft tissues of the neck or mediastinum or a hydropneumothorax in the patient suspected of having a perforation, the diagnosis is almost a certainty. *However, a normal chest roentgenogram does not exclude the possibility of an esophageal perforation.* A contrast study of the esophagus is mandatory both to establish the diagnosis and to demonstrate the exact site of injury so that appropriate therapy can be undertaken.

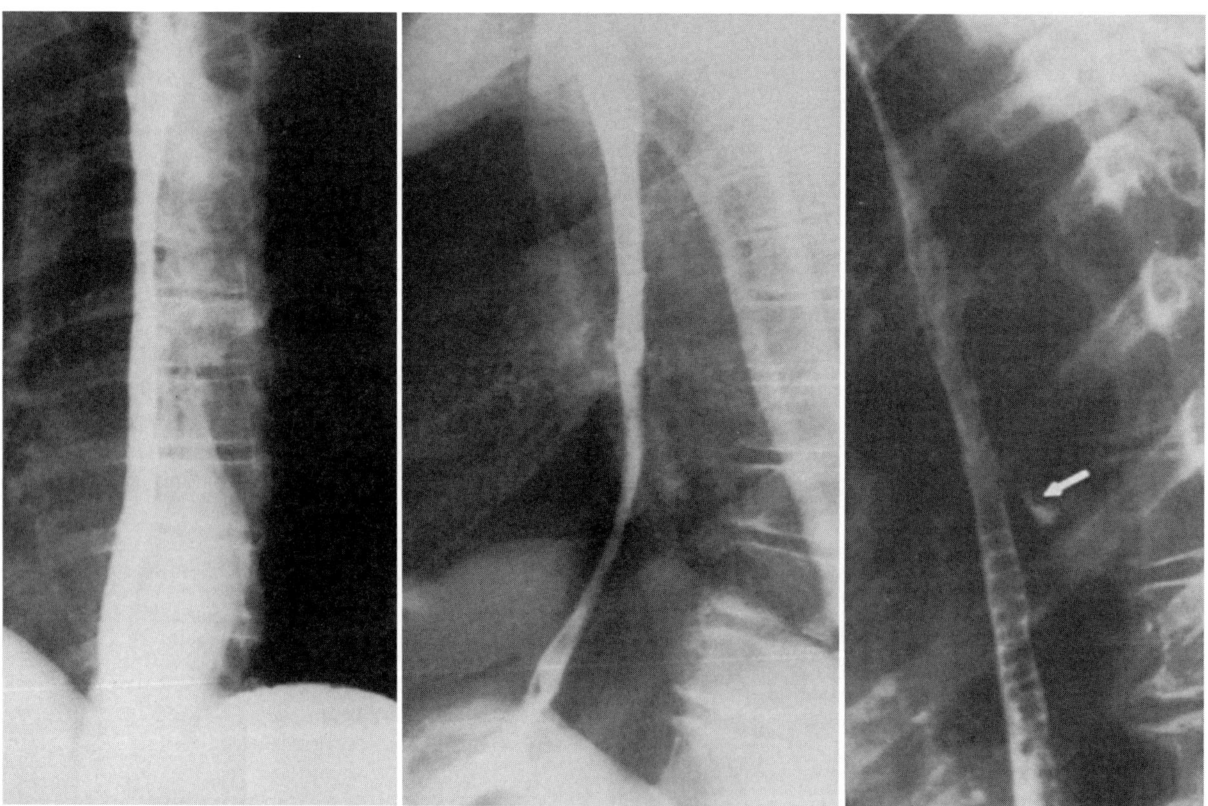

Figure 26–10. Posteroanterior *(left)* and lateral *(center)* views from Gastrografin swallow in a patient with acute caustic injury that was incorrectly dilated prematurely within 10 days of Drano ingestion. There was still acute inflammation in this esophagus, and the patient had a fever and chest pain after the dilation. Despite the negative Gastrografin swallow, dilute barium was administered *(right)*, and a perforation *(arrow)* of the midesophagus was demonstrated. (From Orringer, M.B.: Complications of esophageal surgery and trauma. *In* Greenfield, L.J. [ed.]: Complications in Surgery and Trauma. Philadelphia, J.B. Lippincott, 1984, p. 270, with permission.)

Not every esophageal tear is a full-thickness disruption. A tear of the distal esophageal mucosa and submucosa that occurs during forceful balloon dilatation for achalasia, for example, may appear much more serious than it is, particularly if air insufflation through the flexible esophagoscope results in mediastinal, cervical, or fascial subcutaneous air. The contrast esophagogram frequently shows only intramural dissection of the barium, not free flow into the mediastinum or pleural cavity. Treatment with antibiotics and observation, rather than an emergent thoracotomy to repair the esophagus, is generally successful. A contrast study is warranted whenever a perforation is suspected, because this is the best way to determine the need for surgical intervention.

PATHOPHYSIOLOGY OF ESOPHAGEAL PERFORATION

Dissection of salivary digestive enzymes, oral bacteria, and gastric contents into the fascial planes of the neck and mediastinum initiates both chemical and bacterial inflammatory responses. Negative intrathoracic pressure as well as respiratory movements suck the esophageal and gastric contents into the mediastinum. "Third-space" fluid loss due to this mediastinal burn occurs, and fluid accumulation within the mediastinum may cause displacement of the trachea, heart, or lungs. The tracheobronchial tree may respond to the surrounding mediastinitis with a reflex bronchorrhea that produces copious pulmonary secretions and wet respirations centrally with relatively clear breath sounds peripherally. As circulating extracellular volume is lost into the tissue planes of the neck, mediastinum, or adjacent pericardium, pleura, or peritoneal spaces, hypovolemic shock occurs. When there is pre-existing esophageal obstruction distal to the tear, the process is further aggravated.

The patient with esophageal perforation, then, presents with cervical or thoracic pain, pain or difficulty with swallowing, respiratory distress, and fever. Cervical or high retrosternal pain is more typical of cervicothoracic perforations, whereas mid or distal esophageal tears produce anterior thoracic, posterior, intrascapular, or epigastric pain. Right-sided pleural effusions are more common with tears of the upper or midthoracic esophagus, whereas left pleural effusions are seen with perforations of the distal third.

TREATMENT OF ESOPHAGEAL PERFORATIONS

Once the diagnosis of esophageal perforation is confirmed, oral intake by the patient should stop, and a disposable oral dental suction device at the bedside should be used by the patient to evacuate oral secretions. Aggressive intravenous volume replacement may be necessary if there is hypovolemia associated with an intrathoracic perforation; volume replacement may be facilitated by using either a central venous pressure catheter or pulmonary artery catheter with pressure monitoring. Broad-spectrum intravenous antibiotic coverage with a combination of a cephalosporin (cefazolin or cefamandole, 1 g every 4 hours) and an aminoglycoside (gentamicin or tobramycin, 1 to 1.5 mg/kg every 8 hours) is begun. The presence of carious teeth increases the morbidity risk of an esophageal injury owing to the virulence of swallowed oral bacteria. Thus, oral hygiene, although seemingly unimportant, cannot be neglected in the patient with an esophageal perforation, and frequent brushing of the teeth should be performed. It is not by chance that elderly edentulous patients with few oral bacteria often tolerate a chronic esophageal fistula better than younger patients who have poorer dental hygiene.

There is controversy about the best method of treatment of patients with esophageal perforations. It is clear that all esophageal perforations are not of the same magnitude and that a uniform treatment of all esophageal injuries does not exist. Nonoperative "conservative" therapy is successful in some patients with esophageal perforations, primarily those with pre-existing periesophageal and mediastinal fibrosis that contains the injury.[11,15,71] Thus, for the esophageal disruption in which contrast material extends only a few millimeters from the esophageal lumen and the patient is doing well clinically, antibiotic therapy, chest tube drainage as indicated, and observation may suffice. Unfortunately, many esophageal perforations fail to meet the aforementioned criteria, and a successful outcome requires surgical intervention.

Perforations of the cervical and upper thoracic esophagus are approached through an oblique cervical incision that parallels the anterior border of the left sternocleidomastoid muscle[104] (Fig. 26-11). The sternocleidomastoid muscle and carotid sheath are retracted laterally and the trachea and thyroid gland medially. If the perforation can be identified, it is closed with absorbable polyglycolic acid sutures. If the injury cannot be visualized adequately for repair, the retroesophageal prevertebral space is dissected bluntly with the finger, and the superior mediastinum is drained with two 1-in Penrose drains brought out through the neck wound. Esophageal perforations to the level of the tracheal bifurcation can generally be treated successfully with such a cervical approach. Midthoracic esophageal perforations must be approached through a right thoracotomy, and those of the distal third of the esophagus are approached through a left thoracotomy.

Traditional surgical dogma teaches that esophageal perforations beyond 6 to 12 hours in duration are virtually impossible to repair primarily, the pouting inflamed mucosa at the edge of the tear holding sutures poorly. Isolated reports, however, have emphasized that even after marked delay in repair, successful closure of the esophageal injury may be possible.[5,42,43,46,62] The author has found that the majority of esophageal tears can in fact be repaired successfully using meticulous surgical technique that includes identification of adjacent submucosa by dissecting away the overlying muscle, defining the limits of the mucosal tear, reapproximation of the disrupted mucosa and submucosa with a surgical stapler (Endo-GIA), and reapproximation of the muscle over the

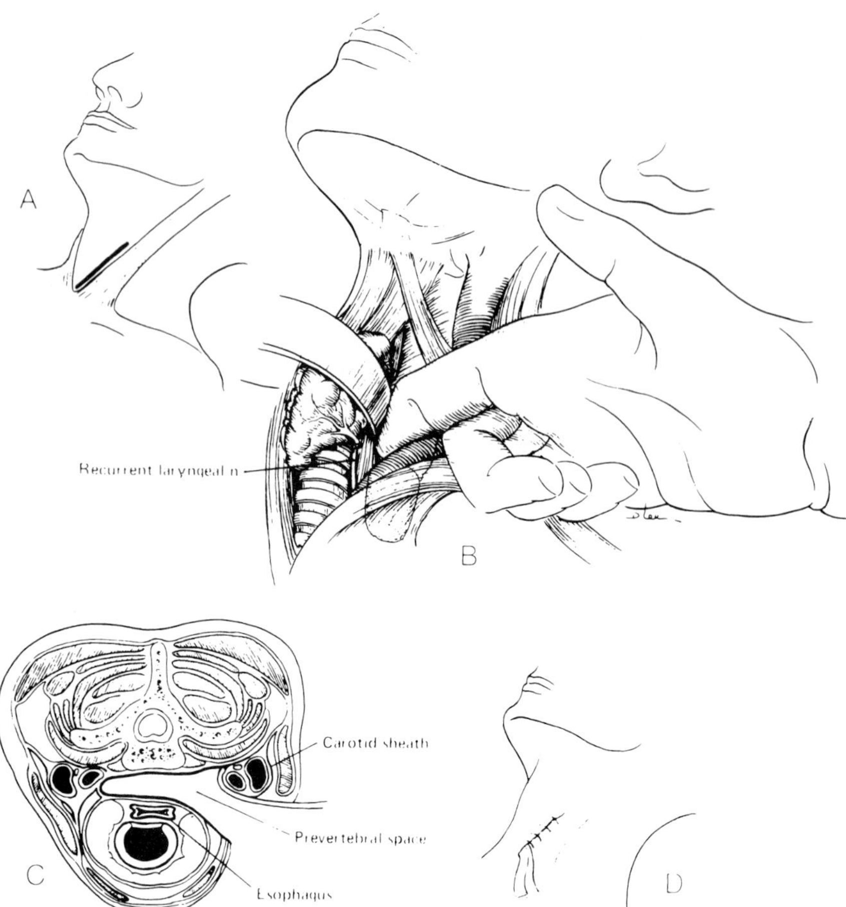

Figure 26–11. Surgical approach to the perforated cervical esophagus. *A,* Skin incision along anterior border of left sternocleidomastoid muscle from the level of the cricoid cartilage to the sternal notch. *B,* Blunt dissection into superior mediastinum along the prevertebral fascia medial to the sternocleidomastoid muscle and carotid sheath. Injury to the recurrent laryngeal nerve in the tracheoesophageal groove must be avoided. *C,* Schematic view of prevertebral space to be drained. *D,* Placement of two 1-in rubber drains to allow establishment of an esophagocutaneous fistula. (From Orringer, M.B.: The mediastinum. *In* Nora, P.F. [ed.]: Nora's Operative Surgery, 3rd ed. Philadelphia, W.B. Saunders, 1990, p. 370, with permission.)

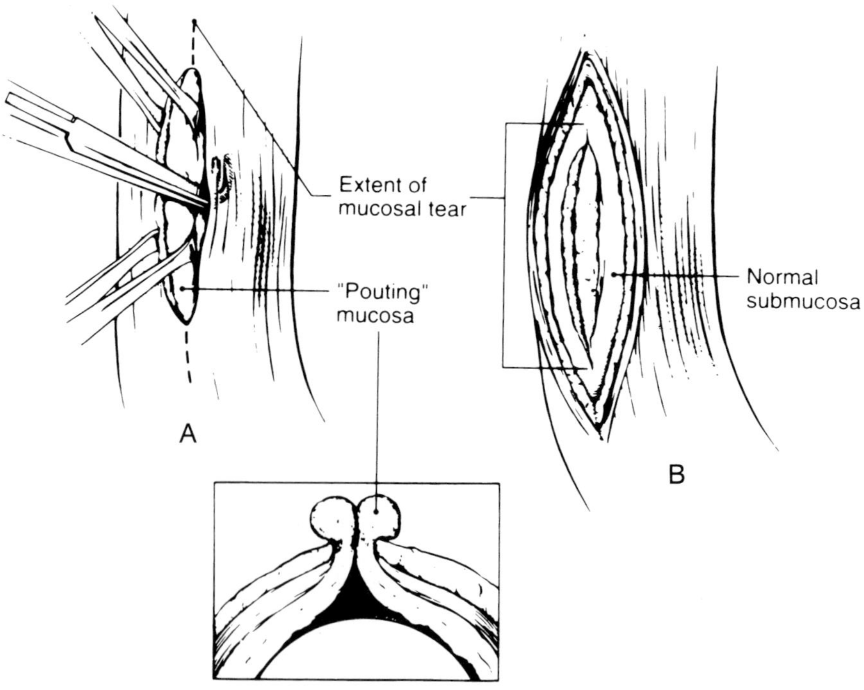

Figure 26–12. Technique of primary repair of esophageal perforation. The pouting mucosa at the site of the tear *(inset)* is grasped with Allis clamps *(A)*, and the adjustment esophageal muscle is mobilized around the entire tear with a right-angle clamp until 1 cm of normal submucosa is exposed around the defect *(B)*. (From Whyte, R.I., Iannettoni, M.D., and Orringer, M.B.: Intrathoracic esophageal perforation: The merit of primary repair. J. Thorac. Cardiovasc. Surg., *109*:140, 1994, with permission.)

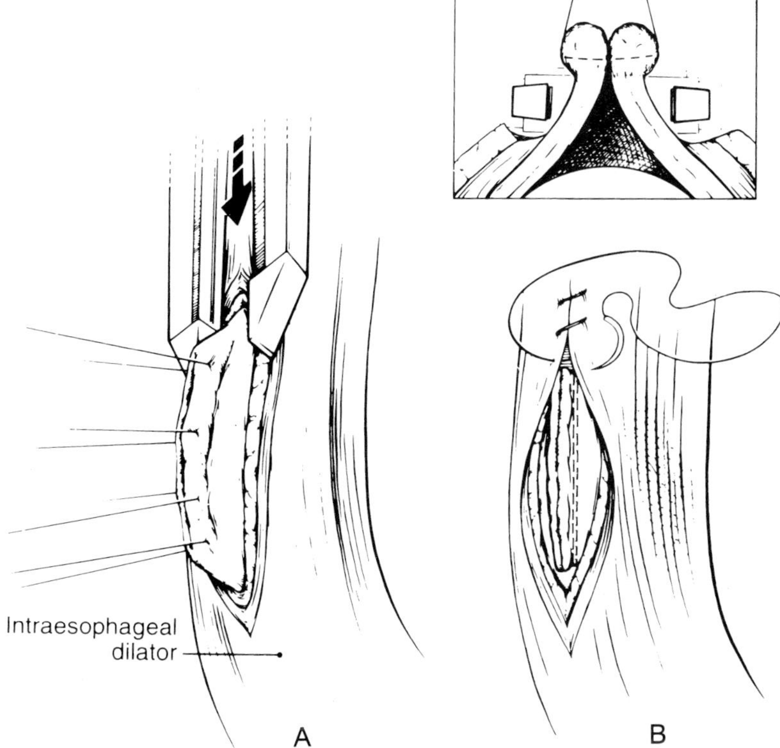

Figure 26–13. Technique of primary repair of esophageal perforation *(continuation of Fig. 26–12).* Traction sutures placed through the inflamed pouting mucosal edge of the tear elevate the submucosa so that an Endo-GIA cartridge can be applied and fixed *(A* and *inset).* The staple suture-line is covered by approximating the adjacent muscle over it from a running absorbable suture *(B).* (From Whyte, R.I., Iannettoni, M.D., and Orringer, M.B.: Intrathoracic esophageal perforation: The merit of primary repair. J. Thorac. Cardiovasc. Surg., *109:*140, 1994, with permission.)

staple suture line (Figs. 26–12 and 26–13).[138] In patients with chronic mediastinitis and pleural reaction, the adjacent mediastinal pleura is thickened and provides an excellent flap with which to reinforce the esophageal suture line.[43] Alternatively, if there is not sufficient parietal pleural thickening to provide adequate support for the suture line, reinforcement with either a pedicled intercostal muscle flap[12,27] (Fig. 26–14), omentum,[76] pericardium[53] (Fig. 26–15), visceral pleura,[80] or diaphragm[59,113,118] may be carried out. The mediastinal pleura must be opened from the apex of the chest to the diaphragm to permit wide drainage of the mediastinum, and after copious irrigation of the mediastinum and pleural cavity and decortication of any acute fibrinous exudate that may have formed over the lung, a large-bore chest tube is left near the esophageal suture line so that if

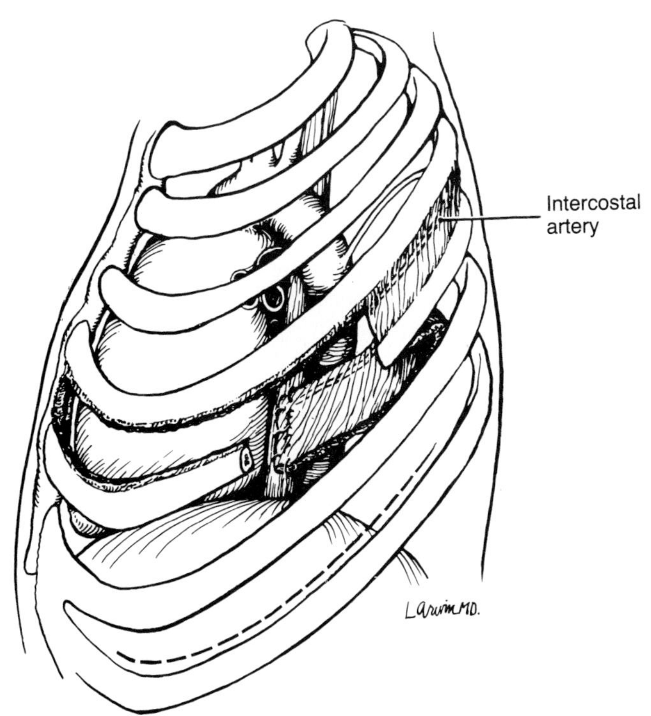

Figure 26–14. Predicted intercostal muscle-flap reinforcement of esophageal suture line. The neurovascular bundle of the intercostal flap must be preserved. The muscle flap is sutured over the esophageal suture line as an "on-lay patch." The intercostal muscle pedicle should not be wrapped around the esophagus lest periosteal regeneration result in annular constriction and obstruction. (For purposes of illustration, a portion of the rib overlying the muscle pedicle has been removed.) (From Orringer, M.B.: Complications of esophageal surgery and trauma. *In* Greenfield, L.J. [ed.]: Complications in Surgery and Trauma. Philadelphia, J.B. Lippincott, 1984, p. 272, with permission.)

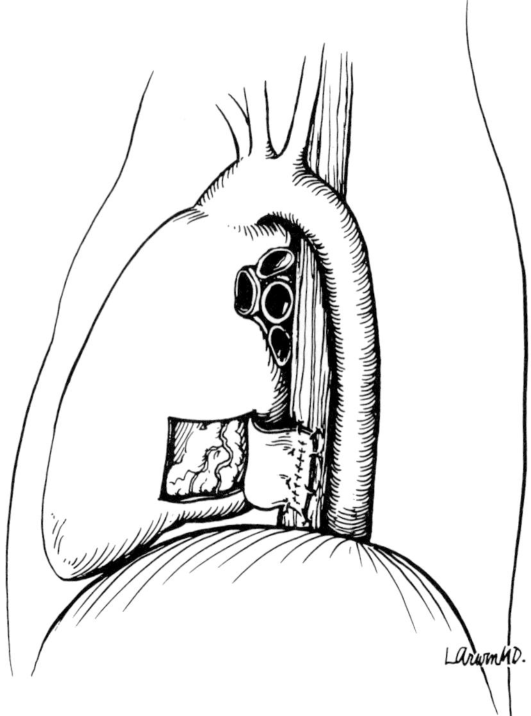

Figure 26–15. Reinforcement of esophageal suture line with pericardial flap. (From Orringer, M.B.: Complications of esophageal surgery and trauma. *In* Greenfield, L.J. [ed.]: Complications in Surgery and Trauma. Philadelphia, J.B. Lippincott, 1984, p. 273, with permission.)

disruption occurs, the result will be an esophagopleural cutaneous fistula.[120]

In treating an esophageal perforation, associated esophageal pathology cannot be ignored. Thus, a perforation proximal to a carcinoma or a caustic or reflux stricture may necessitate an emergent esophagectomy with either primary or delayed esophageal reconstruction.[50,61,101] Alternatively, if it is possible to dilate a benign stricture intraoperatively to relieve the distal obstruction, closure of a proximal esophageal perforation may be successful. A subsequent disruption of the esophageal closure may still eventually heal if dilation of the associated stricture is continued.[88] A perforated pulsion diverticulum of the esophagus may be resected within several hours of the injury, but again, the associated obstruction must be dealt with and the neuromotor esophageal dysfunction responsible for formation of the pouch relieved by performing a concomitant esophagomyotomy.

COMPLICATIONS OF SPECIFIC ESOPHAGEAL OPERATIONS

Esophagoscopy

The enormous recent technologic advances in the development of flexible fiberoptic instruments have facilitated greatly the performance of esophagogastroscopy, resulting in a tremendous increase in the number of these studies being performed on an outpatient basis. Unfortunately, with the greater ease in performing esophagoscopies, an almost cavalier attitude toward this relatively "minor" procedure has emerged. The consequences of esophageal disruption have not changed, however, and perforation during endoscopy occurs in 1 to 2% of patients, even in the hands of the most experienced endoscopist. If this complication of esophagoscopy is to be avoided, certain common principles must be acknowledged and rigidly followed:

1. Adequate preoperative and intraoperative sedation and anesthesia are mandatory. Anxious, combative, or uncooperative patients simply do not tolerate esophagoscopy safely. In some patients, general anesthesia is the only means of creating acceptable conditions for performance of the study for both the patient and the surgeon. The initial dilatation of a tight esophageal stricture is frequently painful, and it is best that the surgeon's attention and concentration be on the operative field and not on a struggling patient.
2. Esophagoscopy should not be carried out unless a prior barium swallow examination has been performed and reviewed by the endoscopist. The films should preferably be displayed in view of the endoscopist at the time of his examination. The current "modern" trend is to perform the flexible endoscopic examination without waiting for the results of a prior barium swallow study and to obtain the contrast study *if* significant pathology is found. This practice is dangerous. Just as the road map alerts the traveler to the road that lies before him, the barium swallow provides information about pre-existing pathology and its expected location (Fig. 26–16). For

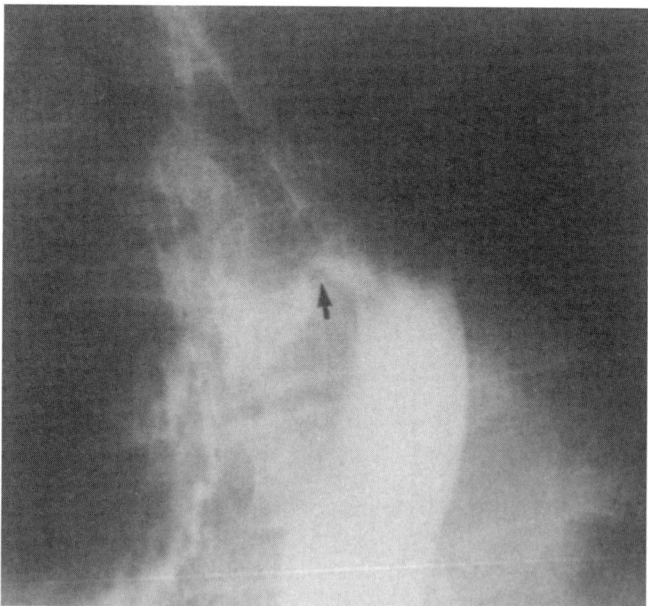

Figure 26–16. Gastrografin swallow showing midesophageal perforation *(arrow)* after rigid esophagoscopy in a patient who had dysphagia. An outside "normal" barium swallow report had been accepted, and esophagoscopy was performed without the endoscopist seeing the contrast study. In this patient, a large subcarinal mass of lymph nodes due to sarcoidosis was displacing the esophagus to the left, as is evident in this posteroanterior view. Without knowledge of this abnormal course of the esophagus in this patient, the esophagoscope was advanced, and a perforation occurred. The surgeon performing esophagoscopy is responsible for seeing the barium swallow examination in the patient *before* he or she passes the esophagoscope.

example, a Zenker's diverticulum identified with a barium esophagogram should be expected to be encountered approximately 15 cm from the upper incisors, the location of the upper esophageal sphincter. A midesophageal carcinoma at the level of the tracheal bifurcation is encountered approximately 25 cm from the upper incisors. An epiphrenic diverticulum located proximal to the esophagogastric junction is encountered before the esophagoscope reaches a point 40 cm from the upper incisors. A perforation of a cervical esophageal diverticulum or a midesophageal stricture cannot be justified because the endoscopist was unaware of these lesions because a prior barium swallow examination was neither obtained nor personally reviewed.

3. Failure to properly introduce the rigid esophagoscope through the upper esophageal sphincter may result in a perforation. The cricopharyngeus muscle originates from the cricoid cartilage, and the natural "pull" of this muscle against the cartilage will result in a posterior perforation unless the larynx is "lifted" anteriorly as the esophagoscope is advanced (Fig. 26–17).

4. The esophagoscope should not be advanced unless the lumen is visible. Preoperative administration of atropine to reduce oral secretions and the availability of adequate suction are important prerequisites for safe endoscopic examination.

5. As the esophagoscope is advanced, adjustment must be made for the natural course of the esophagus. Because the distal esophagus courses anteriorly and to the left as it joins the stomach, particularly when performing rigid esophagoscopy, the instrument must be angled toward the right side of the patient's mouth and the occiput of the head lowered as the esophagoscope is advanced into the distal esophagus.

6. The initial dilatation of a tight esophageal stricture requires adequate sedation and anesthesia, at times general anesthesia (see Chapter 13). This minimizes patient discomfort and allows the surgeon to concentrate on the visual field. When a rigid esophagoscope is used for this initial evaluation, flexible gum-tipped bougies are inserted into the esophagoscope and are passed through the stricture under direct vision, and the pliability and extent of the stenosis are assessed. With a mild "soft" stricture, dilation by advancing the esophagoscope through the stricture may be possible. However, with more firm, high-grade stenoses, it is safer to pass progressively larger dilators through the stricture. This may be achieved through the rigid esophagoscope, as described in Chapter 13, or as is now more often the case, using the Savary-Gilliard guidewire and dilating system. In our experience, the Maloney tapered esophageal dilators are the most reliable and safest instruments for repeated outpatient dilatations of esophageal strictures, and in most cases, their passage requires none of the sedation or anesthesia that are necessary when endoscopic balloon dilations are performed.

Additional minor complications of esophagoscopy, which are more common with rigid esophagoscopes, include fractures of teeth and lip lacerations. These complications are avoided by carefully padding the lips and teeth with a moistened gauze sponge before introducing the esophagoscope into the mouth and by being certain that the upper lip is not compressed between the esophagoscope and the incisor teeth as the esophagoscope is advanced.

Hiatal Herniorrhaphy

Hiatal herniorrhaphy, although conceptually quite simple, can result in a number of serious complications (Table 26-2). The esophagus may be perforated acutely when concomitant esophagoscopy is performed during an antireflux operation or when a distal esophageal stricture

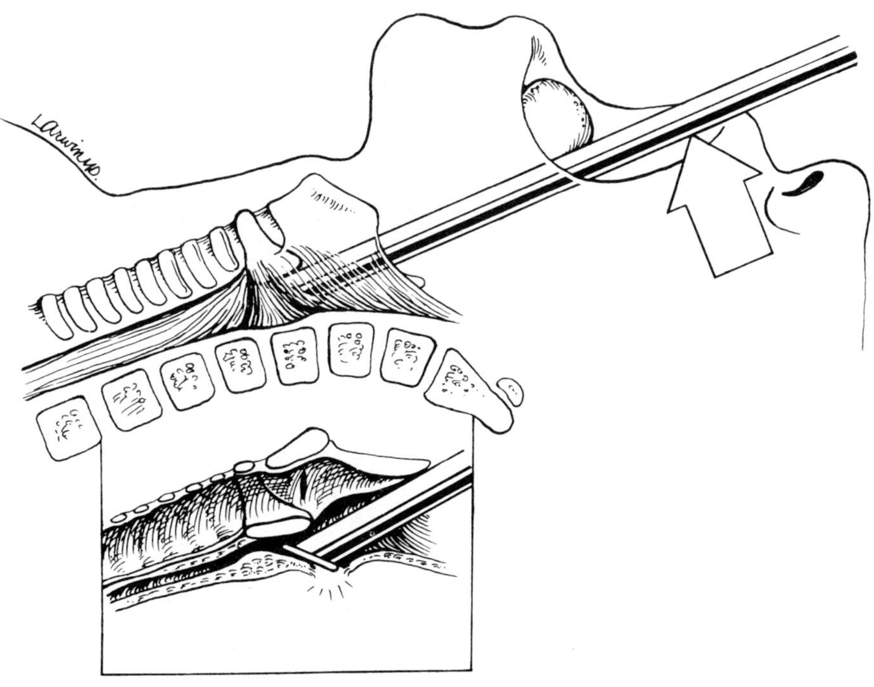

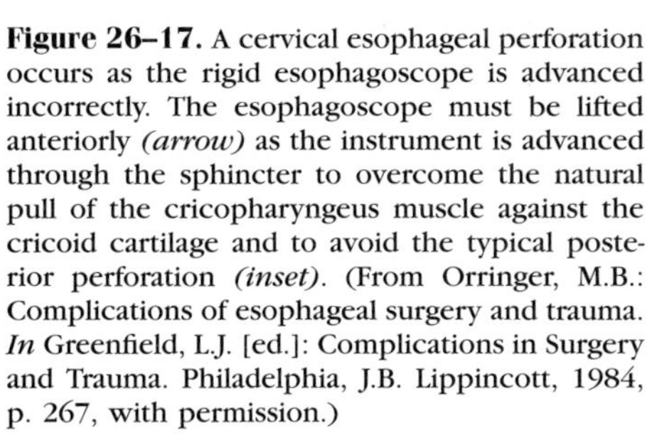

Figure 26–17. A cervical esophageal perforation occurs as the rigid esophagoscope is advanced incorrectly. The esophagoscope must be lifted anteriorly *(arrow)* as the instrument is advanced through the sphincter to overcome the natural pull of the cricopharyngeus muscle against the cricoid cartilage and to avoid the typical posterior perforation *(inset)*. (From Orringer, M.B.: Complications of esophageal surgery and trauma. *In* Greenfield, L.J. [ed.]: Complications in Surgery and Trauma. Philadelphia, J.B. Lippincott, 1984, p. 267, with permission.)

Table 26–2. Complications of Hiatus Hernia Surgery

Intraoperative
Perforation
Endoscopic
During dilation
Vagus nerve injury
Hemorrhage
Splenic injury
Short gastric vessel
Postoperative
Perforation
Stricture
Esophageal suture
Gastric suture
Dysphagia
Transient—"denervation," edema
Mechanical, fundoplication, gastroplasty tube, or hiatus too tight
"Gas bloats"
Gastric atony—pylorospasm
Crural repair disruption
Postvagotomy diarrhea
Chylothorax
Incisional pain

is disrupted during intraoperative dilatation. A delayed perforation, usually within 1 week of surgery, may occur when esophageal sutures placed too deeply during the repair result in local mural necrosis.

Acute esophageal tears recognized before the incision should be approached transthoracically and repaired, and the esophageal suture line reinforced with either the fundoplication if the tear is in the distal esophagus, the pedicled anterior mediastinal fat, or with a pedicled intercostal muscle flap if the tear is higher. When an intercostal muscle pedicle is used to reinforce an esophageal suture line, it should be sutured to the esophagus as an onlay patch, not placed circumferentially around the esophagus; regeneration of bone or cartilage from the perichondrium or periosteum mobilized with the flap may result in a late obstructing ring around the esophagus (Fig. 26–18). When a reflux stricture is perforated during attempted dilation at the time of a planned antireflux operation, unless the involved tissues are relatively healthy and amenable to repair, resectional therapy is generally a better option. Although most reflux strictures can be dilated, and many regress after an antireflux procedure has been carried out, disruption of a stricture during attempted dilation is one of the definitions of an "undilatable" stricture that justifies esophageal resection, and the author's preference in this situation is to proceed with a transthoracic esophagectomy and then reposition the patient supine and carry out a cervical esophagogastric anastomosis.[89] Several additional options for the treatment of a disrupted distal stricture are available. Unfortunately, none is without its associated morbidity. The Thal fundic patch esophagoplasty utilizes adjacent gastric fundus to "patch" the opened narrowed esophagus.[132,133] This procedure not only relies on the healing of the opened, inflamed distal esophagus to which the stomach is sutured but also requires the addition of an intrathoracic fundoplication (Thal-Woodward procedure) to control gastroesophageal reflux—in effect, creation of a man-made paraesophageal hiatal hernia.[73,134,141] The incidence of suture line disruption and mechanical complications associated with this operation condemn its use (Fig. 26–19). For the same reason, we oppose use of an intratho-

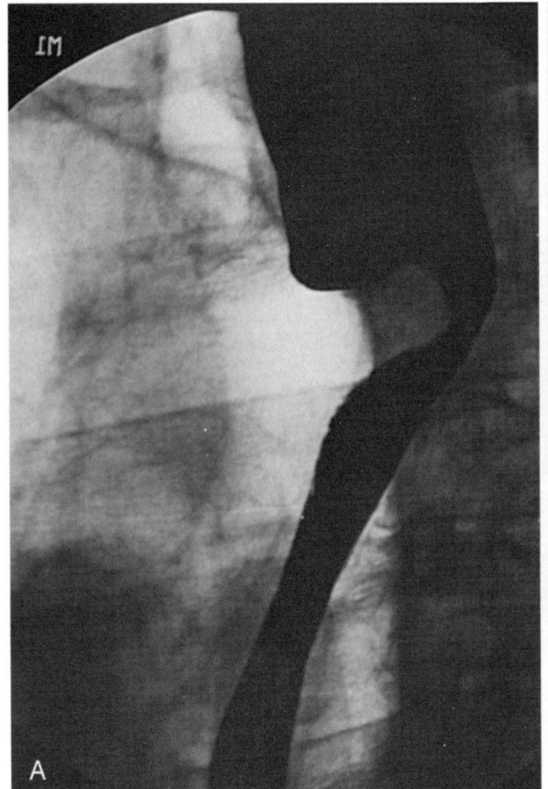

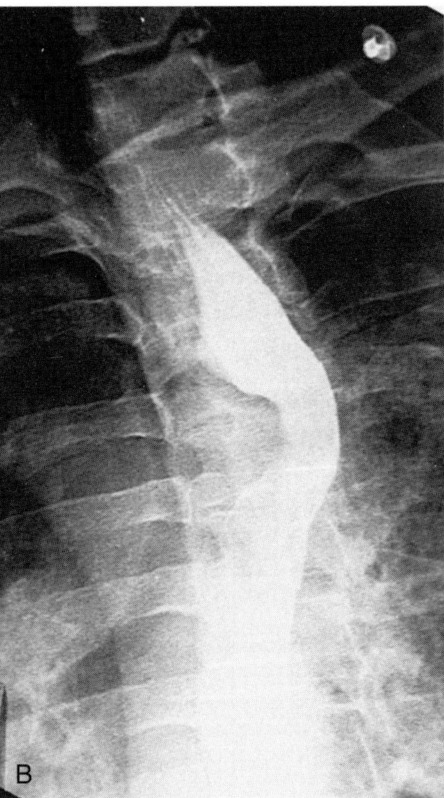

Figure 26–18. *A,* Barium swallow examination in a 49-year-old man who was treated for a gunshot wound of the esophagus and trachea 23 years earlier. At that operation, the tracheal and esophageal holes were débrided and repaired, and the esophagus was incorrectly wrapped circumferentially with a mobilized intercostal muscle pedicle. Subsequent regeneration of cartilage from the perichondrium of the intercostal pedicle resulted in severe dysphagia and the high-grade upper esophageal stenosis with proximal esophageal dilation that is shown. *B,* Postoperative barium swallow after a repeat right thoracotomy and partial resection of the encircling cartilaginous and muscle ring. The lumen was greatly improved, and the dysphagia was relieved.

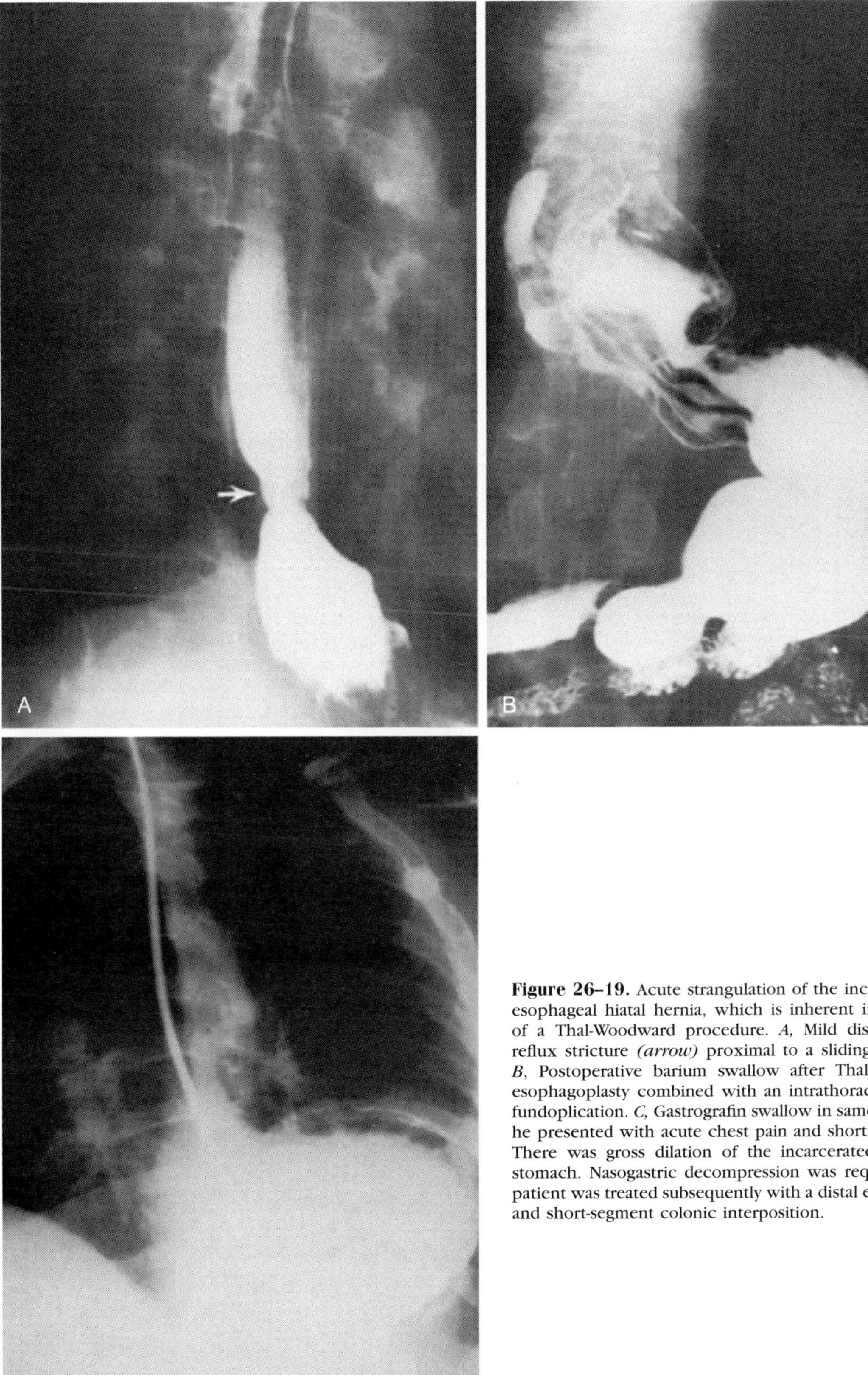

Figure 26–19. Acute strangulation of the incarcerated paraesophageal hiatal hernia, which is inherent in construction of a Thal-Woodward procedure. *A,* Mild distal esophageal reflux stricture *(arrow)* proximal to a sliding hiatal hernia. *B,* Postoperative barium swallow after Thal fundic patch esophagoplasty combined with an intrathoracic Nissen-type fundoplication. *C,* Gastrografin swallow in same patient when he presented with acute chest pain and shortness of breath. There was gross dilation of the incarcerated intrathoracic stomach. Nasogastric decompression was required, and the patient was treated subsequently with a distal esophagectomy and short-segment colonic interposition.

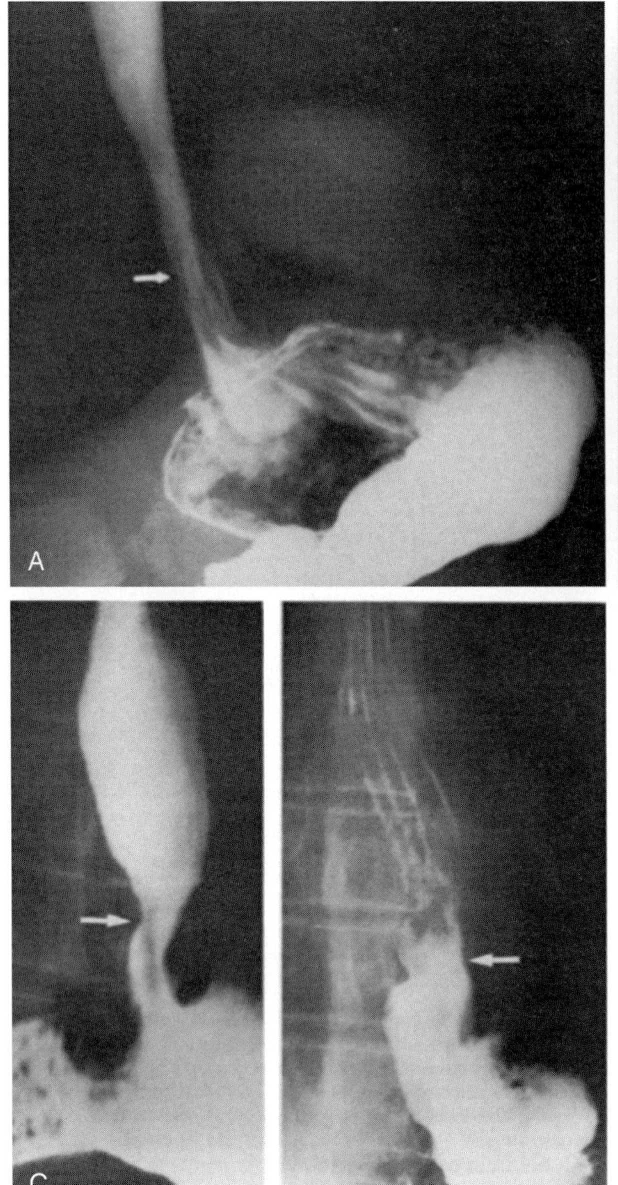

Figure 26–20. Disruption of hiatal hernia repair associated with postoperative gastric dilatation (*arrows* indicate the esophagogastric junction). *A,* Preoperative barium swallow showing a small recurrent hiatal hernia. *B,* Postoperative barium swallow 1 week after Belsey Mark IV repair showing a satisfactory intra-abdominal distal esophageal segment but also gastric dilation and delayed gastric emptying. *C,* After 2 months *(left)* and 4 months *(right)*, the repair has progressively disrupted. The early postoperative delayed gastric emptying, most likely due to inadvertent injury to the vagus nerves, should have been treated with a gastric drainage procedure to minimize the chance of disruption of the repair and recurrence of the hernia. (From Orringer, M.B.: Complications of esophageal surgery and trauma. *In* Greenfield, L.J. [ed.]: Complications in Surgery and Trauma. Philadelphia, J.B. Lippincott, 1984, p. 274, with permission.)

racic fundoplication (without a Thal procedure) to control reflux. The complications of such an approach outweigh its benefits.[74,116,119] Gastric ulceration may complicate 3 to 10% of fundoplications and may occur both in supradiaphragmatic fundic wraps and in intra-abdominal fundoplications.[10,14,109] In the former, one is dealing with a complication of an iatrogenic paraesophageal hiatal hernia, and operative repair is generally indicated. In the latter, ulceration may be due to relative ischemia in the wrap, and treatment with H_2-receptor blockers, proton pump inhibitors, or cytoprotective agents may suffice.

The development of fever, chest pain, or respiratory distress during the first week after a hiatal hernia operation mandates a contrast study, and if a distal esophageal perforation is diagnosed, treatment usually involves reoperation. The site of the perforation is identified intraoperatively, at times by insufflating air through a nasogastric tube. A leak from an intra-abdominal fundoplication suture may be closed and reinforced with adjacent omentum. If the leak is in the chest, pedicled anterior mediastinal fat, intercostal muscle, or pleura is used to reinforce the closure using a transthoracic approach. A jejunostomy feeding tube should be placed to allow nutritional support and unimpeded ambulation in case the repair does not "hold" and an esophageal fistula ensues. Either a large-bore chest tube should be left near the thoracic esophageal repair or a drain should be placed near the transabdominally repaired fundoplication to ensure external drainage of a recurrent fistula.

Low retrosternal dysphagia after an antireflux operation may have one of several causes: (1) distal esophageal edema after intraoperative manipulation; (2) distal esophageal motor dysfunction due to manipulation of the vagus nerves; (3) obstruction due to too tight a fundoplication[125]; or obstruction from excessive closure of the hiatus. Performance of the fundoplication over at least a No. 54 French intraesophageal dilator minimizes the likelihood of this latter complication. Dysphagia after truncal vagotomy has been recognized for more than 40 years, and it is apparent that neuromotor esophageal dysfunction may follow manipulation of the vagus nerves at the level of the distal esophagus.[20,44,45,82] This complication after antireflux surgery is more likely with a transthoracic than with a transabdominal repair because identification and displacement of the main vagal trunks are more routine with the former approach. These patients have dysphagia immediately after the antireflux procedure; on barium swallow examination, the distal esophagus is tapered and empties poorly, resembling the picture of achalasia or esophageal spasm. Reassurance and maintenance of a soft diet for several days usually constitute adequate therapy, although passage of an esophageal dilator is at times required for relief. This problem typically subsides spontaneously, but occasionally reoperation, takedown of the repair, and at times, even esophageal resection may be needed.

Another complication of intraoperative vagus nerve injury occurring during a hiatal hernia repair is impaired gastric motility or pylorospasm resulting in delayed gastric emptying and secondary gastric dilation. This complication has direct implications for the long-term success of the hiatal hernia repair because sustained gastric dilation in combination with a competent distal esophageal sphincter mechanism may eventually result in disruption of the esophageal sutures used to construct the fundoplication and failure of the repair (Fig. 26–20). When the patient who has undergone an antireflux operation develops gastric dilation immediately after operation, a 7- to 10-day trial of gastric decompression with a nasogastric tube is indicated. At times, an anticholinergic (e.g., atropine 0.4 mg either per os or intramuscularly every 4 to 6 hours) may relieve the associated pylorospasm. However, this problem should not be permitted to persist indefinitely, and it is best to perform an early gastric drainage procedure (pyloromyotomy or pyloroplasty) than to risk recurrent gastroesophageal reflux. Finally, vagal nerve injury may result in varying degrees of "dumping syndrome" (e.g., postprandial diarrhea, cramping, abdominal pain, nausea, diaphoresis, palpitations). This problem generally subsides within a few months, but at times long-term management with antidiarrheal medication and dietary restriction may be required.

Before the patient's discharge from the hospital after an antireflux operation, a routine barium swallow examination should be performed to document the postoperative appearance of the reconstructed esophagogastric junction. At times, this contrast study may reveal a "silent" localized extravasation of contrast material at the site of one of the fundoplication sutures that was placed too deeply. If the patient is asymptomatic and the "leak" is very small, no therapy may be required because the supporting fundoplication has prevented a more major disruption. A far more disconcerting radiographic finding on the "routine" postoperative barium swallow obtained prior to discharge is the asymptomatic migration of the fundoplication or gastric fundus into the chest as a result of disruption of the posterior crural repair (Fig. 26–21).

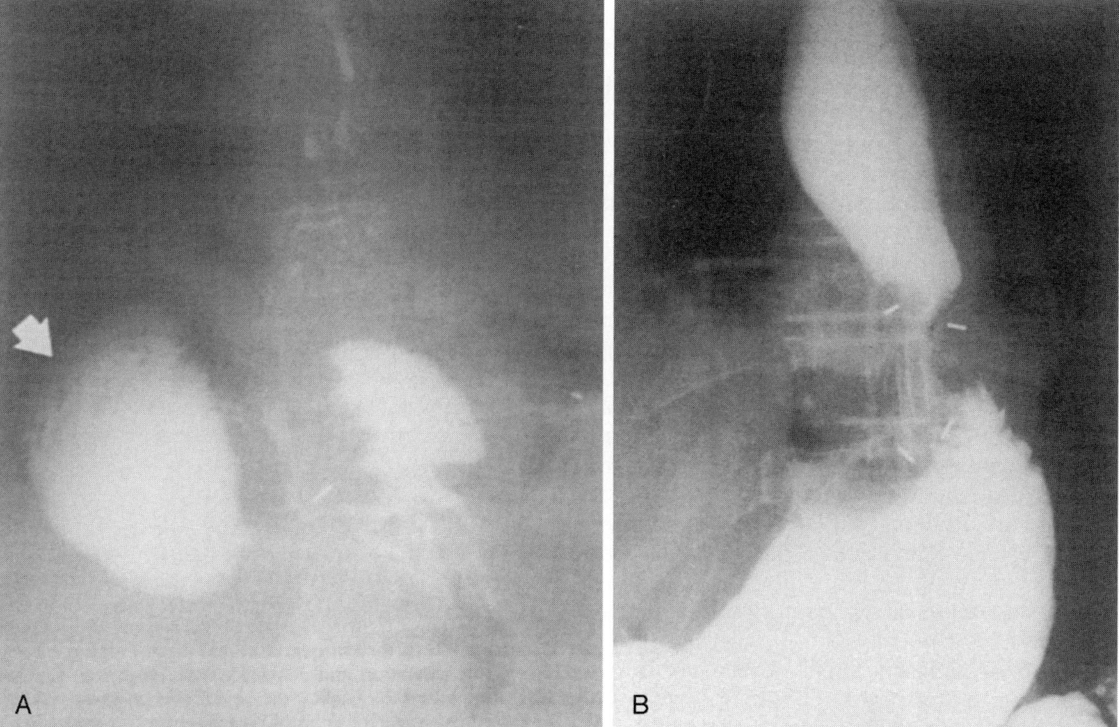

Figure 26–21. *A,* Asymptomatic partial migration of the fundoplication into the chest through the diaphragmatic hiatus 1 week after a Collis-Nissen hiatal hernia repair (*arrow* indicates the portion of fundoplication above the diaphragm). Although asymptomatic, this patient was reoperated on, the fundoplication was reduced and secured below the diaphragm, and the hiatus was narrowed further to prevent later potential complications of this paraesophageal hernia. *B,* After reduction of the fundoplication, the upper silver clips at the level of the diaphragmatic hiatus and the lower set of silver clips at the end of the gastroplasty tube ("neoesophagus") define the length of the fundoplication, which is now below the diaphragm. (From Orringer, M.B.: Complications of esophageal surgery and trauma. *In* Greenfield, L.J. [ed.]: Complications in Surgery and Trauma. Philadelphia, J.B. Lippincott, 1984, p. 275, with permission.)

This iatrogenic paraesophageal hiatal hernia is subject to the same mechanical complications of paraesophageal herniation in the patient who has had no surgery. Reoperation is necessary to reduce the fundoplication back into the abdomen and to replace the posterior crural sutures if they have pulled through the crural muscle (or to narrow the hiatus further if they have not), before postoperative adhesions form between the herniated stomach and adjacent tissues, making any subsequent repair more difficult. It may be difficult to tell the asymptomatic patient recovering from an antireflux operation that reoperation is necessary, but conservative management of this problem is ill-advised.

Chylothorax following an antireflux procedure may result from injury to the thoracic duct, which passes from the abdomen through the aortic hiatus and then courses in the lower chest anterior to the spine between the esophagus and the aorta. Injury may occur during mobilization of the cardia or during placement of the crural sutures. This complication is heralded by prolonged chest tube drainage after a transthoracic repair, and the true cause of this serosanguineous drainage may not become apparent until the patient's diet is liberalized and its fat content increases. If chylothorax is present, the oral administration of 60 to 90 ml of cream for 4 to 6 hours will cause the chest tube drainage to become opalescent and milky chyle. The diagnosis can also be established by staining the fluid with Sudan R, which stains the globules of fat. Determination of the cholesterol and triglyceride levels in the fluid is usually not necessary. A cholesterol/triglyceride ratio of less than 1 is characteristic of a chylous effusion, whereas nonchylous effusions have a ratio of greater than 1. In most cases, a chylothorax following a hiatal hernia repair can be managed conservatively by administering a low-residue elemental diet and maintaining prolonged chest tube suction. If the output of chyle remains significant (>400 to 600 ml per consecutive 8-hour periods) after 7 to 10 days of this treatment, then reoperation with identification and ligation of the injured thoracic duct is indicated.

Acute postoperative hemorrhage after an antireflux operation is most often the result of bleeding from an unsecured divided short gastric vessel along the high greater curvature of the stomach. This possibility should always be borne in mind as the short gastric vessels are divided and ligated before performing a fundoplication. Hemorrhage from these vessels may be a particularly treacherous complication following a transthoracic hiatal hernia repair because the resulting hypovolemic shock may be attributed to other causes (e.g., myocardial infarction) when there is minimal chest tube drainage and the chest roentgenogram shows no hemothorax. Abdominal exploration, evacuation of the blood, and ligation of the bleeding vessel is the proper course of therapy. Splenic injury also occurs in a small percentage of patients undergoing antireflux surgery, particularly in reoperations. The incidence of splenic injury is slightly higher with transabdominal as compared with transthoracic antireflux operations, particularly in obese patients.

The Angelchik antireflux prosthesis was proposed as a simple surgical method of managing gastroesophageal reflux.[3] Although ample laboratory and clinical experience confirmed that this device did in fact control gastroesophageal reflux in most patients in whom it was used, it became apparent that the rate of major complications caused by this prosthesis was at least 10%.[19] Reported complications associated with the Angelchik silicone esophageal collar included disruption and migration of the prosthesis (Fig. 26–22), erosion into or through the esophagus, persistent dysphagia, and pain.[7,32,69,75,81,108,114,127] Complications requiring removal of the prosthesis were frequently catastrophic and necessitated major operative intervention. Erosion of the esophagastric junction caused by the device typically left little possibility of satisfactory reconstruction of the esophagogastric junction that would provide long-term reflux control. Esophageal resection was therefore required, the type of reconstruction depending on the surgeon's experience and preference as well as the patient's general condition. Options included a distal esophagectomy and intrathoracic esophagogastric anastomosis (a poor solution due to the inevitable reflux esophagitis associated with this approach), a distal jejunal or short-segment colonic interposition, or the author's preferred approach of transhiatal esophagectomy with a cervical esophagogastric anastomosis.[99] Esophageal erosion associated with acute mediastinitis at times required initial drainage, esophagectomy, a feeding tube, and cervical or anterior thoracic esophagostomy (Fig. 26–23) until the patient's general condition stabilized sufficiently to permit esophageal reconstruction. In cases in which the prosthesis has obstructed the esophagogastric junction without causing erosion into the esophageal lumen, the goal is to remove the device and then perform a fundoplication to control reflux. Unfortunately, the tough fibrous capsule that develops

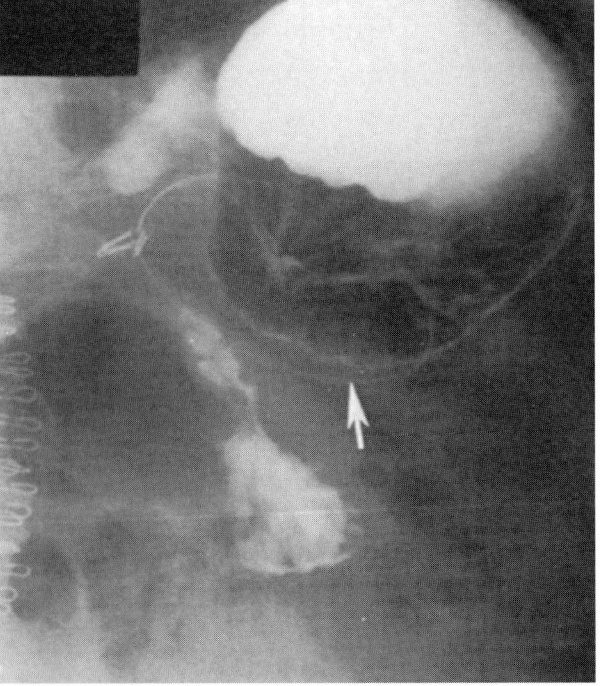

Figure 26–22. Migration of the Angelchik prosthesis *(arrow)* with resultant acute dilation of the gastric fundus. This patient presented with acute upper abdominal pain and required emergent removal of the prosthesis and a fundoplication to control the gastroesophageal reflux.

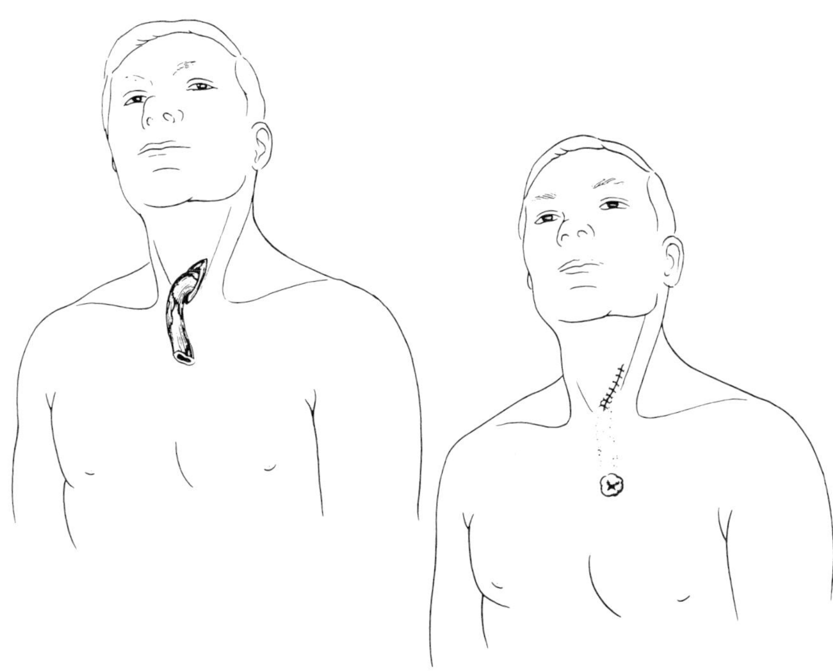

Figure 26–23. Construction of anterior thoracic esophagostomy. When esophageal disruption warrants total esophageal diversion, the intrathoracic esophagus should be mobilized well into the neck through the thoracic incision, and the esophagus should then be delivered out of the neck wound and placed on the anterior chest wall. Viability of the remaining esophagus is maintained through collateral circulation from the inferior thyroid arteries. The esophagus should be tunneled subcutaneously and an anterior thoracic esophagostomy constructed. It is much easier to apply a stomal appliance to the flat surface of the upper chest than to the usual location of a cervical esophagostomy. The remaining esophageal length can be used to advantage when alimentary continuity is reestablished at a later date. (From Orringer, M.B.: Complications of esophageal surgery and trauma. *In* Greenfield, L.J. [ed.]: Complications in Surgery and Trauma, 2nd ed. Philadelphia, J.B. Lippincott, 1990, p. 302, with permission.)

around the prosthesis makes construction of a fundoplication more difficult, and the possibility of injury to the vagus nerves is increased because the presence of the periesophageal fibrosis makes their identification more difficult. The magnitude of the complications associated with the Angelchik prosthesis, even though they were relatively infrequent, has resulted in this device's virtual elimination as an option for antireflux surgery.

Laparoscopic Antireflux/Hiatal Hernia Surgery

Since 1991, when the first reports of laparoscopic antireflux surgery were published, minimally invasive surgical approaches to the diaphragmatic esophageal hiatus have been used with increasing frequency.[112] Although mortality rates for laparoscopic fundoplication have been low (0 to 1.4%), early morbidity rates were acceptable, and conversion rates to the open procedure were from 0 to 14%, the learning curve for this operation is substantial.[122] Unfortunately, lessons that have been learned in the past through the development of the open procedures are often forgotten in the enthusiasm and determination of the minimally invasive surgeon to perform the hiatal hernia repair exclusively with video-assisted technique.

In obese patients, in those with intra-abdominal adhesions from prior surgery, or in those with an unusually large left hepatic lobe, visualization of the operative field may be so difficult that persistence with the "closed" operation may be frankly dangerous. The latter factors remain indications for open transthoracic hiatal hernia repair. Perforations of the distal esophagus or gastric fundus have been reported during laparoscopic fundoplication and warrant conversion to an open procedure for repair. Blind dissection posterior to the esophagus should be avoided to prevent this complication.

Early postoperative dysphagia may result from an overly tight fundoplication, which is more likely to occur with minimally invasive procedures in which tactile sensation is not used to assess the tightness of the wrap. Performance of the fundoplication over at least a size 54 French dilator minimizes the likelihood of this complication. Postoperative dysphagia due to fibrotic stenosis of the muscular esophageal hiatus, attributed to a diathermy injury during the esophageal dissection, has also been reported and treated with laparoscopic hiatal division.[102] Persistent dysphagia after a laparoscopic fundoplication, refractory to dilatation therapy, may necessitate reoperation, takedown of the wrap, and construction of a looser fundoplication. The author's approach for such redo procedures is a transthoracic approach, generally with a combined esophageal lengthening Collis gastroplasty with a Nissen fundoplication (see Figs. 26–7, 26–8, and 26–9).

Additional complications of laparoscopic fundoplication include pneumothorax or pneumomediastinum from CO_2 tracking into the chest during the operation, incisional hernia at a port site, and herniation of the fundoplication through the diaphragmatic hiatus (particularly when the crura were not closed at the time of the original operation).

As enthusiasm for laparoscopic fundoplication has grown, this approach has also been used to repair large paraesophageal hiatal hernias, which are often associated with an attenuated, abnormally wide esophageal hiatus. In 1983, Pearson and associates[105] emphasized that esophageal shortening is common in these patients, most of whom have combined sliding and paraesophageal hiatus hernias, and the authors used the combined Collis gastroplasty-fundoplication operation liberally in this group. With the laparoscopic approach, one cannot assess the degree of tension on the distal esophagus that results from reduction of the esophagogastric junction below the diaphragm, because, again, direct manual palpation of the esophagus is not possible. Furthermore, with the diaphragms pushed abnormally upward by CO_2 instillation into the abdomen during the operation, a false sense of ease of reduction of the esophagogastric junction into the abdomen may occur. The author believes that most large combined sliding and paraesophageal hiatal hernias should be approached through the chest with an open operation, generally a combined Collis-Nissen operation. The increasing number of fundoplications that have "slipped" through the hiatus into the chest after laparoscopic repair likely reflect, at least in part, a lack of recognition by the original surgeon that there was unacceptable tension on the repair. Recurrent herniation of an intact or a partially disrupted fundoplication is the most common reason for failure of laparoscopic fundoplications.[21,54,56,128] Body habitus is another important but often overlooked factor in recurrence after laparoscopic (or any) antireflux operation; obesity is present in a significant number of patients who experience disruption of repairs.[111]

Another laparoscopic technique for the repair of paraesophageal hiatal hernias is the use of mesh to repair the diaphragmatic defect.[33,57,68] This is an ill-conceived operation because the constant diaphragmatic motion against the adjacent esophagus at the hiatus may result in esophageal or gastric erosion and perforation. This approach is mentioned only to condemn its use.

Esophageal Resection and Visceral Esophageal Substitution

In almost every large series of patients undergoing a traditional esophageal resection and substitution with either stomach or intestine, the leading causes of death are (1) respiratory insufficiency associated with the physiologic insult of a combined thoracic and abdominal operation, and (2) sepsis from mediastinitis resulting from disruption of an intrathoracic anastomosis. As a result, the author has adopted a general policy of performing *no intrathoracic esophageal anastomoses* and prefers a cervical esophagogastric anastomosis instead. A cervical esophagogastric anastomotic leak generally represents little more morbidity than a salivary fistula, and spontaneous closure with local wound care is the rule. Use of a stapled esophagogastric anastomosis, generally with a circular EEA stapler, has been recommended by some as one means of decreasing intrathoracic esophageal anastomotic leaks.[103,110] Others have found no difference in leak rate with stapled versus manually sewn anastomoses.[33,112] The author and associates reported a dramatic reduction in the incidence of postoperative cervical esophagogastric anastomotic leak to less than 3% with a side-to-side stapled cervical esophagogastric anastomosis constructed with the Auto Suture Endo-GIA II Stapler (U.S. Surgical Corporation, Auto Suture Company Division, Norwalk, CT).[90] The author has also found that a transhiatal esophagectomy without thoracotomy and a cervical esophagogastric anastomosis is applicable in most patients requiring esophageal resection and reconstruction for both benign and malignant disease (see Chapter 24). This procedure minimizes the operative insult to the patient by avoiding a thoracotomy. The incidence of postoperative pulmonary complications is thereby reduced, and the possibility of mediastinitis resulting from an intrathoracic leak is virtually eliminated. In their extensive collective review of the results of esophagectomy in 76,911 patients with esophageal carcinoma, Muller and associates[83] reported an overall reduction in postoperative mortality rates after esophageal resection by 50% in the 1990s, with the lowest mortality rate (11 ± 8%) in patients undergoing a transhiatal esophagectomy without thoracotomy.

The author recommends a No. 14 French rubber catheter feeding jejunostomy tube secured in place with a Witzel maneuver, not a "needle catheter" jejunostomy, in every patient undergoing esophagectomy and esophageal reconstruction.[40] The jejunostomy tube is regarded as an "insurance policy" if anastomotic disruption necessitates an alternate means of nourishment. If use of the tube is not required postoperatively, it is removed after several weeks. Alternatively, if an anastomotic leak occurs, a feeding jejunostomy tube is safer and more effective in providing calories than intravenous hyperalimentation.

Anastomotic Leak

After completion of a cervical esophageal anastomosis, the neck wound is closed *loosely* with only four or five 4-0 sutures over a ¼-in Penrose drain placed adjacent to the anastomosis (see Chapter 24). If an anastomotic leak does occur, the neck wound is opened at the bedside *in its entirety,* and gentle wound packing with gauze is initiated. The size of the leak can be estimated by having the patient drink water and evaluating the amount that escapes from the neck wound with a disposable bedside suction catheter. Generally, within several days of opening the wound, the drainage diminishes considerably, and the patient may resume oral intake while maintaining steady gentle pressure over the wound to occlude the fistula. Passage of tapered Maloney dilators (generally, Nos. 40 and 46 French) at the bedside during the first week after drainage of the cervical fistula ensures that no element of obstruction from either local edema or spasm contributes to continued drainage of the fistula.[88] More than 98% of cervical esophagogastric anastomotic leaks are small and respond to the open drainage and packing as described. A small proportion, however, are associated with catastrophic complications—major gastric tip necrosis necessitating takedown of the anastomosis, construction of cervical esophagostomy, and resection of nonviable stomach; vertebral body osteomyelitis; epidural abscess with resultant paraplegia; pulmonary microabscesses from an internal jugular vein abscess; and tracheoesophagogastric anastomotic fistula.[58]

When disruption of an intrathoracic esophageal anastomosis occurs during the first 10 critical days after operation, the clinical picture is quite characteristic. The typical symptoms of mediastinitis (fever, chest pain, tachycardia, tachypnea, respiratory distress, peripheral cyanosis, vasoconstriction, hypotension, and shock) associated with a chest roentgenogram that demonstrates hydrothorax or pneumothorax leave little question about the diagnosis, which should nonetheless be documented with a contrast study. An occasional small (<1 cm), contained anastomotic leak detected on a routine postoperative barium swallow in an otherwise asymptomatic patient may require no treatment. In most cases, however, anastomotic disruption warrants immediate reexploration, irrigation of the chest and mediastinum, repair of the fistula, if possible, and chest tube drainage. A localized anastomotic leak with viable adjacent tissue may be amenable to direct suture repair. Reinforcement with a pedicled anterior mediastinal fat or intercostal muscle flap, pleura, or omentum should be carried out. Decompression of the stomach with a nasogastric tube, placement of a jejunostomy tube for nutritional support, and appropriate antibiotics complete the therapy. A barium swallow examination should be performed 10 days later to be certain that healing has occurred, and the chest tube should be removed before this time. If breakdown of the anastomosis occurs again, the goal is to establish a controlled esophagopleural cutaneous fistula. It may be necessary to perform a rib resection in order to position a large-bore drainage tube adjacent to the fistula and ensure that all drainage from the esophageal leak can flow freely out of the chest. Gastric contents that are aspirated through the nasogastric tube can be returned to the alimentary tract through the jejunostomy tube to minimize electrolyte imbalance and to simplify fluid and electrolyte replacement.

If on re-exploration of the chest for a disrupted esophageal anastomosis, extensive local necrosis of the tissue with a major anastomotic dehiscence is found, there is little recourse but to take down the anastomosis, resect the nonviable stomach, and return it to the abdomen. Only nonviable distal esophagus should be resected. The proximal end of the divided intrathoracic esophagus, however, should *not* be oversewn and left in the infected mediastinum while a diverting lateral cervical esophagostomy is carried out. Disruption of the intrathoracic esophageal suture line is not only likely, but if subsequent reconstruction is possible, management of the remaining segment of intrathoracic esophagus presents a considerable technical problem. The best alternative is to circumferentially mobilize the esophagus well into the neck through the thoracic incision and after the thoracotomy is closed, turn the patient supine and construct a formal *end* esophagostomy. As indicated earlier, the submucosal collateral circulation of the esophagus is excellent, and most of the length of the thoracic esophagus will remain viable so long as at least one inferior thyroid artery remains intact. Therefore, after delivering the divided thoracic esophagus out of the neck incision, viable esophagus should not be discarded to "tailor" the remaining esophagus for a standard cervical esophagostomy. Rather, the maximum length of remaining esophagus should be preserved to facilitate later reconstruction. This is achieved by developing a subcutaneous tunnel on the anterior chest wall and constructing an anterior thoracic esophagostomy (see Fig. 26–23). An esophagostomy stoma placed on the relatively flat upper anterior chest wall is much more easily cared for by the patient because a stomal appliance is more readily adapted to this location than to the usual site of a standard cervical esophagostomy. A feeding jejunostomy is, of course, required until later esophageal reconstruction can be performed.

When colon or jejunum has been used to replace the esophagus and necrosis of the graft is documented at reexploration for an anastomotic leak, there is similarly little recourse but to remove the nonviable graft and insert a feeding tube. If the patient survives the sequelae of the mediastinal sepsis, later reconstruction can be considered.

Anastomotic Stricture

The disastrous acute effects of an intrathoracic esophageal anastomotic leak in part prompted the author to begin to use a cervical esophagogastric reconstruction whenever possible after esophagectomy. However, although the management of a cervical anastomotic leak is generally straightforward and seldom associated with death, the long-term sequelae of a cervical leak are far from inconsequential. As many as 50% of cervical esophagogastric anastomotic leaks result in an anastomotic stricture as healing occurs, and this represents an unsatisfactory outcome of an operation that is intended to provide comfortable swallowing. The implications are similar in patients who survive an intrathoracic esophageal anastomotic leak. In their collective review of 46,692 patients undergoing an esophagectomy for cancer, Muller and associates[83] reported that the incidence of anastomotic leakage with an intrathoracic esophagogastric anastomosis was not significantly different for a one-layer (12%) versus a two-layer (12%) anastomosis or for an anastomosis that was performed manually (11%) versus one performed with an EEA surgical stapler (U.S. Surgical Corporation). On the other hand, in a series of 580 esophageal anastomoses, Fok et al.[37] found that a single layer running manually sewn anastomosis was associated with a 5% incidence of leak compared with 3.8% in those with a circular stapled technique ($P = 0.69$), but the stapled anastomoses were associated with a higher number of strictures.

In reviewing the complications of transhiatal esophagectomy in a collective group of 1,353 patients, Katariya et al.[63] reported a mean incidence of cervical anastomotic leaks of 15%, and the same number (15%) of patients developed anastomotic strictures. Dewar et al.[25] reported a 17% incidence of anastomotic leak and a 31% incidence of anastomotic stricture in 169 patients undergoing a cervical esophagogastric anastomosis, and the latter correlated with a prior anastomotic leak ($P = 0.001$). In a review of 131 patients undergoing a transhiatal esophagectomy for carcinoma, the Mayo Clinic group reported a 25% incidence of cervical leaks.[137] In another collective review, cervical anastomotic leaks occurred in 5 to 26% of patients undergoing a transhiatal esophagectomy and cervical esophagogastric anastomosis, and 10 to 15% of the patients developed anastomotic strictures.[39] The anastomotic leak rate averaged 13% in the more than 1,000 transhiatal esophagectomy patients at the University of Michigan, and nearly half of these patients developed subsequent anastomotic strictures.[89] Without question, the prevention of an anastomotic leak is the key to a successful functional outcome in these patients. And the recently reported side-to-side stapled cervical esophagogastric anastomosis, which has been associated with an anastomotic leak rate of less than 3%, has dramatically reduced the need for late postoperative anastomotic dilatations in our patients.[90]

In the patient who has experienced an esophageal anastomotic leak, early passage of a No. 46 French or larger bougie within 1 week of drainage is carried out to maintain a satisfactory lumen and to prevent late high-grade stenosis. A cervical fistula generally heals within 7 to 10 days of external drainage. When the patient returns for follow-up within 2 weeks of discharge, a No. 46 French or larger Maloney bougie is passed through the anastomosis for "calibration." If the patient has no dysphagia and there is no resistance to passage of the bougie, the need for subsequent dilatations is dictated by the return of cervical dysphagia. In patients with anastomotic narrowing that prevents the free passage of a No. 46 French or larger Maloney bougie, a more aggressive program of esophageal dilatation is undertaken—weekly at first. The underlying principle here is that scar tissue stretches, and with an early program of frequent dilatations, anastomotic healing in a patient configuration is often achieved. Patients whose anastomotic stricture produces resistance as the dilator is passed may need more frequent dilatations. In this situation, over several weeks, the patient is taught to pass a No. 46 or 48 French bougie with the assistance of a family member or friend. Once facility with passage of the dilator is achieved, the patient is issued a dilator with instructions to pass it daily for 1 week, then every other day for 1 week, and then at increasingly longer intervals until the longest duration between dilatations without the recurrence of dysphagia can be established. With this aggressive initial program of dilatation, long-term comfortable swallowing with little or no need for subsequent dilatations is generally achieved. Few patients require anastomotic revision. Occasionally, endoscopic injection of steroids into a refractory anastomotic scar facilitates the management of this problem.[65,142]

Pulmonary Complications

Respiratory insufficiency after esophageal resection and reconstruction is exceedingly common and is associated with a mortality rate of up to 40%.[117,123,131] A vital part of minimizing postoperative pulmonary complications after esophageal resection and reconstruction is rigorous preoperative pulmonary physiotherapy. The author insists on total abstinence from cigarette smoking for a minimum of 2 weeks before esophagectomy, and home use of an incentive inspirometer and instruction in deep-breathing exercises are also begun 2 weeks preoperatively. This investment of time and energy in improving the patient's preoperative respiratory status is repeatedly rewarded by a lower incidence of postoperative pulmonary complications after esophageal resection and reconstruction. Adequate postoperative analgesia, particularly epidural anesthesia, is of great value in minimizing postoperative pulmonary problems.

One of the most disastrous complications after esophageal resection is the development of a fistula between the tracheobronchial tree and either the esophagus or esophageal substitute, generally at the anastomotic site. Kron and associates[67] reported a gastrotracheal fistula that followed a transhiatal esophagectomy for carcinoma. Among 207 patients with malignant esophagorespiratory fistulas treated at the Memorial Sloan-Kettering Cancer Center in New York, Burt and associates[13] reported 13 patients who developed their fistulas after resections for esophageal carcinoma. In the author's experience with more than 1,000 transhiatal esophageal resections, the complication of tracheogastric fistula was encountered once; this was in a patient who was discharged with an asymptomatic contained cervical esophagogastric anastomotic leak discovered on a routine postoperative barium esophagogram. Ten days later, the patient was readmitted with a cervical tracheogastric fistula at the anastomosis where the localized infection had eroded through the posterior membranous trachea. The anastomosis was taken down, the intrathoracic stomach returned to the abdomen, and the trachea repaired and buttressed with adjacent muscle. The patient, however, died of progressive pulmonary insufficiency. This occurrence underscores the importance of drainage rather than expectantly following cervical esophageal anastomotic leaks. Once a fistula between the airway and adjacent alimentary tract develops, there is little option other than to prevent continued contamination of the respiratory tree by identifying and dividing the fistula and repairing the airway, generally a major undertaking in a desperately ill patient.

Gastric Outlet Obstruction

The need for a routine gastric drainage procedure following the vagotomy that inevitably accompanies esophagectomy has been debated. It has been shown, for example, that most patients who undergo an esophagectomy and esophagogastric anastomosis *without* a concomitant drainage procedure do not develop difficulty with gastric outlet obstruction.[4,51,55,124] However, in a prospective trial in which 200 patients undergoing esophageal resection were randomized to receive either a pyloroplasty or no gastric drainage procedure, gastric emptying was found to be four times longer in those who did not have a pyloroplasty.[38] Adverse postprandial symptoms were less in those who had a drainage procedure, and there was no morbidity from the pyloroplasty, an observation previously noted.[17] For the occasional patient who does develop significant gastric outlet obstruction after esophageal resection, the outcome may be *disastrous* aspiration pneumonia and impaired nutrition due to inability to eat (Fig. 26–24). Further, reoperation to perform a drainage procedure may be very difficult after the stomach has been mobilized into the chest. For these reasons, the author advocates performance of a gastric drainage procedure in every patient undergoing esophagectomy and esophageal reconstruction preferring a Ramstedt-type extramucosal pyloromyotomy, which avoids the intra-abdominal suture line of a pyloroplasty. After performing the pyloromyotomy, silver clip markers placed at the level of the pylorus aid in interpreting subsequent radiologic studies used to evaluate gastric emptying. In more than 1,000 such pyloromyotomies performed during esopha-

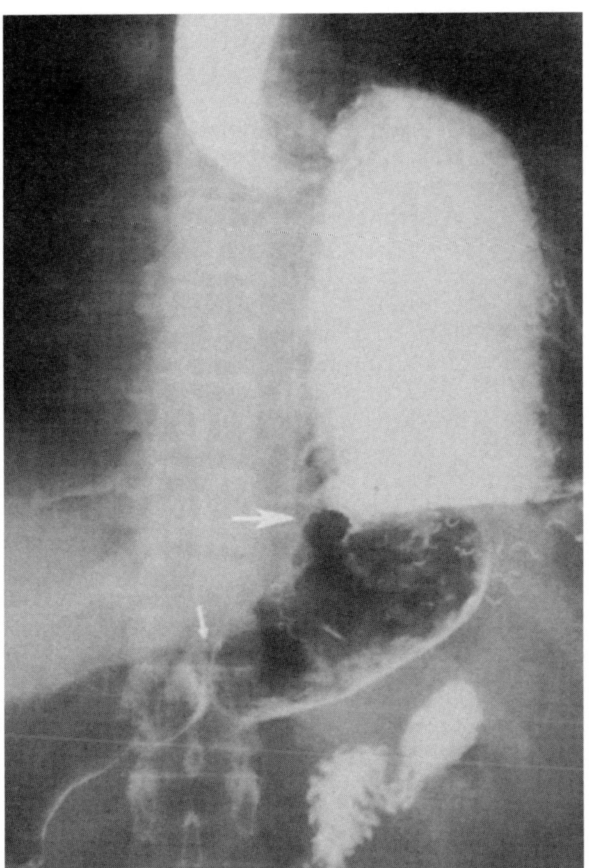

Figure 26–24. Postoperative barium swallow after esophagectomy and an intrathoracic esophagogastric anastomosis for carcinoma. The patient has impaired gastric emptying due to two technical errors: (1) failure to enlarge the diaphragmatic hiatus sufficiently *(large arrow)*, and (2) failure to perform a gastric drainage procedure (the *small arrow* indicates an obstructed gastric outlet). (From Orringer, M.B.: Complications of esophageal surgery and trauma. *In* Greenfield, L.J. [ed.]: Complications in Surgery and Trauma. Philadelphia, J.B. Lippincott, 1984, p. 276, with permission.)

geal bypass or replacement with stomach, the author has experienced one leak postoperatively; this leak resulted in fatal peritonitis. Intrathoracic gastric outlet obstruction may also result from failure to enlarge the diaphragmatic hiatus adequately before mobilizing the stomach into the chest (see Fig. 26–24). The diaphragmatic hiatus should accommodate at least three fingers comfortably alongside the mobilized stomach to prevent this complication.

Diaphragmatic Hiatus Obstruction of Herniation

Not only must the hiatus be enlarged sufficiently to prevent the esophageal substitute from becoming obstructed at the level of the diaphragm, but also the esophageal replacement, whether stomach or intestine, must be carefully sutured to the edge of the diaphragmatic hiatus to prevent subsequent herniation of abdominal viscera through the hiatus and into the chest (Fig. 26–25). This complication may occur acutely within the first several days of operation or years after the esophagectomy. Such a hernia may be an asymptomatic finding on a postoperative chest roentgenogram on which intestinal gas is seen above the level of the hiatus, or the patient may present with vague left upper quadrant abdominal or lower thoracic discomfort, nausea, and vomiting as is the case with chronic traumatic diaphragmatic hernias. Because the risk of incarceration and strangulation of the herniated viscera is substantial, reduction of the hernia is advised. Herniations of intestine through the diaphragmatic hiatus following esophagectomy can generally be repaired transabdominally either in the acute postoperative period or years later. In the case of chronic traumatic diaphragmatic hernias, the opening in the diaphragm is relatively small and the herniated viscera may become adherent to adjacent intrathoracic structures requiring a transthoracic approach for reduction. The majority of herniations of intestine alongside the intrathoracic stomach, on the other hand, occur through a relatively patulous hiatus, and reduction of the hernia and narrowing of the hiatus are readily achieved through the abdomen. As is the case with other complications that follow esophageal surgery, this situation can also generally be prevented. When the esophageal substitute has been brought through the diaphragmatic hiatus and the anastomosis has been completed, several heavy diaphragmatic crural sutures should

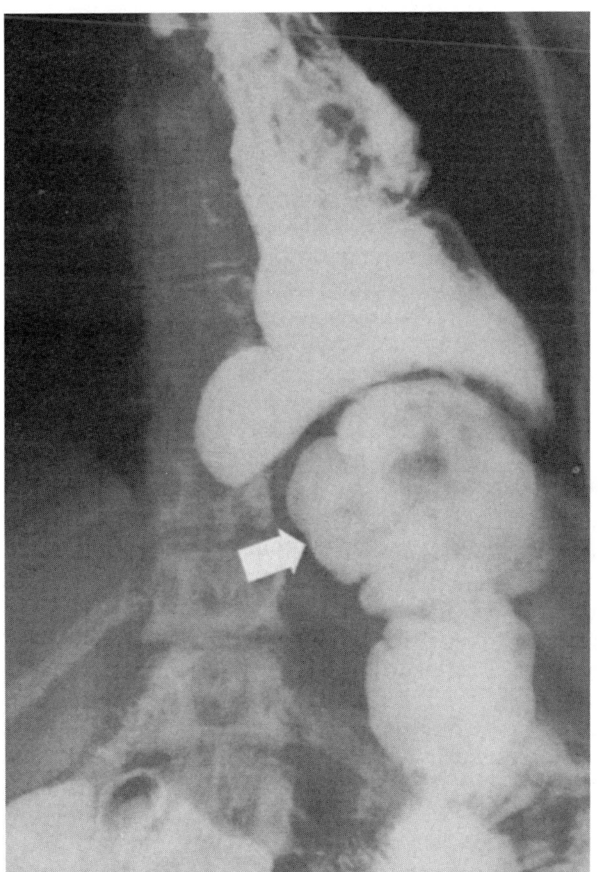

Figure 26–25. Herniation of the splenic flexure of the colon *(arrow)* through the diaphragmatic hiatus after an intrathoracic esophagogastrostomy for a caustic stricture. The stomach had not been sutured to the diaphragmatic hiatus to prevent this complication. (From Orringer, M.B.: Complications of esophageal surgery and trauma. *In* Greenfield, L.J. [ed.]: Complications in Surgery and Trauma. Philadelphia, J.B. Lippincott, 1984, p. 277, with permission.)

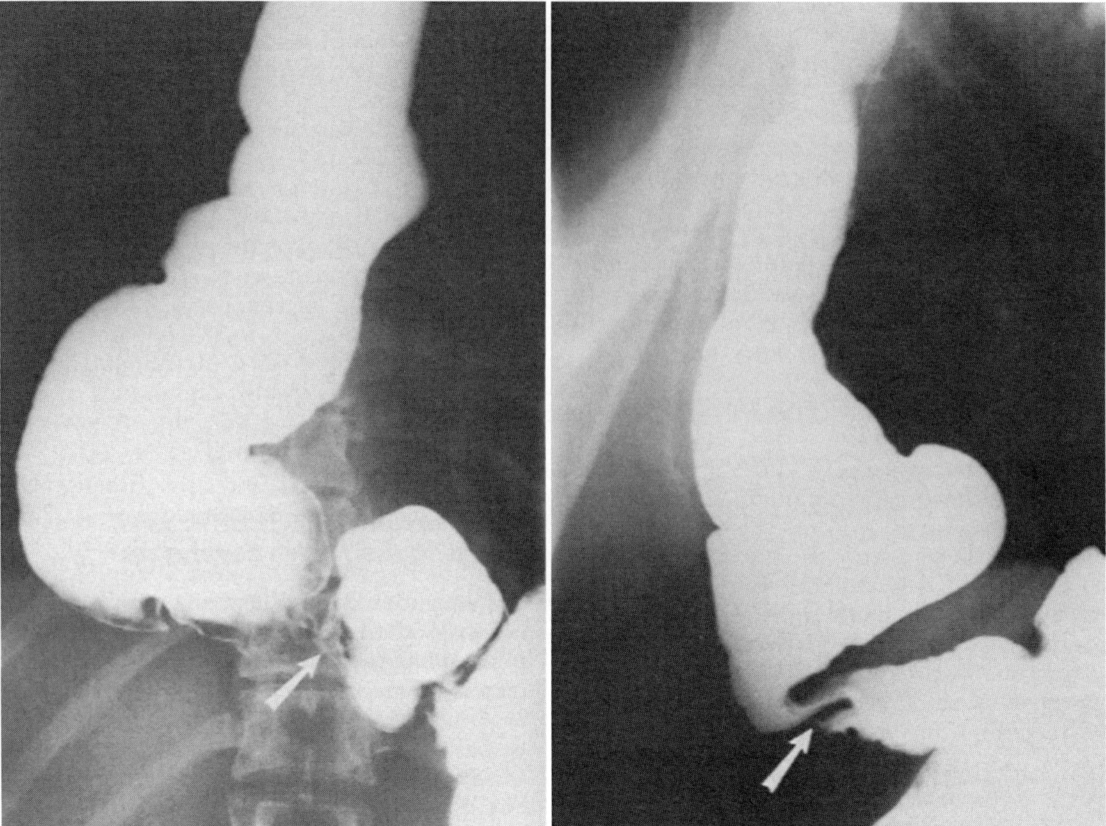

Figure 26–26. Posteroanterior *(left)* and lateral *(right)* views from a barium swallow showing early postoperative obstruction of a retrosternal colonic interposition at the level of the diaphragm *(arrows)* due to failure to create an adequate opening in the diaphragm.

be used to narrow the hiatus so that it admits three fingers alongside the stomach or colon. Then a few interrupted sutures between the edge of the diaphragmatic hiatus and the visceral esophageal substitute should be used to discourage the migration of other intra-abdominal viscera through the hiatus into the chest. Finally, the divided triangular ligament of the mobilized liver should be sutured to the edge of the hiatus to provide one additional barrier to herniation at this site.

Chylothorax

Owing to the proximity of the thoracic duct and the esophagus, chylothorax following esophagectomy is a recognized complication.[9,16] Ligation of the divided periesophageal tissues at the time of esophagectomy minimizes this complication. Compared with the relatively healthy patient who sustains a chylothorax after aortic surgery, however, this complication occurring in the debilitated patient with esophageal obstruction is not well tolerated and has been reported to carry a mortality as high as 50%.[36,70] Patients with chronic esophageal obstruction are already nutritionally depleted, and further loss of protein-rich chyle is not well tolerated. Only a few days should be expended trying to treat this complication conservatively. With aggressive operative intervention and direct ligation of the point of thoracic duct injury, patient salvage is the rule.[87]

Pancreatitis

Postoperative pancreatitis may occur following esophagectomy due to pancreatic injury during either performance of the Kocher maneuver or gastric mobilization. The possibility should be suspected in patients who develop unexplained fever, respiratory distress, or prolonged ileus after esophagectomy. The diagnosis is confirmed by determining serum amylase and calcium levels. Standard treatment of pancreatitis with nasogastric tube decompression of the gastrointestinal tract and intravenous fluids is usually sufficient, although progression to fatal hemorrhagic pancreatitis may occur.

Splenic Injury

Injury to the spleen may occur during esophagectomy, particularly during mobilization of the stomach for esophageal replacement. Careful avoidance of undue traction on the short gastric vessels during gastric mobilization and early division of adhesions between the stomach and the spleen on opening the abdomen minimize this complication. Routine splenectomy as part of the "cancer operation" for esophageal carcinoma is not advocated because splenectomy is associated with a well-documented increased morbidity of its own.[18,22,85]

Peripheral Atheroembolism

Thromboembolic sequelae after transhiatal esophagectomy have been reported in two patients and attributed to inadvertent dislodgement of debris from the diseased aorta in the process of mobilizing the esophagus through the diaphragmatic hiatus.[72] This complication has not

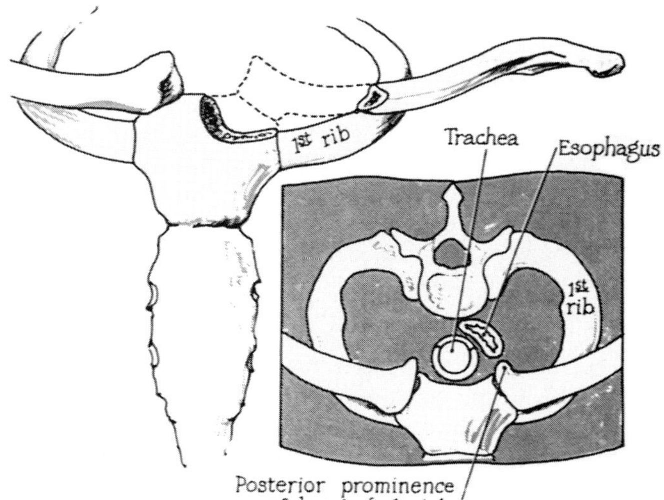

Figure 26–27. The posterior prominence of the head of the clavicle *(inset)* compresses a retrosternal graft brought through the anterior mediastinum at the thoracic inlet. When performing a retrosternal esophageal reconstruction, the medial clavicle and adjacent manubrium *(dotted lines)*, and often the adjacent medial first rib as well, should be resected to prevent obstruction of the graft. (From Orringer, M.B., and Sloan, H.: Substernal gastric bypass of the excluded thoracic esophagus for palliation of esophageal carcinoma. J. Thorac. Cardiovasc. Surg., *70*:836, 1975, with permission.)

been encountered by the author in an experience with more than 1,000 transhiatal esophagectomies.

Complications of Substernal Esophageal Replacement

Several unique complications of esophageal replacement are related to retrosternal placement of the esophageal substitute. The most obvious is potential obstruction at the level of the retrosternal neohiatus due to failure to create an adequate opening (Fig. 26–26). When creating a retrosternal tunnel, it is the author's practice to dilate this space until the entire hand and forearm can be inserted retrosternally, ensuring sufficient room for either the stomach or the colon. Compression and obstruction of the retrosternal esophageal substitute at the superior opening into the anterior mediastinum is a function of the posterior prominence of the clavicular head, which narrows the anterior thoracic inlet (Fig. 26–27). For this reason, when performing a retrosternal interposition of stomach or colon, which requires relocation of the cervical esophagus anteriorly from its usual position to the left and posterior to the trachea, the medial third of the clavicle, the adjacent manubrium, and usually the medial first rib as well should be resected to ensure an adequate opening into the anterior mediastinum (Fig. 26–28).

Complications of Bypassing or Excluding the Native Esophagus

Management of the diseased native esophagus is controversial when performing retrosternal replacement of the

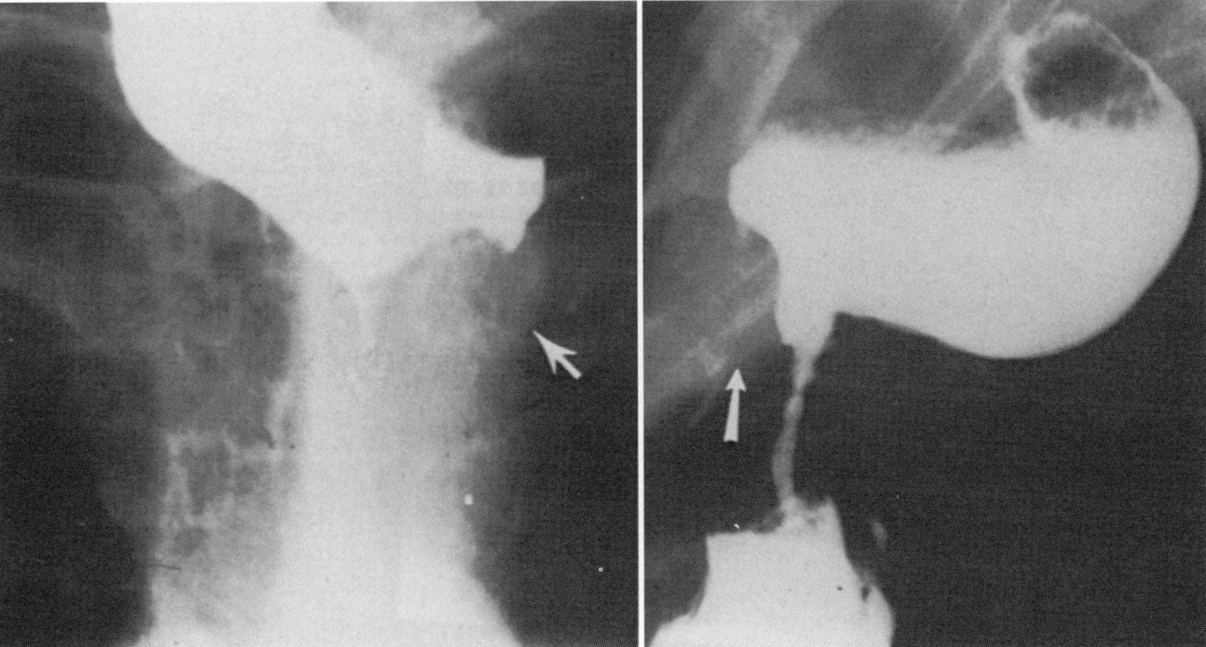

Figure 26–28. Posteroanterior *(left)* and lateral *(right)* views from a barium swallow showing compression of a retrosternal colonic interposition at the level of the unresected left clavicular head *(arrows)*. Enlargement of the anterior opening into the superior mediastinum (as shown in Fig. 26–27) with revision of the anastomotic stricture that had formed was required to relieve the obstruction.

esophagus. An esophagus that is severely strictured from a caustic injury, for example, may simply be left in the posterior mediastinum and bypassed with a retrosternal colon. The potential complications arising from the residual diseased esophagus, however, mandate that it be removed whenever possible. The small but definite increased risk of late development of carcinoma in the caustic strictured esophagus[52,135] is a less compelling reason to resect it than the potential for subsequent reflux esophagitis. A caustic injury may destroy the lower esophageal sphincter mechanism owing to subsequent fibrosis, and such a patient undergoing substernal colon interposition may develop reflux symptoms and severe esophagitis in the native esophagus (Fig. 26–29).

Although substernal bypass of the *excluded* esophagus with either stomach or colon has been used for treatment of both benign and malignant disease,[23,60,98] the complications from such an approach are appreciable. The excluded esophagus may become a giant posterior mediastinal mucocele that causes respiratory distress due to tracheobronchial compression (Fig. 26–30). Of more immediate concern in the postoperative period is the incidence of disruption of the distal end of the excluded esophagus with resultant left subphrenic abscess.[86] When esophageal replacement is necessary for benign disease, the author advocates resection of the esophagus. It is always preferable to place the esophageal substitute in the posterior mediastinum in the original esophageal bed because (1) this is the shortest distance between the neck and the abdominal cavity; (2) if subsequent anastomotic dilation is required, it is far safer and more direct to perform it when one does not have to negotiate the anterior angulation of the cervical esophagus that has been anastomosed to a retrosternal graft; and (3) the incidence of postoperative cervical anastomotic leak is lower. In the original esophageal bed in the neck, the anastomosis is buttressed by adjacent tissues: the spine posteriorly, the carotid sheath laterally, the trachea medially, and the strap muscles anteriorly. An esophageal anastomosis to a retrosternal colon or stomach is basically subcutaneous in the neck and is relatively unsupported. Coughing or a Valsalva maneuver against a closed upper esophageal sphincter results in distention of the retrosternal esophageal substitute with increased pressure on the anastomosis and a higher anastomotic leak rate. If esophageal bypass is performed in patients with unresectable esophageal carcinoma, the distal esophagus should be decompressed into a Roux-en-Y limb or jejunum[1,66,140] rather than excluded.

Esophageal Diverticulectomy

Pulsion diverticula of the esophagus, whether oropharyngeal (Zenker's diverticulum) or intrathoracic, result from associated distal esophageal obstruction, most often neuromotor dysfunction. Thus, if the underlying neuromotor abnormality responsible for the formation of the diverticulum is not addressed at the time of diverticulectomy, failure to relieve the distal obstruction may result in a "blowout" of the suture line[2,24] (Figs. 26–31 through 26–

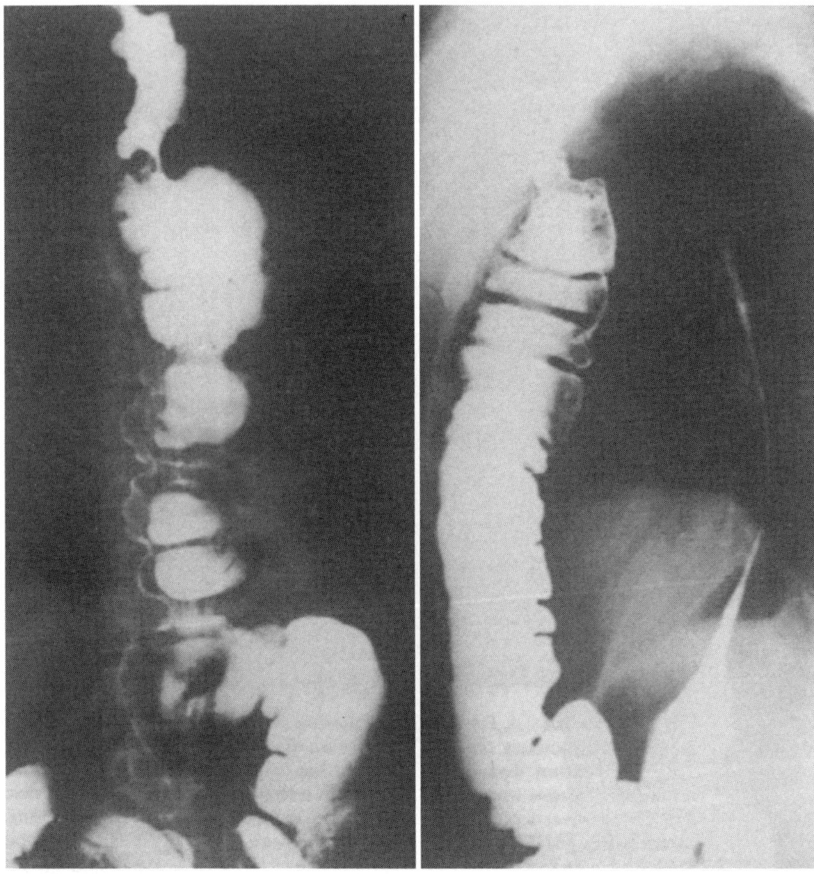

Figure 26–29. Posteroanterior *(left)* and lateral *(right)* views from a barium swallow performed in a patient who had undergone a retrosternal colonic bypass for a caustic esophageal stricture 4 years earlier. This patient had had severe reflux symptoms for 2 years before presenting with upper gastrointestinal bleeding due to reflux esophagitis. The lateral film shows simultaneous opacification of both the colon graft and the native esophagus, which filled as a result of a grossly incompetent lower esophageal sphincter. Resection of the native esophagus was required to relieve the severe reflux esophagitis.

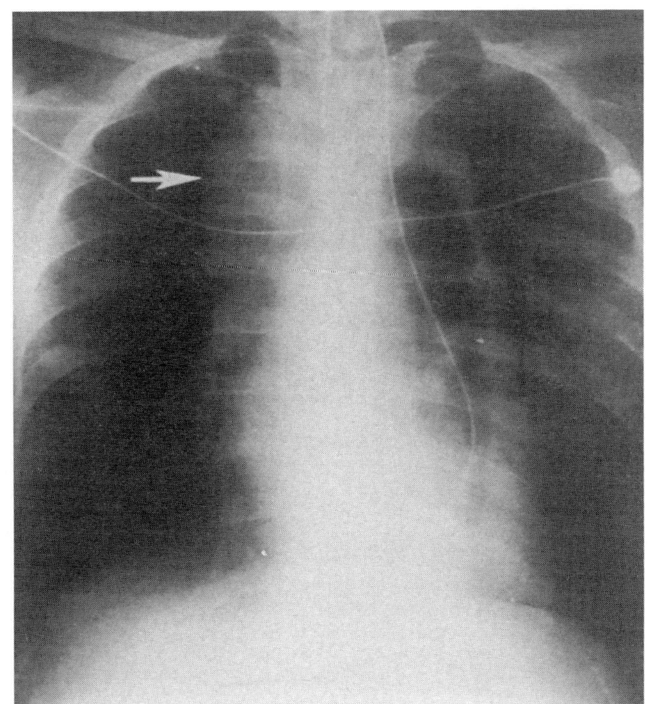

Figure 26–30. Posteroanterior chest roentgenogram in a 27-year-old man who presented with acute respiratory distress 2 years after undergoing substernal gastric bypass of the excluded thoracic esophagus for a caustic stricture. The patient had compression of the tracheobronchial tree by a huge posterior mediastinal mucocele *(arrow)*, which had formed in the excluded esophagus. An endotracheal tube was required to relieve the airway obstruction. A nasogastric tube is seen in the retrosternal stomach. A right-sided thoracotomy and a resection of the dilated esophagus were carried out.

34). Following resection of a diverticulum, the esophagus should be insufflated with air through an indwelling nasogastric tube positioned within the esophagus, and an air leak should be looked for by immersing the pouting esophageal submucosa in saline solution (see Fig. 26–34*D*). The most opportune time to treat such a pinhole leak is at the time of operation, and a single 5-0 stitch may avert a great deal of postoperative morbidity.

Alternatively, if a cervical esophageal leak occurs after diverticulectomy and esophagomyotomy, the neck wound must be opened, irrigated, and drained, as described earlier for the treatment of cervical anastomotic disrup-

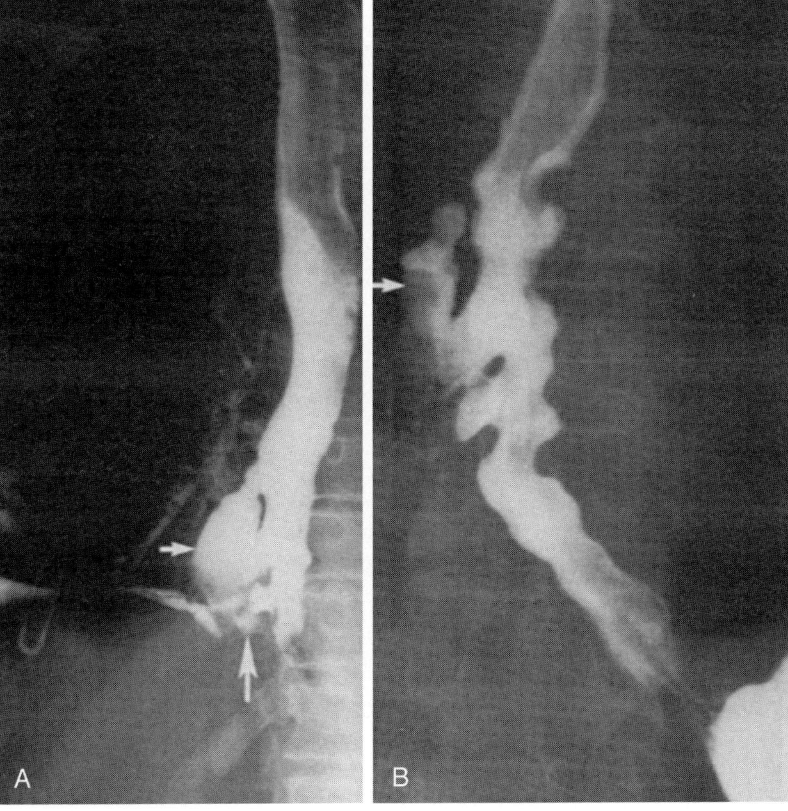

Figure 26–31. *A,* Barium swallow showing an esophagopleurocutaneous fistula *(large arrow)* and a recurrent esophageal diverticulum *(small arrow)* after diverticulectomy *without* an esophagomyotomy. *B,* The persistent underlying neuromotor dysfunction in this patient, as evidenced by this "corkscrew" esophagus, is apparent. Failure to relieve the relative obstruction due to the intermittent esophageal spasm distal to the diverticulum resulted in disruption of the diverticulectomy suture line and recurrence of the diverticulum *(arrow)*. (From Orringer, M.B.: Complications of esophageal surgery and trauma. *In* Greenfield, L.J. [ed.]: Complications in Surgery and Trauma. Philadelphia, J.B. Lippincott, 1984, p. 278, with permission.)

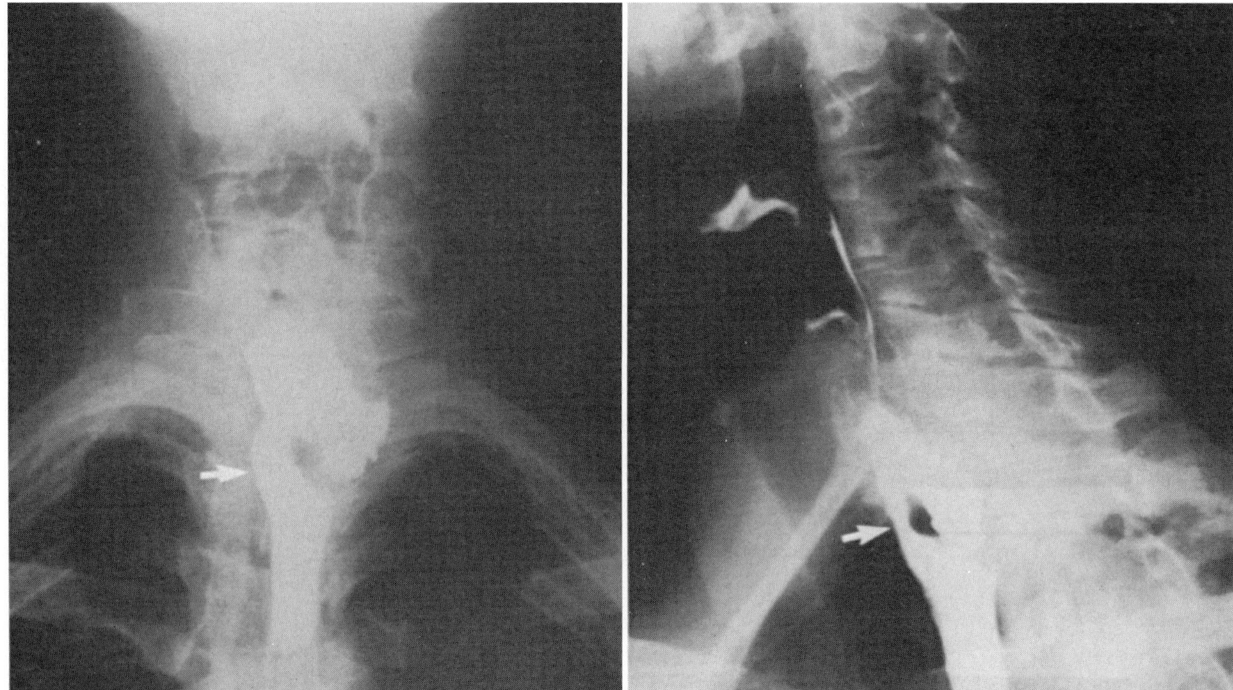

Figure 26–32. Posteroanterior *(left)* and lateral *(right)* views of barium swallow in a patient with a recurrent Zenker's diverticulum after two previous diverticulectomies, each one complicated by disruption of the suture line and an esophagocutaneous fistula. The undivided cricopharyngeus muscle *(arrow)* causing the obstruction distal to the pouch is evident. An esophagomyotomy to relieve this neuromotor dysfunction causing the obstruction had not been performed. A third diverticulectomy, this time combined with an esophagomyotomy, resulted in relief of dysphagia. The diverticulum has not recurred after 10 years of follow-up.

tion. Nutrition may be maintained with feedings through a nasogastric tube or intravenously. Broad-spectrum antibiotics are administered. With an adequate esophagomyotomy that has relieved the distal obstruction, the incidence of leak from a diverticulectomy suture line should be exceedingly low. If a cervical salivary fistula does occur, however, spontaneous closure within 7 to 10 days should be expected. If an intrathoracic esophageal suture line leak occurs within several days of diverticulectomy, immediate re-exploration of the chest with closure of the fistula and reinforcement with adjacent pleura, intercostal muscle, anterior mediastinal fat, or omentum is indicated.

Esophagomyotomy for Achalasia or Esophageal Spasm

The megaesophagus of achalasia may contain 1 to 2 liters of stagnant intraesophageal contents. Induction of general anesthesia in such a patient represents the most

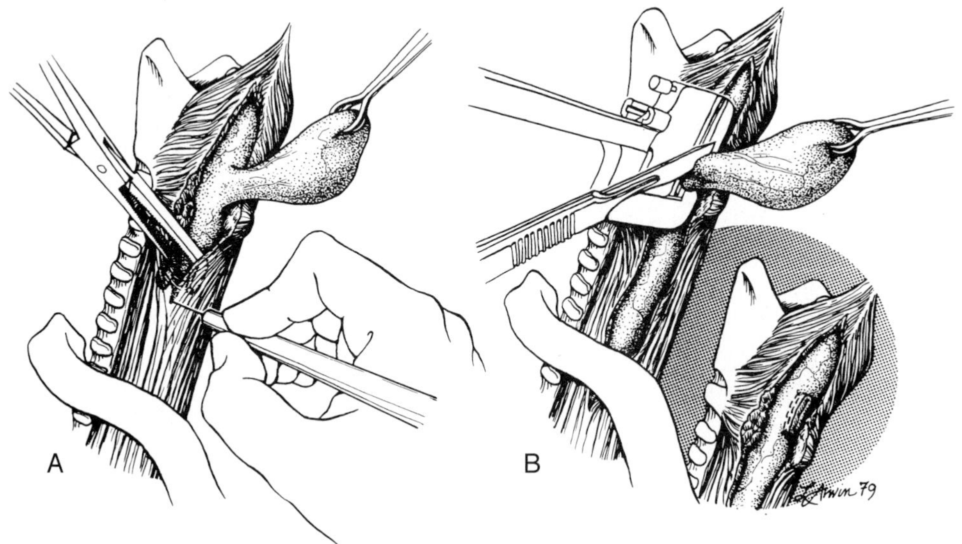

Figure 26–33. Cervical esophagomyotomy is an integral part of Zenker's diverticulectomy. *A,* After mobilization of the diverticulum, the myotomy is performed to relieve the relative distal obstruction responsible for formation of the pouch. *B,* When the esophagomyotomy is completed, the base of the diverticulum is crossed with a surgical stapler, and the pouch is amputated. (From Orringer, M.B.: Extended cervical esophagomyotomy for cricopharyngeal dysfunction. J. Thorac. Cardiovasc. Surg., *80*:669, 1980, with permission.)

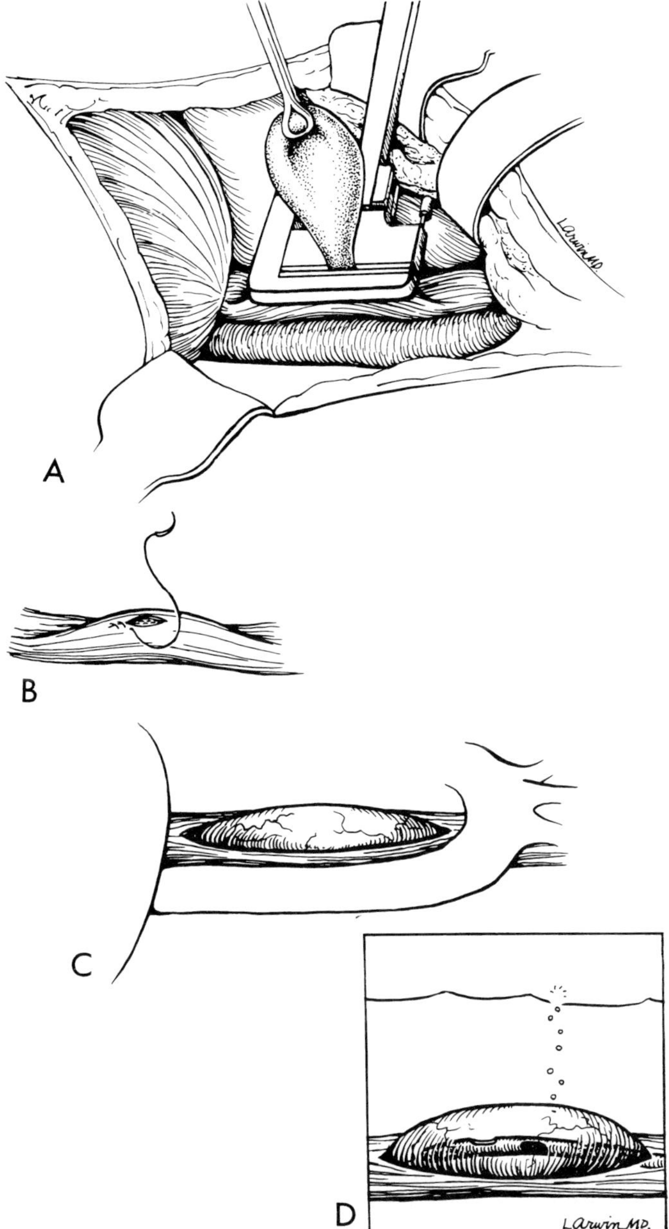

Figure 26–34. Resection of thoracic esophageal diverticulum and concomitant esophagomyotomy. *A,* Mobilized diverticulum is divided at its base and amputated after stapling. *B,* Staple suture line is oversewn. *C,* The esophagus is rotated 180 degrees, and a long esophagomyotomy is performed from the esophagogastric junction to the aortic arch. *D,* Testing for inadvertent esophageal perforation after esophagomyotomy is routine. Insufflation of air through an interesophageal nasogastric tube distends the exposed submucosa. Submersion of the esophagus under saline allows detection of escaping air bubbles and identification and repair of any unsuspected injury that has occurred during performance of the esophagomyotomy. (From Orringer, M.B.: Complications of esophageal surgery and trauma. *In* Greenfield, L.J. [ed.]: Complications in Surgery and Trauma. Philadelphia, J.B. Lippincott, 1984, p. 280, with permission.)

dangerous part of the operation. Because a nasogastric tube interferes with deep breathing and adequate clearing of pulmonary secretions, the author does not use an intraesophageal nasogastric tube to decompress the dilated esophagus for 2 to 3 days before surgery. Rather, the patient is restricted to a clear liquid diet for 2 days before the operation, and then immediately before induction of general anesthesia, with the patient in a sitting position, a nasogastric tube is passed, and the esophagus is aspirated and evacuated. Rapid-sequence "crash" induction of anesthesia is then carried out while constant pressure is maintained on the cricoid cartilage to prevent regurgitation of esophageal contents into the pharynx until the endotracheal tube balloon is inflated. Once the airway is protected, rigid esophagoscopy is carried out, and the esophagus is evacuated and irrigated.

After completion of the esophagomyotomy for either achalasia or esophageal spasm, integrity of the esophageal mucosa is documented by insufflating air into the esophagus through an indwelling intraesophageai nasogastric tube (see Fig. 26–34*D*). As described earlier, identification and closure of an inadvertent esophageal injury at this point is far simpler than when the perforation is detected hours to days after operation.

Controversy exists about the need for a concomitant antireflux procedure with the distal esophagomyotomy, which may render the lower esophageal sphincter incompetent.[6,34,84] Regardless of the approach used, potential complications exist. If a complete distal esophagomyotomy is not performed and the obstruction relieved, dysphagia and regurgitation will continue in the immediate postoperative period and reoperation may be necessary. Alternatively, if the esophagomyotomy is carried onto the stomach to ensure adequate relief of the esophageal obstruction, the incoordinated lower esophageal sphincter may be converted to an incompetent one, and complications of reflux esophagitis may occur.[8,26,44,119] With a few notable exceptions, the majority of esophageal surgeons now advocate some type of fundoplication to prevent the subsequent development of gastroesophageal reflux following esophagomyotomy for achalasia. Either a partial fundoplication of the Belsey or Dorr type,[6,28,41,115] or a very loose, short Nissen fundoplication has been recommended. When performing a fundoplication to ensure lower esophageal sphincter competence in an atonic esophagus, care *must* be exercised to avoid subsequent obstruction due to an overaggressive fundoplication.[31]

Among the more difficult problems of surgery for achalasia is the development of recurrent dysphagia and regurgitation due to esophageal obstruction occurring 1 or more years after a previous esophagomyotomy. Although esophagomyotomy has become the standard surgical approach to patients with achalasia, in those with a tortuous megaesophagus and a supradiaphragmatic pouch of esophagus, delayed esophageal emptying may occur even after a satisfactory esophagomyotomy. Furthermore, the patient who has undergone a previous esophagomyotomy and has recurrent symptoms has only a 40 to 70% chance of experiencing a good result from a "redo" esophagomyotomy. In these patients with either recurrent or persistent symptoms of achalasia with or without associated reflux esophagitis, esophagectomy may provide the best option, eliminating the esophageal obstruction as well as the potential for late development of carcinoma.[88]

References

1. Akiyama, H., and Hiyama, M.: A simple esophageal bypass operation by the high gastric division. Surgery, 75:674, 1974.

2. Allen, T.H., and Clagett, O.T.: Changing concepts in the surgical treatment of pulsion diverticula of the lower esophagus. J. Thorac. Cardiovasc. Surg., *50:*455, 1965.
3. Angelchik, J.P., and Cohen, R.: A new surgical procedure for the treatment of gastroesophageal reflux and hiatus hernia. Surg. Gynecol. Obstet., *14:*246, 1979.
4. Angorn, I.B.: Esophagogastrostomy without a drainage procedure in esophageal carcinoma. Br. J. Surg., *62:*601, 1975.
5. Attar, S., Hankins, J.R., Suter, C.M., et al.: Esophageal perforation: A therapeutic challenge. Ann. Thorac. Surg., *50:*45, 1990.
6. Belsey, R.: Functional diseases of the esophagus. J. Thorac. Cardiovasc. Surg., *52:*164, 1966.
7. Benjamin, S.B., Kerr, R., Cohen, D., et al.: Complications of the Angelchik antireflux prosthesis. Ann. Intern. Med., *100:*570, 1984.
8. Black, J., Vorbach, A.N., and Collis, J.L.: Results of Heller's operation for achalasia of the oesophagus. The importance of hiatal hernia repair. Br. J. Surg., *63:*949, 1976.
9. Bolger, T., Walsh, T., Tanner, W., et al.: Chylothorax after oesophagectomy. Br. J. Surg., *78:*587, 1991.
10. Bremmer, C.G.: Gastric ulcer after the Nissen fundoplication. Surg. Gynecol. Obstet., *148:*62, 1979.
11. Brown, R.H., and Cohen, P.S.: Nonsurgical management of spontaneous esophageal perforation. JAMA, *240:*140, 1978.
12. Bryant, L.R., and Eiseman, B.: Experimental evaluation of intercostal pedicle grafts in esophageal repair. J. Thorac. Cardiovasc. Surg., *50:*626, 1965.
13. Burt, M., Deihl, W., Martini, N., et al.: Malignant esophagorespiratory fistula: Management options and survival. Ann. Thorac. Surg., *52:*1222, 1991.
14. Bushkin, F.L., Woodward, E.R., and O'Leary, J.P.: Occurrence of gastric ulcer after Nissen fundoplication. Am. Surg., *42:*821, 1976.
15. Cameron, J.L., Kieffer, R.H., Hendrix, T.R., et al.: Selective nonoperative management of contained intrathoracic esophageal disruptions. Ann. Thorac. Surg., *27:*404, 1979.
16. Cerfolio, R.J., Allen, M.S., Deschamps, C., et al.: Postoperative chylothorax. J. Thorac. Cardiovasc. Surg. *112:*1361, 1996.
17. Cheung, H.C., Siu, K.F., and Wong, J.: Is pyloroplasty necessary in esophageal replacement by stomach? A prospective randomized controlled trial. Surgery, *102:*19, 1987.
18. Cioffiro, W., Schein, C.J., and Gliedman, M.L.: Splenic injury during abdominal surgery. Arch. Surg., *111:*167, 1976.
19. Condon, R.E.: More misadventures with the esophageal collar. Surgery, *93:*477, 1983.
20. Dagradi, A.E., Stempien, S.J., Seifer, W.H., and Weinberg, J.A.: Terminal esophageal (vestibular) spasm after vagotomy. Arch. Surg., *85:*955, 1962.
21. Dallemagne B., Weerts J.M., Jehaes C., et al.: Causes of failure of laparoscopic antireflux operations. Surg. Endosc. *10:*305, 1996.
22. Danforth, D.N., and Thorbjarnarson, B.: Incidental splenectomy: A review of the literature and the New York Hospital experience. Ann. Surg., *183:*124, 1976.
23. Deaton, W.R., Jr., and Bradshaw, H.H.: The fate of an isolated segment of esophagus. J. Thorac. Surg., *23:*570, 1952.
24. Debas, H.T., Payne, W.S., and Cameron, A.J.: Physiopathology of lower esophageal diverticulum and its implications for treatment. Surg. Gynecol. Obstet., *151:*593, 1980.
25. Dewar, L., Gelford, G., Finley, R.J., et al.: Factors affecting cervical anastomotic leak and stricture formation follow esophagogastrectomy and gastric tube interposition. Am. J. Surg., *163:*484, 1992.
26. Donnelly, R.J., Deverall, P.B., and Watson, D.A.: Hiatus hernia with and without esophageal strictures: Experience with the Belsey Mark IV repair. Ann. Thorac. Surg., *16:*301, 1973.
27. Dooling, J.A., and Zick, H.R.: Closure of an esophagopleural fistula using onlay intercostal pedicle graft. Ann. Thorac. Surg., *3:*553, 1967.
28. Dor, J., Humbert, P., Dor, V., and Figarella, J.: L'intérêt de la technique de Nissen modifiée dans la prévention du reflux après cardiomyotomie extramuqueuse de Heller. Mem. Acad. Chir. (Paris), *88:*877, 1962.
29. Douglas, K., and Nicholson, F.: The late results of Heller's operation for cardiospasm. Br. J. Surg., *47:*250, 1959.
30. Duranceau, A., Jamieson, G., Hurwitz, A.L., and Postlethwait, R.W.: Alteration in esophageal motility after laryngectomy. Am. J. Surg., *131:*30, 1976.
31. Duranceau, A., LaFontaine, E., and Vallieres, B.: Effects of total fundoplication on function of the esophagus after myotomy for achalasia. Am. J. Surg., *143:*22, 1982.
32. Durrans, D., Armstrong, C.P., and Taylor, T.V.: The Angelchik antireflux prosthesis—some reservations. Br. J. Surg., *72:*525, 1985.
33. Edelman, D.S.: Laparoscopic paraesophageal hernia repair with mesh. Surg. Laparosc., *5:*32, 1993.
34. Ellis, F.H., Jr., Gibb, S.P., and Crozier, R.E.: Esophagomyotomy for achalasia of the esophagus. Ann. Surg., *192:*157, 1980.
35. Ellis, F.H., Gibb, S.P., and Watkins, E., Jr.: Esophagogastrectomy: A safe, widely applicable, and expeditious form of palliation for patients with carcinoma of the esophagus and cardia. Ann. Surg., *198:*531, 1983.
36. Ferguson, M.K., Little, A.G., and Skinner, D.B.: Current concepts in the management of postoperative chylothorax. Ann. Thorac. Surg., *40:*542, 1985.
37. Fok, M., Ah-Chong, A., Cheng, S., and Wong, J.: Comparison of a single layer continuous hand sewn method and circular stapling in 580 oesophageal anastomoses. Br. J. Surg., *78:*34, 1991.
38. Fok, M., Cheng, W.K., and Wong, J.: Pyloroplasty versus no drainage in gastric replacement of the esophagus. Am. J. Surg., *162:*447, 1991.
39. Gandhi, S.K., and Naunheim, K.: Complications of transhiatal esophagectomy. Chest Surg. Clin. North Am., *7:*601, 1997.
40. Gerndt, S.J., and Orringer, M.B.: Tube jeujunostomy as an adjunct to esophagectomy. Surgery, *115:*164, 1994.
41. Gerzic, A., Knezevic, J., Milicevic, M., et al.: Results of transabdominal cardiomyotomy with Dor partial fundoplication in the management of achalasia. *In* Siewart, J.R., and Holscher, A.H. (eds.): Diseases of the Esophagus. New York, Springer-Verlag, 1988, p. 970.
42. Gouge, T.H., Depan, H.K., and Spencer, F.C.: Experience with the Grillo pleural wrap procedure in 18 patients with perforation of the thoracic esophagus. Ann. Surg., *209:*612, 1989.
43. Grillo, H.C., and Wilkins, E.W., Jr.: Esophageal repair following late diagnosis of intrathoracic perforation. Ann. Thorac. Surg., *20:*387, 1975.
44. Grimson, K.S., Baylin, G.J., Taylor, H.M., et al.: Transthoracic vagotomy. JAMA, *134:*925, 1947.
45. Guillory, J.R., Jr., and Clagett, O.T.: Postvagotomy dysphagia. Surg. Clin. North Am., *47:*833, 1967.
46. Hardy, J.D., Tompkins, W.C., Jr., Ching, E.C., and Chavez, C.M.: Esophageal perforations and fistulas: Review of 36 cases with operative closure of four chronic fistulas. Ann. Surg., *177:*788, 1973.
47. Henderson, R.D.: Reflux control following gastroplasty. Ann. Thorac. Surg., *24:*206, 1977.
48. Henderson, R.D., Boszko, A., and van Nostrand, S.W.P.: Pharyngoesophageal dysphagia and recurrent laryngeal nerve palsy. J. Thorac. Cardiovasc. Surg., *68:*507, 1974.
49. Henderson, R.D., and Ryder, D.E.: Reflux control following myotomy for diffuse esophageal spasm. Ann. Thorac. Surg., *34:*230, 1982.
50. Hendren, W.H., and Henderson, B.M.: Immediate esophagectomy for instrumental perforation of the thoracic esophagus. Ann. Surg., *168:*997, 1968.
51. Holster, A.H., Voit, H., Siewert, J.R., and Buttermann, G.: Function of the intrathoracic stomach. *In* Siewert, J.R., and Holscher, A.H. (eds.): Diseases of the Esophagus. Berlin, Springer-Verlag, 1988, p. 660.
52. Hopkins, R.A., and Postlethwait, R.W.: Caustic burns and carcinoma of the esophagus. Ann. Surg., *194:*146, 1981.
53. Hopper, C.L., Berk, P.D., and Howes, E.L.: Strength of esophageal anastomosis repaired with autogenous pericardial grafts. Surg. Gynecol. Obstet., *117:*83, 1963.
54. Horgan S., Pohl D., Bogetti D., et al.: Failed antireflux surgery: what have we learned from reoperations? Arch. Surg. *134:*809, 1999.
55. Huang, G.J., Zhang, D.C., and Zhang, D.W.: A comparative study of resection of carcinoma of the esophagus with and without pyloroplasty. *In* DeMeester, T.R., and Skinner, D.B. (eds.): Esophageal Disorders: Pathophysiology and Therapy. New York, Raven Press, 1985, p. 383.
56. Hunter, J.G., Smith C.D., Branum, G.D., et al.: Laparoscopic fundoplication failures: patterns of failure and response to fundoplication revision. Ann. Surg. *230:*595, 1999.

57. Huntington, T.R. Laparoscopic mesh repair of the esophageal hiatus. J. Am. Coll. Surg., *184:*399, 1997.
58. Iannettoni, M.D., Whyte, R.I., and Orringer, M.B.: Catastrophic complications of the cervical esophagogastric anastomosis. J. Thorac. Cardiovasc. Surg., *110:*1493, 1995.
59. Jara, F.M.: Diaphragmatic pedicle flap for treatment of Boerhaave's syndrome. J. Thorac. Cardiovasc., *78:*931, 1979.
60. Johnson, J., Schwegman, C.W., and Kirby, K.K.: Esophageal exclusion for persistent fistula following spontaneous rupture of the esophagus. J. Thorac. Surg., *32:*827, 1956.
61. Johnson, J., Schwegman, C.W., and MacVaugh, H., III: Early esophagogastrostomy in the treatment of iatrogenic perforation of the distal esophagus. J. Thorac. Cardiovasc. Surg., *55:*24, 1968.
62. Jones, W.G., and Ginsberg, R.J.: Esophageal perforation: A continuing challenge. Ann. Thorac. Surg., *53:*534, 1992.
63. Katariya, K., Harvey, J.C., Pina, E., et al.: Complications of transhiatal esophagectomy. Br. J. Surg., *78:*342, 1991.
64. Keighley, M.R.B., Girdwood, R.W., Worler, G.H., et al.: Morbidity and mortality of oesophageal perforation. Thorax, *27:*353, 1972.
65. Kirsch, M., Blue, M., Desai, R.K., et al.: Intralesional steroid injections for peptic esophageal strictures. Gastrointest. Endosc., *37:*180, 1991.
66. Kirschner, M.: Ein neves Verfahren der Oesophagoplastik. Arch. Klin. Chir., *114:*606, 1920.
67. Kron, I., Johnson, A., and Morgan, R.: Gastrotracheal fistula: A late complication after transhiatal esophagectomy. Ann. Thorac. Surg., *47:*767, 1989.
68. Kuster, G.G.R., and Gilroy, S.: Laparoscopic technique for repair of paraesophageal hiatus hernias. J. Laparoendosc. Surg., *3:*331, 1999.
69. Lackey, C., and Potts, J.: Penetration into the stomach: A complication of the antireflux prosthesis. JAMA, *248:*350, 1982.
70. Lam, K.H., Lim, S.T.K., Wong, J., and Ong, G.B.: Chylothorax following resection of the esophagus. Br. J. Surg., *66:*105, 1979.
71. Lyons, W.S., Seremetis, M.G., deGuzman, V.C., et al.: Ruptures and perforations of the esophagus: The case for conservative supportive management. Ann. Thorac. Surg., *25:*346, 1978.
72. Magee, M.J., Landrenegu, R.J., Keenan, R.J., et al.: Peripheral athero-embolism from the aorta complicating transhiatal esophagectomy. Am Surg., *60:*634, 1994.
73. Maher, J.W., Hocking, M.P., and Woodward, E.R.: Long-term follow-up of the combined fundic patch-fundoplication for treatment of longitudinal strictures of the esophagus. Ann. Surg., *194:*64, 1981.
74. Mansour, K.A., Burton, H.G., Miller, J.I., and Heather, C.R., Jr.: Complications of intrathoracic Nissen fundoplication. Ann. Thorac. Surg., *32:*173, 1981.
75. Mansour, K.A., and McKeown, P.P.: Disastrous complications of the Angelchik prosthesis. Am. Surg., *49:*616, 1983.
76. Mathisen, D.J., Grillo, H.C., Vlahakes, G.J., and Daggett, W.M.: The omentum in the management of complicated cardiothoracic problems. J. Thorac. Cardiovasc. Surg., *95:*677, 1988.
77. Mathisen, D.J., Grillo, H.C., Wilkins, E., Jr., et al.: Transthoracic esophagectomy: A safe approach to carcinoma of the esophagus. Ann. Thorac. Surg., *45:*137, 1988.
78. Michel, L., Grillo, H.C., and Malt, R.A.: Esophageal perforation: Collective review. Ann. Thorac. Surg., *33:*203, 1982.
79. Michel, L., Grillo, H.C., and Malt, R.A.: Operative and nonoperative management of esophageal perforations. Ann. Surg., *194:*57, 1981.
80. Middleton, C.J., and Foster, J.H.: Visceral pleural patch for support of esophageal anastomosis. Arch. Surg., *104:*67, 1972.
81. Morris, D.L., Jones, J., and Evans, D.F.: Reflux versus dysphagia: An objective evaluation of the Angelchik prosthesis. Br. J. Surg., *72:*1017, 1985.
82. Moses, W.R.: Critique on vagotomy. N. Engl. J. Med., *237:*603, 1947.
83. Muller, J.M., Erasmi, H., Stelzner, M., et al.: Surgical therapy of esophageal carcinoma. Br. J. Surg., *77:*845, 1990.
84. Murray, G.F., Battaglini, J.W., Keagy, B.A., et al.: Selective application of fundoplication in achalasia. Ann. Thorac. Surg., *37:*185, 1984.
85. Olsen, W.R., and Beaudoin, D.E.: Surgical injury to the spleen. Surg. Gynecol. Obstet., *131:*57, 1970.
86. Orringer, M.B.: Substernal gastric bypass of the excluded esophagus—results of an ill-advised operation. Surgery, *96:*467, 1984.
87. Orringer, M.B., Bluett, M., and Deeb, G.M.: Aggressive treatment of chylothorax complicating transhiatal esophagectomy without thoracotomy. Surgery, *104:*720, 1988.
88. Orringer, M.B., and Lemmer, J.H.: Early dilation in the treatment of esophageal disruption. Ann. Thorac. Surg., *42:*536, 1986.
89. Orringer, M.B., Marshall, B., and Iannettoni, M.D.: Transhiatal esophagectomy: Clinical experience and refinements. Ann. Surg., *230:*392, 1999.
90. Orringer, M.B., Marshall, B., and Iannettoni, M.D.: Eliminating the cervical esophagogastric anastomotic leak with a side-to-side stapled anastomosis. J. Thorac. Cardiovasc. Surg., *119:*277, 2000.
91. Orringer, M.B., and Orringer, J.S.: The combined Collis-Nissen operation: Early assessment of reflux control. Ann. Thorac. Surg., *33:*534, 1982.
92. Orringer, M.B., Skinner, D.B., and Belsey, R.H.R.: Long-term results of the Mark IV operation for hiatal hernia and analyses of recurrences and their treatment. J. Thorac. Cardiovasc. Surg., *63:*25, 1972.
93. Orringer, M.B., and Sloan, H.: An improved technique for the combined Collis-Belsey approach to dilatable esophageal strictures. J. Thorac. Cardiovasc. Surg., *68:*298, 1974.
94. Orringer, M.B., and Sloan, H.: Collis-Belsey reconstruction of the esophagogastric junction. J. Thorac. Cardiovasc. Surg., *71:*295, 1976.
95. Orringer, M.B., and Sloan, H.: Combined Collis-Nissen reconstruction of the esophagogastric junction. Ann. Thorac. Surg., *25:*16, 1978.
96. Orringer, M.B., and Sloan, H.: Complications and failings of the combined Collis-Belsey operation. J. Thorac. Cardiovasc. Surg., *74:*726, 1977.
97. Orringer, M.B., and Sloan, H.: Esophagectomy without thoracotomy. J. Thorac. Cardiovasc. Surg., *76:*643, 1978.
98. Orringer, M.B., and Sloan, H.: Substernal gastric bypass of the excluded thoracic esophagus for palliation of esophageal carcinoma. J. Thorac. Cardiovasc. Surg., *70:*636, 1975.
99. Orringer, M.B., and Stirling, M.C.: Cervical esophagogastric anastomosis for benign disease—functional results. J. Thorac. Cardiovasc. Surg., *96:*687, 1988.
100. Orringer, M.B., and Stirling, M.C.: Esophageal resection for achalasia—indications and results. Ann. Thorac. Surg., *47:*340, 1989.
101. Orringer, M.B., and Stirling, M.C.: Esophagectomy for esophageal disruption. Ann. Thorac. Surg., *49:*35, 1990.
102. Orsoni, P., Berdah, S., Sebag, F., et al.: An unusual cause of dysphagia after lararoscopic fundoplication: A report on two cases. Surgery, *123:*241, 1998.
103. Paterson, I.M., and Wong, J.: Anastomotic leakage: An avoidable complication of Lewis-Tanner oesophagectomy. Br. J. Surg., *76:*127, 1989.
104. Payne, W.S., and Larson, R.H.: Acute mediastinitis. Surg. Clin. North Am., *49:*699, 1969.
105. Pearson, F.G., Cooper, J.D., Ilves, R., et al.: Massive hiatal hernia with incarceration: A report of 53 cases. Ann. Thorac. Surg., *35:*45, 1983.
106. Pearson, F.G., and Henderson, R.D.: Long-term follow-up of peptic strictures managed by dilation, modified Collis gastroplasty, and Belsey hiatus hernia repair. Surgery, *80:*396, 1976.
107. Pearson, F.G., Langer, B., and Henderson, R.D.: Gastroplasty and Belsey hiatus hernia repair. J. Thorac. Cardiovasc. Surg., *61:*50, 1971.
108. Peloso, O.A.: Intra-abdominal migration of an antireflux prosthesis: A cause of bizarre pain. JAMA, *248:*351, 1982.
109. Pennell, T.C.: Supradiaphragmatic correction of esophageal reflux. Ann. Surg., *173:*775, 1981.
110. Peracchia, A., Bardini, R., Ruol, A., et al.: Esophagovisceral anastomotic leak. J. Thorac. Cardiovasc. Surg., *95:*685, 1988.
111. Perez, A.R., Moncure, A.W., and Rattner, D.W.: Obesity is a major cause of failure both for transabdominal and transthoracic antireflux operations (abstract). Gastroenterology, *116:*A1343, 1999.
112. Peters, J.H., Hagen, J.A., DeMeester, S.R., et al.: A decade of laparoscopic Nissen fundoplication. Contemp. Surg., *56:*138, 2000.
113. Petrovsky, B.V.: The use of diaphragm grafts for plastic operations in thoracic surgery. J. Thorac. Cardiovasc. Surg., *41:*348, 1961.
114. Pickleman, J.: Disruption and migration of an Angelchik esophageal antireflux prosthesis. Arch. Surg., *120:*498, 1985.

115. Pinotti, H.W., and Bettarello, A.: Chagasic mega-oesophagus. *In* Jamieson, G.G. (ed.): Surgery of the Oesophagus. London, Churchill Livingstone, 1988, p. 471.
116. Polk, H.C., Jr.: Fundoplication for reflux esophagitis: Misadventures with the choice of operation. Ann. Surg., *183:*645, 1976.
117. Postlethwait, R.: Complications and deaths after operations for esophageal carcinoma. J. Thorac. Cardiovasc. Surg., *85:*627, 1983.
118. Rao, K.V.S., Mir, M., and Cogbill, C.L.: Management of perforations of the thoracic esophagus: A new technique utilizing a pedicle flap of diaphragm. Am. J. Surg., *127:*609, 1974.
119. Richardson, J.D., Larson, G.M., and Polk, H.C.: Intrathoracic fundoplication for shortened esophagus: Treacherous solution to a challenging problem. Am. J. Surg., *143:*29, 1982.
120. Rosoff, L., and White, E.J.: Perforation of the esophagus. Am. J. Surg., *128:*207, 1974.
121. Salama, F.D., and Lamont, G.: Long-term results of the Belsey Mark IV antireflux operation in relation to the severity of esophagitis. J. Thorac. Cardiovasc. Surg., *100:*57, 1990.
122. Sataloff, D.M., Purgnani, K., Hoyo, S., et al.: An objective assessment of laparoscopic antireflux surgery. Am. J. Surg., *174:*63, 1997.
123. Shahian, D., Neptune, W., Ellis, F., and Watkins, E.: Transthoracic versus extrathoracic esophagectomy: Mortality, morbidity, and long-term survival. Ann. Thorac. Surg., *41:*237, 1986.
124. Shapiro, S., Hamlin, D., and Morgenstern, M.: The fate of the pylorus in esophagogastrostomy. Surg. Gynecol. Obstet., *135:*216, 1972.
125. Skinner, D.B.: Complications of surgery for gastroesophageal reflux. World J. Surg., *1:*485, 1977.
126. Skinner, D.B., Little, A.G., and DeMeester, T.R.: Management of esophageal perforation. Am. J. Surg., *139:*760, 1980.
127. Smith, R.S., Chang, F.C., Hayes, K.A., and DeBakker, J.: Complications of the Angelchik antireflux prosthesis. Am. J. Surg., *150:*735, 1985.
128. Soper, N.J., and Dunnegan, D.: Anatomic fundoplication failure after laparoscopic antireflux surgery. Ann. Surg., *229:*669, 1999.
129. Stirling, M.C., and Orringer, M.B.: Continued assessment of the combined Collis-Nissen operation. Ann. Thorac. Surg., *47:*224, 1989.
130. Suefert, R., Schmidt-Matthiesen, A., and Beyer, A.: Total gastrectomy and oesophagojejunostomy—a prospective randomized trial of a hand-sutured versus mechanically stapled anastomosis. Br. J. Surg., *77:*50, 1990.
131. Tam, P., Fok, M., and Wong, J.: Re-exploration for complications after esophagectomy for cancer. J. Thorac. Cardiovasc. Surg., *98:*1122, 1989.
132. Thal, A.P.: A unified approach to surgical problems of the esophagogastric junction. Ann. Surg., *168:*542, 1968.
133. Thal, A.P., and Hatafuku, T.: Improved operation for esophageal rupture. JAMA, *188:*626, 1964.
134. Thomas, H.F., Clarke, J.M., Rayl, J.E., and Woodward, E.R.: Results of the combined fundic patch-fundoplication operation in the treatment of reflux esophagitis with stricture. Surg. Gynecol. Obstet., *135:*240, 1972.
135. Ti, T.K.: Oesophageal carcinoma associated with corrosive injury: Prevention and treatment by oesophageal resection. Br. J. Surg., *70:*223, 1983.
136. Trus, T.L., Bax, T., Richardson, W.S., et al.: Complications of laparoscopic paraesophageal hernia repair. J. Gastrointest. Surg., *1:*221, 1997.
137. Vigneswaran, W.T., Trastek, V.F., Pairolero, P.C., et al.: Transhiatal esophagectomy for carcinoma of the esophagus. Ann. Thorac. Surg., *56:*836, 1993.
138. Whyte, R.I., Iannettoni, M.D., and Orringer, M.B.: Intrathoracic esophageal perforation: The merit of primary repair. J. Thorac. Cardiovasc. Surg., *109:*140, 1994.
139. Wingfield, H.V., and Karwowski, A.: The treatment of achalasia by cardiomyotomy. Br. J. Surg., *59:*281, 1972.
140. Wong, J., Lam, K.W., Wei, W.I., and Ong, G.B.: Results of the Kirschner operation. World J. Surg., *5:*547, 1981.
141. Woodward, E.R.: Sliding esophageal hiatal hernia and reflux peptic esophagitis. Mayo Clin. Proc., *50:*523, 1975.

VOLUME

I

Trauma

CHAPTER

27 Esophageal Trauma

MARK D. IANNETTONI • MARK B. ORRINGER

The immediate concern with any esophageal injury is the possibility of perforation and mediastinal soilage. Although late complications of esophageal trauma such as stricture can occur, these are rare and usually related to esophageal perforation. Approximately 75% of esophageal perforations are iatrogenic in origin, the majority caused by instrumentation or paraesophageal surgery. About 25% of esophageal perforations are caused by external trauma, barogenic trauma, corrosive injuries, or swallowed foreign bodies.[4] Extraluminal injury to the esophagus accounts for approximately 20% of esophageal perforations, with the majority of these being due to blunt or penetrating trauma (Table 27-1). Esophageal perforation from whatever cause has a common pathophysiology after the rupture has occurred. The constant egress of swallowed salivary juices combined with oral bacteria and refluxed gastric contents occurs through the tear into the periesophageal tissues in the neck, mediastinum, or abdomen. Respiratory movements and negative intrathoracic pressure tend to exacerbate the problem by increasing the spillage of material outside the esophagus. The clinical consequences of the chemical "burn" (volume loss, tissue necrosis) and the sepsis resulting from bacterial contamination are devastating. Esophageal perforations are one of the most serious perforations of the gastrointestinal tract, with mortality rates ranging from 15 to 34% in collected series with varying forms of treatment.[1,16,17,51,65,71,99] The morbidity and mortality rates from esophageal perforation are dependent on three important factors: (1) the location of injury, (2) the type of injury, and (3) the duration of injury.

Table 27-1. Traumatic Causes of Esophageal Perforation

Traumatic Causes of Esophageal Perforation
Instrumental
Endoscopy
Dilation
Intubation
Sclerotherapy
Laser therapy
Non-instrumental
Barogenic trauma
Postemetic (Boerhaave's syndrome)
Other (e.g., labor, convulsions, defecation, blunt trauma)
Penetrating neck, chest, or abdominal trauma
Operative trauma (vagotomy, pulmonary resection, esophageal reconstruction)
Caustic injuries
Swallowed foreign bodies

The key to reducing morbidity and mortality rates from esophageal perforations is early diagnosis. Perforations treated within six hours have about the same mortality rate as that associated with controlled operative esophagotomy. The reported mortality rate from esophageal perforation diagnosed in less than 24 hours was 5%, and the rate for those diagnosed after more than 24 hours was 14%. This significant improvement in mortality and morbidity rates does not condone a delay in immediate surgical treatment, because such delays have a negative effect on favorable outcomes in these patients. However, delays in the diagnosis of esophageal perforations continue to be the rule rather than the exception for injuries due to both iatrogenic and noniatrogenic causes. All suspected esophageal injuries must be evaluated vigorously with the aggressive use of esophagography and, when indicated, esophagoscopy.

The contrast biplane esophagogram has long been the "gold standard" for evaluation of suspected perforations of the esophagus. This study can be performed easily and rapidly and provides a diagnosis of perforation in most cases. However, there are instances in which the esophagogram may be equivocal or clinical suspicion overrules the findings of a negative study. In these cases, contrast-enhanced computed tomography (CT) may lead to the correct diagnosis of esophageal perforation, particularly in patients in whom there is a high clinical suspicion and there are other associated injuries.[7] However, the more important use of CT scanning in the diagnosis of esophageal perforation is in those patients with atypical symptoms or those in whom the diagnosis is in question. Diagnostic CT findings may include the presence of extraesophageal air, thickening of the esophagus, or a small pleural effusion with thickening of the mediastinal tissues and may result in earlier treatment.[7]

The treatment of esophageal perforations, especially those diagnosed later (after 24 hours), is challenging, controversial, and still evolving. However, many thoracic surgeons believe that primary repair is the treatment method of choice for esophageal perforations regardless of the duration of perforation.[114] Although general guidelines are helpful, treatment must be carried out on an individual basis. The clinician must select the best of several treatment options and apply it to a patient faced with a high likelihood of complications or death should the treatment fail. The first part of this chapter describes the various causes of esophageal trauma and their incidence, pathophysiology, and clinical features. Aspects of treatment unique to each of the different causes of esophageal trauma are also addressed. The second part of the chapter examines in detail the general problem of management of the perforated esophagus.

CAUSES OF ESOPHAGEAL TRAUMA

Instrumental Trauma

Iatrogenic instrumentation is the most common cause of esophageal perforation, accounting for approximately 45% of cases.[51] Although most instrumental perforations of the esophagus occur during endoscopy with or without dilation, almost all varieties of tubes used for both intended and inadvertent intubation of the esophagus, such as nasogastric tubes, endotracheal tubes, Sengstaken-Blakemore tubes, and tubes placed for palliation of esophageal carcinoma, have been reported to cause perforation (Figs. 27-1 and 27-2).[41,66,70,74,75,96,98] Sclerotherapy for variceal hemorrhage may also result in esophageal perforation due to necrosis of the esophageal wall presumably caused by the sclerosant.[8,100] Laser therapy has emerged as another cause of iatrogenic esophageal perforation,[4] especially when combined with photodynamic therapy for the treatment of inoperable esophageal malignancy.

The more widespread use of endoscopy has led to an increase in the actual number of esophageal perforations. Upper gastrointestinal endoscopy alone results in a perforation rate of 0.03 to 0.35%, perforation being more likely to occur when the examination is performed for esophageal disease than for gastric or duodenal disease.[66,70] Dilation of esophageal strictures causes perforation in 0.25 to 0.38% of cases.[66,70] Forceful pneumatic or hydrostatic dilation for achalasia has a perforation rate of 4%, making this the second most common cause of instrumental perforation and accounting for 25% of these injuries. The frequency of other instrumental perforations is shown in Figure 27-3.[51]

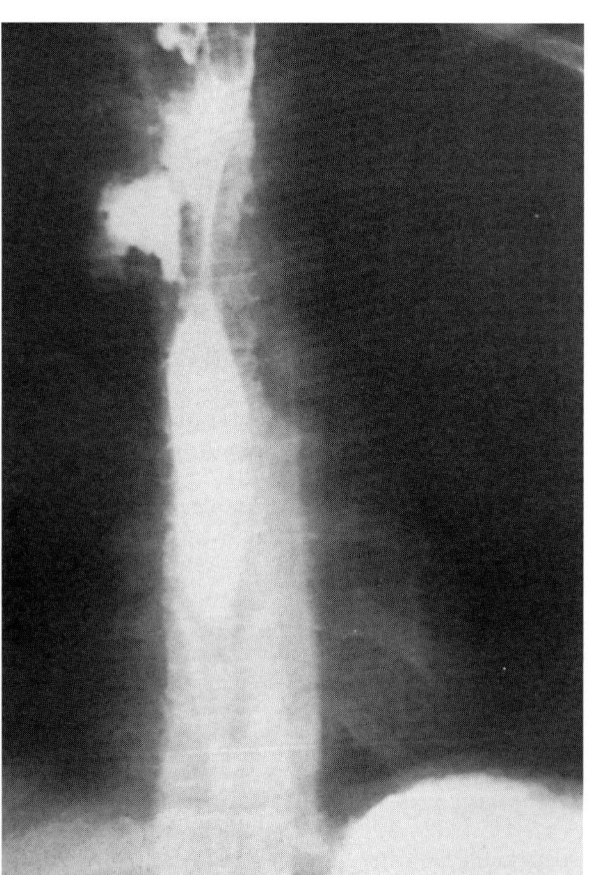

Figure 27-1. Esophageal perforation due to attempted emergency endotracheal intubation. Contrast extravasates at the level of the cricopharyngeus muscle, and the abscess cavity extends inferiorly to just above the carina.

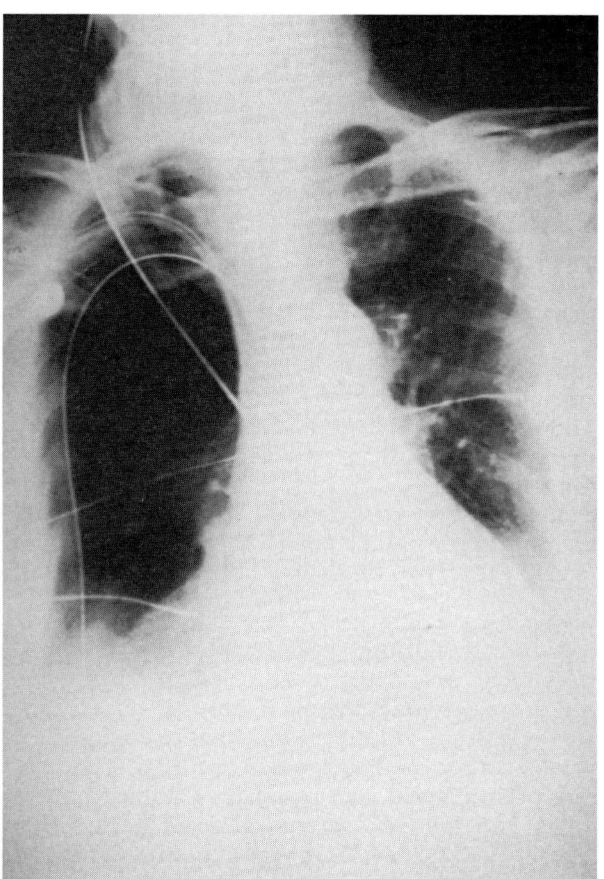

Figure 27-2. Esophageal perforation resulting from nasogastric tube passage. The tube is visible in the right pleural cavity, and a large associated pneumothorax is present.

Iatrogenic injuries can be minimized by proper performance of esophageal instrumentation. Certain basic principles deserve emphasis. In the opinion of the authors, no esophagoscope should ever be passed without reviewing a prior barium swallow. Lack of appreciation of existing esophageal pathology can have serious consequences (e.g., the perforation of an unsuspected cervical esophageal diverticulum during esophagoscopy for symptoms of heartburn). Esophagoscopy should not be performed in anxious, combative, or noncooperative patients, and general anesthesia may be preferable for the initial evaluation of obstructing esophageal lesions in such patients. This allows use of the rigid esophagoscope, through which one can obtain better (larger) biopsies and perform dilation under direct vision. Subsequent

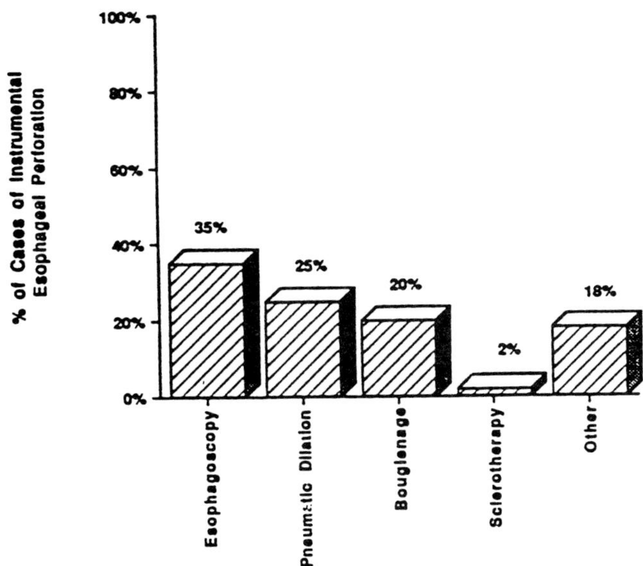

Figure 27–3. Distribution of instrumental perforations in 511 iatrogenic esophageal injuries depicted by procedure. (From Jones, W.G., II, Ginsberg, R.J., and Jones, W.G.: Esophageal perforation: A continuing challenge. Ann. Thorac. Surg., *53*:534, 1992, with permission.)

"blind" dilations can then be performed more safely (see Chap. 13).

The most common sites of instrumental esophageal perforation are at the level of the cricopharyngeus muscle, followed by the relatively fixed area of the esophagus just proximal to the hiatus, and, last, at the level of the aortic arch and left main bronchus. The cricopharyngeal area is at greatest risk of perforation because it is the most narrow portion of the esophageal lumen, and the region of the transition from the oblique thyropharyngeus fibers to the horizontal cricopharyngeus fibers (Killian's triangle) at the level of the C5 and C6 vertebrae is covered only by fascia with no muscular support posteriorly. Proper introduction of the rigid esophagoscope through this upper esophageal sphincter requires anterior displacement to the larynx by the advancing instrument. Otherwise, a posterior perforation can occur. The esophageal lumen must be visualized at all times as the endoscope is advanced during the examination. Although it is assumed that the rate of perforation is increased with rigid esophagoscopy, one series comparing both methods when used for diagnosis and biopsy has demonstrated no perforations in either group. However, the diagnostic success rate with rigid esophagoscopy was superior to that achieved with flexible esophagoscopy.[89]

The most common clinical finding after instrumental perforation is pain.[96] Fever and leukocytosis occur early in approximately two thirds of patients. Palpable cervical crepitance and mediastinal emphysema seen on chest roentgenogram occur less often but are very helpful diagnostic signs when present. Dysphagia, odynophagia, and respiratory distress after esophageal instrumentation suggest rupture of the esophagus. New pleural effusions can occur, especially after perforations of the thoracic esophagus.

Unfortunately, diagnostic delays are common in cases of iatrogenic instrumental esophageal perforation; in up to 40% of cases, diagnosis occurs after 24 hours.[57] Any patient with pain, fever, or any other finding suggestive of esophageal rupture after instrumentation should undergo an immediate contrast study of the esophagus. Dilute barium is the initial study preferred at our institution, because water-soluble agents frequently provide a false-negative result. If the dilute barium esophagram is negative for a perforation, this is followed by a definitive full-strength barium contrast study. Almost all cases of instrumental perforation can be diagnosed in this manner.

The management of instrumental perforation of the esophagus is discussed later in the section "Management of Esophageal Perforation." However, one type of iatrogenic esophageal perforation deserves special consideration—the postintubation tracheoesophageal fistula.[37,61] This condition is caused by indwelling endotracheal or tracheostomy tubes, which can cause full-thickness pressure necrosis of the tracheal and esophageal walls. Most patients also have indwelling esophageal tubes. Tracheoesophageal fistula is heralded by the appearance of copious secretions and tube feedings in the tracheobronchial tree, associated pneumonia, and gastric distention. Repair, which is best deferred until the patient is weaned from the ventilator, involves resection of the damaged portion of the trachea and primary reanastomosis, esophageal closure, and interposition of pedicled strap muscle between the two organs.[61] A ventilator-dependent patient can usually be managed by removing indwelling esophageal tubes, placing a low-pressure cuffed tube in the trachea, and making use of a draining gastrostomy and feeding jejunostomy until independence from the ventilator is achieved. Rarely, ventilator-dependent patients with a tracheoesophageal fistula have such a massive air leak into the gastrointestinal tract that effective ventilation is not possible. Ligation or division of the esophagus both proximal and distal to the fistula may prove lifesaving in this situation.

Barogenic Trauma

In 1724, Boerhaave described a fatal case of postemetic esophageal rupture in the Dutch Admiral Baron DeWassenaer.[24] This clinical entity has subsequently been called Boerhaave's syndrome, or spontaneous rupture of the esophagus. The term "spontaneous rupture," which simply means esophageal perforation unassociated with external trauma, internal instrumental trauma, or ingested foreign bodies or corrosives, is inaccurate because almost all spontaneous ruptures are associated with conditions that can cause abrupt, severe increases in intraesophageal pressure. Thus, it seems most appropriate to classify Boerhaave's syndrome as a type of barogenic esophageal rupture.

Although vomiting is the precipitating event in most cases of barogenic esophageal rupture, many other causes have been reported, including straining at defecation, childbirth, blunt trauma, seizures, heavy lifting, and forceful swallowing.[108] These entities, when superimposed on an underlying esophageal obstruction caused by acute secondary spasm due to gastroesophageal reflux, chronic motility disorder, or other pre-existing esophageal disease, can generate the sudden explosive rise in intraluminal pressure necessary to rupture the esophagus. It is possible, for example, that prolonged vomiting may fatigue the vomiting center in the brain stem, leading to discoordination of the vomiting reflex and spasm of the esophageal muscle with obstruction of the esophageal lumen. Barogenic perforation may also be associated with organic intraluminal or extraluminal obstruction associated with abrupt increases in intraluminal pressure.[108]

Perforation resulting from barogenic trauma is located in the lower third of the esophagus on the left side in more than 90% of cases, although ruptures of the proximal esophagus and involvement of the right side have been reported. The tear is usually longitudinal and often has clean-cut edges, as though the esophagus had been "cut with a knife." The length of the tear averages about 3 cm but varies from a tiny opening to a 10-cm rent.[52,108] Ruptures may either be contained within the mediastinum or extend through the mediastinal pleura into the pleural cavity. Relatively greater mediastinal and pleural contamination is seen with barogenic rupture than with other causes of esophageal perforation because of the great force with which esophageal contents are propelled through the tear. The Mallory-Weiss syndrome is a closely related clinical entity caused by vomiting and characterized by a mucosal tear on the gastric side of the esophagogastric junction. This condition is often associated with major gastrointestinal hemorrhage; however, esophageal perforation does not occur.[104]

The clinical features of spontaneous or barogenic esophageal rupture have been well described.[21,24,35,52,60,81,106,108] The condition is most commonly seen in men between the ages of 35 and 55, about half of whom have a history of alcoholism. Excruciating pain in the precordium or epigastrium that *follows* vomiting (commonly the precipitating event) is the most prominent and common symptom, although some patients have minimal pain. The pain may radiate to the back of the shoulders and is generally made worse by swallowing and inspiration. As the process continues, the pain becomes more widespread and severe. Dyspnea may or may not be a feature depending on the presence and severity of associated hydropneumothorax. Severe thirst is a frequent symptom. Hematemesis is rarely of significance in contrast to its predominance in the Mallory-Weiss syndrome.

After perforation, fluid is rapidly lost into the mediastinum and pleural cavities, causing progressively severe shock with tachycardia, hypotension, cyanosis, and cold, clammy extremities. This process is exacerbated by progressive sepsis resulting from superimposed bacterial contamination. However, it should be noted that fever is often absent early in the course of the disease. Upper abdominal tenderness and rigidity are commonly present and often create diagnostic confusion. Swallowed air leaving the esophagus can result in pneumothorax (usually on the left) if the pleura is torn and may also track along mediastinal tissue planes up into the neck, causing cervical subcutaneous emphysema (in approximately one third of patients) and "nasal" changes in the voice as air dissects into the nasopharyngeal soft tissues. Mediastinal air can sometimes be appreciated by auscultation (Hamman's crunch).

Mackler identified the triad of vomiting, low thoracic pain, and cervical emphysema as almost pathognomonic of Boerhaave's syndrome.[60] However, many patients do not present with these classic features.[81] Spontaneous rupture of the esophagus may occur without pain, vomiting, or subcutaneous emphysema.

The plain chest radiograph may provide important diagnostic information. Mediastinal emphysema suggests esophageal rupture. Other possible findings include pneumothorax, pleural effusions (unilateral or bilateral), and patchy lower lobe infiltrates due to chemical pleuritis. Although thoracentesis often reveals a foul brown fluid with an elevated amylase level, this procedure is not essential and should never delay the definitive diagnostic test, the contrast esophagogram. This study typically shows a "jutting out" of contrast agent from the lower left esophagus (Fig. 27-4); contrast may either be contained in the mediastinum or track freely into one of the pleural cavities. An immediate contrast study should be performed in all patients with a history suggestive of esophageal rupture or with suspicious physical or radiographic findings, especially subcutaneous or mediastinal emphysema.

The presentation of a perforated peptic ulcer may closely mimic that of spontaneous esophageal rupture. Lack of free air under the diaphragms on an upright chest radiograph and the presence of pleural or mediastinal air

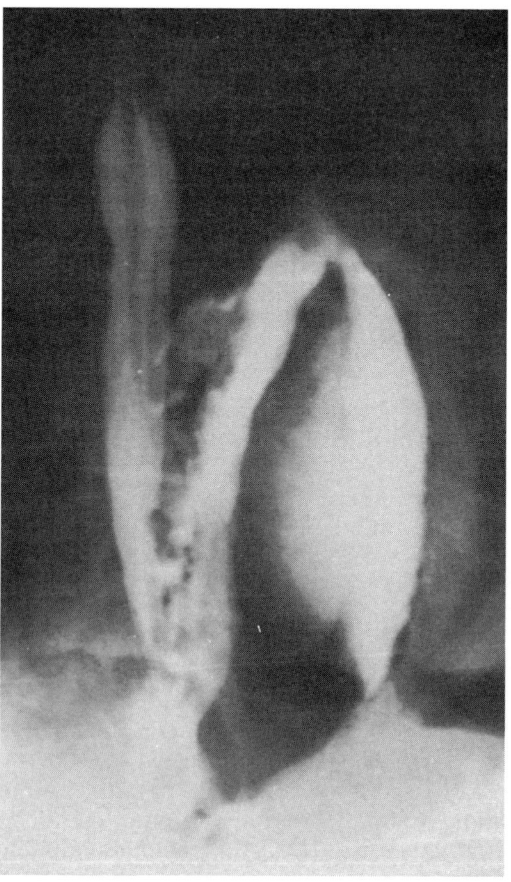

Figure 27-4. Postemetic esophageal rupture. Water-soluble contrast esophagogram showing marked extravasation of contrast from the left lower esophagus.

in association with intrathoracic pain are the most helpful differentiating features. Acute aortic dissection, pancreatitis, and myocardial infarction may also be confused with spontaneous esophageal perforations, as may any intrathoracic or abdominal catastrophe.

The treatment of barogenic rupture of the esophagus does not differ significantly from the management of esophageal perforations in general and is discussed subsequently. However, it is important to remember that the mucosal tear that occurs in barogenic esophageal rupture often extends beyond the muscular tear. Therefore, when closure is attempted, it is imperative to visualize the full extent of the muscular layer.[114] A recent report of primary repair for Boerhaave's syndrome demonstrated an 80% success rate for primary repair and a 14% mortality rate.[58] The report shows a marked improvement over previous series, which is consistent with improvements in primary repair for all situations.

External Trauma

Blunt trauma is a rare cause of esophageal perforation. The mechanisms by which blunt trauma can cause esophageal rupture are not completely clear. Blunt trauma to the chest or abdomen, combined with conditions that cause esophageal obstruction (e.g., acute spasm due to reflux), can result in explosive increases in intraesophageal pressure and barogenic rupture, usually of the lower left thoracic esophagus as described earlier. Blunt trauma to the cervical region may injure the esophagus directly, as may whiplash injuries.[38,92,101] Rupture of the distal thoracic esophagus has recently been reported after motor vehicle accidents associated with improper positioning of seat belts and sudden deceleration injury. Esophageal ruptures due to blunt trauma occur most frequently in the cervical esophagus and are commonly associated with injuries to other organs, usually the trachea.[31,53,102]

Penetrating esophageal injuries resulting from stab wounds and gunshot wounds are more frequent than esophageal injuries caused by blunt trauma but are still uncommon. As with blunt trauma, penetrating trauma more commonly injures the cervical esophagus, and serious associated injuries are found in almost every case.[23,31,80,83,105,107] High-caliber gunshot wounds can cause extensive esophageal tissue necrosis, which complicates the surgical management of this problem. Cervical esophageal disruption from trauma frequently heals without complication after repair or drainage. However, esophageal fistula associated with penetrating trauma to the cervical esophagus occurs in almost 10% of patients with gunshot wounds. The method of closure (i.e., whether a single-layer or multilayer closure was performed) has been shown to have no influence on the rate of fistula formation, and all fistulas eventually closed with nonoperative management.[115]

Clinical and plain roentgenographic findings in patients with esophageal rupture resulting from external trauma are nonspecific, often subtle, and frequently overshadowed by serious injuries to other organs. Patients with esophageal injuries may have subcutaneous emphysema, respiratory distress, hoarseness, dysphagia, and blood in the nasogastric tube. Neck tenderness, hematomas, and decreased mobility may also be seen with cervical esophageal injuries. Perforations of the intra-abdominal esophagus due to external trauma are rare and are associated with abdominal tenderness and signs of peritoneal irritation. Plain chest radiographs may show cervical or mediastinal air, mediastinal widening, pneumothorax, or hemothorax. Retropharyngeal swelling on lateral neck films may denote the presence of an injury to the cervical esophagus.

Because signs of esophageal injury are nonspecific and often subtle in the setting of trauma, a high index of suspicion is essential if esophageal perforations are to be detected early. Suspicion of esophageal disruption should be aroused whenever any of the physical signs or plain radiographic features described earlier are present. The diagnosis should be considered in all patients with bullet or knife wounds that may have traversed the mediastinum and those who present with a missile in close proximity to the esophagus.

The diagnostic approach to suspected traumatic esophageal perforation varies somewhat according to the urgency of associated injuries.[87] In trauma patients who must undergo immediate neck, chest, or abdominal exploration, careful and thorough intraoperative examination of the accessible esophagus should be performed. If this is not possible or is inadequate, intraoperative esophagoscopy should be performed. Emergent intraoperative esophagoscopy has been shown to have a sensitivity of 100% and a specificity of 80% in detecting penetrating injury to the esophagus in this setting.[45] Air-insufflation through a flexible esophagoscope is very helpful in identifying esophageal tears intraoperatively. Postoperative contrast esophagograms should be considered if concern remains that an injury may have been missed during exploration. Patients who do not require immediate exploratory surgery should undergo an urgent contrast esophagogram. Because 10 to 20% of contrast esophagograms are falsely negative in the setting of external trauma, negative esophagograms should be followed by endoscopic examination if esophageal injury is suspected.[23,31,53,80,87,101] Again, the use of contrast-enhanced CT may be diagnostic in those patients undergoing evaluation for multisystem trauma.[7,113] Evaluation of the esophagus should be an integral part of this examination when the search for other unsuspected injuries is being performed.

Management of esophageal perforation due to external trauma does not differ significantly from the management of other types of esophageal perforation except that the associated injuries must also be treated. Repairs of concomitant tracheal injuries should be separated from esophageal suture lines by the interposition of normal tissues, such as strap muscles in the neck or intercostal muscle or pleura in the thorax. Extensive devitalization from gunshot wounds is uncommon but may preclude primary esophageal repair (see later section, "Management of Esophageal Perforation").

Operative Trauma

Inadvertent injury to the esophagus may occur during esophageal or periesophageal operations such as hiatal hernia repair, vagotomy, esophagomyotomy, or pneumonectomy.[2,11,26,62,84,116] Most antireflux operations involve placement of suture through the esophageal muscular layers. A tear of the esophageal wall may result when these sutures are placed too deeply.[66] Disruption of the esophagus may also occur during operative dissection to expose the esophagus, particularly if dissection is rendered difficult by inflammatory adhesions resulting from previous surgery or infection.[62,84,116] When the esophagus is obscured by adhesions, identification can be greatly facilitated by placing a dilator in the esophagus through the mouth or, even more effectively, by leaving a flexible endoscope in the esophagus with the light on. During vagotomy, the esophagus should be handled with great care, minimizing traction and blind dissection.

Esophagopleural fistula after pneumonectomy results from direct operative trauma to the esophageal wall or from devascularization and subsequent mural necrosis.[11,26] Most cases of esophagopleural fistula have occurred after pneumonectomy for tuberculosis, particularly on the right side, and pre-existing esophageal traction diverticula are thought to be a predisposing factor. This serious complication is now rarely seen.

Esophageal surgeons should adopt an aggressive posture toward the diagnosis of esophageal perforations. Acute intraoperative injuries, if recognized, can usually be satisfactorily repaired with little risk of postoperative morbidity. Whenever any significant possibility of esophageal injury exists, the esophagus should be carefully and thoroughly examined. For example, after the completion of an esophagomyotomy for achalasia or spasm, the integrity of the esophageal mucosa should be ascertained by having the anesthesiologist fill the esophagus with air insufflated through an intraesophageal nasogastric tube. The esophagus is then submerged in saline and observed carefully for the escape of air bubbles (Fig. 27-5). If a small mucosal rupture is discovered, it can usually be satisfactorily closed with a stapler as described in subsequent sections.

Unrecognized intraoperative esophageal injuries may present in the postoperative period with fever, leukocytosis, pain, cervical or mediastinal emphysema, pleural effusions, or pneumothorax. Fever often is the earliest and most helpful sign of postoperative esophageal leak. After esophageal or periesophageal surgery, fever that is not clearly attributable to other sources should be considered indicative of an esophageal perforation until proved otherwise by a negative contrast esophagogram. The management of postoperative esophageal leak is discussed later.

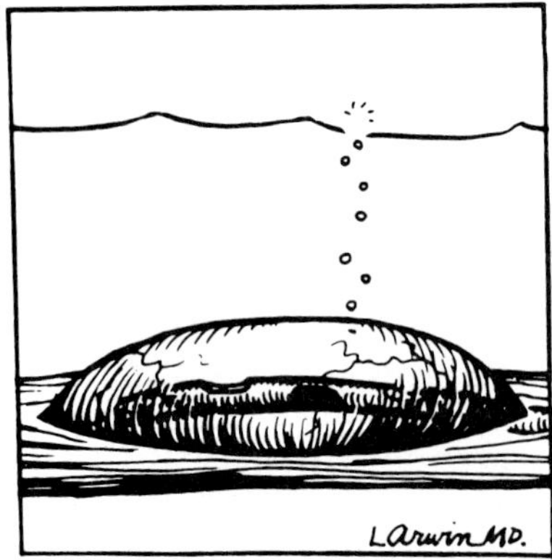

Figure 27-5. Method of testing for inadvertent esophageal perforation after esophagomyotomy. The esophagus is inflated with air through a nasogastric tube and is submerged in saline. Air bubbles indicate a perforation. (From Orringer, M.B.: Complications of esophageal surgery and trauma. *In* Greenfield, I.J. [ed.]: Complications in Surgery and Trauma. Philadelphia, J.B. Lippincott, 1984, with permission.)

Caustic Injuries

Swallowed chemicals are a major source of damage to the upper gastrointestinal tract. Caustic substance ingestion tends to occur in two groups of patients—children less than 5 years old who accidentally swallow these agents, and adults who attempt suicide. It is estimated that more than 5,000 caustic ingestions occur each year in the United States.[69] The major agents responsible are alkalis, acids, bleach, and detergents containing sodium tripolyphosphate. Detergents and bleach virtually always cause only mild esophageal irritation, which heals without adverse sequelae. Acids and alkalis, however, are capable of producing devastating injuries ranging from chronic esophageal and gastric strictures to acute multiorgan necrosis and perforation. Alkalis are the most destructive, causing liquefaction necrosis that facilitates deep penetration, whereas acids typically produce coagulation necrosis that tends to limit, to some extent, the depth of the injury.[40]

Before 1967, alkali (lye) was generally available only in solid form. In solid form, lye tends to adhere to the mucosa of the oropharynx and upper esophagus, producing burns in patches or linear streaks. Solid alkali rarely reaches the stomach in sufficient quantity to cause damage to it.[27] The introduction in the United States of concentrated liquid alkali preparations (e.g., Drano, Liquid-Plumr) in 1967 drastically changed the nature and extent of caustic esophageal injuries. These agents are the most common cause of severe caustic injuries today. The high viscosity of liquid alkali preparations tends to prolong the contact of these substances with mucous membranes and contributes to their rapid passage into the stomach. Extreme damage to the esophagus and stomach and adjacent organs such as the trachea, colon, small bowel, pancreas, and aorta frequently results. Ingested acids tend to cause significant gastric damage with relative sparing of the esophagus, although severe esophageal injuries can occur.[32] Reflex pyloric spasms occurring in response to contact with a corrosive agent causes pooling of both acids and alkalis in the gastric antrum, resulting in severe damage that can lead to antral stenosis or an hourglass type of deformity (Fig. 27-6). Experimental studies in dogs have shown that both cricopharyngeal and pyloric spasm occur after concentrated lye instillation into the esophagus. Contractions of the esophagus and stomach then propel the contents back and forth between the two organs for several minutes until gastric and esophageal atony occur after extensive damage to both organs.[90]

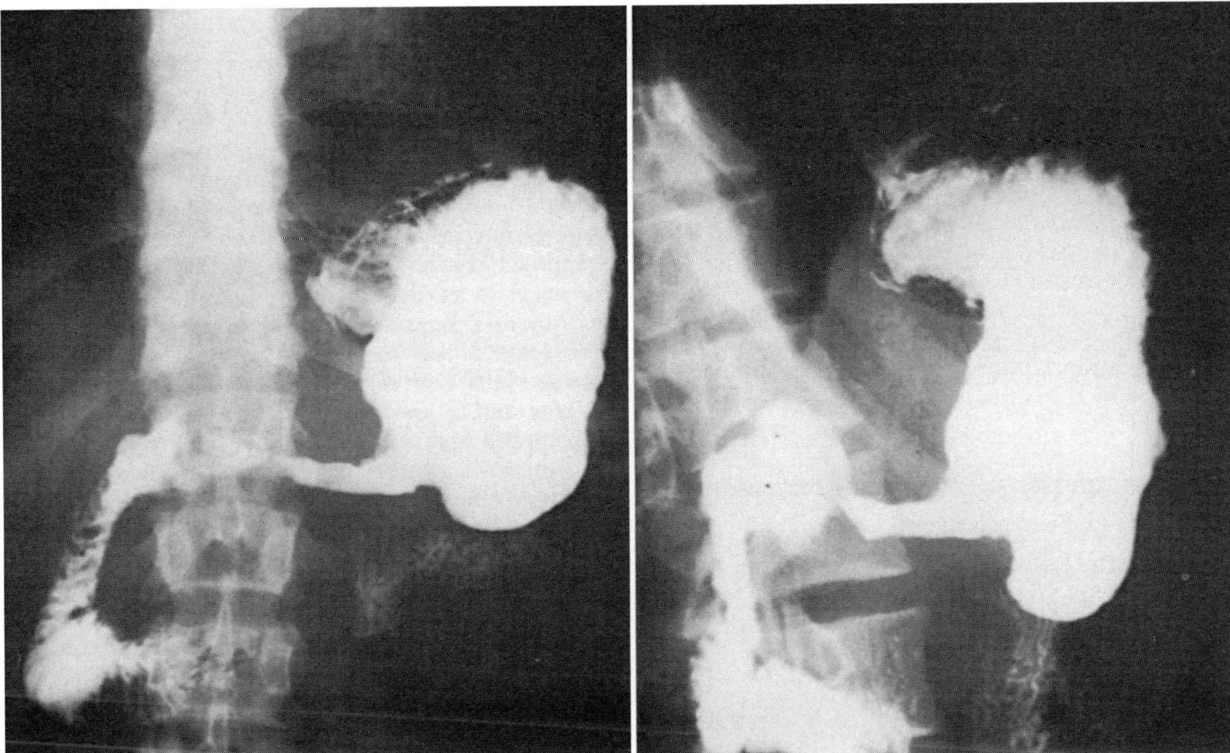

Figure 27–6. Caustic injury of the stomach. Severe antral stenosis is present with relative sparing of the body of the stomach and the duodenum.

Clinical Manifestations

Clinical manifestations vary slightly according to the amount and character of caustic agent ingested.[32] Mild burns of the pharynx, esophagus, and stomach may be virtually asymptomatic. *Solid alkali* usually causes burns of the mouth, pharynx, and upper esophagus as mentioned earlier. The severe pain caused by these burns usually induces immediate expectoration so that little is swallowed. Such burns commonly induce excessive salivation as well. Examination of the mouth and oropharynx reveals areas of mucosa that are replaced by white to gray-black pseudomembranes. Hoarseness, stridor, aphonia, and dyspnea suggest the presence of laryngotracheal edema or actual destruction. *Liquid alkali* is usually swallowed rapidly, causing less injury to the mouth and pharynx but extensive damage to the esophagus, stomach, or both. Dysphagia, odynophagia, and aspiration may be present. Severe substernal, back, and abdominal pain and peritoneal signs suggest that mediastinitis or peritonitis have resulted from an esophageal or gastric perforation. As noted earlier, with *acid ingestion*, injury to the stomach is more common, and therefore symptoms and signs are often more localized to the abdomen.

Although controversial, examination of the oropharynx is invaluable in patients with caustic ingestion, especially children. Of these patients with severe laryngeal burns, more than 70% have esophageal burns as well, and more importantly, all patients with severe esophageal burns have pharyngeal burns. The associated symptom complex in patients with alkaline ingestion, however, is less than diagnostic. Patients presenting with vomiting or respiratory distress have a high incidence of significant esophageal burns. However, in a review of a large group of patients with severe esophageal burns, only 30% had severe symptoms. It has been emphasized, therefore, that no single group of initially reported signs or symptoms can identify patients with potentially serious esophageal burns.[5]

Severe caustic injuries that result in esophageal or gastric perforation are associated with progressively severe septic and hypovolemic shock until appropriate therapy is instituted. When perforation of the stomach or esophagus does not occur, the acute clinical manifestations usually resolve within several days. Resolution is followed by a period of clinical improvement generally lasting several weeks. Symptoms due to stricture formation in the esophagus or stomach then become manifest. Strictures occur in only 10 to 25% of patients after ingestion of solid alkali.[27] However, most patients who have ingested liquid alkali have severe esophageal (and often gastric) damage that frequently progresses to stricture formation. Acid ingestion is more likely to result in stricture or contracture of the antrum or pylorus.

Immediate Diagnostic and Treatment Measures

Patients with acute caustic ingestion should be admitted to the hospital. Early management is directed toward ensuring an adequate airway, providing hemodynamic stabilization, and assessing the severity of the injury. Vomiting should not be induced. Because of the nearly instantaneous nature of most current caustic injuries, attempts to dilute the agent by having the patient drink water are of little value. In fact, this may increase the problem by creating gastric distention or inducing vomiting. Oral intake is withheld, and hypovolemia is treated with appropriate intravenous infusions. Patients are carefully observed for signs of airway obstruction. Endotracheal intubation or tracheostomy may be necessary because of laryngeal edema or actual laryngeal destruction. Antibiotics should be started as soon as the diagnosis of significant esophageal injury is established to decrease the risk of pulmonary infection from aspiration and bacterial invasion through the damaged esophageal wall.[29,32,52,54,73] Steroids have been advocated in the acute phase of caustic ingestion to prevent stricture formation.[40] However, their efficacy has never been established, and their use may obscure signs of sepsis and visceral perforation and impair healing. In a retrospective collective review, it has been suggested that steroids may be of benefit in those children with severe third-degree esophageal burns.[46] However, in a recent prospective randomized study that evaluated children over an 18-year period after caustic injection, steroids had no significant benefit in the prevention of caustic stricture.[5] The use of steroids for caustic injury cannot at the present be recommended.[5,32,46,54,73]

Radiographic contrast examination of the upper gastrointestinal tract can provide valuable information in the patient with a caustic injury and should be performed initially in most patients.[55] Esophageal mucosal injuries are seen on radiographs as blurred irregular margins with linear streaking of contrast in deeper ulcers. Scalloped or straightened esophagogastric margins may represent submucosal edema. Dilatation of the esophagus and stomach may be apparent, as may gastric ulcerations, air in the gastric wall, or frank extravasation of contrast agent. Contrast esophagography is the best way to make the diagnosis of esophageal perforation and should be performed whenever this entity is suspected, either at the time of admission to the hospital or subsequently.

Management

Early endoscopy is indicated in virtually every patient with a suspected caustic esophageal injury.[27,32,54,69,73,95] Endoscopy establishes whether a significant esophageal injury has taken place, and its findings can be used to grade the severity of injury (Table 27-2).[27] Endoscopic examination alone, however, cannot determine the actual depth of the burn. The risk of endoscopic perforation is minimized if the examination is performed by an experienced endoscopist using general anesthesia and a flexible pediatric endoscope. Flexible endoscopy can also be safely performed in conscious patients if adequate sedation is used to prevent retching and movement by the patient. Formerly, it was believed that the endoscope should not be advanced beyond the first burned area.[54,72] More recently, however, complete examination of the esophagus and stomach has been recommended, particularly if severe burns are not present proximally.[20,32,95,103]

Table 27-2. Endoscopic Evaluation of Caustic Injuries

Extent of Injury	Endoscopic Findings
First degree	Mucosal hyperemia and edema
Second degree	Mucosal ulceration with blisters and exudates; pseudomembrane formation
Third degree	Deep ulceration with charring and eschar formation; massive edema obliterating the esophageal lumen

After the initial supportive and diagnostic measures described earlier have been taken, management of patients with caustic injuries is generally expectant. Patients with no more than first-degree burns need no specific treatment other than observation for 24 to 48 hours. Subsequent esophageal narrowing is uncommon in patients with mild burns. Patients with second- or third-degree burns must be observed more carefully for a longer period of time for evidence of esophageal or gastric necrosis occurring in the acute phase of the injury. Full-thickness caustic necrosis of the esophagus, stomach, or other organs requires emergency resection. The challenge is to determine on the basis of clinical, endoscopic, and radiographic information when full-thickness necrosis has occurred. Surgical exploration is mandatory in patients with free intraperitoneal or mediastinal air, extravasation of contrast material from the stomach or esophagus, peritoneal signs, and sepsis that apparently arises in the abdomen or mediastinum. The need for surgical exploration is also suggested by severe, persistent back or substernal pain (indicating mediastinitis) and by metabolic acidosis (indicating extensive visceral necrosis). Likewise, the finding of a gastric pH greater than 7 suggests severe gastric damage and the need for exploration, although this finding is not reliable in the presence of a significant amount of blood in the stomach.[54,116]

Emergency surgical exploration in the setting of liquid caustic ingestion generally should be performed through the abdomen. This approach allows accurate assessment of damage to intra-abdominal organs and resection of areas of full-thickness gastric necrosis. Obviously, only the lower portion of the esophagus is well visualized through a laparotomy. However, when esophageal resection is necessary, transhiatal esophagectomy can be relatively easily performed through a combined cervical and abdominal approach.[34,76,77] Transhiatal esophagectomy without thoracotomy is the ideal technique for esophageal resection in the setting of acute caustic injury because it spares these critically ill patients a thoracotomy. Remarkably, the transhiatal esophageal dissection is often facilitated rather than hindered by the periesophageal edema resulting from the caustic burn.

Alimentary reconstruction after emergency gastric or esophageal resection for acute transmural caustic injury should be deferred until mucosal healing has occurred and the severity of chronic stricture occurring in retained organs is clearly evident. Most patients with severe gastric burns from either acid or alkali also have significant associated esophageal injuries.[27,54] Therefore, when gastric resection is required, esophageal resection is usually required as well. Even when concomitant esophageal resection is not required, it is generally unwise to leave the closed esophagus as a blind tube in the mediastinum, and therefore transhiatal dissection of the esophagus should be performed at the time of gastrectomy. The mobilized thoracic esophagus is delivered out of the cervical incision, and any necrotic portion is resected. Sparing as much potentially viable esophagus as possible, the end of the remaining esophagus is tunneled subcutaneously on the lower neck or, preferably, the anterior chest wall, where a stoma is constructed. (See the later section "Intrathoracic Esophageal Perforation" for a more complete description of this technique.)

In contrast with the standard expectant method for managing acute caustic injuries, Estrera and colleagues[27] recommend a more aggressive approach. All patients in whom second- or third-degree injuries are seen at endoscopy undergo immediate exploratory laparotomy. Patients with full-thickness injuries are treated by resection, usually esophagogastrectomy. When full-thickness injury has not occurred, a silicone stent is positioned in the esophagus and left in place for about 3 weeks to prevent stricture formation. Early results with this approach appear very promising, although further experience is necessary to define its role clearly in the management of acute caustic esophageal injury.

Severe but less than full-thickness esophageal injuries are very likely to progress to stricture formation. Dilation is the standard therapy for chronic caustic esophageal strictures. Because early dilations are associated with an increased risk of perforation, dilation should not be instituted until at least 6 to 8 weeks after the injury, when re-epithelialization as documented endoscopically has occurred.[54] A perforation resulting from dilation of a caustic esophageal stricture is best treated by esophagectomy because more conservative procedures invariably fail to salvage the esophagus as a functional organ, and repair of a perforation to a stricture is usually doomed to failure. Strictures that are not dilatable or that remain refractory to dilation after 6 to 12 months necessitate esophageal substitution, usually with colon. Although the stomach is generally not an acceptable esophageal substitute in these patients because of the gastric scarring and contracture resulting from the original injury, caustic gastric burns limited to the prepyloric area may be resected, preserving the right gastric and gastroepiploic vascular arcades and still permitting a cervical esophagogastrostomy and distal gastrojejunostomy.

When esophageal substitution is required for a stricture resulting from caustic ingestion, the need for concomitant resection of the damaged esophagus is controversial. Whenever possible, however, the esophagus should be resected. This has the advantages of preventing the development of (1) a retention cyst or abscess in the retained esophagus, (2) reflux esophagitis if the retained esophagus is left attached to the stomach, and (3) esophageal carcinoma. Resection of the esophagus also allows placement of the esophageal substitute in the posterior mediastinum in the original esophageal bed, the shortest and most direct route between the neck and the abdominal cavity. In this position, resection of the head of the clavicle and adjacent sternum to enlarge the superior opening into the anterior mediastinum is *not* required in contrast to retrosternal placement of the graft. There is a 1,000-fold increased risk of developing esophageal carcinoma after caustic injury, with an incidence of 0.8 to 4%, often after a latent period of 20 to 40 years.[1] Patients who have a retained esophagus with a caustic stricture should be followed carefully for the development of this complication for the rest of their lives.

Swallowed Foreign Bodies

Ingested material may become lodged in the esophagus and lead to obstruction, abrasion, or perforation. Failure of ingested substances to pass through the esophagus may be the result of underlying organic or functional (neuromotor) obstruction. Small children and psychiatric patients are especially prone to ingest foreign bodies. In small children, the offending object is most frequently a coin (69%), but tacks, bones, and buttons are commonly found as well. In adults, bones and buttons are the most common offenders.[18,43,64] Adult patients who wear upper dentures may have impaired ability to sense foreign objects in the mouth, thus leading to inadvertent ingestion. Occasionally, pieces of dentures or bridge work are swallowed (Fig. 27-7). Esophageal perforation after foreign body ingestion may result from direct penetration of the esophageal wall by a sharp edge, from pressure necrosis, or from endoscopic attempts to remove the foreign body.[10,34,63]

A history of foreign body ingestion is often not obtainable; children and psychiatric patients are frequently poor historians, and normal adults may be unaware that they have swallowed a foreign object. Diagnosis of an esophageal foreign body therefore requires a high index of suspicion. The most common symptoms are dysphagia and odynophagia. Large cervical esophageal foreign bodies may cause signs and symptoms of associated upper airway obstruction. A few patients have the clinical symptoms and signs of esophageal perforation (fever, chest pain, cervical crepitance) as the first manifestation of an esophageal foreign body.[64]

The diagnosis of radiopaque esophageal foreign bodies can be made by plain roentgenograms of the neck and chest. Posteroanterior roentgenograms of the neck should be taken with the neck in hyperextension because the manubrium tends to obscure the esophageal inlet in the neutral position. If plain films do not reveal a suspected foreign body, thin barium should be given orally; most foreign bodies are seen with this technique. Rarely, esophagoscopy is necessary to diagnose small foreign bodies or to differentiate symptomatic esophageal abrasions from small foreign bodies.

Esophageal foreign bodies should be removed because of the risks of obstruction and perforation, unlike gastric foreign bodies, which often do not require removal. Smaller, smooth-edged foreign bodies such as coins can often be removed with a Foley catheter, passing the catheter past the object, inflating the balloon, and withdrawing the catheter and object together.[14,72] However, when this technique is used, extreme care must be taken to prevent the patient from aspirating the foreign body into the airway as it is brought out past the epiglottis. Esophagoscopy is necessary for larger, smooth, and all sharp objects. Although some objects can be removed with the flexible instrument, rigid esophagoscopy using general anesthesia is usually preferable because of its

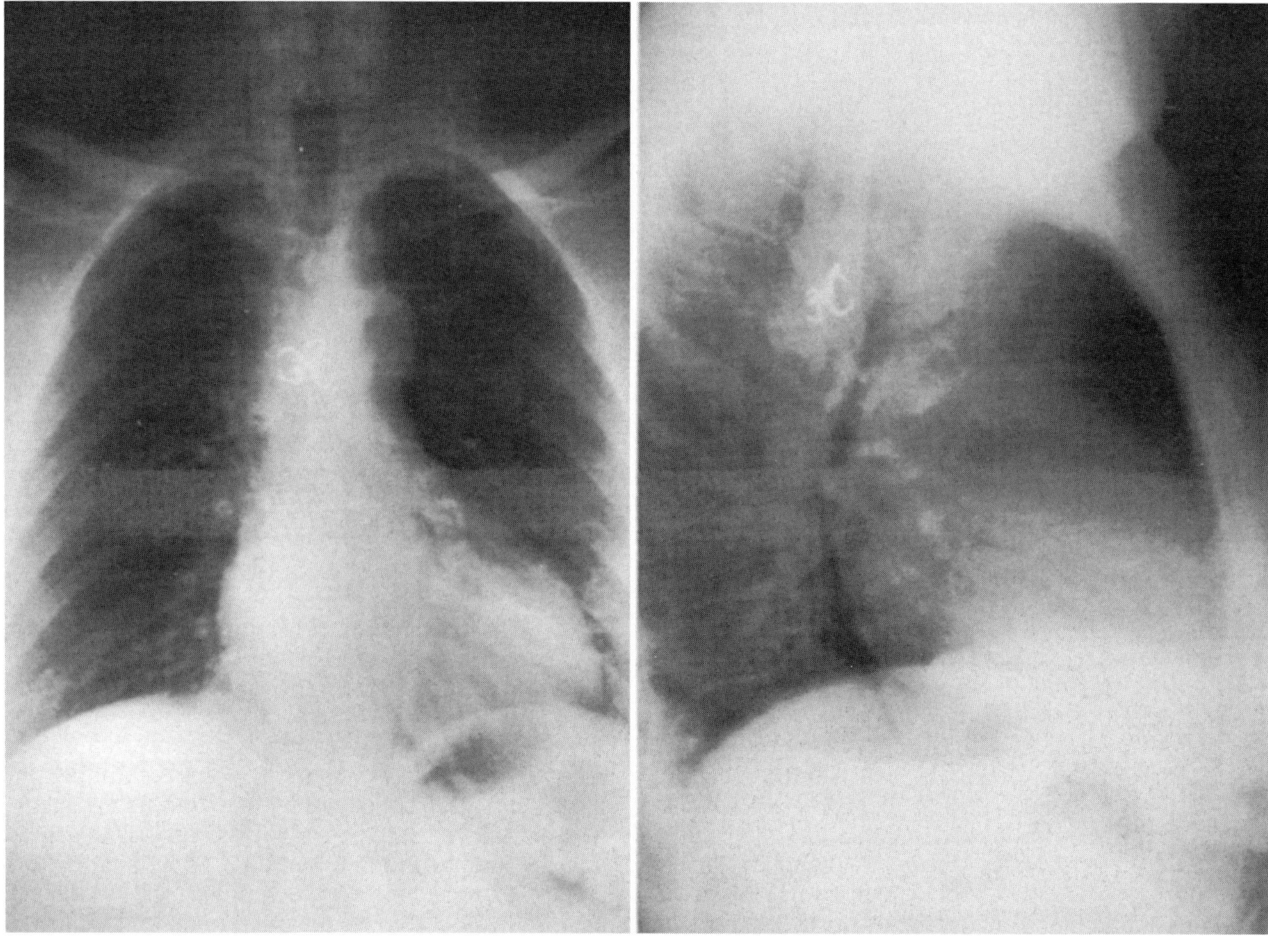

Figure 27–7. Inadvertently swallowed bridgework. Attempted endoscopic removal resulted in extensive esophageal laceration and perforation, which was shown by the presence of mediastinal air. At exploratory thoracotomy, repair of the esophagus was not possible, and an esophagectomy with cervical esophagogastric anastomosis was carried out.

greater safety and effectiveness. We do *not* recommend using the esophagoscope to push the object into the stomach. This maneuver carries a significant risk of esophageal perforation and should be attempted only with smooth objects and when a distal esophageal obstruction is known not to be present. Esophagograms should be done routinely after foreign body removal to enhance early diagnosis of esophageal perforations and to exclude underlying esophageal disease.

Occasional patients give a reliable history of meat ingestion immediately preceding symptoms of esophageal obstruction. This problem may at times be treated by having the patient ingest a dilute enzymatic solution containing papain (e.g., meat tenderizer) to digest the impacted meat partially and permit it to pass into the stomach. Brooks recommends a dose of 5 ml of 20% papain in 10% alcohol every 5 minutes for 1 hour.[18] Both the presence and the resolution of the meat impaction should be documented by barium esophagography.

Esophageal foreign bodies that cannot be safely or effectively removed with the rigid esophagoscope require esophagotomy for removal. Objects in the distal esophagus (below 35 cm) should be approached through a left thoracotomy, whereas a right thoracotomy should be used for foreign bodies in the more proximal thoracic esophagus. Perforations that result from foreign bodies or their attempted removal require operative intervention, as discussed in the next section.

MANAGEMENT OF ESOPHAGEAL PERFORATION

The immediate resuscitative treatment of acute esophageal perforation is directed toward decreasing bacterial and chemical contamination of the mediastinum and restoring associated intravascular volume losses. Broad-spectrum intravenous antibiotics with activity against oral flora should be started as soon as possible. All oral intake should be stopped, and vigorous intravenous hydration should be instituted. Nasogastric tube decompression of the stomach is indicated in most patients to lessen soilage through the esophageal defect from gastroesophageal reflex. However, a nasogastric tube may be counterproductive in some patients, particularly those with well-contained proximal perforations.

Definitive management of the esophageal perforation should be undertaken as soon as possible after institution of the general supportive measures described previously. Proper treatment of thoracic esophageal tears *always* involves adequate drainage of the mediastinum and repair of the esophageal tear whenever feasible. However, the therapy of esophageal perforation is influenced by the location of the tear, its size and cause, the length of delay in diagnosis, the extent of mediastinal and pleural contamination, and the presence of underlying esophageal disease. Because so many factors must be taken into consideration when treating esophageal ruptures, treatment must be instituted on an individual basis. Nonetheless, effective and practical approaches to most patients with esophageal perforation have emerged from previous clinical experience.

Non-operative Therapy

Operative intervention is indicated in virtually all cases of esophageal perforation. However, a few carefully selected patients may be appropriately and successfully managed non-operatively.[19,65] Candidates for non-operative therapy should have (1) locally contained disruption without pleural contamination, (2) evidence on contrast study of drainage of the localized perforation back into the esophagus, (3) minimal symptoms, and (4) minimal clinical evidence of sepsis. Such patients usually have proximal esophageal tears caused by esophagoscopy or intramural dissections that have occurred during dilation of a stricture.

Pneumatic balloon dilatation can result in esophageal perforation in up to 10% of patients. When these injuries are confined to linear mucosal tears without significant mediastinitis, they can be managed successfully with observation.[68] However, if increasing signs of sepsis or hemodynamic instability occur, a more aggressive approach must be adopted. Treatment in these patients consists of cessation of oral intake, administration of antibiotics, and intravenous hydration until the disruption heals or until the certainty of eventual healing is made manifest by a decrease in the size of the cavity. Optimal oral hygiene is essential to minimize further contamination by swallowed oral bacteria. Brushing of the teeth four to six times a day is instituted. A nasogastric tube for drainage is usually not necessary. During healing, nutrition must be maintained by nasogastric, gastrostomy, or jejunostomy tube feedings or by intravenous hyperalimentation until oral intake can be resumed, usually within 1 to 3 weeks after the injury.

When selecting candidates for non-operative therapy, it is essential that the cavity resulting from the perforation is both well contained and well drained internally into the esophagus. Unfortunately, it is usually not possible to be certain that the leak is well contained in patients who present early (<24 hours) after injury, and mediastinal sepsis may progress during the ensuing hours if surgery is delayed. Thus, non-operative therapy of esophageal perforations is most appropriate for selected patients who present late (>24 hours) after the injury, have no systemic evidence of infection, and have obviously contained, internally drained leaks. Most other patients should be treated operatively.

Operative Therapy

Cervical and Upper Thoracic Esophageal Perforations

Perforation of the cervical esophagus leads to progressive contamination of the mediastinum because of the dependent spread of infection along fascial planes from the neck.[82] Death from mediastinitis ensues unless adequate drainage is achieved. Most cervical and upper thoracic esophageal perforations (down to the level of the carina or the fourth thoracic vertebral body) can be effectively treated by placing drains in the retroesophageal space through a *cervical approach*.[17,18,59,65,66,82] This is accomplished by making a skin incision parallel to the anterior border of the sternocleidomastoid muscle (see Fig. 26–11). Dissection is then continued posteriorly (medial to the sternocleidomastoid muscle and carotid sheath and lateral to the thyroid gland and strap muscles). The omohyoid muscle, the middle thyroid vein, and occasionally the inferior thyroid artery are divided until the prevertebral fascia is reached. Blunt dissection with the finger in the retroesophageal prevertebral space then gives access to the abscess cavity and allows placement of the drains, which are then brought out through the skin incision.

Closure of the proximal esophageal laceration is not mandatory because spontaneous healing after a few days invariably occurs if distal obstruction is not present. However, suture closure of accessible early perforations may be performed in addition to drainage. Regardless of whether simple drainage or surgical closure is used for cervical perforations, the outcome is the same, with both groups having a 6% reported mortality rate.[51] Some even advocate observation without exploration until evidence of extension or significant symptoms develop.[109] Oral nutrition can usually be resumed after 5 to 7 days, when the perforation has either healed or significantly decreased in size so that fistula output is minimal. Nutrition during the first few days is maintained with nasogastric tube feedings. Cervical esophageal perforations that involve either pleural cavity or extend into the lower mediastinum are inadequately drained by the cervical approach and require transthoracic drainage (Fig. 27–8).

Intrathoracic Esophageal Perforation

Esophageal perforations that are diagnosed early (within approximately 24 hours) are more easily treated and have a better prognosis than those diagnosed late (after 24 hours). As time passes after the injury, the edges of the esophageal disruption become progressively more inflamed and friable, making them less likely to hold repair sutures. Prompt surgical treatment is therefore indicated in all patients with early esophageal disruption.

It is generally agreed that early thoracic esophageal perforations *not associated with intrinsic esophageal*

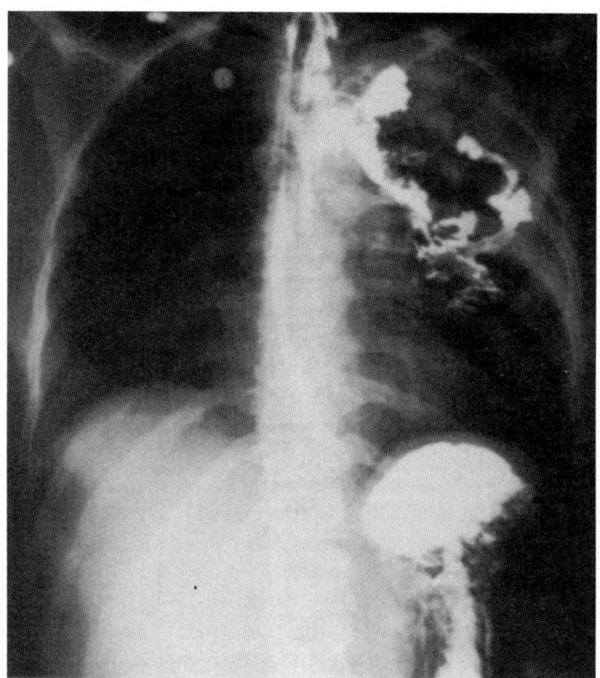

Figure 27–8. Delayed recognition of cervical esophageal perforation after attempted endotracheal intubation. The large abscess in the upper left thorax required transthoracic drainage.

disease should be treated with primary repair of the defect combined with wide mediastinal drainage.[1,13,16,17,65,66,71,91,93,99] Increasing experience, however, suggests that regardless of the duration of the injury primary, repair should be attempted, for with meticulous technique, the results will frequently be good.[11] For primary repair to be successful, regardless of the length of the delay in diagnosis, it is imperative that the entire length of the mucosal injury be exposed. This requires extension of the muscular defect approximately 1 to 2 cm proximally and distally beyond the extent of the mucosal tear (Fig. 27–9). Only minimal débridement of the inflamed mucosal edges of the defect should be performed. With a No. 40 to 46 French Hurst-Maloney bougie within the esophagus, a meticulous two-layer closure is performed, approximating the mucosal defect with a linear stapling device and the muscular layer with absorbable suture (Fig. 27–10).[119] Wide mediastinal drainage is mandatory in addition to the repair. Drainage is achieved by opening the mediastinal pleura above and below the level of the tear from the thoracic inlet to the diaphragm, irrigating the mediastinum, and then draining the mediastinum transpleurally using a large-bore chest tube. Perforations of the lower third of the esophagus are generally best approached through a left-sided thoracotomy, and perforations of the more proximal thoracic esophagus are approached through a right thoracotomy. Perforations of the intra-abdominal esophagus without intrapleural contamination may be approached through the abdomen. However, the authors generally prefer a transthoracic exposure.[13]

Reinforcement or buttressing of the repair with pedicled flaps of adjacent normal tissues is an important adjunct in reducing postoperative suture-line disruption.[16,65,71,88,91] A variety of tissues have been used to buttress esophageal repairs, including parietal pleura, gastric fundus, intercostal or diaphragmatic muscle, lung, and omentum. A report is available of primary repair followed by wrapping of the esophagus in absorbable mesh covered with fibrin glue that indicated extremely good results when there was no other alternative.[9] Re-

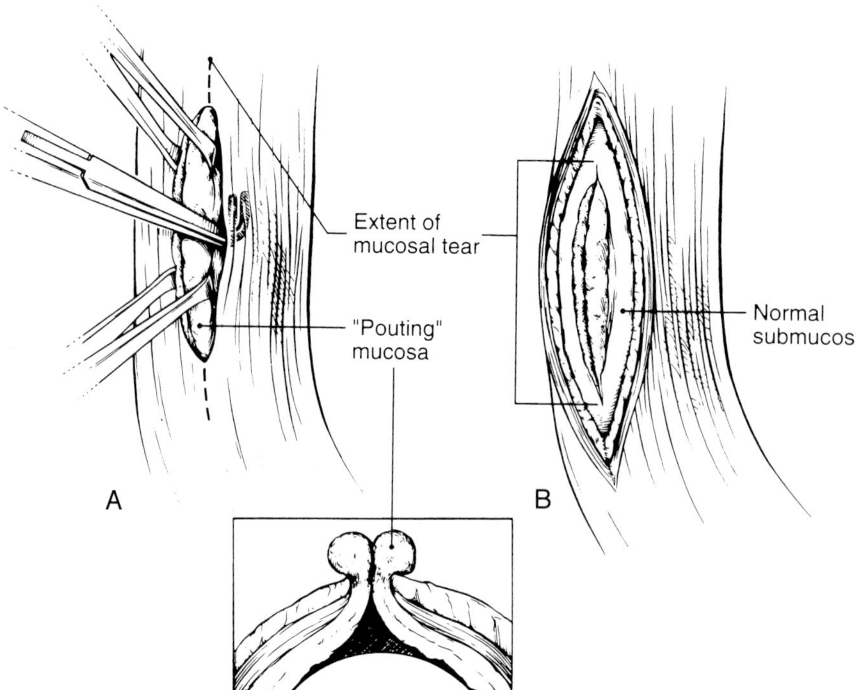

Figure 27–9. Primary repair of esophageal perforation illustrating exposure of the esophageal perforation. *A*, Extension of the muscular tear proximal and distal to the injury to allow complete exposure of the mucosal defect. The *inset* demonstrates the damaged pouting mucosa initially seen on inspection of the injury. *B*, Mobilization of the submucosa away from the muscular coat to allow exposure of the defect surrounded by normal submucosa and both the proximal and distal extent of the mucosal injury by extension of the muscular tear. (From Whyte, R.I., Iannettoni, M.D., and Orringer, M.B.: Intrathoracic esophageal perforation: The merit of primary repair. J. Thorac. Cardiovasc. Surg., *109:*140, 1995.)

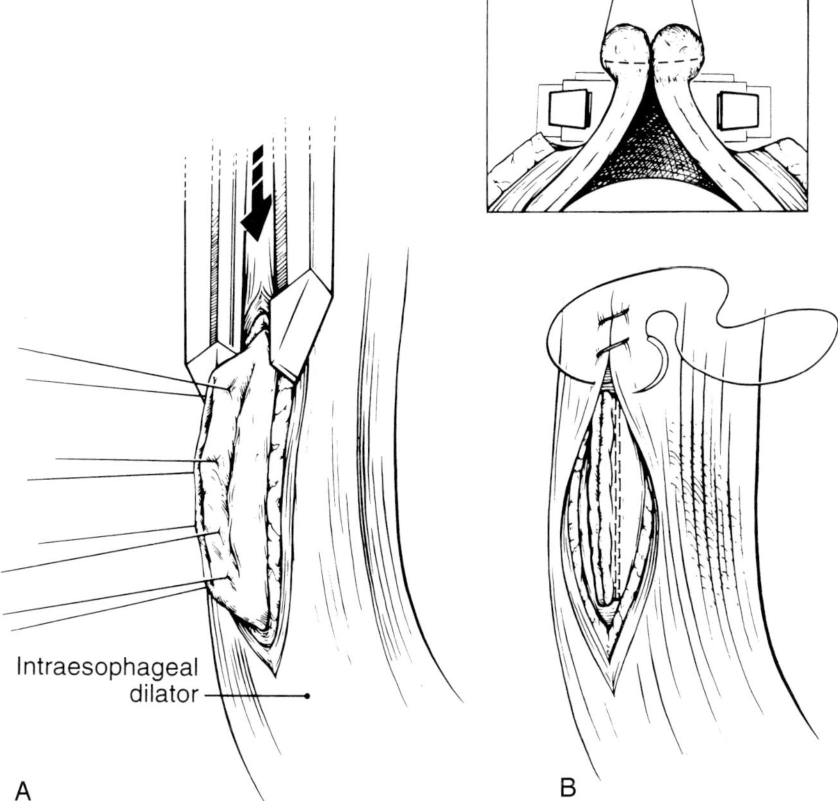

Figure 27–10. Technique of primary repair of esophageal perforation illustrating (*A*) closure of the defect with GIA surgical stapler after mobilization and exposure of the mucosal and submucosal tear beyond the muscular tear, and (*B*) approximation of the muscular coat over the suture line with a running absorbable suture. The stapler is applied over an intraesophageal bougie (*inset*) to healthy mucosa and submucosa, not to the inflamed edges of the defect. (From Whyte, R.I., Iannettoni, M.D., and Orringer, M.B.: Intrathoracic esophageal perforation: The merit of primary repair. J. Thorac. Cardiovasc. Surg., *109*:140, 1995.)

pairs of perforations of the lower esophagus (e.g., postemetic rupture) are ideally reinforced by wrapping the fundus of the stomach around the repair (Fig. 27–11). This fundoplication should be reduced below the diaphragm to prevent complications of an iatrogenic paraesophageal hernia. Repairs in the more proximal esophagus can generally be buttressed with intercostal muscle or parietal pleura.[25,36] Omentum may be used to buttress abdominal esophageal perforations in addition to or instead of the gastric fundus or may be mobilized into the chest to virtually any level of the esophagus. Pericardium has occasionally been used to buttress repairs of thoracic esophageal perforations, but this is not recommended by the authors, because its use carries a risk of purulent pericarditis. Pedicled flaps of diaphragm have also been used.[85,112]

After esophageal repair and drainage, a nasogastric tube is used to treat any postoperative paralytic ileus. Thereafter, the nasogastric tube can be used to give enteral feedings until oral intake is resumed. It is wishful thinking to assume that a patient who is swallowing no food has a "protected" esophageal suture line, because saliva containing digestive enzymes and oral bacteria begins to traverse the esophagus from the moment the patient awakens from general anesthesia. Thus, oral liquids may be resumed once the intestinal ileus has subsided. There is no convincing evidence that swallowing a liquid diet results in a higher incidence of subsequent esophageal suture-line disruption. Well-drained esophagocutaneous fistulas resulting from breakdown of the esophageal repair usually heal spontaneously if there is no associated distal obstruction. Such fistulas are not a contraindication to oral alimentation if they are small, well drained, and not associated with distal obstruction.[78]

Late Esophageal Perforation

Traditional teaching holds that closure of a nonmalignant esophageal perforation after 24 hours is associated with appreciable morbidity and mortality rates, and as a result, a variety of operations to divert, drain, or exclude the esophagus with a late-diagnosed perforation have evolved. However, the results of primary repair of intrathoracic esophageal perforations have improved considerably, so that currently in those with minimal intrinsic esophageal disease, primary repair of esophageal perforations is recommended regardless of the duration of the injury. Patients with intrinsic esophageal disease represent a distinct subset and are discussed subsequently.

In a prospective study, 22 patients with nonmalignant esophageal perforations deemed to have an otherwise salvageable esophagus at the time of presentation were treated by the authors with a primary two-layer repair regardless of the duration of the tear.[114] There was no significant difference in morbidity or mortality rates between patients who underwent repair in less than 24 hours (13 of 22, or 59%) and patients who underwent repair at greater than 24 hours (9 of 22, or 41%). The four patients who developed recurrent esophageal fistulas (one who had a repair less then 24 hours after the injury and three who had a repair of more than 24 hours) were all managed conservatively with either tube thoracostomy

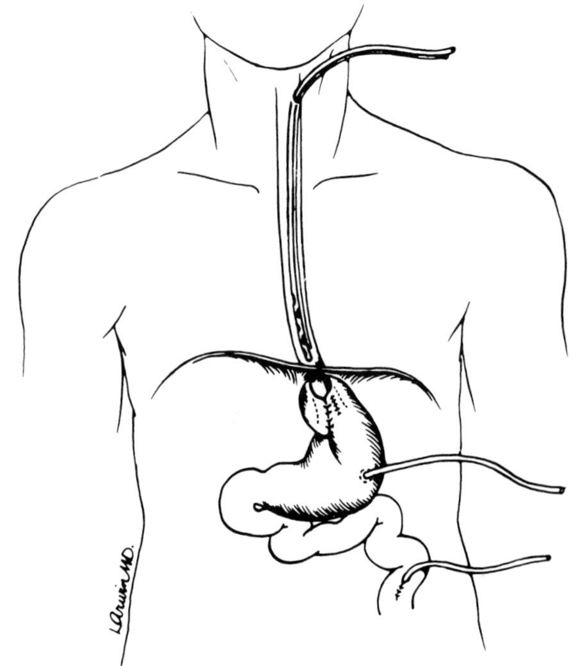

Figure 27–11. Repair of a distal esophageal perforation and reinforcement with fundoplication. The fundoplication has been reduced below the diaphragm to prevent complications of a paraesophageal hernia. A nasogastric tube, decompressing gastrostomy, and feeding jejunostomy have been added. (From Orringer, M.B.: Complications of esophageal surgery and trauma. *In* Greenfield, L.J. [ed.]: Complications in Surgery and Trauma. Philadelphia, J.B. Lippincott, 1984, with permission.)

drainage (two patients) or rib resection and drainage (two patients). All patients subsequently had healed perforations, and none have required further related operative therapy. The authors did not routinely buttress the esophageal repairs; however, five patients received some type of fundoplication. The authors believe that primary repair, whenever possible, is preferable to resection and one-stage reconstruction or delayed reconstruction, and the occasional esophagopleural cutaneous fistulas after primary repair seem to be easily controlled with simple drainage and heal if distal obstruction has been relieved, and intrinsic esophageal pathology can be controlled and treated.

The other available options for the treatment of late esophageal perforations include wide drainage alone, exclusion and diversion, and non-operative management. The use of these different methods of treatment is somewhat controversial and is influenced by the experience of the surgeon, the condition of the patient, and the surgeon's assessment of the quality of the esophageal tissue at the site of injury. In virtually all patients with delayed recognition of esophageal perforation, a feeding jejunostomy tube should be inserted. Wide drainage is the mainstay of treatment of delayed esophageal perforation and should be instituted in all cases regardless of the other therapeutic options used.[88] Adequate drainage of perforations of the thoracic esophagus below the level of the fourth thoracic vertebra generally requires a thoracotomy with opening of the mediastinal pleura over the perforated esophagus and transpleural drainage with large chest tubes. Transpleural drainage of course necessitates a degree of ongoing contamination of the pleural cavity, but this is usually well tolerated if appropriate antibiotic therapy is administered until a chronic controlled esophagopleurocutaneous fistula is established. Alternatively, for treatment of esophageal perforations, Santos and Frater[94] advocated chest tube drainage alone and continuous irrigation of the mediastinum and pleural cavity by having the patient swallow water. Posterior mediastinotomy is another alternative that allows extrapleural drainage of abscesses confined to the mediastinum and is an excellent option in a select number of patients.[97] Wide drainage alone has been recommended for patients who can tolerate some degree of pleural contamination and in whom closure of the defect does not appear to be feasible. The authors do not recommend this approach, however, and drainage alone is best applied to cervical esophageal perforations.[51]

The decision about whether to attempt closure of perforations diagnosed late must be made at the time of thoracotomy when the quality of the esophageal tissue at the edges of the defect can be assessed. But with increasing experience, the majority of these patients are undergoing successful closure of their esophageal perforations even after delayed recognition of the injury.[28,36,71] Some esophageal defects are too large to permit direct closure without tension. On occasion, these larger defects can be closed by using pedicled adjacent tissue flaps as a patch, which is sutured to the edges of the defect (Fig. 27–12).[36] Closure of esophageal perforations should always be accompanied by adequate drainage and should never be performed in the setting of unrelieved distal obstruction.[7]

Esophageal Perforations Associated With Esophageal Disease

The management of *esophageal perforations associated with intrinsic esophageal disease causing distal obstruction* is more complex, even when they are diagnosed early. Primary repair combined with drainage is inadequate because the repair invariably breaks down in the presence of distal obstruction. Whenever possible in these cases, relief of the associated obstruction should be achieved at the time of repair and drainage.[56,66,96] Thus, patients with achalasia who incur perforation during attempted dilation should be treated with suture repair, esophagomyotomy, and a partial fundoplication to buttress the tear if possible. Small perforations above *readily dilatable* esophageal reflux strictures can be treated with suture repair, dilation of the stricture to relieve the obstruction, and an antireflux operation. We evaluated the functional results in 42 patients with esophageal perforation, 25 of whom underwent primary repair; one-third (8 of 25) required further therapy with either esophageal dilatation or reconstruction.[47] These latter patients all had either pre-existing esophageal strictures or diffuse motility disorders.

Esophageal resection is the best option for perforation occurring with intrinsic esophageal disease (neoplasm, nondilatable stricture, caustic injury, extensive devitalization) that cannot be treated effectively by more conservative measures.[17,42,50,56,65,99] Patients with perforations in

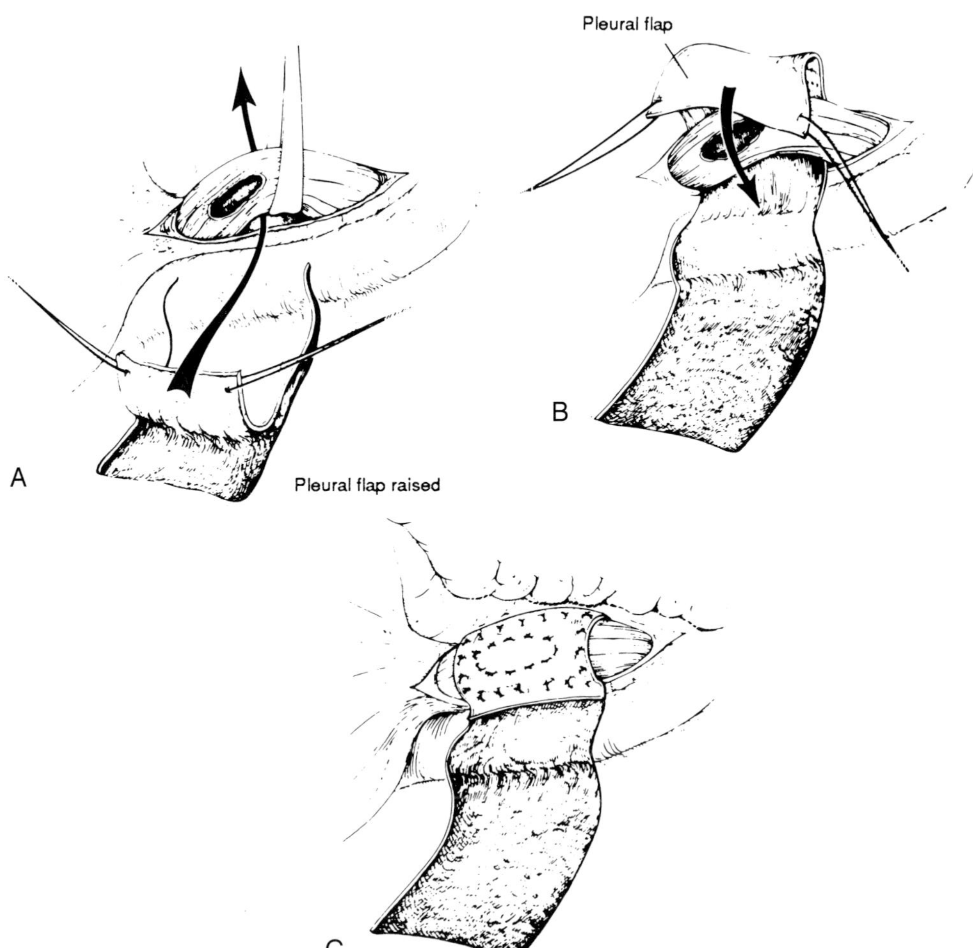

Figure 27–12. Pleural flap patch closure of a large esophageal defect. *A*, After mobilization of the esophagus, a pleural flap is raised. *B*, The flap is placed around the esophagus, covering the perforation. *C*, The flap is sutured to itself. Sutures are placed above and below at the margins of the flap and also the perforation itself, tacking the pleura firmly to the esophageal muscularis. (From Gricco, H.C., and Wilkins, F.W.: Esophageal repair following late diagnosis of intrathoracic perforation. Ann. Thorac. Cardiovasc. Surg., *20*:337, 1975, by permission of The Society of Thoracic Surgeons.)

association with cancer or nondilatable benign strictures are best treated by resection, as are patients with perforations sustained after caustic injury. Extensive esophageal revitalization that occurs with some high-velocity gunshot wounds may also necessitate resection. Patients with benign esophageal strictures that fracture during attempted dilation are also probably best managed by resection. It is generally unwise to attempt to salvage a diseased esophagus simply because esophagectomy is considered to be too major an undertaking. When esophagectomy is necessary, a total thoracic esophagectomy has advantages compared with a more limited resection because it completely eliminates the source of mediastinal and pleural sepsis and is well tolerated by most patients, especially those with perforations that are diagnosed early. Reports of transhiatal esophagectomy with primary reconstruction in such patients have documented excellent overall survival rates and definitive treatment of the esophageal pathology.[3,39,79]

Immediate reconstruction of the alimentary tract is possible in many patients who require esophagectomy for a promptly diagnosed perforation. This approach, however, is best undertaken when an intact, healthy stomach is available for esophageal substitution utilizing a cervical esophagogastric anastomosis. Immediate esophageal substitution with unprepared colon has been advocated by some but is not recommended by the authors. Patients with esophageal perforations caused by acute caustic injuries and unstable or severely ill patients should undergo esophagectomy followed by later reconstruction. Immediate reconstruction is best performed by placing the mobilized, elongated stomach in the posterior mediastinum in the native esophageal bed and performing a cervical esophagogastrostomy (Fig. 27–13). A feeding jejunostomy is performed routinely.

When severe caustic injuries with uncertain respiratory tract involvement or cardiovascular instability from associated sepsis preclude immediate esophagectomy and reconstruction for acute perforation, the esophagogastric junction is divided through an abdominal approach and the divided cardia carefully oversewn. Working through the diaphragmatic hiatus and a separate cervical incision, the intrathoracic esophagus is then completely mobilized and the entire thoracic esophagus is delivered into the neck wound. *Only devitalized or extensively damaged esophagus should be resected.* The esophageal hiatus should be closed to avoid herniation of abdominal viscera into the chest. The maximal length of esophagus is preserved and tunneled subcutaneously onto the left anterior chest wall, where the stoma is constructed (Fig. 27–14). An esophagostomy stoma is much easier to care for at this site than at its usual location on the neck, and the extra length of remaining esophagus may facilitate later reconstructive efforts using substernal stomach or colon.

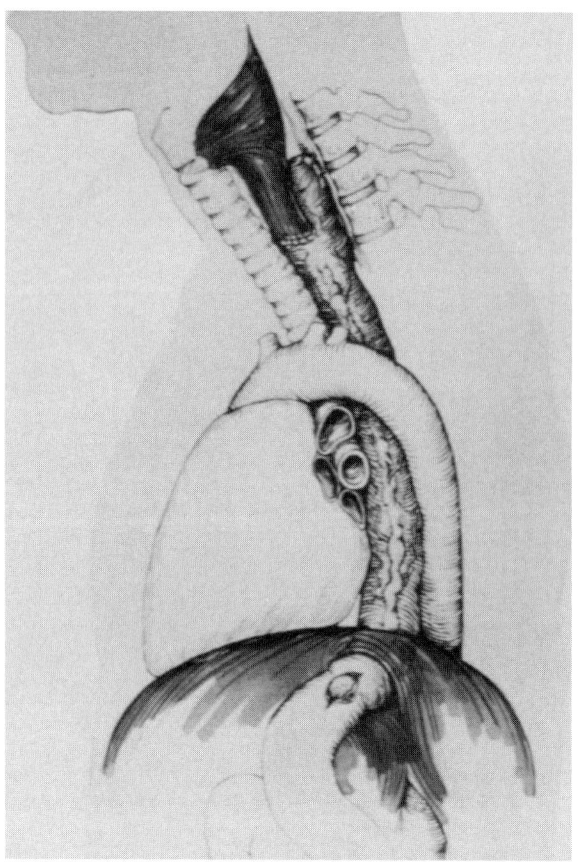

Figure 27–13. Esophageal replacement with stomach in the native esophageal bed. A cervical esophagogastrostomy has been performed. (From Orringer, M.B., and Sloan, H.: Esophagectomy without thoracotomy. J. Thorac. Cardiovasc. Surg., *76*:643, 1978, with permission.)

A feeding jejunostomy is constructed to allow enteral alimentation until reconstruction is performed at a later date. A gastrostomy tube should also be inserted because gastric atony or pylorospasm may occur after the vagotomy that inevitably accompanies esophagectomy. If the stomach proves to empty well after several days, gastrostomy feedings may be used in preference to jejunostomy tube feedings, which are less amenable to bolus administration and are thus less convenient for the patient.

Certain types of intrinsic esophageal pathology make it impossible or unlikely that the perforated esophagus can be salvaged as a functional alimentary organ. Esophagectomy is the best option in the majority of these patients, even after delayed recognition of the esophageal perforation. Reconstruction is best deferred, depending on the condition of the patients and the availability of an esophageal substitute.

The concept of esophageal exclusion for esophageal perforation was first described in 1956.[49] The originally described technique involved division and closure of the distal thoracic esophagus through a thoracotomy or laparotomy, division of the distal cervical esophagus, and a proximal end-cervical esophagostomy. This technique successfully decreases mediastinal contamination but results in major difficulties with subsequent esophageal reconstruction. With the intent of alleviating the problems with esophageal reconstruction after a previous exclusion, Urschel et al.[110] developed the technique of esophageal diversion and exclusion in continuity. This procedure involves placing a ligature around the distal thoracic esophagus to control reflux and performing a side-cervical esophagostomy to divert oropharyngeal secretions (Fig. 27–15).

Despite the conceptual appeal of this approach, significant problems re-establishing comfortable swallowing after this procedure have persisted, control of mediastinal contamination has not been absolute, and the authors do not use this technique.[51,88] The use of absorbable staples to temporarily exclude the ruptured esophagus has been described. This technique has been followed by healing of the perforation and by spontaneous reversal of the esophageal obstruction after 3 to 4 weeks without stricture formation in several patients.[44] Further experience

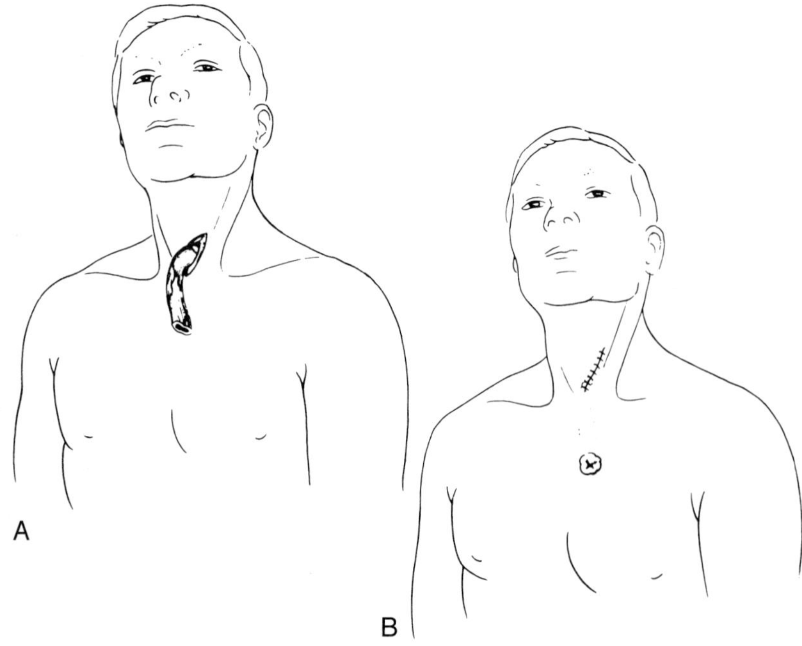

Figure 27–14. Construction of an anterior thoracic esophagostomy to preserve maximal length of esophagus. *A*, The mobilized thoracic esophagus is placed on the anterior chest wall to determine the location of the stoma. *B*, The esophagus is then tunneled subcutaneously and the esophagostomy is constructed. Stomal appliances are easily applied to the flat surface of the chest, and the additional esophageal length provided by the technique often facilitates later reconstruction. (From Orringer, M.B.: Complications of esophageal surgery and trauma. *In* Greenfield, L.J. [ed.]: Complications in Surgery and Trauma. Philadelphia, J.B. Lippincott, 1984, with permission.)

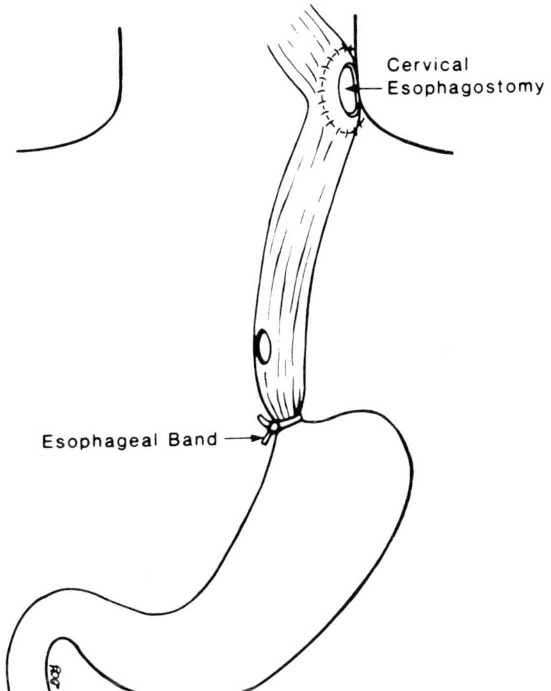

Figure 27–15. Technique of esophageal exclusion. A side cervical esophagostomy diverts oral secretions. Reflux of gastric and biliary secretions is prevented by an umbilical tape tied at the gastroesophageal junction. The tape is tied tightly enough to obstruct the lumen but not tight enough to cause mural ischemia. The vagus nerves are not included in the tie but lie superficial to it. (From Brewer, I.A., Carter, R., Mulder, G.A., and Stiles, Q.R.: Options in the management of perforations of the esophagus. Am. J. Surg., *152*:62, 1986, with permission.)

may demonstrate the efficiency of this method of esophageal exclusion. Similarly, the reported use of esophageal stenting for the treatment of perforations not amenable to repair or resection[15] may merit further evaluation.

SUMMARY

Esophageal perforation is virtually always an indication for surgery except in patients with well-contained leaks with good internal drainage. A minority of patients with poorly contained disruptions have been treated successfully non-operatively with tube thoracostomy for drainage or tube thoracostomy combined with esophageal intubation to occlude the esophageal tear.[12,48] Despite occasional success with these conservative methods, nonoperative therapy is contraindicated in most patients with esophageal disruption, and an aggressive approach, if necessary using an esophagectomy in those with intrinsic esophageal disease, is often less "radical" treatment in the long run. Meticulous primary repair of esophageal disruption, regardless of the duration of the tear, is an established principle in the management of this disastrous injury.

References

1. Ajalat, G.M., and Mulder, D.G.: Esophageal perforations: The need for an individualized approach. Arch. Surg., *119*:1318, 1984.
2. Albin, J., Noel, T., Allan, K., et al.: Intrathoracic esophageal perforation with the Angelchik antireflux prosthesis: Report of a new complication. Gastrointest. Radiol., *10*:330, 1985.
3. Altorjay, A., Kiss, J., Voros, A., et al.: The role of esophagectomy in the management of esophageal perforations. Ann. Thorac. Surg., *65*:1433, 1998.
4. Ancona, E., Gayet, B.: Etiology, diagnostic localization and symptoms: A GEEMO questionaire. *In* Siewert, J.R., and Holscher, A.H. (eds.). Diseases of the Esophagus. Berlin, Springer-Verlag, 1988, p. 1327.
5. Anderson, K.D., Rouse, T.M., and Randolph, J.G.: A controlled trial of corticosteroids in children with corrosive injury of the esophagus. N. Engl. J. Med., *323*:637, 1990.
6. Appelqvist, P., and Salmo, M.: Lye corrosion carcinoma of the esophagus: A review of 63 cases. Cancer, *45*:2655, 1980.
7. Backer, C.L., LoCicero, J.D., Hartz, R.S., et al.: Computed tomography in patients with esophageal perforation. Chest, *98*:1078, 1990.
8. Bacon, B.R., Camara, D.S., and Duffy, M.C.: Severe ulceration and delayed perforation of the esophagus after endoscopic variceal sclerotherapy. Gastrointest. Endosc., *33*:311, 1987.
9. Bardaxoglou, E., Manganas, D., Meunier, B., et al.: New approach to surgical management of early esophageal thoracic perforation: Primary suture repair reinforced with absorbable mesh and fibrin glue. World J. Surg., *21*:618, 1997.
10. Benda, T.J.: Perforating foreign body of the esophagus. Laryngoscope, *79*:470, 1969.
11. Benjamin, I., Olsen, A.M., and Ellis, F.H., Jr.: Esophagopleural fistula: A rare postpneumonectomy complication. Ann. Thorac. Surg., *7*:139, 1969.
12. Berger, R.L., and Donato, A.T.: Treatment of esophageal disruption by intubation: A new method of management. Ann. Thorac. Surg., *13*:27, 1972.
13. Berne, C.J., Shader, A.E., and Doty, D.B.: Treatment of effort rupture of the esophagus by epigastric celiotomy. Surg. Gynecol. Obstet., *129*:277, 1969.
14. Bigler, F.C.: The use of a Foley catheter for removal of blunt foreign bodies from the esophagus. J. Thorac. Cardiovasc. Surg., *51*:759, 1966.
15. Bisgaard, T., Wojdemann, M., Heindorff, H., et al.: Nonsurgical treatment of esophageal perforations after endoscopic palliation in advanced esophageal cancer. Endoscopy, *29*:155, 1997.
16. Bladergroen, M.R., Lowe, J.E., and Postlethwait, R.W.: Diagnosis and recommended management of esophageal perforation and rupture. Am. Thorac. Surg., *43*:235, 1986.
17. Brewer, L.A., Carter, R., Mulder, G.A., et al.: Options in the management of perforations of the esophagus. Am. J. Surg., *152:* 62, 1986.
18. Brooks, J.W.: Foreign bodies in the air and food passages. Ann. Surg., *175*:720, 1972.
19. Cameron, J.L., Kieffer, R.F., Hendrix, T.R., et al.: Selective nonoperative management of contained intrathoracic esophageal disruptions. Ann. Thorac. Surg., *27*:404, 1979.
20. Chung, R.S., and DenBesten, L.: Fiberoptic endoscopy in treatment of corrosive injury of the stomach. Arch. Surg., *110*:725, 1975.
21. Curci, J.J., and Horman, M.J.: The importance of early diagnosis and treatment. Ann. Surg., *145*:30, 1983.
22. Davies, A.P., and Vaughan, R.: Expanding mesh stent in the emergency treatment of Boerhaave's syndrome. Ann. Thorac. Surg., *67:* 1482, 1999.
23. Defore, W.W., Jr., Mattox, K.L., Hansen, H.A., et al.: Surgical management of penetrating injuries of the esophagus. Am. J. Surg., *134*:734, 1977.
24. Derbes, V.J., and Mitchell, R.E.: Hermann Boerhaave's "Atrocis, nec descripti prius, morbi historia." First translation of classic case report of rupture of esophagus, with annotations. Bull. Med. Lib. Assoc. *43*:217, 1955.
25. Dooling, J.A., and Zick, H.R.: Closure of an esophagopleural fistula using onlay intercostal pedicle graft. Ann. Thorac. Surg., *3*:553, 1967.
26. Engleman, R.M., Spencer, F.C., and Berg, P.: Postpneumonectomy esophageal fistula: Successful one-stage repair. J. Thorac. Cardiovasc. Surg., *59*:871, 1970.
27. Estrera, A., Taylor, W., Mills, L.J., et al.: Corrosive burns of the esophagus and stomach: A recommendation for an aggressive surgical approach. Ann. Thorac. Surg., *41*:276, 1986.
28. Finley, R.J., Pearson, F.G., Weisel, R.D., et al.: The management of

nonmalignant intrathoracic esophageal perforations. Ann. Thorac. Surg., *30:*575, 1980.
29. Foley, M.J., Ghahremani, G.G., and Rogers, L.F.: Reappraisal of contrast media used to detect upper gastrointestinal perforations: Comparison of ionic water-soluble media with barium sulfate. Radiology, *144:*231, 1982.
30. Gayett, B., and Ancona, E.: Esophageal perforations: High risk group patients and treatment. A GEEMO questionnaire. In Siewert, J.R., Holscher, A.H. (eds.): Diseases of the Esophagus. Berlin, Springer-Verlag, 1988, p. 1331.
31. Glatterer, M.S., Jr., Toon, R.S., Ellestad, C., et al.: Management of blunt and penetrating external esophageal trauma. J. Trauma, *25:*784, 1985.
32. Goldman, L.P., and Weigert, J.M.: Corrosive substance ingestion: A review. Am. J. Gastroenterol., *79:*85, 1984.
33. Gorman, R.L., Khin-Maung-Gyi, M.T., Klein-Schwartz, W., et al.: Initial symptoms as predictors of esophageal injury in alkaline corrosive ingestions. Am. J. Emerg. Med., *10:*189, 1992.
34. Gossot, D., Sarfati, E., and Celerier, M.: Early blunt esophagectomy in severe caustic burns of the upper digestive tract. J. Thorac. Cardiovasc. Surg., *84:*188, 1987.
35. Graeber, G.M., Niezgoda, J.A., Albus, R.A., et al.: A comparison of patients with endoscopic esophageal perforations and patients with Boerhaave's syndrome. Chest, *92:*995, 1987.
36. Grillo, H.C., and Wilkins, E.W., Jr.: Esophageal repair following late diagnosis of intrathoracic perforation. Ann. Thorac. Surg., *20:*387, 1975.
37. Grillo, H.C., Moncure, A.C., and McEnany, M.T.: Repair of inflammatory tracheoesophageal fistula. Ann. Thorac. Surg., *22:*112, 1976.
38. Gulbrandson, R.N., and Gaspard, D.J.: Steering wheel rupture of the pharyngoesophagus: A solitary injury. J. Trauma, *17:*74, 1977.
39. Gupta, N.M.: Emergency transhiatal oesophagectomy for instrumental perforation of an obstructed thoracic oesophagus. Br. J. Surg., *83:*1007, 1996.
40. Haller, J.A., Jr., Andrews, H.G., White, J.J., et al.: Pathophysiology and management of acute corrosive burns of the esophagus: Results of treatment in 285 children. J. Pediatr. Surg., *6:*578, 1971.
41. Hankins, J.R., Cole, F.N., and Attar, S.: Palliation of esophageal carcinoma with intraluminal tubes: Experience with 30 patients. Ann. Thorac. Surg., *28:*224, 1976.
42. Hendren, W.H., and Henderson, B.M.: Immediate esophagectomy of instrumental perforation of the thoracic esophagus. Ann. Surg., *68:*997, 1968.
43. Henry, K., Toro, C., and Crossley, K.B.: Perforation of the esophagus by chicken bones: A report of two cases and a review of the literature. Minn. Med., *70:*459, 1987.
44. Holzinger, F., Metzger, A., Barras, J.P., et al.: Temporary exclusion of the perforated esophagus using a linear vascular stapler: A new surgical treatment. Hepatogastroenterology, *43:*155, 1996.
45. Horwitz, B., Krevsky, B., Buckman, R.F., Jr., et al.: Endoscopic evaluation of penetrating esophageal injuries. Am. J. Gastroenterol., *88:*1249, 1993.
46. Howell, J.M., Dalsey, W.C., Hartsell, F.W., et al.: Steroids for the treatment of corrosive esophageal injury: A statistical analysis of past studies. Am. J. Emerg. Med., *10:*421, 1992.
47. Iannettoni, M.D., Vlessis, A.A., Whyte, R.I., et al.: Functional outcome after surgical treatment of esophageal perforation. Ann. Thorac. Surg., *64:*1606; discussion 1609, 1997.
48. Imre, J.: Plastic tube prosthesis for the surgical treatment of perforations in esophageal strictures. Ann. Thorac. Surg., *15:*275, 1973.
49. Johnson, J., Schwegman, C.W., and Kirby, C.K.: Esophageal occlusion for persistent fistula following spontaneous rupture of the esophagus. J. Thorac. Cardiovasc. Surg., *32:*827, 1956.
50. Johnson, J., Schwegman, C.W., and MacVaugh, H.: Early esophagogastrostomy in the treatment of iatrogenic perforation of the distal esophagus. J. Thorac. Cardiovasc. Surg., *55:*24, 1968.
51. Jones, W.G., and Ginsberg, R.J.: Esophageal perforation: A continuing challenge. Ann. Thorac. Surg., *53:*534, 1992.
52. Keighley, M.R., Girdwood, R.W., Ionescu, M.I., et al.: Spontaneous rupture of the oesophagus: Avoidance of postoperative morbidity. Br. J. Surg., *59:*649, 1972.
53. Kelly, J.P., Webb, W.R., Moulder, P.V., et al.: Management of airway trauma. II: Combined injuries of the trachea and esophagus. Ann. Thorac. Surg., *43:*160, 1987.
54. Kirsh, M.M., Peterson, A., Brown, J.W., et al.: Treatment of caustic injuries of the esophagus: A ten year experience. Ann. Surg., *188:*675, 1978.
55. Kuhn, J.R., and Tunell, W.P.: The role of initial cineesophagography in caustic esophageal injury. Am. J. Surg., *146:*804, 1983.
56. Larsson, S., and Pettersson, G.: Advisability of concomitant immediate surgery for perforation and underlying disease of the esophagus. Scand. J. Thorac. Cardiovasc. Surg., *18:*275, 1984.
57. Lawrence, D.R., Moxon, R.E., Fountain, S.W., et al.: Iatrogenic oesophageal perforations: A clinical review. Ann. R. Coll. Surg. Engl., *80:*115, 1998.
58. Lawrence, D.R., Ohri, S.K., Moxon, R.E., et al.: Primary esophageal repair for Boerhaave's syndrome. Ann. Thorac. Surg., *67:*818, 1999.
59. Loop, F.D., and Groves, L.K.: Esophageal perforations. Ann. Thorac. Surg., *10:*571, 1970.
60. Mackler, S.A.: Spontaneous rupture of the esophagus. Surg. Gynecol. Obstet., *95:*345, 1952.
61. Mathisen, D.J., Grillo, H.C., Wain, J.C., et al.: Management of acquired nonmalignant tracheoesophageal fistula. Ann. Thorac. Surg., *52:*759, 1991.
62. McBurney, R.P.: Perforation of the esophagus: A complication of vagotomy or hiatal hernia repair. Ann. Surg., *169:*851, 1969.
63. McLaughlin, R.T., Morris, J.D., and Haight, C.: The morbid nature of the migrating foreign body in the esophagus. J. Thorac. Cardiovasc. Surg., *55:*188, 1968.
64. Meislin, H., and Kobernick, M.: Corn chip laceration of the esophagus and evaluation of suspected esophageal perforation. Ann. Emerg. Med., *12:*455, 1983.
65. Michel, L., Grillo, H.C., and Malt, R.A.: Operative and nonoperative management of esophageal perforations. Ann. Surg., *194:*57, 1981.
66. Michel, L., Grillo, H.C., and Malt, R.A.: Esophageal perforation. Ann. Thorac. Surg., *33:*203, 1982.
67. Micon, L., Geis, L., Siderys, H., et al.: Rupture of the distal thoracic esophagus following blunt trauma: Case report. J. Trauma, *30:*214, 1990.
68. Molina, E.G., Stollman, N., Grauer, L., et al.: Conservative management of esophageal nontransmural tears after pneumatic dilation for achalasia. Am. J. Gastroenterol., *91:*15, 1996.
69. Moore, W.R.: Caustic ingestions. Pathophysiology, diagnosis, and treatment. Clin. Pediatr. (Phila.), *25:*192, 1986.
70. Nashef, S.A., and Pagliero, K.M.: Instrumental perforation of the esophagus in benign disease. Ann. Thorac. Surg., *44:*360, 1987.
71. Nesbitt, J.C., and Sawyers, J.L.: Surgical management of esophageal perforation. Am. Surg., *53:*183, 1987.
72. Nixon, G.W.: Foley catheter method of esophageal foreign body removal: Extension of applications. AJR Am. J. Roentgenol., *132:*441, 1979.
73. Oakes, D.D., Sherck, J.P., and Mark, J.B.: Lye ingestion. Clinical patterns and therapeutic implications. J. Thorac. Cardiovasc. Surg., *83:*194, 1982.
74. Ogilvie, A.L., Dronfield, M.W., Ferguson, R., et al.: Palliative intubation of oesophagogastric neoplasms at fibreoptic endoscopy. Gut, *23:*1060, 1982.
75. Okike, N., Payne, W.S., Neufeld, D.M., et al.: Esophagomyotomy versus forceful dilation for achalasia of the esophagus: Results in 899 patients. Ann. Thorac. Surg., *28:*119, 1979.
76. Orringer, M.B.: Technical aids in performing transhiatal esophagectomy without thoracotomy. Ann. Thorac. Surg., *38:*128, 1984.
77. Orringer, M.B.: Transhiatal esophagectomy for benign disease. J. Thorac. Cardiovasc. Surg., *90:*649, 1985.
78. Orringer, M.B., and Lemmer, J.H.: Early dilation in the treatment of esophageal disruption. Ann. Thorac. Surg., *42:*536, 1986.
79. Orringer, M.B., and Stirling, M.C.: Esophagectomy for esophageal disruption. Ann. Thorac. Surg., *49:*35, discussion 42, 1990.
80. Pass, L.J., LeNarz, L.A., Schreiber, J.T., et al.: Management of esophageal gunshot wounds. Ann. Thorac. Surg., *44:*253, 1987.
81. Patton, A.S., Lawson, D.W., Shannon, J.M., et al.: Reevaluation of the Boerhaave syndrome. A review of fourteen cases. Am. J. Surg., *137:*560, 1979.
82. Pearse, H.E.: The operations for perforations of the cervical esophagus. Surg. Gynecol. Obstet., *56:*192, 1933.
83. Popovsky, J.: Perforations of the esophagus from gunshot wounds. J. Trauma, *24:*337, 1984.
84. Postlethwait, R.W., Kim, S.K., and Dillon, M.L.: Esophageal complications of vagotomy. Surg. Gynecol. Obstet., *128:*481, 1969.

85. Rao, K.V., Mir, M., and Cogbill, C.L.: Management of perforations of the thoracic esophagus: A new technic utilizing a pedicle flap of diaphragm. Am. J. Surg., *127:*609, 1974.
86. Reeder, L.B., DeFilippi, V.J., and Ferguson, M.K.: Current results of therapy for esophageal perforation. Am. J. Surg., *169:*615, 1995.
87. Richardson, J.D., Flint, L.M., Snow, N.J., et al.: Management of transmediastinal gunshot wounds. Surgery, *90:*671, 1981.
88. Richardson, J.D., Martin, L.F., Borzotta, A.P., et al.: Unifying concepts in treatment of esophageal leaks. Am. J. Surg., *149:*157, 1985.
89. Ritchie, A.J., McGuigan, J., McManus, K., et al.: Diagnostic rigid and flexible oesophagoscopy in carcinoma of the oesophagus: A comparison. Thorax, *48:*115, 1993.
90. Ritter, F.N., Newman, M.H., and Newman, D.E.: A clinical and experimental study of corrosive burns of the stomach. Ann. Otol. Rhinol. Laryngol., *77:*830, 1968.
91. Rosoff, L. Sr., and White, E.J.: Perforation of the esophagus. Am. J. Surg., *128:*207, 1974.
92. Rotstein, O.D., Rhame, F.S., Molina, E., et al.: Mediastinitis after whiplash injury. Can. J. Surg., *29:*54, 1986.
93. Safavi, A., Wang, N., Razzouk, A., et al.: One-stage primary repair of distal esophageal perforation using fundic wrap. Am. Surg., *61:*919, 1995.
94. Santos, G.H., and Frater, R.W.: Transesophageal irrigation for the treatment of mediastinitis produced by esophageal rupture. J. Thorac. Cardiovasc. Surg., *91:*57, 1991.
95. Sarfati, E., Gossot, D., Assens, P., et al.: Management of caustic ingestion in adults. Br. J. Surg., *74:*146, 1987.
96. Sarr, M.G., Pemberton, J.H., and Payne, W.S.: Management of instrumental perforations of the esophagus. J. Thorac. Cardiovasc. Surg., *84:*211, 1982.
97. Seybold, W.D., and Johnson, M.A., III: Perforation of the esophagus: An analysis of 50 cases and an account of experimental studies. Surg. Clin. North Am., *30:*1155, 1950.
98. Silvis, S.E., Nebel, O., Rogers, G., et al.: Endoscopic complications: Results of the 1974 American Society for Gastrointestinal Endoscopy Survey, JAMA *235:*928, 1976.
99. Skinner, D.B., Little, A.G., and DeMeester, T.R.: Management of esophageal perforation. Am. J. Surg., *139:*760, 1980.
100. Soderlund, C., and Wiechel, K.L.: Oesophageal perforation after sclerotherapy for variceal haemorrhage. Acta Chir. Scand., *149:*491, 1983.
101. Splener, C.W., and Benfield, J.R.: Esophageal disruption from blunt and penetrating external trauma. Arch. Surg., *111:*663, 1976.
102. Stothert, J.C., Jr., Buttorff, J., and Kaminski, D.L.: Thoracic esophageal and tracheal injury following blunt trauma. J. Trauma, *20:*992, 1980.
103. Sugawa, C., Mullins, R.J., Lucas, C.E., et al.: The value of early endoscopy following caustic ingestion. Surg. Gynecol. Obstet., *153:*553, 1981.
104. Sugawa, C., Benishek, D., and Walt, A.J.: Mallory-Weiss syndrome. A study of 224 patients. Am. J. Surg., *145:*30, 1983.
105. Symbas, P.N., Tyras, D.H., Hatcher, C.R., Jr., et al.: Penetrating wounds of the esophagus. Ann. Thorac. Surg., *13:*552, 1972.
106. Symbas, P.N., Hatcher, C.R., Jr., and Harlaftis N: Spontaneous rupture of the esophagus. Ann. Surg., *187:*634, 1978.
107. Symbas, P.N., Hatcher, C.R. Jr., and Vlasis, S.E.: Esophageal gunshot injuries. Ann. Surg., *191:*703, 1980.
108. Tesler, M.A., and Eisenberg, M.M.: Spontaneous esophageal rupture. Int. Abstr. Surg., *117:*1, 1963.
109. Tilanus, H.W., Bossuyt, P., Schattenkerk, M.E., et al.: Treatment of oesophageal perforation: A multivariate analysis. Br. J. Surg., *78:*582, 1991.
110. Urschel, H.C. Jr., Razzuk, M.A., Wood, R.E., et al.: Improved management of esophageal perforation: Exclusion and diversion in continuity. Ann. Surg., *179:*587, 1974.
111. Vergauwen, P., Moulin, D., Buts, J.P., et al.: Caustic burns of the upper digestive and respiratory tracts. Eur. J. Pediatr., *150:*700, 1991.
112. Westaby, S., Shepherd, M.P., and Nohl-Oser, H.C.: The use of diaphragmatic pedicle grafts for reconstructive procedures in the esophagus and tracheobronchial tree. Ann. Thorac. Surg., *33:*486, 1982.
113. White, C.S., Templeton, P.A., and Attar, S.: Esophageal perforation: CT findings. AJR Am. J. Roentgenol., *160:*767, 1993.
114. Whyte, R.I., Iannettoni, M.D., and Orringer, M.B.: Intrathoracic esophageal perforation. The merit of primary repair. J. Thorac. Cardiovasc. Surg., *109:*140, discussion 144, 1995.
115. Winter, R.P., and Weigelt, J.A.: Cervical esophageal trauma. Incidence and cause of esophageal fistulas. Arch. Surg., *125:*849; discussion 851, 1990.
116. Wirthlin, L.S., and Malt R.A.: Accidents of vagotomy. Surg. Gynecol. Obstet., *135:*913, 1972.

VOLUME I

Esophageal Varices

CHAPTER

28 Esophageal Varices

FREDERIC E. ECKHAUSER • JAMES A. KNOL • GEORGE A. SAROSI

Esophageal varices are thin-walled submucosal veins that develop most commonly in the lower esophagus and gastric cardia in response to elevated pressure in the portal circulation. Acute bleeding is the only clinical manifestation of esophageal varices and can be torrential. Management of variceal hemorrhage requires a thorough knowledge of the various treatment options, astute clinical judgment, and timely interventions.

Our understanding of the pathophysiology, diagnosis, and management of variceal bleeding has changed somewhat in the past several decades. The use of early fiberoptic upper gastrointestinal endoscopy for diagnosis and possibly intervention is now routine practice. Balloon tamponade, pharmacologic control of bleeding, percutaneous variceal obliteration, and injection sclerotherapy are important steps in the initial management of these patients. All of these modalities offer temporary control of bleeding with acceptable morbidity. The respective roles of nonselective and selective portasystemic shunt procedures are now more clearly defined, and nonshunt procedures have been refined for use in patients with variations in venous anatomy or severely compromised liver function that would preclude a portal decompressive shunt.

PATHOGENESIS

A variety of collateral venous channels form between the portal and systemic circulations in response to portal hypertension (Fig. 28-1). Communications occurring at the gastroesophageal junction are extremely complex. Until recently, the normal anatomy of this venous network and its response to portal hypertension have been poorly understood. In a series of elegant studies using three complementary techniques (radiology, corrosion casting, and morphometry), Vianna and colleagues[4] defined four distinct zones of venous drainage at the gastroesophageal junction: (1) a gastric zone; (2) a palisade zone; (3) a perforating zone; and (4) a truncal zone. The gastric zone consists of a circular band of veins oriented longitudinally within the submucosa in the proximal stomach. At the distal end of this zone, veins within the submucosa join to form larger trunks that communicate with the portal vein through the left gastric or coronary vein and with the splenic vein through the short gastric veins. The palisade zone is a cephalic continuation of the gastric zone extending 2 to 3 cm above the gastroesophageal junction. Gastric zone vessels pierce the muscularis mucosae just below the gastroesophageal junction to form a network of parallel and longitudinally oriented veins that lie within the lamina propria of the palisade zone. There are frequent anastomoses between and within these groups of vessels. Above the palisade zone vessels again pierce the muscularis mucosae to lie within the submucosa. The perforating zone located 3 to 5 cm above the gastroesophageal junction consists of longitudinal trunks formed by the confluence of vessels from the palisade zone. These vessels perforate the esophageal wall and fuse extramurally to form the external esophageal veins. Last, the truncal zone extends for 8 to 10 cm proximal to the perforating zone. Large venous trunks running longitudinally with the submucosal folds predominate in this zone and communicate at irregular intervals with the external esophageal veins through perforating veins.

In patients with portal hypertension, this venous network has to accommodate a greatly increased venous flow, redirecting across the diaphragm as much as 400 to 500 ml/min of portal blood. The area of maximum resistance to blood flow through the intrinsic network of the gastroesophageal venous plexus occurs in the palisade zone. High pressures occurring below this zone account for the appearance of gastric varices. Veins within the palisade zone may dilate in response to increased collateral flow from vessels located inferiorly in the gastric zone and from additional communications located superiorly in the truncal zone. The superficial location of this venous plexus within the lamina propria may predispose the patient to acute rupture or erosion with catastrophic bleeding.

Portal pressure is implicated as the chief factor in the pathogenesis of variceal bleeding, although its exact role is not known. Previous studies have shown a fairly good correlation between the "extent" or "size" of varices demonstrated with endoscopy or portography and the extent of portal pressure elevation. However, Lebrec and associates[2] failed to show a clear relationship between variceal size or the likelihood of rebleeding and the degree of portal hypertension. Portal pressure is not static. In fact, there is an approximate linear relationship between portal pressure and blood volume. There is also an excellent correlation between wedged hepatic vein pressure and free portal vein pressure, except when the portal hypertension is presinusoidal or extrahepatic in origin. Based on hemodynamic measurements in patients with portal hypertension, we now believe that an absolute portal pressure or portohepatic gradient (wedged hepatic vein pressure minus free hepatic vein pressure) of 12 mm Hg or less in a patient with cirrhosis is rarely associated with variceal bleeding.

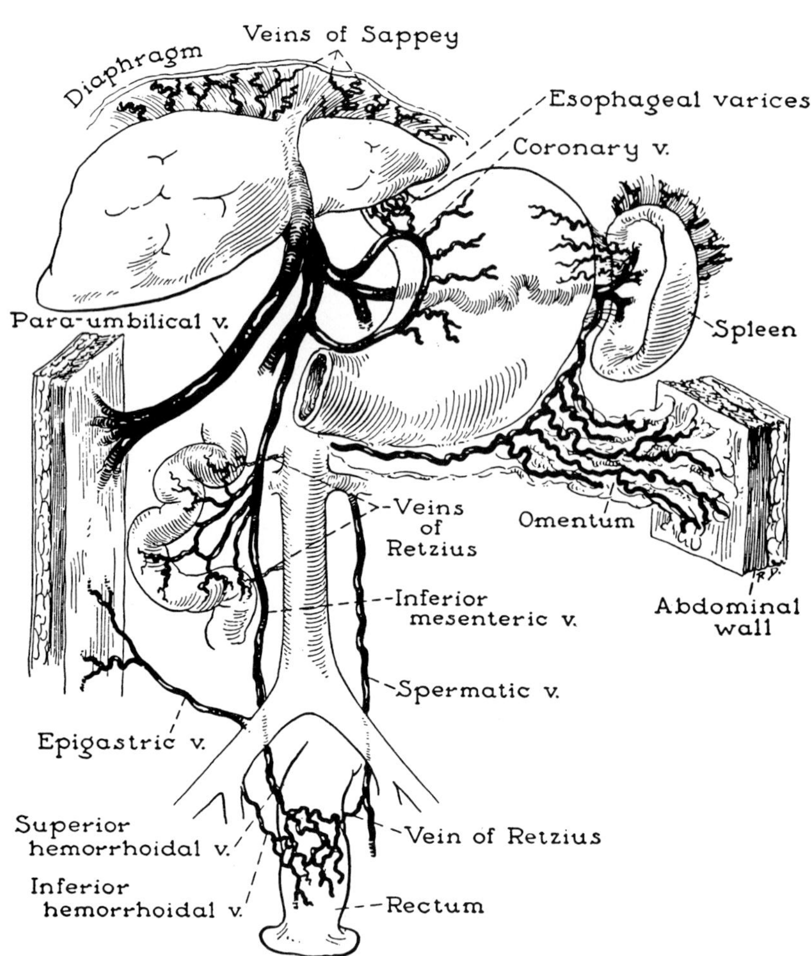

Figure 28–1. Collateral venous channels that may develop in obstruction of the portal system. (From Gray, H.K., and Whitsell, F.B., Jr.: Hemorrhage from esophageal varices: Surgical management. Ann. Surg., *132*:798, 1950, with permission.)

Conn[1] observed serial decrements in portal pressure among patients studied at intervals of 2 weeks after an acute episode of variceal bleeding. Others, including Leevy and associates,[3] noted the tendency of varices to wax and wane during periods of intensive medical management and documented reductions in portal pressure among patients with mild to moderate cirrhosis. Although it would be tempting teleologically to assume that resistance to portal flow, and therefore portal pressure, decreases during periods of clinical improvement, the evidence available to support this assumption is largely circumstantial.

Regardless of the influence of outside factors, the key to our understanding of the pathogenesis of variceal bleeding is portal hypertension and its effect on the venous anatomy at the gastroesophageal junction. In theory, acute elevations of portal pressure above some critical level might cause excessive wall stress at some weak point in the venous collateral network, resulting in rupture analogous to rupture of an aortic aneurysm. Laplace's law states that the tension in the wall of a vessel equals the pressure times the internal radius of the vessel (T = Pr) and is truly applicable only to thin-walled vessels. According to the study of Vianna and associates[4] of the venous anatomy at the gastroesophageal junction, the highest resistance to flow in this network occurs in the fine interdigitating vessels of the palisade zone, which lie superficially within the lamina propria. Because these high-resistance, thin-walled vessels are not supported by surrounding connective tissue, including muscularis mucosae, any increase in portal pressure might result in acutely increased wall tension and rupture, giving rise to what Conn[1] described as the "exploding volcano phenomenon."

ETIOLOGY

Portal hypertension generally develops because of an obstruction to portal venous flow. Rare exceptions include arterioportal communications resulting from trauma or rupture of congenital, arteriosclerotic, or inflammatory aneurysms. Obstruction of portal flow can occur at many levels. To avoid confusion, a classification system relating the level of obstruction anatomically to the hepatic sinusoid (presinusoidal, sinusoidal, or postsinusoidal) was developed. This type of classification is useful from a prognostic standpoint because presinusoidal causes of portal hypertension are generally not associated with impaired hepatic reserve. On the other hand, cirrhosis or hepatic veno-occlusive disease (Budd-Chiari syndrome) may have a profound effect on hepatic function.

Presinusoidal extrahepatic portal hypertension is due primarily to intra-abdominal infections. Appendicitis with para-appendiceal abscess and pyelophlebitis is a classic cause of portal pyemia, pyogenic liver abscesses, and portal vein thrombosis. Perinephric and other intra-abdominal abscesses can also cause portal vein thrombosis. Typically, there is a latent period of several years between the occurrence of the abscess and the development of esophageal varices. Portal vein thrombosis also occurs after splenectomy performed for trauma, Hodgkin's disease and lymphoma staging, and hematologic disorders. Thrombus occurring at or near the ligated or oversewn end of an excessively long splenic vein stump after splenectomy may propagate distally, causing complete or incomplete thrombosis of the portal or mesenteric veins.

The paradigm of presinusoidal intrahepatic portal vein obstruction is schistosomiasis. Schistosomiasis is not a common problem in the United States except in certain immigrant populations. However, it is endemic in many parts of the world, including Africa and the Middle East. Ova are released by the parasite into the portal circulation and lodge in the intrahepatic portal venules where they evoke a cell-mediated response. The resultant inflammatory response causes obstruction to portal blood flow. Other, less common causes of presinusoidal intrahepatic block include congenital hepatic fibrosis and hepatoportal sclerosis.

Cirrhosis is the most common cause of portal hypertension. Among Western patients with cirrhosis, chronic alcoholism is the leading cause. Alcoholic liver disease can present with a spectrum of histologic findings, including steatosis, alcoholic hepatitis, and cirrhosis. Steatosis (fatty liver) is an early, reversible stage in which portal hypertension is caused by cell swelling and by compression of intrahepatic venules.[7] Alcoholic hepatitis develops after chronic ingestion and is characterized histologically by ballooning degeneration, liver cell necrosis, an inflammatory cell infiltrate, Mallory bodies (intracytoplasmic inclusion bodies whose significance is uncertain), and fibrosis. The fibrosis is caused by deposition of collagen, primarily in the central venule areas, and causes impaired portal flow as well as capillarization of sinusoids. The latter inhibits passage of essential nutrients into the spaces of Disse by occluding the fenestrations between endothelial cells.[6]

Micronodular cirrhosis (Laënnec's cirrhosis) is the end-stage lesion seen in patients with alcoholic liver disease. Morphologically, cirrhosis is characterized by variably sized regenerating pseudolobules of liver parenchyma surrounded by delicate but diffuse fibrosis. The resultant distortion of the intrahepatic vascular anatomy (particularly the venous architecture) causes increased resistance to portal blood flow and results in elevated portal pressures. Other causes of cirrhosis include postnecrotic as well as primary and secondary forms of biliary cirrhosis. Additional diseases such as sclerosing cholangitis, cystic fibrosis, and alpha$_1$-antitrypsin deficiency all may cause liver injury leading to portal hypertension.

Postsinusoidal causes of portal hypertension are relatively uncommon but, from a pathophysiologic standpoint, are fascinating. Diseases of the hepatic veins and inferior vena cava predominate in this group. The Budd-Chiari syndrome, described originally in the mid nineteenth century, is caused by thrombosis of the main hepatic veins. Hepatic vein thrombosis may result from trauma, myeloproliferative syndromes, tumors arising in organs adjacent to the liver and vena cava (kidney and adrenal), pregnancy, and use of oral contraceptives. About half of these lesions are cryptogenic in origin. The Budd-Chiari syndrome usually presents as a subacute or chronic illness with ascites, hepatomegaly, upper abdominal discomfort, and variceal bleeding as the chief clinical manifestations. Early operative intervention is indicated to prevent irreversible fibrosis and hepatic parenchymal atrophy. In patients with a patent inferior vena cava, portacaval anastomosis is recommended.[9] However, almost complete or total obstruction of the inferior vena cava may necessitate construction of a mesoatrial shunt.[5]

Hepatic veno-occlusive disease results most commonly from endophlebitis of centrilobular and intraparenchymal hepatic veins secondary to ingestion of "herbal remedies" containing pyrrolidizine alkaloids. However, similar lesions have been noted in patients undergoing chemotherapy, hepatic irradiation, and bone marrow transplantation. The pathophysiologic changes, clinical features, and management of these patients are similar to those of patients with Budd-Chiari syndrome.

Peliosis hepatis is an increasingly frequent hepatic disease related to ingestion of anabolic steroids (androgens).[8] The characteristic histologic lesion is widespread dilatation of hepatic sinusoids, often associated with confluent cystic changes and loss of intervening parenchyma. The pathogenesis of peliosis hepatis is unclear. Fatalities resulting from liver failure or hemorrhage into the abdominal cavity have been reported in patients with peliosis.

PATHOPHYSIOLOGY: IMPLICATIONS FOR TREATMENT

Esophageal varices develop as a result of complex derangements in local and systemic physiology. Pressure in the portal circulation varies in accordance with Ohm's law:

$$P = Q \times R$$

where P = intravascular pressure, Q = flow, and R = resistance. According to current ideology, increased resistance to portal flow at presinusoidal, sinusoidal, or postsinusoidal levels in addition to splanchnic hypervolemia resulting from an expanded plasma volume and a hyperdynamic circulation contribute to the development of portal hypertension.

Total liver blood flow in an adult averages about 1.5 l/min and accounts for almost 25% of the cardiac output. In cirrhosis, cardiac output may increase threefold or fourfold above normal levels.[10] Several contributing factors have been identified in cirrhotic patients with a hyperdynamic circulation, including elevated levels of circulating vasodilators and opening of widespread arteriovenous communications.

Increased resistance in portal collaterals has also been implicated in the development of portal hypertension and may be more important quantitatively than circulatory derangements.[11] Attempts to decrease portal resistance have led to various therapeutic approaches, including vasodilator therapy, portal-caval shunting procedures, and splenic transposition or splenopneumopexy to encourage development of additional portasystemic collaterals. Nonshunt procedures are discussed later in this chapter.

NATURAL HISTORY OF CIRRHOSIS AND VARICEAL BLEEDING

Esophageal varices are asymptomatic until they bleed. Hemorrhage from varices is painless, sudden, and in many cases catastrophic. Until recently, the natural history of cirrhosis and that of variceal bleeding were uncertain. We now know that about 12% of cirrhotic patients develop varices that are demonstrable with conventional imaging and endoscopic techniques. Of these patients, one third experience an episode of bleeding at some time with an associated mortality rate that is almost 60%. Those who survive the initial bleed have about a 30 to 50% risk of rebleeding within 6 weeks if no further therapy is given.[12] The risk of dying appears to be the same with each episode of variceal bleeding. The relationships are shown in Figure 28–2. If a patient survives an episode of variceal bleeding and the ensuing high-risk period (6 to 8 weeks), the subsequent risk of late rebleeding is similar to that reported for unselected cirrhotic patients or for cirrhotic patients with demonstrated varices. It is clear that if we hope to alter the natural history of cirrhosis and variceal bleeding, we must concentrate our efforts on reducing the "early" mortality associated with bleeding. It is toward this end that many if not all of our recent therapeutic endeavors have been directed.

DIAGNOSIS

Variceal bleeding is often massive and is associated with hemodynamic instability. Initial diagnosis must be integrated with ongoing efforts at resuscitation. Rapid stabilization of the patient in an intensive care unit setting is important to reverse hypotension and avoid the sequelae of prolonged hepatic hypoperfusion. Physiologic monitoring of hemodynamic parameters such as pulse, blood pressure, urine output, and central venous pressure should be performed routinely. An oximetric Swan-Ganz catheter should be inserted whenever feasible to monitor central venous oxygen saturation and cardiovascular parameters such as cardiac output, pulmonary artery wedge pressure, and systemic vascular resistance. After the patient has been resuscitated, a large-bore evacuation tube should be used to empty the stomach of clots. Endoscopy should be performed expediently to determine the source of bleeding and to intervene therapeutically if indicated. This is especially important because up to 40% of patients with upper gastrointestinal bleeding and signs of chronic liver disease have a nonvariceal source of bleeding. Nonvariceal sources of bleeding include peptic ulcerations of the stomach or duodenum, Mallory-Weiss tears caused by vigorous retching, and erosive gastritis

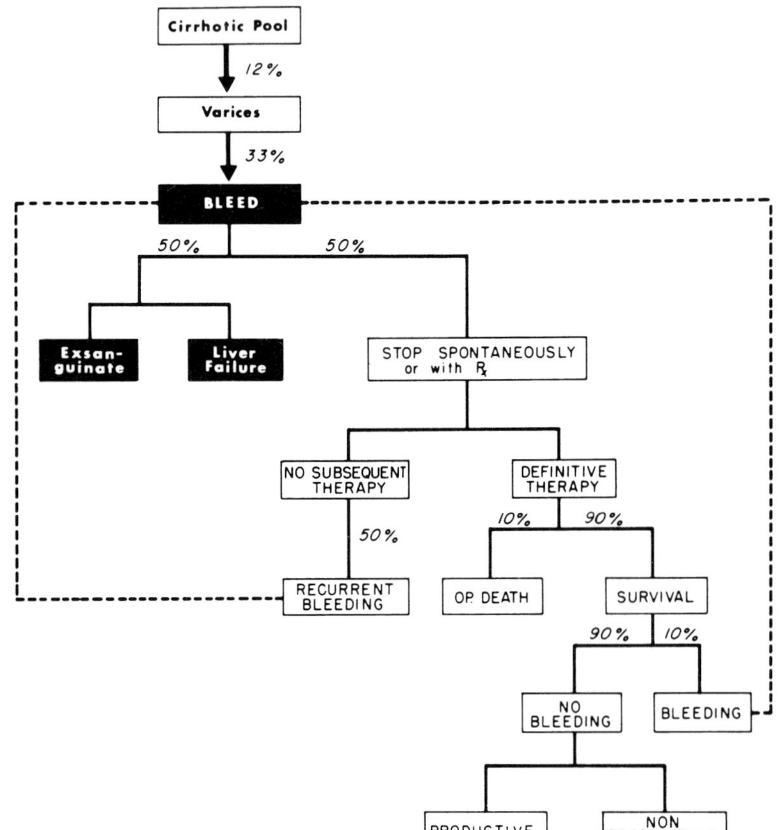

Figure 28–2. Natural history of cirrhosis and bleeding esophageal varices. (From Voorhees, A.B.: Portal hypertension as I see it. *In* Child, C.G., III [ed.]: Portal Hypertension. Philadelphia, W.B. Saunders, 1974, p. 63, with permission.)

resulting from ingestion of alcohol or drugs that cause mucosal injury. Congestive gastritis associated with portal hypertension has been recognized as a frequent source of upper gastrointestinal bleeding in cirrhotic patients. The prognosis and management of patients with bleeding from portal hypertensive gastritis or varices are generally similar. However, erosive gastritis and portal hypertensive gastritis require entirely different therapeutic approaches. In patients with portal hypertensive gastritis, procedures such as partial gastrectomy, which would ordinarily be adequate to treat erosive gastritis, are without value, and a portal-systemic shunt is frequently required to control bleeding.[17]

Other modalities are becoming increasingly important in the evaluation of the patient with portal hypertension and esophageal varices. Ultrasound is rapid, noninvasive, and portable and may provide useful information about the patency of the portal circulation and the direction of portal blood flow.[16] Newer, more sensitive tests of hepatic functional reserve have been developed and may assist in planning surgical therapy. Of these, the aminopyrine test, measurements of galactose elimination capacity, and blood clearance of indocyanine green show the greatest promise as predictors of hepatic reserve and outcome after surgery.[13,14] Panhepatic angiography should be obtained whenever shunt procedures are contemplated to define the vascular anatomy and to obtain baseline pressure measurements that may be useful for comparison after surgery. Measurement of portal hemodynamic parameters is generally of little value in patient management, except when a presinusoidal etiology is suspected.[15] For example, isolated left-sided portal hypertension with variceal bleeding can be caused by splenic vein thrombosis due to chronic pancreatitis or pancreatic tumors. These patients rarely have concomitant liver disease and can be cured by splenectomy.

PHARMACOLOGIC THERAPY

Vasopressin

Vasopressin is a nonapeptide derived from the posterior pituitary. When administered systemically, it causes a number of physiologic effects, including nonspecific constriction of vascular smooth muscle and increased gut peristalsis. The basis for using vasopressin in the management of variceal bleeding is evidence that intravenous administration causes a reduction in portal vein flow and pressure.[25] Alternative explanations have been presented to explain why variceal bleeding stops in some patients receiving vasopressin without demonstrable evidence of reduced portal flow or pressure. The most tenable of these explanations is based on the observation that vasopressin can cause constriction of esophageal smooth muscle, thus cutting off flow to the varices.[18]

Intravenous vasopressin controls hemorrhage in 50 to 70% of patients with variceal bleeding. However, complications occur in up to 75% of patients, and almost half are significant. It was hoped that administration of vasopressin directly into the superior mesenteric artery would reduce the dose necessary to control bleeding, thus lowering drug toxicity. However, results from two major clinical trials failed to demonstrate the superiority of the intra-arterial route of vasopressin administration.[22,24] In addition, catheter-related complications, such as intimal dissection of major visceral arteries, pseudoaneurysm formation at the site of catheter insertion, in situ arterial thrombosis, and distal embolization of fragments of fibrin dislodged from the catheter tip, occur with surprising frequency. There is also evidence that vasopressin may have an adverse effect on hepatic metabolism.[19] Vasopressin analogues and nitroglycerin have been investigated as ways of overcoming this problem. Nitroglycerin administered by either the intravenous, transdermal, or sublingual route appears to ameliorate the cardiovascular side effects of vasopressin and may have a secondary beneficial effect on portal pressure.[23] Glypressin is a vasopressin analogue that is equally effective in stopping bleeding and has less cardiac toxicity.[28]

Vasopressin administration may be useful to control acute bleeding but should not be considered a form of definitive treatment. Because the drug has significant cardiac toxicity, it should be administered only in an intensive care unit setting. We prefer the intravenous route and advocate a high initial rate of infusion (0.4 to 0.6 units/min or 24 to 36 units/hr). After bleeding has stopped, the dose should be reduced to below 0.4 units/min and maintained for several additional hours before being stopped. Vasopressin should be coadministered with intravenous nitroglycerin to avoid the potential cardiotoxic effects of vasopressin. If rebleeding occurs, the vasopressin infusion can be started again, but one should also consider the use of other modalities, such as balloon tamponade, transhepatic variceal obliteration, or sclerotherapy.

Somatostatin

Somatostatin is a naturally occurring 14-amino-acid polypeptide that is broadly distributed throughout both the gastrointestinal tract and the central nervous system. It has been shown to reduce splanchnic blood flow in both normal and cirrhotic subjects[20] without producing systemic vasodilatation. This decrease in blood flow is mediated by both a direct action on mesenteric vascular smooth muscle and decreasing serum glucagon levels. Octreotide, an 8-amino-acid longer half-life synthetic analogue of somatostatin, has also been shown to decrease portal venous blood flow.

Initial studies comparing somatostatin to placebo in controlling acute variceal hemorrhage produced conflicting results.[25] However, seven randomized, controlled trials have subsequently compared somatostatin to vasopressin, and another trial compared octreotide to vasopressin. In these studies somatostatin produced a 60 to 90% rate of control of bleeding, with a much lower complication rate (0 to 18%) than vasopressin. Two recent meta-analyses[26,27] demonstrated that somatostatin is more effective than vasopressin in controlling variceal bleeding, and this result approaches statistical significance.

Both somatostatin and octreotide are administered by

intravenous drip, typically over a period of 3 to 5 days, to reduce rebleeding rates. Somatostatin is given as a 250-μg bolus followed by a 250 μg/hr drip. Octreotide is given as a 50-μg bolus followed by a 50 μg/hr drip.

Propranolol and Nitrate Therapy

Propranolol is a noncardioselective beta-blocker that has been well studied as a pharmacologic manipulation to prevent variceal bleeding in cirrhotic patients. Beta-blockers were first used for the prevention of variceal bleeding because of their ability to reduce portal pressures. They reduce portal pressure by reducing cardiac output and producing splanchnic vasoconstriction mediated by blockade of $beta_2$-receptors. Beta-blockers have been shown to prevent both initial bleeds in cirrhotic patients and recurrent variceal bleeding in patients with a history of variceal bleeding.

In a recent meta-analysis of nine controlled trials of beta-blockers versus nonactive treatment, beta-blockers were shown to reduce the rate of initial bleeding by almost 50%.[26] In addition to reducing the rate of first variceal bleeding, this meta-analysis suggested that beta-blocker therapy appeared to reduce mortality rates by about 25%. Although the reduction in bleeding incidence was statistically significant, the decrease in mortality rate was not. Because most patients in these studies had Child's class A or B cirrhosis, these results may need to be qualified with regard to class C cirrhosis.[27]

The use of beta-blockers to prevent rebleeding in cirrhotic patients with a prior history of bleeding has also been well studied. In a recent meta-analysis of 12 controlled trials, Bernard and colleagues demonstrated a 21% decrease in the rate of variceal rebleeding with beta-blocker therapy.[29] In addition, this meta-analysis demonstrated a 5% increase in mean survival attributable to beta-blocker therapy.

In light of the relatively low incidence of side effects, beta-blocker therapy is an important tool in the prevention of variceal bleeding and should be used in all cirrhotic patients without contraindications. Contraindications to beta-blockers include congestive heart failure, severe chronic obstructive lung disease, asthma, and insulin-dependent diabetes mellitus. For patients with contraindications, long-acting nitrates, such as isosorbide mononitrate, may be a reasonable alternative. In a single randomized controlled trial, it has been shown to be as effective as propranolol.[30] Beta-blocker therapy or nitrates need to be continued indefinitely once started because cessation of treatment after 2 years is associated with a return of the risk for bleeding.[31]

BALLOON TAMPONADE

Balloon tamponade is an effective method for controlling acute variceal bleeding. The mechanism of action is thought to be compression of submucosal varices in the distal esophagus and gastric fundus. A variety of tubes are available for use, but the two used most commonly are the Blakemore-Sengstaken (BS) tube and the Minnesota tube. The BS tube is a triple-lumen device with gastric and esophageal balloons and a port for aspirating gastric secretions (Fig. 28–3). Inflation of one or both balloons causes complete esophageal obstruction and requires that an additional tube be positioned proximal to the esophageal balloon for aspiration of swallowed oropharyngeal secretions. The Minnesota tube is softer and thus may be more difficult to pass than the BS tube, has a slightly larger gastric balloon (500 ml versus 200 to 400 ml), and has an additional port for aspirating the esophagus. Both tubes are equally effective and temporarily control bleeding in about 80% of patients. Rebleeding occurs in up to one third of patients but can usually be controlled with reinflation of the balloons. Simultaneous use of a vasoconstrictor such as vasopressin results in higher control rates for variceal bleeding and may be beneficial in reducing the balloon-inflation time required for hemostasis.[33]

The chief disadvantage of balloon tamponade is a high rate of complications. The most common complication, aspiration pneumonia, occurs in 5 to 10% of patients and can be prevented. We advocate endotracheal intubation in *all* patients who require balloon tamponade for control of bleeding. Other potential complications include migration of the gastric balloon with encroachment on the tracheal bifurcation and esophageal rupture due to inadvertent inflation of the gastric balloon in the esophagus. The latter complication can be avoided by confirming the position of the gastric balloon in the stomach radiographically before inflating. Some authors have cited serious complication rates of 15 to 35% depending on the type of tube used, the experience of the physician inserting the tube, and the care taken to maintain it properly until it is removed.[32] Others, such as Sarin and

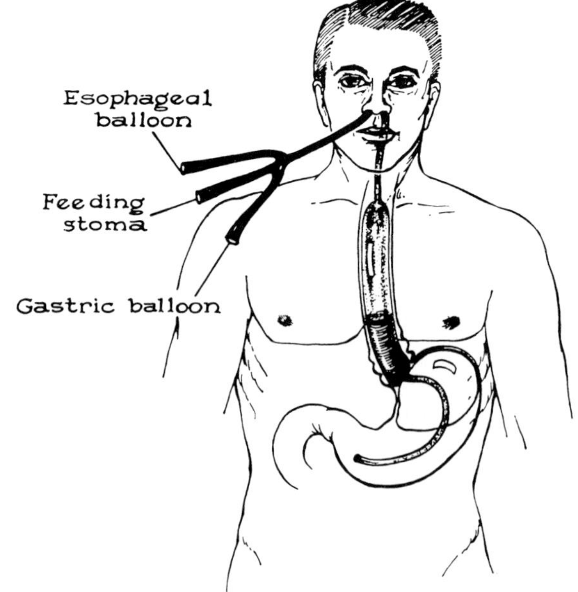

Figure 28–3. Diagrammatic placement of the Sengstaken-Blakemore tube. (From Hermann, R.E., and Traul, D.: Experience with the Sengstaken-Blakemore tube for bleeding esophageal varices. Surg. Gynecol. Obstet., *130*:879, 1970, by permission of Surgery, Gynecology and Obstetrics.)

Mundy,[34] have reported excellent control of bleeding (75%) in patients treated with balloon tamponade with no tube-related mortality. Nonfatal but potentially serious complications were noted in one third of patients.

One additional modification of the tube deserves mention. Reynaert and colleagues[35] reported the results of a retrospective, comparative study using a Linton-Nachlas tube in 35 patients and a Michel tube in 48 patients. The Linton tube consists of a single large gastric balloon and two aspirating channels for the stomach and esophagus. The Michel tube has a lightbulb-like configuration and compresses the distal esophagus and gastric fundus without the need for traction. Better bleeding control and fewer complications were encountered with the Michel tube. Although there is little experience in the United States with the Michel tube, the reported safety and efficacy of this device compared with more traditional tubes seems to warrant further study.

TRANSHEPATIC VARICEAL OBLITERATION

The original technique of transhepatic variceal obliteration (TVO) was introduced by Lunderquist and Vang in 1974[36]; it included transhepatic catheterization of the portal vein and embolization of the coronary vein with glucose and thrombin. Since then, transumbilical and transjugular approaches have been described, and new sclerosing agents have been used to reduce the unacceptably high incidence of recanalization and recurrent bleeding observed with glucose and thrombin.

TVO successfully controls bleeding in 60 to 80% of patients.[37] Rebleeding occurs in up to two thirds of patients after TVO, but a 2- to 3-week bleeding-free interval can usually be anticipated. This allows time to improve hepatic function if further definitive treatment is required. Treatment failures most commonly result from inability to catheterize the portal vein, formation of new varices, and recanalization of obliterated veins.

The complication rate associated with TVO varies from 25 to 40% and is highest in patients undergoing emergency intervention. Portal vein thrombosis occurs in up to 25% of patients and is the most serious complication for several reasons. First, sudden cessation of portal blood flow can precipitate irreversible hepatic failure. Second, thrombosis of the portal vein eliminates the possibility of subsequent portacaval shunt and may preclude any form of portal-systemic shunt if the clot propagates to involve the superior mesenteric and splenic veins. Third, further consideration of liver transplantation may be eliminated. Hemoperitoneum is another complication of TVO, especially in patients with severe clotting abnormalities and thrombocytopenia.

There are relatively few controlled trials of TVO compared with other treatment options in patients with variceal bleeding. In one study, Terabayashi and associates[38] randomized 66 patients to either elective TVO or endoscopic sclerotherapy. Patients were treated electively after variceal bleeding had stopped following treatment with vasopressin and balloon tamponade. Six patients (18%) in the sclerotherapy group and 21 patients (64%) in the TVO group rebled at least once during the follow-up period. The cumulative variceal bleeding rate was considerably lower in the sclerotherapy group, and fewer patients in the sclerotherapy group died of recurrent variceal bleeding. This study consisted of *elective* intervention in patients with *nonalcoholic* cirrhosis and therefore may be flawed by selection bias. Nonetheless, these data suggest that TVO offers little long-term protection against variceal rebleeding and should be limited to patients in whom other nonsurgical forms of treatment have failed and to those who refuse surgery or for whatever reason are considered to be unsuitable for surgery.

SCLEROTHERAPY

Injection sclerotherapy is a relatively old technique that has experienced an explosive rebirth. This technique was initially reported by Craaford and Frenckner in 1939; they employed general anesthesia, a rigid esophagoscope, and a quinine-based sclerosant.[39] Despite widespread early enthusiasm, large trials were not undertaken because portal-systemic shunt surgery had become the predominant therapy for variceal bleeding in many countries. Several decades and multicenter trials later, it became apparent that the protection against variceal bleeding conferred by portal-systemic shunt procedures was largely offset by an increased morbidity and mortality associated with encephalopathy and accelerated hepatic failure. Dissatisfaction with the results of portal-systemic shunting procedures led to a resurgence of interest in endoscopic injection sclerotherapy. This was aided by the development of flexible fiberoptic endoscopes that made sclerotherapy easier and safer and avoided the need for general anesthesia.

During the past several decades, a wealth of information has been accumulated concerning the role of variceal sclerotherapy in the long-term management of variceal bleeding. Eight randomized clinical trials have compared the effects of serial sclerotherapy versus conventional medical treatment on the long-term survival of patients with documented variceal bleeding. Six trials showed improved long-term survival following sclerotherapy, and two did not. To help resolve this controversy, the results of eight independent trials, which totaled 1,111 patients were combined to perform a meta-analysis.[26] In general, sclerotherapy was added to some form of medical therapy or compared to medical treatment alone. A variety of different esophagoscopes, injection techniques, and sclerosants were used. To assess the effect of sclerotherapy, the mortality rates and control of bleeding rates were assessed for each clinical trial and combined to provide an estimate of the overall risk difference. The results of the study suggested that sclerotherapy performed early and in conjunction with other medical measures is associated with improved long-term survival compared to medical treatment alone. In addition, a marked decrease in the rate of rebleeding from esophageal varices was demonstrated. The protective effect of serial injection sclerotherapy—that is, its ability to reduce mortality and improve long-term survival—is only moderate. However, this observation has potential clinical relevance because the mortality rate associated with variceal hemorrhage is high (up to 40% in some series).[52]

Complications of sclerotherapy can be classified as early or late. Early complications occur in about 30% of patients. The most common immediate complications include fever, retrosternal pain after the injection procedure, and hemorrhage from the injection site requiring either reinjection or balloon tamponade. Other, less common early complications include esophageal necrosis with perforation and mediastinitis (about 4%), bleeding due to ulceration and sloughing of the associated eschar (about 12%), and aspiration with pneumonia (about 6%). Late complications include rebleeding and esophageal stricture (about 11%).[56] In a study, Minoli analyzed 822 complications observed among 1,192 patients who underwent a total of 4,550 endoscopic injection sclerotherapy treatments by members of the New Italian Endoscopic Club.[59] Overall, 583 patients (49%) developed at least one complication, and 16% developed multiple complications. Nonconfluent and confluent ulcerations were observed in 33% and 8.5% of patients, respectively. Although most postinjection ulcerations cause no problems, there have been reports of severe bleeding and even fatalities.[47]

Sclerotherapy-induced esophageal strictures can be a major source of patient morbidity. These strictures usually cause variable degrees of dysphagia, are commonly solitary, and generally occur in the distal esophagus. The worldwide incidence varies widely, but 10 to 12% appears to be a reasonable estimate.[56] The major determinant is thought to be tissue reaction to the sclerosant solutions, but other factors, including alterations in esophageal motility and acid reflux, may be contributory. Kochhar and associates recently evaluated 129 sclerotherapy patients followed over a 4-year period and documented a 15.5% incidence of persistent esophageal stricture.[57] A number of possible pathogenetic factors were evaluated, including the etiology of portal hypertension, the severity of underlying liver disease, the type of sclerosant used, and the intensity of variceal sclerosis judged by the volume of sclerosant injected and the number of sclerotherapy sessions. There was no demonstrable correlation between the type of sclerosant used, the volume of injectate, or the number of injection sessions and adverse outcome. However, they did demonstrate an increased incidence of stricture formation in patients with large or persistent ulcers. Other studies have yielded contradictory results. Guynn and colleagues recently assessed risk factors and prognosis associated with postsclerotherapy strictures among 117 patients who underwent variceal sclerosis at a single teaching institution.[54] The risk of stricture formation correlated with the cumulative amount of sclerosant used and the number of injection sessions, but not with the volume of sclerosant injected per treatment or the number of previous bleeds.

Sclerotherapy-induced esophageal strictures can usually be treated with dilation, but up to half of patients require two or more dilations to achieve satisfactory results.[54] Despite successful dilation, 10 to 15% of patients may experience persistent dysphagia. The proposed explanation is sclerotherapy-induced intramural fibrosis and secondary esophageal dysmotility.[58] The risk of sclerotherapy-induced complications appears to be largely operator dependent. One can standardize many variables, but the depth of injection is difficult to assess and even more difficult to control. Overzealous intravariceal injection may rupture a submucosal varix, leading to extravasation and dissection with the wall of the esophagus. Deep intramural injection may lead to focal necrosis and perforation of the esophagus with resulting mediastinitis.[46] To minimize the morbidity of injection sclerotherapy, we and others strongly advocate multiple, small-volume injections rather than limited numbers of high-volume injections.

ENDOSCOPIC LIGATION OF VARICES

In 1988, Stiegmann and Goff described a preliminary clinical experience with endoscopic varix ligation (EVL).[61] The technique is similar to that used for elastic band ligation of internal hemorrhoids. Feasibility studies in a canine model of EVL showed that endoscopic elastic band ligation produced focal areas of ischemic necrosis with formation of shallow ulcers that healed with obliteration of underlying venous channels.[63] These experiments indicated that EVL might be useful as an alternative to injection sclerotherapy in patients with variceal bleeding.

The technique is performed with a device that consists of an outer cylinder affixed to the end of a standard flexible fiberoptic gastroscope and an inner cylinder fitted with a clasp and tripwire (Fig. 28–4).[87] An elastic O ring is attached over the inner cylinder, and tripwire is exited through the biopsy channel port of the endoscope. The varix to be ligated is approached en face by the endos-

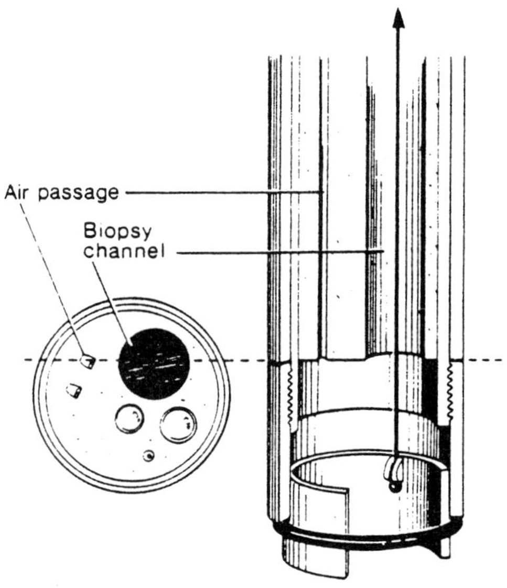

Figure 28–4. Transparent view of the endoscopic ligating device and distal gastroscope. The prototype device was built with threaded ends to attach directly to the endoscope. Note the tripwire *(arrow)*, which runs retrograde through the biopsy channel and exits the biopsy channel entry port. The elastic O ring is positioned at the far end of the inner cylinder. (From Van Stiegmann, G., and Goff, S.F.: Endoscopic esophageal varix ligation: Preliminary clinical experience. Gastrointest. Endosc., *34*:113, 1988, with permission.)

copist. By applying suction, the varix is drawn into the inner cylinder, causing a sudden obscuration of vision, or "red out." The tripwire is pulled, moving the inner cylinder toward the endoscope and discharging the O ring around the base of the varix. The ligated varix is disgorged, the scope is withdrawn through an outer tube used to facilitate reintroduction of the instrument, the inner cylinder is reloaded with another O ring, and the process is repeated (Fig. 28-5).

Stiegmann's early experience consisted of 132 EVL procedures performed during 44 separate sessions in 14 patients.[61] Up to six ligations were performed during the initial session, and up to six sessions were sometimes necessary to achieve complete variceal obliteration. Two patients died (14%) after EVL, but neither death was procedure related. No major complications developed, and there were no treatment failures. Complete eradication of esophageal varices was achieved in 10 surviving patients (83%). Follow-up endoscopy within 4 to 10 days of EVL showed the development of shallow, circular ulcers at each treatment site. The ulcers reproducibly measured 10 to 12 mm in diameter and were distinctly more superficial than ulcers created by injection sclerotherapy. By 21 days, most of the ulcers had healed with re-epithelialization of the treatment sites leaving small, shallow depressions in the mucosa.

Endoscopic varix ligation has been shown to control active bleeding and eradicate varices when sessions are repeated. Proponents cite fewer local and systemic complications compared with injection sclerotherapy. To compare and characterize the ulcerations produced by endoscopic ligation versus injection sclerotherapy, Young and associates randomized 23 patients to serial treatment and follow-up.[64] Both procedures were rigidly standardized and repeated at 7- to 10-day intervals until obliteration of all variceal channels had been achieved. The presence of ulcerations, including the location, number, size, and color, were recorded at each subsequent endoscopy. EVL produced shallow, circular ulcerations with a large surface area that healed in about 14 days. By comparison, endoscopic sclerotherapy produced linear, deep ulcerations that took about 21 days to resolve. Fewer EVL sessions were required to achieve complete obliteration of variceal channels. No significant intergroup differences were noted with regard to stricture formation or death.

Randomized Clinical Trial Results for Control of Acute Variceal Bleeding

Cello and co-workers[41] recently randomized 52 patients with severe cirrhosis to sclerotherapy or portacaval shunt. Intravariceal sclerotherapy was performed with a flexible endoscope using 5% sodium morrhuate as the sclerosant. Initial injections were made at or just proximal to the gastroesophageal junction and later were followed

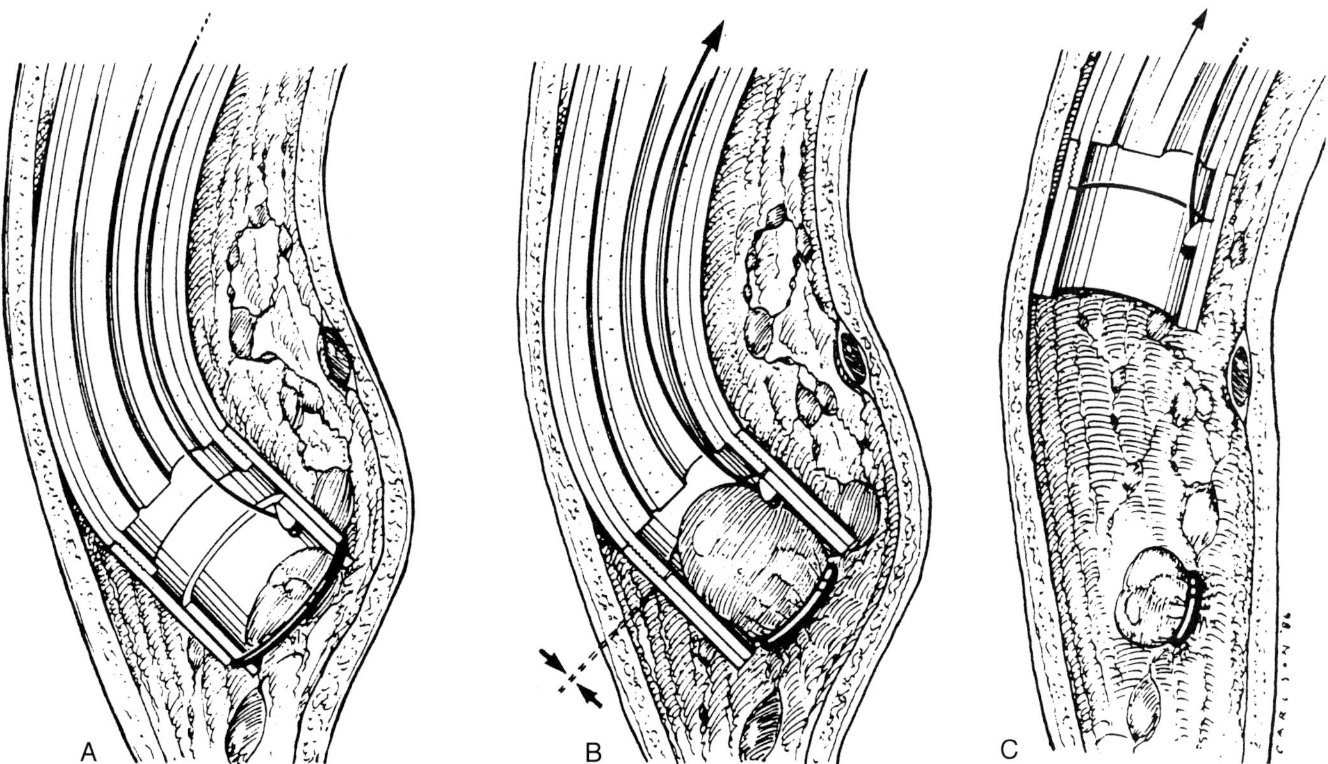

Figure 28-5. *A*, The endoscopist approaches the target varix and obtains 360-degree tissue contact between the target and the end of the inner cylinder. Endoscopic suction is activated at this point. *B*, Endoscopic suction has drawn the target varix fully inside the inner (ligating) cylinder. Once endoscopic "red-out" has occurred, the tripwire is pulled, moving the inner cylinder toward the endoscope and releasing the elastic O ring around the neck of the varix. *C*, The ligated varix is discharged from the cylinder by withdrawing the endoscope 2 to 3 cm and insufflating air. The endoscope and device are withdrawn and reloaded and further ligations are performed. This sequence is facilitated by use of an endoscopic overtube. (From Van Stiegmann, G., and Goff, S.F.: Endoscopic esophageal varix ligation: Preliminary clinical experience. Gastrointest. Endosc., *34*:113, 1988, with permission.)

by repeated injections at prescribed intervals. Half of the patients in both study groups died during the initial hospitalization, but recurrent hemorrhage was a more frequent cause of death in the sclerotherapy group than in the portacaval shunt group. Rehospitalization was more frequently necessary in the sclerotherapy group to control recurrent bleeding. Long-term survival determined by Kaplan-Meier survival function estimates was uniformly poor, and no significant difference was observed between the sclerotherapy and shunt groups.

The results of the Copenhagen multicenter trial comparing sclerotherapy with conventional treatment with balloon tamponade and vasopressin were equally discouraging.[40] The paravariceal injection technique was done using 3% polidocanol in 55% ethanol as the sclerosant. This controlled prospective trial showed that sclerotherapy increased long-term survival by reducing the risk of recurrent bleeding but offered no initial advantages over conventional therapy for stopping variceal hemorrhage and had no significant effect on early survival.

It has become increasingly clear that early and long-term survival in cirrhotic patients with variceal bleeding correlated more closely with the severity of the underlying liver disease than with the type of intervention used to control bleeding. In a study from the Mayo Clinic, DiMagno and associates[42] reviewed the effect of sclerotherapy on survival compared with survival in the presclerotherapy era. When the survival rates and bleeding-free intervals were analyzed according to hepatic risk classification, no discernible differences between patients receiving sclerotherapy and historic controls were found.

Although EVL appears to be relatively safe compared with endoscopic sclerotherapy, serious complications, including esophageal laceration and perforation, have been reported. Esophageal perforation associated with the use of overtubes has been attributed to either varix laceration from excessive force or pinching of the mucosa between the endoscope and the inner channel of the overtube. To avoid the latter problem, Goldschmiedt and colleagues recommended backloading the overtube onto a tapered dilator and intubating the esophagus over the dilator rather than an endoscope.[51]

Comparison of Sclerotherapy and Ligation of Varices

To date, three prospective clinical trials comparing endoscopic variceal ligation with endoscopic sclerotherapy have been conducted in the United States, Japan, and the United Kingdom.[50,55,62] Overall, 143 patients were randomized to endoscopic variceal ligation, and 139 patients were randomized to endoscopic sclerotherapy. The United States study, which included 129 patients, demonstrated that EVL achieved better initial control of bleeding and required fewer mean treatments to eradicate varices. By comparison, the mortality rate, the risk of rebleeding, and the incidence of complications were all higher for the endoscopic sclerotherapy group.[62] The incidence of ulcerations was comparable after both interventions, but most ulcers in the banding group were small and rarely associated with symptoms. The stricture rate in the United Kingdom study was significantly lower than that reported by Stiegmann (0% versus 12%).[60] The Japanese study randomized 50 patients and demonstrated virtually identical results except for a slightly reduced complication rate in the EVL group.[53]

Endoscopic variceal ligation was developed in an attempt to provide a treatment equivalent in efficacy to endoscopic sclerotherapy but with fewer local and systemic complications. Although the United States trial was unblinded and possibly biased, EVL was shown to be at least as effective as endoscopic sclerotherapy for both arresting acute hemorrhage and for preventing variceal rebleeding. Compared with endoscopic sclerotherapy, EVL has been shown to confer at least equal survival benefit and in one study demonstrated improved survival, especially among patients with good or moderate hepatic reserve (Child's class A and B patients). Although the definition of postprocedural complications varies widely, EVL appears to be associated with a lower incidence of complications than endoscopic sclerotherapy. EVL is a technically straightforward procedure for experienced endoscopists and results in a more standardized and reproducible degree of tissue injury. Complications related to insertion of the overtube can be largely avoided by backloading and introducing it over a tapered dilator rather than the endoscope. Procedural costs for EVL are comparable to endoscopic sclerotherapy,[49] but EVL ultimately may be more cost-effective because it requires fewer treatment sessions to eradicate varices.[64] This may have particular benefit for less compliant patients and for patients who live in remote geographic areas where medical expertise may not be readily available.

Transjugular Intrahepatic Portal-Systemic Shunts

A new investigational therapy (transjugular intrahepatic portal-systemic shunt [TIPS]) has shown considerable promise for managing variceal hemorrhage. This technique establishes an artificial fistula between branches of the portal vein and the systemic circulation within the substance of the liver, in essence creating an intrahepatic portal-systemic shunt. The concept of creating an intrahepatic portal-systemic shunt was proposed more than 20 years ago by Rosch, Hanafee, and Snow.[80] Using a transjugular approach in dogs, the authors established and then dilated a parenchymal tract between branches of the portal and hepatic veins. Unfortunately, the early thrombosis rate was high because of the natural tendency of the hepatic parenchyma to collapse in animals with normal portal pressure. Colapinto was the first to successfully establish an intrahepatic portal-systemic shunt in a human subject with cirrhosis and bleeding varices in the early 1980s.[66] It soon became apparent that successful shunts could be established in most patients. However, over time, a high incidence of stenosis was observed despite repeated attempts at balloon dilation.

The development of an implantable, expandable metal stent by Palmaz and colleagues in 1985 was a major advance that enhanced the potential applicability of this technology for treatment of variceal bleeding in humans.[75] These investigators created an iatrogenic fistula between the anterior wall of the inferior vena cava and the portal vein in a series of 12 dogs. They observed a high rate of stent thrombosis that was attributed to normal portal pressures and hence low flows across the fistula. Later studies in dogs with portal hypertension created by an alcohol-polyvinyl embolization technique showed long-term stent patency of up to 3.5 years with histologic evidence of minimal tissue reaction and partial endothelialization of the luminal surface of the fistula.[74]

The TIPS technique currently employed worldwide is now fairly standardized with minor variations and is a direct outgrowth of modifications originally described by Ring and colleagues in 1992.[79] Two stents have been used, including the Palmaz balloon expandable stent (Johnson & Johnson, New Brunswick, NJ) and the Wallstent (Schneider U.S. Stent Division, Pfizer Hospital Products Group, Plymouth, MN). The Palmaz stent is relatively rigid and can be expanded to 12 to 16 mm ID. The Wallstent is self-expanding, more flexible, and therefore easier to insert. The technique of TIPS placement can briefly be summarized as follows (Fig. 28-6): The suprahepatic inferior vena cava and hepatic veins are identified and cannulated with a conventional angiography catheter introduced through a transjugular approach. The angiography catheter is replaced with a Colapinto needle, which is directed forward toward the hilum of the liver. Puncture of a portal vein branch is confirmed by aspiration of blood and subsequent injection of contrast material (see Fig. 28-6*A*). A guidewire is threaded through the needle, which is then withdrawn and replaced with an angiography catheter advanced into the superior mesenteric vein (see Fig. 28-6*B*). An angioplasty balloon catheter is then positioned across the parenchymal tract and inflated with contrast medium to a diameter of 10 mm (see Fig. 28-6*C*). The balloon catheter is withdrawn and replaced with a delivery catheter to which is mounted a Wallstent enclosed by a retractable plastic sheath (see Fig. 28-6*D*). Depending on the length of the parenchymal tract, a 42- or 68-mm stent is employed. The stent is deployed to cover the entire intraparenchymal tract and ideally should extend about 5 mm into the lumen of the portal and hepatic veins. Correct placement of the stent is confirmed to ensure adequate portal decompression (see Fig. 28-6*E*). If the stent is too short, a second overlapping stent can be deployed. If decompression is inadequate, the stent can be dilated slightly to 10 mm. Occasionally, a second stent is required to achieve adequate portal decompression.

A number of clinical studies worldwide have demonstrated the feasibility and safety of TIPS in patients with portal hypertension and variceal bleeding. Two investigators and their colleagues (Ring and Rossle) have now performed more than 100 TIPS procedures. These data were summarized by Conn in 1993.[67] Both groups were able to successfully implant stents in about 90% of patients, with a 50% reduction in portal pressure and an overall 30-day mortality rate of 8%. The higher mortality rate reported by the American group can be partly attributed to the higher percentage of poor-risk cirrhotic patients included in the study. TIPS achieved hemostasis in 90% of patients with active bleeding and successfully controlled ascites in 70% of patients.

There are now reproducible data that TIPS is safe and effective treatment for selected patients with variceal bleeding. Because TIPS is hemodynamically equivalent to a side-to-side portacaval anastomosis, it should theoretically be of value in patients with refractory ascites or hydrothorax. Preliminary reports indicate that ascites or hydrothorax either resolves or becomes more responsive to diuretic therapy after TIPS.[77,78,88] In one study, TIPS was used to treat refractory ascites in 19 patients.[77] Although ascites became more responsive to diuretic therapy in 15 patients (79%), eight patients died, and five additional patients developed disabling encephalopathy during follow-up of 3 to 18 months. Although TIPS may prove to be good palliation for refractory ascites, its survival benefit remains questionable.

Some preliminary data suggest that TIPS may be useful for treatment of Budd-Chiari syndrome.[73] In one report, transluminal venous angioplasty and placement of a Gianturco expandable, metallic stent resulted in significant immediate- and short-term clinical improvement of ascites in a 26-year-old man with documented Budd-Chiari syndrome.[73] The role of TIPS in these patients is unclear because portacaval and mesoatrial shunts, as well as orthotopic liver transplantation, have been used with reasonable success. However, TIPS may be especially useful in patients with high-grade obstruction of the intrahepatic inferior vena cava that precludes mesocaval or portacaval shunt or in patients with well-preserved hepatic function that contraindicates liver transplantation. There is also preliminary evidence that TIPS may be useful in patients with congestive gastropathy.[76] In four patients reported by Peine and associates, bleeding ceased, and the need for further blood transfusion was eliminated. Follow-up endoscopy at a mean of 5 weeks showed either complete resolution or marked improvement in gastric mucosal pathology.[76]

In addition to controlling acute variceal bleeding, TIPS may prove to be most useful as a bridge to hepatic transplantation. Treatment options in patients with variceal bleeding unresponsive to medical measures include sclerotherapy or endoscopic ligation or both, portal-systemic shunt procedures, and liver transplantation.[89] Liver transplantation performed in the setting of acute or ongoing variceal bleeding is associated with increased morbidity and mortality.[73] Portal-systemic shunts of various types effectively reduce portal pressure and prevent variceal rebleeding but are associated with considerable risks, including progressive deterioration of hepatic function and encephalopathy. TIPS is easier and safer to perform than a portal-systemic shunt and facilitates subsequent liver transplantation by eliminating the potential for troublesome adhesions and the need to dismantle the shunt. Several studies have shown that liver transplantation in the presence of a portal-systemic shunt is associated with longer operating times, increased intraoperative blood loss, longer hospital stay, and possible decreased survival.[65,72] In one recent study, Somberg and co-workers reported follow-up data on 192 TIPS patients, of whom 83 were evaluated as candidates for orthotopic liver transplantation.[86] All patients had complications of portal hy-

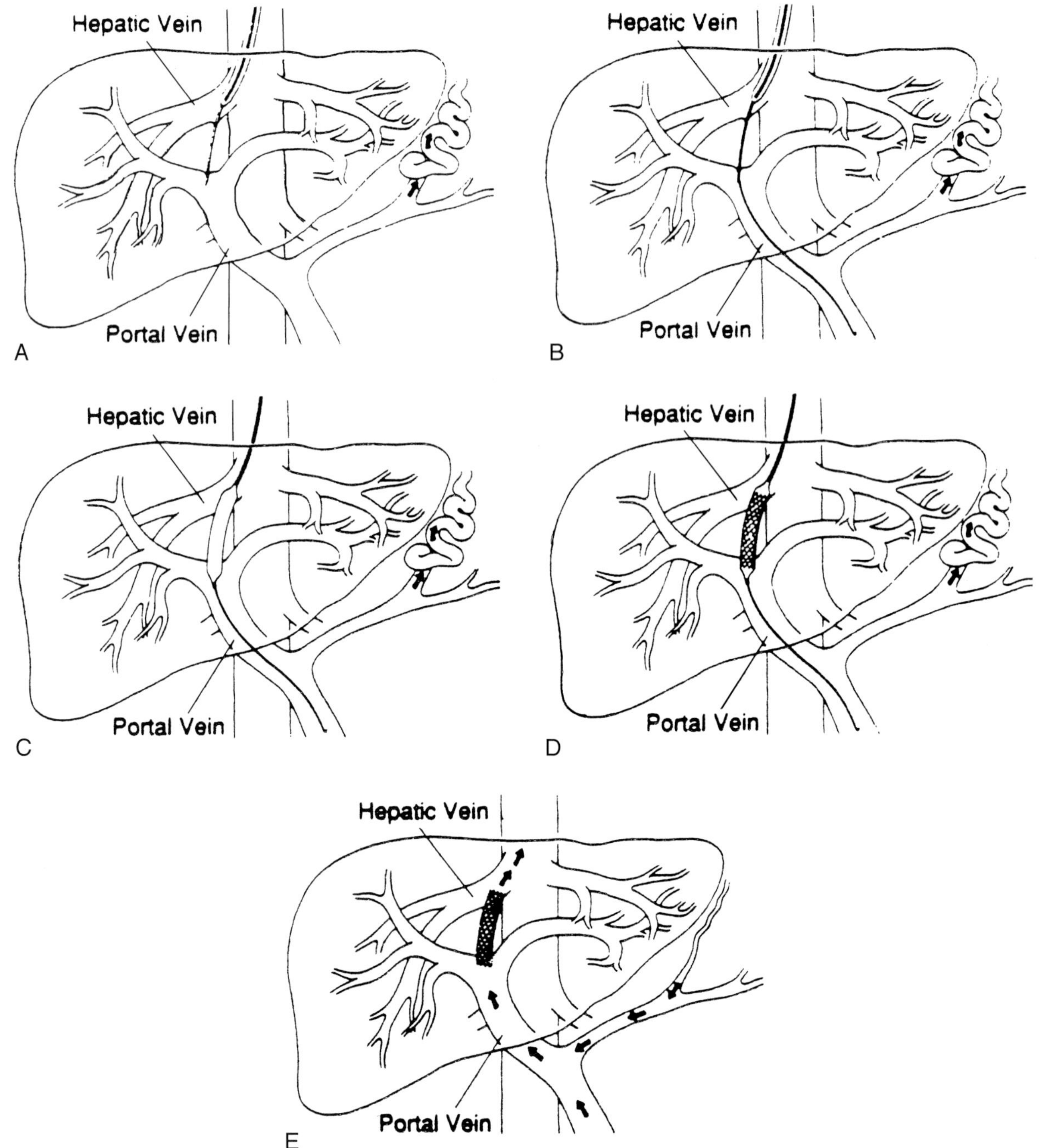

Figure 28–6. *A*, Modified Ross needle is advanced from a hepatic to a portal vein via a transjugular approach (*arrows* indicate hepatofugal flow in an enlarged coronary vein). *B*, Guidewire is advanced through the needle into the superior mesenteric vein. *C*, An 8-mm angioplasty balloon is advanced over the guidewire and expanded across hepatic parenchymal tract. *D*, Palmaz stent, mounted on an 8-mm angioplasty balloon, is expanded to bridge hepatic and portal veins. *E*, Final appearance of stent resulting in an intrahepatic shunt from portal to hepatic vein. Coronary vein is smaller and demonstrates return to hepatopetal flow. (From Zemel, G., Katzen, B.T., Becker, G.J., et al.: Percutaneous transjugular portosystemic shunt. JAMA, *266:*390, 1991, with permission.)

pertension and marked synthetic dysfunction. Liver transplantation was performed in 37 of 83 (45%) patients a mean of 58 days after TIPS placement. Of the remaining 39 patients, 1 patient died, 11 patients remain as potential transplantation candidates, and 27 patients (33%) are well and do not require transplantation. Many physicians are concerned that TIPS placement in patients with poor hepatic reserve will accelerate hepatic dysfunction because of decreased portal venous perfusion. However, initial reports have not validated this concern.[90] It has been shown that TIPS is associated with a 10 to 25% risk of hepatic encephalopathy, but this complication is usually manageable with protein restriction and lactulose.

The principal complications of TIPS include encephalopathy and stenosis or occlusion of the stent. Encephalopathy has been reported in 10 to 20% of patients after TIPS, usually occurs within 1 month of the procedure, and is relatively easy to manage with protein restriction and lactulose.[81] Investigators have observed that the incidence of encephalopathy after TIPS correlates with increasing age of the patient and increased mean shunt diameter and shunt flow.[85] Preliminary data suggest that TIPS may reduce the risk of hepatic encephalopathy as compared with surgical portacaval anastomosis. The severity of the underlying liver disease may not be as important as the size or diameter of the intrahepatic shunts. Several decades ago, complete decompression of the portal circulation was deemed desirable, and large-diameter shunts were routinely constructed. However, the resulting 40% incidence of hepatic encephalopathy significantly altered the patient's quality of life and detracted from the overall usefulness of the procedure. Dissatisfaction with the high incidence of encephalopathy after standard portacaval anastomosis led to the development of "selective" portal decompression with the distal splenorenal or Warren shunt and "partial" portal decompression with the small-caliber H-graft interposition portacaval or Sarfeh shunt. Both Sarfeh and colleagues[83] and Johansen[70] used 8- and 10-mm grafts to reduce portal pressure below a critical threshold necessary to prevent further variceal hemorrhage while retaining partial prograde portal flow and mesenteric portal hypertension, thereby reducing the risk of encephalopathy. Radiologically placed intrahepatic stents generally vary from 7 to 10 mm in diameter and appear to have the same physiologic consequences as surgically constructed small-caliber interposition H-grafts.

The second most common TIPS complication is stenosis or thrombosis. Preliminary studies indicated a stenosis rate of 5 to 15%, with progression to thrombosis in 5 to 10% of patients.[67] In one recent study, 22% of TIPS patients ultimately required revision to correct a technical failure.[69] Aside from purely technical factors such as angulation or kinking of the stent, or placement of a stent that incompletely covers the intraparenchymal tract, the most plausible explanation for progressive stent occlusion is the development of excessive neointimal hyperplasia.[71] Histologically, this lesion is characterized by the early deposition of pseudomyxomatous granulation tissue with a variable number of inflammatory cells. The pseudointima appears to be thickest at the central portion of the parenchymal tract and does not appear to involve the intravenous portions of the stents.

The development of pseudointimal hyperplasia is unpredictable. As the shunt diameter is progressively compromised, the portal-systemic pressure gradient increases, as does the risk of recurrent variceal hemorrhage. Clinical bleeding after TIPS placement indicates the need for vigorous assessment of stent patency and function. Color duplex ultrasonography has been shown to be a reliable noninvasive method for assessing stent patency and blood flow.[68] In one series, Haag and colleagues utilized color duplex ultrasonography to document changes in stent flow over time in 42 patients who underwent TIPS placement.[68] Over a 6-month observation period, they noted stable stent flow in 20% of patients, progressive reduction to 30% of baseline with subsequent stabilization in 60% of patients, and progressively decreasing flow with flow reversal indicating the need for restenting in 20% of patients. Regardless of the cause, progressive stent occlusion is a real clinical problem that may result in serious morbidity and even death in patients with severe, recurrent variceal bleeding. All TIPS patients should be followed with serial duplex ultrasound examinations to assess stent patency and flow. Equivocal results should prompt angiographic evaluation with direct measurement of the portal-systemic pressure gradient and contrast injection to identify potential technical problems. Deployment of a second stent inside the original stent or placement of a second stent through a new and separate parenchymal tract may be necessary to prevent rebleeding.

Less common complications of TIPS include embolization of the stent to the pulmonary artery, inadvertent puncture of the gallbladder or laceration of the liver capsule with resulting intraperitoneal hemorrhage, hemobilia, bacteremia with septic shock, and contrast-induced oliguric renal failure. Intravascular hemolysis has also been reported after TIPS.[82] The authors attributed the observed coagulopathy to damage of erythrocytes exposed to the wire mesh of the stent.

The current status of TIPS in the overall management of patients with liver disease and portal hypertension complicated by bleeding from varices or congestive gastropathy or by refractory ascites or hydrothorax is unclear. We are again indebted to Harold Conn for his succinct assessment of the status of TIPS in modern medicine[67]:

> The results so far reported represent rays of sunlight in a field that has long been dominated by doom and gloom. Nevertheless, in my opinion, TIPS should continue to be an experimental procedure until its efficacy and safety are unequivocally established. It should only be used in institutions at which sufficient experience has been accumulated to perform the procedure safely and well. . . . After 40 years of working in this field, I believe that TIPS is a major breakthrough that deserves careful, objective, large-scale clinical assessment so that we can provide definitive answers to a host of questions.

Randomized Clinical Trial Results for Elective Control of Variceal Bleeding

Three randomized clinical trials of sclerotherapy versus portal-systemic shunt in the elective management of variceal bleeding have been published. Rikkers and colleagues[43] studied 57 patients randomized to shunt surgery or sclerotherapy and observed a threefold higher incidence of rebleeding among sclerotherapy patients who were followed for a mean of 25 months. Of the patients treated surgically, 85% underwent distal splenorenal shunt. Two-year survival rates were similar for both groups of patients, and there were no significant differences in encephalopathy, quantitative liver function, or cumulative medical costs. However, the disconcerting observation that only 20% of patients in whom sclerotherapy had failed could be salvaged by surgery led the authors to conclude that sclerotherapy is an "acceptable, but not superior, alternative to shunt surgery for treatment of variceal hemorrhage."

Data from the Emory University randomized clinical trial comparing elective sclerotherapy in 36 patients with distal splenorenal shunt (DSRS) in 35 patients led to different conclusions.[45] Rebleeding occurred more frequently after sclerotherapy compared with DSRS (53% versus 3%, respectively), but bleeding in only one third of the sclerotherapy patients could not be controlled with additional sclerotherapy; these patients were designated as treatment failures. Two-year survival was significantly better in the sclerotherapy group (84%) than in the DSRS group (59%). It should be noted that survival analysis of the sclerotherapy group included treatment failures who subsequently underwent shunt surgery. Hepatic function as determined by serial measurements of galactose elimination capacity was also better maintained after sclerotherapy. Based on these data, the authors recommended that sclerotherapy be used as initial treatment for variceal bleeding in cirrhotic patients, reserving selective shunt for sclerotherapy treatment failures. In another large randomized clinical trial of 112 Child's class A or B patients, Teres and associates[44] concluded that sclerotherapy is a good alternative to DSRS for elective management of variceal bleeding, especially in patients likely to develop encephalopathy. Rebleeding occurred more frequently in the sclerotherapy group, whereas encephalopathy was more common in the shunt group.

These studies have helped to define better the role of sclerotherapy in the treatment of variceal bleeding. In patients with acute bleeding, the results of sclerotherapy are perhaps marginally better than those of alternative forms of medical treatment, but there is no distinct advantage in terms of bleeding control or early survival. However, there is valid evidence from three randomized clinical trials conducted by reputable investigators that sclerotherapy is an equally effective and possibly better elective treatment for variceal bleeding than distal splenorenal shunt because it preserves hepatic function and lessens the risk of encephalopathy. Additional randomized clinical trials comparing sclerotherapy with splenic transposition and gastroesophageal devascularization procedures are needed to ascertain the role of these modalities in the treatment of variceal bleeding.

SPLENIC TRANSPOSITION

Thoracic transposition of the spleen was introduced clinically by Nylander and Turunen[96] in 1955 with the expectation that newly formed vascular anastomoses between the spleen and thoracic cavity and chest wall would relieve portal hypertension and prevent variceal hemorrhage. Three debilitated patients underwent operation with no operative mortality and remained well for up to 2 years without variceal rebleeding or encephalopathy.

Turcotte and associates[99] demonstrated that new collaterals originate primarily from veins of the splenic hilum and drain through intercostal, phrenic, cardiophrenic, and undefined mediastinal veins into the superior vena cava system through the azygos and hemiazygos veins. Extensive venous collaterals between the splenic parenchyma and branches of the pulmonary venous circulation were rarely observed. The formation of collaterals was attributed to the pressure gradient between the portal and systemic venous circulations across the diaphragm, which in turn is influenced by respiration. To test this hypothesis, Turunen and Autio[100] transposed the spleen to the thoracic cavity and retroperitoneum in dogs and observed diminished splenocaval collateral formation below the diaphragm.

The splenic capsule and overlying peritoneum serve as an effective barrier to the formation of parenchymal collaterals. Efforts to enhance collateral formation include mechanical abrasion of the splenic capsule and topical application of asbestos powder. Turcott and colleagues[99] showed that decapsulation of the spleen produces abundant splenic adhesions; they further documented the functionality of these collaterals with radionuclides and colored dyes by demonstrating reversal of splenic vein flow after thoracic transposition. Turcotte and associates further showed that these neocollaterals shunt not only splenic artery blood but also some portal vein blood.

During the 1960s, several modifications of splenic transposition were developed. Bourgeon and Mouiel[93] described splenopexy, which included resection of part of the left hemidiaphragm to produce vascular adhesions between the spleen and the intrathoracic structures. Splenopneumopexy, aimed at producing splenopulmonary shunts by implanting part of the decapsulized superior pole of the spleen into the left lung, was later introduced by Auvert and associates.[92] These investigators all realized that effective thoracic splenocaval decompression of varices depended on the development of venous collaterals and recognized that 4 to 8 weeks was required for development of an adequate venous collateral network. To reduce the risk of early variceal hemorrhage during the period of splenothoracic collateral development, several authors, including Turunen, combined esophagotomy and varix ligation with splenic transposition. However, this practice was soon abandoned because of increased mortality and morbidity related to esophageal leak, empyema, and pleurocutaneous fistulas.

By 1970, 123 cases of splenic transposition had been reported in the literature. Authors repeatedly emphasized the technical ease and safety of this procedure even in poor-risk patients. In addition to decreasing the risk of recurrent variceal hemorrhage, splenic transposition was also found to have a favorable effect on the management of hypersplenism and ascites. Akita and Sakoda[91] used a two-stage procedure to produce portopulmonary shunts by splenopneumopexy in 15 patients with Budd-Chiari syndrome and reported effective control of variceal hemorrhage and ascites with no cardiopulmonary, hepatic, or neurologic complications.

In a classic study published in 1971, Hastbacka reported his results in 37 patients with portal hypertension treated by splenic transposition or resection-transposition during a 17-year period.[95] The causes of portal hypertension included intrahepatic or sinusoidal block in 26 patients and prehepatic block in 11 patients. In most cases, splenic transposition was performed as an elective procedure after variceal bleeding had been controlled with conservative measures. The original technique, consisting of splenic transposition without partial splenectomy, was performed in 23 patients. After 1966, the resection-transposition technique was adopted and used in an additional

11 patients. The operative mortality rate for the entire series was 11%. Survival was affected primarily by the presence of portal hypertension and by the severity of the underlying liver disease. There were no postoperative deaths in the group of 11 patients with presinusoidal block. By comparison, 4 of 26 cirrhotic patients (15%) died as a result of the operation. Mortality among poor-risk patients with cirrhosis (older than 60 years of age and severely impaired liver function) was even higher (27%). Significant complications, including diaphragmatic hernia, pleurocutaneous fistula, and hemothorax, developed in 16% of patients. Encephalopathy was uncommon.

According to Hastbacka's study,[95] the major shortcoming of the original splenic transposition or resection-transposition techniques was an unexpectedly high incidence of recurrent variceal bleeding. Early rebleeding was observed in 14 of 37 patients (38%) but was fatal in only one case (7%). Late rebleeding occurred in 10 of 30 patients (33%) surviving longer than 6 months. However, only two of these patients required operative management, and none died of exsanguinating hemorrhage.

Because splenic transposition reduces the risk of variceal rebleeding without altering portal pressure, one must speculate about the mechanism of protection afforded by this procedure. Hastbacka obtained serial venographic studies in a group of patients who underwent secondary splenic artery ligation for either rebleeding or hypersplenism with thrombocytopenia. Intraoperative studies performed after splenic artery ligation showed enhanced venous flow toward splenothoracic collaterals and away from the portal vein. Late studies obtained 3 months to 2 years after the operation suggested that better visualization of splenothoracic collaterals was evident compared with earlier examinations. Portal pressure decreased by an average of 5 to 10 cm H_2O after splenic artery ligation, and these changes persisted over time. The author concluded that splenic transposition exerts a protective effect against rebleeding by acting as "a pressure-equalizing system which decreased the chance of any sudden pressure rise in esophageal veins." Radiographic studies showing more effective venous decompression after secondary splenic artery ligation suggest that relieving the collateral network of a considerable portion of its arterial blood load may be a crucial element in this approach.

Hastbacka emphasized certain physiologic similarities between splenic transposition and the selective portal decompression afforded by the distal splenorenal or Warren shunt.[101] The procedures are shown in Figure 28–7, which is reproduced from Hastbacka's article in 1971. Both procedures transform the spleen into a more effective capacitor by either directly (splenorenal vein anastomosis) or indirectly (production of splenothoracic collaterals) reducing splenic venous outflow resistance. Both maintain prograde portal flow and intestinal venous hypertension by somewhat different mechanisms, thus preserving liver function. After splenic transposition, contiguity of the splenic vein with the rest of the portal circulation is preserved. Therefore, depending on the extent of the collaterals that develop after this procedure, the potential exists to siphon a portion of portal blood into the systemic circulation analogous to a central splenorenal shunt.

Multistaged splenic transposition procedures as described earlier cause greater morbidity than a single operation because two general anesthetics are required and two body cavities are violated. Ono and colleagues[97] from Japan described an approach to esophageal varices that involves injection sclerotherapy, transcatheter left gastric and splenic arterial embolization, and splenopneumopexy and eliminates the need for multiple surgical procedures. The technique is based on Akita's demonstration in 1980 that effective portopulmonary shunts develop after splenopneumopexy in the management of Budd-Chiari syndrome.

The objectives of transarterial artery embolization (TAE) deserve to be emphasized and can be summarized as follow: TAE effectively eliminates the splenic component of portal blood flow, thereby reducing portal pressure and the risk of recurrent variceal bleeding. Eliminating the major component of splenic arterial blood flow greatly reduces blood loss during the splenic decapsulation phase of splenopneumopexy and decreases the risk of operation. Improvement of hypersplenism with resolution of thrombocytopenia is frequently seen after TAE and may be beneficial in decreasing the risk of spontaneous variceal rebleeding or surgical bleeding at the time of operation.[94,98] Finally, TAE provides a relatively risk-free interval of 2 to 3 weeks during which the patient's liver function and nutritional status can be improved in preparation for splenopneumopexy.

Although opinion differs about the need for an abdominal phase in this approach, there is uniform agreement about the thoracic phase of the operation. The technical aspects of splenopneumopexy are shown in the drawings that accompany the text. The left pleural cavity is entered through an eighth intercostal space incision that extends posteriorly to the midscapular line. The left diaphragm is palpated gently to determine the position of the superior pole of the spleen. The peritoneal cavity is entered by creating a small incision in the muscular portion of the diaphragm away from the spleen tip. A circular segment of diaphragm measuring about 10 cm in diameter is excised. Hemostasis along the cut edge of the diaphragm is achieved by using a continuous nonabsorbable suture. Interrupted sutures are placed between the cut edge of the diaphragm and the spleen to prevent herniation of intra-abdominal contents into the chest (Fig. 28–8*A*). These sutures should be overlapped slightly to minimize leakage of postoperative ascites into the pleural space and should be placed with care to ensure that 4 to 6 cm of spleen protrudes above the diaphragm into the thoracic cavity.

The next step involves removing the splenic capsule and the overlying visceral peritoneum. Akita recommends using multiple rectangular incisions and stripping away as much of the splenic capsule as is easily accessible. We have found that sutures placed between the splenic parenchyma and lung do not hold securely and have adopted a slightly different approach. Rather than stripping the entire exposed splenic capsule, we create multiple 1- to 1.5-cm wide furrows of bare splenic parenchyma separated by thin bridges of intact splenic capsule and

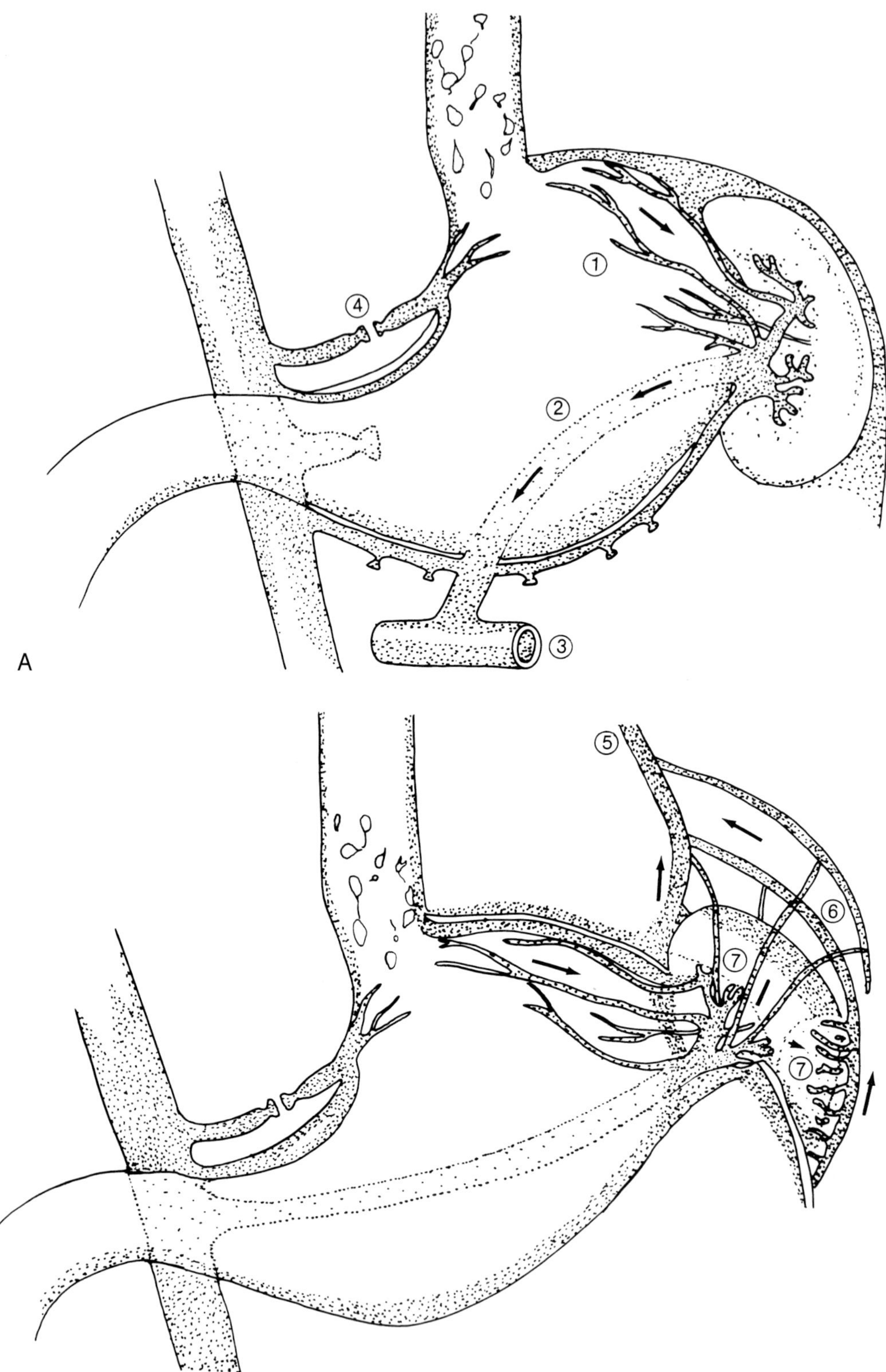

Figure 28–7. Selective transplenic decompression of gastroesophageal varices via *(A)* distal splenorenal shunt or *(B)* splenic transposition. Analogy between the two techniques is illustrated by the schematic drawings. (From Hastbacka, J.: Thoracic transposition of the spleen in portal hypertension. Ann. Chir. Gynaecol., *60*:54, 1971, with permission.)

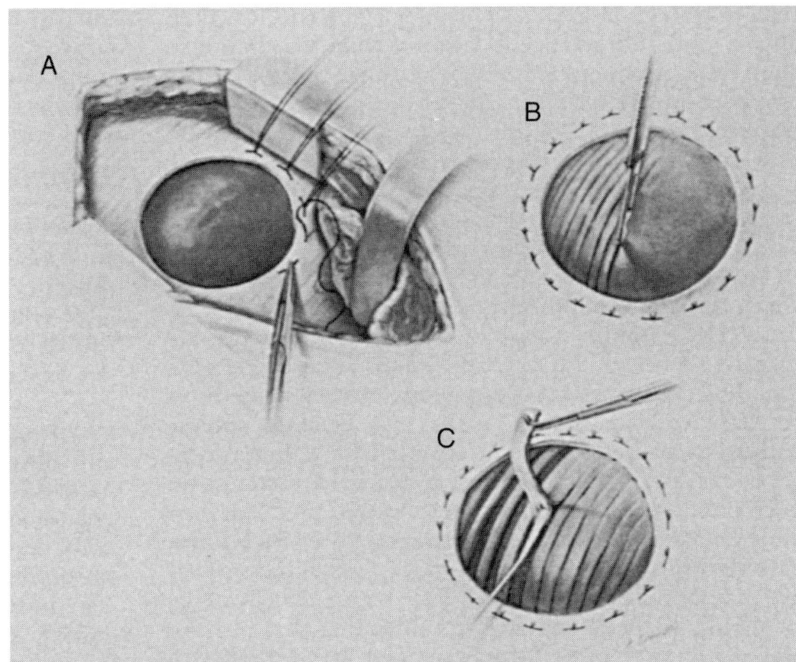

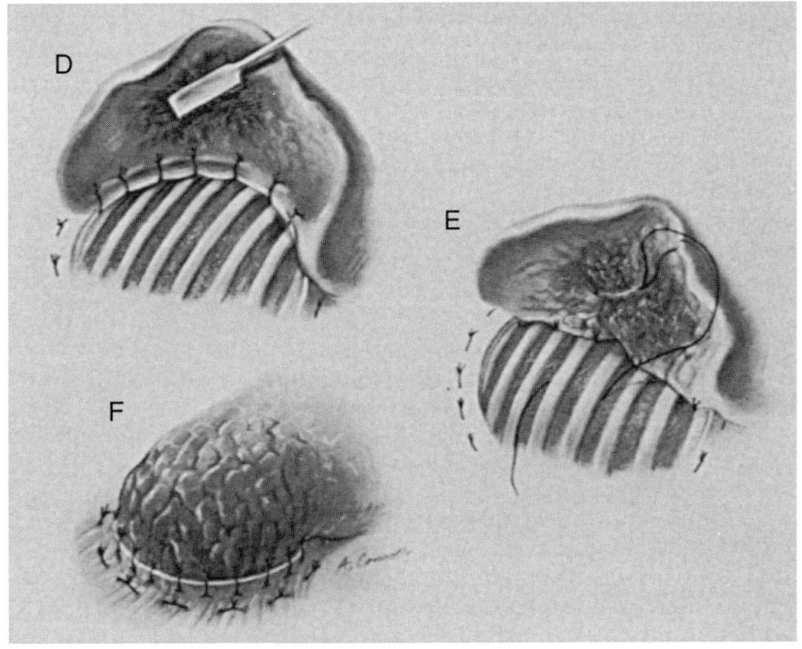

Figure 28–8. The technique of splenopneumopexy establishes splenothoracic collaterals in patients with portal hypertension and gastroesophageal varices. *A*, A 10-cm circular segment of diaphragm is excised, exposing the superior pole of the spleen. The spleen is sutured circumferentially to the diaphragm to decrease ascites leak or herniation of intra-abdominal contents into the thoracic cavity. *B* and *C*, Multiple longitudinal furrows are created by excising the splenic capsule and overlying peritoneum. Strips of retained capsule help to secure the sutures placed between the splenic parenchyma and lung. *D*, A rim of lung tissue is sutured to the posterior aspect of a previously created defect in the diaphragm. The lung is abraded with a bone rasp to produce moderate bleeding and air leakage. *E*, Ten to 12 deep, absorbable sutures are placed between the lung tissue and the splenic parenchyma to ensure close apposition of these surfaces, thus encouraging the formation of collaterals. *F*, The anterior and lateral lung edges are secured to the cut edge of the corresponding section of diaphragm.

peritoneum (see Fig. 28–8*B* and *C*). This technique ensures direct apposition of the abraded undersurface of the lung with the spleen surface and facilitates formation of collaterals. Bleeding from the cut surface of the spleen is rarely excessive and can be easily controlled by compression with gauze moistened in warm saline.

After the spleen has been decapsulated, attention is then turned toward the lung. The undersurface of the left lower lobe is abraded vigorously with a bone rasp to produce mild bleeding and air leakage (see Fig. 28–8*D*). The mediastinal and posterior edges of the lung are invaginated beneath the cut edge of the diaphragm and secured with interrupted sutures. About 10 to 12 interrupted sutures of 2-0 Vicryl are then placed between the apposing surfaces of the spleen and lung and tied securely (see Fig. 28–8*E*). It is important to incorporate large bites of tissue in these sutures to prevent tearing and distraction of the surfaces. The anterior and lateral lung edges are then secured to the cut edge of the corresponding sections of diaphragm (see Fig. 28–8*F*). A chest tube is placed, and the thoracic wound is closed.

Preliminary results reported by Ono and colleagues[97] using this multimodality approach in 16 patients have been encouraging. Thirteen patients (81%) were cirrhotic; of these, 10 (77%) had moderate or severely impaired liver function (Child's class B or C). The estimated average blood loss during surgery was less than 400 ml, and the average operating time was 3 hours. There were no operative deaths or major postoperative complications. Recurrent variceal bleeding occurred in only 1 patient (6.3%) during a mean follow-up period of 16 months. There was one late death from liver failure, and encephalopathy was not a problem. Repeat endoscopy showed marked improvement or disappearance of varices in the remaining patients.

The advantages of splenic transposition compared with portal-systemic shunt procedures include a lower operative risk, a more physiologic outcome, and the absence of significant late complications, such as encephalopathy. Subsequent portal-systemic shunt procedures are technically feasible, if necessary, because splenic transposition does not sacrifice any major tributaries of the portal circulation. Finally, portal vein thrombosis, which is an acknowledged complication of portal-systemic shunt and devascularization or transection procedures, is avoided with splenic transposition, thus allowing liver transplantation if it is needed.

DEVASCULARIZATION AND TRANSECTION PROCEDURES

A wide variety of "ablative" procedures have been devised to manage variceal bleeding. The primary objective of these procedures is to interrupt extraesophageal and intramural venous collaterals between the portal circulation and the variceal watershed at the esophagogastric junction.[102,108] Splenectomy is frequently performed as well to decongest the portal circulation. It is difficult to reconcile the widely differing results reported from the United States and other parts of the world. These disparities reflect the heterogeneity of the patient groups involved as well as differences in the etiology and severity of the underlying disease processes and the multitude of procedures we are attempting to compare. The various ablative procedures currently performed can be conveniently classified into three groups: esophageal transection with reanastomosis and gastroesophageal devascularization with and without transection.

Esophageal Transection With Reanastomosis

Esophageal transection and reanastomosis with autosuture devices or hand suture techniques adequately prevents acute rebleeding, but operative mortality and late rebleeding rates are unacceptably high. In one series of 20 patients, Wanamaker and colleagues[110] used the EEA stapling instrument to control bleeding esophageal varices. A transabdominal approach was used. All patients underwent concomitant coronary vein ligation, and 9 patients underwent splenectomy. Almost all patients were poor-risk cirrhotic patients, and 75% required urgent or emergent operation. The overall operative mortality rate was 60%, but the rate increased considerably (89%) among patients requiring emergency operation. The addition of splenectomy slightly prolonged the operation but did not alter mortality. The duration of follow-up varied from 10 to 60 months with a mean of 31 months. Although rebleeding did not occur in the postoperative period, late rebleeding occurred in 4 of 8 surviving patients (50%), 2 of whom died of hemorrhage. One additional patient died of liver failure, resulting in a long-term, unadjusted survival rate of 25% in this group of patients. Although no postoperative esophageal leaks occurred, the authors commented on the high frequency of technical problems encountered intraoperatively with the use of the EEA stapling instrument.

Gouge and Ranson[105] reported their experience with the thoracic phase of the Sugiura procedure (equivalent to esophageal transection and reanastomosis) in 15 cirrhotic patients, nearly all of whom were alcoholics. In all cases, a transthoracic approach was used, and the esophageal anastomosis was hand sewed. Eleven patients (73%) required urgent or emergent operation to control bleeding. The hospital mortality rate among these patients was 53%. Bleeding was uniformly controlled in the postoperative period, but complications, many of which were significant, developed in 86% of surviving patients. Excluding 1 patient who later underwent the abdominal phase of the Sugiura procedure, the remaining patients all died 5 to 35 months after the operation. Late rebleeding occurred in 4 of 7 (67%) survivors and was the principal cause of death in 3 of these patients.

Devascularization Without Transection

The major disadvantage of esophageal transection or reanastomosis procedures is their ineffectiveness in preventing rebleeding. A number of devascularization procedures have been described to control variceal bleeding without impairing portal blood flow. Hassab from Egypt[106] described an operation that includes splenectomy, ligation of the left gastric artery, and devascularization of the distal esophagus and proximal portion of the stomach. The operation was performed in 605 patients, of whom 65% had documented schistosomal hepatic fibrosis. The operative mortality rate for elective procedures was 10%, and patients with hepatic failure were excluded. A subset of 232 patients with 1- to 12-year follow-up was reviewed to evaluate long-term survival and the risk of rebleeding. Of these patients, 44 (18%) died during the study period. Only 3% died of bleeding, and there was virtually no encephalopathy. Hassab's results are unequivocally excellent. However, it is difficult to compare his results in patients with schistosomiasis to Western studies of patients with predominantly alcoholic and posthepatitic cirrhosis.

Several Western surgeons have attempted to adopt and modify the technique of esophageal transection and paraesophagogastric devascularization described by Sugiura in 1973. Estes and Pierce[104] described a transthoracic approach in which the proximal stomach was devascularized by transecting the short gastric, left gastroepiploic, coronary, and left gastric vessels immediately adjacent to the stomach and a 12- to 18-cm segment of distal esophagus was skeletonized. Splenectomy was performed only when required to devascularize the greater curvature of the stomach safely. A Nissen fundoplication was performed to prevent gastroesophageal reflux. The authors emphasized the importance of completely interrupting the portal-systemic collaterals between the esophagogastric watershed, the diaphragm, and the azygous system.

All of Estes and Pierce's patients who were treated by extended devascularization were moderately high-risk (Child's class B or C), and 10 of the 12 (83%) were alcoholics. Eight patients underwent emergency operation, and four patients had surgery on a semielective basis. There were two postoperative deaths (17%). Four late deaths occurred from 30 to 48 months after operation, including two from massive variceal bleeding and two from liver failure. The six surviving patients had no evidence of rebleeding an average of 54 months after surgery. The unadjusted 5-year survival rate in this group of patients is 50%.

These results are good considering the patient population. Estes and Pierce presupposed that effective control of variceal bleeding depended chiefly on extensive interruption of all external portal-systemic collaterals from the level of the inferior pulmonary vein superiorly to the right gastric artery on the lesser curvature and beyond the midpoint of the greater curvature inferiorly. Esophageal transection was deleted in the belief that interruption of intramural venous collaterals in the distal esophagus and gastric cardia was less important than external portal disconnection of the azygous system. Splenectomy was not performed routinely, but it is unclear from the text how many patients underwent this procedure at the time of devascularization.

Devascularization With Transection

The objectives of this approach include interruption of all extraesophageal portal venous collaterals, partial or complete esophageal transection with reanastomosis to obliterate intramural venous communications, and frequently splenectomy to decongest the splanchnic venous circulation. The gold standard against which other procedures are compared is the Sugiura procedure. The original technique, described by Sugiura and Futagawa[109] in 1973, consisted of thoracic and abdominal phases performed through separate incisions. The operation was designed to be performed in one or two stages depending on the urgency of the case and on the patient's hepatic risk status. The authors emphasized the importance of preserving the major coronary–azygous communications and dividing only "shunting" veins between these vessels and the esophagus. In 1984, Sugiura reported his results in 671 patients operated on between 1967 and 1984. About 23% of the patients had cirrhosis, and of these, alcoholism was a cause in only one third. Therapeutic procedures were performed in 468 patients. The operative mortality rate was 3% in 363 elective cases and 13% in 135 emergency cases. The operative mortality rate correlated directly with the patient's preoperative hepatic risk status but was not affected significantly by the presence or etiology of cirrhosis. The incidence of recurrent varices after the complete Sugiura procedure was 5%, and rebleeding occurred in only 1.4% of patients. By comparison, almost 60% of patients developed recurrent varices, and rebleeding occurred in 15% when only the abdominal phase of the procedure had been completed. The actuarial 10-year survival rate was 55% in emergency cases and 72% in elective cases. Major complications, including esophageal leak, anastomotic stricture, and portal vein thrombosis, developed in 60 patients (8.9%). Most esophageal leaks resolved with nonoperative treatment, but septic complications developed in five patients (13%), who subsequently died. Portal vein thrombosis occurred in five patients and was uniformly fatal. Anastomotic strictures were managed effectively with endoscopic dilatation.

A number of Western surgeons have tried to adopt Sugiura's technique with variable results. However, of the four major series reviewed, only Gouge and Ranson in the United States used the procedure intact without modification.[105] Of the 35 patients studied by these authors, 83% were alcoholic, and about 50% had severely compromised liver function. Fifteen patients underwent only the thoracic phase of the operation, with a 53% operative mortality rate and a 67% late rebleeding rate among surviving patients. This group consisted of patients with an advanced stage of disease (poor hepatic risk, urgent or emergent operation) in whom a lengthy operation violating two body cavities was judged inadvisable. In comparison, 20 patients underwent the complete operation, with an operative mortality rate of 9.5% and a late rebleeding rate of 37%. The operation effectively controlled variceal bleeding in all patients during the early postoperative period. However, the incidence of late rebleeding appears to be dictated by the "completeness" of the operation. Long-term survival in this group was also poor, and all except 1 of the original 15 patients (94%) died after an average of 19 months (range, 5 to 35 months). Of the 21 patients who underwent the complete procedure, 8 (38%) were alive after an average follow-up of 29 months (range, 9 to 52 months).

The three remaining Western studies all used modifications of the original Sugiura procedure. Barbot and Rosato[103] from the United States used a transthoracic approach with transection of all significant portal azygous collaterals, ligation of the right gastric artery, splenectomy and interruption of the lesser curvature vessels at the omental level rather than along the gastric wall, and transection or reanastomosis of the esophagus with the EEA stapling instrument. Because of technical difficulties related to the esophageal anastomosis, transection was later omitted in favor of injection sclerotherapy. Twenty-eight patients were treated, with a 32% operative mortality rate and a long-term survival rate of 67%. About 25% of patients experienced late rebleeding, but only one proved to have a variceal source. Encephalopathy was a problem in two patients, both of whom had similar symptoms before operation. This series contained a smaller percentage of poor-risk patients with alcoholic cirrhosis than that in Gouge and Ranson's study, and this difference may explain the observed differences in early and late mortality.

Orozco and colleagues[107] published their experience in Mexico with 45 patients using a one- or two-staged procedure similar to that advocated by Barbot and Rosato. Operative mortality for urgent or emergent and elective cases was 41% and 11%, respectively. The actuarial 3-year survival rate was 40% for urgent or emergent cases and

83% for elective cases. No rebleeding was encountered in patients who survived the operation. This series contained a high percentage (32%) of patients with noncirrhotic portal hypertension (schistosomal fibrosis and extrahepatic portal vein occlusion), and 82% of the group was classified as low risk. As such, it differs considerably from the "typical" United States experience with high-risk alcoholics and makes valid comparison of results more difficult.

Abouna and co-workers[102] from Kuwait published the Middle Eastern experience with the Sugiura procedure. The patient composition in this study was comparable to that of Orozco's series and consisted mostly of patients with schistosomal fibrosis and nonalcoholic forms of cirrhosis. It is the only Western series to use a transabdominal approach and conceptually is analogous to the original Sugiura procedure. The crucial elements of the procedure are illustrated in Figures 28-9 through 28-11. The abdomen is entered through an upper midline incision. The relationships of the upper abdominal viscera before devascularization or transection are shown in Figure 28-9. The upper half of the greater curvature of the stomach is devascularized along with the lesser curvature down to the area of the "crow's foot," and highly selective vagotomy is performed. The entire abdominal esophagus and 6 to 8 cm of the thoracic esophagus are devascularized by dividing "shunting" veins and preserving major coronary azygous collaterals. Splenectomy is performed routinely. The extent of devascularization before esophageal transection is shown in Figure 28-10. The final step of the procedure includes transection of the esophagus with an EEA stapling instrument introduced through a gastrotomy. To prevent tearing or perforation of the esophagus, it is important to select an EEA stapler of the appropriate size. The esophagus is transected about 2 cm above the gastroesophageal junction, and the ring of tissue excised by the stapler is inspected for completeness (Fig. 28-11). The use of closed-suction drainage after completion of the procedure is a matter of personal preference.

Abouna and associates treated 26 patients with the modified Sugiura procedure during a 5-year period. Schistosomal fibrosis and extrahepatic portal vein occlusion were identified as pathologic causes of portal hypertension in almost 50% of the cases. Only 12% of patients were classified as poor risk (Child's class C). The operative mortality rate was 7.7%. No encephalopathy and no late deaths occurred in the series. Only one patient had late rebleeding. Upper gastrointestinal series obtained 3 months to 2 years after the operation showed complete disappearance of varices in the majority of patients.

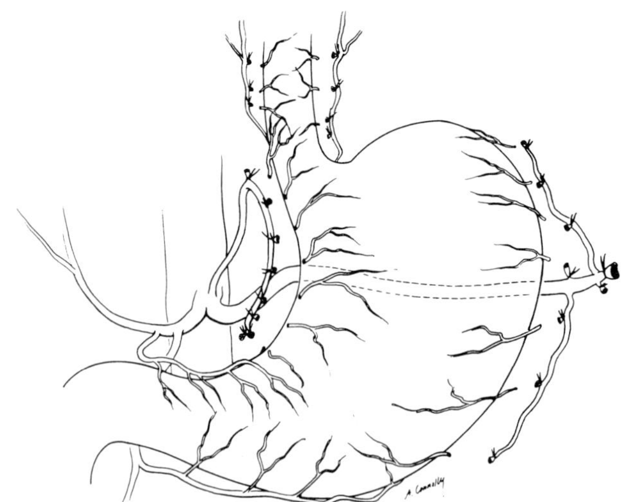

Figure 28–10. The anatomy of the upper abdomen after extensive paraesophagogastric devascularization and splenectomy. The entire abdominal esophagus and 6 to 8 cm of thoracic esophagus are devascularized by dividing the "shunting" veins and by preserving the major portal azygous collaterals. The stomach is devascularized distally to the level of the crow's foot along the lesser curvature and to the midpoint of the greater curvature. Splenectomy is performed routinely with this particular technique.

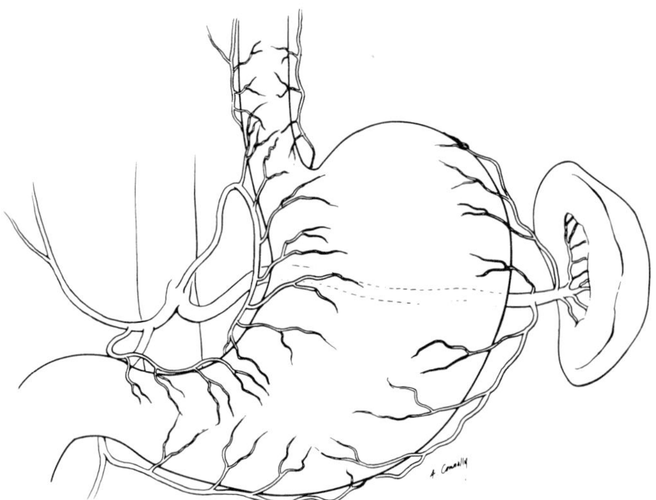

Figure 28–9. Normal anatomy of the upper abdomen and gastroesophageal area before devascularization.

Some authors have concluded that "ablative" operations for the treatment of esophageal varices are associated with prohibitive risks of operative mortality and recurrent bleeding and should *not* be used except in patients who cannot undergo a decompressive shunt. It is true that the operative mortality rate for patients undergoing urgent to emergent or "incomplete" procedures varies from 40 to 55%. In this setting, the severity of the underlying disease may be a more important determinant of survival than the type of operation performed. The operative mortality rate following "complete" devascularization or transection procedures under elective circumstances in nonalcoholic cirrhotic patients or in patients with noncirrhotic etiologies of portal hypertension varies from 3 to 12% in most reported series and compares favorably with the results of nonselective or selective shunt procedures. The average 3-year survival rate reported for the latter groups of patients is 61%, and the range is 38 to 83%. In Sugiura's series, the 10-year survival rate was 72% for patients who underwent "complete" elective operation. These figures are comparable with the results achieved after selective shunting. Encephalopathy is uncommon after ablative procedures, and on careful review it was usually found to be present before operation or occurred during an episode of recurrent bleeding.

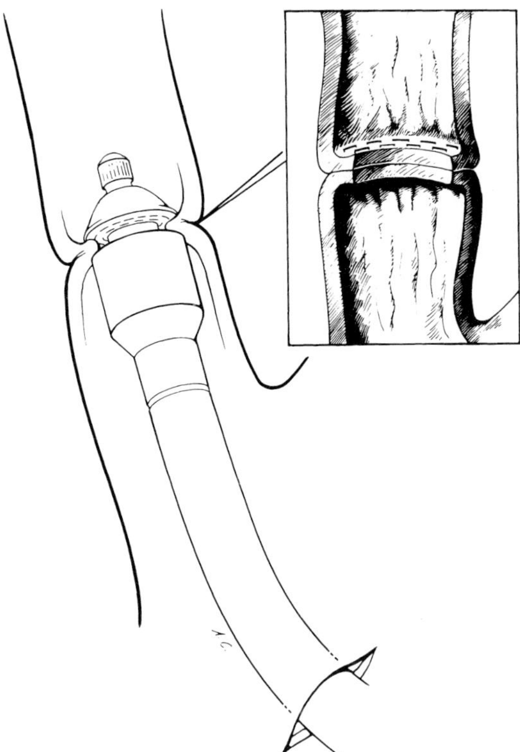

Figure 28–11. The technique of esophageal transection and reanastomosis. An EEA stapling instrument is inserted through a proximal gastrotomy incision. The esophagus is transected approximately 2 cm above the gastroesophageal junction. The excised rings of tissue should be inspected carefully for completeness. The gastrotomy incision is closed in layers.

The major disadvantage of ablative procedures is the risk of rebleeding. In studies involving predominantly nonalcoholic cirrhotic patients and patients with noncirrhotic forms of portal hypertension, rebleeding rates ranging from 0 to 8% have been reported. In contrast, rebleeding rates of 25 to 37% have been reported in Western studies consisting primarily of poor-risk alcoholics. Although the risk of death from rebleeding after devascularization or transection is high, it is not substantially greater than the risk incurred by an untreated cirrhotic patient at the time of the initial bleeding episode.

References

Pathogenesis

1. Conn, H.O.: The volcano varix connection (Editorial). Gastroenterology, *79:*1333, 1980.
2. Lebrec, D., De Fleurry, P., Reuff, B., et al.: Portal hypertension, size of esophageal varices, and the risk of gastrointestinal bleeding in alcoholic cirrhosis. Gastroenterology, *79:*1139, 1980.
3. Leevy, C.M., Zinke, M., Baber, J., et al.: Observations on the influence of medical therapy on portal hypertension in hepatic cirrhosis. Ann. Intern. Med., *49:*837, 1958.
4. Vianna, A., Hayes, P.C., Moscosco, G., et al.: Normal venous circulation of the gastroesophageal junction. A route to understanding varices. Gastroenterology, *98:*876, 1987.

Etiology

5. Cameron, J.L., and Maddrey, W.: Meso-atrial shunt: A new treatment for Budd-Chiari syndrome. Ann. Surg., *187:*402, 1978.
6. Huet, P.M., Villineuve, J.P., and Pomier-Layrargues, G.: Hepatic circulation in cirrhosis. Clin. Gastroenterol., *14:*155, 1985.
7. Leevy, C.M.: Fatty liver: A study of 270 patients with biopsy-proven fatty liver and a review of the literature. Medicine, *41:*249, 1982.
8. Nadell, J., and Kosek, J.: Peliosis hepatis: Twelve cases associated with oral androgen therapy. Arch. Pathol. Lab. Med., *101:*405, 1977.
9. Orloff, M., and Johansen, K.: Treatment of Budd-Chiari syndrome by side-to-side portacaval shunt: Experimental and clinical results. Ann. Surg., *188:*494, 1978.

Pathophysiology: Implications for Treatment

10. Siegel, J.H., Giovannini, I., Coleman, B., et al.: Death after portal decompressive surgery: Physiologic state, metabolic adequacy and the sequence of development of the physiologic determinants of survival. Arch. Surg., *116:*1330, 1981.
11. Zimmon, D.S., and Kessler, R.E.: Effect of portal venous blood flow diversion on portal pressure. J. Clin. Invest., *65:*1388, 1980.

Natural History of Cirrhosis and Variceal Bleeding

12. Graham, D.Y., and Smith, J.L.: The course of patients after variceal hemorrhage. Gastroenterology, *80:*800, 1981.

Diagnosis

13. Gill, R.A., Goddman, M.W., Golfus, G.R., et al.: Aminopyrine breath test predicts surgical risk for patients with liver disease. Ann. Surg., *198:*701, 1983.
14. Henderson, J.M., Kutner, M.H., and Bain, R.P.: First order clearance of plasma galactose: The effect of liver disease. Gastroenterology, *83:*1090, 1982.
15. McLeod, M.K., Eckhauser, F.E., and Turcotte, J.G.: Significance of corrected sinusoidal pressure (CSP) in patients with cirrhosis and portal hypertension. Ann. Surg., *194:*562, 1981.
16. Moriyasu, F., Nishida, O., Ban, N., et al.: Measurement of portal vascular resistance in patients with portal hypertension. Gastroenterology, *90:*710, 1986.
17. Sarfeh, I.J., Juler, G.L., Stemmler, E.A., et al.: Results of surgical management of hemorrhagic gastritis in patients with gastroesophageal varices. Surg. Gynecol. Obstet., *155:*167, 1982.

Pharmacologic Therapy

18. Aronse, K.F., and Nylander, G.: The mechanism of vasopressin hemostasis in bleeding esophageal varices: An angiographic study in the dog. Acta Chir. Scand., *131:*443, 1966.
19. Barbare, J.C., Poupon, R., Jaillon, P., et al.: The influence of vasoactive agents on the metabolic activity of the liver in cirrhosis: A study of the effects of posterior pituitary extract, vasopressin and somatostatin. Hepatology, *4:*59, 1984.
20. Bosch, J., Kravetz, D., and Rodes, J.: Effects of somatostatin on hepatic hemodynamics in patients with cirrhosis of the liver: Comparison with vasopressin. Gastroenterology, *80:*518, 1981.
21. Chojkier, M., Groszmann, R., Atterbury, C., et al.: A controlled comparison of continuous intra-arterial and intravenous infusion of vasopressin in hemorrhages from esophageal varices. Gastroenterology, *77:*540, 1979.
22. Groszmann, R.J., Kravetz, D., Bosch, J., et al.: Nitroglycerin improves the hemodynamic response to vasopressin in portal hypertension. Hepatology, *2:*562, 1982.
23. Johnson, W., Widrich, W., Ansell, J., et al.: Control of bleeding varices by vasopressin: A prospective, randomized study. Ann. Surg., *180:*369, 1977.
24. Kehne, J., Hughes, F., and Gompertz, M.: The use of pituitrin in the control of esophageal varix bleeding: An experimental study and report of two cases. Surgery, *39:*917, 1956.
25. Valenzuela, J.E., Schubert, T., Fogel, M.R., et al.: A multicenter randomized double blind trial of somatostatin in the management of acute hemorrhage from esophageal varices. Hepatology, *10:*958, 1989.
26. D'Amico, G., Pugliaro, L., and Bosch, J.: The treatment of portal hypertension: A meta-analytic review. Hepatology, *22:*332, 1995.
27. Grace, N.D.: Diagnosis and treatment of gastrointestinal bleeding

secondary to portal hypertension. Am. J. Gastroenterol., *192:*1081, 1997.
28. Vosmik, J., Jedlicka, K., Mulder, J., et al.: Action of the homonogen of vasopressin (glypressin) in patients with liver cirrhosis and bleeding esophageal varices. Gastroenterology, *72:*605, 1977.
29. Bernard, B., Lebrec, D., Mathurin, P., et al.: Beta-adrenergic antagonists in the prevention of gastrointestinal rebleeding in patients with cirrhosis: A meta-analysis. Hepatology, *25:*63, 1997.
30. Angelico, M., Lurli, R., Pruit, C., et al.: Isosorbide 5 mononitrate versus propranolol for prevention of first bleeding in cirrhosis. Gastroenterology, *104:*1460, 1993.
31. Grace, N.D., Conn, H.O., Groszmann, R.J., et al.: Propranolol for the prevention of first variceal hemorrhage: A lifetime of commitment? Hepatology, *12:*407, 1990.

Balloon Tamponade

32. Chojkier, M., and Conn, H.O.: Esophageal tamponade in the treatment of bleeding varices. Dig. Dis. Sci., *25:*267, 1980.
33. Gimson, A.E.S., Westaby, D., Hegarty, J., et al.: A randomized trial of vasopressin and vasopressin plus nitroglycerin in the control of acute variceal hemorrhage. Hepatology, *6:*410, 1986.
34. Sarin, S.K., and Mundy, S.: Balloon tamponade in the management of bleeding esophageal varices. Ann. R. Coll. Surg. Engl., *66:*30, 1984.
35. Reynaert, M., Zilic, M., Marion, E., et al.: Traitement de l'hemorrhagie par rupture de varices oesophagiennes au moyen da la sonde de Michel. Acta Gastroenterol. Belg., *46:*142, 1983.

Transhepatic Variceal Obliteration

36. Lunderquist, A., and Vang, J.: Transhepatic catheterization of the coronary vein in patients with portal hypertension and esophageal varices. N. Engl. J. Med., *291:*646, 1974.
37. Smith-Laing, G., Scott, J., Long, R.G., et al.: Role of percutaneous transhepatic obliteration of varices in the management of hemorrhage from gastroesophageal varices. Gastroenterology, *80:*1031, 1981.
38. Terabayashi, H., Ohnishi, K., Tsunoda, T., et al.: Prospective controlled trial of elective endoscopic sclerotherapy in comparison with percutaneous transhepatic obliteration of esophageal varices in patients with nonalcoholic cirrhosis. Gastroenterology, *93:*1205, 1987.

Sclerotherapy

39. Craaford, C., and Frenckner, P.: New surgical treatment of varicose veins of the esophagus. Acta Otolaryngol., *27:*422, 1939.
40. Andersen, B., Burcharth, F., Matzen, P., et al.: Sclerotherapy after first variceal hemorrhage in cirrhosis: A randomized multicenter trial. N. Engl. J. Med., *311:*1594, 1984.
41. Cello, J.P., Grendell, J.H., and Crass, R.A.: Endoscopic sclerotherapy versus portacaval shunt in patients with severe cirrhosis and variceal hemorrhage. N. Engl. J. Med., *311:*1589, 1984.
42. DiMagno, E.P., Zinsmeister, A.R., Larson, D.E., et al.: Influence of hepatic reserve and cause of esophageal varices on survival and rebleeding before and after the introduction of sclerotherapy: A retrospective analysis. Mayo Clin. Proc., *60:*149, 1985.
43. Rikkers, L.F., Burnett, D.A., and Volentine, G.D.: Shunt surgery versus endoscopic sclerotherapy for long-term treatment of variceal bleeding. Ann. Surg., *206:*261, 1987.
44. Teres, J., Bordas, J.M., Bravo, D., et al.: Sclerotherapy vs. distal splenorenal shunt in the elective treatment of variceal hemorrhage: A randomized controlled trial. Hepatology, *7:*430, 1987.
45. Warren, W.D., Henderson, J.M., Millikan, W.J., et al.: Distal splenorenal shunt versus endoscopic sclerotherapy for long-term management of variceal bleeding. Ann. Surg., *203:*454, 1986.
46. Barsoum, M.S., Khattar, N.Y., and Riskl-Allah, M.A.: Technical aspects of injection sclerotherapy of acute variceal hemorrhage as seen by radiography. Br. J. Surg., *65:*588, 1978.
47. Craaford, C., and Frenckner, P.: New surgical treatment of varicose veins of the esophagus. Acta Otolaryngol., *27:*422, 1939.
48. deDombal, F.T., Clarke, J.R., Clamp, S.E., et al.: Prognostic factors in UGI bleeding. Endoscopy, *18*(Suppl. 2):6, 1986.
49. Gilbert, G.A., Beulow, R.G., Chung, R.S.K., et al.: Technology assessment status evaluation: Endoscopic band ligation of varices. Gastrointest. Endosc., *37:*670, 1991.
50. Gimson, A.E., Ramage, J.K., Panos, M.Z., et al.: Randomized trial of variceal banding ligation versus injection sclerotherapy for bleeding esophageal varices. Lancet, *342:*391, 1993.
51. Goldschmiedt, M., Haber, G., and Kandel, G.: A safety maneuver for placing overtubes during endoscopic variceal ligation. Gastrointest. Endosc., *38:*399, 1992.
52. Graham, D.Y., and Smith, J.L.: The course of patients after variceal hemorrhage. Gastroenterology, *80:*800, 1981.
53. Guady, H., Rosman, A., and Korssen, M.: Prevention of stricture formation after endoscopic sclerotherapy of esophageal varices. Gastrointest. Endosc., *35:*377, 1989.
54. Guynn, T.P., Eckhauser, F.E., Knol, J.A., et al.: Injection sclerotherapy-induced esophageal strictures: Risk factors and prognosis. Am. Surg., *53:*567, 1991.
55. Hashizume, M., Ohta, M., Ueno, K., et al.: Endoscopic ligation of esophageal varices compared with injection sclerotherapy: A prospective randomized trial. Gastrointest. Endosc., *39:*123, 1993.
56. Infante-Rivard, C., Esnaola, S., and Villineuve, J.-P.: Role of endoscopic variceal sclerotherapy in the long-term management of variceal bleeding: A meta-analysis. Gastroenterology, *96:*1087, 1989.
57. Kochhar, R., Goenka, M.K., and Mehta, S.K.: Esophageal strictures following endoscopic variceal sclerotherapy: Antecedents, clinical profile and management. Dig. Dis. Sci., *37:*347, 1992.
58. Larson, G.M., Vandertoll, D.J., Netscher, D.T., and Polk, H.C.: Esophageal motility: Effects of injection sclerotherapy. Surgery, *96:*703, 1984.
59. Minoli, G.: Complications of endoscopic sclerotherapy of esophageal varices. Gastrointest. Endosc., *39:*221A, 1993.
60. Polson, R., Westaby, D.W., and Gimson, A.E.S.: Sucralfate for the prevention of early rebleeding following injection sclerotherapy for esophageal varices. Hepatology, *109:*279, 1989.
61. Stiegmann, G.V., and Goff, J.S.: Endoscopic esophageal varix ligation: Preliminary clinical experience. Gastrointest. Endosc., *34:*113, 1988.
62. Stiegmann, G.V., Goff, J.S., Michaletz-Onody, P.A., et al.: Endoscopic sclerotherapy compared with endoscopic ligation for bleeding esophageal varices. N. Engl. J. Med., *326:*1527, 1992.
63. Stiegmann, G.V., Sun, J.H., and Hammond, W.: Results of experimental endoscopic esophageal varix ligation. Am. Surg., *53:*246A, 1987.
64. Young, M.F., Sanowski, R.A., and Rasche, R.: Comparison and characterization of ulcerations induced by endoscopic ligation of esophageal varices versus endoscopic sclerotherapy. Gastrointest. Endosc., *39:*119, 1993.
65. Brems, J.J., Hiatt, J.R., and Klein, A.S.: Effect of a prior portosystemic shunt on subsequent liver transplantation. Ann. Surg., *209:*51, 1989.
66. Colapinto, R.F., Stronell, R.D., Gildiner, M., et al.: Formation of an intrahepatic portosystemic shunt using balloon dilatation catheter: Preliminary clinical experience. Am. J. Roentgenol., *140:*709, 1983.
67. Conn, H.O.: Transjugular intrahepatic portosystemic shunt: The state of the art. Hepatology, *17:*148, 1993.
68. Haag, K., Noeldge, G., and Sellinger, M.: Transjugular portosystemic shunt (TIPS): Monitoring of function by color duplex ultrasonography. Gastroenterology, *102:*817A, 1992.
69. Helton, W.S., Belshaw, A., Althaus, S., et al.: Critical appraisal of the angiographic portacaval shunt. Am. J. Surg., *165:*566, 1993.
70. Johansen, K.H.: Partial portal decompression for variceal hemorrhage. Am. J. Surg., *157:*479, 1989.
71. LaBerge, J.M., Ferrell, L.B., and Ring, E.J.: Histopathologic study of transjugular intrahepatic portosystemic shunts. J. Vasc. Intervent. Radiol., *2:*549, 1991.
72. Langnas, A.N., Marujo, W.C., Stratta, R.J., et al.: Influence of a prior portosystemic shunt on outcome after liver transplantation. Am. J. Gastroenterol., *87:*714–718, 1992.
73. Lopez, R.R., Benner, K.C., Hall, L., et al.: Expandable venous stents for treatment of Budd-Chiari Syndrome. Gastroenterology, *100:*1435, 1991.
74. Palmaz, J., Garcia, F., Sibbitt, R.R., et al.: Expandable intrahepatic portocaval shunt stents in dogs with chronic portal hypertension. Am. J. Roentgenol., *147:*1251, 1986.

75. Palmaz, J., Sibbitt, R.R., Reuter, S.R., et al.: Expandable intrahepatic portacaval stents: Early experience in the dog. Am. J. Roentgenol., *145:*821, 1985.
76. Peine, C.J., Freeman, M.L., Miller, R.P., et al.: Resolution of congestive gastropathy using transjugular intrahepatic portosystemic shunts. Hepatology, *16:*801A, 1992.
77. Pomier-Layragues, G., Legault, L., Roy, L., et al.: TIPS for treatment of refractory ascites: A pilot study. Hepatology, *18:*187A, 1993.
78. Reynolds, T.B., Donovan, A.J., Mikkelson, W.P., et al.: Results of a 12 year randomized trial of portacaval shunt in patients with alcoholic disease and bleeding varices. Gastroenterology, *80:*1005, 1981.
79. Ring, E.J., Lake, J.R., and Roberts, J.P.: Using transjugular intrahepatic portosystemic shunts to control variceal bleeding before liver transplantation. Ann. Intern. Med., *116:*304, 1992.
80. Rosch, J., Hanafee, W.N., and Snow, H.: Transjugular portal venography and radiological portosystemic shunt: An experimental study. Radiology, *92:*1112, 1969.
81. Sanyal, A.J., Freedman, A.M., and Shiffman, M.L.: Portosystemic encephalopathy following transjugular intrahepatic portosystemic stent (TIPS): A controlled study. Hepatology, *16:*85A, 1992.
82. Sanyal, A.J., Freedman, A.M., and Purdum, P.P.: Ann. Intern. Med., *117:*443, 1992.
83. Sarfeh, I.J., Rypins, E.B., and Mason, G.R.: A systematic appraisal of portacaval H-graft diameters: Clinical and hemodynamic perspective. Ann. Surg., *204:*356, 1986.
84. Schuman, B.M., Beckman, J.W., Tedesco, F.J., et al.: Complications of endoscopic injection sclerotherapy: A review. Am. J. Gastroenterol., *82:*823, 1987.
85. Sellinger, M., Haag, K., Ochs, A., et al.: Factors influencing the incidence of hepatic encephalopathy in patients with transjugular intrahepatic portosystemic stent-shunt (TIPS). Hepatology, *16:*122A, 1992.
86. Somberg, K.A., Lake, J.R., Doherty, M.H., et al.: The clinical course following TIPS in liver transplant candidates. Hepatology, *18:*186, 1993.
87. Stiegmann, G.V., Cambee, T., and Sun, J.H.: A new endoscopic elastic band ligating device. Gastrointest. Endosc., *32:*230, 1986.
88. Strauss, R.M., Martin, L.G., Kaufman, S.L., et al.: Role of TIPS in the primary management of refractory hydrothorax. Hepatology, *16:*162A, 1992.
89. Wood, R.P., Shaw, B.W., and Rikkers, L.F.: Liver transplantation for variceal hemorrhage. Surg. Clin. North. Am., *70:*449, 1990.
90. Woodle, E.S., Darcy, M., White, H.M., et al.: Intrahepatic portosystemic vascular stents: A bridge to hepatic transplantation. Surgery, *113:*344, 1993.

Splenic Transposition

91. Akita, H., and Sakoda, K.: Portopulmonary shunt by splenopneumopexy as a surgical treatment of Budd-Chiari syndrome. Surgery, *87:*85, 1980.
92. Auvert, J., Le Brigand, H., Seringe, P., et al.: Possibilities therapeutiques de la splenopexie intra-pulmonaire. Ann. Chir. Thorac. Cardiovasc., *5:*83, 1966.
93. Bourgeon, R., and Mouiel, J.: La chirurgie conservatrice de la rate: Splenorraphic, splenectomie partielle. Presse Med., *74:*303, 1966.
94. Del Guercio, L.R.M., Hodgson, W.J.B., and Morgan, J.C.: Splenic artery and coronary vein occlusion for bleeding esophageal varices. World J. Surg., *8:*680, 1984.
95. Hastbacka, J.: Thoracic transposition of the spleen for portal hypertension. Ann. Chir. Gynaecol., *60*(Suppl.):1, 1971.
96. Nylander, P.E.A., and Turunen, M.: Transposition of the spleen into the thoracic cavity in cases of portal hypertension. Ann. Surg., *142:*954, 1955.
97. Ono, J., Katsuki, T., and Kodama, Y.: Combined therapy for esophageal varices: Sclerotherapy, embolization and splenopneumopexy. Surgery, *101:*535, 1987.
98. Porter, B.A., Frey, C.F., Link, D.P., et al.: Splenic embolization monitored by video dilution technique. Am. J. Roentgenol., *141:*1063, 1983.
99. Turcotte, J.G., O'Neal, R.M., Zuidema, G.D., et al.: The effect of splenic transposition on the portal circulation. J. Surg. Res., *1:*299, 1961.
100. Turunen, M., and Autio, L.: Experimentelle und klinische Beobachtungen zur Verlagerung der Milz in die Brusthohle bei Pfortaderstauung. Zbl. Chir., *92:*1515, 1967.
101. Warren, W.D., Zeppa, R., and Fomon, J.J.: Selective trans-splenic decompression of gastroesophageal varices by distal splenorenal shunt. Ann. Surg., *166:*437, 1967.

Devascularization and Transection

102. Abouna, G.M., Baissony, H., Al-Nakib, B.M., et al.: The place of Sugiura operation for portal hypertension and bleeding esophageal varices. Surgery, *101:*91, 1987.
103. Barbot, D.J., and Rosato, E.F.: Experience with the esophagogastric devascularization procedure. Surgery, *101:*685, 1987.
104. Estes, N.C., and Pierce, G.E.: Late results of an extended devascularization procedure for patients with bleeding esophageal varices. Am. Surg., *50:*381, 1984.
105. Gouge, T.H., and Ranson, J.H.C.: Esophageal transection and paraesophagogastric devascularization for bleeding esophageal varices. Am. J. Surg., *151:*47, 1986.
106. Hassab, M.A.: Nonshunt operations in portal hypertension without cirrhosis. Surg. Gynecol. Obstet., *131:*648, 1970.
107. Orozco, H., Juarez, F., Uribe, M., et al.: Sugiura procedure outside Japan: The Mexican experience. Am. J. Surg., *152:*539, 1986.
108. Sugiura, M., and Futagawa, S.: A new technique for treating esophageal varices. J. Thorac. Cardiovasc. Surg., *56:*677, 1973.
109. Sugiura, M., and Futagawa, S.: Esophageal transection with paraesophagogastric devascularization in the treatment of esophageal varices. World J. Surg., *8:*673, 1984.
110. Wanamaker, S.R., Cooperman, M., and Carey, L.C.: Use of the EEA stapling instrument for control of bleeding esophageal varices. Surgery, *94:*621, 1983.

VOLUME

I

Miscellaneous Conditions

CHAPTER

29 Miscellaneous Conditions of the Esophagus

RICHARD I. WHYTE • ABE DEANDA, JR • MARK B. ORRINGER

PHARYNGOESOPHAGEAL OR CRICOPHARYNGEAL DYSFUNCTION (OROPHARYNGEAL DYSPHAGIA)

A variety of terms have been used to define a symptom complex in which a presumed functional abnormality of the upper esophageal, or cricopharyngeal, sphincter causes cervical dysphagia or a sensation of a "lump in the throat." In the past, terms such as *cricopharyngeal chalasia, achalasia*, or *spasm* have little more objective basis than the diagnosis of "globus hystericus" because standard esophageal manometry using perfused polyvinyl catheters have failed to demonstrate either true hypotonicity or hypertonicity of the upper esophageal sphincter (UES) or failure to relax with swallowing (achalasia). Technical advances in catheter design, with the development of balloon, directly transducing, and directional catheters, have improved the physiologic characterization of the region surrounding the UES.[92,144] Using these catheters, the length, position, and function of the cricopharyngeal sphincter can be characterized, and, based on these data, appropriate therapy can be chosen.[116,124] Manometric data can be combined with radiographic evaluation to better characterize the swallowing disorder. Because standard barium esophagograms often fail to demonstrate the rapid events of early deglutition, cineradiography should be employed. The combination of manometric and radiographic evaluation can now be used to identify patients with abnormal cricopharyngeal tonicity and coordination.

The anatomy and innervation of the UES is complex but explains much of the dysfunction encountered clinically. There appears to be a disparity between the anatomic location of the cricopharyngeus and the manometric high-pressure zone. The cricopharyngeus muscle appears to correspond to the distal third of the high-pressure zone, and the peak high-pressure zone appears to be located proximal to the cricopharyngeus muscle.[66] The UES is generally closed at all times, except during normal swallowing. It is composed of striated muscle, which has both sympathetic and parasympathetic innervation. The sympathetic fibers are branches of the cervical sympathetic chain. Parasympathetic innervation is derived from the vagus and includes branches from the recurrent laryngeal, glossopharyngeal, and bulbar roots of the spinal accessory nerves. Henderson has emphasized that a variety of disorders of the pharynx, cricopharynx, and upper third of the esophagus have common presenting symptoms because they involve the pharyngoesophageal junction as a unit.[84] He has classified pharyngoesophageal disorders into primary and secondary problems (Table 29-1).

The underlying cause of pharyngoesophageal dysphagia is often neurologic. Oculopharyngeal muscular dystrophy is a familial disease that often presents in late life with dysphagia and ptosis.[19,49,186] In these patients, the greatest problem is with poor pharyngeal contraction, although there is also abnormal cricopharyngeal function and upper esophageal motility. Impairment of swallowing with secondary choking and aspiration may follow strokes, particularly those involving the brain stem. Although swallowing may return to normal either spontaneously or with rehabilitation, some patients have persistent dysphagia. Nonvascular central nervous system abnormalities that may produce oropharyngeal dysphagia include amyotrophic lateral sclerosis,[102,109] bulbar poliomyelitis,[51] Parkinson's disease,[29,95] the Riley-Day syndrome, and, in children, Chiari malformations.[153]

Recurrent laryngeal nerve injury resulting from any cause—infectious neuritis, head and neck surgery (e.g., during thyroidectomy, laryngectomy, or mobilization of the cervical esophagus), radiation therapy, or recurrent tumor—interrupts vagal innervation of the UES and may result in incapacitating cervical dysphagia and/or aspiration[47,140] (Figs. 29-1 and 29-2).

In myasthenia gravis, particularly the bulbar form, impaired neural transmission to the skeletal muscle of the pharyngoesophageal junction results in cervical dyspha-

Table 29-1. Disorders of the Pharyngoesophageal Junction

- I. Primary
  - A. Myogenic
    - 1. Myotonia (muscular dystrophy)
    - 2. Thyrotoxic
  - B. Neurogenic
    - 1. Congenital: Riley-Day syndrome
    - 2. Acquired central
      - a. Stroke
      - b. Bulbar poliomyelitis
    - 3. Acquired peripheral-recurrent laryngeal nerve injury or neuritis
  - C. Myoneurogenic: myasthenia gravis
- II. Secondary
  - A. Gastroesophageal reflux
  - B. Caustic burns

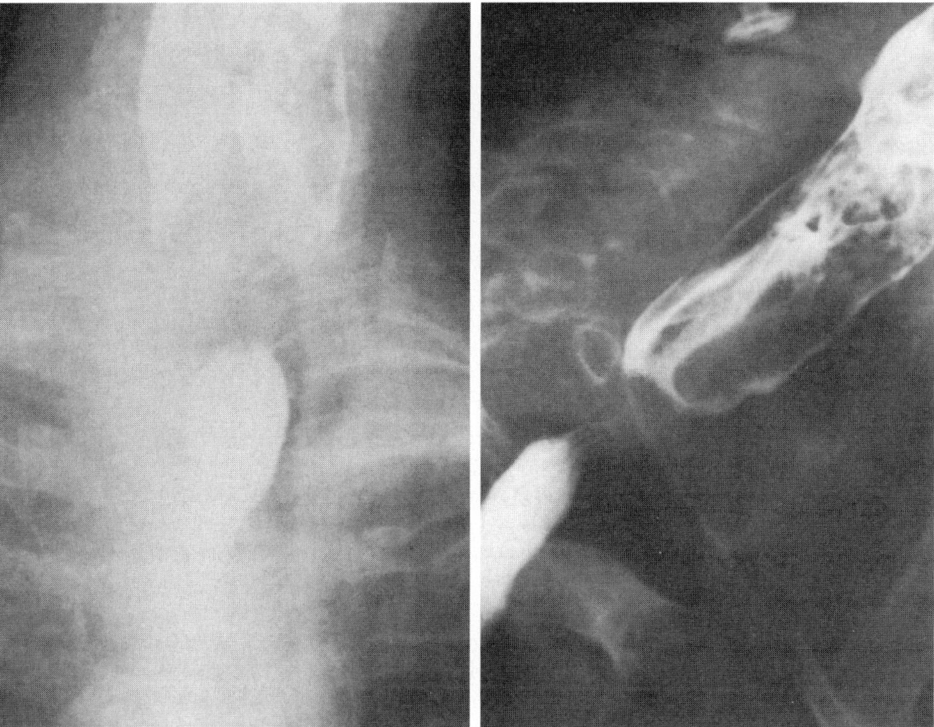

Figure 29–1. Cervical esophagogram in a patient with severe cervical dysphagia after a radical neck dissection with resection of the left recurrent laryngeal nerve. The posteroanterior *(left)* and lateral *(right)* views show marked constriction of the esophagus at the level of the C6 to C7 vertebral bodies, initially misdiagnosed as recurrent tumor. This patient had cricopharyngeal neuromotor dysfunction on the basis of injury to the recurrent laryngeal nerve.

gia with aspiration and nasopharyngeal regurgitation. Swallowing symptoms, like the muscle weakness elsewhere in the body, frequently become more noticeable as the day progresses. Successful treatment of the myasthenia with cholinergic drugs or thymectomy may relieve the difficulty swallowing.

In 10 to 15% of patients with gastroesophageal reflux, cervical dysphagia or a feeling of a lump in the throat is the presenting symptom. This discomfort may be referred from the distal esophagus, or it may represent reflex cricopharyngeal motor dysfunction (spasm) resulting from the reflux.

Dysphagia may also be a result of metabolic disorders and may be the presenting complaint of 5% of patients with thyrotoxicosis. In such cases, the abnormal cricopharyngeal motor function may be reversed with antithy-

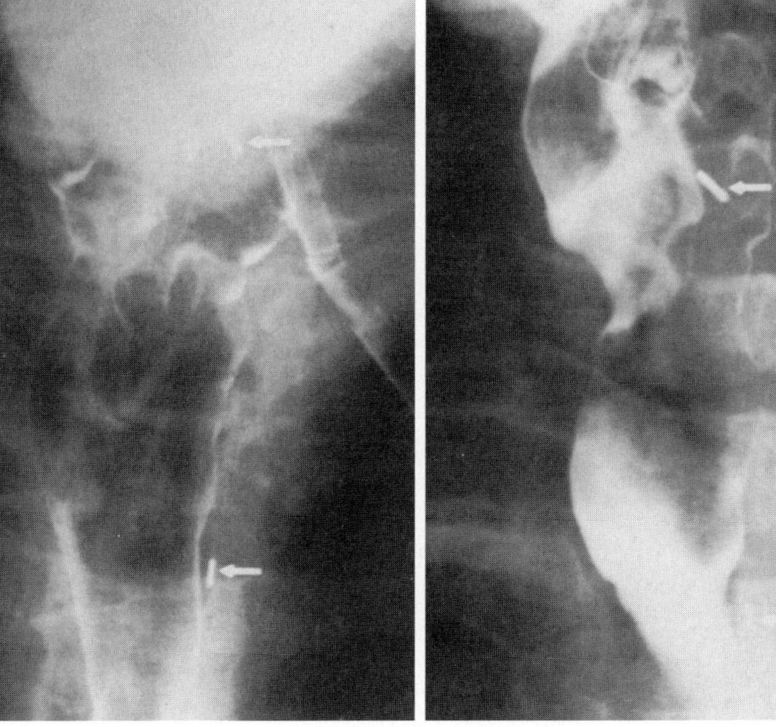

Figure 29–2. Cervical esophagogram after cervical esophagomyotomy in patient shown in Figure 29-1. Silver clips *(arrows)* mark the superior and inferior extents of the myotomy. The obstruction has been relieved.

roid medication.[24] Finally, when evaluating any patient with cervical dysphagia, however, other local causes for this complaint must be excluded: *extrinsic* compression of the esophagus by thyroid or parathyroid tissue (Figs. 29–3 and 29–4), cervical lymphadenopathy, or hyperostosis of the cervical spine (Fig. 29–5) and *intrinsic* compromise of the esophageal lumen by tumor, web, stricture, or abscess.

Regardless of the etiology, patients with cricopharyngeal dysfunction frequently present with a characteristic symptom complex: cervical dysphagia, expectoration of excessive saliva, intermittent hoarseness, and weight loss. Hoarseness may be caused by spasm of the inferior pharyngeal constrictor muscle, which acts on the alae of the thyroid cartilage and lengthens and tenses the vocal cords, and contraction of the cricopharyngeus, which pulls the cricoid cartilage posteriorly and stretches the vocal cords. Alternatively, hoarseness may be due to irritation of the vocal cords due to repeated episodes of aspiration.

The standard barium examination in the patient with cricopharyngeal dysfunction may reveal a spectrum of findings: an intermittently prominent upper sphincter (Fig. 29–6), a prominent posterior cricopharyngeal bar (Fig. 29–7), or Zenker's diverticulum. Although each of these findings may occur in patients without symptoms, even the more sensitive video-fluoroscopic examination may be normal in many patients with cervical dysphagia.[14]

The primary surgical therapy for cricopharyngeal dysphagia is cricopharyngeal myotomy. The operation is performed through a 5- to 6-cm long incision, centered at the level of the cricoid cartilage and paralleling the anterior border of the left sternocleidomastoid muscle (Fig. 29–8). The sternocleidomastoid muscle and carotid sheath are retracted laterally. A No. 40 French Maloney dilator in the esophagus aids in defining the posterolateral esophageal wall on which the subsequent myotomy is performed, well away from the recurrent laryngeal nerve in the tracheoesophageal groove. The vertical esophageal muscle fibers are incised initially for 1 to 2 cm, and a fine-tipped right angle clamp is then used to dissect the circular muscle fibers away from the submucosa as a needle-tip point electrocautery divides the muscle. Because the length of the upper esophageal sphincter is variable on manometric evaluation (and may be up to 5 to 7 cm long), a 7- to 10-cm extended esophagomyotomy should be performed to ensure complete relief of the functional obstruction (Fig. 29–9).

In appropriately selected patients, cervical esophagomyotomy may provide excellent relief of symptomatic cricopharyngeal dysfunction. Mason and colleagues pointed out that the best results are obtained when there is manometric evidence of defective sphincter opening and increased intrabolus pressure.[116] Poirier reported improved symptoms in 75% of 40 patients with myotomy and incapacitating oropharyngeal dysphagia of neurologic origin.[149a] In addition, he demonstrated decreased resting and closing pressures of the cricopharyngeal sphincter as a result of the myotomy. In cases of oculopharyngeal muscular dystrophy, cricopharyngeal myotomy cannot restore the strength of pharyngeal contraction; however, it

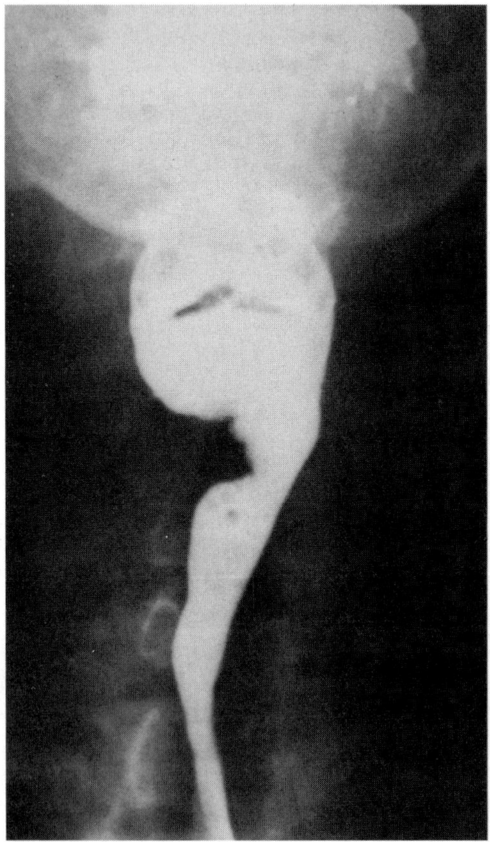

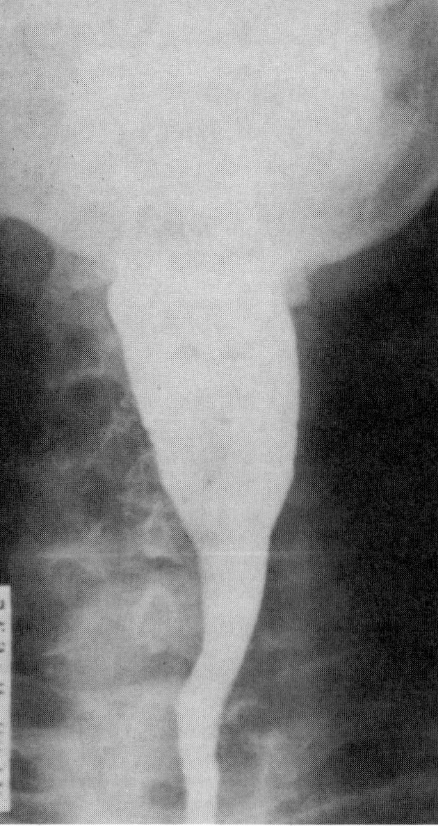

Figure 29–3. Cervical esophagogram showing an extrinsic right lateral mass *(left)*. An aberrant right lobe of the thyroid gland, which extended posterolateral to the esophagus, was found at exploration. After a right thyroid lobectomy *(right)*, the dysphagia was relieved. (From Orringer, M.B.: Diverticula and miscellaneous conditions of the esophagus. *In* Sabiston, D.C., Jr. [ed.]: Textbook of Surgery, Philadelphia, W.B. Saunders, 1986, p. 731, with permission.)

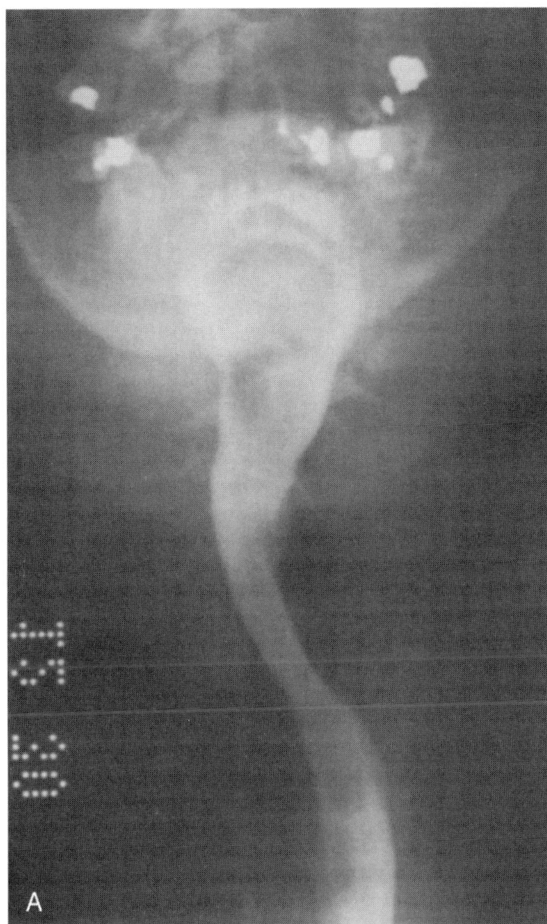

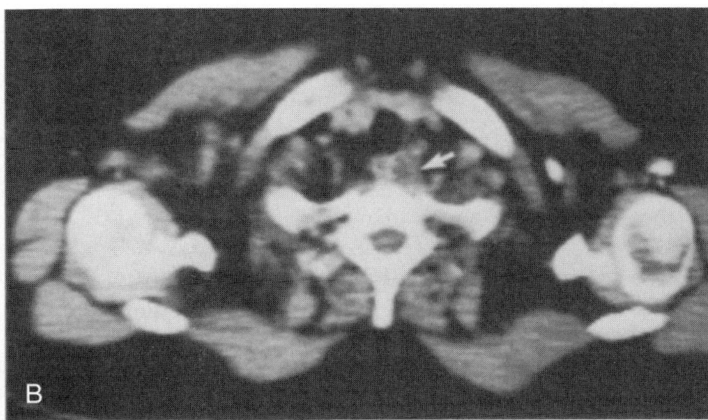

Figure 29–4. *A*, Cervical esophagogram in a young woman with cervical dysphagia. There is deviation of the esophagus toward the right side. *B*, Computed tomography scan shows a soft tissue mass *(arrow)* adjacent to the esophagus. This proved to be a parathyroid cyst, which was resected with a good result.

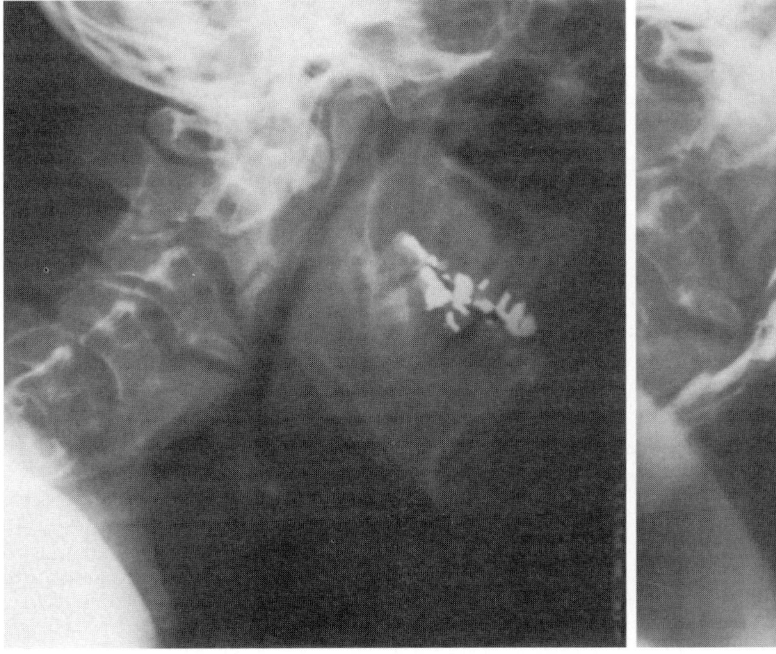

Figure 29–5. Anterior cervical vertebral osteophytes are evident on the lateral soft tissue view of the neck *(left)*. The barium esophagogram *(right)* shows the posterior impression on the cervical esophagus by the osteophytes. (From Orringer, M.B.: Diverticula and miscellaneous conditions of the esophagus. *In* Sabiston, D.C., Jr. [ed.]: Textbook of Surgery, Philadelphia, W.B. Saunders, 1986, p. 731, with permission.)

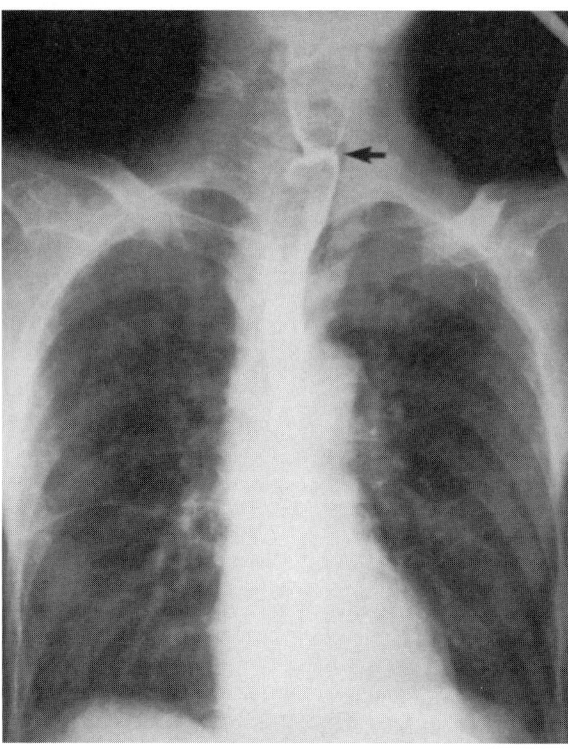

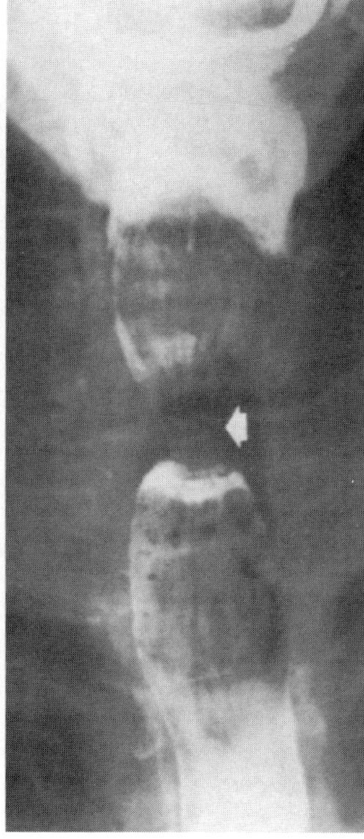

Figure 29–6. Barium esophagogram showing intermittent prominence of the cricopharyngeal sphincter *(arrows)* in a patient with cervical dysphagia and symptomatic gastroesophageal reflux. Cervical symptoms responded to an intensive anti-reflux medical regimen. (From Orringer, M.B.: Extended cervical esophagomyotomy for cricopharyngeal dysfunction. J. Thorac. Cardiovasc. Surg., *80*:669, 1980, with permission.)

can produce gratifying symptomatic improvement.[48,130,145] Furthermore, cricopharyngeal myotomy has repeatedly been helpful in cases of prolonged cervical dysphagia after stroke and in Parkinson's disease.[22,23,28,61,139]

In cases of amyotrophic lateral sclerosis (ALS), cricopharyngeal myotomy has been used with less predictable results. In a comparison of 13 ALS patients and controls, MacDougall and colleagues found no differences in pharyngoesophageal motility; however, in a subset of ALS patients with dysphagia, there was significantly reduced UES aftercontraction amplitude during water and bread swallows.[112] They concluded that the dysphagia of ALS may not be due to UES spasm and that treatment by cricopharyngeal myotomy may be inappropriate.

Cricopharyngeal dysphagia in the setting of gastroesophageal reflux often responds to a conservative antireflux medical regimen or a successful antireflux procedure. In 50% of 200 consecutive patients with symptomatic gastroesophageal reflux, Henderson found symptomatic pharyngoesophageal dysphagia that responded to antireflux surgery.[82] A subsequent cricopharyngeal myotomy for persistent cervical dysphagia was required in only 8 of 490 patients undergoing a hiatal hernia repair. Although Belsey has warned against performing cervical esophagomyotomy in a patient with gastroesophageal reflux because of the potential for massive aspiration from unrestrained reflux, Henderson achieved good relief of cervical dysphagia in five patients with

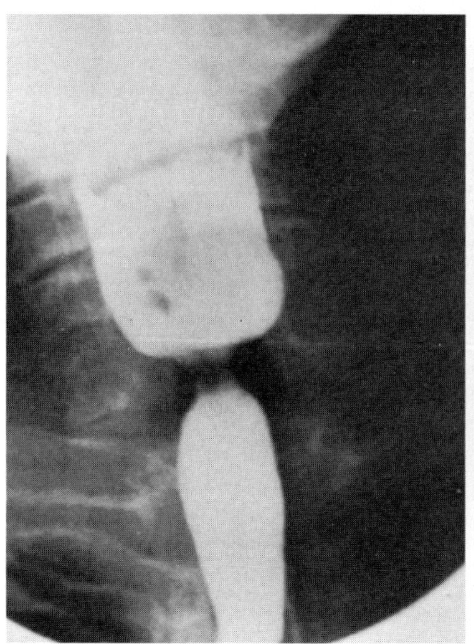

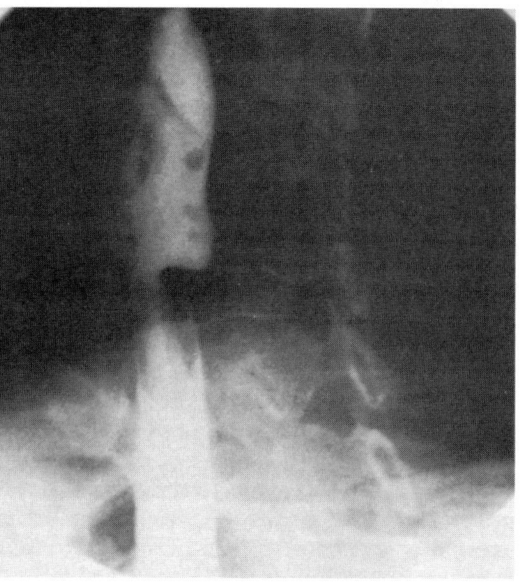

Figure 29–7. Posteroanterior *(left)* and lateral *(right)* barium swallow views showing a prominent cricopharyngeus sphincter. The criocopharyngeal bar extending from the posterior esophageal wall as seen on the lateral view is characteristic. (From Orringer, M.B.: Extended cervical esophagomyotomy for cricopharyngeal dysfunction. J. Thorac. Cardiovasc. Surg., *80*:669, 1980, with permission.)

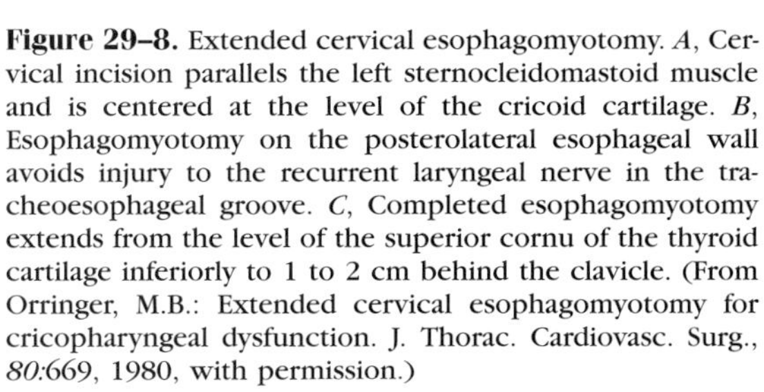
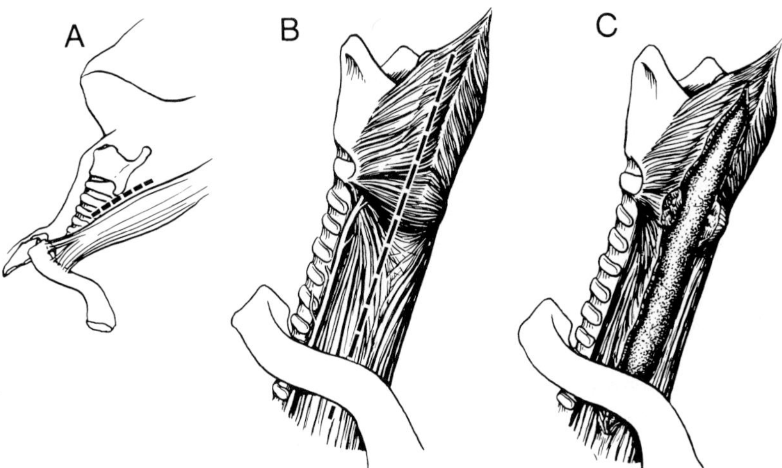

Figure 29–8. Extended cervical esophagomyotomy. *A*, Cervical incision parallels the left sternocleidomastoid muscle and is centered at the level of the cricoid cartilage. *B*, Esophagomyotomy on the posterolateral esophageal wall avoids injury to the recurrent laryngeal nerve in the tracheoesophageal groove. *C*, Completed esophagomyotomy extends from the level of the superior cornu of the thyroid cartilage inferiorly to 1 to 2 cm behind the clavicle. (From Orringer, M.B.: Extended cervical esophagomyotomy for cricopharyngeal dysfunction. J. Thorac. Cardiovasc. Surg., *80*:669, 1980, with permission.)

gastroesophageal reflux who were either too ill for an antireflux operation or had dominant cervical dysphagia with minimal symptoms of reflux.[18,83] In addition, Orringer reported seven patients with cervical dysphagia and abnormal gastroesophageal reflux who underwent a cervical esophagomyotomy, with either good or excellent results in six patients and no subsequent aspiration.[139] He indicated that only the minority of patients with gastroesophageal reflux actually regurgitate gastric contents to the level of the pharynx. Therefore, in some patients with objectively documented gastroesophageal reflux, cricopharyngeal dysfunction may be treated with a cervical esophagomyotomy and a strict antireflux medical regimen, resorting to an antireflux operation only if pulmonary symptoms from aspiration occur.

Other treatment options for cricopharyngeal dysphagia exist. Although dilational therapy has been employed in the past, there is now documented evidence of its efficacy both in improving dysphagia and in reducing UES pressures.[79] While dilation may produce less durable benefit that cricopharyngeal myotomy, the ease of the procedure may make it more desirable in certain patients. Another new therapy, injection of botulinum toxin, has been used successfully in small series of patients with cricopharyngeal dysphagia.[11,162] Finally, endoscopic laser myotomy was reported to be safe and effective in a series of 44 patients with cricopharyngeal dysfunction without Zenker's diverticulum.[107]

ESOPHAGEAL WEBS AND RINGS

Sideropenic Dysphagia (Plummer-Vinson or Patterson-Kelly Syndrome)

The term *sideropenic dysphagia* refers to the occurrence of cervical dysphagia in patients with iron deficiency

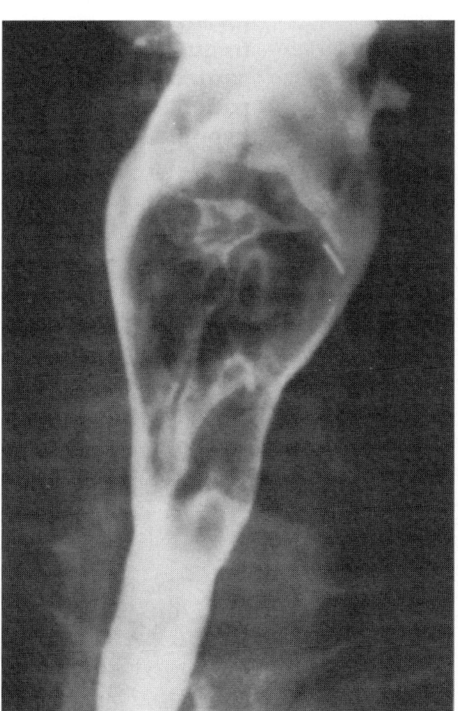
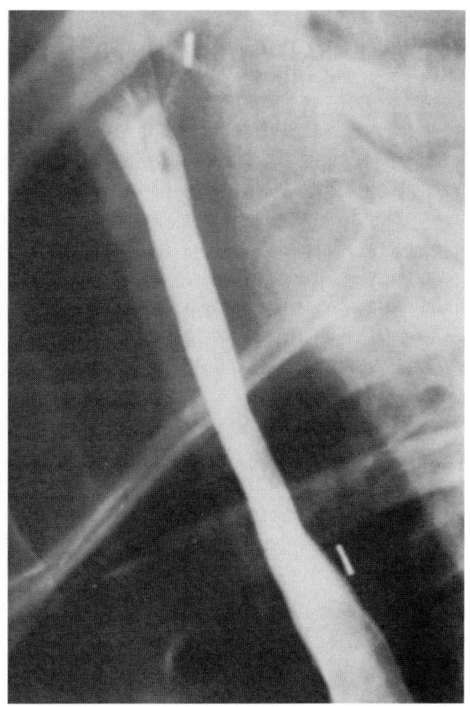

Figure 29–9. Barium esophagogram. Posteroanterior *(left)* and lateral *(right)* views in a patient with cricopharyngeal dysfunction (also shown in Figure 29–2) after extended cervical esophagomyotomy. The silver clips mark the superior and inferior limits of the myotomy. The obstructing posterior cricopharyngeal bar is no longer evident.

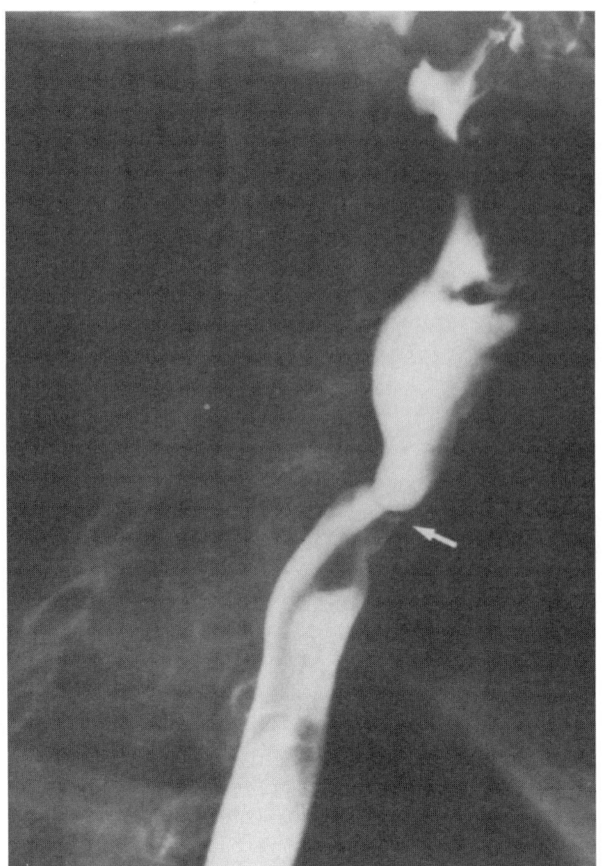

Figure 29–10. Cervical esophageal web *(arrow)* extending from the anterior esophageal wall. (From Orringer, M.B.: Diverticula and miscellaneous conditions of the esophagus. *In* Sabiston, D.C., Jr. [ed.]: Textbook of Surgery. Philadelphia, W.B. Saunders, 1986, p. 729, with permission.)

anemia. This condition was initially described by Brown Kelly[94] and Patterson[143] in England in 1919 and was then reported in the United States by Vinson (1922).[187] Plummer's role in the description of this condition is elusive, although his name has been associated with it since 1926.[169] The occurrence of a cervical esophageal web in many of these patients was recognized about 10 years later.[88] Recently, the incidence of Plummer-Vinson syndrome has declined—perhaps because of improved nutrition—and the very existence of a syndrome of sideropenic dysphagia has been questioned on the basis of a lack of convincing epidemiologic data.[15,34]

Although the syndrome may occur in men, most patients are postmenopausal women who are edentulous and have impaired oral intake. They develop iron deficiency anemia and demonstrate a smooth, reddened tongue (glossitis). The patients frequently present with cheilosis (fissures at the angles of the mouth). Atrophic oral mucosa and brittle spoon-shaped fingernails (koilonychia), achlorhydria, and splenomegaly were formerly common when poor dietary intake was responsible for vitamin deficiency. More recently, however, because patients can obtain adequate caloric intake with readily available liquid diet supplements, many of the changes of impaired nutrition are not seen with this syndrome. This syndrome has a high frequency in Scandinavia and Great Britain and is regarded as a premalignant lesion because nearly 10% of patients with this condition develop malignancies of the hypopharynx, oral cavity, or esophagus. The cause of dysphagia in patients with this syndrome is generally considered to be mechanical obstruction due to the upper esophageal web; however, some data suggest that altered pharyngeal and esophageal motility may also play a role.[41]

The radiographic demonstration of a cervical esophageal web may be extremely difficult because of the rapid passage of barium through the cervical esophagus with swallowing. The webs are typically demonstrated only in the active phase of swallowing and appear as thin membranous projections from the *anterior* esophageal wall near the cricopharyngeus sphincter (Fig. 29–10). They should not be confused with the cricopharyngeus muscle impression, which always presents as a posterior impression on the esophageal lumen (see Fig. 29–7).

The treatment of this condition is rupture of the web, using either bougienage or rigid endoscopy with dilation, and correction of the underlying nutritional deficiency, although resolution of symptoms may occur with iron replacement alone. Esophageal brushings and biopsies are warranted to exclude early carcinoma. Periodic esophageal dilations should be performed if dysphagia recurs, and surveillance esophagoscopy is indicated to monitor for the development of carcinoma.

Distal Esophageal Web (Schatzki's Ring)

Distal esophageal webs are frequently seen on esophageal contrast studies at the esophagogastric junction in patients with a sliding hiatal hernia. They give the appearance of an annular stricture projecting into the lumen at right angles to the long axis of the esophagus (Fig. 29–11). This radiographic abnormality was initially described by Templeton (1944), Schatzki and Gary (1953), and Ingelfinger and Kramer (1953).[90,161,177] Although many patients with this abnormality are asymptomatic, dysphagia may occur when the diameter of the ring is 20 mm or less and invariably occurs when the diameter is 13 mm or less.

On the basis of histologic studies of Schatzki's rings that were resected with the intent of relieving dysphagia, it is known that the rings characteristically occur at the squamocolumnar epithelial junction.[150] The upper surface of the ring is covered by squamous epithelium and the lower surface by columnar epithelium. The mucosa is mildly abnormal, showing acanthosis and occasional hyperkeratosis, but no ulceration. The greatest histologic changes occur deeper where there is submucosal infiltration of lymphocytes and plasma cells, increased vascularity, and distortion and fragmentation of the muscularis mucosa. Panmural fibrosis, as seen in reflux strictures, is not characteristic of Schatzki's rings.

Because the ring occurs at the squamocolumnar junction, the fact that it can be radiographically demonstrated above the diaphragm indicates that a hiatal hernia exists. A Schatzki's ring therefore indicates *only* that there is a hiatal hernia, not that there is either gastroesophageal

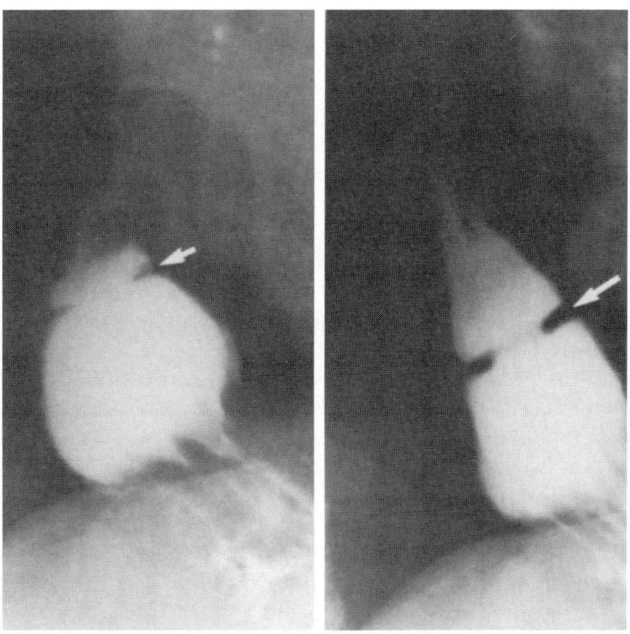

Figure 29–11. Distal esophageal (Schatzki's) ring *(arrows)* occurring at its characteristic location at the esophagogastric junction above a sliding hiatal hernia. (From Orringer, M.B.: Diverticula and miscellaneous conditions of the esophagus. *In* Sabiston, D.C., Jr. [ed.]: Textbook of Surgery. Philadelphia, W.B. Saunders, 1986, p. 729, with permission.)

reflux or esophagitis. It may be difficult to differentiate a Schatzki's ring from a localized reflux stricture.

In patients with symptomatic rings and minimal or no reflux symptoms, excellent results are obtained with intermittent esophageal dilatation. The addition of an antireflux medical regimen is also necessary. In patients whose reflux symptoms fail to respond to conservative therapy or in whom dilations are not well tolerated, intraoperative dilation in association with an antireflux procedure provides excellent results. Resection of the ring alone without repair of the associated hiatal hernia *should not* be carried out.

Multiple Esophageal Webs

The condition of multiple esophageal webs is uncommon and does not have a clear etiology. Although occurring as isolated cases, we have seen one case of familial multiple esophageal webs (Fig. 29–12), a condition that has been reported only once in the literature.[78] Generally, multiple esophageal webs respond well to dilation; however, our patient presented with a distal esophageal perforation after dilation and underwent successful esophagectomy.

MALLORY-WEISS SYNDROME (EMETOGENIC MUCOSAL LACERATION)

In the process of forceful vomiting against the closed glottis, the rapid increase in intra-abdominal pressure is transmitted to the esophagus, where a mucosal laceration at the esophagogastric junction may occur.[113,190] This condition, called *Mallory-Weiss syndrome*, has been reported in children through patients in their 80s, but most patients are in their 40s. It occurs three to five times more commonly in men and is responsible for 5 to 15% of the cases of acute upper gastrointestinal hemorrhage.[97,174] Although alcoholic debauch and vomiting were originally incriminated as causative factors in this condition, it is now recognized that neither vomiting nor alcohol consumption need be present for these mucosal tears to occur. Thus, Mallory-Weiss syndrome has been reported after vigorous coughing, status asthmaticus, childbirth, epileptic seizure, or closed chest cardiac massage. Vomiting is still the leading precipitating event, and this has been attributed to alcohol (or other drug ingestion), peptic ulcer disease, uremia, pancreatitis, cholecystitis, upper gastrointestinal endoscopy, myocardial infarction, and pregnancy. Cadaver studies have documented esophageal mucosal tears with an intragastric pressure of 150 mm Hg.[10] Mucosal tears occur before esophageal muscular tears.[108] Underlying mucosal disease, such as atrophic gastritis or reflux esophagitis, may predispose to the tear, and about 30% of patients have a history of recent use of nonsteroidal anti-inflammatory drugs. The typical Mallory-Weiss laceration is longitudinal and extends through the mucosa and into the submucosa. Although usually single,

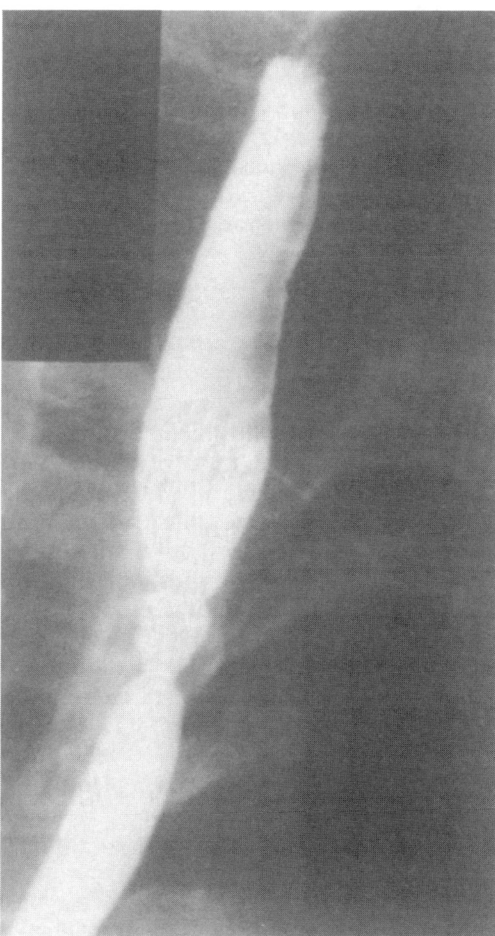

Figure 29–12. Lateral esophagogram of a 19-year-old man with familial multiple esophageal webs. His two upper thoracic esophageal webs are shown.

two to three tears may occur. Most lacerations occur just distal to the esophagogastric junction, although about 10% extend into the esophagus. Rarely is the tear confined to the esophagus.

Hematemesis occurs in 85% of patients with Mallory-Weiss syndrome. Furthermore, about half of patients have an antecedent history of vomiting.[77] Unlike Boerhaave's syndrome, bleeding from Mallory-Weiss tears is usually painless.

After stabilization of the patient, fiberoptic gastroscopy should be performed to evaluate the cause of upper gastrointestinal hemorrhage. In 50 to 80% of patients, active bleeding has stopped by the time of endoscopy. Radiographic evaluation, such as a barium contrast study, rarely provides diagnostic information, although other potential causes of bleeding may be discovered. At times, selective celiac arteriography demonstrates the bleeding site if the rate of blood loss is great enough at the time of the study.

Treatment of most patients with Mallory-Weiss syndrome consists of intravenous volume replacement, nasogastric tube decompression of the stomach, and treatment with histamine-2 blockers or proton pump inhibitors to allow the mucosal laceration to heal. In patients who have active bleeding at the time of endoscopy, bleeding can usually be controlled with cauterization, heater probe application, or injection sclerotherapy.[16,142,175] Other procedures that have been tried with varying degrees of success include systemic vasopressin[42,123,179] and transcatheter embolization.[31,105] Placement of a Sengstaken-Blakemore tube has been advocated in the past but now is thought to be contraindicated for fear of propagating the mucosal tear.

In the relatively small percentage of patients with massive hemorrhage from a Mallory-Weiss tear, the operative approach is a transabdominal one using a table-mounted upper-hand retractor to facilitate exposure of the esophagogastric junction. The distal esophagus and upper stomach are mobilized, and a proximal gastrotomy is performed for inspection of the cardia. After evacuation of the clots, the tear is identified and oversewn. Identification of the tear may be facilitated by intraoperative gastroscopy or use of a laparoscope passed through the gastrotomy. Surgical treatment of Mallory-Weiss syndrome is highly effective, and recurrence of bleeding is unusual. The reported overall mortality rate for Mallory-Weiss syndrome is less than 5%. It is significantly higher, however, in patients requiring operative control of bleeding—perhaps because this represents a select group of patients, some with coexistent liver disease resulting in coagulopathy and portal hypertension.

DISSECTING INTRAMURAL HEMATOMA (ESOPHAGEAL APOPLEXY)

Hemorrhage can occur within the wall of the esophagus and result in an intramural hematoma. When this occurs spontaneously, the term *esophageal apoplexy* has been used,[176] although development of an intramural hematoma can also be due to trauma, such as with foreign-body impaction (food or pills) or injection sclerotherapy. Spontaneous intramural esophageal hemorrhage was first described in 1968[114] and has been reported sporadically since. The condition is frequently associated with a history of gastroesophageal reflux but may be due to propagation of a Mallory-Weiss tear. There is also an association between intramural hematoma and abnormal coagulation.[9,33]

The clinical presentation of esophageal apoplexy is one of substernal or epigastric pain and dysphagia. Hypotension, tachycardia, and diaphoresis may be present, but these signs are more suggestive of mediastinitis secondary to an esophageal perforation. The barium esophagogram may demonstrate a double-barrel appearance corresponding to the true and false lumens of the esophagus, or may simply show a mass-like obstruction.[63] Endoscopy may demonstrate an area of bulging mucosa or discoloration from submucosal bleeding. Treatment is generally nonoperative, and patients can be managed with intravenous hydration and the withholding of oral intake until healing of mucosal tear has occurred and lack of further progression of the hematoma has been documented with an esophagogram.[146] Endoscopic treatment involving internal drainage of the hematoma has also been reported.[13]

INFECTIOUS ESOPHAGITIS

Infectious esophagitis, rare in healthy people, is generally associated with debilitation, immunosuppression, or prolonged antibiotic usage. The most common form of infectious esophagitis is that caused by *Candida albicans*; however, with the progression of the acquired immunodeficiency syndrome (AIDS) epidemic, esophageal infections caused by other fungi (*Torulopsis* and *Histoplasma* species), viruses (cytomegalovirus [CMV], herpes simplex virus [HSV], and Epstein-Barr virus), mycobacteria, and protozoa (*Cryptosporidia* and *Pneumocystis* species) have been reported.[134,193] Finally, the role of *Helicobacter pylori* in reflux esophagitis is under investigation.[74]

Monilial Esophagitis

C. albicans, a fungus that is normally a commensal inhabitant of the mouth, oropharynx, and gastrointestinal tract, may become pathogenic in severely debilitated or immunosuppressed patients and produce esophagitis. In its initial stages, acute monilial esophagitis with oropharyngeal involvement generally presents with painful swallowing. Progression of the disease into the thoracic esophagus results in abnormal esophageal peristalsis and often spasm. Inflammation and edema of the submucosa result in the "cobblestone" pattern of luminal nodularity seen radiographically.[65,69] As acute monilial esophagitis progresses, mucosal ulceration with an irregular, shaggy appearing, narrowed esophageal lumen due to mucosal and submucosal edema and pseudomembrane formation can be seen on the barium swallow examination. Endoscopically, the esophageal mucosa is initially erythematous and non-ulcerated and has an overlying whitish exudate or pseudomembrane. With progression of the inflammatory reaction into the wall of the esophagus, the mucosa becomes more granular and friable. Panmural invasion of the esophageal wall can be controlled by antifungal therapy, but healing of the inflamed esophagus may result in chronic stricture formation.[138,166] Because submucosal esophageal glands tend to be more numerous in the upper half of the esophagus, the inflammatory reaction that involves these glands is responsible for the greater frequency of monilial esophageal strictures in the upper half of the thoracic esophagus. The term *intramural esophageal pseudodiverticulosis* has been used to describe the dilation and outpouching of the esophageal submucosal glands that are inflamed from associated infection, stasis, or distal obstruction[121,191] (Fig. 29-13).

Acute monilial esophagitis should be considered in debilitated, postoperative, and immunosuppressed patients with odynophagia. Treatment depends on the patient's immune status and the extent of the infection. For infections that are mild or that occur in normal or minimally immune-suppressed patients, initial therapy consists of clotrimazole, 100 mg three to five times daily, or nystatin suspension, 1 to 3 million units every 6 hours. This generally relieves symptoms and controls the infection within 1 week. Acceptable alternatives include oral amphotericin lozenges, ketoconazole, and fluconazole. For more advanced infections or those occurring in more immune-suppressed patients (i.e., those with AIDS), higher doses of fluconazole (100 to 200 mg orally once daily) or itraconazole are indicated. For patients with fluconazole-resistant candidal infection, itraconazole and amphotericin B oral suspension can be used.[185] Intravenous fluconazole or amphotericin may be necessary for granulocytopenic patients.[119]

Other Forms of Infectious Esophagitis

After candidal esophagitis, viral infection is the second most common cause of infectious esophageal disease. Cytomegalovirus is the most common viral infection in human immunodeficiency virus (HIV)-positive patients, whereas in immunosuppressed transplant recipients, HSV is more common.[193] Viral infections of the esophagus typically produce mucosal ulceration, and as with other forms of esophagitis, dysphagia and odynophagia are common symptoms. In patients with viral esophagitis, the barium esophagogram may show single or multiple discrete ulcerations with areas of intervening normal mucosa. CMV esophageal ulcers are frequently large, whereas HSV ulcers are generally small (less than 1.5 cm). Endoscopic evaluation is crucial for an accurate diagnosis because specimens can be taken for histology, cytology, and viral culture. Mycobacterial disease of the esophagus is rare but may be caused by either *Mycobacterium tuberculosis* or *Mycobacterium avium-intracellulare*.[57,129]

Surgical Complications of Esophageal Infection

Surgical complications of esophageal infection include bleeding (from ulceration), perforation, and development of a bronchoesophageal fistula.[4,36,60] Because of the possibility of the development of an esophageal stricture after an acute monilial esophageal infection of the esophagus, patients recovering from severe acute monilial esophagitis should be followed during the first year to ensure the earliest possible detection of a developing stricture as

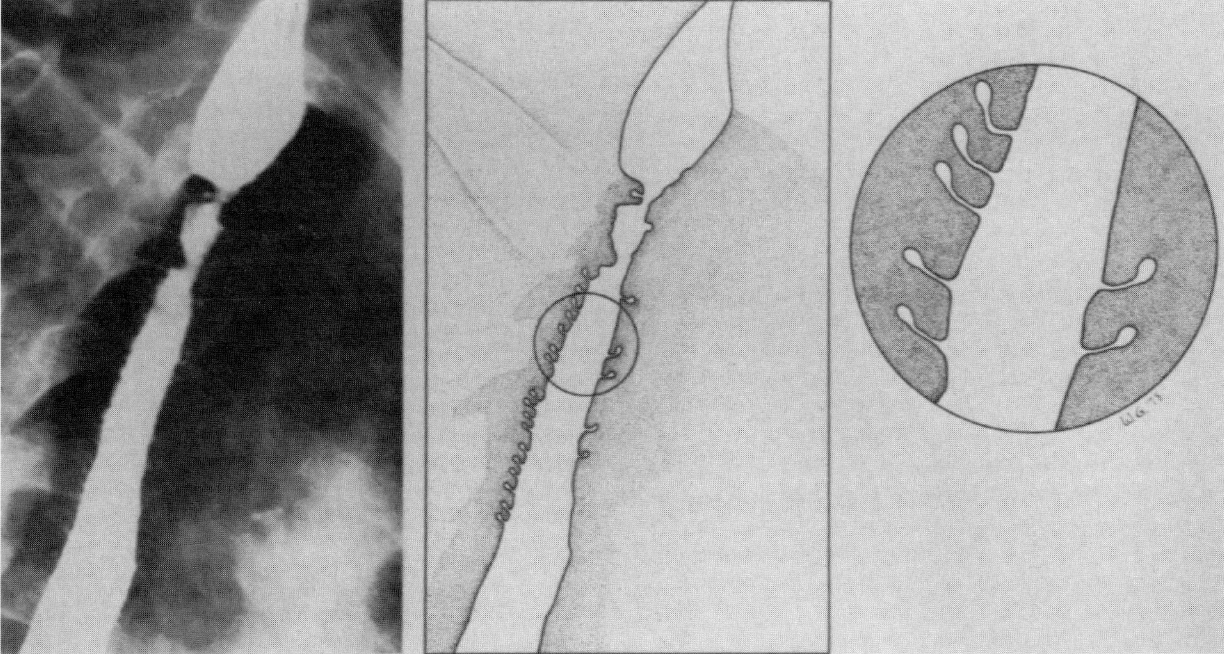

Figure 29-13. Esophagogram *(left)* and line-drawing interpretation *(center* and *right)* of irregular upper thoracic esophageal stricture due to monilial esophagitis. The small outpouchings (intramural pseudodiverticulosis) are dilated submucosal esophageal glands. (From Orringer, M.B., and Sloan, H.: Monilial esophagitis: An increasingly frequent cause of esophageal stenosis? Ann. Thorac. Surg., *26*:364, 1978, with permission.)

well as prompt institution of dilation therapy. In AIDS patients with ulcerative esophagitis, esophageal strictures are rare.[192]

GIANT FIBROEPITHELIAL ESOPHAGEAL POLYP

Esophageal polyps follow leiomyoma as the second most common benign tumor of the esophagus.[148,151] Nearly 80% arise in the cervical esophagus and develop a progressively longer stalk as peristaltic action pulls the polyp distally. These polyps may grow to unusually large size and may have a dramatic clinical presentation when regurgitated into the posterior pharynx, larynx, or mouth. Respiratory obstruction may result. The patient typically presents with dysphagia and regurgitation. The barium swallow shows a huge filling defect, which may simulate an extensive malignancy (Fig. 29–14). Because the polyp is covered by normal mucosa and is soft and mobile, it may be missed at esophagoscopy. Histologically, these tumors contain loose fibrous and myxomatous cells and fat and may be designated fibrovascular polyps, fibroma, myxoma, fibrolipoma, or hamartoma. Treatment is complete removal of the polyp, including the base of the stalk. Although small polyps may be removed using an endoscopic snare and coagulation, this approach is inap-

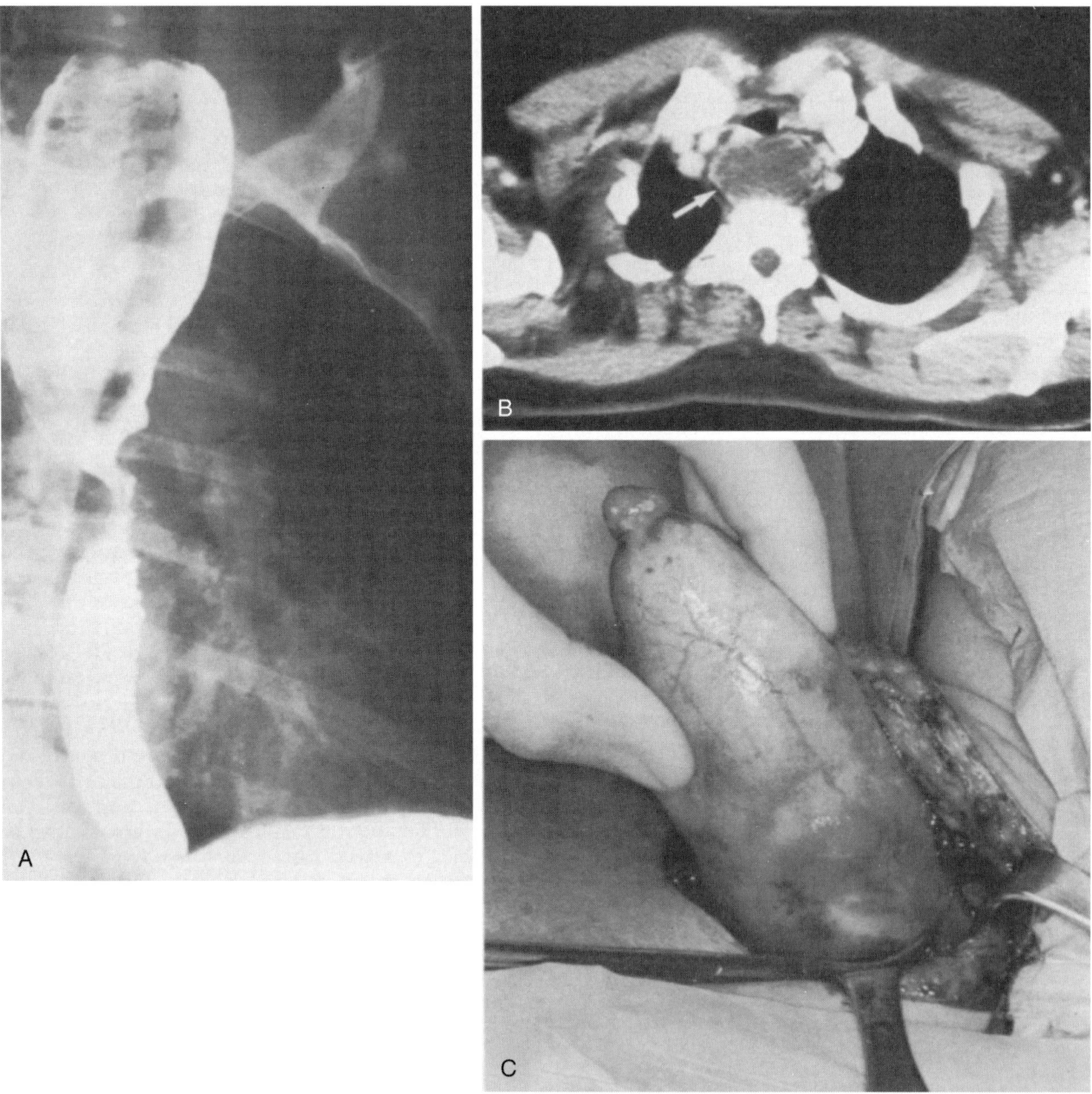

Figure 29–14. *A*, Barium esophagogram in a 37-year-old woman with progressive cervical dysphagia. A large intraluminal mass distending the cervical and upper thoracic esophagus is seen. *B*, Computed tomography scan shows a huge mass in the esophagus *(arrow)*. *C*, Operative photograph of the patient shown in *A* and *B* showing a giant benign fibroepithelial polyp delivered out of the left cervical incision. The patient's head is toward the right, and the retractors are against the sternocleidomastoid muscle. The hemostat points to the base of the polyp, which was elliptically excised.

propriate for giant polyps, which require an esophagostomy. Resection is curative if total removal of the base, which may be quite wide, is achieved.

CARDIOVASCULAR CAUSES OF DYSPHAGIA

Dysphagia may be the result of esophageal compression by vascular rings, cardiac enlargement, and aortic aneurysms (Fig. 29–15). Vascular rings are developmental abnormalities of the aorta and great vessels that form a circle (either complete or incomplete) and constrict the esophagus and trachea. Although there are numerous anatomic variations, the most common types involve right arch with aberrant left subclavian artery and double aortic arch.[35,53,71] The term *dysphagia lusoria* was used by Bayford in 1794 in reference to a patient who died of starvation secondary to severe dysphagia and, at autopsy, was found to have an anomalous right subclavian artery originating from the descending aorta and coursing between the esophagus and trachea. More commonly associated with dysphagia is a left arch with an anomalous right subclavian artery coursing behind the esophagus. Although not a true vascular ring, the esophagus can be compressed with resulting dysphagia.

The diagnosis of a vascular ring can generally be made by an esophagogram.[35] The characteristic finding of an aberrant right subclavian artery on barium swallow examination is an indentation of the posterior esophagus high in the thorax caused by the artery. Angiography, computed tomography, echocardiography, or magnetic resonance imaging may also be useful. The treatment of vascular rings generally involves a left thoracotomy; thorough mobilization of the aortic arch, subclavian artery, and ligamentum arteriosum (or patent ductus arteriosus); and division of the ring. This essentially always involves division of the ligamentum arteriosum but may also involve division of a double aortic arch. The initially described approach to patients with a left arch and an aberrant right subclavian artery involved ligation and division of the aberrant artery.[70] Although this treatment is still applicable in infants, adults so treated may develop subclavian steal syndrome, and reimplantation of the artery is indicated.[128] In adults, the anomaly can be corrected through a median sternotomy or thoracotomy.[12,104]

Another cardiovascular cause of dysphagia is left atrial enlargement due to rheumatic mitral valvular disease. In such cases, medical management may relieve the symptoms.[43] Esophageal obstruction due to left ventricular enlargement compressing the esophagus against a tortuous thoracic aorta has also been reported.[103] Tortuosity or aneurysmal dilatation of the descending thoracic aorta can also cause esophageal obstruction; treatment is directed to repair of the aneurysm.[37,75,93,100,159]

CERVICAL VERTEBRAL EXOSTOSES

Cervical dysphagia may be caused by anterior displacement of the esophagus by cervical vertebral body osteo-

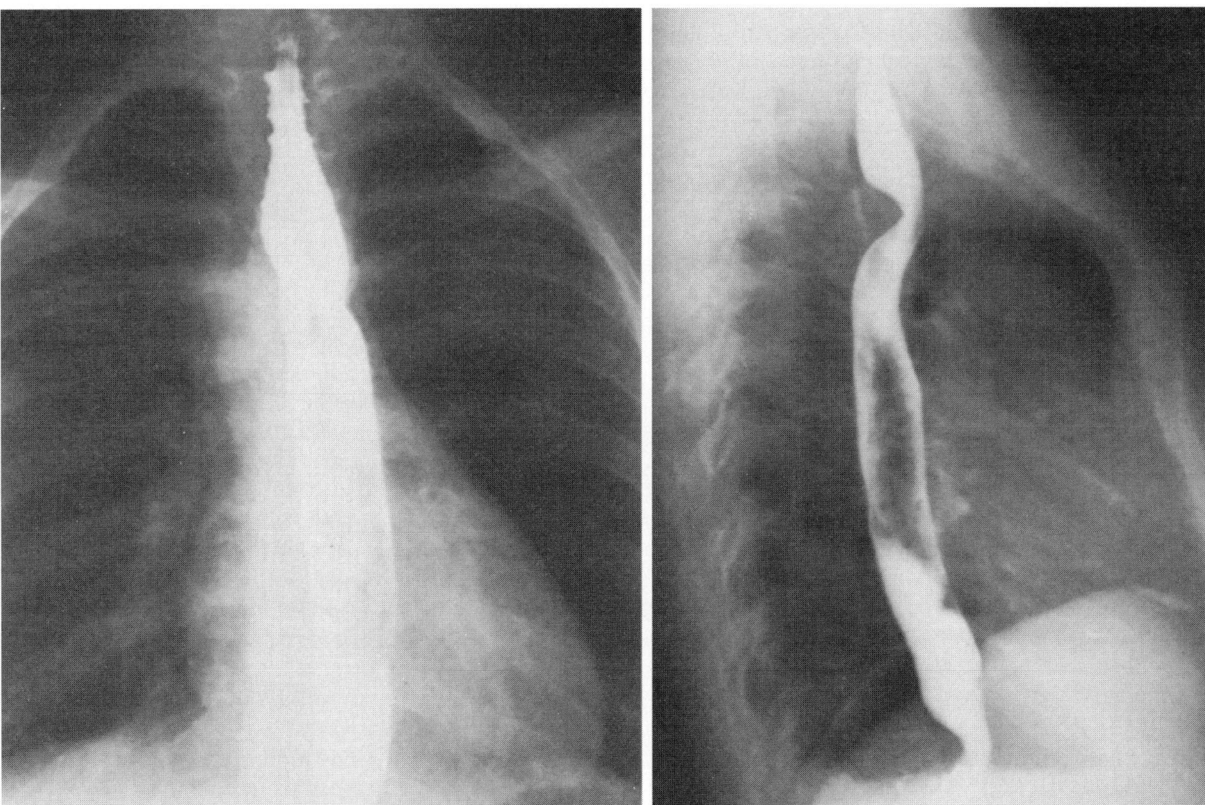

Figure 29–15. Posteroanterior *(left)* and lateral *(right)* barium esophagogram views in a young woman with dysphagia and a right-sided aortic arch from which the left subclavian artery arose. The posterior impression on the esophagus by the aberrant blood vessel is seen on the lateral view.

phytic spurs.[17,30,80,132,152] These exostoses generally arise from the fifth, sixth, and seventh cervical vertebral bodies and displace the esophagus from behind. The earliest report of dysphagia associated with cervical exostosis was by Mosher in 1926.[132] Painful swallowing and hoarseness can also result.[17,80] Injury to the cervical esophagus during performance of rigid esophagoscopy in such patients is obviously more dangerous; however, perforation with the flexible fiberoptic esophagoscope has also been described.[194] These patients typically complain of cervical dysphagia that is worse when the neck is extended. There may be associated pain on swallowing that occasionally radiates to the shoulders and arms. The lateral cervical spine views demonstrate the exostoses, and impingement on the esophageal lumen is demonstrated with the barium swallow (see Fig. 29-10). These patients are frequently elderly, and before attributing symptoms of dysphagia to degenerative changes in the cervical spine, the presence of an esophageal tumor must be excluded. Resection of the vertebral body exostosis through an anterior cervical approach has been reported to provide excellent results.[30,120,152]

INVOLVEMENT OF THE ESOPHAGUS BY SECONDARY MALIGNANCIES

Secondary involvement of the esophagus by nonesophageal neoplasms, a topic reviewed by Herrera, is a relatively uncommon occurrence.[85] Although both direct invasion by an adjacent extraesophageal neoplasm and metastasis from a more distant primary tumor are possible, the former is significantly more common.[180] Many tumors are capable of metastasizing to the esophagus, although carcinomas of the breast, stomach, and lung predominate. Other tumors that have been reported to metastasize to the esophagus include tumors of the pharynx, prostate, bladder, kidney, and ovary. Subcarinal lymph node metastases, from bronchogenic carcinoma or breast cancer, may secondarily involve, or displace, the esophagus and produce dysphagia[171] (Fig. 29-16).

Metastases to the esophagus may be insidious in their clinical presentation because there are few early signs of invasion of the esophageal wall from without and because these tumors tend to remain intramural. Thus, endoscopic biopsies of the overlying intact mucosa may fail to establish the diagnosis. Finally, in breast and ovarian tumors, the interval between the primary tumor and development of esophageal metastases may be several decades.[8,127,184] Consequently, in women with a history of breast carcinoma, no matter how remote, a complaint of dysphagia should raise the possibility of metastasis to mediastinal lymph nodes or to the wall of the esophagus.[86,99,149] Lymphomatous involvement of the esophagus may result in a tracheoesophageal fistula; more recently, mycosis fungoides of the esophagus has been reported.[68,156,164]

ESOPHAGEAL INVOLVEMENT IN MEDIASTINAL FIBROSIS

Mediastinal fibrosis, a sclerosing fibrous reaction of the tissues of the mediastinum, is a poorly understood condition that has been described by a variety of terms, including idiopathic mediastinal fibrosis, fibrosing mediastinitis, chronic fibrous mediastinitis, sclerosing fibrosis, and sclerosing mediastinitis.[73,111,173] A variety of etiologies have been incriminated in this process, including syphilis, tuberculosis, histoplasmosis, coccidioidomycosis, asbestos exposure, autoimmune disease, hypersensitivity reaction, drug reaction to methysergide taken for migraine headache, and periaortitis from advanced arteriosclerotic disease.[44,67,91,106,126,188] Pathologically, the mediastinum is infiltrated by dense fibrous tissue containing hyalinized collagen, numerous fibroblasts, and scattered inflammatory cells.[3] The fibrous tissue may involve adjacent blood vessels, fat, and nerves. Calcification and dense hyalinization of the collagen occur in the late stages of the disease.[26] Patients typically present with symptoms related to compression of a vital mediastinal organ. Superior vena caval obstruction,[26,54] left ventricular failure,[141,147] chylothorax,[25] constrictive pericarditis,[7,21] coronary artery occlusion,[157] tracheobronchial obstruction,[106] and dysphagia due to esophageal obstruction[3,46,73] have been reported. The etiology of the obstruction seen on barium swallow and endoscopy is difficult to diagnose because it is extrinsic to the esophagus. Mediastinoscopy and biopsy of the abnormal fibrous tissue may help to exclude neoplasm, but in the presence of superior vena caval obstruction, great care must be taken to avoid hemorrhage. There is no reliably successful medical therapy for this condition, although ketaconazole and tamoxifen have been reported to be successful in a few patients.[160,181] Surgical treatment involves resection of associated mediastinal granulomas and mobilization of the encased esophagus.[3,73] Involvement of other vital structures is generally the life-limiting aspect of this condition.

ESOPHAGEAL INVOLVEMENT IN DERMATOLOGIC DISORDERS

Squamous epithelium of the esophagus, like that of the skin, may be affected by a number of dermatologic disorders.[20,62,76,155,165,167] Vesiculation with subsequent formation of thin webs has been reported in pemphigus vulgaris, bullous pemphigoid, and benign mucous membrane pemphigoid. Esophageal dilation should be instituted early in the course of the disease when the patient complains of dysphagia or painful swallowing to prevent the late development of dense, more severe strictures. Similar vesiculobullous lesions of the esophagus have been reported in patients after bone marrow transplantation—probably as a result of graft-versus-host disease.[125] Epidermolysis bullosa dystrophica is a rare genetic skin disease that, unlike other of the bullous dermatoses, is inherited and typically begins early in life. Severe blistering of the mucous membranes may ultimately result in stricture formation, is frequently associated with dysphagia, and may result in esophageal perforation.[89] Dilation therapy is extremely important in the maintenance of comfortable swallowing.

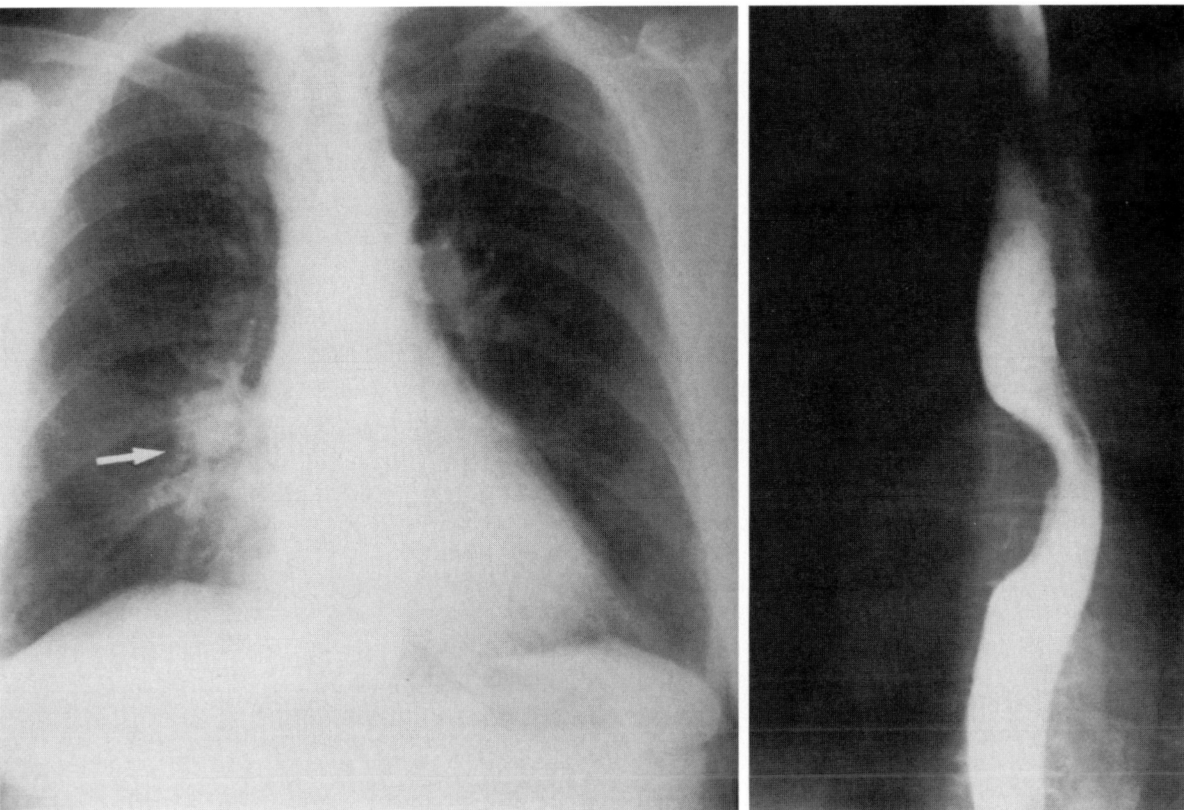

Figure 29–16. Chest radiograph *(left)* of a 60-year-old smoker who presented with dysphagia and a right infrahilar mass *(arrow)*. He had bronchogenic adenocarcinoma with metastases to subcarinal lymph nodes, which were displacing the mid esophagus, as seen on the barium esophagogram *(right)*.

ACQUIRED TRACHEOESOPHAGEAL FISTULAS

Nonmalignant Fistulas

Acquired fistulas between the esophagus and the tracheobronchial tree are relatively rare and are generally due to malignant disease.[72] Nonmalignant fistulas may result from erosion of contiguous infected subcarinal or mediastinal lymph nodes (e.g., tuberculosis, histoplasmosis, syphilis, actinomycosis); trauma (e.g., caustic ingestion, penetrating or blunt chest trauma, intubation, erosion of aspirated foreign body, dilation of esophageal stricture); late sequelae of a chronic mid esophageal traction diverticulum; or, as most frequently occurs, a complication of chronic ventilatory support and erosion by an endotracheal or tracheostomy tube cuff.[117,178,182,196] The clinical presentation is characteristic, with paroxysmal coughing occurring while the patient is eating, and swallowed food or liquid enters the tracheobronchial tree. Patients who are being mechanically ventilated may have copious tracheal secretions, difficulty with ventilation due to loss of inspired air into the gastrointestinal tract or out of the mouth, or gastric distention. If the patient is taking oral or tube feedings, the feedings may be retrieved from the trachea on suctioning. Regurgitation of gastric contents may cause rapid and progressive aspiration pneumonia.

When a fistula is suspected, a contrast esophagogram should be obtained. This generally establishes the diagnosis as well as localizes and determines the size of the communication. Because of the hygroscopic and irritating pulmonary effects of water-soluble contrast agents, it is preferable to use dilute barium sulfate for this study; barium is inert and, in small amounts, will cause no harm to the lungs. A computed tomography (CT) scan of the chest delineates associated mediastinal adenopathy or tumor mass and should be obtained in the preoperative evaluation. Endoscopic assessment of the tracheobronchial tree and esophagus is always indicated to exclude a malignant etiology and to assess the size and location of the fistula. Both the tracheal and esophageal sides of the fistula are biopsied and brushed for cytologic evaluation. Bronchography is occasionally helpful in assessing a fistula due to an infectious etiology because it may also define diseased pulmonary parenchyma that may require resection at the time of repair of the fistula.

Benign acquired intrathoracic esophagotracheobronchial fistulas are generally best approached through a right posterolateral thoracotomy in the fourth or fifth intercostal space. The fistulous tract is divided, and the opening in the esophagus is débrided and closed. The opening in the respiratory tract is similarly repaired, although at times, a pulmonary resection may be required. Viable adjacent tissue, mediastinal fat, pleura, pericardium, or a rotated intercostal muscle pedicle, must be interposed between the tracheobronchial and esophageal suture lines to prevent recurrence of the fistula. The long-term results are excellent, and recurrence of a properly repaired fistula is rare.[117]

Patients who develop a tracheoesophageal fistula while on a ventilator constitute a unique, high-risk population. It is always preferable to defer repair of the fistula until the patient has been weaned from the ventilator. Immediate management consists of removing any esophageal tube present and replacing the endotracheal tube with another with a large-volume, low-pressure cuff gently inflated below the fistula, if possible. A decompressing gastrostomy is inserted to prevent gastroesophageal reflux, and a feeding jejunostomy is used for alimentation. It is preferable not to divide the cervical esophagus (to achieve diversion of swallowed saliva) because this greatly complicates subsequent esophageal reconstruction. However, this is sometimes necessary to restore adequate ventilation.[101]

Cervical fistulas (e.g., those following intubation trauma) are approached through a cervical collar or oblique incision anterior to the sternocleidomastoid muscle. The fistula is divided after developing the tracheoesophageal groove. Closure of the tracheal and esophageal openings is achieved with absorbable sutures, and sternohyoid muscle is detached from the hyoid bone, rotated over the esophageal suture line, and sutured in place to prevent fistula recurrence.

Tracheoesophageal fistulas due to cuff injuries are generally associated with circumferential tracheal damage that requires resection. This can be performed in a single stage through a cervical collar incision, dividing the damaged trachea, and intubating the distal end. The esophageal opening is sutured closed and covered with mobilized sternocleidomastoid muscle. The area of tracheal damage is resected, and a primary tracheal anastomosis is performed. No tracheal tube is left in place postoperatively if possible. The results of operation for such cuff-injury tracheoesophageal fistulas have been excellent.[117]

Endoscopic closure of tracheoesophageal fistulas has been reported; however, this technique has not yet gained widespread acceptance.[6,183]

Malignant Tracheoesophageal Fistulas

Most malignant tracheoesophageal fistulas occur as a result of either esophageal or tracheal carcinoma (Fig. 29–17). Martini and associates have reported an incidence of tracheoesophageal fistulas of 4.9% in 1,943 patients with esophageal cancer, 0.16% in 5,714 with lung cancer, and 14.75% in 41 with tracheal cancer.[115] About one fifth of patients with middle-third esophageal cancers associated with radiographically demonstrable abnormalities of the posterior tracheal wall eventually develop a tracheoesophageal fistula.[40] Clearly, not all malignant fistulas between the esophagus and respiratory tree involve the trachea, the fistulas being tracheoesophageal in about 55%, bronchoesophageal in about 40%, and between the esophagus and peripheral lung parenchyma in about 10%.[5,27] About 80% of patients with this condition die within 3 months of the onset of the fistula formation, and the cause of death in 85% is aspiration pneumonia, not distant metastatic disease.[27] For the most part, a malignant tracheoesophageal fistula represents incurable disease, and the aggressiveness of treatment must be balanced against the short-term gain that is possible in these patients. Curative resection has been attempted,[135] but the tremendous operative mortality has caused general abandonment of such an approach.

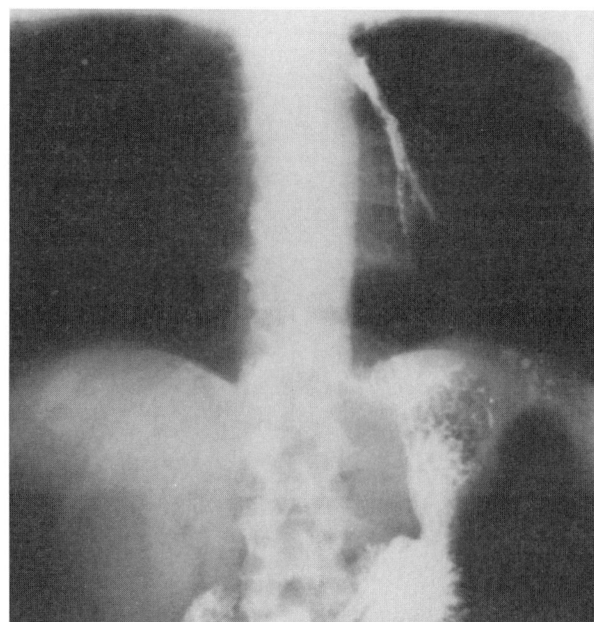

Figure 29–17. Barium esophagogram in a patient with a malignant tracheoesophageal fistula showing the characteristic simultaneous opacification of the gastrointestinal tract and the left main-stem bronchus. (From Orringer, M.B., and Sloan H.: Substernal gastric bypass of the excluded thoracic esophagus for palliation of esophageal carcinoma. J. Thorac. Cardiovasc. Surg., *70*:836, 1975, with permission.)

Palliative therapy for malignant tracheoesophageal fistulas has included intubation, stenting, placement of feeding tubes with or without concomitant diverting cervical esophagostomy, esophageal exclusion with simultaneous or delayed bypass procedures, and radiation therapy. Intubation, involving placement of a rigid prosthesis to occlude the fistula, can be performed using either pulsion or traction techniques. With pulsion intubation, successful control of pulmonary soilage is accomplished in about 75% of cases.[5,39,81] Pull-through, or traction, intubation can be performed using Celestin, Mousseau-Barbin, or Fell tubes and is associated with a mortality rate ranging from 12 to 64%.[39,81,110]

More recently, expansile covered metal stents have become a standard form of treatment for unresectable malignant strictures and esophagorespiratory fistulas[45,98] (see Chap. 22). In numerous series, albeit with fairly small numbers of patients, placement of such stents was highly effective in occluding malignant esophagorespiratory fistulas and palliating dysphagia.[55,118,131,133,154,189,195] In fact, the major issues now are not whether to place a stent but which type of stent to use and whether to place an esophageal stent only or to place parallel tracheal and esophageal stents.[56,58]

Laser vaporization, dilation of the malignant stricture, and placement of an endoesophageal prosthesis have also been used successfully in the treatment of a malignant

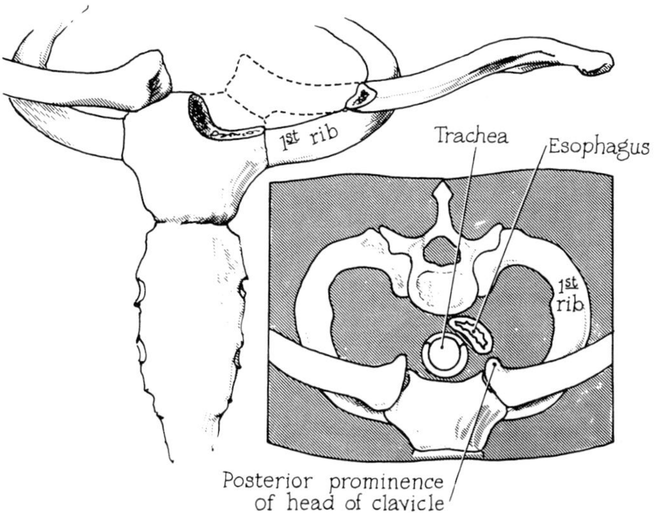

Figure 29–18. Enlargement of the superior opening into the anterior mediastinum, which is recommended whenever an esophageal substitute is placed in the retrosternal position. The posterior prominence of the clavicular head *(inset)* can compress and obstruct the retrosternal stomach or colon; therefore, resection of the medial clavicle, sternoclavicular joint, upper corner of the manubrium *(dotted lines)*, and the adjacent first rib is performed in these procedures. (From Orringer, M.B., and Sloan H.: Substernal gastric bypass of the excluded thoracic esophagus for palliation of esophageal carcinoma. J. Thorac. Cardiovasc. Surg., *70*:836, 1975, with permission.)

esophagorespiratory fistula.[64] The use of radiation therapy for the treatment of malignant tracheoesophageal fistulas is controversial. It is generally thought that tumor necrosis produced by radiation therapy may precipitate a malignant tracheoesophageal fistula; however, radiation therapy can be part of the treatment. Ahmed and colleagues described a small series of patients in whom malignant esophagorespiratory fistulas closed with a combination of chemotherapy and radiation.[1]

There are a number of surgical options in the management of malignant tracheoesophageal fistulas. Gastrostomy or jejunostomy alone achieves improved nutrition but does not address the problem of persistent tracheobronchial aspiration, which is the most immediate threat to the patient's life. Thus, 60% of 92 collected patients so treated died in the immediate postoperative period, primarily of pulmonary complications.[50] Performing an end-cervical esophagostomy at the time of insertion of a feeding tube achieves a means of alimentation as well as diversion of saliva from the esophagus, so long as gastroesophageal reflux does not occur. A feeding jejunostomy, rather than a gastrostomy, is therefore a better alternative in this situation. Alimentary continuity with extracorporeal esophagogastric tubes placed between the cervical esophagostomy and stomach have been used to allow these "excluded" patients to swallow.[163,168] These devices, for the most part, are cumbersome and do not permit satisfactory alimentation. The patient is still left with a feeding tube and a wet, excoriated neck around the cervical esophagostomy. This is clearly less than ideal palliation.

The Kirschner operation, substernal gastric interposition,[96] has been used by several surgeons in an attempt to bypass malignant tracheoesophageal fistulas.[136,137,158,172,196] Orringer has advocated enlargement of the anterior thoracic inlet (Figs. 29–18 and 29–19) when performing any type of esophageal replacement using the retrosternal route.[137] Because of dissatisfaction with the results of excluding the esophagus that contains an unresectable tumor (disruption of the distal esophageal closure in 17% of patients), Orringer and Sloan[137] advocated decompressing the divided distal esophagus into a Roux-en-Y jejunal loop, as originally proposed by Kirschner[96] and more recently by Akiyama and Hiyama.[2] Although substernal gastric bypass of the excluded thoracic esophagus may provide excellent palliation for the patient with a malignant tracheoesophageal fistula, the average survival of these patients is only 6 months, and this poor prognosis must be weighed against the appropriateness of performing such a procedure that carries an operative mortality rate of 20 to 61%.[50,122] The results of using long segments of jejunum[135] or colon[110,115] to bypass malignant tracheoesophageal fistulas are equally dismal. The potential for a good functional result here has difficulty outweighing an operative mortality rate in excess of 33%.[52] Isolated case reports, however, suggest that radiation therapy may in fact result in healing of the fistula.[59,115]

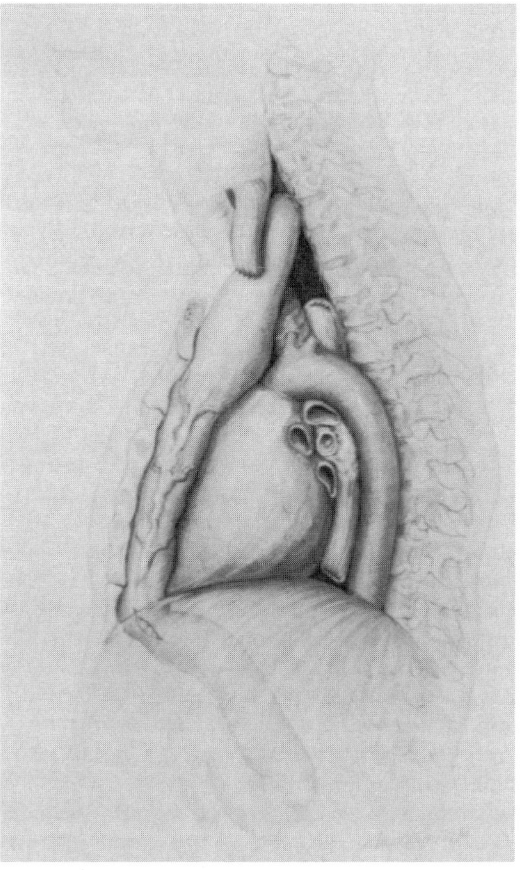

Figure 29–19. Lateral view of the completed substernal gastric bypass of the excluded thoracic esophagus. The gastric fundus is suspended from the cervical prevertebral fascia, an end-to-side cervical esophagogastrostomy is constructed, and the esophagus, with its unresectable tumor, is excluded in the posterior mediastinum. (From Orringer, M.B., and Sloan H.: Substernal gastric bypass of the excluded thoracic esophagus for palliation of esophageal carcinoma. J. Thorac. Cardiovasc. Surg., *70*:836, 1975.)

Burt reviewed the experience at the Memorial Sloan-Kettering Cancer Center with this morbid condition and found a 3-month survival rate of 13% when supportive care alone was employed, 17% when the esophagus was excluded, 21% in cases of esophageal intubation, 30% when radiation therapy was employed, and 46% when the esophagus was bypassed. The 30-day mortality rates also demonstrate the poor survival with operative intervention: 55% in patients undergoing exclusion, 43% with intubation, 25% with esophageal bypass, and 60% with resection. Statistical analysis indicated that survival was significantly prolonged in patients treated with radiation therapy or esophageal bypass compared with those treated with other modalities.[27]

In summary, no single treatment of malignant tracheoesophageal fistulas has emerged as being clearly superior. Regardless of the operative approach, when a patient with unresectable esophageal cancer is treated, the morbidity and mortality rates are high, and the benefits, if any, are short-lived. Only the relatively healthy patient whose fistula develops abruptly before weight loss and inanition have become established may warrant a major operative procedure to bypass the excluded esophagus. At times, the esophageal surgeon's enthusiasm to provide palliation of dysphagia must be tempered by surgical judgment and knowledge of the poor survival associated with a malignant tracheoesophageal fistula.

AORTOESOPHAGEAL FISTULA

Aortoesophageal fistula is a rare condition that carries an extremely high mortality rate. This condition is most commonly seen in association with thoracic aortic aneurysms but may also be due to foreign-body ingestion, esophageal malignancy, reflux esophagitis, tuberculous infection, postoperative intrathoracic anastomotic leak, erosive esophagitis from lye ingestion, and anomalies of the aortic arch.[38,87] Presentation is that of massive upper gastrointestinal hemorrhage, and the characteristic constellation of mid thoracic pain, sentinel arterial hemorrhage, and finally, exsanguination after a symptom-free period has been termed *Chiari's triad*.[197]

Survival after development of an aortoesophageal fistula is uncommon; however, direct suturing of the aortic defect, extra-anatomic bypass with resection of the diseased esophagus, and placement of a Dacron interposition graft with esophageal resection have all been reported to be successful in the treatment of this condition.[32,38,170] We have treated two patients with intrathoracic aortogastric fistulas occurring after esophagectomy and esophagogastrostomy for carcinoma. The first of these, who had also undergone radiation therapy, was treated with primary repair of the stomach and patch angioplasty of the aorta using cryopreserved allograft. This approach failed because the aortic repair dehisced several days postoperatively. The second patient with a similar history was managed successfully with resection of the intrathoracic stomach, esophageal diversion, suture closure of the small aortic bleeding point, and delayed colon interposition. A third patient with an aortoesophageal fistula secondary to a thoracic aortic aneurysm has been successfully managed by aortic interposition grafting with temporary esophageal exclusion.

Although experience with this condition is limited, survival appears to depend on exclusion, if not resection, of the involved esophagus. If the aortic lesion is small, it can be repaired directly; however, larger areas of aortic involvement, such as those occurring with an aneurysm, should be managed either with interposition grafting and lifelong antibiotics or with an extra-anatomic bypass and resection of the involved aorta.

References

1. Ahmed, H.F., Hussain, M.A., Grant, C.E., and Wadleigh, R.G.: Closure of tracheoesophageal fistulas with chemotherapy and radiotherapy. Am. J. Clin. Oncol., *21:*177, 1998.
2. Akiyama, H., and Hiyama, M.: A simple esophageal bypass operation by the high gastric division. Surgery, *75:*674, 1974.
3. Albrechtsen, D., and Nygaard K.: Idiopathic mediastinal fibrosis. Acta Chir. Scand., *147:*219, 1981.
4. Allen, C.M., Craze, J., and Grundy, A.: Tuberculous broncho-esophageal fistula in the acquired immunodeficiency syndrome. Clin. Radiol., *43:*60, 1991.
5. Angorn, I.B.: Intubation in the treatment of carcinoma of the esophagus. World J. Surg., *5:*535, 1981.
6. Antonelli, M., Cicconetti, F., Vivino, G., and Gasparetto, A.C.F.: Closure of a tracheoesophageal fistula by bronchoscopic application of fibrin glue and decontamination of the oral cavity. Chest, *100:*578, 1991.
7. Arnett, E N., Bacos, J.M., Macher, A.M., et al.: Fibrosing mediastinitis causing pulmonary arterial hypertension without pulmonary venous hypertension. Am. J. Med., *632:*634, 1977.
8. Asamura, H., Goya, T., Hirata, K., et al.: Esophageal and pulmonary metastases from ovarian carcinoma: A case report of long-term survival following metastatic resections. Jpn. J. Clin. Oncol., *21:*211, 1991.
9. Ashman, F.C., Hill, M.C., Saba, G.P., and Diaconis, J.N.: Esophageal hematoma associated with thrombocytopenia. Gastrointest. Radiol., *3:*115, 1978.
10. Atkinson, M., Bottrill, M.B., Edwards, A.T., et al.: Mucosal tears at the oesophagogastric junction (the Mallory-Weiss syndrome). Gut, *2:*1, 1961.
11. Atkinson, S.I., and Rees, J.: Botulinum toxin for cricopharyngeal dysphagia: Case reports of CT-guided injection. J. Otolaryngol., *26:*273, 1997.
12. Austin, E.H., and Wolfe, W.G.: Aneurysm of aberrant subclavian artery with a review of the literature. J. Vasc. Surg., *2:*571, 1985.
13. Bak, Y.T., Kwon, O.S., Yeon, J.E., et al.: Endoscopic treatment in a case with extensive spontaneous intramural dissection of the oesophagus. Eur. J. Gastroenterol. Hepatol., *10:*969, 1998.
14. Baredes, S., Shah, C.S., and Kaufman, R.: The frequency of cricopharyngeal dysfunction on videofluoroscopic swallowing studies in patients with dysphagia. Am. J. Otolaryngol., *18:*185, 1997.
15. Baron, J.H.: The Paterson-Brown Kelly syndrome of sideropenic dysphagia does not exist. J. R. Coll. Physicians Lond., *25:*361, 1991.
16. Bataller, R., Llach, J., Salmeron, J.M., et al.: Endoscopic sclerotherapy in upper gastrointestinal bleeding due to the Mallory-Weiss syndrome. Am. J. Gastroenterol., *89:*2147, 1994.
17. Beahrs, O.H., and Schmidt, H.W.: Dysphagia caused by hypertrophic changes in the cervical spine: Report of two cases. Ann. Surg., *149:*297, 1959.
18. Belsey, R.: Functional disease of the esophagus. J. Thorac. Cardiovasc. Surg., *52:*162, 1966.
19. Bender, M.D.: Esophageal manometry in oculopharyngeal dystrophy. Am. J. Gastroenterol., *62:*215, 1976.
20. Benedict, E.B., and Leve, W.F.: Stenosis of the esophagus in benign mucous membrane pemphigus. Ann. Otol. Rhinol. Laryngol., *61:*1120, 1952.
21. Bindelglass, I.L., and Trubowitz, S.: Pulmonary vein obstruction. Ann. Intern. Med., *48:*876, 1958.

22. Bonavina, L., Khan, N.A., and DeMeester, T.R.: Pharyngoesophageal dysfunctions: The role of cricopharyngeal myotomy. Arch. Surg., *120*:541, 1985.
23. Born, L., Harned, R.H., Rikkers, L.F., et al.: Cricopharyngeal dysfunction in Parkinson's disease: Role in dysphagia and response to myotomy. Mov. Disord., *11*:53, 1996.
24. Branski, D., Levey, J., Globus, M., et al.: Dysphagia as a primary manifestation of hyperthyroidism. J. Clin. Gastroenterol., *6*:437, 1984.
25. Bristo, L.D., Mandal, A.K., Oparah, S.S., and Bauer, H.M.: Bilateral chylothorax associated with sclerosing mediastinitis. Int. Surg., *68*:273, 1983.
26. Buckberg, G.D., Dilley, R B., and Longmire, W.D., Jr.: The protean manifestations of sclerosing fibrosis. Surg. Gynecol. Obstet., *423*:729, 1966.
27. Burt, M., Diehl, W., Martini, N., et al.: Malignant esophagorespiratory fistula: Management options and survival. Ann. Thorac. Surg., *52*:1222, 1991.
28. Butcher, R.B.: Treatment of chronic aspiration as a complication of cerebrovascular accident. Laryngoscope, *92*:681, 1982.
29. Calne, D.B., Shaw, D.G., Spiers, A.S.D., and Stern, G.M.: Swallowing in parkinsonism. Br. J. Radiol., *43*:456, 1970.
30. Carlson, M.J., Stauffer, R.N., and Payne, W.S.: Ankylosing vertebral hyperostosis causing dysphagia. Arch. Surg., *109*:567, 1974.
31. Carsen, G.M., Casarella, W.J., and Spiegel, R.M.: Trans-catheter embolization for treatment of Mallory-Weiss tears of the esophagogastric junction. Radiology, *128*:309, 1978.
32. Carter, R., Mulder, G.A., Snyder, E.N., Jr., and Brewer, L.A.: Aortoesophageal fistula. Am. J. Surg., *136*:26, 1978.
33. Chen, P., Lebowitz, R., and Lewicki, A.M.: Spontaneous hematoma of the esophagus: A complication of uremia. Radiology, *100*:281, 1971.
34. Chen, T.S., and Chen, P.S.: Rise and fall of the Plummer-Vinson syndrome. J. Gastroenterol. Hepatol., *9*:654, 1994.
35. Chun, K., Colombani, P.M., Dudgeon, D.L., and Haller, J.A., Jr.: Diagnosis and management of congenital vascular rings: A 22-year experience. Ann. Thorac. Surg., *53*:597, 1992.
36. Cirillo, N.W., Lyon, D.T., and Schuller, A.M.: Tracheoesophageal fistula complicating herpes esophagitis in AIDS. Am. J. Gastroenterol., *88*:587, 1992.
37. Conte, B.A.: Dysphagia caused by an aneurysm of the descending thoracic aorta. N. Engl. J. Med., *274*:956, 1966.
38. Cronen, P., Snow, N., and Nightingale, D.: Aortoesophageal fistula secondary to reflux esophagitis. Ann. Thorac. Surg., *33*:78, 1982.
39. Cusumano, A., Ruol, A., Segalin, A., et al.: Push-through intubation: Effective palliation in 409 patients with cancer of the esophagus and cardia. Ann. Thorac. Surg., *53*:100, 1992.
40. Daffner, R.H., Postlethwait, R.W., and Putman, C.E.: Retrotracheal abnormalities in esophageal carcinoma: Prognostic implications. Am. J. Roentgenol., *130*:719, 1978.
41. Dantas, R.O., and Villanova, M.G.: Esophageal motility impairment in Plummer-Vinson syndrome—correction by iron treatment. Dig. Dis. Sci., *38*:968, 1993.
42. Dill, J.E., and Wells, R.F.: Use of vasopressin in the Mallory-Weiss syndrome. N. Engl. J. Med., *284*:852, 1971.
43. Dines, D.E., and Anderson, M.W.: Giant left atrium as a cause of dysphagia. Ann. Intern. Med., *65*:759, 1966.
44. Dines, D.E., Payne, W.S., Bernatz, P.E., and Pairolero, P.C.: Mediastinal granuloma and fibrosing mediastinitis. Chest, *75*:320, 1979.
45. Do, Y.S., Sond, H.-Y., Lee, B.H., et al.: Esophagorespiratory fistula associated with esophageal cancer: Treatment with a Gianturco stent tube. Radiology, *187*:673, 1993.
46. Dukes, R.J., Vaughn, S.C., Dines, D.E., et al.: Esophageal involvement with mediastinal granuloma. J.A.M.A., *236*:2313, 1976.
47. Duranceau, A., Jamieson, G.G., Hurwitz, A.L., et al.: Alteration in esophageal motility after laryngectomy. Am. J. Surg., *131*:30, 1976.
48. Duranceau, A., Forand, M.D., and Fanteux, J.P.: Surgery in oculopharyngeal muscular dystrophy. Am. J. Surg., *139*:33, 1980.
49. Duranceau, A., Beauchamp, G., Jamieson, G.G., and Barbeau, A.: Oculopharyngeal dysphagia and oculopharyngeal muscular dystrophy. Surg. Clin. North Am., *63*:825, 1983.
50. Duranceau, A., and Jamieson, G.G.: Malignant tracheoesophageal fistula—collective review. Ann. Thorac. Surg., *37*:346, 1984.
51. Duranceau, A., Lafontaine, L., and Taillefer, R.: Oropharyngeal dysphagia. *In* Jamieson, G. G. (ed.): Surgery of the Oesophagus. Edinburgh, Churchill Livingstone, 1988, p. 413.
52. Eastridge, C.E., Greenberg, B.E., Hughes, F.A., and Aslam, P.A.: Cancer of the esophagus. South. Med. J., *63*:1135, 1970.
53. Edwards, J.E.: Malformations of the aortic arch system manifested as "vascular rings." Lab. Invest., *2*:56, 1953.
54. Effler, D.B., and Groves, L.K.: Superior vena caval obstruction. J. Thorac. Cardiovasc. Surg., *43*:574, 1962.
55. Ell, C., May, A., and Hahn, E.G.: Gianturco-Z stents in the palliative treatment of malignant esophageal obstruction and esophagotracheal fistulas. Endoscopy, *27*:495, 1995.
56. Ellul, J.P., Morgan, R., Gold, D., et al.: Parallel self-expanding covered metal stents in the trachea and oesophagus for the palliation of complex high tracheo-oesophageal fistula. Br. J. Surg., *83*:1767, 1996.
57. Eng, J., and Sabanathan, S.: Tuberculosis of the esophagus. Dig. Dis. Sci., *36*:536, 1991.
58. Freitag, L., Tekolf, E., Steveling, H., et al.: Management of malignant esophagotracheal fistulas with airway stenting and double stenting. Chest, *110*:1155, 1996.
59. Fry, W.A., Griem, M.L., and Adams, W.E.: Malignant tracheoesophageal fistula treated by combined radiotherapy and surgical excision. Dis. Chest., *54*:384, 1968.
60. Gaissert, H.A., Breuer, C.K., Weissburg, A., and Mermel, L.: Surgical management of necrotizing Candida esophagitis. Ann. Thorac. Surg., *67*:231, 1999.
61. Gay, I., Chisin, R., and Elidan, J.: Myotomy of the cricopharyngeal muscle: A treatment for dysphagia and aspiration in neurologic disorders. Rev. Laryngol., *105*:271, 1984.
62. Gedde-Dahl, T.J.: Epidermolysis Bullosa: A Clinical, Genetic, and Epidemiological Study. Baltimore, The Johns Hopkins Press, 1971.
63. Geller, A., and Gostout, C.J.: Esophagogastric hematoma mimicking a malignant neoplasm: Clinical manifestations, diagnosis, and treatment. Mayo Clin. Proc., *73*:342, 1998.
64. Ghazi, A., and Nussbaum, M.: A new approach to the management of malignant esophageal obstruction and esophagorespiratory fistula. Ann. Thorac. Surg., *41*:531, 1986.
65. Goldberg, H.I., and Dodds, W.J.: Cobblestone esophagus due to monilial infection. Am. J. Roentgenol., *104*:608, 1968.
66. Goyal, R.K., Martin, S.B., Shapiro, J., and Spechler, S.J.: The role of cricopharyngeus muscle in pharyngoesophageal disorders. Dysphagia, *8*:252, 1993.
67. Graham, J.R., Suby, H.I., LeCompte, P.R., and Sadowsky, N.L.: Fibrotic disorders associated with methysergide therapy for headache. N. Engl. J. Med., *274*:359, 1966.
68. Greven, K.M., and Evans, L.S.: The occurrence and management of esophageal fistulas resulting from Hodgkin's disease. Cancer, *69*:1031, 1992.
69. Grieve, N.W. T.: Monilial esophagitis. Br. J. Radiol., *37*:551, 1964.
70. Gross, R.E.: Surgical treatment for dysphagia lusoria. Ann. Surg., *124*:532, 1946.
71. Gross, R.E.: Arterial malformations which cause compression of the trachea and esophagus. Circulation, *11*:124, 1955.
72. Gudovsky, L.M., Koroleva, N.S., Biryukov, Y.B., et al.: Tracheoesophageal fistulas. Ann. Thorac. Surg., *55*:868, 1993.
73. Hache, L., Woolner, L.B., and Bernatz, P.E.: Idiopathic fibrous mediastinitis. Dis. Chest, *41*:9, 1962.
74. Hackelsberger, A., Schultze, V., Grunther, T., et al.: The prevalence of Helicobacter pylori gastritis in patients with reflux oesophagitis: A case-control study. Eur. J. Gastroenterol. Hepatol., *10*:465, 1998.
75. Hanna, E.A., and Derrick, J.R.: Dysphagia caused by tortuosity of the thoracic aorta. J. Thorac. Cardiovasc. Surg., *57*:134, 1969.
76. Hardy, K.M., Perry, H.O., Pingree, G.C., and Kirby, T.J., Jr.: Benign mucous membrane pemphigoid. Arch. Dermatol., *104*:467, 1971.
77. Harris, J.M., and DiPalma, J.A.: Clinical significance of Mallory-Weiss tears. Am. J. Gastroenterol., *88*:2056, 1993.
78. Harrison, C.A., and Katon, R.M.: Familial multiple congenital esophageal rings: Report of an affected father and son. Am. J. Gastroenterol., *87*:1813, 1992.
79. Hatlebakk, J.G., Castell, J.A., Spiegel, J., et al.: Dilatation therapy for dysphagia in patients with upper esophageal sphincter dysfunction—manometric and symptomatic response. Dis. Esophagus, *11*:254, 1998.
80. Heck, C.V.: Hoarseness and painful deglutition due to massive cervical exostoses. Surg. Gynecol. Obstet., *102*:657, 1956.
81. Hegarty, M.M., Angorn, I.B., Bryer, J.V., et al.: Palliation of malignant esophagorespiratory fistulae by permanent indwelling prosthetic tube. Ann. Surg., *185*:88, 1977.

82. Henderson, R.D.: Disorders of the pharyngoesophageal junction. *In* Motor Disorders of the Esophagus. Baltimore, Williams & Wilkins, 1976, p. 184.
83. Henderson, R.D., and Maryatt, G.: Cricopharyngeal myotomy as a method of treating cricopharyngeal dysphagia secondary to gastroesophageal reflux. J. Thorac. Cardiovasc. Surg., *74:*721, 1977.
84. Henderson, R.E.: The Esophagus: Reflux and Primary Motor Disorders. Baltimore, Williams & Wilkins, 1980, p. 223.
85. Herrera, J.L.: Case report: Esophageal metastasis from breast carcinoma presenting as achalasia. Am. J. Med. Sci., *303:*321, 1992.
86. Herrera, J.L.: Benign and metastatic tumors of the esophagus. Gastroenterol. Clin. North Am., *20:*775, 1991.
87. Hollander, J.E., and Quick, G.: Aortoesophageal fistula: A comprehensive review of the literature. Am. J. Med., *91:*279, 1991.
88. Hoover, W.B.: The syndrome of anemia, glossitis, and dysphagia: Report of cases. N. Engl. J. Med., *213:*394, 1935.
89. Horan, T.A., Urshel, J.D., MacEachern, N.A., et al.: Esophageal perforation in recessive dystrophic epidermolysis bullosa. Ann. Thorac. Surg., *57:*1027, 1994.
90. Ingelfinger, F.J., and Kramer, P.: Dysphagia produced by a contractile ring in the lower esophagus. Gastroenterology, *23:*419, 1953.
91. Jenkins, D.W., Fisk, D.E., and Byrd, R.B.: Mediastinal histoplasmosis with esophageal disease. Gastroenterology, *70:*109, 1976.
92. Kahrilas, P.J., Clouse, R.E., and Hogan, W.J.: American Gastroenterological Association technical review on the clinical use of esophageal manometry. Gastroenterology, *107:*1865, 1994.
93. Keates, P.G., and Magidson, O.: Dysphagia associated with sclerosis of the aorta. Br. J. Radiol., *28:*184, 1955.
94. Kelly, A.B.: Spasm at entrance to oesophagus. J. Laryngol. Rhinol. Otol., *34:*285, 1919.
95. Kilman, W.J., and Goyal, R.K.: Disorders of pharyngeal and upper esophageal sphincter motor function. Arch. Intern. Med., *136:*592, 1976.
96. Kirschner, M.B.: Ein neues Verfahren der Oesophagoplatik. Arch. Klin. Chir., *114:*606, 1920.
97. Knauer, C.M.: Mallory-Weiss syndrome: Characterization of 75 Mallory-Weiss lacerations in 528 patients with upper gastrointestinal hemorrhage. Gastroenterology, *71:*51, 1976.
98. Knyrim, K., Wagner, H.-J., Bethge, N., et al.: A controlled trial of an expansile metal stent for palliation of esophageal obstruction due to inoperable cancer. N. Engl. J. Med., *329:*1302, 1993.
99. Laforet, E., and Kondi, E.: Postmastectomy dysphagia. Am. J. Surg., *121:*368, 1971.
100. Lambert, A.: Surgical correction of esophageal obstruction due to tortuosity of the aorta. J. Thorac. Cardiovasc. Surg., *62:*973, 1971.
101. Landreneau, R.J., Hazelrigg, S.T., Boley, T.M., et al.: Management of an extensive tracheoesophageal fistula by cervical esophageal exclusion. Chest, *99:*777, 1991.
102. Lebo, C.P., Kwei Sang, U., and Norris, F.H.: Cricopharyngeal myotomy in amyotrophic lateral sclerosis. Laryngoscope, *86:*862, 1976.
103. LeRoux, B., and Williams, M.A.: Dysphagia megalatriensis. Thorax, *24:*603, 1969.
104. Lichter, I.: The treatment of dysphagia lusoria in the adult. Br. J. Surg., *50:*793, 1963.
105. Lieberman, D.A., Keller, F.S., Katon, R.M., and Rosch, J.: Arterial embolization for massive upper gastrointestinal tract bleeding in poor surgical candidates. Gastroenterology, *86:*876, 1984.
106. Light, A.M.: Idiopathic fibrosis of mediastinum: A discussion of three cases and review of the literature. J. Clin. Pathol., *31:*78, 1978.
107. Lim, R Y.: Endoscopic CO_2 laser cricopharyngeal myotomy. J. Clin. Laser Med. Surg., *13:*241, 1995.
108. Lion-Cachet, J.: Gastric fundal mucosal tears. Br. J. Surg., *50:*985, 1963.
109. Loizou, L.A., Small, M., and Dalton, G.A.: Cricopharyngeal myotomy in motor neurone disease. J. Neurol. Neurosurg. Psychiatry, *43:*42, 1980.
110. Lolley, D.M., Jefferson, F.R., III, Ransdell, H.T., et al.: Management of malignant esophagorespiratory fistula. Ann. Thorac. Surg., *25:*516, 1978.
111. Longmire, W.J., Goodwin, W.E., and Buckberg, G.D.: Management of sclerosing fibrosis of the mediastinal and retroperitoneal areas. Ann. Surg., *165:*1013, 1967.
112. MacDougall, G., Wilson, J.A., Pryde, A., and Grant, R.: Analysis of the pharyngoesophageal pressure profile in amyotrophic lateral sclerosis. Otolaryngol. Head Neck Surg., *112:*258, 1995.
113. Mallory, G.K., and Weiss, S.: Hemorrhages from lacerations of the cardiac orifice of the stomach due to vomiting. Am. J. Med. Sci., *178:*506, 1929.
114. Marks, I.N., and Keet, A.D.: Intramucosal rupture of the esophagus. Br. Med. J., *3:*536, 1968.
115. Martini, N., Goodner, J.T., D'Angio, G.J., and Beattie, E.J.: Tracheoesophageal fistula due to cancer. J. Thorac. Cardiovasc. Surg., *59:*319, 1970.
116. Mason, R.J., Bremner, C.G., DeMeester, T.R., et al.: Pharyngeal swallowing disorders: Selection for and outcome after myotomy. Ann. Surg., *228:*598, 1998.
117. Mathisen, D.J., Grillo, H.C., Wain, J.C., and Hilgenberg, A.D.: Management of acquired nonmalignant tracheoesophageal fistula. Ann. Thorac. Surg., *52:*759, 1991.
118. May, A., and Ell, C.: Palliative treatment of malignant esophagorespiratory fistulas with Gianturco-Z stents: A prospective clinical trial and review of the literature on covered metal stents. Am. J. Gastroenterol., *93:*532, 1998.
119. McDonald, G.: Esophageal disease caused by infection, systemic illness, medications, and trauma. *In* Sleisenger, M. S. (ed.): Gastrointestinal Disease, 5th ed. Philadelphia, W. B. Saunders, 1993, p. 427.
120. Meeks, L.W., and Renshaw, T.S.: Vertebral osteophytosis and dysphagia: Two case reports of the syndrome recently termed ankylosing hyperostosis. J. Bone Joint Surg., *55-A:*197, 1973.
121. Mendl, K., McKay, J.M., and Tanner, C.H.: Intramural diverticulosis of the esophagus and Rokitanski-Aschoff sinuses of the gallbladder. Br. J. Radiol., *33:*496, 1960.
122. Meunier, B., Spiliopoulos, Y., Stasik, C., et al.: Retrosternal bypass operation for unresectable squamous cell cancer of the esophagus. Ann. Thorac. Surg., *62:*373, 1996.
123. Michel, L., Serrano, A., and Malt, R.A.: Mallory-Weiss syndrome: Evolution of diagnostic and therapeutic patterns over two decades. Ann. Surg., *192:*716, 1980.
124. Migliore, M., Payne, H.R., and Jeyasingham, K.: Pharyngo-oesophageal dysphagia: Surgery based on clinical and manometric data. Eur. J. Cardiothorac. Surg., *10:*365, 1996.
125. Minocha, A., Mandanas, R.A., Kida, M., and Jazzar, A.: Bullous esophagitis due to chronic graft-versus-host disease. Am. J. Gastroenterol., *92:*529, 1997.
126. Mitchinson, M.J., Wight, D.G.D., Arno, J., and Milstein, B.B.: Chronic coronary periarteritis in two patients with chronic periaortitis. J. Clin. Pathol., *37:*32, 1984.
127. Mizobuchi, S., Tachimori, Y., Kato, H., et al.: Metastatic esophageal tumors from distant primary lesions: Report of three esophagectomies and study of 1835 autopsy cases. Jpn. J. Clin. Oncol., *27:*410, 1997.
128. Mok, C.K., Cheung, K.C., Kong, S.M., and Ong, G.B.: Translocating the aberrant right subclavian artery in dysphagia lusoria. Br. J. Surg., *66:*113, 1979.
129. Mokoena, T., Shama, D.M., Ngakane, H., and Bryer, J.V.: Oesophageal tuberculosis: A review of eleven cases. Postgrad. Med. J., *68:*110, 1992.
130. Montgomery, W.W., and Lynch, J.P.: Oculopharyngeal muscular dystrophy treated by inferior constrictor myotomy. Trans. Am. Acad. Ophthalmol. Otolaryngol., *75:*986, 1971.
131. Morgan, R.A., Ellul, J.P., Denton, E.R., et al.: Malignant esophageal fistulas and perforations: Management with plastic-covered metallic endoprostheses. Radiology, *204:*527, 1997.
132. Mosher, H.P.: Exostoses of the cervical vertebrae as a cause for difficulty in swallowing. Laryngoscope, *36:*181, 1926.
133. Nelson, D.B., Axelrad, A.M., Fleischer, D.E., et al.: Silicone-covered Wallstent prototypes for palliation of malignant esophageal obstruction and digestive-respiratory fistulas. Gastrointest. Endosc., *45:*31, 1997.
134. Noyer, C.M., and Simon, D.: Oral and esophageal disorders. Gastroenterol. Clin. North Am., *26:*241, 1997.
135. Ong, G.B., and Kwong, K.H.: Management of malignant esophagobronchial fistula. Surgery, *67:*293, 1970.
136. Ong, G.B.: The Kirschner operation: A forgotten procedure. Br. J. Surg., *60:*221, 1973.
137. Orringer, M.B., and Sloan, H.: Substernal gastric bypass of the excluded thoracic esophagus for palliation of esophageal carcinoma. J. Thorac. Cardiovasc. Surg., *70:*836, 1975.

138. Orringer, M.B., and Sloan, H.: Monilial esophagitis: An increasingly frequent cause of esophageal stenosis? Ann. Thorac. Surg., *26:*364, 1978.
139. Orringer, M.B.: Extended cervical esophagomyotomy for cricopharyngeal dysfunction. J. Thorac. Cardiovasc. Surg., *80:*669, 1980.
140. Orringer, M.B., and Stirling, M.C.: Cervical esophagogastric anastomosis for benign disease-functional results. J. Thorac. Cardiovasc. Surg., *96:*887, 1988.
141. Pang, J., Vicary, F.R., and Beck, E.R.: Coexisting retroperitoneal and mediastinal fibrosis. Postgrad. Med. J., *59:*450, 1983.
142. Papp, J.P.: Electrocoagulation of actively bleeding Mallory-Weiss tears. Gastrointest. Endosc., *26:*128, 1980.
143. Patterson, D.R.: A clinical type of dysphagia. J. Laryngol. Rhinol. Otol., *34:*289, 1919.
144. Pera, M., Yamada, A., Hiebert, C.A., and Duranceau, A.: Sleeve recording of upper esophageal sphincter resting pressures during cricopharyngeal myotomy. Ann. Surg., *225:*229, 1997.
145. Perie, S., Eymard, B., Laccourreye, L., et al.: Dysphagia in oculopharyngeal muscular dystrophy: A series of 22 French cases. Neuromuscul. Disord., 7(Suppl 1):S96, 1997.
146. Phan, G.Q., and Heitmiller, R.F.: Intramural esophageal dissection. Ann. Thorac. Surg., *63:*1785, 1997.
147. Pick, R.A., Joswig, B.C., and Bloor, C.M.: Recurrent cardiac constriction after pericardiectomy. J. Thorac. Cardiovasc. Surg., *144:*2061, 1969.
148. Plachta, A.: Benign tumors of the esophagus. Am. J. Gastroenterol., *38:*639, 1962.
149. Polk, H.C., Camp, F.A., and Walker, A.W.: Dysphagia and esophageal stenosis—manifestation of metastatic mammary cancer. Cancer, *20:*2002, 1967.
149a. Poirier, N.C., Bonavina, L., Taillefer, R., et al.: Cricopharyngeal myotomy for neurogenic oropharyngeal dysphagia. J. Thorac. Cardiovasc., *113:*233, 1997.
150. Postlethwait, R.W.: Surgery of the Esophagus. New York, Appleton-Century-Crofts, 1979, p. 259.
151. Postlethwait, R.W.: Benign tumors and cysts of the esophagus. Surg. Clin. North Am., *63:*925, 1983.
152. Prince, D.S., Luna, R.F., Cohn, M.G., and Sabiston, W.R.: Osteophyte-induced dysphagia: Occurrence in ankylosing hyperostosis. J.A.M.A., *234:*77, 1975.
153. Putnam, P.E., Orenstein, S.R., Pang, D., et al.: Cricopharyngeal dysfunction associated with Chiari malformations. Pediatrics, *89:*871, 1992.
154. Raijman, I., Siddique, I., Ajani, J., and Lynch, P.: Palliation of malignant dysphagia and fistulae with coated expandable metal stents: Experience with 101 patients. Gastrointest. Endosc., *48:*172, 1998.
155. Raque, C.J., Stein, K.M., and Samitz, M.H.: Pemphigus vulgaris involving the esophagus. Arch. Dermatol., *102:*371, 1970.
156. Redleaf, M.I., Moran, W.J., and Gruber, B.: Mycosis fungoides involving the cervical esophagus. Arch. Orolaryngol. Head Neck Surg., *119:*690, 1993.
157. Reed, W.G., and Stinely, R.W.: Massive periaortic and periarterial fibrosis: Report of a case. N. Engl. J. Med., *261:*320, 1959.
158. Roeher, H.D., and Horeyseck, G.: The Kirschner operation: A palliation for complicated esophageal carcinoma. World J. Surg., *5:*543, 1981.
159. Sakiyalak, P., Bellon, E.M., David, P., and Ankeney, J.L.: Esophageal obstruction due to saccular aneurysm of the distal thoracic aorta. J. Thorac. Cardiovasc. Surg., *64:*959, 1972.
160. Savelli, B.A., Parshley, M., and Morganroth, M.L.: Successful treatment of sclerosing cervicitis and fibrosing mediastinitis with tamoxifen. Chest, *111:*1137, 1997.
161. Schatzki, R., and Gary, J.E.: Dysphagia due to diaphragm-like localized narrowing in lower esophagus (lower esophageal ring). Am. J. Roentgenol., *70:*911, 1953.
162. Schneider, I., Thumfart, W.F., Pototschnig, C., and Eckel, H.E.: Treatment of dysfunction of the cricopharyngeal muscle with botulinum A toxin: Introduction of a new, noninvasive method. Ann. Otol. Rhinol. Laryngol., *103:*31, 1994.
163. Schreiber, H., and Pories, W.J.: External diversion for palliative treatment of malignant tracheoesophageal or bronchoesophageal fistulas. Am. J. Surg., *131:*775, 1976.
164. Sharpe, D.A.C., Sendegeya, S.Z., Parry, D.H., and Drakeley, M.J.: Tracheoesophageal fistula after chemotherapy for lymphoma. Ann. Thorac. Surg., *54:*366, 1992.
165. Shearman, D.J.C., and Finlayson, N.D.C.: Diseases of the Gastrointestinal Tract and Liver. Edinburgh, Churchill Livingstone, 1982, p. 114.
166. Sheft, D.J., and Shrago, G.: Esophageal moniliasis: The spectrum of the disease. J.A.M.A., *213:*1859, 1970.
167. Shklar, G., and McCarthy, P.L.: Oral lesions of mucous membrane pemphigoid: A study of 85 cases. Arch. Otolaryngol., *93:*354, 1971.
168. Skinner, D.B., and DeMeester, T.R.: Permanent extracorporeal esophagogastric tube for esophageal replacement. Ann. Thorac. Surg., *22:*107, 1976.
169. Slater, S.D.: The Brown Kelly-Paterson or Plummer-Vinson syndrome: An old score finally settled. J. R. Coll. Physicians Lond., *25:*57, 1991.
170. Snyder, D M., and Crawford, E.S.: Successful treatment of primary aorta-esophageal fistula resulting from aortic aneurysm. J. Thorac. Cardiovasc. Surg., *85:*457, 1983.
171. Stankey, R.M., Roshe, J., and Sogocio, R.M.: Carcinoma of the lung and dysphagia. Chest, *55:*13, 1969.
172. Steiger, A., Nickel, W.O., Wilson, R.F., and Arbulu, A.: Far advanced carcinoma of the esophagus treated with substernal bypass using stomach. Gastrointest. Res., *5:*136, 1979.
173. Strimlan, C.V., Dines, D.E., and Payne, W.S.: Mediastinal granuloma. Mayo Clin. Proc., *50:*702, 1975.
174. Sugawa, C., Benishek, D., and Walt, A.J.: Mallory-Weiss syndrome: A study of 224 patients. Am. J. Surg., *145:*30, 1983.
175. Sugawa, C., Shier, M., Lucas, C.E., and Walt, A.J.: Electrocoagulation of bleeding in the upper part of the gastrointestinal tract. Arch. Surg., *110:*975, 1975.
176. Talley, N.A., and Nicks, R.: Spontaneous submucosal haematoma of the esophagus: "Oesophageal apoplexy." Med. J. Aust., *2:*146, 1969.
177. Templeton, F.E.: X-Ray Examination of the Stomach: A Description of the Roentgenologic Anatomy, Physiology and Pathology of the Esophagus, Stomach, and Duodenum. Chicago, University of Chicago Press, 1944.
178. Thomas, A.N.: The diagnosis and treatment of tracheoesophageal fistula caused by cuffed tracheal tubes. J. Thorac. Cardiovasc. Surg., *65:*612, 1973.
179. Thomas, E., and Reddy, K.R.: Systemic vasopressin therapy for Mallory-Weiss bleeding. South. Med. J., *75:*691, 1982.
180. Torenson, W.E.: Secondary carcinoma of the esophagus as a cause of dysphagia. Arch. Pathol., *38:*82, 1944.
181. Urschel, H.C., Jr., Razzuk, M.A., Netto, G.J., et al.: Sclerosing mediastinitis: Improved management with histoplasmosis titer and ketoconazole. Ann. Thorac. Surg., *50:*215, 1990.
182. Utley, J.R., Dillon, M.L., Todd, E.P., et al.: Giant tracheoesophageal fistula-management by esophageal diversion. J. Thorac. Cardiovasc. Surg., *75:*373, 1978.
183. Vandenplas, Y., Helven, R., Derop, H., et al.: Endoscopic obliteration of recurrent tracheoesophageal fistula. Dig. Dis. Sci., *38:*374, 1993.
184. Varanasi, R.V., Saltzman, J.R., Krims, P., et al.: Breast carcinoma metastatic to the esophagus: Clinicopathological and management features of four cases, and literature review. Am. J. Gastroenterol., *90:*1495, 1995.
185. Vazquez, J.A.: Options for the management of mucosal candidiasis in patients with AIDS and HIV infection. Pharmacotherapy, *19:*76, 1999.
186. Victor, M., Hayes, R., and Adams, R.D.: Oculopharyngeal muscular dystrophy, a familial disease of late life characterized by dysphagia and progressive ptosis of the eyelids. N. Engl. J. Med., *267:*1267, 1962.
187. Vinson, P.P.: Hysterical dysphagia. Minn. Med., *5:*107, 1922.
188. Weider, S., and Rabinowitz, J.G.: Fibrous mediastinitis: A late manifestation of mediastinal histoplasmosis. Radiology, *125:*305, 1977.
189. Weigert, N., Neuhaus, H., Rosch, T., et al.: Treatment of esophagorespiratory fistulas with silicone-coated self-expanding metal stents. Gastrointest. Endosc., *41:*490, 1995.
190. Weiss, S., and Mallory, G.K.: Lesions of the cardiac orifice of the stomach produced by vomiting. J.A.M.A., *98:*1353, 1932.
191. Wightman, A.J.A., and Wright, E.A.: Intramural esophageal diverticulosis: A correlation of radiological and pathological findings. Br. J. Radiol., *47:*496, 1974.
192. Wilcox, C.M.: Esophageal strictures complicating ulcerative esophagitis in patients with AIDS. Am. J. Gastroenterol., *94:*339, 1999.

193. Wilcox, C.M.: Esophageal disease in the acquired immunodeficiency syndrome: Etiology, diagnosis, and management. Am. J. Med., *92:*412, 1992.
194. Wright, R.: Upper esophageal perforation with flexible endoscopy secondary to cervical osteophytes. Dig. Dis. Sci., *25:*66, 1980.
195. Wu, W.C., Katon, R.M., Saxon, R.R., et al.: Silicone-covered self-expanding metallic stents for the palliation of malignant esophageal obstruction and esophagorespiratory fistulas: Experience in 32 patients and a review of the literature. Gastrointest. Endosc., *40:*22, 1994.
196. Wychulis, A.R., Ellis, F.H., Jr., and Anderson, H.A.: Acquired nonmalignant esophagotracheobronchial fistula: Report of 3 cases. J.A.M.A., *196:*117, 1966.
197. Yonago, R.H., Iben, A.B., and Mark, J.B.D.: Aortic bypass in the management of aortoesophageal fistula. Ann. Thorac. Surg., *7:*235, 1969.

Index

Note: Page numbers in *italics* refer to illustrations; page numbers followed by t refer to tables.

ISBN 0 7216 8204 9